Public Health Administration

Principles for Population-Based Management

Edited by

Lloyd F. Novick, MD, MPH
Commissioner of Health
Onondaga County, New York

Professor
Department of Medicine
SUNY Upstate Medical University

Glen P. Mays, MPH, PhD
Visiting Postdoctoral Fellow
Department of Health Care Policy
Harvard Medical School

Research Fellow
School of Public Health
The University of North Carolina at Chapel Hill

Senior Public Health Advisor
Georges C. Benjamin, MD
Secretary of Health and Mental Hygiene
State of Maryland

JONES AND BARTLETT PUBLISHERS
Sudbury, Massachusetts
BOSTON TORONTO LONDON SINGAPORE

World Headquarters
Jones and Bartlett Publishers
40 Tall Pine Drive
Sudbury, MA 01776
978-443-5000
info@jbpub.com
www.jbpub.com

Jones and Bartlett Publishers Canada
6339 Ormindale Way
Mississauga, Ontario
L5V 1J2

Jones and Bartlett Publishers International
Barb House, Barb Mews
London W6 7PA
UK

Jones and Bartlett's books and products are available through most bookstores and online booksellers. To contact Jones and Bartlett Publishers directly, call 800-832-0034, fax 978-443-8000, or visit our website, www.jbpub.com.

Substantial discounts on bulk quantities of Jones and Bartlett's publications are available to corporations, professional associations, and other qualified organizations. For details and specific discount information, contact the special sales department at Jones and Bartlett via the above contact information or send an email to specialsales@jbpub.com.

ISBN: 0-7637-3552-1
ISBN: 0-7637-4078-0

Production Credits
Publisher: Michael Brown
Editorial Assistant: Kylah Goodfellow McNeill
Production Director: Amy Rose
Production Editor: Renée Sekerak
Associate Marketing Manager: Wendy Thayer
Manufacturing and Inventory Coordinator: Amy Bacus
Printing and Binding: Hamilton Printing
Cover Printing: Hamilton Printing

Printed in the United States of America
08 07 06 05 10 9 8 7 6 5 4 3

Table of Contents

Contributors

Lu Ann Aday, PhD
Professor
Behavioral Sciences and Management and Policy Sciences
School of Public Health
The University of Texas
Houston, Texas

Tim E. Aldrich, PhD, MPH
Adjunct Associate Professor
Department of Epidemiology and Biostatistics
University of South Carolina
Columbia, South Carolina

Michael S. Ascher, MD, FACP
Chief
Viral and Rickettsial Disease Laboratory
Division of Communicable Disease Control
California Department of Health Services
Berkeley, California

Elizabeth A. Baker, PhD, MPH
Assistant Professor
Department of Community Health
School of Public Health
Saint Louis University
St. Louis, Missouri

Scott J. Becker, JD, CPA
Executive Director
Association of Public Health Laboratories
Washington, D.C.

Steven M. Becker, PhD
Assistant Professor
Social and Behavioral Sciences and Public Health
University of Alabama at Birmingham
Birmingham, Alabama

Richard A. Bissell, PhD
Associate Professor
Department of Emergency Health Services
University of Maryland Baltimore County
Baltimore, Maryland

Eric C. Blank, MPH, DrPH
Director
State Public Health Laboratory
Missouri Department of Health
Jefferson City, Missouri

Ross C. Brownson, PhD
Professor
Department Chair
Department of Community Health
School of Public Health
Saint Louis University
St. Louis, Missouri

Thomas A. Burke, PhD, MPH
Associate Professor
Department of Health Policy and Management
School of Hygiene and Public Health
The Johns Hopkins University
Baltimore, Maryland

Willard Cates, Jr., MD, MPH
President
Family Health International
Research Triangle Park, North Carolina

Brad Christensen
U.S. Marketing/Communications Director
AMEC Earth and Environmental
Past-President
National Public Health Information Coalition
Former Communications Director
Arizona Department of Health Services
Phoenix, Arizona

Lynne Doner, MA
Social Marketing Consultant
Arlington, Virginia

Anne M. Gadomski, MD, MPH
Research Scientist
Attending Pediatrician
Bassett Hospital
Cooperstown, New York

Kristine M. Gebbie, DrPH, RN
Associate Professor of Nursing
Director
Center for Health Policy
Columbia University School of Nursing
New York, New York

Robert B. Gerzoff, MS
Statistical Analyst
Public Health Practice Program Office
Division of Public Health Systems
Centers for Disease Control and Prevention
Atlanta, Georgia

Sholom Glouberman, PhD
Philosopher in Residence
Baycrest Centre for Geriatric Care
Toronto, Ontario, Canada

Bruce Gordon, MD
Co-Chair
Institutional Review Board
Associate Professor
Pediatrics
University of Nebraska Medical Center
Omaha, Nebraska

Lawrence O. Gostin, JD, LLD (Hon.)
Professor of Law
Georgetown University
Professor of Public Health
The Johns Hopkins University
Co-Director
The Georgetown/Johns Hopkins Program on Law and Public Health
Georgetown University Law Center
Washington, D.C.

Lawrence W. Green, DrPH
Distinguished Fellow/Visiting Scientist
Office on Smoking and Health
National Center for Chronic Disease Prevention and Health Promotion
Centers for Disease Control and Prevention
Atlanta, Georgia

Paul K. Halverson, DrPH
Director
National Public Health Performance Standards Program
Public Health Program Office
Centers for Disease Control and Prevention
Atlanta, Georgia

Arden S. Handler, DrPH
Associate Professor of Community Health Sciences
Division of Community Health Sciences
School of Public Health
University of Illinois at Chicago
Chicago, Illinois

Michael T. Hatcher, MPH
Health Scientist
Division of Public Health Systems
Public Health Practice Program Office
Centers for Disease Control and Prevention
Atlanta, Georgia

Theresa Hatzell, PhD, MPH
Senior Research Associate
Family Health International
Research Triangle Park, North Carolina

Douglas Hirano, MPH
Chief
Bureau of Health Systems Development
Arizona Department of Health Services
Phoenix, Arizona

Nadia Shalauta Juzych, ScD, MS
Research Consultant
Pew Environmental Health Commission
Baltimore, Maryland

Arnold D. Kaluzny, PhD
Professor
Department of Health Policy and Administration
Director
Public Health Leadership Program
School of Public Health
University of North Carolina at Chapel Hill
Chapel Hill, North Carolina

Stephanie A. Kennan, MA
Senior Health Policy Advisor to U.S. Senator Ron Wyden (D-OR)
Washington, D.C.

Linda Young Landesman, DrPH, MSW
Assistant Vice President
Office of Professional Services and Affiliations
New York City Health and Hospitals Corporation
New York, New York

C. Virginia Lee, MD, MPH, MA
Chief
Spatial Analysis and Information Dissemination Section
Agency for Toxic Substances and Disease Registry
Atlanta, Georgia

Perri S. Leviss, MPM
Director of Government Services
Healthcare Services Group
American Express Tax and Business Services Inc.
New York, New York

Stephen H. Linder, PhD
Associate Professor
Management and Policy Sciences
School of Public Health
The University of Texas
Houston, Texas

Patricia A. MacCubbin, MS
Director
Institutional Review Boards
University of Utah
Salt Lake City, Utah

Josephine Malilay, PhD, MPH
Epidemiologist
Health Studies Branch
Division of Environmental Hazards and Health Effects
Centers for Disease Control and Prevention
Atlanta, Georgia

Robert Martin, DrPH, MPH
Director
Division of Laboratory Systems
Public Health Practice Program Office
Centers for Disease Control and Prevention
Atlanta, Georgia

Glen P. Mays, MPH, PhD
Visiting Postdoctoral Fellow
Department of Health Care Policy
Harvard Medical School
Boston, Massachusetts
Research Fellow
School of Public Health
The University of North Carolina at Chapel Hill
Chapel Hill, North Carolina

Alan L. Melnick, MD, MPH
Director
Joint Residency in Family Medicine/Public Health and General Preventive Medicine
Oregon Health Sciences University
Portland, Oregon

Ray M. Nicola, MD, MHSA
Senior Advisor
Centers for Disease Control and Prevention Assignee
Turning Point National Program Office
Seattle, Washington

Lloyd F. Novick, MD, MPH
Commissioner of Health
Onondaga County, New York
Professor
Department of Medicine
SUNY Upstate Medical University
Syracuse, New York

Judith M. Ottoson, EdD, MPH
Associate Professor
Andrew Young School of Policy Studies
Applied Research Center
Public Administration and Urban Studies
Georgia State University
Atlanta, Georgia

Stephen Parente, PhD, MPH
Department of Health Policy and Management
School of Public Health
University of Minnesota
Minneapolis, Minnesota

Ernest D. Prentice, PhD
Co-Chair
Institutional Review Board
Associate Dean for Research
University of Nebraska Medical Center
Omaha, Nebraska

Beth E. Quill, MPH
Associate Professor
Management and Policy Sciences
School of Public Health
The University of Texas
Houston, Texas

Les Roberts, PhD, MSPH
Lecturer
Whiting School of Engineering
The Johns Hopkins University
Baltimore, Maryland

William L. Roper, MD, MPH
Dean
School of Public Health
Professor
Department of Health Policy and Administration
University of North Carolina at Chapel Hill
Chapel Hill, North Carolina

Euichul Shin, MD, PhD
Assistant Professor
Department of Preventive Medicine
The Catholic University of Korea
Seoul, Korea

Michael Siegel, MD, MPH
Associate Professor
Social and Behavioral Sciences Department
Boston University School of Public Health
Boston, Massachusetts

Michael Skeels, PhD, MPH
Director
Oregon State Public Health Laboratory
Oregon Health Division
Portland, Oregon

William A. Sollecito, DrPH
Research Professor
Department of Health Policy and Administration
Associate Director
Public Health Leadership Program
School of Public Health
University of North Carolina at Chapel Hill
Chapel Hill, North Carolina

Anton M. Somlai, MAT, EdD
Associate Professor
Director of the Intervention Support and Dissemination Core
Center for AIDS Intervention Research (CAIR)
Department of Psychiatry and Behavioral Medicine
Medical College of Wisconsin
Milwaukee, Wisconsin

Michael A. Stoto, PhD
Professor and Chair
Department of Epidemiology and Biostatistics
School of Public Health and Health Services
The George Washington University
Washington, D.C.

Lee Thielen, MPA
Associate Director (retired)
Colorado Department of Public Health and Environment
Denver, Colorado

Bernard J. Turnock, MD, MPH
Clinical Professor of Community Health Sciences
Division of Community Health Sciences
School of Public Health
University of Illinois at Chicago
Chicago, Illinois

Vaughn Mamlin Upshaw, DrPH, EdD
Clinical Assistant Professor
Department of Health Policy and Administration
School of Public Health
University of North Carolina at Chapel Hill
Chapel Hill, North Carolina

Foreword

This book could be the last text on public health administration and the first on population-based management. Persons who read it at the beginning of their careers can learn why their professional lives can differ from those of most public health practitioners in the past. Readers in mid-career will find chapters that help to explain the turmoil in public health of recent years. Senior public health managers can read the text as a surrogate collective autobiography of the achievements and legacy of their generation.

Population-based management is more than a fashionable way to talk about the traditional practice of public health. Two significant characteristics of a population health perspective are emerging in health policy and management in the United States and many other countries.

The first characteristic is that the theory of population health—although not yet its practice—encompasses a broader array of determinants of health than the field of public health has previously addressed. The emerging theory and practice of population health incorporate the traditional concerns of public health. Assessing the burden of disease, preventing and treating it, and protecting against environmental hazards still matter in the emerging era of population health. But a population health perspective accords high priority to such issues as the effects on health status of—for example—relative income and social status, racial and gender disparities, and educational achievement.

Moreover, a population health perspective addresses changes in health status that result from the preferences of individuals as well as of decision makers in government and business. Both individuals and decision makers, for instance, usually assign higher priority than public health professionals do to maintaining and increasing jobs and personal income. In the years ahead a critical challenge for health programs managers in the public, private, and nonprofit sectors will be to maximize the positive effects of economic growth and productivity on the health status of populations.

The second significant characteristic of a population health perspective is that persons who embrace it acknowledge that responsibility for population health is diffuse and that it is likely to remain so. Many organizations are partially accountable for the health of any population. In the United States, for example, government on all levels, private employers, unions, and individuals purchase health services for particular populations. State and local public health agencies are responsible for preventing particular communicable and chronic diseases, for providing personal health services for persons in defined populations, and in many jurisdictions, for preventing illnesses that result from toxins in the environment.

Many public health leaders call this diffusion of responsibility fragmentation and deplore it. The emerging population health perspective, in contrast, accepts diffusion of responsibility for health as the norm of American political and economic life. If diffusion is the norm, the fundamental political and management problem of professionals in population health is how to increase the incentives of individuals and organizations to more effectively address the multiple determinants of health.

This first text intended to embrace and clarify the transition from a public to a population health perspective is edited and written by experienced persons. Each chapter is authoritative. More than a few of them are compelling and imaginative. The authors combine enthusiasm for their subjects with optimism about prospects for improving the health of populations. They articulate and advocate high standards for management during a transition that is likely to occur with increasing speed in the next few decades.

Daniel M. Fox, PhD
President
Milbank Memorial Fund

Preface

Improving health within communities and population groups is hard work. The difficulties of improving health at the population level persist despite society's growing knowledge about disease and human behavior, and despite its growing armamentarium of pharmaceutical, biologic, behavioral, and information technologies in health. In fact, the growing complexity of public health practice is one of the most challenging aspects of achieving population health improvement.

The challenge of complexity in public health is fundamentally a managerial issue rather than a scientific, clinical, or technological issue. Public health professionals must decide how best to organize and apply society's scarce health resources to address population health needs. Professionals face many more degrees of freedom in making these managerial decisions than previously, due to such factors as the expanding availability of health information to support these decisions, the expanding set of intervention opportunities created by new health knowledge and technologies, and the growing constellation of institutions and individuals that engage in population health issues—including medical care providers, health plans, employers, community-based organizations, and health care consumers. Moreover, public health managers face mounting uncertainty and risk in their decision-making responsibilities due to continual changes in population health status caused by emerging diseases and evolving health threats. Increasingly, the risks involved in managerial decisions entail both health and economic consequences. The complexity, uncertainty, and risk that characterize contemporary public health practice effect fundamental changes in how public health interventions are defined, organized, and carried out. These developments also drive fundamental changes in the set of institutions and individuals that comprise the nation's de facto public health system. In this environment, optimal managerial decision making in public health is rarely straightforward.

This book provides a comprehensive overview of concepts and strategies for contemporary public health administration. We examine the theoretical and philosophical underpinnings of managerial decision making in public health, as well as the practical knowledge, tools, and strategies required by organizations to navigate the contemporary public health environment. The concept of *population-based management* provides the key organizing principle and unifying theme for this text. This concept describes managerial strategies for maximizing expected health and well-being across the entire community or population involved, as opposed to strategies for maximizing performance within individual programs and organizations. Population-based management requires public health professionals to optimize their decisions and actions across multiple interventions, institutions, and risk groups—rather than within them. This concept reflects the fact that in the emerging health system, an increasing amount of public health activity is organized and managed not within individual institutions, but between them. As a consequence, public health professionals require the ability to manage partners rather than subordinates to achieve populationwide gains in health. More than any other single attribute, the concept of population-based management is what distinguishes this text from the larger body of literature on the theory and practice of health administration.

Consistent with the theme of population-based management, we use broad and inclusive criteria to identify the types of organizations and professionals that make up the public health system. As a consequence, current and prospective professionals should find this book helpful for managerial decision making in a variety of practice settings. The concepts and strategies explored in this text are highly relevant for governmental public health agencies at local, state, and federal levels; however, this material should also be immediately useful to professionals managing population-based programs within managed care plans, hospitals, community-based organizations, foundations, employer coalitions, and many other organizational and interorganizational settings. Although many applications described within the text focus on domestic practice settings, the managerial concepts and strategies examined herein are equally applicable to global and international health initiatives.

This text focuses on management strategies for the emerging public health environment, and as such, we have designed the book to be particularly useful for graduate students in public health, health administration, and community health programs. Nonetheless, practicing public health professionals should also find this text to be a key professional reference and a source for new ideas and insight concerning contemporary management issues. Although designed with the public health manager in mind, this book should also be of interest to individuals in the policy arena who are seeking current perspectives on organizational behavior and decision making within public health institutions and programs. Likewise, public health researchers should find this book helpful for developing new areas of scholarship and, perhaps even more importantly, for translating new discoveries into practice. Our coverage of topics in the management of public health research initiatives should also be of particular interest to the scientific community.

This text presents the work of a multidisciplinary team of public health scholars and practitioners who have been assembled to address the broad set of topics and issues that make up modern public health administration. The work is organized into four parts.

- Part I examines the underlying theoretical and structural elements of public health administration that shape contemporary decision making and practice. These chapters examine key historical developments and basic philosophical tenets that provide rationale and direction for modern public health initiatives. These chapters also provide an overview of the basic structural elements that make up the nation's public health system, including its organizational and interorganizational structures, its work force, its political and legal framework, and its ethical context.
- Part II examines managerial issues related to key operations that are carried out by public health organizations. These operations include data acquisition and surveillance, information systems design and management, public health assessment, health education and health promotion intervention, program evaluation, and public health research.
- Part III moves beyond operational issues to explore core managerial strategies for public health professionals to use across functional areas and organizational boundaries. These strategies involve human resources management, financial management, performance measurement and improvement, communications and media relations, marketing, constituency building, academic partnerships, legislative relations, and leadership.
- Part IV examines applications of contemporary managerial decision making in a va-

riety of specific practice settings. Although it would be impossible to cover all of the relevant practice settings in a single text, we selected settings that would reflect the diversity of issues and activities that make up modern public health practice. These applications include community-based prevention initiatives, environmental health programs, public health laboratory settings, disaster preparedness and response initiatives, human immunodeficiency virus (HIV) prevention and control programs, and public health responses to managed care and the uninsured. These chapters demonstrate how core managerial concepts and strategies can be used to address a variety of specific public health problems and issues.

The organization and content of the book is designed to stimulate critical thinking about modern public health issues while also communicating state-of-the-art management techniques and perspectives. Continued progress in improving population health will require new ways of approaching persistent public health problems, as well as creative ways of adapting current technologies to emerging health threats. We hope this book will help to inspire new and innovative strategies for managing the public's health.

Acknowledgments

My wife, Carole, encouraged and motivated me to develop this text and was a constant support throughout, also providing for the research and documentation of Chapters 1 and 2.

I am grateful for the assistance of Joe D. Kimbrell, Executive Director of the Louisiana Public Health Institute, for his assistance in the initial planning of this text.

—L.F.N.

This text was made possible through the foresight, enthusiasm, and commitment to excellence of acquisitions editor Kalen Conerly, who worked with the Editors on a daily basis throughout the eighteen months of development to bring the effort to fruition.

The Editors also express their gratitude to Denise Coursey, senior editor, for her invaluable assistance in developing this publication.

—L.F.N & G.P.M.

Part I

Conceptual and Structural Elements of Public Health Administration

The modern public health organization is in many ways a product of its unique historical development and its position within the current political, economic, and technological environment. Public health organizations are also shaped by the prevailing philosophical and ethical views that motivate modern public health initiatives. The chapters in Part I examine the underlying theoretical and structural elements of public health administration that shape current decision making and practice. Chapters 1 and 2 review historical and contemporary trends that define the scope and nature of public health practice. As part of this review, the author develops a conceptual framework for delineating the core activities involved in modern public health administration and explores the importance of this framework in designing, managing, and evaluating public health organizations and programs. Chapter 3 provides an overview of the basic institutional structure for public health in the United States, with emphasis on both organizational and interorganizational elements. Issues of organizational design and behavior in public health are explored in this chapter. The public health work force is profiled in Chapter 4, including a discussion of work force development needs and strategies faced by public health organizations. Chapter 5 profiles the legal framework that supports the nation's public health system and examines the implications of this framework for public health organizations. Finally, the ethical context for public health administration and practice is explored in Chapter 6. Together, these chapters characterize the intellectual and structural landscape in which modern public health decision making occurs.

CHAPTER 1

Defining Public Health: Historical and Contemporary Developments

Lloyd F. Novick

Public health practice comprises organized efforts to improve the health of communities. Public health prevention strategies are targeted to populations rather than to individuals. Throughout history, public health effort has been directed to the control of transmissible disease, reduction of environmental hazards, and provision of safe drinking water. The historic emphasis on protecting communities from infectious disease and environmental threats is now expanding to counter risks from behaviors and lifestyles that lead to chronic disease. Population-based prevention has resulted in major gains in life expectancy during the twentieth century. Because social, environmental, and biologic factors interact to determine health, public health practice must utilize a broad set of skills and interventions.

DEFINING PUBLIC HEALTH

Public health consists of organized efforts to improve the health of communities. The operative components of this definition are that public health efforts are *organized* and *directed to communities* rather than to individuals. Public health practice does not rely on a specific body of knowledge and expertise; rather, a combination of science and social approaches is used. The definition of public health reflects its central goal—the reduction of disease and the improvement of health in the community.

Population-based strategies for improving community health include efforts to control epidemics, ensure safe water and food, reduce vaccine-preventable diseases, improve maternal and child health, and conduct surveillance of health problems (Exhibit 1–1). In addition to long-standing efforts to protect communities from contagious and environmental health threats, the public health arena is expanding to counter new and contemporary risks: adolescent pregnancy, injury, violence, substance abuse, sexually transmitted disease (STD), and human immunodeficiency virus (HIV) infection. To be successful, the population-based approach to improving health must interact with clinical preventive activities directed at the individual, as presented in Figure 1–1.

Ample evidence for the importance of influencing population-based determinants of health is shown by the increase in life expectancy from 45 to 75 years for individuals living in industrialized countries during the twentieth century. The majority of this gain, 25 of the 30 years, can be attributed to public health measures such as better nutrition, sanitation, and housing.[1] Medical care focusing on individual patients, though important, only contributed five years of the life-expectancy gain.

Public health differs from clinical medicine by emphasizing prevention and keying interventions to multiple social and environmental determinants of disease. Clinical medicine focuses on the treatment of the individual. However, interaction between public health and medicine is necessary because individual health and com-

Exhibit 1–1 Public Health Activities

- Prevents epidemics
- Protects the environment, workplaces, housing, food, water
- Monitors health status of population
- Mobilizes community action
- Responds to disasters
- Assures quality, accessibility, accountability of medical care
- Reaches out to link high-risk and hard-to-reach people to needed services
- Researches to develop new insights and innovative solutions
- Leads the development of sound health policy and planning

Source: Reprinted from *For a Healthy Nation: Returns on Investments in Public Health,* Executive Summary, 1994, U.S. Department of Health and Human Services, Public Health Services.

munity health are not discrete phenomena but rather elements of a continuum. Tuberculosis (TB), HIV infection, STD, lead toxicity, vaccine-preventable disease, and many other health problems are dealt with in both clinical and population settings.

The relevance of public health and clinical collaboration is underscored by estimates that 50 percent of premature deaths are preventable and influenced by personal behaviors—the abuse of tobacco and other substances, poor diet, and sedentary lifestyles.[2] Changes in health status can best be achieved through partnership between clinical efforts focusing on individual patients and communitywide public health interventions addressing environmental and educational determinants of these health risks.

In 1920, C.-E.A. Winslow provided a definition of public health practice.

> Public health is the science and art of preventing disease, prolonging life, and promoting physical health and efficiency through organized community efforts for the sanitation of the environment, the control of community infections, the education of the individual in principles of personal hygiene, the organization of medical and

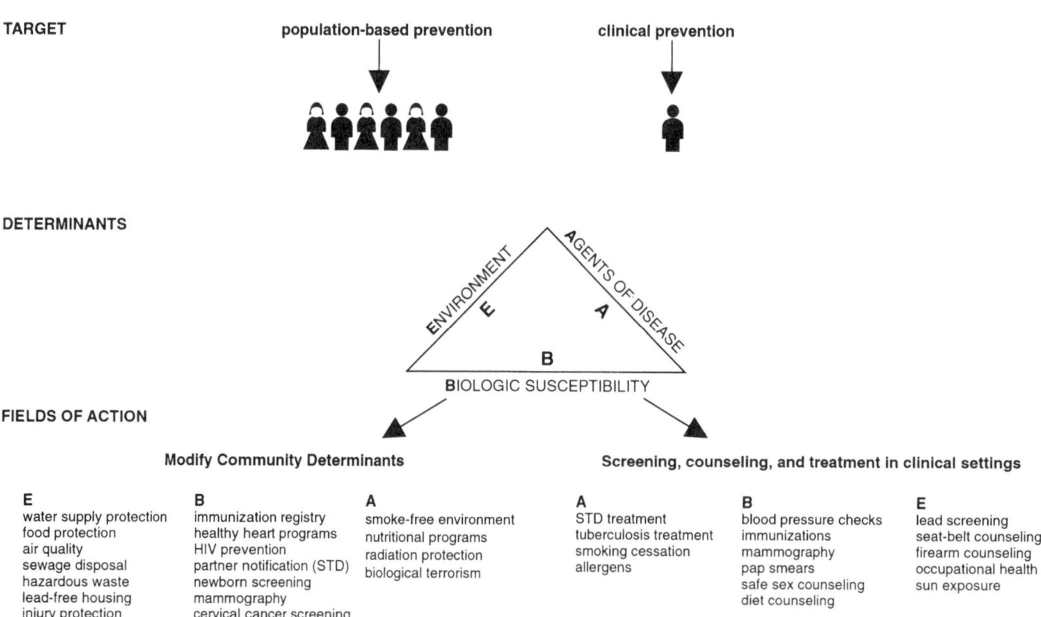

Figure 1–1 Public Health Approaches to Improving Health. *Source:* Copyright © 2000, L.F. Novick.

> nursing services for the early diagnosis and preventive treatment of disease, and the development of social machinery which will ensure to every individual in the community a standard of living adequate for the maintenance of health.[3(p.34)]

In 1988, the Institute of Medicine (IOM) published a classic report, *The Future of Public Health,* similarly defining public health as an "organized community effort to address the public interest in health by applying scientific and technical knowledge to prevent disease and promote health."[4(p.7)] The mission of public health, then, is to ensure conditions to promote the health of the community.

Both science and socioeconomic factors form the basis for public health intervention. Successfully eradicating a vaccine-preventable disease from a community requires more than development of the vaccine itself. Use of the vaccine in the community is dependent on a successful public health initiative providing public information and facilitating delivery. Too often, scientific advances are not translated into community health improvement. Congenital syphilis remains a health problem despite the scientific means, penicillin, to eradicate it. Ensurance of adequate prenatal care for at-risk women is a public health approach that combines the science with practical approaches to address socioeconomic factors important to the improvement of birth outcomes.

Recently, a community in upstate New York experienced an outbreak of TB among 12 homeless men attending the same shelter. Anti-TB medications and sophisticated diagnostic methods were combined with an approach incorporating outreach and incentives for directly observed therapy tailored for the social factors associated with this homeless group. Protecting the health of the community was more than the sum of the individual treatment of the 12 men; it involved identification of hundreds of possibly exposed individuals. This effort can be defined as a public health activity by the primary objective—the prevention of transmission to others in this risk group and the community.

Even with attention provided to the unique social factors of this homeless group, a number of individuals with active pulmonary TB did not agree to treatment, thereby jeopardizing not only themselves but others. The local public health agency obtained court orders requiring hospitalization and treatment of these individuals. The definition of public health is keyed to organized efforts to protect the health of the community even when these efforts conflict with the autonomy of the individual.

ACCOMPLISHMENTS OF PUBLIC HEALTH

The efficacy of public health practice derives from its ability to extend effective preventive interventions to a community. Unlike clinical approaches that target individual patients, public health deals with a wide range of antecedent environmental, social, and lifestyle risks and mounts activities to modify or eliminate these factors. Health issues result from interactions among individuals, disease agents, and the broader environment. In the example previously described, *mycobacteria tuberculum* was the agent responsible for the outbreak of TB. But the occurrence of the health issue was triggered by important host susceptibility conditions as well as environmental, behavioral, and social factors. Concomitant HIV infection, alcohol and substance abuse, homelessness, and inadequate ventilation of the shelter were all determinants of this outbreak. Addressing the multiple determinants was required in resolving this community health problem.

Defining public health in terms of its goal of community health improvement leads to an examination of the success or accomplishments of this endeavor. Interventions have improved sanitation, water purity, nutrition, control of infectious disease, and immunization.[5] Major gains in our nation's health have occurred over the last 125 years. Life expectancy has increased by greater than 30 years, and the quality of life is remarkably improved. But the public may not recognize many of these gains because it has become accustomed to the accrual of long-standing benefits from communal efforts to protect against hazards to health. Quentin Young, former president of the American Public Health Association, remarked: "Turning on any kitchen faucet for a glass of drinking water without hesitation of peril is a silent homage to public health success, which would not have been possible at the start of the twentieth century."[6(p.1)]

Individuals living in the United States have an unquestioned reliance on their water quality. Similarly, they are likely to be unaware of the recent progress in the last 100–150 years with respect to leading causes of death, particularly infectious disease. Absent the threat or recognition of the accomplishment, the importance of public health activity cannot be credited.

For example, a remarkable gain in population health status in New York City was attributed to the 50 years of public health activity dating from 1873. The death rate from all causes in New York City was 31 per thousand in 1824, 41 per thousand in 1851, and 29 per thousand in 1875. This rate fell to 12 per thousand in 1925—a reduction of three-fifths in 50 years. In 1879–80, the average life span in New York–Brooklyn was 36 years; by 1919–20, individual life expectancy had increased to 53 years for New York City. This is an increase of 47 percent in a 40-year period.[7] Marked reductions in the prevalence of infectious disease were documented in New York City (Table 1–1). And as pointed out by Winslow and others, public health activities in reducing environmental and infectious disease threats were responsible: "Our achievements were almost wholly based on the organized application of the sciences of sanitary engineering and bacteriology."[7(p.1079)]

Public health has provided the basis for health improvements for the last century. In this century, this activity has been important to the: (1) substantial decrease in cigarette smoking, (2) decline in the rates of heart disease mortality and motor vehicle–associated fatalities, (3) control of infectious diseases, and (4) improved quality of the workplace.[8]

Exhibit 1–2 lists the 10 great public health achievements.

It is ironic that the very accomplishments in population-based prevention have probably resulted in decreased visibility for public health

Table 1–1 Mortality from Certain Causes and from all Causes per 100,000 Population

	Manhattan and Bronx 1873–75	*Greater New York 1923–25*	*Percent Change*
Scarlet fever	80	1	–99
Diphtheria and croup	235	11	–95
Diarrhea under five years	335	22	–93
Diseases of the nervous system	252	39	–85
Pulmonary tuberculosis	404	84	–79
All other causes not listed	874	316	–64
Acute respiratory diseases	352	164	–53
All causes	2,890	1,220	–42
Bright's disease and nephritis	100	69	–31
Violence	120	85	–27
Cancer	41	113	+176
Heart disease	89	255	+187
Diseases of the arteries	8	61	+650

Source: Reprinted with permission from C. -E.A. Winslow, Public Health at the Crossroads, *American Journal of Public Health,* Vol. XVI, No. 11, p. 1077, © 1926, American Public Health Association.

Exhibit 1–2 Ten Great Public Health Achievements

1. **Vaccines:** Few treatments were effective in the prevention of infectious diseases in 1900. Now, smallpox, measles, diphtheria, pertussis, rabies, typhoid, cholera, and the plague are preventable through widespread use of vaccines.
2. **Recognition of tobacco use as a health hazard:** Since the 1964 surgeon general's report on risks associated with smoking, smoking among adults has decreased, saving lives.
3. **Motor vehicle safety:** Improved engineering of vehicles and roads plus the use of seat belts, car seats, and helmets have reduced the number of deaths, as has decreased drinking and driving.
4. **Safer workplaces:** A 40 percent decrease in fatal occupational injuries (since 1980) has resulted through efforts to control work-related diseases such as pneumoconiosis (black lung) and silicosis, which are associated with coal mining, and to improve safety in manufacturing, construction, transportation, and mining.
5. **Control of infectious diseases:** Efforts to protect the water supply and keep it clean with improved sanitation methods have greatly improved health, particularly curbing the spread of cholera and typhoid. The discovery of antimicrobial therapy has helped to control tuberculosis and sexually transmitted diseases (STDs).
6. **Fewer deaths from heart disease and stroke:** Smoking cessation, blood pressure control, early detection, and better treatments have resulted in a 51 percent decrease in death rates for coronary heart disease since 1972.
7. **Safer and healthier foods:** Major nutritional deficiency diseases such as rickets, goiter, and pellagra have been virtually eliminated in the United States through greater recognition of essential nutrients, increases in nutritional content, food fortification, and decreases in microbial contamination.
8. **Healthier mothers and babies:** Better hygiene, nutrition, access to health care, antibiotics, and technologic advances have helped to reduce infant mortality by 90 percent and maternal mortality by 99 percent.
9. **Family planning and contraceptive services:** These services have altered the social and economic roles of women. Access to counseling and screening has resulted in fewer infant, child, and maternal deaths. Contraceptives have provided protection from human immunodeficiency virus and other STDs.
10. **Fluoridation of drinking water:** Nearly 150 million people have access to treated water, a safe and effective way to prevent tooth decay. Fluoridation has helped to reduce tooth decay in children by 40–70 percent and tooth loss in adults by 40–60 percent.

Source: Adapted from Ten Great Public Health Achievements—United States, 1900–1999, *Morbidity and Mortality Weekly Report,* Vol. 48, No. 12, pp. 1–3, 1999, Centers for Disease Control and Prevention.

activities in our communities. If these protective activities work well, illnesses from water, food, and environmental toxins will not occur. Without experiencing problems, the public knows little about the methods of assurance, and collective support for public health resources and programs will be minimal. Yet, the line of protection for health hazards can be breached, resulting in significant numbers of illnesses in our community. In 1997, contamination of a drinking water source at a ski area in New York State resulted in gastrointestinal illnesses in 1,400 individuals. Numerous episodes of *E. Coli*—infections from contaminated meat and water—have occurred. As public health activities expand into new arenas, complacency in performing traditional functions needs to be avoided.

Abundant examples demonstrate the continued threat of infectious disease outbreaks associated with environmental problems and requiring vigorous public health action. In 1999, more than 1,000 individuals became ill with *E. Coli* after drinking water from a contaminated well at a county fair in Washington County, New York. A short time later, an outbreak of encephalitis in New York City was identified as being caused by West Nile Virus, never previously identified in the Western Hemisphere. This infection, with birds as a reservoir and mosquitoes as a vector, initiated a classic public health response of protection of the community, employing methods of surveillance, information dissemination, and vector control.

CHANGING SCOPE OF PUBLIC HEALTH PRACTICE

Attempts to replicate the successes achieved with infectious and environmentally related disease have been extended to the contemporary health challenges of nutrition, injury prevention, violence, substance abuse, HIV infection, and tobacco-related and other chronic diseases. Winslow argued early for this extension in a speech delivered before the American Public Health Association in Buffalo in 1926.

> We may . . . say that the health officer should concern himself only with communicable disease. That is a logical position, though a narrow one. Or we may combine this etiological criterion with another based on age and say that the field of the health department includes all the health problems of the infant and the child plus the communicable diseases of the adult. This is a second clear and defensible position and one that approximates current-day practice. Or we may take a still wider view and say that the health program must envisage the whole field of the prevention of disease and the promotion of physical and mental health and efficiency.[7(p.1080)]*

A critical issue is the feasibility of the extension of the scope of public health practice to the set of twenty-first-century public health challenges. Infectious disease, although still of critical importance, no longer causes the majority of deaths. One hundred years ago, public health activities were initiated in response to a markedly different pattern of community health, as shown in Table 1–2 and Figure 1–2. National data show the same transition to chronic disease (Figure 1–3). Tobacco, alcohol, illicit drugs, firearms,

**Source:* Reprinted with permission from C. -E.A. Winslow, Public Health at the Crossroads, *American Journal of Public Health,* Vol. XVI, No. 11, p. 1080, © 1926, American Public Health Association.

Table 1–2 Most Prominent Causes of Death in Residents of Syracuse, NY, from 1891 to 1900

Reported Cause	*1891*	*1892*	*1893*	*1894*	*1895*	*1896*	*1897*	*1898*	*1899*	*1900*
Consumption	228	247	234	220	180	181	246	253	136	184
Heart disease	63	89	113	101	121	132	76	74	117	162
Pneumonia	104	122	153	109	80	115	155	134	110	127
Bright's disease	32	27	42	45	54	57	46	39	76	103
Cancer	43	38	47	47	59	52	36	34	46	78
Old age	67	69	59	57	62	80	69	83	76	67
Cholera infantum	123	98	92	92	92	71	72	104	91	49
Meningitis	38	36	50	57	61	56	46	54	43	43
Bronchitis	53	62	73	59	75	46	64	65	51	38
Typhoid fever	40	33	34	35	31	27	24	47	20	29
Apoplexy	25	31	30	28	32	24	31	27	33	24
Diphtheria	18	51	97	54	22	23	1	41	43	21
Peritonitis	24	39	21	25	24	21	30	32	32	19
Dysentery	12	15	9	12	9	2	21	5	5	23
Marasmus	9	17	19	26	32	32	19	9	35	22

Source: Onondaga County Department of Health, 1999, Onondaga County, New York.

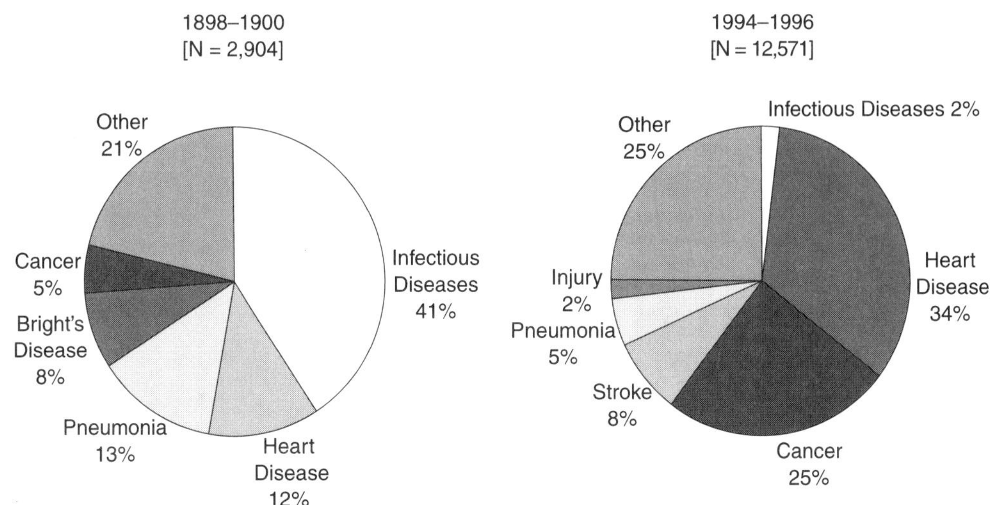

Figure 1–2 Leading Causes of Death in Syracuse, NY, from 1898 to 1900 and from 1994 to 1996. *Source:* Onondaga County Department of Health, 1999, Onondaga County, New York.

motor vehicles, diet, activity levels, and sexual behaviors are responsible for nearly half the deaths in the United States.[2] Monitoring deaths and injuries related to firearms and motor vehicles, studying associations between environmental factors and diseases, and surveying sexual and substance abuse behaviors of adolescents are now staples of local public health activity.

Contemporary public health emerged to control communicable diseases related to nineteenth and twentieth century industrialization and urbanization. Epidemics of chronic disease were the next target of public health activities, including atherosclerotic heart disease, cancer, chronic obstructive lung disease, and diabetes. Now a third group of problems has appeared: HIV/acquired immune deficiency syndrome (AIDS), domestic and street violence, and substance abuse.[9]

Local and state health departments are on the front line protecting the public health of communities, providing resources, monitoring performance, and providing technical assistance and surveillance. Can the successes achieved in life expectancy and quality of life by public health methods in the early twentieth century be extended to impact the now wide array of contemporary problems?

The IOM report, *The Future of Public Health,* identified the basic challenge for public health as determining methods and implementing activities to resolve a group of health issues that are quite different than contamination of water by a microbial agent.[4] Infant mortality, HIV infection, and violence are examples of contemporary health issues facing the nation's local health departments. Determinants are a complex mixture of social, environmental, and educational factors. As described in this text, public health methods are being adapted to include new types of collaborative partnerships and community-based prevention that hold the promise of increased effectiveness with our current health problems.

EARLY COLLECTIVE ACTION TO IMPROVE HEALTH

The evolving definition of public health activity is forged by hazards requiring collective action. Throughout history, attention has been directed to controlling transmissible disease, improving the environment, and providing safe drinking water. Toilets drained by covered sewers have been found in excavations of civilizations dating to 4,000 years ago in the Indus Val-

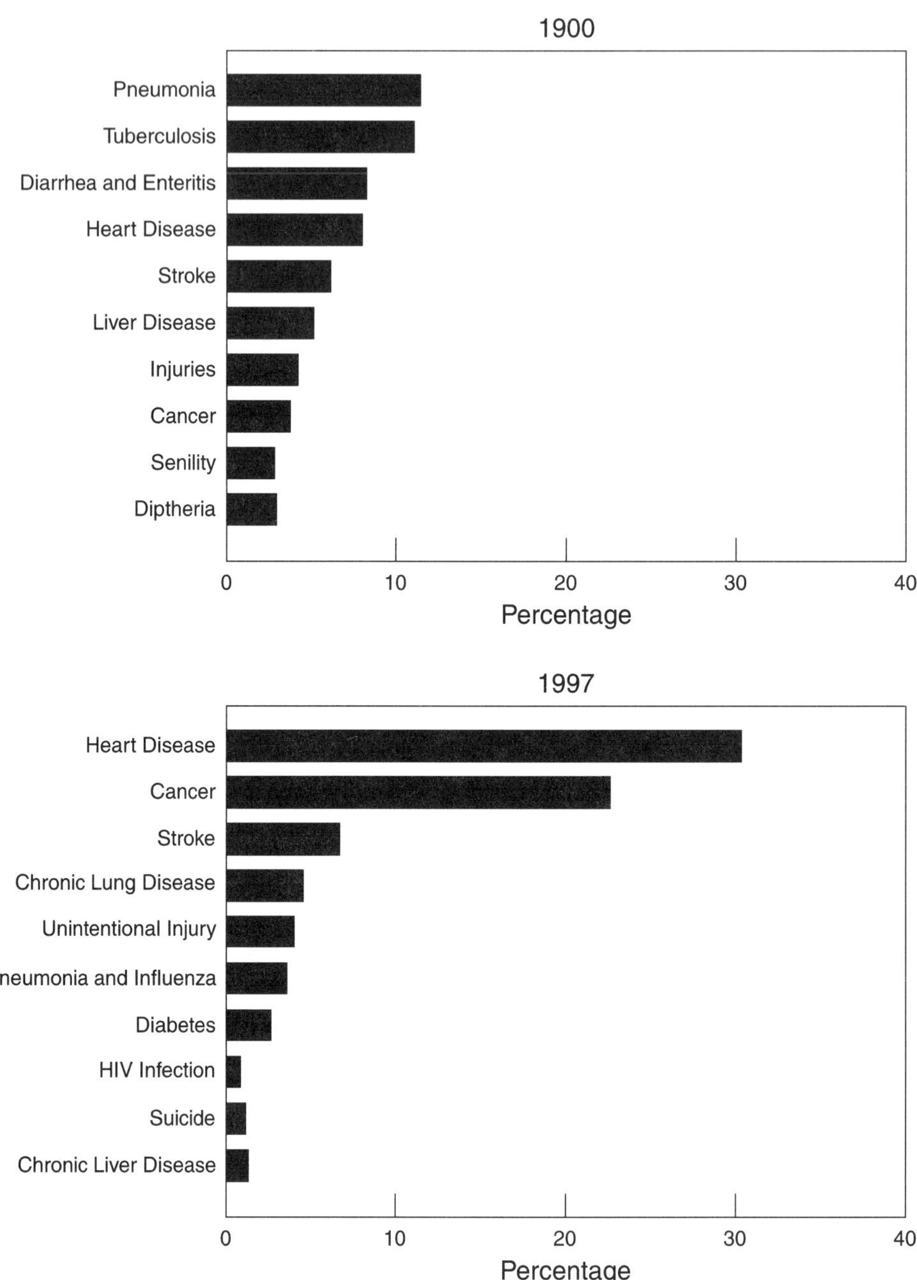

Figure 1–3 The 10 Leading Causes of Death as a Percentage of All Deaths in the United States in 1900 and 1997. *Source:* Adapted from *Morbidity and Mortality Weekly Report,* Vol. 48, No. 29, July 30, 1999, Centers for Disease Control and Prevention.

ley. In 2000 BC, cities, including Troy, had highly developed water supply systems.[10] At the time of Joshua when Israelites settled in the Holy Land, there were rules governing the water supply. There could not be a cemetery, animal slaughterhouse, tannery, or furnace within 50 cubits (approximately 25 meters) of a village water supply.[11] In the Western Hemisphere, impressive ruins of sewers and baths document the achievements of the Incas in public health engineering.[10]

The Greeks believed that ill health developed from an imbalance between man and his environment, not unlike contemporary public health theories of multifactorial disease causation, in which environment plays a prominent role. The Hippocratic book *On Airs, Waters and Places* summarizes factors important to disease, including climate, soil, water, mode of life, and nutrition.[12]

Most important, Hippocrates provided guidance to the location of Greek colonies as they expanded eastward to Italy and Sicily. Houses were to be located on elevated and sunny areas, avoiding marshes and swamps with their vector-borne illnesses.[10] The Romans also made the connection between swamps and disease (specifically, malaria), and determining salubrity was an important component of the selection of places for habitation. Ancient terms describing disease are still in use, including endemic (background or usual occurrence) and epidemic (excessive occurrence).

In the Middle Ages, epidemics of infectious disease spurred collective activities by communities to promote the public health, presaging the later formation of boards of health and public health departments in the nineteenth century. The Middle Ages (AD 500–1500) were marked by two major epidemics—the Plague of Justinian (543) and the Black Death (1348)—with smaller outbreaks of various diseases in the intervening period, including leprosy, smallpox, tuberculosis, and measles.[10] During this period, lepers were considered public menaces and were expelled from the community. This is a stark example of deprivation of individual civil rights in a quest to protect the health of the public. This precedent remains relevant and controversial in contemporary public health practice. The Black Death, a plague pandemic, was regarded as a communicable disease, and the countermeasure employed, similar to leprosy, was isolation of the ill individual. Patients had to be reported to the authorities—a forerunner of the basic public health functions of disease reporting and surveillance. Quarantine measures were instituted to stop the entry of plague from outside regions. In 1348, Venice, a chief port of entry for commerce from the Orient, was the first to institute quarantine, inspecting and segregating suspected ships and individuals. In 1423, Venice erected a pesthouse or *lazaretto* to detain individuals suspected of harboring infection (*lazaretto* is derived from the name of the Biblical character Lazarus, who was a leper). These detention areas were used for isolation in many types of pestilence.[13] Similar to other cities, Venice also set up a council of three men to supervise the health of the city—a forerunner of boards of health that were implemented centuries later.[10] These interactions are diagrammed in Figure 1–4.

Medieval cities were run by councils who were charged with routine community administration as well as the supervision of disease prevention, sanitation, and protection of the community health. Measures were instituted to control the transmission of infections, including isolation and disinfection. Food inspection and regulation of waste disposal protected citizens.[10] These collective actions to protect public health that were implemented in the Middle Ages exhibit patterns that are very much in existence in our current public health programs for communities. These include a population-based focus for interventions, involvement of government, prominence of environmental interventions, and potential for infringement of individual rights to protect the public.

COLLECTIVE ACTIVITIES TO PROTECT HEALTH IN THE UNITED STATES

The early American colonists struggled with hunger and malnutrition, scurvy, and infectious diseases, including smallpox, cholera, measles, diphtheria, and typhoid fever.[14] Smallpox was the epidemic disease of the colonies in the seventeenth century, yellow fever became prominent in the eighteenth century, and the dread disease of the nineteenth century was cholera.[13] The major important public health function of the colonies was the control of communicable diseases. Enactment of sanitary laws by the colonies included regulating such matters as privies, the disposal of wastes, and the disposition of animals. The colonies consisted principally of a se-

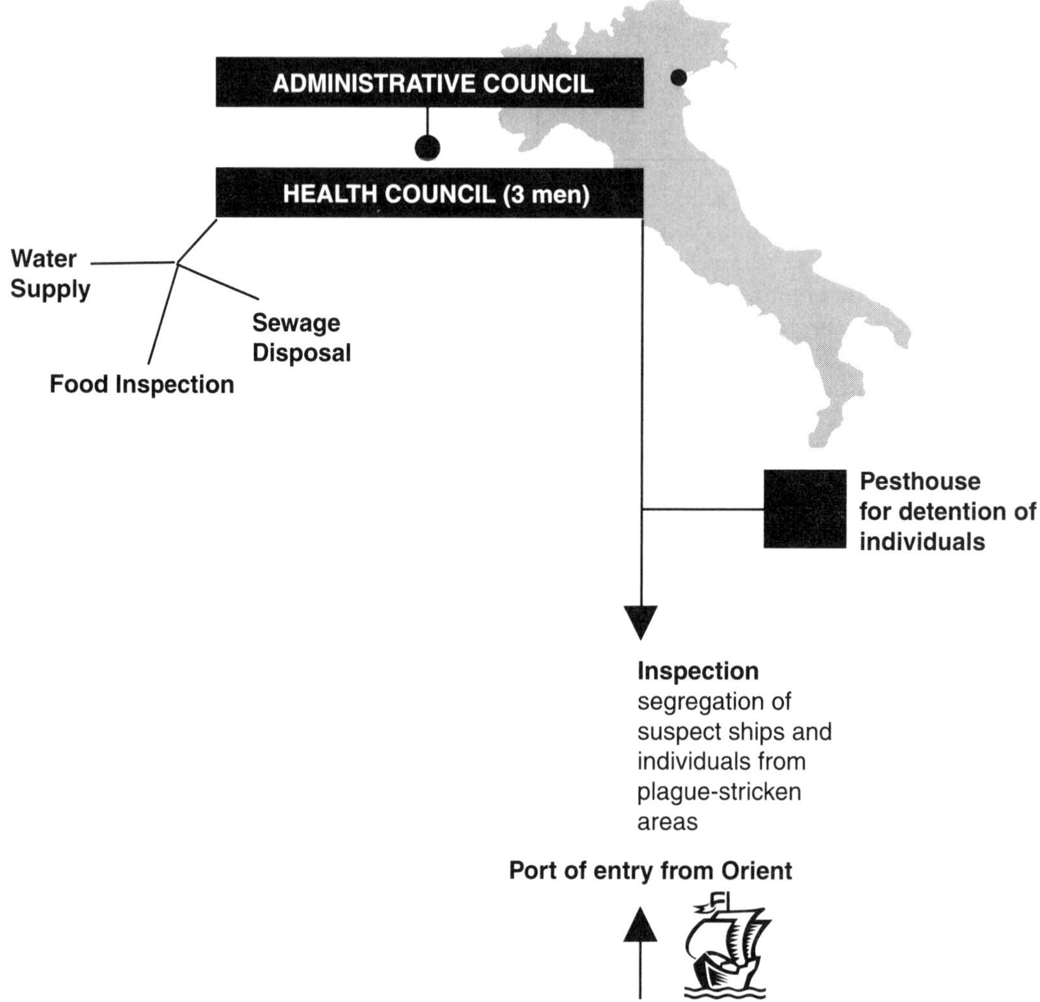

Figure 1–4 Medieval Model for Public Health Practice: Venice, 1300–1500. *Source:* Copyright © 2000, L.F. Novick.

ries of seaports connected by ships. Quarantine laws were enacted in all major towns along the eastern seaboard. The foundation for this activity was established by the Massachusetts Quarantine Act of July 1701, which required parties bringing infectious diseases within the colony to pay all costs and damages and compelled confinement of individuals who were infected with pestilential illnesses. In 1699, William Penn, concerned about yellow fever in the colony he had established, passed an Act to Prevent Sickly Vessels from Coming into This Government.[13]

The notable public health intervention of the colonial period was smallpox inoculation. Reverend Cotton Mather had earlier provided an account of the smallpox epidemic of 1689–90 in New England: "In about a twelvemonth, one thousand of our neighbors have been carried to their long home."[13(p.22)] The total population of Boston at that time was only 6,000. In a smallpox epidemic of Boston in 1721, Cotton Mather suggested smallpox inoculation. As with many public health interventions, initially there was considerable controversy concerning smallpox inoculation. But when smallpox again struck Massachusetts in 1792, the death rate was 14 percent in individuals who were not vaccinated and 1.8 percent in those who were.[13]

Yellow fever was the scourge of the eighteenth century. Yellow fever is an acute viral infectious disease of short duration and varying severity.[15] Following importation of the disease from St. Thomas of the Virgin Islands, New York City bore the brunt of the epidemic in 1702. Philadelphia and New York experienced repeated epidemics. Norfolk, Charleston, New Orleans, Boston, and other cities were also affected by this epidemic illness. Philadelphia experienced 4,044 deaths in 1793 and 3,506 deaths in 1798. Nearly 50,000 people contracted yellow fever in 1793.[16] Later in this same century, yellow fever epidemics were experienced in New Orleans, Atlanta, Memphis, and Jacksonville.[17] Transmission of the virus is by the bite of an *Aedes aegypti* mosquito. The disease only occurred in summer in the northern part of America after ships entered from ports where the disease was occurring. When the October frost arrived, the epidemics ended. The importance of environment in epidemic disease underscores the opportunity and necessity for public health measures.

Consequently, to nineteenth-century New Yorkers, the word epidemic was all too clearly understood and experienced in the form of cholera, smallpox, yellow fever, and typhoid (Table 1–3).[16]

The nature of these contagions or threats to health from infection defines the approach to public health. These threats cannot be countered successfully by addressing the ill individual. They can only be countered in terms of population-based efforts focused on the causal or underlying environmental and social conditions. Public health workers had a different working definition of health improvement than clinicians. David Rosner has observed that "while physicians saw sick patients and sought to identify the cause of disease and treat its symptoms, public health workers addressed the problem of environmental control, developing a perspective that emphasized personal and public hygiene."[16]

Table 1–3 The Great Epidemics of New York City during the Nineteenth Century

Year	*Disease*	*Total Deaths*	*Deaths per 100,000*
1832	Cholera	3,513	1,561
1849	Cholera	5,071	1,014
1851	Dysentery	1,173	221
1854	Cholera	2,509	395
1866	Cholera	1,137	113
1872	Smallpox	1,666	118
1881	Diphtheria	4,894	266
1887	Diphtheria	4,509	226

Source: Reprinted from Bulletin New York City Department of Health, p. 6, March 1953.

SOCIAL AND ENVIRONMENTAL FACTORS ARE BASIC TO PUBLIC HEALTH ACTION

Epidemics transmitted through food and water can be addressed by removing their environmental causes. Similarly, social and environmental factors can be causally linked to the occurrence of TB, the leading cause of death in the nineteenth century. Nearly one out of every four dwellings in New York City in 1890 experienced a death from TB. The toll was much higher in poorer neighborhoods, leaving these communities devastated by disease.[16]

Lemuel Shattuck was the foremost American advocate for community action in this area of environmental health. In an early report, *Census of Boston*, Shattuck reported on a high mortality, infant, and maternal mortality with prevalent communicable disease and TB.[10] He described these findings as directly related to living conditions and low income. In his 1850 report, Shattuck recommended the establishment of a state health department and local boards of health in each town.[18]

Early public health interventions in the United States followed a similar pattern of collective action, often requiring government authority to address environmental factors thought to be compromising the health of communities. From 1832, repeated cholera epidemics stimulated the creation of boards of health in the eastern United States, and port cities instituted a 40-day quarantine of ships entering harbors.[19] Various claims have been made asserting the community formation of the first board of health in the United States. Baltimore, Charleston, Petersburg, New York City, and Philadelphia are contenders. New York City established a board of health in 1796, consisting of three commissioners and a health officer. The term health officer designates responsibilities as a quarantine officer.

In 1865, the Association of New York issued a report, *Sanitation of the City,* pressuring New York (both city and state) to organize a Metropolitan Board of Health the following year.[16] The report documented the intimate relationship between social and economic forces creating ill health. A newly organized New York City Department of Public Health followed and soon became a model for others to emulate. The focus was on cleaning the streets, regulating sewage and waste disposal, and mandating tenement reforms.[16] The continuing environmental problems necessitating interventions were described in a 1912 annual report. The department removed 20,000 dead horses, mules, donkeys, and cattle from the streets and also nearly half a million smaller animals such as pigs, hogs, calves, and sheep. Disposal of more than five million pounds of spoiled poultry, fish, pork, and beef was accomplished. There were records of 343,000 complaints from the public of poor ventilation and waste disposal and unlicensed manure dumps.[16]

Throughout its history, the definition of public health has been characterized by a premium on prevention in protecting and promoting health. A multifactorial approach is employed, addressing environment, individual health risks, and agents of disease. Historical forces that molded public health were related to infectious disease and influenced by environmental conditions. The current scope of activities is expanding to include additional health risks, but unchanged is the fundamental of a population-based approach targeting the social and environmental determinants of health.

OTHER FORMATIVE INFLUENCES

Public health activities in both England and the United States were greatly influenced by growing urbanization and industrialization. Public health organization in the United States has English antecedents. In the early 1800s, people came to the cities for work, creating urban slums and conditions fostering ill health. London more than tripled in size from approximately 200,000 inhabitants in 1600 to 674,000 in 1700. During the eighteenth century, London grew only by approximately one-third and still had less than one million residents. But within the first 40 years of the nineteenth century, London doubled in size to nearly two million residents.[20] Malnutrition, crowding, filth, and poor working conditions contributed to severe disease outbreaks.[9] Similarly in New York City, a large number of immigrants in the 1840s and 1850s exacerbated the rise of typhus as a significant cause of death. The rise of tenements changed typhus into an endemic slum disorder but, because it affected the poorest group of individuals, it was said to have aroused little public concern.[21]

In 1842, Chadwick published the *General Report on the Sanitary Condition of the Laboring Population of Great Britain.*[10] In 1850, Shattuck published a report, already referred to, describing health and social conditions in Massachusetts.[18] These classic public health documents stimulated sanitary awakening and social reforms.[9–11,13] Edwin Chadwick described the prevalence of disease among the laboring people, showing that the poor exhibited a preponderance of disease and disability compared to more affluent individuals.[13] The conclusion of the report was that the cause of poor health of working people was the unsanitary environment. Disease was attributed to miasma and bad odors.[13] Epidemic diseases such as typhus, typhoid, and cholera were secondary to filth, stagnant pools, rotting animals and vegetables, and garbage.[20]

Chadwick was the chief administrator of the Poor Law Commission and responsible for relief to the impoverished in England and Wales. He became the champion of sanitary reform, which became the basis for public health activities at that time in both Great Britain and the United States. The "sanitary idea" is public health through public works. The prevention of infectious disease is accomplished through providing water that is pure and sewers for waste disposal. This theory of public health antedated the germ theory, which did not become dominant until the end of the nineteenth century.[22]

Chadwick was also the chief architect of the 1848 Public Health Act, which created a general board of health empowered to establish local boards of health and appoint an officer of health.[10,23] The latter was required to be a medically qualified medical practitioner and inspector of nuisances and sanitary conditions. But the board of health incurred the opposition of property interests that were opposed to proposals for improvement of drainage and water supplies. In 1854, after only five years of operation, Parliament refused to renew the Public Health Act and the first national board of health ended.[10]

Despite its repeal, the 1848 Public Health Act was instrumental in improving public health and remains relevant to current population-based preventive efforts.[23] The act identified all major public health issues of the time and assigned responsibility to local people. These issues were poverty, housing, water, sewerage, the environment, safety, and food. Organization of public health in England and Wales was addressed with the purpose of improving sanitary conditions of the towns. The background to this act was data-based mortality and morbidity rates.[23] The national and local boards included inspectors and officers of health. The drafters of the 1848 Public Health Act were clearly concerned with population health, assigning that responsibility to national and local government.[23]

In this same time period, John Snow, a physician who had provided anesthesia at Queen Victoria's childbirth, investigated London cholera epidemics in 1849 and 1854.[10] He demonstrated through epidemiologic analysis that cholera was transmitted through water contaminated with sewage.[13] Although this theory of waterborne cholera was not fully accepted, the London Board of Health did attempt to avoid disease by obtaining nonpolluted water.[13] The same concepts were followed in the United States.[13] These events in Great Britain shaped the development of public health practice in America. Early health reformers, including Henry Griscom of New York and Lemuel Shattuck of Boston, identified environmental improvement to prevent epidemic disease as a moral mission.[24] Shattuck's *General Plan for the Promotion of Public and Personal Health,* published in 1850, extolled "the sanitary movement abroad."[18] Sewage, refuse, and waste disposal and drainage were priority public health activities; of these, sewage disposal was most important.[25] Winslow characterized sanitation—ensuring healthful environmental conditions—as the first stage in public health. He stated, "To a large section of the public, I fear that the health authorities are still best known as the people to whom one complains of unpleasant accumulations of rubbish in the back yard of a neighbor—accumulations which possess such offensive characteristics which somehow can only originate in a neighbor's yard and never in one's own."[3(p.5)]

THE NEW PUBLIC HEALTH: BACTERIOLOGY

Scientific advances, particularly in microbiology, during the latter part of the nineteenth and early twentieth century, ushered in a new dimension for the field of public health.[9] This second or bacteriologic phase of the public health movement was ushered in by the discoveries of Pasteur and Koch, leading to a "germ theory" of disease. Initially studying fermentation, Pasteur discovered aerobic and anaerobic organisms and began to consider the possibility of a causal relationship between germs and disease. Robert Koch, a country physician, worked with the bacillus responsible for anthrax and demonstrated that the disease was transmissible in mice. With methods developed by Koch, various problems of infectious disease were revealed between 1880 and 1900, including relapsing fever, typhoid, leprosy, TB, and diphtheria. New horizons were now available for the control of infectious disease, including improved diagnosis and understanding of carrier states and vectors important to transmission. Preparation of antitoxin against diphtheria and development of immunizations against this disease, beginning in New York City in 1920, were harbingers of the abilities of organized public health programs to prevent a wide range of diseases.[10]

The bacteriologic discoveries of Pasteur, working on yeast and rabies, became a marker between the "old" and the "new" public health.[26] The identification of bacteria identified the enemy as specific organisms and drew attention away from the sanitary problems of water supply, street cleaning, housing, and living conditions of the poor.[16,19,26] A disease-oriented approach to public health became important for health officers and local health agencies.[19] Transmission of typhoid fever by polluted water was demonstrated, and methods were developed to measure bacteria in air, water, and milk.[26] At the same time, public health professionals continued to stress social reform and that disease could not be separated from living and working conditions.[16]

By the end of the nineteenth and early twentieth century, the stage had been set for the forerunners of our contemporary public health agencies. The initial spurs to community action were threats from the environment, water, and food, resulting in epidemic disease. Options for collective action had been used for centuries, including isolation, quarantine, and waste disposal. The momentum for organized public health activities increased with urbanization and population increases that exacerbated outbreaks of disease and unsatisfactory health. In the nineteenth century, the twin models of organized sanitary practices and government structures for public health activities developed in England also became of major importance for the United States.

Local public health agencies in the United States developed from local boards of health dating to the eighteenth century.[27] Subsequent development was sporadic until around 1910, when severe epidemics of typhoid fever occurred at a number of locations, including Yakima, Washington, leading to a recommendation from the federal government that full-time local health departments be formed. The first state board of health was established by the Louisiana State Legislature in 1855 in response to yellow fever, but this proved not to be a functional organization. The first board of health is thus stated to have been legislated in Massachusetts in 1869[13] following a recommendation made by Shattuck in his 1850 report.[18] Other states quickly followed: California (1870), Minnesota (1872), Virginia (1872), Michigan (1873), Maryland (1874), and Alabama (1875). By 1900, all but eight states had boards of health. With New Mexico forming this organization in 1919, all states had boards.[13]

CONCEPT OF HEALTH: THE BASIS FOR ACTION

Health has multiple determinants. Factors important to health, illness, and injury are social, economic, genetic, perinatal, nutritional, behavioral, infectious, and environmental.[28] The broad definition developed by the IOM is that "health is a state of complete physical, mental and social well-being and not merely the absence of disease or infirmity."[29(p.41)]

The IOM Committee on Using Performance Monitoring To Improve Community Health worked with a definition of health that relies on community participation: "Health is a state of well-being and the capability to function in the face of changing circumstances—Health is, therefore, a positive concept emphasizing social and personal resources as well as physical capabilities. Improving health is a shared responsibility of health providers, public health officials, and a variety of other actors in the community who can contribute to the well being of individuals and populations."[29(p.41)]

Interaction of social, environmental, and biologic factors determines the health of individuals and populations (Figure 1–5). Environment includes physical environment, conditions of living, and the presence of toxic and infectious agents. Social factors of importance include poverty, education, and cultural environments, including isolation. Biologic factors include genetics and other influences, including behaviors, that determine the susceptibility of the indi-

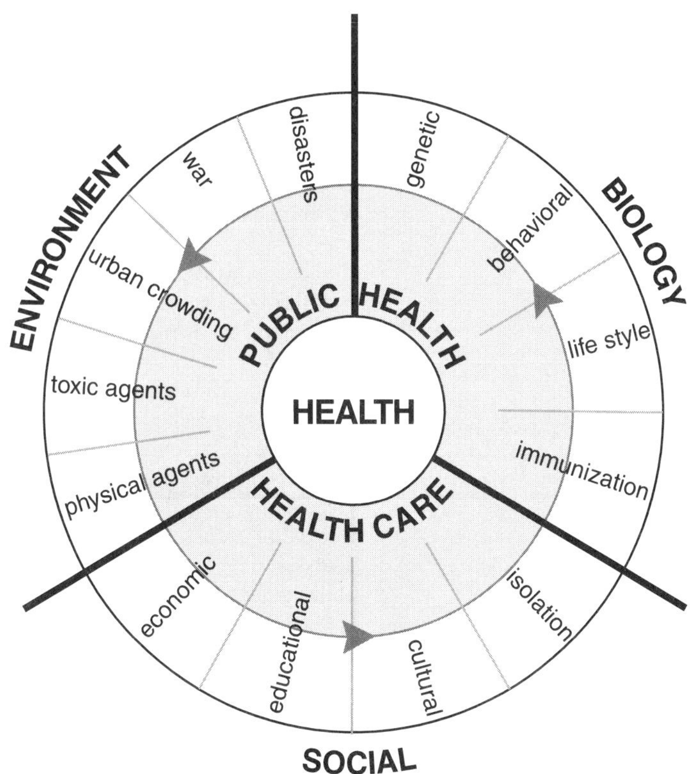

Figure 1–5 Determinants of Health. *Source:* Copyright © 2000, L.F. Novick.

vidual to disease. This formulation is derived from a basic public health and epidemiologic model, explaining ill health as a product of an interaction between the host, the agent, and the environment.

The epidemiologic distribution of disease is determined by factors that: (1) influence contact with disease agents and (2) determine the susceptibility of the individual. The availability of the susceptible individual or host and the presence of the agent both are influenced by the environment. This fundamental interaction producing ill health is true for both infectious agents and noninfectious disease. In this model, agents can include nutritional deficiencies or excesses, toxins, substances, firearms, and so forth. The critical contribution of this model is that effects on health are produced by interactions of multiple factors, as shown in Exhibit 1–3.

For example, the transmission of HIV in a community is determined by: (1) infection of individuals with the infectious *agent* HIV, (2) susceptible *host individuals* with risk behaviors related to unprotected sex or needle-sharing drug use, and (3) the presence of an *environment* that does not constrain the development of risk behaviors and provides opportunity for interaction between the infected and vulnerable individuals. The agent–host–environment model facilitates public health intervention because disease can be interdicted by addressing any one of these factors, as shown in Figure 1–6. Reducing the transmission of HIV through needle exchange is a successful strategy based on environmental intervention. Successful development of a vaccine would modify host susceptibility. Attempts to change the infectivity of this agent would be far more difficult but have been important in curtailing the transmission of other infectious diseases.

Physical Environment

Housing, urbanization, overcrowding, and the availability of quality water have been described

Exhibit 1–3 Classification of Agent, Host, and Environmental Factors That Determine the Occurrence of Diseases in Human Populations

I. Agents of Disease: Etiological Factors	*Examples*
A. Nutritive elements	
Excesses	Cholesterol
Deficiencies	Vitamins, proteins
B. Chemical agents	
Poisons	Carbon monoxide, carbon tetrachloride, drugs
Allergens	Ragweed, poison ivy, medications
C. Physical agents	Ionizing radiation, mechanical
D. Infectious agents	
Metazoa	Hookworm, schistosomiasis, onchocerciasis
Protozoa	Amoebae, malaria
Bacteria	Rheumatic fever, lobar pneumonia, typhoid, Tuberculosis, syphilis
	Histoplasmosis, athlete's foot
Rickettsia	Rocky Mountain spotted fever, typhus
Viruses	Measles, mumps, chickenpox, smallpox, poliomyelitis, rabies, yellow fever
II. Host Factors (Intrinsic Factors): Influence Exposure, Susceptibility, or Response to Agents	
A. Genetic	Sickle cell disease
B. Age	
C. Sex	
D. Ethnic group	
E. Physiologic state	Fatigue, pregnancy, puberty, stress, nutritional state
F. Prior immunologic	
Experience	Hypersensitivity, protection
Active	Prior infection, immunization
Passive	Maternal antibodies, gamma globulin prophylaxis
G. Intercurrent or preexisting disease	
H. Human behavior	Personal hygiene, food handling, diet, interpersonal contact, occupation, recreation, utilization of health resources
III. Environmental Factors (Extrinsic Factors): Influence Existence of the Agent, Exposure, or Susceptibility to Agent	
A. Physical environment	Geology, climate
B. Biologic environment	
Human populations	Density
Flora	Sources of food, influence on vertebrates and arthropods as a source of agents
Fauna	Food sources, vertebrate hosts, arthropod vectors
C. Socioeconomic Environment	
Occupation	Exposure to chemical agents
Urbanization and economic development	Urban crowding, tensions, and pressures; cooperative efforts in health and education
Disruption	Wars, floods

Source: From *Foundations of Epidemiology, Third Edition* by David E. Lilienfeld and Paul D. Tolley, copyright 1994 by Oxford University Press, Inc. Used by permission of Oxford University Press, Inc.

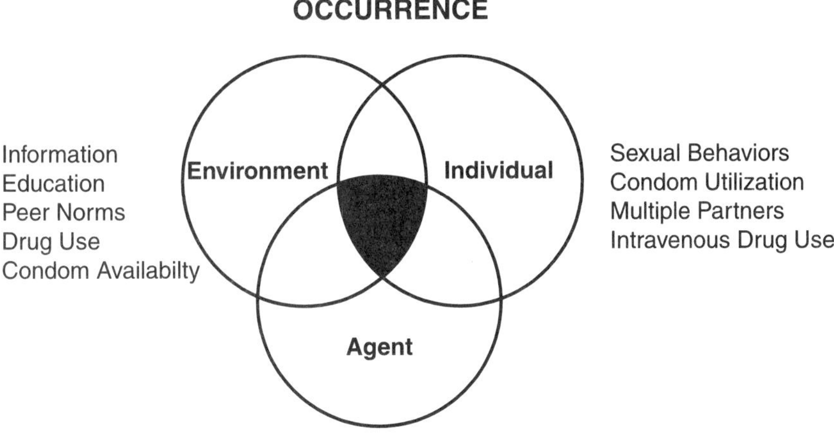

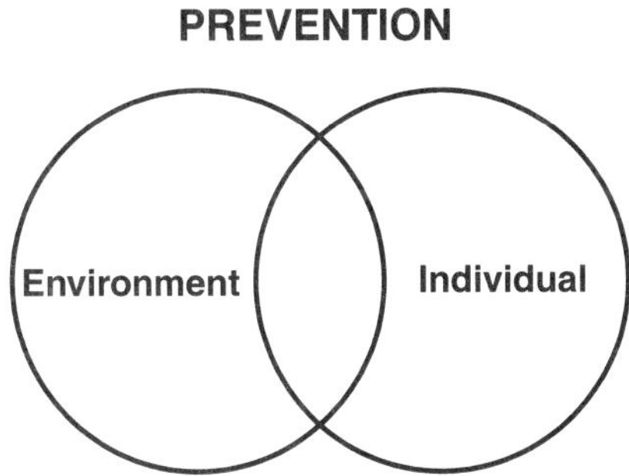

Partner Notification / Needle exchange / Safe Sex / Condoms

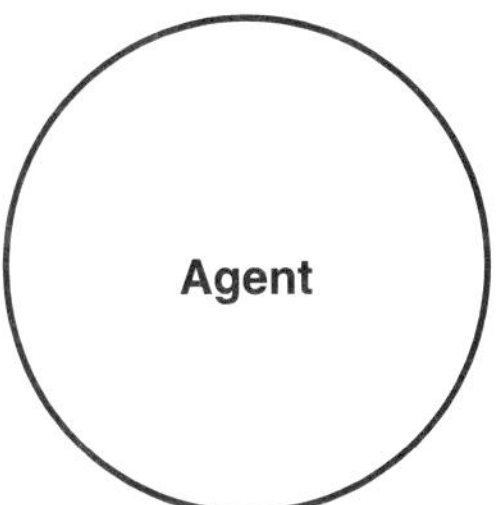

Figure 1–6 Community Prevalence of HIV Infection. *Source:* Copyright © 2000, L.F. Novick.

as being critically important to the health of the public and were a focus of early community efforts. A wide array of problems, including infectious diseases, injuries, and chronic illnesses, can be partly attributed to poor environmental conditions.[30] With the diminished prevalence of infectious diseases as a cause for mortality, there has been a rise in chronic conditions, including cancer, cardiovascular disease, and chronic lung disease. Environmental exposures, including those in the workplace, are important to the increased occurrences of these conditions.[31] Also important is that environmental effects on mortality and morbidity may occur only after long lag times because of the latency periods of these exposures.

Concern with the environment extends far beyond sanitation. Physical and chemical factors are important in the ecosystem and directly influence health. Air pollution containing potentially hazardous chemicals, biologic and chemical contamination of foods, home accidents, and environmental carcinogens are all important to the health of the community.[32] Exposures to pesticides are a major environmental problem where the risks from such exposures need to be better understood. Issues that constitute environmental health priorities for action include wastewater treatment, safe drinking and recreational water sources, ambient air standards, childhood asthma, lead toxicity, indoor air quality, foodborne illness, and household and industrial chemicals.[33]

Socioeconomic Factors

Social and economic factors and their influence on life processes are among the most powerful influences on health.[34] The health disadvantage of those in lower socioeconomic groups cannot be explained in terms of only one or two diseases. Elevated death rates for the poor are evident in almost all of the major causes of death and in each major group of diseases, including infectious, nutritional, cardiovascular, injury, metabolic, and cancers. The only exceptions are breast and skin cancer. The latter is related to exposure from the sun.[34]

The relationship between health status and education, a measure of socioeconomic level, for selected causes of death is shown in Figure 1–7.[26] Heart disease is the leading cause of death in the United States. During the period 1979–89, among men 25–64 years of age, heart disease mortality for those men with incomes less than $10,000 was 2.5 times that for those men with incomes of $25,000 or more, as shown in Figure 1–8.[27]

Life expectancy appears more related to income inequalities than to average income or wealth.[35] In a study of the relationship between total and cause-specific mortality with income distribution for households of the United States, a Robin Hood index measuring inequality was calculated and found to be strongly associated with infant mortality, coronary heart disease, malignant neoplasms, and homicide.[36] Growing inequalities in income and wealth over the last two decades will be a key determinant of disparities of health in the next decade.[37] Widening disparities are occurring in mortality rates by education and income level despite the overall decrease in mortality. Mortality rates for children and adults are related both to poverty and to the distribution of income inequality.[37]

This socioeconomic gradient in health is important to the health of mothers and children—a priority target of public health efforts. Adolescent childbearing, a risk factor for poor health in childhood, is more common in women of lower socioeconomic status as measured by educational attainment (Figure 1–9). Children whose usual activities such as playing and going to school are limited by chronic health problems are shown in Figure 1–10. Again, activity limitation is increased among the poor. Elevated blood lead among children one to five years of age and smoking in pregnancy also vary by family income or education (Figure 1–11 and Figure 1–12).

Other social factors, including avoidance of social exclusion, are vital to the maintenance of health. Social exclusion results in not only social, but also economic and psychological isolation.[38] Disruptive effects when individuals migrate and change cultures have also been described as having a deleterious impact on health.[39] Social support systems have a positive influence, and persons with extensive networks generally have longer life expectancies.[40]

Lifestyle

Personal behaviors play critical roles in the development of many serious diseases and injuries.[41] Behavioral factors largely determine the patterns of disease and mortality of the twentieth-century populations of the United States.[42] The 1964 surgeon general's report, *Smoking and Health,* concluded that cigarette smoking causes lung cancer, chronic bronchitis, and emphysema.[43] Smoking is responsible for approxi-

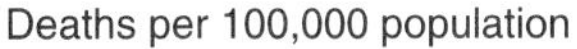

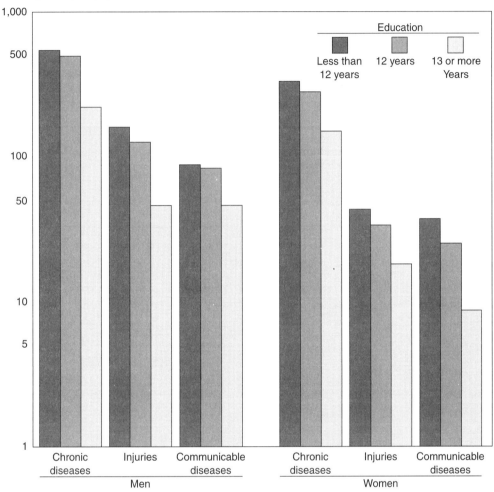

Notes: Death rates are age adjusted. "Injuries" include homicide, suicide, unintentional injuries, and death from adverse effects of medical procedures. Rates are plotted on a log scale.

Figure 1–7 Death Rates for Selected Causes for Adults 25–64 Years of Age by Educational Level and Sex: Selected States, 1995. *Source:* Reprinted from *Health United States, 1998 Socioeconomic Status and Health Chart Book,* p. 91, U.S. Department of Health and Human Services.

mately 20 percent of premature deaths in the United States.[2] The Framingham study showed the role of cigarette smoking, high serum cholesterol, and hypertension in ischemic heart disease.[44] Risk factors including smoking, lack of exercise, substance abuse, and consumption of diets high in fat and calories have increased since the early part of the twentieth century, resulting in epidemics of cardiovascular disease, lung cancer, chronic obstructive lung disease, and diabetes.[42] *Our Healthier Nation,* a 1998 United Kingdom report presented to Parliament by the secretary of state for health, stated that the causes of ill health were complex and included lifestyle as a predominant factor: "How people live has an important impact on health. Whether people smoke, whether they are physically active, what and how much they eat and drink; their sexual behavior and whether they take illicit drugs—all of these factors can have a dramatic and cumulative influence on how healthy people are and how long they will live."[38(p.5)]

Socioeconomic disparities occur for smoking, obesity, and sedentary lifestyles.[37] Individuals below the poverty level are more likely to smoke than those above the poverty level (32.5 percent vs. 23.8 percent).[37] The importance of these risks or personal behaviors is shown in a study by McGinnis and Foege, who calculated their relation to preventable causes of death.[2] Smoking emerged as the largest preventable cause of death (Figure 1–13).

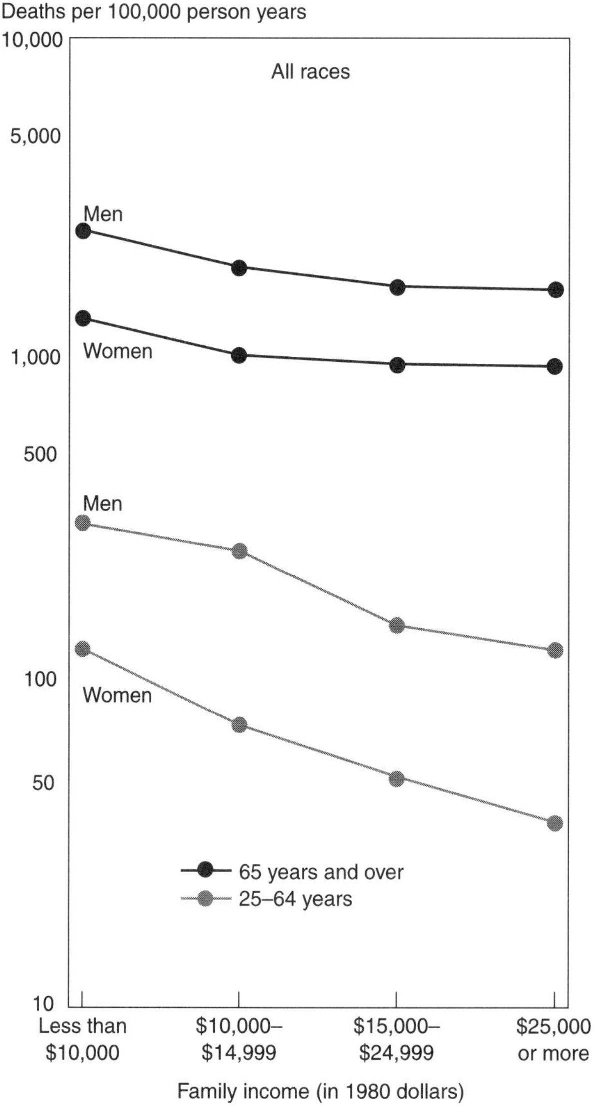

Figure 1–8 Heart Disease Death Rates among Adults 25–64 Years of Age and Older by Family Income and Sex: United States, Average Annual 1979–89. *Source:* Reprinted from *Health United States, 1998 Socioeconomic Status and Health Chart Book,* p. 92, U.S. Department of Health and Human Services.

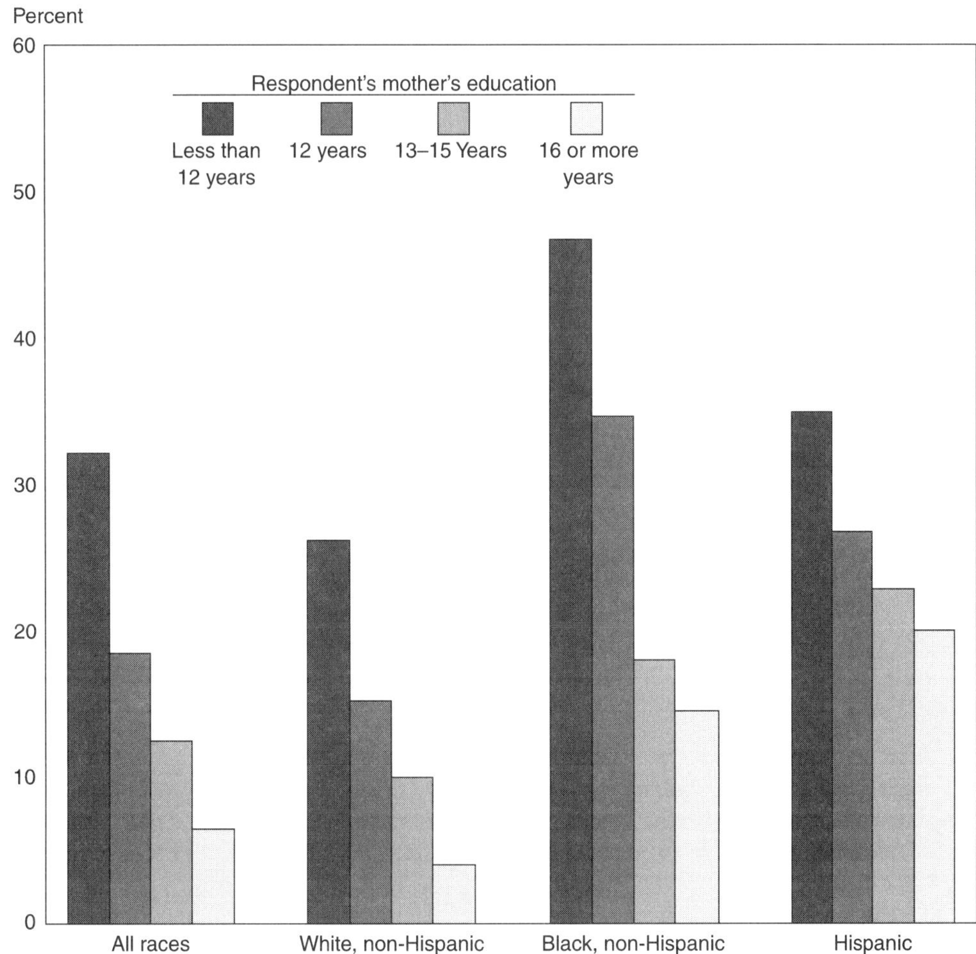

Figure 1–9 Percentage of Women 20–29 Years of Age Who Had a Teenage Birth by Respondent's Mother's Education, Respondent's Race, and Hispanic Origin: United States, 1995. *Source:* Reprinted from *1995 Survey of Family Growth,* Centers for Disease Control and Prevention, National Center for Health Statistics.

POPULATION-BASED PREVENTION STRATEGY

The public health strategy of prevention begins with the recognition that the health of the community is dependent on an interaction between behavioral and environmental factors affecting the entire population. The target for intervention is not framed in terms of individual clinical interactions or groups enrolled at health care facilities or public health service activities. Rather, the target is a geographic or otherwise defined population. Individuals seeking care from practitioners and groups attending health facilities or using public health services are viewed in this strategy as components or subgroups of the larger population.

Using a population as an organizing principle for preventive action has considerable benefit because of the broad distribution of most diseases and health determinants. However, this basic preventive concept is frequently misunderstood not only by the public, but also by public health workers who manage preventive initia-

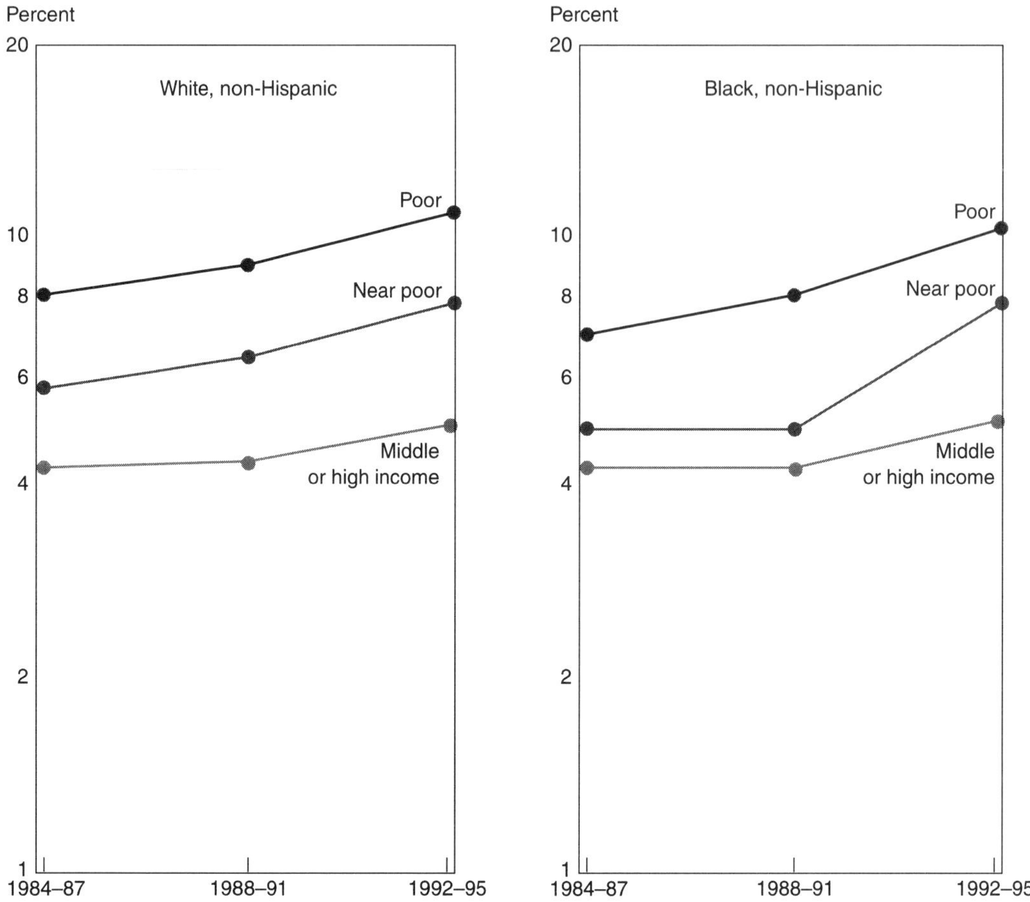

Figure 1–10 Activity Limitation among Children 18 Years of Age by Family Income, Race, and Hispanic Origin: United States, Average Annual 1984–87, 1988–91, and 1992–95. *Source:* Reprinted from *National Health Interview Survey,* Centers for Disease Control and Prevention, National Center for Health Statistics. (See related *Health United States, 1998,* table 60.)

tives in terms of facility enrollees or high-risk individuals already identified, thus reducing the potential for health enhancement. As Geoffrey Rose has stated, "A large number of people exposed to a small risk may generate many more cases than a small number exposed to a high risk."[45(p.24)] Therefore, widespread problems call for a widespread response, i.e., for a population strategy. A preventive policy targeted at high-risk individuals may benefit these individuals, but its impact on the total burden of disease in the community will be disappointing. For example, more heart disease problems arise from the many people who are at low risk than the relatively smaller number who are at high risk. The population-based strategy will be directed toward changing the prevalence of risk factors for the entire community rather than toward identifying those at high risk through screening for interventions. Population-based and individual targeted preventive strategies are not exclusive but complementary. Strategies involving screening can also be populationwide, such as screening for metabolic diseases, lead toxicity, mammography, and pap smears.

A strategy for populationwide prevention based on the interaction between health determinants is shown in Table 1–4. This contract is based on a populationwide target for the United Kingdom—to reduce the death rate from heart

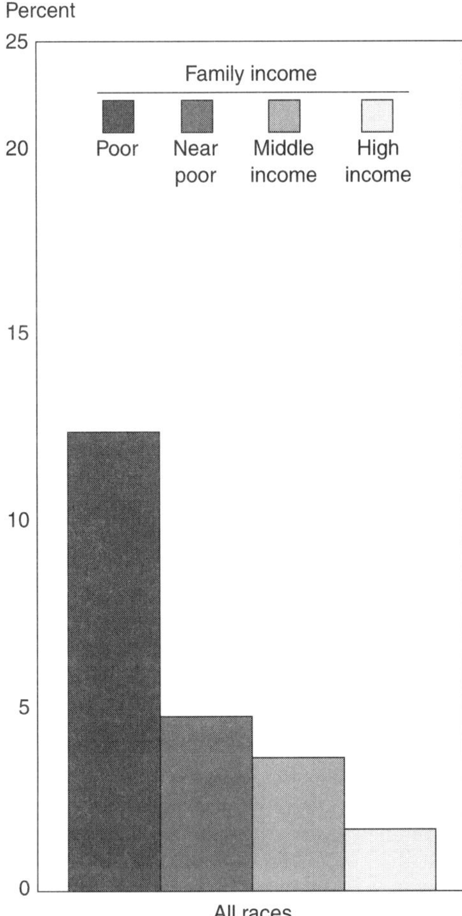

Figure 1–11 Elevated Blood Lead among Children 1–5 Years of Age by Family Income: United States, Average Annual 1988–94. *Source:* Reprinted from *Health United States, 1998 Socioeconomic Status and Health Chart Book,* p. 62, U.S. Department of Health and Human Services.

disease and stroke and related illnesses among people under 65 years by at least a further third (33%) by 2010 from a baseline of 1996.[38]

Two North American reports both published in the 1970s set the stage for population-based preventive activities. *A New Perspective on the Health of Canadians* (Lalonde report) was issued in 1974,[46] and *Healthy People: The Surgeon General's Report on Health Promotion and Disease Prevention* was published in 1979.[41]

Lalonde Report

The Lalonde report sets forth a field concept patterned after the determinants of health. Four broad elements are included in this concept: human biology, environment, lifestyle, and health care organization. *Human biology* includes genetic inheritance and the processes of aging and disease. *Environment* includes matters related to health and external to the individual (including the social environment) and over which the individual has no control. *Lifestyle* includes personal decisions and habits of the individual, which have an adverse impact on health. *Health care organization* refers to the health care system.[46]

> Until now, most of society's efforts to improve health and the bulk of direct health care expenditures have been focused on the *health care organization.* Yet, when we identify the present main causes of sickness and death in Canada, we find that they are rooted in the three other elements of the concept: *human biology, environment* and *lifestyle.* It is apparent, therefore, that vast sums are being spent treating diseases that could have been prevented in the first place.[46(p.32)]

The Lalonde report proposed five strategies for health improvement.

1. a *health promotion strategy* aimed at informing, influencing, and assisting both individuals and organizations so that they will accept more responsibility and be more active in matters affecting mental and physical health
2. a *regulatory strategy* aimed at using federal regulatory powers to reduce hazards to mental and physical health, and at encouraging and assisting provinces to use their regulatory powers to the same end
3. a *research strategy* designed to yield knowledge needed to solve mental and physical health problems
4. *health care efficiency strategy,* the objective of which will be to help the provinces reorganize the system for delivering mental and physical health care so that the

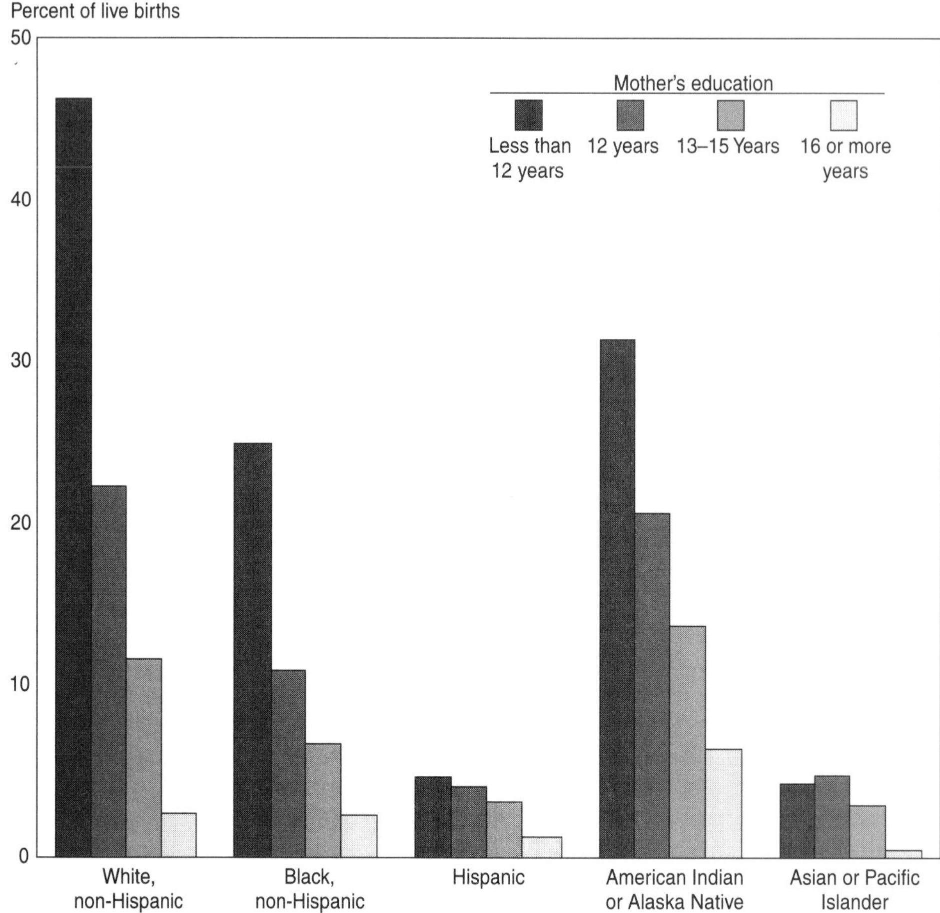

Figure 1–12 Cigarette Smoking during Pregnancy among Mothers 20 Years of Age and Over by Mother's Education, Race, and Hispanic Origin: United States, 1996. *Source:* Reprinted from *National Vital Statistics System,* Centers for Disease Control and Prevention, National Center for Health Statistics. (See related *Health United States, 1998,* table 10.)

three elements of cost, accessibility, and effectiveness are balanced in the interest of Canadians

5. a *goal-setting strategy,* the purpose of which will be to set, in cooperation with others, goals for raising the level of the mental and physical health of Canadians and improving the efficiency of the health care system[46]

Healthy People

In 1979, *Healthy People* marked a turning point in the approach and strategy for public health in the United States. Joseph Califano, Secretary of the Department of Health, Education and Welfare, wrote:

> And let us make no mistake about the purpose of this, the first Surgeon General's Report on Health Promotion and Disease Prevention. Its purpose is to encourage a second public health revolution in the history of the United States. And let us make no mistake about the significance of this document. It represents an emerging consensus among scientists and the

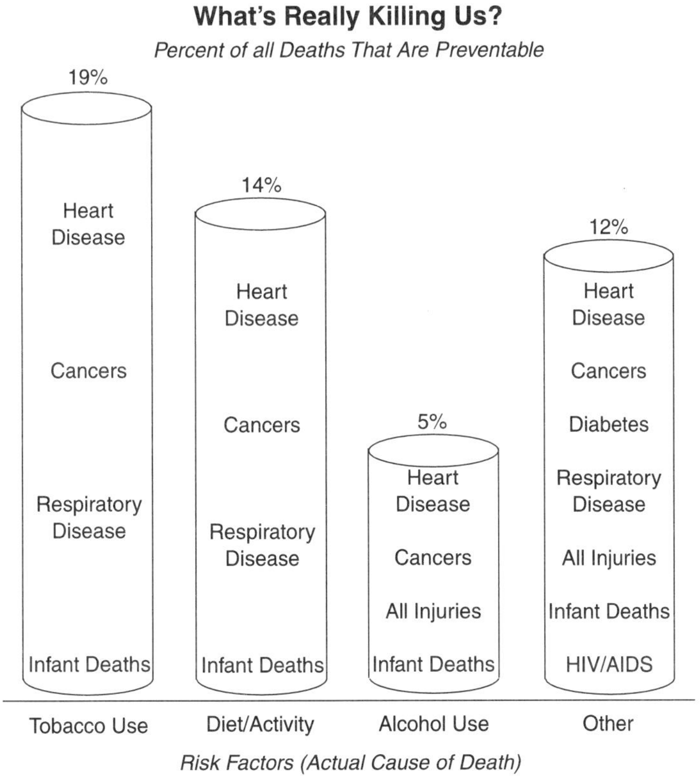

What's Really Killing Us?

Percent of all Deaths That Are Preventable

Tobacco Use — 19%: Heart Disease, Cancers, Respiratory Disease, Infant Deaths

Diet/Activity — 14%: Heart Disease, Cancers, Respiratory Disease, Infant Deaths

Alcohol Use — 5%: Heart Disease, Cancers, All Injuries, Infant Deaths

Other — 12%: Heart Disease, Cancers, Diabetes, Respiratory Disease, All Injuries, Infant Deaths, HIV/AIDS

Risk Factors (Actual Cause of Death)

Figure 1–13 Percent of Preventable Deaths. *Source:* Reprinted from *Health Status Report,* Draft (version 8) January 2000, p. 3, U.S. Department of Health and Human Services.

> health community that the Nation's Health strategy must be dramatically recast to emphasize the prevention of disease.[41(p.vii)]

The first public health revolution was the struggle against infectious disease in the late nineteenth and early twentieth century, which involved sanitation and immunization. The second revolution was spurred by the prevalence of chronic disease, including heart disease and cancer. The key to *Healthy People* was the premise that the personal habits and behaviors of individuals determined "whether a person will be healthy or sick, live a long life or die prematurely."[41(p.viii)] The report urged Americans to adopt simple measures to enhance health.

- elimination of cigarette smoking
- reduction of alcohol misuse
- moderate dietary changes to reduce the intake of excess calories, fat, salt, and sugar
- moderate exercise
- periodic screening (at intervals to be determined by age and sex) for major disorders such as high blood pressure and certain cancers
- adherence to speed laws and the use of seat belts

The role of the individual and personal lifestyle choices were emphasized. This was a change from earlier public health approaches, including the actions undertaken to protect health in the nineteenth century. Geoffrey Rose observed, "Actions such as the provision of clean water supplies and sanitation were undertaken for people rather than by people. They have been followed in this century by further centrally provided and regulated measures to protect or improve health, including the

Table 1–4 A National Contract on Heart Disease and Stroke

A National Contract on Heart Disease and Stroke	*Government and National Players Can:*	*Local Players and Communities Can:*	*People Can:*
Social and economic	Continue to make smoking cost more through taxation. Tackle joblessness, social exclusion, low educational standards, and other factors that make it harder to live a healthier life.	Tackle social exclusion in the community, which makes it harder to have a healthy lifestyle. Provide incentives to employees to cycle or walk to work, or leave their cars at home.	Take opportunities to better their lives and their families' lives, through education, training, and employment.
Environmental	Encourage employers and others to provide a smoke-free environment for nonsmokers.	Through local employers and others, provide a smoke-free environment for nonsmokers. Through employers and staff, work in partnership to reduce stress at work. Provide safe cycling and walking routes.	Protect others from secondhand smoke.
Lifestyle	End advertising and promotion of cigarettes. Enforce prohibition of sale of cigarettes to youngsters. Develop Healthy Living Centers. Ensure access to, and availability of, a wide range of foods for a healthy diet. Provide sound information on the health risks of smoking, poor diet, and lack of exercise.	Encourage the development of healthy schools and healthy workplaces. Implement an integrated transport policy, including a national cycling strategy and measures to make walking more of an option. Target information about a healthy life on groups and areas where people are most at risk.	Stop smoking or cut down, watch what they eat, and take regular exercise.
Services	Encourage doctors and nurses and other health professionals to give advice on healthier living. Ensure catering and leisure professionals are trained in healthy eating and physical activity.	Provide help to people who want to stop smoking. Improve access to a variety of affordable food in deprived areas. Provide facilities for physical activity and relaxation and decent transport to help people get to them. Identify those at high risk of heart disease and stroke and provide high-quality services.	Learn how to recognize a heart attack and what to do, including resuscitation skills. Have their blood pressure checked regularly. Take medicine as it is prescribed.

Source: Reprinted from *A National Contract on Heart Disease and Stroke,* presented to Parliament by the Secretary of State for Health, February 1998, © 1998, The Stationery Office, United Kingdom. Crown copyright material is reproduced with the permission of the Controller of Her Majesty's Stationery Office.

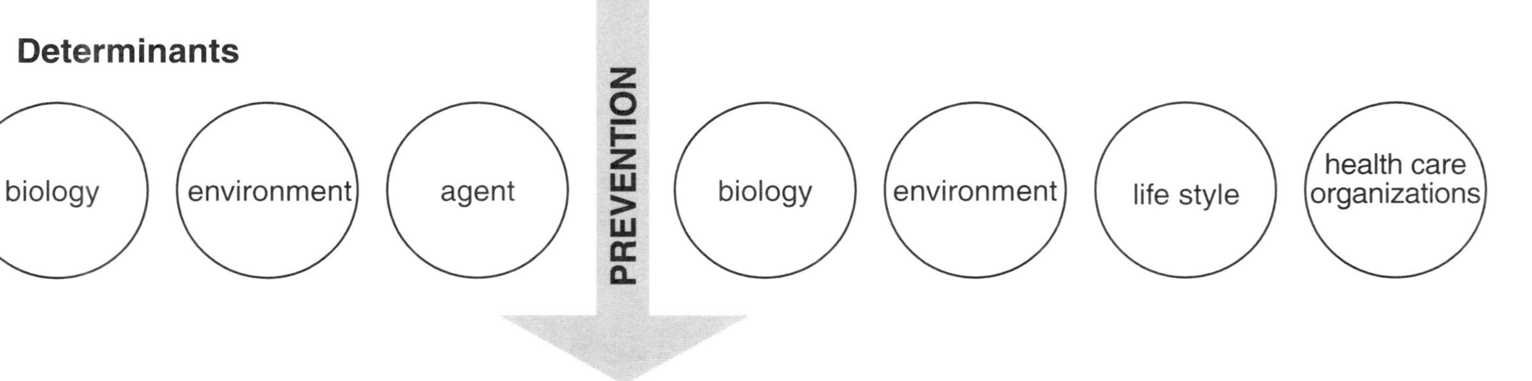

Figure 1–14 Public Health Approach: Before and after Lalonde and *Healthy People* Reports. *Source:* Copyright © 2000, L.F. Novick.

Table 1–5 Leading Causes of Death by Age Category in Onondaga Co, NY, 1994–1996 in Relation to Upstate NY, 1995

		Age-Proportionate Mortality			
		Onondaga Co. 1994–1996		*Upstate NY 1995*	
Age	*Cause*	*Percent*	*Frequency*	*Percent*	*Frequency*
<1 Yr.	All causes	100	176	100	972
	Cond. orig. in perinatal per	55	97	50	488
	Congenital anomalies	20	35	23	227
	Sudden infant death syndrome	9	16	8	82
	Pneumonia	4	7	2	20
	Oth. ill-def. & unk. causes	3	6	—	—
1–9 Yrs.	All causes	100	44	100	312
	Malignant neoplasms	16	7	8	25
	Congenital anomalies	11	5	11	33
	Drownings	9	4	5	16
	Cerebrovascular disease	7	3	2	7
	Motor vehicle	7	3	12	36
10–19 Yrs.	All causes	100	74	100	532
	Motor vehicle	26	19	34	183
	Suicide	18	13	13	67
	Homicide and legal interven.	10	7	8	44
	Malignant neoplasms	8	6	9	46
	Diseases of the heart	7	5	3	15
20–24 Yrs.	All causes	100	68	100	496
	Motor vehicle	27	18	28	137
	Suicide	19	13	17	82
	Homicide and legal interven.	13	9	12	61
	Malignant neoplasms	9	6	8	41
	AIDS	3	2	3	13
25–44 Yrs.	All causes	100	614	100	5,008
	Malignant neoplasms	20	123	17	833
	AIDS	19	116	19	947
	Diseases of the heart	11	70	12	625
	Suicide	11	65	7	350
	Motor vehicle	7	40	8	390
45–64 Yrs.	All causes	100	1,869	100	14,693
	Malignant neoplasms	38	714	38	5,651
	Diseases of the heart	29	546	28	4,157
	Cerebrovascular disease	5	84	4	519
	"Chr. airway obstr., not else spec."	3	53	2	340
	Cirrhosis of liver	3	49	3	369
65+ Yrs.	All causes	100	9,726	100	75,411
	Diseases of the heart	37	3,630	40	30,288
	Malignant neoplasms	23	2,250	23	17,617
	Cerebrovascular disease	9	841	7	5,254
	Pneumonia	6	544	5	3,620
	"Chr. airway obstr., not else spec."	5	442	4	3,050

Source: Reprinted from Bureau of Biometrics, New York State Department of Health.

immunization of infants and children, fluoridation of water, control of food quality and additives, and (limited) cleaning up of the environment."[45(p.103)] *Healthy People* recognized that individuals did not have complete control or responsibility over their health status because of socioeconomic and environmental determinates.[41] Yet, healthy behaviors were seen as an individual responsibility with an important influence on health (Figure 1–14).

A major thrust of the report was a focus on age-related risk. The health problems that affect children change in adolescence and early adulthood and again in old age. At each stage in life, there are different problems and different preventive actions. Table 1–5 shows the change in leading causes of death by stage of life. Accidents and violence predominate in adolescence; chronic disease is the major problem in later adulthood and old age. Public health program planning must be attuned to the age-specific diversity of health problems. *Healthy People* set out five goals in 1977 that were age-specific.[41]

1. Continue to improve infant health and, by 1990, reduce infant mortality by at least 35 percent to fewer than 9 deaths per 1,000 live births.
2. Improve child health, foster optimal child development, and, by 1990, reduce deaths among children 1 to 14 years by at least 20 percent, to fewer than 34 per 100,000.
3. Improve the health and health habits of adolescents and young adults and, by 1990, reduce deaths among people ages 15–24 by at least 20 percent, to fewer than 93 per 100,000.
4. Improve the health of adults and, by 1990, reduce deaths among people ages 25–64 by at least 25 percent, to fewer than 400 per 100,000.
5. Improve the health and quality of life for older adults and, by 1990, reduce the average annual number of days of restricted activity due to acute and chronic conditions by 20 percent, to fewer than 30 days per year for people aged 65 and older.

These goals with specific objectives were reformulated by a second report issued by the surgeon general in the fall of 1980.[47] *Promoting Health/Preventing Disease: Objectives for the Nation* established quantifiable objectives to reach the broad goals of *Healthy People.* This objective-based population preventive strategy continues today with year 2000 and 2010 objectives. As will be described, some progress has been made in the nation's health, as measured by at least some of these goals that were formulated more than two decades ago. For example, the infant mortality rate has declined steadily for 20 years and was 7.6 deaths per 1,000 live births in 1995, exceeding the expectation of the *Healthy People* goal. However, the rate among African American infants was 2.4 times that of Caucasian infants. Although infant mortality rates have decreased, the proportional discrepancy between African Americans and Caucasians remains.[37]

• • •

Public health as a field of practice has evolved in tandem with historic and contemporary trends in science, disease, and social and environmental conditions. Modern public health practice now extends far beyond the historic focus on infectious disease and environmental threats. To achieve meaningful improvements in population health, contemporary public health organizations engage in a broad scope of activities, many of which now focus on affecting changes in human behavior. The nation's public health system has achieved notable improvements in population health throughout the twentieth century. Continued progress will likely hinge on the ability of public health organizations and professionals to mount broad-based, multisectoral health interventions that address the diffuse social and ecological pathways to population health.

CHAPTER REVIEW

1. Operative components of the definition of public health are *organized* and *community effort.*
2. The majority of the gain in life expectancy in the twentieth century (25 of 30 years) can be attributed to public health measures such as better nutrition, sanitation, and housing.

3. For scientific advances to be translated into community health improvement, the following factors are important:
   - public information
   - community acceptance
   - design of a delivery system for the intervention
4. Health issues are an interaction of the following elements:
   - host
   - agent
   - environment
5. The changing scope of public health practice initially concerned with infectious and environmentally related disease has been extended to nutrition, injury prevention, violence, substance abuse, and tobacco-related and other chronic diseases.
6. Lemuel Shattuck was a foremost advocate for public health action in the eighteenth century, recommending environmental improvement and the formation of public health agencies.
7. Public health activities in both England and the United States were greatly influenced by growing urbanization and industrialization.
8. Scientific advances, particularly microbiology, ushered in a new dimension for the field of public health in the latter part of the nineteenth and early twentieth century.
9. The interaction of social, environmental, and biologic factors determines the health of individuals.
10. The public health strategy of prevention begins with the recognition that the health of the community is dependent on an interaction between behavioral and environmental factors.
11. Two North American reports both published in the 1970s set the stage of population-based preventive activities.
    - *A New Perspective on the Health of Canadians* (Lalonde report)
    - *Healthy People: The Surgeon General's Report on Health Promotion and Disease Prevention*

REFERENCES

1. J. Bunker, "Improving Health: Measuring Effects of Medical Care," *The Milbank Quarterly* 72 (1994): 225–258.
2. J. McGinnis and W. Foege, "Actual Causes of Death in the United States," *Journal of the American Medical Association 270,* no. 18 (1993): 2,207–2,212.
3. C.-E.A. Winslow, *The Untilled Fields of Public Health* (New York: Health Service, New York County Chapter of the American Red Cross, 1920).
4. Institute of Medicine, *The Future of Public Health* (Washington, DC: National Academy Press, 1988).
5. C. Kivlahan, "Public Health in the Next Century," *Missouri Medicine 91,* no. 1 (1994): 19–23.
6. Q. Young, "Public Health: A Powerful Guide," *Journal of Health Care Finance 25,* no. 1 (1998): 1–4.
7. C. Winslow, "Public Health at the Crossroads," *American Journal of Public Health* 16 (1926): 1,075–1,085.
8. U.S. Department of Health and Human Services, Public Health Service, *For a Healthy Nation: Returns on Investment in Public Health. Executive Summary* (Washington, DC: U.S. Government Printing Office, 1994).
9. A. Affi and L. Breslow, "A Maturing Paradigm of Public Health," *Annual Review of Public Health* 15 (1994): 223–235.
10. G. Rosen, *A History of Public Health* (New York: MD Publications, 1958).
11. S. Kottek, "Gems from the Talmud: Public Health I—Water Supply," *Israel Journal of Medical Science* 31 (1995): 255–256.
12. Hippocrates, *On Airs, Waters and Places.* Translated and republished in *Medical Classics* 3 (1938): 19–42.
13. W. Smillie, *Public Health: Its Promise for the Future* (New York: The Macmillan Co., 1955).
14. J. Duffy, *Epidemics in Colonial America* (Baton Rouge, LA: Louisiana State University Press, 1953).
15. A. Benenson, ed., *Control of Communicable Diseases in Man* (Washington, DC: American Public Health Association, 1990).

16. D. Rosner, *Hives of Sickness* (New Brunswick, NJ: Rutgers University Press, 1995).
17. J. Ellis, "Businessmen and Public Health in the Urban South during the Nineteenth Century: New Orleans, Memphis, and Atlanta." *Bulletin of the History of Medicine 44,* no. 4 (1970): 346–371.
18. L. Shattuck, *General Plan for the Promotion of Public and Personal Health* (Boston: Dutton & Wentworth, State Printers, 1850).
19. E. Fee, "The Origins and Development of Public Health in the United States," in *Oxford Textbook of Public Health,* eds. W. Holland et al. (Oxford, New York, Toronto: Oxford University Press, 1991), 3–21.
20. W. Bynum and R. Porter, *Living and Dying in London* (London: Wellcome Institute for the History of Medicine, 1991).
21. J. Duffy, *A History of Public Health in New York City, 1866–1966* (New York: Russell Sage Foundation, 1968).
22. C. Hamlin and S. Sheard, "Revolutions in Public Health: 1848, and 1998?" *British Medical Journal* 317 (1998): 587–591.
23. J. Ashton and I. Sram, "Millennium Report to Sir Edwin Chadwick," *British Medical Journal* 317 (1998): 592–596.
24. E. Porter, "The History of Public Health and the Modern State, Introduction (editorial)." *Clio Medica* 26 (1994): 1–44.
25. H. Kramer, "Agitation for Public Health Reform in the 1870's," *Journal of the History of Medicine* Autumn (1948): 473–488.
26. E. Fee, "Public Health and the State: The United States," *Clio Medica* 26 (1994): 224–275.
27. J. Jeckel, "Health Departments in the U.S. 1920–1988: Statements of Mission with Special Reference to the Role of C.-E.A. Winslow," *The Yale Journal of Biology and Medicine* 64 (1991): 467–479.
28. G. Omenn, "Health Status and its Determinants in Urban Populations" *Journal of Urban Health, Bulletin of New York Academy of Medicine 75,* no. 2 (1998): 222.
29. Institute of Medicine, *Improving Health in the Community* (Washington, DC: National Academy Press, 1997).
30. R. Jackson, "Habitat and Health: The Role of Environmental Factors in the Health of Urban Populations," *Journal of Urban Health, Bulletin of New York Academy of Medicine 75,* no. 2 (1998): 258–262.
31. P. Lehman, "Improving the Quality of the Work Environment," in *Healthy People: The Surgeon General's Report on Health Promotion and Disease Prevention—Background Papers* [DHEW Publication #79–55071A] (Washington, DC: U.S. Government Printing Office, 1979), 387–407.
32. World Health Organization, "The Human Environment," *Promoting Health in the Human Environment* (Geneva, Switzerland, 1975), 17–29.
33. V. Lafronza, "The Evolution of Environmental Health," *Transformations in Public Health 2,* no. 2 (1999): 1–4.
34. R. Wilkinson, *Unhealthy Societies* (London: Routledge, 1997).
35. R. Wilkinson, "Class Mortality Differentials, Income Distribution and Trends in Poverty 1921–1981," *Journal of Social Policy* 18 (1989): 307–335.
36. B. Kennedy et al., "Income Distribution and Mortality: Cross Sectional Ecological Study of the Robin Hood Index in the United States," *British Medical Journal* 312 (1996): 1,004–1,007.
37. U.S. Department of Health and Human Services, Office of Public Health and Science, *Healthy People 2010 Objectives, Draft for Public Comment* (Washington, DC: U.S. Government Printing Office, 1998).
38. Office of Secretary of State for Health, *Our Healthier Nation* (London: The Stationery Office, 1998).
39. R. Evans et al., eds., *Why Are Some People Healthy and Others Not?* (New York: Aldine de Gruyter, 1994).
40. J. Last, "Social and Behavioral Determinants of Health," *Public Health and Human Ecology* (East Norwalk, CT: Appleton & Lange, 1987), 211–242.
41. U.S. Department of Health, Education and Welfare, *Healthy People: The Surgeon General's Report on Health Promotion and Disease Prevention* (Washington, DC: U.S. Government Printing Office, 1979).
42. L. Breslow, "Behavioral Factors in the Health Status of Urban Populations," *Journal of Urban Health, Bulletin of New York Academy of Medicine 75,* no. 2 (1998): 242–249.
43. Surgeon General's Advisory Committee on Smoking and Health, *Smoking and Health* (Washington, DC: U.S. Government Printing Office, 1964).
44. J. Last, "Health Information and Epidemiology," *Public Health and Human Ecology* (East Norwalk, CT: Appleton & Lange, 1987), 27–102.
45. G. Rose, *The Strategy of Preventive Medicine* (New York: Oxford University Press, 1992).
46. M. Lalonde, *A New Perspective on the Health of Canadians—A Working Document* (Ottawa, Canada: Government of Canada, 1974).
47. U.S. Department of Health and Human Services, *Promoting Health/Preventing Disease: Objectives for the Nation* [DHHS (PHS) Publication No. 79–55071] (Washington, DC: U.S. Government Printing Office, 1980).

CHAPTER 2

A Framework for Public Health Administration and Practice

Lloyd F. Novick

Activities performed by health departments have evolved throughout the last century. A persistent unanswered question has been whether the scope of public health work should include the actual delivery of personal health services. In 1988, a pivotal report of the Institute of Medicine (IOM), *The Future of Public Health*, established recommendations for a new way of organizing public health activities that places expanded emphasis on population-based efforts rather than on personal health care delivery. Three core public health functions were identified, denoted as assessment, policy development, and assurance. Several years later, a federally sponsored task force developed another taxonomy of public health activity that centered around Ten Essential Services of Public Health. Contemporary public health activities have been shaped not only by efforts to redefine the conceptual basis of public health practice, but also by efforts to redefine specific public health goals. Federal health agencies have developed national health objectives for the years 1980, 1990, and 2000, and now for the year 2010. Recent efforts to improve the processes and outcomes of public health practice have emphasized strategies for increasing the public's quality and years of life, eliminating health disparities, and building infrastructure of public health efforts.

PUBLIC HEALTH FUNCTIONS

Before 1908, no county in the United States had a full-time health officer with the exception of New York City.[1] In 1910–11, multiple epidemics of typhoid fever, including one in Yakima, Washington, prompted a strong federal recommendation for the creation of full-time local health departments.[2] Rapid growth of these agencies began in the following decade. Between 1908 and 1934, more than a quarter of the counties in the nation had public health services under the direction of a full-time health officer for some part of that period.[2]

In 1933, an American Public Health Association statement* listed two primary goals for public health agencies: (1) the control of communicable diseases and (2) the promotion of child health. Specific services were also listed, including: (1) laboratory, (2) sanitation, (3) public health education, (4) public health nursing, (5) vital statistics, and (6) research in disease prevention.[3] This basic categorization described the public health role as fundamentally preventive, with a clear separation from the provision of medical care.

Local Health Units for the Nation, another report by Haven Emerson, produced a similar listing of six basic functions of a health department (Exhibit 2–1).[1]

A survey published by Mountin in 1941 of the 48 then-existing state health agencies showed a

*The 1933 statement was developed by a subcommittee of the American Public Health Association (APHA), Committee on Administrative Practice (CAP), and signed by Haven Emerson and by other committee members, including C.-E.A. Winslow.[2]

Exhibit 2–1 Six Basic Functions of a Local Health Department

1. Vital statistics, or the recording, tabulation, interpretation, and publication of the essential facts of births, deaths, and reportable diseases
2. Control of communicable diseases, including tuberculosis, the venereal diseases, malaria, and hookworm disease
3. Environmental sanitation, including supervision of milk and milk products, food processing and public eating places, and maintenance of sanitary condition of employment
4. Public Health laboratory services
5. Hygiene of maternity, infancy, and childhood, including supervision of the health of the school child
6. Health education of the general public so far as not covered by the functions of departments of education

Source: Reprinted from H. Emerson, *Local Health Units for the Nation,* 1945, The Commonwealth Fund, New York.

similar constellation of interests, including vital statistics, communicable disease and tuberculosis (TB) control, maternal and child health (MCH) services, health education, and environmental activities.[4] Again, the role of public health was targeted to prevention with a focus on the indigent. It did not include the provision of medical care except to treat TB and sexually transmitted diseases (STDs).

In the last half-century, new influences have shaped the development of basic public health functions. Also in this period, a major question for public health has been the merit of continuing to provide preventive services for the indigent versus assuming responsibility for the actual delivery of medical care. Should prevention and medical care be delivered separately but coordinated? Or, should prevention and medical care be integrated into one system?

New federal programs beginning in the 1960s highlighted this choice and influenced the evolution of public health functions. The Maternal and Infant Care (MIC) Program was passed in 1965 (part of Title V of the Social Security Act), as was the Community Mental Health Act. In the same year, additional legislation enacted as part of the "Great Society" included Medicare, Medicaid, and the Children and Youth Program (C&Y), as well as Comprehensive Health Planning (CHP) and Regional Medical Planning (RMP).[2] In some instances, these programs changed the structure of governmental agencies. To participate in Medicaid, states were required to designate a single state agency to administer the program, often setting up a dichotomy between public health services and Medicaid activities.[5] Comprehensive health planning legislation resulted in the creation of new planning bodies at state and local levels. These new entities also had populationwide agendas, with a wide base of provider and consumer participation.

Federal programs of the 1960s did to some extent spur growth of health services in local health departments. Local health departments sponsored approximately 13 percent of the neighborhood health centers, nearly 30 percent of the child and youth projects, and 76 percent of the maternal and infant care projects.[6] But predominantly, federal funds bypassed state and local government and fostered the growth of community agencies and health centers. These health activities often were not coordinated with local public health agencies, whose role remained more narrowly defined in terms of the traditional functions of vital statistics, communicable disease, health education, and MCH activities. Local health departments were weakened by competing "mini-health departments," including community health centers and community health agencies.[2] The health-planning role was now performed by the Comprehensive Health Planning agencies. Also, many environmental responsibilities were transferred from public health to new state environmental agencies fostered by the creation of the federal Environmental Protection Agency (EPA) in 1970.

During the 1960s, an increased number of local health departments were providing personal health services to indigent individuals. Many local and state public health agencies were providers of last resort to the poor, uninsured, and

Medicaid clients.[5] In communities with substantial numbers of uninsured, public health agencies attempted to provide a "safety net," but generally services were inadequate and not comprehensive. As early as 1949, Terris and Kramer noted that local health departments were moving beyond prevention and into treatment services.[7] A 1968 study by the Public Health Service documented that local health departments were offering medical care services.[8] Involvement of local health departments in providing medical care continued to increase over the next several decades.[6] Health departments in the Sun Belt, Pacific, and Mountain areas were most involved in the provision of medical services.[6] In response to the question of whether a health department should provide assurance of care and act as a guarantor versus actually engaging in the delivery of medical care, the 1988 report by the IOM strongly recommended the assurance role rather than actual delivery. The responsibility of providing medical care to the poor was seen as draining resources and attention away from disease prevention and health promotion activities that benefit the entire community. It was believed that government had the responsibility to provide access and services, but by another mechanism.[5]

CORE PUBLIC HEALTH FUNCTIONS

In 1988, the pivotal report, *The Future of Public Health,* had set out recommendations for a new categorization of public health functions.[5] These functions were recommended to counter the attrition of public health vigilance in protecting the public. Lack of agreement concerning mission, politicized decision making, and unsatisfactory linkages with private medicine were cited as underlying difficulties. Little attention to management and the lack of development of leaders were also described as root causes of ineffective public health action. Recommendations included designating central responsibility to state health departments and grouping all primarily health-related functions there. State delegation of this responsibility to local government was foreseen. The IOM report provided a new categorization of public health functions, which has become widely adopted. Functions were denoted as assessment, policy development, and assurance.[5]

Assessment

> The committee recommends every public health agency regularly and systematically collect, assemble, analyze, and make available information on the health needs of the community, including statistics on health status, community health needs, and epidemiological and other studies of health problems.[5(p.7)]

Policy Development

> The committee recommends that every public health agency exercise its responsibility to serve the public interest in the development of comprehensive public health policies by promoting the use of the scientific knowledge base in decision making about public health and by developing public health policy. Agencies must take a strategic approach, developed on the basis of a positive appreciation for the democratic political process.[5(p.8)]

Assurance

> The committee recommends that public health agencies assure their constituents that services necessary to achieve agreed upon goals are provided, either by encouraging actions by other entities (private or public sector), by requiring such action through regulation, or by providing services directly.
>
> The committee further recommends that each public health agency involve lay policymakers and the general public in determining a set of high-priority personal and community-wide health

> services that governments will guarantee to every member of the community. This guarantee should include subsidization or direct provision of high-priority personal health services for those unable to afford them.[5(p.8–9)]

Specific public health activities have been identified for each of these functions as indicated in Exhibit 2–2. Categorization of assessment, policy development, and assurance have become a commonly used rubric to describe public health activities. A number of states have adopted this format in organizing their public health systems. For example, Washington State used the core public health functions to develop their Public Health Improvement Plan (PHIP). By grouping public health functions into an overall population-based health improvement mission, plans can address specific activities to improve community health status.[9] A difficulty, however, with this type of format is that public health activities are described in general categories but are not readily identifiable, especially to those not in the public health field, such as legislators and the public. A remedy for this can be the concomitant use of examples that point to specific activities, such as linking the core as-

Exhibit 2–2 Activities of Six State Agencies

I. Assessment	
A. Data Collection	
Vital records	6
Morbidity	3
Health facilities	4
Health manpower	5
Health system funds	5
Health interview surveys	2
Health trends analysis	3
Health status assessment	5
B. Epidemiology	
Communicable disease	6
Health screening	6
Laboratory analysis	6
C. Research	
Research projects	4
Laboratory research	1
II. Policy Development	
A. Policy	
Goals developed through health assessments	1
Standards for local health agencies	5
B. Health Planning	
State health planning	2
Categorical plans	5
Certificate of need	5
III. Assurance	
A. Inspection	
Food and milk control	6
Product safety, substance control	3
Housing, public lodging, recreational facility safety	6
Health facility safety	5
B. Licensing	
C. Health Education	
Education	5
Health promotion, disease prevention	2
D. Environment	
Air quality	3
Occupational health and safety	5
Radiation control	6
Solid waste management	3
Hazardous waste management	3
Public water supply	5
Individual water supply	4
Sewage disposal	5
E. Personal Health	
Maternal and child health	6
Home health	4
Immunizations	6
Dental health	6
Mental health	5
Alcohol abuse	5
Drug abuse	5
Chronic disease	6
Inpatient facilities	2
F. Resources Development	6

Source: Copyright © 1986, Public Health Foundation.

sessment function to a specific activity such as behavioral risk surveys (Figure 2–1).

THE 10 ORGANIZATIONAL PRACTICES

Although the core functions described the role of public health activities in broad terms, more specific delineation of public health functions was needed. In 1989 the Centers for Disease Control and Prevention (CDC) convened a meeting with public health practice organizations. This "brainstorming" session resulted in the identification of more than 140 essential activities or functions. At additional meetings, 10 groups of organizational practices were determined.[10]

- **Assessment**
  1. Assess the health needs of the community.
  2. Investigate the occurrence of health effects and hazards in the community.
  3. Analyze the determinants of identified health needs.
- **Policy Development**
  4. Advocate for public health, build constituencies, and identify resources in the community.
  5. Set priorities among health needs.
  6. Develop plans and policies to address priority health needs.
- **Assurance**
  7. Manage resources and develop organizational structure.
  8. Implement programs.
  9. Evaluate programs and provide quality assurance.
  10. Inform and educate the public.

These 10 practices provided a basis for both implementing and measuring the performance of the three core functions. Studies determining the allocation of effort among these functions by local health agencies showed that the assurance function received the majority of time and resources, whereas few resources were being devoted to assessment and policy development.[11]

HEALTH CARE REFORM AND PUBLIC HEALTH

Further impetus for describing public health activities in more specific terms followed the introduction in October of 1993 of the Health Se-

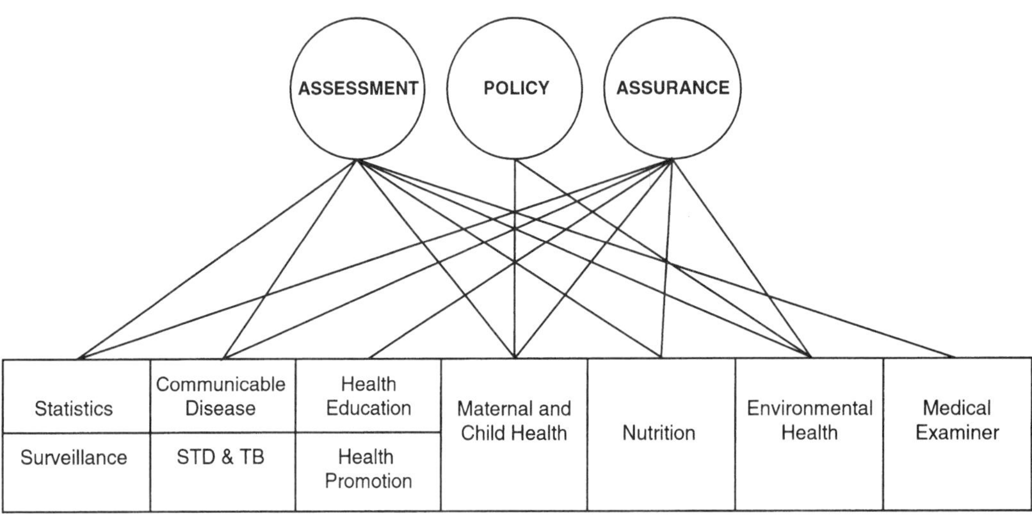

Figure 2–1 The Core Functions of Assessment, Policy, and Assurance Targeted to Specific Areas of a Local Health Department. *Source:* Copyright © 2000, L.F. Novick.

curity Act in the 103rd Congress.[12] This legislation was designed to provide universal access to health services by providing entry to all individuals and their families to a health care plan. In addition to medical care, these plans were to provide a schedule of clinical preventive services including immunization, serum cholesterol measurement every five years, and screening for cervical cancer and mammography for women.[12]

Although this act ultimately failed to pass, the prospect of this legislation raised a number of questions for public health practice. With provisions for clinical prevention and medical care by managed care plans, these activities would not also be required of public health agencies. Questions were raised concerning a need for public health services under a reformed system of health care. But an important role remained in the provision of population-based preventive functions.

In 1993, a core functions group of the Public Health Service, chaired by the assistant secretary for health and the surgeon general, vigorously supported the necessary role of public health and population-based programs for a reformed health care insurance system in the United States. They emphasized the core public health functions needed to address the health needs and conditions of populations, as distinct from individuals.[13] Only one percent of aggregate national health expenditures was used to support population-based health functions. Included in the Health Security Act is Subtitle D–Core Functions of Public Health Programs Regarding Preventive Health, which is adapted in Exhibit 2–3. This legislation also provided for resources to perform the core functions ($750 million by year 2000). The legislation failed to be enacted, but not without great impact on the future role of public health. Amplified by the subsequent growth of managed care, public health was slotted into assuming responsibility for population-based prevention but not direct provision of medical services (Figure 2–2). Important exceptions or variations to this theme do exist, including the provision of medical care by a number of large health departments, particularly in the Southeast, and for those local health departments participating as providers in managed care plans.

Exhibit 2–3 Core Functions of Public Health Proposed by the Health Security Act of 1993

1. Data collection activities related to population health measurement and outcomes monitoring
2. Activities to protect the environment and to ensure the safety of housing, workplaces, food, and water
3. Investigation and control of adverse health conditions, including improvements in emergency treatment preparedness, cooperative activities to reduce violence levels in communities, and activities to control the outbreak of disease
4. Public information and education programs to reduce risks to health such as use of tobacco, alcohol, and other drugs; sexual activities that increase the risk of HIV transmission and sexually transmitted diseases; poor diet; physical inactivity; and low childhood immunization levels
5. Accountability and quality assurance activities, including monitoring the quality of personal health services furnished by health plans
6. Provision of public health laboratory services
7. Training and education to ensure provisions of care by all health professionals, with special emphasis placed on the training of public health professionals
8. Leadership, policy development, and administration activities, including needs assessment, the setting of public health standards, the development of community public health policies, and the development of community public health coalitions

Source: Adapted from Health Security Act: 103rd Congress of the United States.

ESSENTIAL HEALTH SERVICES

The 10 essential health services represent a further development of the core functions and

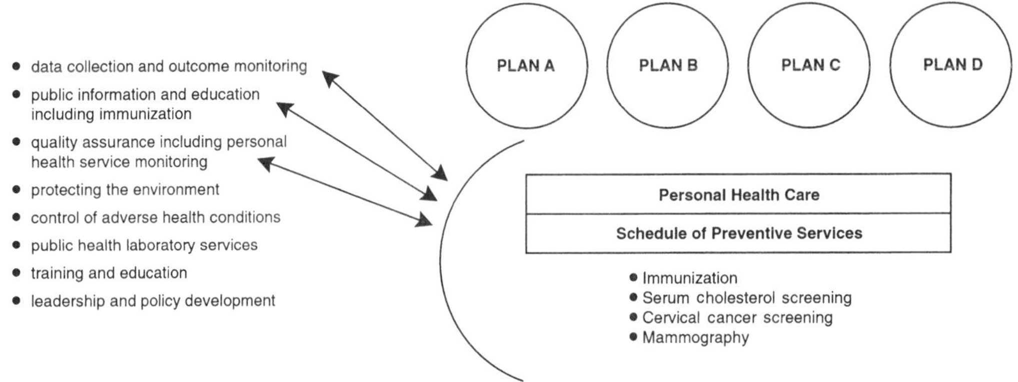

Figure 2–2 Population-Based and Individual Prevention as Proposed in the Health Security Act of 1993. *Source:* Copyright © 2000, L.F. Novick.

organization practices. This is the current taxonomy most often used to describe public health functions. The Public Health Service (Public Health Functions Steering Committee) issued a vision and mission statement listing these essential health services in the fall of 1994 (Exhibit 2–4). This essential service framework has gained momentum and is commonly used both by public health practitioners and by policy makers. Cost studies by the Public Health Foundation have been performed to determine expenditures by function for state and local departments of health.[14] This format provides a common vocabulary and expresses the mission of public health in terms of communitywide health improvement. But the essential service framework groups activities into categories that are abstract and not immediately recognizable for budget officers, legislators, and the public, who are expecting service activities. A similar difficulty was previously described with the core public health functions. A crosswalk prepared by the Public Health Foundation is useful because it matches essential health services with specific service activity (Table 2–1).

A framework of essential services can also be applied to a specific area of public health, as in the dissemination of the document *Public MCH Program Functions Framework: Essential Public Health Services To Promote Maternal and Child Health in America.*[15] Table 2–2 shows the core function and essential services for MCH. This framework was reported to be useful for public health agencies in Delaware, Maryland, South Carolina, and Wyoming among others, particularly in reference to communicating public health activities to managed care organizations.[16] The Division of Reproductive Health of the CDC has offered its activities in the assessment and monitoring of MCH status, mobilization of community partnerships, and research for innovative solutions as examples of providing essential services.[17] The success of performance evaluation is tied to uniform measures based on appropriate formats such as essential services.[18]

CORE FUNCTIONS AND ESSENTIAL HEALTH SERVICES: IMPLEMENTATION

Surveys of state public health agencies in both 1989 and 1996 revealed virtually all respondents adopting and agreeing with the importance of the core functions.[19,20] A high proportion indicated that their operations included performance of these functions: assessment (80%), policy development (49%), and assurance (42%).[19] As recommended earlier by the IOM report, there

Exhibit 2–4 Public Health in America

Vision:
Healthy People in Healthy Communities
Mission:
Promote Physical and Mental Health and Prevent Disease, Injury, and Disability

Public Health

- Prevents epidemics and the spread of disease
- Protects against environmental hazards
- Prevents injuries
- Promotes and encourages healthy behaviors
- Responds to disasters and assists communities in recovery
- Assures the quality and accessibility of health services

Essential Public Health Services

1. Monitor health status to identify community health problems
2. Diagnose and investigate health problems and health hazards in the community
3. Inform, educate, and empower people about health issues
4. Mobilize community partnerships to identify and solve health problems
5. Develop policies and plans that support individual and community health efforts
6. Enforce laws and regulations that protect health and ensure safety
7. Link people to needed personal health services and assure the provision of health care when otherwise unavailable
8. Assure a competent public health and personal health care workforce
9. Evaluate effectiveness, accessibility, and quality of personal and population-based health services
10. Research for new insights and innovative solutions to health problems

Source: Adopted Fall 1994, Public Health Functions Steering Committee Members (July 1995): American Public Health Association; Association of Schools of Public Health; Association of State and Territorial Health Officials; Environmental Council of the States; National Association of County and City Health Officials; National Association of State Alcohol and Drug Abuse Directors; National Association of State Mental Health Program Directors; Public Health Foundation; U.S. Public Health Service—Agency for Health Care Policy and Research; Centers for Disease Control and Prevention; Food and Drug Administration; Health Resources and Services Administration; Indian Health Service; National Institutes of Health; Office of the Assistant Secretary for Health; Substance Abuse and Mental Health Services Administration.

was evidence of outreach by state health agencies with increasing legislative activity and relationships with voluntary health agencies.[19] Another IOM recommendation was the divestiture of public health agencies from direct provision of personal health services. However, the survey documented an increase in delivery of personal services from 58 percent in 1989 to 83 percent in 1996.[20] The question was still unresolved. Should the public health entity be the guarantor or the actual provider of medical care? The increase in delivery of services reported by this survey was attributed to an increase in the number of uninsured, with the public health system acting as a "safety net."[19]

A similar survey of local public health agencies performed in 1996 demonstrated almost universal agreement with the core functions and an increasing proportion of health departments in which these functions are operative. However, less than 50 percent reported these functions to be currently operative and available in their communities.[21]

An expanding area of interest is the extent to which nongovernmental entities can provide essential health services. Private sector health care

Table 2–1 State/Local Health Department Crosswalk of Program Activities to Essential Services

Essential Service	*Includes but Is Not Limited To:*	*Does Not Include:*
1. Monitor health status to identify community health problems.	• Disease and injury registries • Epidemiology (surveillance, disease reporting, sentinel events), including injury epidemiology, mental health epidemiology, and substance abuse epidemiology • Population-based/community health needs assessments • State/community report cards/development of health status indicators • Vital statistics • Environmental epidemiology • Immunization status tracking • Public Health Laboratory Information System (PHLIS) • Linkages of data sets for population-based applications • Population-based health interview surveys (e.g., BRFSS or other state surveys)	• Management of client-based data systems should be included under #7b. Cost of accessing client-based data systems to evaluate accessibility and quality of care should be included under #9.
2. Diagnose and investigate health problems and health hazards in the community.	• Communicable disease detection (case finding) • Chronic disease detection (case finding) • Injury detection • HIV/AIDS prevention: –Counseling and testing –Partner notification • Outbreak investigation and control (including immunizations as part of outbreak control) • EPSDT • Population-based screening services (e.g., cholesterol), including follow-up counseling (e.g., nutrition and exercise) • Contact tracing (e.g., STD or TB) • Environmental risk assessment • Environmental sampling • Lead investigation • Radon detection • Asbestos detection • Diagnostic laboratory services (e.g., bacteriology, parasitology, virology, immunology, clinical chemistry) in support of population-based health activities • Environmental laboratory services (e.g., environmental microbiology samples, environmental chemistry samples, and occupational safety and health samples)	• Primary care services • Treatment of STD, TB, and other communicable diseases • CD4+ testing • Dental health services (including topical fluoride treatments in schools) • Treatment of diabetes, lupus, hemophilia, sickle cell anemia, epilepsy, Alzheimer's disease, and other chronic diseases • Genetic disease services • Home health care services • Purchase and provision of AZT/other drugs • Prenatal/perinatal care • Services for premature and newborn infants and preschool-aged children • Services to children with special health care needs • Immunizations, except as part of outbreak control (Note: All the above activities should be included under #7b.)

continues

Table 2–1 continued

Essential Service	*Includes but Is Not Limited To:*	*Does Not Include:*
3. Inform, educate, and empower people about health issues.	• Comprehensive school health education • Populationwide health promotion/risk reduction programs: –Injury prevention education and promotion –Parenting education –Physical activity and fitness –Population-based risk reduction programs –Seat belt education/promotion –Sexuality education –Tobacco use prevention and cessation • Nutrition education (e.g., Five-A-Day programs) • Nutrition education as part of WIC • School campaigns (e.g., "Say No to Drugs Day") • Substance abuse prevention • Public education campaigns • Worksite health promotion • HIV education/information • Educational activities as part of outreach • Educational activities related to enforcement of laws and regulations (i.e., education of tobacco vendors)	• Counseling and education as part of personal health services (e.g., nutrition counseling as part of prenatal care [include under #7b])
4. Mobilize community partnerships and action to identify and solve health problems. (See #5 for planning and policy development activities.)	• Coalition building • Collaboration with outside agencies/ organizations • Forming community partnerships to solve health problems (e.g., task forces, multidisciplinary advisory groups) • Advocacy and budget justification (e.g., testifying at hearings) • Technical assistance to facilitate mobilization of local health agencies or community groups • HIV community planning (include portion, if any, that involves building community partnerships; planning portion should be included under #5)	• Development of legislation, policies, or plans (include under #5)
5. Develop policies and plans that support individual and community health efforts. (See #4 for collaborative activities.)	• Agenda setting • Development of policies and guidelines • Legislative activities (e.g., drafting legislation, developing agency budgets) • Planning (including certificate of need) • *Healthy People 2000* objective-setting activities • APEX *PH* Parts I and II/Healthy Communities/PATCH/other planning models • HIV community planning (include portion related to planning; portion supporting community partnerships should be included under #4)	• Forming partnerships to solve health problems (include under #4)

continues

Table 2–1 continued

Essential Service	*Includes but Is Not Limited To:*	*Does Not Include:*
6. Enforce laws and regulations that protect health and ensure safety.	• Air quality (indoor and outdoor) • Asbestos control • Consumer protection and sanitation • Food sanitation • General sanitation • Housing • Public lodging • Recreational sanitation • Shellfish sanitation • Substance control/product safety • Vector/rodent control • Fluoridation services • Hazardous materials management (accidents, transportation spill, etc.) • Occupational health and safety • Radiation control • Lead abatement • Radon mitigation • Waste management—sewage, solid, and toxic • Water quality control (public/private drinking water, groundwater protection, etc.) • Emergency response teams to toxic spills, product recalls, and response to natural disasters (including the maintenance and development of emergency systems) • Medical examiner, toxicology, and other forensic medicine • Enforcement activities related to compliance with youth access to tobacco regulations • Enforcement activities related to the agency's police authority (e.g., quarantine, forcing patients to take medications)	• Construction of facilities and physical plans (this is generally funded through special capital accounts)
7a. Link people to needed personal health services.	• Case management/care coordination services • Information and referral hotlines • Outreach services related to linking individuals to personal health services • School health outreach, case-finding, and referral services • Transportation and other enabling services • Development of primary care services in underserved communities	• Direct health care services • School-based clinical services (include under #7b)
7b. Ensure the provision of care when otherwise unavailable.	• Personal health services, including: –Primary care services –Treatment of STD, TB, and other communicable diseases	• Population-based health services

continues

Table 2–1 continued

Essential Service	*Includes but Is Not Limited To:*	*Does Not Include:*
	–CD4+ testing –Dental health services (including topical fluoride treatments in schools) –Treatment of diabetes, lupus, hemophilia, sickle cell anemia, epilepsy, Alzheimer's disease, and other chronic diseases –Genetic disease services –Home health care –Hospitals –Purchase and provision of AZT/other drugs –Prenatal/perinatal care –Services for premature and newborn infants and preschool-aged children –Services to children with special health care needs • Clinical preventive services (e.g., routine immunizations, family planning) • School-based clinical services • Management of client-based data systems that support the services above	
8. Ensure a competent public health and personal health care work force.	• Required continuing education • Recruitment and retention of health professionals • Professional education and training • Health and environmental professionals licensing • Leadership training/programs	• Facilities licensing (include under #9) • Quality improvement (include under #9)
9. Evaluate effectiveness, accessibility, and quality of personal and population-based health services.	• Facilities licensing • Health care systems monitoring • Hospital outcomes data • Personal health services monitoring (including analysis and use of client-based data) • Program evaluation • Data systems related to service availability, utilization, cost, and outcome • Laboratory regulation and quality control services • Regulation of EMS personnel/services • Quality assurace/quality improvement activities (implementation)	• Management of client-based data systems (include under #7b) • Development (vs. implementation) of a quality improvement plan/policy (see #5)

continues

Table 2–1 continued

Essential Service	*Includes but Is Not Limited To:*	*Does Not Include:*
10. Research for new insights and innovative solutions to health problems.	• Biomedical, preventive, and clinical investigations • Health services research • Research and monitoring about the effects of the changing health care environment and unique strategies employed by public health agencies • Demonstration programs • Methods development • Research grants to others • Innovative technologies	
General administration	• Stand-alone administration activities (e.g., accounting, legal, or personnel activities) • Office of the health director • Computer support • Maintenance of buildings and grounds • Reporting requirements	

Source: The Public Health Expenditures Project Team, 1998: Public Health Foundation; National Association of County and City Health Officials; National Association of Local Boards of Health; Association of State and Territorial Health Officials; with funding from the Office of Disease Prevention and Health Promotion, Department of Health and Human Services.

providers, previously involved with inpatient care, are evolving into consolidated and integrated health care systems. Enrollment in health maintenance organizations has rapidly increased. These changes in the health care marketplace potentially could lead to interest in providing essential public health services.[22] Listed in Table 2–3 are eight exemplary private sector entities, all nonprofit health care systems and health plans, that were studied in 1995–96 to determine if their activities included the three core public health functions and the 10 essential health services. These eight plans were determined to be conducting 44 activities addressing core functions and essential health services, as shown in Table 2–4. The authors of this study concluded that private sector organizations are willing to perform public health activities and that local health departments will further their mission by forging collaborative partnerships.[22]

The World Health Organization (WHO) has decided to employ the essential public health functions (EPHFs) as a tool for implementing "Health for All in the 21st Century."[23] This initiative began in May 1981 when WHO members agreed to pursue health gains for their countries.[24] To achieve consensus on this approach, 145 public health leaders, managers, teachers, and practitioners were convened during February and March 1997 for a Delphi exercise. The Delphi methodology employs a group of knowledgeable individuals to achieve consensus on a group of complex issues. The essential public health categories and functions that resulted from this process are similar to those described earlier that were developed by the Core Functions Steering Committee, but differ somewhat in format. Exhibit 2–5 displays these functions and also a prioritization as to their importance.

It was strongly agreed by the participants in this process that public health functions might be performed by nongovernmental entities, including the private sector. The rationale advanced was that because the determinants of health status are not confined to the health sector, essential health services can be carried out in other areas. More importantly, however, the implementation of EPHFs needs to be monitored by government agencies.[23]

Table 2–2 MCH Core Functions and Practices Framework

Function	*Practice*	*Definition*
Assessment	Assess	Collect and analyze data on demographic, health status, and behavioral characteristics of MCH populations.
	Investigate	Investigate health hazards and problems that impact women, children, and youth.
	Analyze	Identify determinants and contributing factors to MCH outcomes.
Policy development	Mobilize	Develop and support MCH community action programs.
	Prioritize	Select key endpoints for focused intervention activity.
	Promote	Initiate and support laws, policies, regulations, and standards that ensure the health and safety of women, children, and youth.
Assurance	Link	Triage and refer women, children, and youth to needed population-based and personal health services.
	Ensure	Support the competency and quality of MCH interventions at varied community settings.
	Evaluate	Systematically examine the effectiveness, accessibility, and quality of MCH services.
	Inform	Educate and empower the public and families about MCH to promote positive attitudes and behaviors.

Source: Reprinted from J. Mayer, *Journal of Public Health Management and Practice,* Vol. 3, No. 5, 1997, Aspen Publishers, Inc.

NATIONAL HEALTH OBJECTIVES

National health objectives for the United States grew out of a health strategy initiated with the publication in 1979 of *Healthy People: The Surgeon General's Report on Health Promotion and Disease Prevention.*[25] This was expanded with the 1980 publication of *Promoting Health/ Preventing Disease: Objectives for the Nation,* which contained an agenda and targets for the next 10 years leading up to 1990.[26] The report was organized into five broad health status goals keyed to the various stages of the life cycle, from healthy infants, healthy children, healthy adolescents and young adults, and healthy adults, to healthy older adults. There were 15 priority areas in three categories of preventive health services, health protection, and health promotion, as shown in Exhibit 2–6. There were 226 objectives in these 15 priority areas. Examining the risk factors responsible for the preponderance of morbidity and mortality for each age group and also assessing the feasibility of successful public health intervention identified the 15 priority areas. The basis for this health promotion effort was the multiple determinants of health involving biologic, social, environmental, and behav-

Table 2–3 Case Study Organizations

Name	*Location*
Allina Health System	Minneapolis, MN
Baptist Health	Little Rock, AR
BJC Health System	St. Louis, MO
Cambridge Hospital Community Health Network	Cambridge, MA
Harvard Pilgrim Health Care	Boston, MA
Henry Ford Health System	Detroit, MI
Mt. Sinai Health System	Chicago, IL
Riverside Methodist Hospitals*	Columbus, OH

*Merged with its sister facility, Grant Hospital, in September 1995 to become Grant/Riverside Methodist Hospitals.

Source: Reprinted from Centers for Disease Control and Prevention, *Private Sector Health Care Organizations and Public Health: Potential Effects on the Practice of Local Public Health,* March 1996, Macro International, Atlanta, Georgia.

Table 2–4 Distribution of Activities by Primary Core Public Health Function

Essential Public Health Service (EPHS)	*Number of activities addressing EPHSs*	
	Predominantly	*Total*
Assessment		
Monitor	6	18
Investigate	2	6
Policy development		
Inform	7	15
Mobilize	4	9
Plan	—	6
Assurance		
Enforce	—	—
Link	21	27
Competent work force	3	6
Evaluate	1	5
Research and development	—	2
Total	44	94*

*Each of the 44 activities could address more than one essential public health service.

Source: Reprinted from Centers for Disease Control and Prevention, *Private Sector Health Care Organizations and Public Health: Potential Effects on the Practice of Local Public Health,* March 1996, Macro International, Atlanta, Georgia.

ioral factors. Prevention and risk reduction strategies need to be aimed at the individual susceptibilities and behavior, agents of disease, environmental factors, and particularly the interaction between these determinations. As discussed in Chapter 1, *Healthy People* emphasized the importance of personal behaviors of the individual in determining health status and also recognized the role of environmental factors.[25]

After preliminary work by U.S. Public Health Service agencies, 167 nongovernmental experts were convened at a conference in 1979 and organized into 15 working groups who developed the draft objectives for the priority areas.[24] This resulted in the publication of *Promoting Health/ Preventing Disease,* which, as stated earlier, set 226 goals to be achieved by 1990.[26] A measurement taken in 1987 showed that nearly half of the objectives had been reached. An additional one-quarter were not achieved and data were not available for monitoring the objectives in the remaining quarter. Priority areas where considerable progress was documented included high blood pressure control, immunization, control of infectious diseases, unintentional injury prevention, and control of smoking, alcohol, and drugs. Areas where progress lagged included pregnancy and infant health, nutrition, physical fitness, family planning, STDs, and occupational safety and health.[27] Major declines in the death rates for heart disease, strokes, and unintentional injury during this 1980–90 period gave hope for progress in succeeding decades, spurring the next installment of objectives: *Healthy People 2000: National Health Promotion and Disease Prevention Objectives.*[27]

HEALTHY PEOPLE 2000

Eight regional hearings with testimony from more than 750 individuals and organizations became the primary resource material for crafting the *Healthy People 2000* objectives.[27] The resulting report presents a national prevention strategy. *Healthy People 2000* identifies three broad goals and 319 objectives. The goals are increasing the span of life, reducing health disparities, and achieving access to preventive services. The objectives are organized into 22 priority areas as shown in Exhibit 2–7. The first 21 of these areas are in three broad categories: health promotion, health protection, and preventive services.[27]

Health promotion strategies focus on lifestyle and personal behaviors including physical activity, nutrition, tobacco, and alcohol. *Health protection* strategies include environmental and regulatory activities. *Preventive services* include counseling, screening, and immunization. A special category was established in *Healthy People 2000* for *data and surveillance activities* (priority area 22). Each priority area is assigned to a government lead agency, as shown in Table 2–5.

Healthy People 2000 was designed to offer a vision for the new century based on achieving reductions in preventable disability and death. When work on this report began in 1987, a new health threat had appeared and was already responsible for substantial decrements in health. Human immunodeficiency virus (HIV) infection is priority area 18. A summary of the objectives

Exhibit 2–5 Essential Public Health Categories and Functions (Resulting from the International Delphi Survey of 1997, Rank out of 37)

1. **Prevention, surveillance, and control of communicable and noncommunicable diseases**
    - Immunization (1)
    - Disease outbreak control (3)
    - Disease surveillance (4)
    - Prevention of injury (20)
2. **Monitoring the health situation**
    - Monitoring of morbidity and mortality (2)
    - Monitoring the determinants of health (6)
    - Evaluation of the effectiveness of promotion, prevention, and service programs (10)
    - Assessment of the effectiveness of public health functions (11)
    - Assessment of population needs and risks to determine which subgroups require service (12)
3. **Health promotion**
    - Promotion of community involvement in health (5)
    - Provision of information and education for health and life skill enhancement in school, home, work, and community settings (9)
    - Maintenance of linkages with politicians, other sectors and the community in support of health promotion, and public health advocacy (14)
4. **Occupational health**
    - Setting occupational health and safety standards (18)
5. **Protecting the environment**
    - Production and protection of, and access to, safe water (7)
    - Control of food quality and safety (8)
    - Provision of adequate drainage, sewerage, and solid waste disposal services (15)
    - Control of hazardous substances and wastes (16)
    - Provision of adequate vector control measures (17)
    - Ensuring protection of water and soil resources (29)
    - Ensuring environmental health aspects are addressed in development policies, plans, programs, and objects (32)
    - Prevention and control of atmospheric pollution (33)
    - Ensuring adequate prevention and promotive environmental services (34)
    - Ensuring adequate inspection, monitoring, and control of environmental hazards (35)
    - Controlling radiation (36)
6. **Public health legislation and regulations**
    - Reviewing formulation and enactment of health legislation, regulations, and administrative procedures (13)
    - Ensuring adequate legislation to protect environmental health (22)
    - Health inspection and licensing (23)
    - Enforcement of health legislation, regulations, and administrative procedures (24)
7. **Public health management**
    - Ensuring health policy, planning, and management (19)
    - Use of scientific evidence in the formulation and implementation of public health policy (21)
    - Public health and health systems research (30)
    - International collaboration and cooperation in health (37)
8. **Specific public health services**
    - School health services (25)
    - Emergency disaster services (27)
    - Public health laboratory services (28)
9. **Personal health care for vulnerable and high-risk populations**
    - Maternal health and family planning (26)
    - Infant and child care (31)

Source: Reprinted with permission from D. Bettcher et al., Delphi Study, *World Health Statistics Quarterly,* 51, p. 49,

in this priority area appears in Exhibit 2–8. The objectives are grouped as health status objectives, risk reduction objectives, and service and protection objectives.

Health status objectives set outcome targets. Progress in combating HIV infection is measured by annual incidence and prevalence for the general population, with additional targets for at-risk groups of special populations such as gay and bisexual males or intravenous drug users. These targets are set nationally and their utility for local use is limited because of the question of comparability

Exhibit 2–6 Priority Areas of Preventive Services for 1990

Preventive health services for individuals
- High blood-pressure control
- Family planning
- Pregnancy and infant health
- Immunization
- Sexually transmitted diseases

Health protection for population groups
- Toxic-agent and radiation control
- Occupational safety and health
- Accident-prevention and injury control
- Fluoridation and dental health
- Surveillance and control of infectious diseases

Health promotion for population groups
- Smoking and health
- Misuse of alcohol and drugs
- Nutrition
- Physical fitness and exercise
- Control of stress and violent behavior

Source: Reprinted from U.S. Department of Health and Human Services, *Promoting Health/Preventing Disease,* (PHS) Publication No. 79-55071, 1980, U.S. Government Printing Office.

Exhibit 2–7 *Healthy People 2000* Priority Areas

Health Promotion
1. Physical activity and fitness
2. Nutrition
3. Tobacco
4. Alcohol and other drugs
5. Family planning
6. Mental health and mental disorders
7. Violent and abusive behavior
8. Educational and community-based programs

Health Protection
9. Unintentional injuries
10. Occupational safety and health
11. Environmental health
12. Food and drug safety
13. Oral health

Preventive Services
14. Maternal and infant health
15. Heart disease and stroke
16. Cancer
17. Diabetes and chronic disabling condition
18. HIV infection
19. Sexually transmitted diseases
20. Immunization and infectious diseases
21. Clinical preventive services

Surveillance and Data Systems
22. Surveillance and data systems

Source: Reprinted from National Health Promotion Disease Prevention Objectives, *Healthy People 2000,* p. 7, U.S. Department of Health and Human Services, Public Health Service.

of local populations, including the prevalence of at-risk groups, to these national projections.

Risk reduction objectives focus on the presence of risk behaviors associated with HIV prevalence, such as nonprotected sexual activity and the use of shared needles. For these behaviors, targets are set in reducing the risk activity. Setting of the target certainly has a highly speculative basis, but the issue is measurable reduction in the risk and not reaching a precise number. Another problem with using these targets locally is the paucity of small-area measurements on these risk activities.

Whereas the initial objectives measured health outcomes or intermediate outcomes, *services and protection objectives* set targets for specific process activities such as HIV testing and counseling and school education and outreach. These objectives provide a menu of recommendations to be implemented in an HIV prevention program. Measurement of these objectives would, at least theoretically, be possible at the local level.

Similar to the progress report described for the 1990 objectives, the Public Health Service has issued midcourse reviews on *Healthy People 2000* with the final review available for 1998–99. Fifteen percent of the objectives have met the year 2000 targets, with an additional 44 percent showing movement toward the targets and 18 percent moving in a direction away from the targets. Eleven percent of the objectives lacked data for measurement. The remainder showed mixed results or no change.[28]

Table 2–5 Priority Area Lead Agencies for *Healthy People 2000*

Priority Area	*Lead Agency*
1. Physical activity and fitness	President's Council on Physical Fitness and Sports
2. Nutrition	National Institutes of Health Food and Drug Administration
3. Tobacco	Centers for Disease Control and Prevention
4. Substance abuse: alcohol and other drugs	Substance Abuse and Mental Health Services Administration
5. Family planning	Office of Population Affairs
6. Mental health and mental disorders	Substance Abuse and Mental Health Services Administration and the National Institutes of Health
7. Violent and abusive behavior	Centers for Disease Control and Prevention
8. Educational and community-based programs	Centers for Disease Control and Prevention Health Resources and Services Administration
9. Unintentional injuries	Centers for Disease Control and Prevention
10. Occupational safety and health	Centers for Disease Control and Prevention
11. Environmental health	National Institutes of Health Centers for Disease Control and Prevention
12. Food and drug safety	Food and Drug Administration
13. Oral health	National Institutes of Health Centers for Disease Control and Prevention
14. Maternal and infant health	Health Resources and Services Administration
15. Heart disease and stroke	National Institutes of Health
16. Cancer	National Institutes of Health
17. Diabetes and chronic disabling condition	National Institutes of Health Centers for Disease Control and Prevention
18. HIV infection	Centers for Disease Control and Prevention
19. Sexually transmitted diseases	Centers for Disease Control and Prevention
20. Immunization and infectious diseases	Centers for Disease Control and Prevention
21. Clinical preventive services	Health Resources and Services Administration Centers for Disease Control and Prevention
22. Surveillance and data systems	Centers for Disease Control and Prevention

Source: Reprinted from *Healthy People 2000 Review 1998–99*, p. 230, U.S. Department of Health and Human Services.

HEALTHY PEOPLE 2010 OBJECTIVES

Healthy People 2010 now establishes the nation's prevention agenda and a scorecard for monitoring health status.[29] Development of a small set of leading health indicators was seen as critical to improving the planning process and communicating with the public. *Healthy People 2010* has two broad types of objectives—measurable and developmental. The *measurable objectives*, similar to the majority of the preceding *Healthy People 2000* objectives, have baselines

Exhibit 2–8 HIV Infection

Health Status Objectives

18.1 Confine manual incidence of diagnosed AIDS cases to no more than 98,000 cases. (Baseline: An estimated 44,000 to 50,000 diagnosed cases in 1989)

Special Population Targets

	Diagnosed AIDS Cases	*1989 Baseline*	*2000 Target*
18.1a	Gay and bisexual men	26,000–28,000	48,000
18.1b	Blacks	14,000–15,000	37,000
18.1c	Hispanics	7,000–8,000	18,000

Note: Targets for this objective are equal to upper bound estimates of the incidence of diagnosed AIDS cases projected for 1993.

18.2 Confine the prevalence of HIV infection to no more than 800 per 100,000 people. (Baseline: An estimated 400 per 100,000 in 1989)

Special Population Targets

Estimated Prevalence of HIV Infection (per 100,000)

		1989 Baseline	*2000 Target*
18.2a	Homosexual men	2,000–42,000†	20,000
18.2b	Intravenous drug abusers	30,000–40,000‡	40,000
18.2c	Women giving birth to live-born infants	150	100

†Per 100,000 homosexual men aged 15 through 24 based on men tested in selected sexually transmitted disease clinics in unlimited surveys; most studies find HIV prevalence of between 2,000 and 21,000 per 100,000

‡Per 100,000 intravenous drug abusers aged 15 through 24 in the New York City vicinity; in areas other than major metropolitan centers, infection rates in people entering selected drug treatment programs tested in unlinked surveys are often under 500 per 100,000

Risk Reduction Objectives

18.3 Reduce the proportion of adolescents who have engaged in sexual intercourse to no more than 15 percent by age 15 and no more than 40 percent by age 17. (Baseline: 27 percent of girls and 33 percent of boys by age 15; 50 percent of girls and 66 percent of boys by age 17; reported in 1988)

18.4 Increase to at least 50 percent the proportion of sexually active, unmarried people who used a condom at last sexual intercourse. (Baseline: 19 percent of sexually active, unmarried women aged 15 through 44 responded that their partners used a condom at last sexual intercourse in 1988)

Special Population Targets

	Use of Condoms	*1989 Baseline*	*2000 Target*
18.4a	Sexually active young women aged 15–19 (by their partners)	60%	26%
18.4b	Sexually active young men aged 15–19	57%	75%
18.4c	Intravenous drug abusers	—	60%

Note: Strategies to achieve this objective must be undertaken sensitively to avoid indirectly encouraging or condoning sexual activity among teens who are not yet sexually active.

18.5 Increase to at least 50 percent the estimated proportion of all intravenous drug abusers who are in drug abuse treatment programs. (Baseline: An estimated 11 percent of opiate abusers were in treatment in 1989)

18.6 Increase to at least 50 percent the estimated proportion of intravenous drug abusers not in treatment who use only uncontaminated drug paraphernalia ("works"). (Baseline: 25 to 35 percent of opiate abusers in 1989)

18.7 Reduce to no more than 1 per 250,000 units of blood and blood components the risk of transfusion-transmitted HIV infection. (Baseline: 1 per 40,000 to 150,000 units in 1989)

continues

Exhibit 2–8 continued

Services and Protection Objectives

18.8 Increase to at least 80 percent the proportion of HIV-infected people who have been tested for HIV infection. (Baseline: An estimated 15 percent of approximately 1,000,000 HIV-infected people had been tested at publicly funded clinics in 1989)

18.9 Increase to at least 75 percent the proportion of primary care and mental health care providers who provide age-appropriate counseling on the prevention of HIV and other sexually transmitted diseases. (Baseline: 10 percent of physicians reported that they regularly assessed the sexual behaviors of their patients in 1987)

Special Population Targets

Counseling on HIV and STD Prevention	*1989 Baseline*	*2000 Target*
18.9a Providers practicing in high incidence areas	—	90%

Note: Primary care providers include physicians, nurses, nurse practitioners, and physician assistants. Areas of high AIDS and sexually transmitted disease incidence are cities and states with incidence rates of AIDS cases, HIV seroprevalence, gonorrhea, or syphilis that are at least 25 percent above the national average.

18.10 Increase to at least 95 percent the proportion of schools that have age-appropriate HIV education curricula for students in 4th through 12th grade, preferably as part of quality school health education. (Baseline: 66 percent of school districts required HIV education but only 5 percent required HIV education in each year for 7th through 12th grade in 1989)

Note: Strategies to achieve this objective must be undertaken sensitively to avoid indirectly encouraging or condoning sexual activity among teens who are not yet sexually active.

18.11 Provide HIV education for students and staff in at least 90 percent of colleges and universities. (Baseline data available in 1995)

18.12 Increase to at least 90 percent the proportion of cities with populations over 100,000 that have outreach programs to contact drug abusers (particularly intravenous drug abusers) to deliver HIV risk reduction messages. (Baseline data available in 1995)

Note: HIV risk reduction messages include messages about reducing or eliminating drug use, entering drug treatment, disinfection of infection equipment if still injecting drugs, and safer sex practices.

18.13 Increase to at least 50 percent the proportion of family planning clinics, maternal and child health clinics, sexually transmitted disease clinics, tuberculosis clinics, drug treatment centers, and primary care clinics that screen, diagnose, treat, control, and provide (or refer for) partner notification services for HIV infection and bacterial sexually transmitted diseases (gonorrhea, syphilis, and chlamydia). (Baseline: 40 percent of family planning clinics for bacterial sexually transmitted diseases in 1989)

18.14 Extend to all facilities where workers are at risk for occupational transmission of HIV regulations to protect workers from exposure to bloodborne infections, including HIV infection. (Baseline data available in 1992)

Note: The Occupational Safety and Health Administration (OSHA) is expected to issue regulations requiring worker protection from exposure to bloodborne infections, including HIV, during 1991. Implementation of the OSHA regulations would satisfy this objective.

Source: Reprinted from *Healthy People 2000,* p. 637, 1990, U.S. Department of Health and Human Services, Public Health Service.

and available data for national measurement purposes. *Developmental objectives* represent a desired outcome or health status for which current surveillance systems cannot yet provide data. *Healthy People 2010* has two goals: (1) increase quality and years of life and (2) eliminate health disparities.

Increase Quality and Years of Healthy Life

Objectives for the first goal are shown in Exhibit 2–9. This first goal of 2010 is to increase the quality and not just the years of healthy life. A healthy life means a full range of functional capacity throughout each life stage. A range of measures

Exhibit 2–9 Goal 1, Increase Quality and Years of Life

Number	*Objective*
1.	Total mortality
2.	Adolescent and young adult deaths
3.	Adult deaths
4.	Life expectancy
5.	Years of potential life lost
6.	People with good, very good, or excellent health
7.	Healthy days
8.	Able to do usual activities
9.	Years of health life
10.	Years of health life, older adults

Source: Reprinted from *Healthy People 2010 Objectives,* Draft for Public Comment, Goal 1, U.S. Department of Health and Human Services, Office of Public Health and Science.

will be used for this goal, relying on morbidity, mortality, and quality. With success in extending life expectancy, more attention is now being focused toward improving the quality of life (QOL). Health-related quality of life (HRQOL) includes both physical and mental health and their determinants.[29] HRQOL has a relationship to individual perception and ability to function. On a community basis, HRQOL includes all aspects that have an influence on health (Table 2–6).

Eliminate Health Disparities

Eliminating disparities was a goal of *Healthy People 2000,* which had special population targets for some objectives. These targets did not aim at eliminating health disparities by the year 2000. *Healthy People 2010* has the goal of eliminating these disparities during the next decade.[29] In February 1998, President William Clinton called for eliminating disparities between racial and minority groups in six areas: infant mortality, cancer, cardiovascular disease, diabetes, HIV/acquired immune deficiency syndrome (AIDS), and immunizations. Exhibit 2–10 lists *Healthy People 2000* objectives where there is a disparity of 25 percent or greater between the general population and at least one select population.

PUBLIC HEALTH INFRASTRUCTURE

For the first time, *Healthy People 2010* includes the area of infrastructure, with the goal of ensuring capacity to provide the essential public health services at federal, state, and local levels. Objectives for this area are shown in Exhibit 2–11.

Infrastructure has been described as the basic support for the delivery of public health activities. Five components of infrastructure are skilled work force, integrated electronic information systems, public health organizations, resources, and research. The need for infrastructure was pointed out by the IOM report in 1988.[5] Keeping pace with information technology, availability of a trained work force, and availability of resources for local public health problems are infrastructure priorities. This infrastructure chapter is a new focus area that does not target health outcomes but rather increased capacity to deliver public health services. As

Table 2–6 Health-Related Quality of Life (HRQOL)

"Health"	*vs. HRQOL*	*vs. QOL*
Individual level		
Death	Functional status	Happiness
Disease	Well-being	Life satisfaction
Community level		
Life expectancy	Environment	Participation
	Livability	Sustainability

Source: Reprinted from *Healthy People 2010 Objectives,* Draft for Public Comment, Goal 7, 1998, U.S. Department of Health and Human Services, Office of Public Health and Science.

Exhibit 2–10 Health Disparities of 25 Percent in *Healthy People 2000**

Race/Ethnicity

coronary heart disease deaths (1.1)
sedentary lifestyle (1.5)
cancer deaths (2.2)
overweight (2.3)
growth retardation among low-income children (2.4)
colorectal cancer deaths (2.23)
prevalence of diabetes (2.25)
cigarette smoking (3.4)
smokeless tobacco use (3.9)
stroke deaths (3.18)
alcohol-related motor vehicle deaths (4.1)
cirrhosis deaths (4.2)
drug-related deaths (4.3)
teen pregnancies (5.1)
planned pregnancies (5.2)
infertility (5.3)
suicides (6.1)
homicide (7.1)
firearm-related deaths (7.3)
high school completion rates (8.2)
unintentional injury deaths (9.1)
motor-vehicle crash deaths (9.3)
drowning deaths (9.5)
residential fire deaths (9.6)
asthma hospitalizations (11.1)
dental caries (13.1)
diagnosis/treatment of dental caries (13.2)
gingivitis (13.5)
oral cancer deaths (13.7)
regular dental visits (13.14)
infant deaths (14.1)
fetal deaths (14.2)
maternal mortality (14.3)
fetal alcohol syndrome (14.4)
severe complications of pregnancy (14.7)
low birth weight incidence (14.5)
breast-feeding in the first 6 months (14.9)
prenatal care in the first trimester (14.11)
end-stage renal disease (15.3)
female breast cancer deaths (16.3)
cervical cancer deaths (16.4)
diabetes deaths (17.9)
HIV infection incidence (18.1)
adolescent sexual intercourse (18.3)
gonorrhea infection incidence (19.1)
primary and secondary syphilis (19.3)
congenital syphilis (19.4)
hospitalizations for pelvic inflammatory ds. (19.6)
viral hepatitis cases (20.3)
tuberculosis cases (20.4)
influenza vaccine in last 12 months > 65 yrs (21.2)
pneumococcal vaccine in lifetime > 65 yrs (21.2)
tetanus booster in last 10 yrs (21.2)
preventive services receipt (21.4)

Socioeconomic Status (income, education, and employment related)

vigorous physical activity (1.4)
sedentary lifestyle (1.5)
cigarette smoking (3.4)
smoking initiation by children and adolescents (3.5)
smoking cessation during pregnancy (3.7)
work-related injury deaths (10.1)
nonfatal work-related injuries (10.2)
cumulative trauma disorders (10.4)
diagnosis/treatment of dental caries (13.2)
complete tooth loss for 65 years or older (13.4)
breast cancer screening (16.11)
limitation in major activity (17.2)

Disability

sedentary lifestyle (1.5)
overweight (2.3)

Gender

smokeless tobacco use (3.9)
suicides (6.1)
diagnosis/treatment of depression (6.15)
homicide (7.1)
unintentional injury deaths (9.1)
drowning deaths (9.5)
hip fractures among adults 65 yrs and older (9.7)
nonfatal spinal cord injuries (9.10)
oral cancer deaths (13.7)

Age

sedentary lifestyle (1.5)
alcohol-related motor vehicle deaths (4.1)
homicide (7.1)
motor-vehicle crash deaths (9.3)
fall-related deaths (9.4)
drowning deaths (9.5)
residential fire deaths (9.6)
hip fractures among adults 65 yrs and older (9.7)
nonfatal poisoning (9.8)
asthma hospitalizations (11.1)
cervical cancer screening (16.12)
gonorrhea infection incidence (19.1)
hospitalizations for pelvic inflammatory ds. (19.6)
tetanus booster in last 10 yrs (21.2)

Geographic Location

regular dental visits (13.14)
preventive services receipt (21.4)

*25 percent or greater disparity as reported in *Healthy People 2000 Review, 1997.*

( ) Numbers in parentheses indicate the number for this objective in *Healthy People 2000: National Health Promotion and Disease Prevention Objectives.*

Source: Reprinted from *Healthy People 2010 Objectives,* Draft for Public Comment, Goal 22, 1998, U.S. Department of Health and Human Services, Office of Public Health and Science.

Exhibit 2–11 Public Health Infrastructure

Number	*Objective*
1.	Competencies for public health workers
2.	Training in essential public health services
3.	Continuing education and training by public health agencies
4.	Use of Standard Occupational Classification System
5.	Onsite access to data
6.	Access to public health information and surveillance data
7.	Tracking *Healthy People 2010* objectives for select populations
8.	Data collection for *Healthy People 2010* objectives
9.	Use of geocoding in health data systems
10.	Performance standards for essential public health services
11.	Health improvement plans
12.	Access to laboratory services
13.	Access to comprehensive epidemiology services
14.	Model statutes related to essential public health services
15.	Data on public health expenditures
16.	Collaboration and cooperation in prevention research efforts
17.	Summary measures of population health and the public health infrastructure

Source: Reprinted from *Healthy People 2010 Objectives,* Draft for Public Comment, Public Health Infrastructure 14-1, 1998, U.S. Department of Health and Human Services, Office of Public Health and Science.

such, the objectives currently lack data systems to monitor progress, but these will be developed. Apart from building work force competency and increasing training and continuing education opportunities, the majority of infrastructure objectives directly address the capacity of state and local health agencies by calling for increases in the use of technology, scientific disciplines, planning, and improved organization of services. For example, a target of 90 percent is set for the proportion of state and local public health agencies that use electronic data and on-line information for data to improve their operations. Additionally, geocoding is to be incorporated into databases so that federal, state, and local entities will have geographic information system capability to make maps showing disease, risk factors, environmental hazard, and service delivery.[29] Another objective targets the availability of individuals with epidemiology skills for local and state public health agencies. States and local public health jurisdictions are also expected to develop health improvement plans to monitor and meet performance standards for the essential public health services.

Placement of the infrastructure objectives in *Healthy People 2010* signifies the importance of a core capacity for population-based activities as provided by local, state, and federal public health agencies in collaboration with communities and other providers in the public and private sectors. Public health departments responsible for the health of communities need the basic tools: skilled workers and the resources to perform their task. This noncategorical approach focuses on the skills, manpower, and technology available to these agencies, not for specific programmatic use, but for the array of public health functions.

Creating infrastructure objectives will not lead to their realization without the commitment for implementation and the necessary resources. The resource question is particularly thorny because funding sources are not specified in *Healthy People 2010.* Requests for infrastructure funding of federal, state, or local governments suffer from being generic and lacking immediate relevance to activities that deal with visible health issues such as infectious disease, maternal and child health, and environmental hazards. Various approaches to this difficulty can be used, including reattaching and integrating infrastructure with program budgets. No approach to this issue is more than partially satisfactory, and the availability of resources is the major factor that will determine whether the infrastructure objectives in *Healthy People 2010* will be achieved over the next decade.

GOVERNMENTAL AND NONGOVERNMENTAL ASPECTS OF PUBLIC HEALTH

Relationships that support core public health functions have been described in four categories: (1) between different health agencies at various levels of government, (2) between health agencies and other public agencies, (3) between health agencies and the private sector, and (4) among private and voluntary organizations.[5] All of these interactions occur regularly in practice so that public health cannot be categorized as strictly governmental or nongovernmental activity, but rather as a network of functions involving both sectors. Relationships between health agencies occur at multiple levels, including, for example, the funding and guidance offered by state public health agencies to local health departments. Information and recommendations are a two-way exchange between these levels and also with federal health agencies including the CDC, Human Resources Services Agencies (HRSA), and Food and Drug Administration (FDA).

Relationships between governmental public health agencies and the private and voluntary sector are also manifold. Local health departments work with both nonprofit and investor-owned organizations, including hospitals and businesses interested in mounting health promotion activities. Voluntary associations like the American Heart Association and the American Cancer Association act in the private sector, often in cooperation with governmental activities. The government's role has been central to the provision of health protection for the community because the genesis of public health activities was in addressing environmental and disease threats. Countering these hazards to health required a governmental presence as manifested by statutory protection, regulation, inspection, and enforcement.

Even in the early development of public health efforts, governmental authority did not act separately from private sector involvement, including business, medicine, and voluntary associations. As public health practice has evolved with a broader definition of scope extending beyond infectious disease, private sector involvement in these community preventive activities has grown more important. The IOM report of 1988 characterized the official public health agency as "the place where the health buck stops" in making decisions concerning preventive health functions.[5] This report, as previously described, characterized the government's role in terms of the functions of assessment, policy development, and assurance.[5] However, the role of government is shaped by community priorities that often originate in nongovernmental sectors. The functions of assessment, policy development, and assurance—a basic responsibility of governmental public health agencies—are also carried out by nongovernmental entities.

The role of governmental activity in public health is not constant but varies with larger political and social trends. There was a growth of federal activities in public health from the 1930s through 1970s as part of Roosevelt's New Deal and Johnson's Great Society. The Shepard-Towner Act of 1922 was the first legislation to provide funding to the states for personal health services by establishing MCH programs. The Social Security Act of 1935 included funding to the states for public health services and training.[5] New programs were funded during the 1960s and 1970s, including Medicaid, Medicare, maternal and infant care projects, family planning services, Head Start, and the Special Supplemental Food Program for Women, Infants, and Children. But in the 1980s, the new federalism of the Reagan administration shifted the locus of responsibility to the states. Less money for programs was available, and funds of categorical programs were consolidated into the Maternal and Child Health Block Grant and the Preventive Services Block Grant.[30] The MCH block grant consolidated programs for sudden infant death syndrome (SIDS), lead poisoning, and adolescent pregnancy while also imposing an overall reduction in funds from the totals of these programs in previous years. This new federalism has motivated much of the recent effort to refocus the mission of public health toward population-based core functions. Increased state authority to implement mandatory managed care for Medicaid enrollees has led to reductions in demand for clinical services.[31] A substantial portion of the personal health care and clinical preventive services now provided by public health departments is being transferred to the private health sector and managed care.[32] This change is being hastened by grants from the federal government to states for the Child Health Insurance Program. A dominant element of public policy with respect to public health activities is devolution—the shift of responsibilities from the federal government to the state and then to the localities and often to private vendors.[33]

Fox has pointed to four limitations of government in the public health arena.[34] These heighten the importance of participation by the community, including the private sector, in health improvement. The limitations of government, compromising its role in public health, include a reduced probability of success for interventions, management by crisis, fragmentation, and competing governmental agencies. Many current public health issues and interventions do not inspire governmental action as did the nineteenth-century threats from diseases such as diphtheria and TB, where the proposed actions had high probabilities of success at limited costs. A second limitation is that public health crises have been associated with public management of the problem but not long-term policy changes. A third limitation is the fragmentation of health responsibilities among a number of different public agencies using separate approaches to public health problems.[34] Fourth, competition for resources between governmental agencies, including welfare, corrections, and police, leaves public health agencies at a disadvantage, particularly because their activities are not perceived as being of similar critical importance to their counterparts.

A COMMUNITY PERSPECTIVE

The domain of public health extends beyond the range of governmental activities. Many individuals, organizations, and other entities are directly or indirectly involved with community health.[35] In addition to public health agencies, stakeholders include individual health providers, purchasers of care, and voluntary and community organizations.[36] Even agencies without an explicit health designation, including schools and businesses, can have important health-related roles. This broad net of those entities abetting public health purposes is warranted but makes a single definition of public health practice or designation of the public health work force complex. Director of the Public Health Practice Program Office at the CDC Edward Baker has emphasized this broader approach: "We present a re-definition of public health practice that extends well beyond the usual government efforts and aggressively seeks out and embraces the skills and resources of many new nontraditional players. While in no way diminishing the importance of public health agencies, we foresee a significantly greater participation by the private sector, particularly the personal medical care system in the future."[37(p.1276)]

The interaction between governmental public health agencies and the private sector is currently in flux. The increase in the number of organized health care delivery systems, including managed care plans, is making it possible for governmental health agencies to ensure access to care directly rather than to deliver personal health services directly. As reported in the 1996 IOM report, *Healthy Communities: New Partnerships for the Future of Public Health*, there is a question of how many elements of public health can or should be subsumed by the private sector.[36] The number could be considerable. An earlier study was described of nonprofit organizations performing essential public health services.[22] A range of for-profit and nonprofit organizations are already involved in activities that incorporate public health practices using any definition. Notable examples include Henry Ford Health System, Parkland Health and Hospital System, and Beth Israel Deaconess Medical Center, briefly described below.

The Henry Ford Health System (HFHS) is a major comprehensive nonprofit organization serving seven counties in southeastern Michigan. Based in Detroit, the system provides care to the insured and uninsured in areas with high rates of poverty, unemployment, and violence. Principles used in operation include a definition of health as more than the absence of disease, participation in community prevention, and use of the *Healthy People 2000* goals.[38]

The Parkland Health and Hospital System (PHHS) is one of the nation's largest teaching hospitals and has served as a safety net for Dallas for more than 100 years.[39] A Community Oriented Primary Care System (COPC) serves more than 300,000 individuals annually with nine centers. Care is also provided in nontraditional settings, including care for the homeless. Measurements of health outcomes are used to evaluate the program's effectiveness. Health outcomes are calculated using preexisting morbidity based on morbidity and mortality rate data in the served community. The assumption is that the delivery of preventive care will improve the health of the community.[39]

Beth Israel Deaconess Medical Center in Boston operates a WELL (Women Enjoying Longer Lives) Program designed to increase the delivery of preventive services to inner-city women between the ages of 40–65. The program is described as applying a population perspective to medical practice.[40] These programs all illustrate the extension of public health practice into nongovernmental spheres. These programs are based on the health improvement targeted for a population or community and on multiple determinants of ill health. Successful public health efforts are increasingly based on broad partnerships including both governmental public health agencies and multiple community entities.

MEDICINE AND PUBLIC HEALTH

Medicine and public health have operated separately in the United States, pursuing different approaches to health improvement. Public health practitioners worked in governmental and social agencies, in contrast to the activities of medicine in the private sector. These activities were focused on the individual, employing a set of biologic disciplines and subspecialties.[41] The Flexnerian reforms in medical education made medical practice more dependent on scientific knowledge and a relationship with hospital settings, resulting in less physician interest in community and preventive activity.[42] Public health focused on populations and determinants of health. The separation of medicine and public health has been associated with conflict. For example, when public health clinics started treating indigent patients in the 1920s and 1930s, it raised the issue of competition with private medicine.[41] Viseltear, a public health historian, has described fundamental differences between the two professions, which have resulted in an "impenetrable barrier" between medicine and public health.[43]

> One difference was based on the economic imperative which held that, as the medical profession was concerned primarily with cure and reimbursed on a fee-for-service basis, the public health profession perforce must be relegated entirely to providing those services in which the private physician had no interest; and the second was the rise of the basic sciences, which led to the emergence of medical specialties and the enthronement of reductionist medicine, upon which the medical schools and medical profession justified as their primary mission sickness and not health, the patient and not the community, cure and not prevention—all principles which are at variance with the public health ethos.[43(p.148)]

In the nineteenth and early twentieth century, there was a supportive relationship between physicians and public health, with leaders of the profession playing important roles in community health improvement.[44] Leaders in the two sectors overlapped, and many physicians were actively involved in public health activities.[45] At this time, medical interventions were largely ineffective in treating infectious disease, increasing support for public health measures.[45] But private physicians resisted early twentieth-century efforts in compulsory TB reporting and in the role of public health laboratories in testing for diphtheria and antitoxin production.[42,46] Some physicians also resisted development of well-baby clinics, health centers, and immunization programs.[46,47] Physician interest in public health waned until the growth of therapeutic armamentarium and antibiotics later in the twentieth century and the growth of reimbursement mechanisms for diagnostic and therapeutic interventions.[45] The medical profession moved from strong support of public health activities to ambivalence or even hostility.[46]

More recently, several factors have emerged that may improve the dysfunctional relationship between medicine and public health. The growth of managed care and the increased recognition of the value of partnerships and collaboration by public health entities has led to efforts by both sectors to bridge this historical separation. In March of 1994, the leaders of both the American Medical Association and the American Public Health Association met for this purpose, and a working partnership was established with support of the Josiah Macy, Jr. and the W.K. Kellogg foundations.[41] In March of 1996, a historic congress brought together nearly 400 leaders of the professional organizations representing those in practice, education, and research in public health and medicine.[41] Seven elements[41] were agreed on:

1. Engage the community.
2. Change the educational process.
3. Create joint research efforts.
4. Devise a shared view of health and illness.
5. Work together in health care provision.
6. Develop health care assessment measures.
7. Create local and national networks.

The American Medical Association and the American Public Health Association have made a long-term commitment to this medicine/public health initiative.

• • •

A variety of administrative and policy frameworks now exist to assist public health institutions in defining, organizing, managing, and evaluating their core activities. Nonetheless, important differences remain in how institutions conceptualize and practice public health. A key point of contention involves the role of public health organizations in delivering personal health services. Despite differences of opinion in certain process-related issues, public health organizations appear to be reaching consensus about the larger public health mission, goals, and objectives. A key area of consensus involves core functions that should be performed by public health organizations in both governmental and private settings. Another area of consensus concerns the importance of cooperation between public and private organizations and between medical practice and public health practice. The growing acceptance of these shared goals and objectives promises to improve performance among individual public health organizations and within the public health system as a whole.

CHAPTER REVIEW

1. An issue for local health departments is whether their scope of functions should include medical care services in addition to their preventive responsibilities.
2. *The Future of Medicine,* a 1988 IOM report, characterized the functions of public health as *assessment, policy,* and *assurance.* These were designated as core functions and have been widely used to describe the activities of health agencies.
3. In 1994, a listing of 10 essential services was developed, representing a further development of the core functions. This is the current taxonomy most often used to describe public health activities.
4. The issue of health care reform has crystallized the constellation of functions of public health. With the provision of health services through structured organized plans such as managed care, the functions of the health agency are less in service provision and more in population-based health protection and promotion, as described in the essential functions.

5. National health objectives for the United States grew out of a health strategy initiated with the publication of *Healthy People* in 1979. Starting with the publication of objectives for 1990 and followed by objectives for 2000, objectives for 2010 are the currently available set.
6. Objectives for *Healthy People 2010* focus on: (1) eliminating health disparities, (2) increasing quality and years of life, and (3) developing infrastructure for public health activities. The set of objectives as a whole constitutes an agenda for health improvement and monitoring progress.
7. The interaction between governmental health agencies and the private sector is currently in flux. With the increase in organized health delivery systems, including managed care, the role of government is moving to assurance rather than delivery of personal services.

REFERENCES

1. H. Emerson, *Local Health Units for the Nation* (New York: The Commonwealth Fund, 1945).
2. J. Jekel, "Health Departments in the U.S. 1920–1988: Statements of Mission with Special Reference to the Role of C.-E. A. Winslow," *The Yale Journal of Biology and Medicine* 64 (1991): 467–479.
3. American Public Health Association, "An Official Declaration of Attitude of the American Public Health Association on Desirable Standard Minimum Functions and Suitable Organization of Health Activities," *American Journal of Public Health Yearbook for 1933,* 6–11.
4. W. Mountin, "Distribution of Health Services in the Structure of State Government," *Public Health Reports,* no. 34 (1941): 1,674–1,698.
5. Institute of Medicine, *The Future of Public Health* (Washington, DC: National Academy Press, 1988).
6. A. Miller and M.K. Moos, *Local Health Departments: Fifteen Case Studies* (Washington, DC: American Public Health Association, 1981).
7. M. Terris and N. Kramer, "Medical Care Activities of Full Time Health Departments," *American Journal of Public Health* 39 (1949): 1,129–1,135.
8. B. Meyers et al., "The Medical Care Activities of Local Health Units," *Public Health Reports* 83 (1968): 757–769.
9. National Association of County and City Health Officials, *1992–93 National Profile of Local Health Departments* (Washington, DC: NACCHO, 1995).
10. W. Dyal, "Ten Organizational Practices of Public Health: A Historical Perspective," *Research and Measurement in Public Health Practice* (supplement to the *American Journal of Preventive Medicine),* no. 6 (1995): 6–8.
11. J. Studnicki et al., "Analyzing Organizational Practices in Local Health Departments," *Public Health Reports 109,* no. 4 (1994): 485–490.
12. Health Security Act of 1993, 103rd Cong., 1st sess.
13. Core Functions Project, U.S. Public Health Service, "Health Care Reform and Public Health: A Paper on Population-Based Core Functions," *Journal of Public Health Policy 19,* no. 4 (1998): 394–419.
14. K. Eilbert et al., "Public Health Expenditures: Developing Estimates for Improved Policy Making," *Journal of Public Health Management and Practice 3,* no. 3 (1997): 1–9.
15. H.A. Grason and B. Guyer, *Public MCH Program Functions Framework: Essential Public Health Services To Promote Maternal and Child Health in America* (Baltimore: Johns Hopkins University, 1995).
16. H.A. Grason, "Use of MCH Functions Framework as a Tool for Strengthening Public Health Practice," *Journal of Public Health Management and Practice 3,* no. 5 (1997): 14–15.
17. L. Wilcox, "Important Directions in Public Health Surveillance and Community-Based Research in Maternal and Child Health: A CDC Perspective," *Journal of Public Health Management and Practice 3,* no. 5 (1997): 17–19.
18. R. Gerzoff, "Comparisons: The Basis for Measuring Public Health Performance," *Journal of Public Health Management and Practice 3,* no. 5 (1997): 20–21.
19. H. Scott, "The Future of Public Health: A Survey of States," *Journal of Public Health Policy 11,* no. 3 (1990): 296–304.
20. F. Scutchfield et al., "A Survey of State Health Department Compliance with the Recommendations of the Institute of Medicine Report, *The Future of Public Health,*" *Journal of Public Health Policy 18,* no. 2 (1997): 13–29.
21. F. Scutchfield, "Compliance with the Recommendations of the Institute of Medicine Report, *The Future of Public Health:* A Survey of Local Health Departments," *Journal of Public Health Policy 18,* no. 2 (1997): 155–166.

22. T. Chapel, "Private Sector Health Care Organizations and Essential Public Health Services: Potential Effects on the Practice of Local Public Health," *Journal of Public Health Management and Practice 4,* no. 1 (1999): 36–44.
23. D. Bettcher et al., "Delphi study," *World Health Statistics Quarterly* 51 (1998): 44–55.
24. J. McGinnis et al., "Objectives-Based Strategies for Disease-Prevention," in *Oxford Textbook of Public Health,* eds. W. Holland et al. (New York: Oxford University Press, 1991), 127–144.
25. U.S. Department of Health, Education and Welfare, *Healthy People: The Surgeon General's Report on Health Promotion and Disease Prevention* (Washington, DC: U.S. Government Printing Office, 1979).
26. U.S. Department of Health and Human Services, *Promoting Health/Preventing Disease: Objectives for the Nation* (Washington, DC: U.S. Government Printing Office, 1980).
27. U.S. Department of Health and Human Services, Public Health Service, *Healthy People 2000: National Health Promotion and Disease Prevention Objectives* (Washington, DC: U.S. Government Printing Office, 1990).
28. U.S. Department of Health and Human Services, Centers for Disease Control and Prevention, *Healthy People 2000 Review* (Washington, DC: U.S. Government Printing Office, 1998–99).
29. U.S. Department of Health and Human Services, Office of Public Health and Science, *Healthy People 2010 Objectives, Draft for Public Comment* (Washington, DC: U.S. Government Printing Office, 1998).
30. G. Omenn, "What's Behind Those Block Grants in Health?" *New England Journal of Medicine 306,* no. 17 (1982): 1,057–1,060.
31. S. Wall, "Transformations in Public Health Systems," *Health Affair 17,* no. 3 (1998): 64–80.
32. J. Lumpkin, "Impact of Medicaid Resources on Core Public Health Responsibilities of Local Health Departments in Illinois," *Journal of Public Health Management and Practice 4,* no. 6 (1998): 69–78.
33. R. Baxter, "The Roles and Responsibilities of Local Public Health Systems in Urban Health," *Journal of Urban Health 75,* no. 2 (1998): 322–329.
34. D. Fox, "Accretion, Reform, and Crisis: A Theory of Public Health Politics in New York City," *The Yale Journal of Biology and Medicine 64* (1991): 455–466.
35. D. Patrick and T. Wickizer, "Community and Health," in *Society and Health,* eds. B. Amick et al. (New York: Oxford Press, 1995), 46–92.
36. M. Stoto et al., eds., *Healthy Communities: New Partnerships for the Future of Public Health* (Washington, DC: Institute of Medicine, 1996).
37. E. Baker et al., "Health Reform and the Health of the Public," *Journal of the American Medical Association 272,* no. 16 (1994): 1,276–1,282.
38. N. Whitelaw et al., "Current Efforts toward Implementation of an Urban Health Strategy: The Henry Ford Health System," *Journal of Urban Health 75,* no. 2 (1998): 356–366.
39. R. Anderson et al., "Toward a New Urban Health Model: Moving beyond the Safety Net To Save the Safety Net—Resetting Priorities for Health Communities," *Journal of Urban Health 75,* no. 2 (1998): 367–378.
40. M. Raskin, "Current Efforts toward Implementation of an Urban Health Strategy: Boston," *Journal of Urban Health 75,* no. 2 (1998): 383–390.
41. S. Reiser, "Medicine and Public Health," *Journal of the American Medical Association 276,* no. 17 (1996): 1,429–1,430.
42. E. Fee, "The Origins and Development of Public Health in the US," in *Oxford Textbook of Public Health,* eds. W. Holland et al. (New York: Oxford University Press: 1991), 3–22.
43. A. Viseltear, "The Ethos of Public Health," *Journal of Public Health Policy 11,* no. 2 (1990): 146–150.
44. E. Fee, "Public Health and the State: The United States," *Clio Medica* 26 (1994): 224–275.
45. R. Lasker, *Medicine & Public Health: The Power of Collaboration* (New York: The New York Academy of Medicine, 1997).
46. J. Duffy, "The American Medical Profession and Public Health: From Support to Ambivalence," *Bulletin of the History of Medicine* 53 (1979): 1–22.
47. Council on Scientific Affairs, "The IOM Report and Public Health," *Journal of the American Medical Association 264,* no. 4 (1990): 508–509.

CHAPTER 3

Organization of the Public Health Delivery System

Glen P. Mays

A complex array of institutions and interorganizational structures supports the delivery of public health services in the United States. Governmental and private organizations factor prominently in the nation's public health system, yet there is no definitive division of labor among the institutions that make up this system. This chapter examines the defining organizational and structural characteristics of public health activities in the United States, with special emphasis given to the intergovernmental and interorganizational arrangements that increasingly support these activities. Effective management of public health organizations in any setting requires a thorough understanding of these basic structural elements.

The administration and practice of public health in the United States encompass a broad and evolving scope of activities. In view of this broad scope, it is difficult to imagine a simple and static institutional structure to support these endeavors. The constellation of organizations involved in public health administration is complex and changing, reflecting historical and contemporary trends in health, politics, economics, and social structures. A clear division of labor among the different types of public health organizations does not exist. Governmental health agencies factor prominently in this mix of institutions, and their responsibilities mirror the federalist system of government from which they derive. Nongovernmental organizations also play vital roles in public health delivery at local, state, national, and international levels. Many public health activities are organized not within institutions but between them, through an array of interorganizational and intergovernmental structures. Adding to the complexity, the organization of public health activities varies widely across communities, states, and regions. The organizational infrastructure extant in any given locale is shaped by the confluence of public priorities and values, available health resources and financing mechanisms, specific political processes and interest groups, and unique historical and environmental conditions.[1]

This chapter examines the defining organizational and structural characteristics of public health activities in the United States. Some observers contend that these characteristics sufficiently constitute a delivery system for public health activities, whereas others argue that the institutions supporting such activities do not yet function as a coherent system. Although a definitive answer to this question is not possible, this chapter highlights the structural elements that support the delivery of public health services in the United States—elements that provide a foundation for public health system devel-

Source: © *Joint Commission Journal on Quality Improvement,* Vol. 24, No. 10. Oakbrook Terrace, IL: Commission on Accreditation of Healthcare Organizations. 1998, pp. 518–540. Adapted with permission.

opment and improvement. The effective management of public health programs, services, and organizations in any setting requires a thorough understanding of these structural elements. This chapter therefore profiles the public and private institutions—and the intergovernmental and interorganizational relationships—that comprise an emerging if not extant public health delivery system.

GOVERNMENTAL PUBLIC HEALTH ORGANIZATIONS

Governmental responsibilities in public health evolve in response to public needs and demands as well as political will. Economic theory has long provided a rationale for decisions concerning the most appropriate governmental roles in public health service delivery. Those services that represent *public goods* with high *externalities* are often underproduced by private actors despite the fact that such goods improve social welfare; therefore, governmental involvement in the provision of these services is essential for social well-being.[2] One public policy challenge lies in determining which public health activities constitute public goods such that consumption of the good by one individual does not reduce the ability of others to consume the good (e.g., the benefits of production accrue to a broad cross section of the population) and which activities entail high externalities (e.g., beneficial side effects are received by those not directly involved in the production or consumption of the good). In a federalist system of government such as the United States has, another challenge lies in determining the appropriate roles of each level of governmental authority in carrying out public health activities.

The organization of governmental public health activities in the United States flows directly from this limited federalist system of government based on national, state, and local levels of authority. States occupy pivotal positions within this system because they maintain the governmental authority that is not expressly reserved for the federal government through constitutional provisions and legislative power. States, in turn, choose whether to exercise this authority directly or delegate it to local governmental bodies in accordance with state constitutional and legislative provisions. In the domain of public health, the federal government exercises authority primarily through policy development, public health financing, and, to a lesser extent, regulatory enforcement. By comparision, state government agencies typically play a larger role in public health regulatory activities while also carrying out substantial responsibilities in public health program administration and resource allocation. Local governmental agencies often shoulder the primary responsibilities for implementing public health activities within communities. States vary markedly in the volume and scope of public health activities that are delegated to local governmental control, and both historical and contemporary trends in state–local political relationships contribute to this variation.[3,4] Specific organizational structures used to support public health activities at federal, state, and local levels are examined in the following paragraphs.

Federal Agencies Contributing to Public Health

Federal health agencies are important actors in the public health arena because of their ability to formulate and implement a national health policy agenda and to allocate health resources across broad public priorities.[5] Both executive agencies and legislative institutions engage in federal health policy and resource allocation activities. As part of the policy development and administration process, many federal health agencies provide information and technical assistance to other organizations involved in public health activities, including state and local agencies as well as nongovernmental organizations.[6] In some cases, federal agencies also engage directly in implementing public health activities within specific communities or populations. Direct federal involvement in public health practice typically occurs only for narrowly defined public health activities such as the investigation and control of major health threats, the study of new public health interventions, or the response to major disasters and emergencies. A 1998 study of the nation's largest local public health jurisdictions found that federal agencies were directly involved in implementing public health activities in less than half of the jurisdictions examined.[7] In those jurisdictions having some direct federal involvement, federal agencies were involved in only 7 percent of the public health activities examined in the study. Federal agencies were most frequently involved in activities concerning adverse health events investigation, public health laboratory testing, and support and communications functions for public health interventions.

Federal agencies undertake public health activities using a variety of policy and administrative instruments. Agencies that are part of the executive branch of federal government use instruments that include regulatory development and enforcement, resource allocation, information production and dissemination, and policy advocacy and agenda setting. The specific set of policy instruments used by a given agency for a given public health issue depends on the authority granted to the agency by Congress, as well as the administrative and political environment in which the agency operates.

Federal Policy and Administrative Instruments for Public Health

Regulatory Development and Enforcement

Federal agencies receive their regulatory power either through congressional legislation or, less frequently, through presidential executive order. Often this authority involves a directive to establish the administrative procedures and infrastructure necessary to enforce a specific regulatory provision enacted by Congress. For example, a federal law passed in 1996 charges the U.S. Department of Health and Human Services (DHHS) to enforce a regulatory provision requiring managed care plans to offer women undergoing childbirth at least 48 hours of inpatient hospitalization coverage following a normal delivery. Alternatively, federal agencies may be empowered to develop standards and regulations within a broad domain of activity, subject to a public review and evaluation process. Many of the environmental health regulations enforced by the U.S. Environmental Protection Agency (EPA), for example, are developed by the agency itself under broad regulatory authority established by federal laws such as the National Environmental Policy Act of 1969 and the Clean Water Act of 1977.

Whether an agency is given broad latitude or a specific mandate for regulatory development, the process of creating a regulation is relatively uniform at the federal level. To develop a regulation, agencies first research the issue thoroughly, including the regulatory intent of the authorizing body (either Congress or the president). A proposed rule is then developed by the agency and published in the *Federal Register* for review and comment by the public. In many cases, the most active reviewers of proposed federal regulations are those organizations and individuals likely to be affected by or covered under the regulation, as well as those policy makers involved in authorizing the regulatory action. After a specified comment period, the agency evaluates the comments and revises the rule accordingly. Revised rules reappear in the *Federal Register* until the agency has decided on a final form for the rule. At that point, the regulation is codified by being published in the *U.S. Code of Federal Regulations.*

In the domain of public health, federal health agencies make relatively limited use of regulatory powers. The most active federal regulatory activities occur in the areas of food protection, drug and device development, occupational health and safety, and environmental health protection. For example, federal regulations concerning the manufacture, processing, and labeling of food products are carried out as consumer protection activities through agencies such as the U.S. Food and Drug Administration (FDA) and the U.S. Department of Agriculture. Similarly, federal regulations concerning the development, manufacture, distribution, and marketing of pharmaceutical products and medical devices are extensive, with the FDA requiring rigorous scientific proof of the safety and efficacy of these products in human populations before they are licensed for distribution in the United States. By comparison, the federal government historically has been reluctant to engage in regulatory activities in the field of medical practice and health care financing—preferring to delegate these tasks to state agencies and to the health professions themselves. Federal involvement in this area has increased in recent years as public concern has grown concerning the quality of medical care and health insurance under managed care plans.[8,9] Examples of recent federal regulatory activity include the minimum 48-hour hospital stay provision for childbirth, the requirement that health plans establish equal benefit levels for medical and mental health services (so-called mental health parity legislation of 1996), and the requirement that health plans offer renewable and portable individual health insurance to individuals who lose coverage from a group insurance plan (the Health Insurance Portability and Accountability Act of 1996).[10]

Health Resource Allocation

Another powerful public health instrument wielded by federal agencies is the authority to distribute program funds in pursuit of national public health goals and objectives. Most federal public health programs are not carried out through direct provision of public health services, but rather through financial and technical support provided to programs that are maintained by other public health organizations. Federal agencies allocate financial resources to public health programs through two principal avenues: categorical grants-in-aid and block granting. *Categorical grant programs* are targeted at specific public health services and population groups; *block grants* allocate financial resources to broad domains of activity that are largely determined by the grant recipients. All block grants and many categorical grants are allocated exclusively to state governments, which are charged with disbursing funds appropriately to specific programs and providers. Some categorical grants to states formalize this process by including "pass-through" provisions that require states to allocate resources for specific purposes using a predetermined formula or other mechanism. Categorical grants allow federal agencies to exercise more control over how public health funds are spent than do block grants, which allow greater levels of state discretion in resource use.

Categorical and Block Grant Programs. Categorical grants are often criticized as a resource allocation vehicle for their tendency to encourage public health organizations to operate in accordance with federal funding streams rather than in accordance with public health needs and priorities in the populations served. A public health agency might, for example, invest heavily in a cancer screening program in order to draw down federal grant funds, even though population health needs might indicate that priority should be given to maternal and child health (MCH) services. Block grants are often viewed as a strategy for preventing such perverse resource allocation decisions. Critics of block grant strategies argue, however, that these funding vehicles may allow important but low-visibility programs and health needs—including many public health services—to be de-emphasized in times of financial crisis. Critics also maintain that block grants can be used to mask overall reductions in federal support for public health activities. Nevertheless, federal block grants for health services have grown steadily over the past two decades and now include the Preventive Health and Health Services Block Grant, the Maternal and Child Health Block Grant, the Community Mental Health Services Block Grant, and the Prevention and Treatment of Substance Abuse Block Grant.

Entitlement and Discretionary Programs. Several of the largest federal categorical grant-in-aid programs in the domain of public health confer program benefits to broad classes of individuals and therefore constitute entitlement programs. Both of these programs—Medicaid and the State Child Health Insurance Program (S-CHIP)—provide funds to states for the purchase of health care services for low-income families and children. (Another federal entitlement program in health, the Medicare program, does not function through a grant-in-aid process at all but rather is administered directly at the federal level.) Most of the outlays for these programs fund the delivery of medical care, long-term care, and mental health services; nonetheless, these programs are important sources of financing for public health services. The Medicaid program, for example, finances the delivery of clinical preventive services, prenatal care, maternal support and case management services, communicable disease screening and treatment services, family planning services, childhood developmental screening services, and Medicaid outreach and enrollment services for low-income individuals eligible for the program. These programs function as entitlements because funds are allocated to states in amounts based on a proportion of the expenditures incurred by states in serving eligible recipients. Funding levels are therefore determined by program eligibility and utilization, rather than by explicit policy decisions concerning the allocation of federal resources to specific program areas.

Most other grant-in-aid programs that support public health activities are discretionary programs that operate through a fixed appropriation of federal revenue that is subject to periodic updates, adjustments, and revisions. Discretionary programs are generally much more sensitive to political bargaining and governmental financing obligations than are entitlement programs. As a result, many of these programs experience periodic fluctuations in funding levels and scope of authority as they come due for reauthorization and reappropriation decisions in Congress. Prominent examples of federal discretionary programs in public health include the following:

- The *Preventive Health and Health Services Block Grant* supports initiatives such as the national breast and cervical cancer screening program through grants to state health agencies from the U.S. Centers for Disease Control and Prevention (CDC).
- The *Community Health Centers Program* and the *Migrant Health Centers Program* (Sections 330 and 329 of the Public Health Service Act), both categorical grant-in-aid programs, support comprehensive primary care centers operating in medically underserved areas through direct federal grants to health centers from the U.S. Health Resources and Services Administration (HRSA).
- The *Maternal and Child Health Services Block Grant* supports an array of services involving family planning, maternity support, prenatal care, high-risk pregnancy support, well-child care, and developmental screening through grants to state health agencies from the HRSA.
- The *Special Supplemental Food Program for Women, Infants, and Children* (WIC) funds state health agencies to operate nutritional support programs for low-income pregnant women and women with young children.

Matching Requirements. Many federal grant-in-aid programs include a requirement that grantees contribute a specified amount of nonfederal funds in order to secure federal funding under the program. Matching requirements allow federal agencies to leverage their limited federal funds in order to secure larger investments of public funds in priority areas. Matching requirements also allow federal agencies and their grantees to share the financial risks associated with investments in public programs—an arrangement that potentially creates additional incentives for the grantee to achieve desirable program performance. Both the Medicaid and the S-CHIP entitlement programs include a federal matching component that requires the state grantees to contribute a specified amount of state funds in order to secure federal funds through the program. In Medicaid, the proportion of funds that derive from the federal government varies across states from a minimum of 50 percent to a maximum of 77 percent because the state matching requirement is determined by a formula that compares each state's per capita personal income level with the nation's per capita income level. A similar formula is used to determine the state matching requirement under the S-CHIP program.

Competitive and Performance-Based Allocation. Increasingly, federal agencies are adopting competitive systems for allocating resources to public health activities, including performance-based funding strategies. In one example of this approach, research and demonstration grants are used by federal agencies to develop and test innovative models for public health service delivery that may eventually be suitable for widespread dissemination and use. Under these types of grants, federal agencies solicit competitive proposals from prospective grantees and select those proposals that hold the greatest potential for success while also meeting budgetary and programmatic requirements. If successful program models are identified through the initial set of funded projects, federal agencies may allocate resources to additional grantees for replication and expansion of successful program features.

A good example of this resource allocation approach can be found in the Healthy Start Initiative administered by the Bureau of Maternal and Child Health Services within the HRSA. Through a competitive proposal process, the HRSA initially funded 15 community-based projects designed to reduce infant mortality and improve MCH outcomes in communities with high rates of infant mortality and morbidity. All of the selected programs were required to include certain common features such as maternity support and case management services, but all were also allowed to implement additional features based on local needs and capacities. After an initial three-year demonstration period, the HRSA has begun to support dissemination and expansion programs that are designed to replicate successful program features in other communities. Many other federal agencies that support public health programs also include competitive features as part of their resource allocation processes.

More recently, many federal agencies have moved to adopt performance-based resource allocation systems for public health programs. Under the Government Performance and Results Act of 1993 (GPRA), federal agencies are now required to measure routinely the performance and outcomes of the programs they administer, and to demonstrate accountability for the federal funds they use to support these programs. In response to these requirements, federal funds for public health programs are increasingly allocated on the basis of objective performance measures rather than simply on the basis of need or program potential. For example, states that receive funds under the Maternal and Child Health Services Block Grant now report performance measures that document the effects of programs supported under the previous cycle of awards. Several of these performance measures are based on a set of 10 essential public health services identified by a task force of the DHHS. Similarly, the DHHS is rapidly moving toward implementation of performance partnerships grants with state health agencies, another outgrowth of the GPRA. This initiative, which is already underway in some states, allows state health agencies to establish action plans and performance objectives as part of their contracts with the DHHS for federal public health funding.[11] As part of this initiative, a special panel commissioned by the DHHS recently identified performance measures that are appropriate for key public health, mental health, and substance abuse services.[12] This initiative places additional emphasis on the ability of state health agencies to measure public health performance at state and local levels and to demonstrate accountability for federal funds.

Information Production and Dissemination

A third type of policy instrument used by federal agencies involves the production and dissemination of information. In the domain of public health, this information is often produced through federally financed research efforts, surveillance systems, and policy studies. All of the major federal health agencies maintain units devoted to research efforts, but the dominant federal agencies for health-related research include the National Institutes of Health (NIH), the Agency for Health Care Research and Quality (AHRQ), and the CDC. Agencies carry out data collection and research efforts both through internal activities and through extramural relationships with universities, professional associations, and contract research organizations. The public health impact of these federal activities is substantial but highly variable. For example, biomedical research supported by NIH is leading to the development of new clinical technologies and practices that can be used for health promotion and disease prevention. Genetic information produced through NIH's Human Genome Project is fueling the development of new screening and early detection technologies for chronic diseases having an identifiable genetic basis, such as breast cancer. Likewise, health services research supported through the AHRQ and the CDC produces information about effective strategies for encouraging physicians to deliver clinical preventive services and for encouraging health care consumers to comply with these services. Other federal research efforts produce valuable information regarding public health effects and public health interventions in areas such as nutrition, physical activity, social behaviors, and environmental conditions.

The public health impact of federal activities in health information production often hinges on the effectiveness of federal efforts to disseminate this information appropriately. Federal agencies pursue an array of dissemination strategies that includes making data resources available to outside organizations for further analysis and application as well as informing the producers and consumers of public health services about the implications of new research findings. This first approach is actively used by the CDC, as many state and local public health organizations use data from its birth, mortality, health risk factor, and infectious disease surveillance systems to identify public health needs and evaluate the impact of local public health interventions. Similarly, many health researchers and policy analysts make use of data from the CDC's numerous national health surveys for scientific investigations of health status, health behavior, and health care delivery.

Certain federal health agencies also actively engage in educating relevant organizations and individuals about the public health implications of new health information. In some cases, this approach serves as an alternative to the use of regulatory power by federal agencies. Agencies use the quality of the available information, together with the visibility and authority of their federal office, to educate and influence behavior. The EPA, for example, maintains an array of "industry partnerships" through which it encourages voluntary compliance with strategies to reduce the production and release of harmful pollutants. Similarly, the CDC supports an initiative to encourage the voluntary adoption of community-based preventive services among public health organizations across the nation. In some cases, it may be the implicit threat of federal regulation or resource reallocation, rather than the influential power of information and education, that encourages voluntary compliance with such strategies. Nevertheless, federal agencies often are able to use the visibility and authority of their offices to draw public attention to important public health issues, to convene important public health stakeholders around such issues, and to lend credibility to new public health information.

Policy Advocacy and Agenda Setting

A final policy instrument used by federal health agencies in the public health arena involves policy advocacy and agenda setting in the legislative process. The U.S. Constitution's separation of powers doctrine ensures that agencies in the executive branch of the federal government have no formal legislative authority. Nonetheless, these agencies often play important roles in placing public health issues on Congress' legislative agenda and in garnering support for public health legislative proposals at the federal level.[13] These roles are perhaps carried out most frequently by informing members of Congress and their staff about important public health issues using tools such as legislative briefings, testimony, and conferences. Additionally, federal health agencies often carry out more direct roles in agenda setting by participating in the design of model legislation and by recruiting legislators to sponsor these proposals. Finally, federal health agencies may play roles in garnering legislative support (or opposition) for proposals under consideration in Congress through informal lobbying efforts and direct appeals to professional associations, political interest groups, and members of the public. Through these types of activities, federal health agencies can exert a strong voice in legislative decisions that have implications for public health activities—including resource allocation issues as well as regulatory issues.

The U.S. Congress also has its own internal structures for acquiring information about public health programs, policies, and resource needs. These federal legislative agencies should be recognized for their important roles in public health policy development and implementation at the federal level. The U.S. General Accounting Office (GAO) is known as the investigative arm of Congress, and it conducts policy analysis, program evaluation, and financial auditing activities for all federal agencies and federally funded programs. Most often, these activities are initiated in response to requests from specific congressional bodies or members of Congress. A division within the GAO specializes in federal public health and health care programs and generates periodic reports and congressional testimony on major public health programs. As a source of policy information and evaluation, the GAO plays a critical role in the policy development process and can have an important impact on public health policy decisions. For example, during the 1990s, a series of GAO evaluations of the federal vaccine purchasing program Vaccines for Children led many members of Congress to consider reforms in this program.[14] More recently, an unflattering GAO analysis of federal lead poisoning prevention programs is leading legislators to consider policy changes.[15] Other federal legislative agencies that perform important functions in the policy development process include the Congressional Budget Office, which examines the effects of current and proposed policies on federal spending, and the Congressional Research Service, which produces summaries and policy briefs on a wide range of policy issues of interest to Congress.

Overview of Federal Agencies with Public Health Responsibilities

Many of the federal agencies that contribute to public health activities are organized within the DHHS (Figure 3–1). This cabinet-level department in the executive branch of federal government administers programs involving public health services, medical care financing and delivery, mental health and substance abuse services, and social services, including income support and child welfare programs. Several of these agencies make up the U.S. Public Health Service, a functional division of the DHHS that is devoted to public health activities. Eight separate agencies form the U.S. Public Health Service, each of which is described in the following paragraphs.

The CDC

The CDC operates 11 administrative units devoted to preventing and controlling specific disease, injury, and disability risks on a national level through research, epidemiologic surveillance and investigation, and program development and dissemination activities. The CDC carries out this mission through a staff of more than 7,500 and an annual budget that totals $2.6 billion (FY 1999). The CDC maintains a strong intramural research program that uses state-of-the-art laboratory and field resources to examine disease risks, transmission routes, and intervention strategies for a wide range of public health threats. Additionally, the CDC maintains an extensive extramural research program that uses a broad network of university-based research centers for the scientific investigation of public health risks and opportunities for prevention and control.

Historically, the CDC's research and development initiatives have emphasized laboratory and epidemiologic methods for investigating disease transmission, control, and prevention mechanisms. In recent decades, the CDC's scientific agenda in public health has grown to include an expanded emphasis on the behavioral and social sciences in studying public health issues such as the adoption and diffusion of prevention practices among health care providers and populations at risk, and the cost-effectiveness of community-level interventions such as health education campaigns. As evidence of this new emphasis, the CDC created a Program for Prevention Effectiveness Research in 1991 to foster

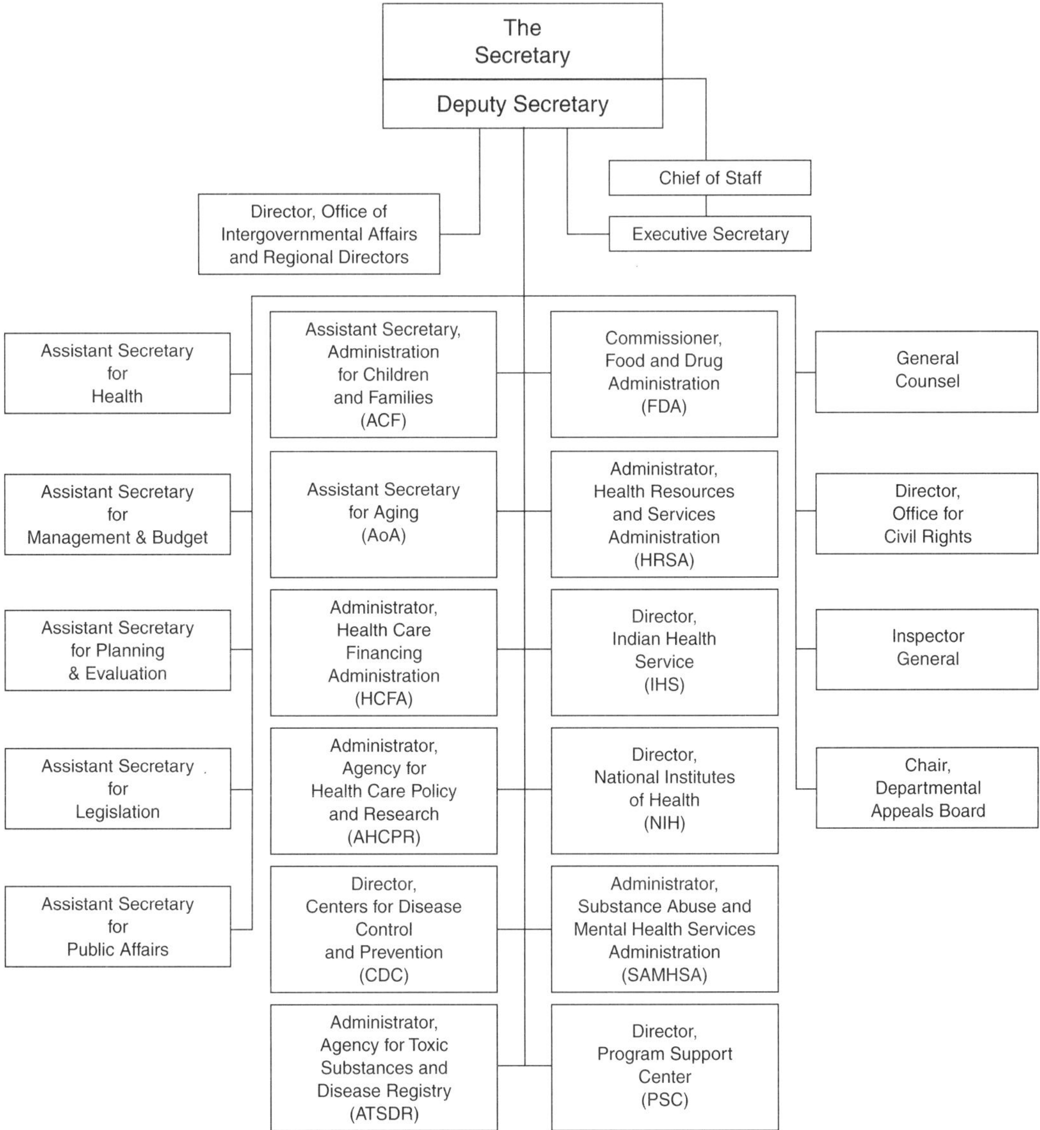

Figure 3–1 Agencies within the U.S. Department of Health and Human Services. *Source:* U.S. Department of Health and Human Services.

the development and application of social science methods for the study of public health intervention performance in real-world settings. Nevertheless, most of the centers within the CDC are organized around specific disease processes and intervention opportunities (Figure 3–2). These centers include the following:

- The *National Center for Chronic Disease Prevention and Health Promotion* fields research and development activities involving chronic disease prevention and early intervention for health issues such as cancer, cardiovascular disease, diabetes, arthritis, and the special health concerns of maternal,

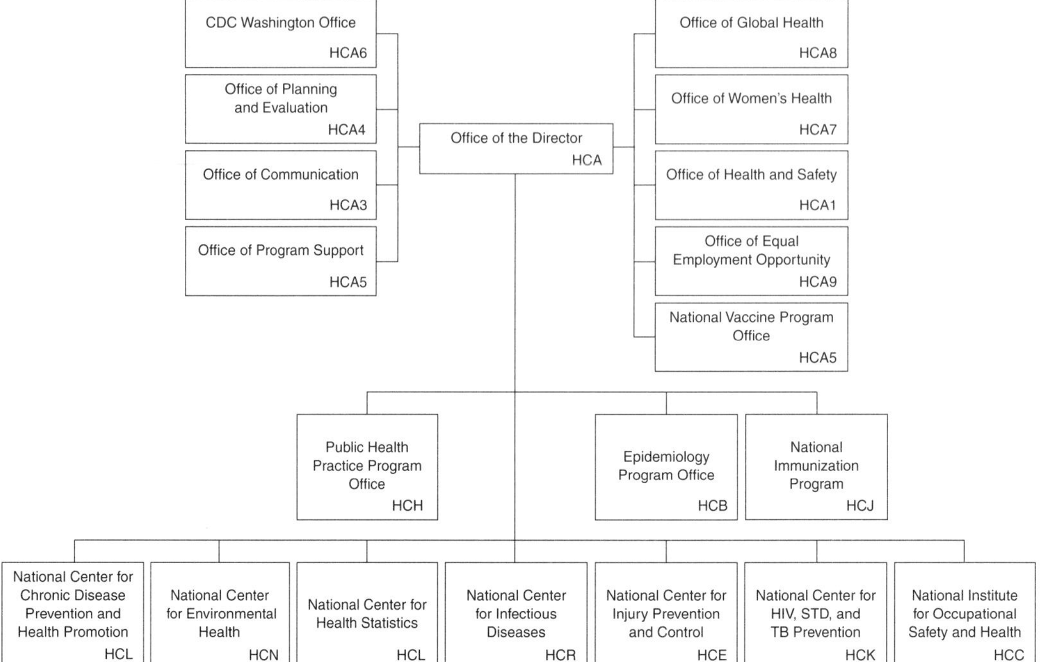

Figure 3–2 Agencies within the U.S. Centers for Disease Control and Prevention. *Source:* U.S. Centers for Disease Control and Prevention.

infant, and adolescent populations. Among other activities, this center fields the Behavioral Risk Factor Surveillance System, which collects periodic national and state-level data on adult health risk factors.

- The *National Center for HIV, STD, and TB Prevention* administers surveillance and disease prevention and control programs that target the transmission of the serious and often interrelated communicable diseases of human immunodeficiency virus (HIV), other sexually transmitted diseases (STDs), and tuberculosis (TB).
- The *National Center for Infectious Diseases* sponsors research and program development activities designed to prevent and control a wide array of existing, emerging, and resurgent infectious diseases—including those that pose unique health threats due to drug resistance or intentional transmission through bioterrorist acts.
- The *National Center for Injury Prevention and Control* designs and fields research and intervention programs that focus on the prevention of both unintentional and intentional injuries occurring outside the workplace.
- The *National Institute for Occupational Safety and Health* supports scientific investigations of workplace health threats and designs prevention and control programs to improve safety and wellness and reduce health risks within occupational settings.
- The *National Center for Environmental Health* fields research and intervention efforts designed to forestall illness, disability, and death due to human interaction with harmful environmental substances such as indoor and outdoor air pollutants, hazardous wastes, waterborne pathogens and pollutants, foodborne pathogens, and lead exposure.

Additionally, the CDC includes several agencies that address national public health resource and infrastructure needs that cut across specific disease areas and populations. These agencies include the following:

- The *National Center for Health Statistics* functions as the nation's public health data repository by fielding national surveys of health status, health behavior, and health care practices and by maintaining vital and health statistics databases. Among the periodic national surveys and surveillance systems fielded by the center are the National Health Care Survey, the National Immunization Survey, the National Health Interview Survey, and the National Health and Nutrition Examination Survey. The center also maintains efforts for tracking national statistics on prenatal care, births, and deaths through the National Vital Statistics System.
- The *Public Health Practice Program Office* performs research, technical assistance, program development, and evaluative activities designed to strengthen the nation's public health infrastructure and improve the organization and operation of state and local public health systems. This office sponsors initiatives that target the development of state and local public health agencies and administrators, public health laboratories, public health information systems, and global public health work force and infrastructure capacities.
- The *Epidemiology Program Office* supports the development and use of epidemiologic surveillance systems, analytic methods, and tools throughout the CDC and the public health organizations with which it interacts. Among other activities, this office maintains the National Notifiable Diseases Surveillance System, which tracks the incidence of 52 high-priority infectious diseases among U.S. residents.
- The *National Immunization Program* oversees national and state-based efforts to expand age-appropriate vaccination coverage rates for children, adolescents, and adults. This agency has been heavily involved in the development of immunization registries and tracking systems at the provider level, the community level, and the state level.

Among all of the federal health agencies, the CDC is arguably the most heavily invested in intergovernmental relationships with state and local public health organizations. Many of the CDC's initiatives in disease surveillance and control depend on activities carried out by state public health agencies and their affiliated local health departments. For example, the National Notifiable Diseases Surveillance System and the Behavioral Risk Factor Surveillance System depend on data that are collected and reported by state agencies (as well as local agencies in the former case). Likewise, state and local agencies frequently depend on the specialized expertise and technology maintained at the CDC for activities such as laboratory analysis of newly detected unknown pathogens and control of particularly potent infectious disease outbreaks. To address these mutual dependencies, the CDC maintains a series of efforts to equip state and local public health work forces with the necessary expertise and technology to carry out public health activities of national importance. For example, the CDC assigns trained staff to work in each of the nation's state public health agencies, as well as many local health departments, carrying out disease surveillance and control activities as well as special research and demonstration initiatives. Perhaps the oldest and largest of these initiatives, the CDC's Epidemiologic Intelligence Service (EIS), has placed health professionals in state health departments around the nation since 1951 to carry out two-year fellowships devoted to epidemiologic investigation. The CDC also maintains a number of work force development initiatives that range from training and continuing education programs to staff exchange programs—all designed to strengthen state and local public health agency capacities for implementing core public health activities.

Finally, the CDC routinely develops cooperative agreements with state and local agencies as well as professional associations for the development of specific programs and tools to enhance public health capacity. For example, the CDC's National Public Health Practice Program Office has worked collaboratively with the National Association for County and City Health Officials (NACCHO) for nearly a decade in developing self-assessment tools for local public health organizations, including the widely used *Assessment Protocol for Excellence in Public Health.* Similarly, this CDC office is currently developing a national performance measurement system for public health organizations in collaboration with the NACCHO, the Association of State and Territorial Health Officials, and several individual state and local health agencies.

Other Agencies of the U.S. Public Health Service

The CDC effectively functions as the federal government's lead agency for both scientific and practice-based public health activities. Nevertheless, a number of other federal agencies within the U.S. Public Health Service carry out critical public health functions that largely complement those of the CDC. These agencies include the following:

- The *HRSA* administers nearly $4 billion in federal programs designed to expand public access to health care professionals and facilities, particularly in underserved areas. The Maternal and Child Health Bureau within the HRSA administers an array of services and programs designed to increase the timely delivery and uptake of prenatal, infant, and child health services in order to ensure the health of children and their families. The bureau administers grants to states through the Maternal and Child Health Services Block Grant, which supports programs designed to reduce infant mortality; provide comprehensive care for women before, during, and after pregnancy and childbirth; reduce adolescent pregnancy; improve childhood vaccination coverage; and meet the nutritional and developmental needs of children and their families. The bureau also administers categorical grant programs that support the provision of emergency medical services for children and the delivery of abstinence education services to children and adolescents.

  The Bureau of Primary Health Care within the HRSA provides funding and technical assistance to agencies that provide comprehensive primary care services in medically underserved areas, including local health departments as well as nonprofit community health centers. The HRSA's Bureau of Health Professions maintains programs for monitoring and improving the accessibility of health professionals within the United States, including the National Health Services Corps, which sponsors professionals to practice in medically underserved communities. Other initiatives sponsored by this bureau are designed to address training needs and potential work force shortages and surpluses of health professionals in various fields of specialization and practice settings. A Bureau of HIV/AIDS Services administers funding and technical assistance to programs that provide primary medical care and support services to individuals with HIV and AIDS, and to programs that conduct clinical research on HIV services. Finally, a special programs division within the HRSA manages a variety of health resource programs that include: (1) the Hill-Burton program to ensure that health facilities funded through the federal Hill-Burton Act meet their obligations to provide adequate levels of free and reduced-fee care to low-income populations and (2) the federal Organ Procurement and Transplantation Network that coordinates organ and tissue donation activities.
- The nation's leading agency for funding and administering health care research and demonstration initiatives is *NIH.* The Institutes that comprise NIH conduct intramural as well as extramural research activities in areas of public health importance. NIH contributes to local public health practice

by leading investigations of public health threats, conducting demonstrations of public health interventions, and supporting the public health research interests of local health departments and other community organizations. Consisting of 25 separate research institutes and centers, NIH is the lead federal agency for biomedical research, and therefore emphasizes both laboratory research and, to a lesser but growing extent, clinical research. Medical schools and academic health centers across the country depend on NIH for most of their research funding because NIH operates with a total budget of nearly $16 billion (FY 1999). The single largest NIH research effort, the Human Genome Project, endeavors to characterize the human genome through a complete mapping and sequencing of the human DNA—an initiative that could have profound public health applications through disease prevention and early detection strategies. Other NIH units with a particular public health focus include the National Cancer Institute; the National Institute of Allergy and Infectious Diseases; the National Institute of Child Health and Human Development; the National Heart, Lung, and Blood Institute; and the National Institute of Environmental Health Sciences.

- The *Agency for Healthcare Research and Quality (AHRQ)* administers a much smaller research enterprise by comparison to NIH. The agency's sponsored research generally focuses on the organization, delivery, and financing of health services—which includes prevention and public health services but often emphasizes medical care services. Issues of health care quality and accessibility are additional research areas with particular relevance to public health activities. The agency is especially active in the development of clinical practice guidelines and strategies for evidence-based clinical practice grounded in sound scientific research. Through its information dissemination activities, the agency maintains strong relationships with major health profession organizations and health care financing organizations.
- The *FDA* functions as the nation's largest consumer protection agency by administering regulatory programs to ensure the safety of food, cosmetics, medicines, medical devices, and radiation-emitting products. Veterinary food and medications also fall under the regulatory purview of the FDA. As specified in the Food, Drug and Cosmetics Act of 1962 and the FDA Modernization Act of 1997, the FDA's responsibility in drug and device regulation involves ensuring the safety as well as the efficacy of these products. For all of the products monitored by the FDA, the agency ensures accurate labeling, marketing, and consumer information. In carrying out these activities, the FDA inspects food and drug manufacturing facilities, tests products, reviews scientific evidence in support of safety and efficacy claims, and monitors labeling and marketing practices. The FDA enforces its regulatory authority through both governmental influence and legal sanction. The agency frequently encourages manufacturers of products to undertake voluntary corrections or institute voluntary product recalls when problems are identified. When necessary, the agency can obtain court orders to prohibit the manufacture and sale of products or to seize and destroy existing products. The agency can also pursue criminal penalties against manufacturers and distributors.
- The *Indian Health Service* administers programs that provide health services to federally recognized American Indian and Alaska Native tribes. This Public Health Service agency provides health services directly and by contract with tribal organizations. Federally operated facilities consist of 37 hospitals, 64 health centers, 50 health stations, and five school-based health clinics. The health organizations supported through Indian Health Service funds provide both medical and public health services to native populations.

- The *Agency for Toxic Substances and Disease Registry* (ATSDR) operates programs to prevent and control exposure to hazardous substances. With strong administrative ties to the CDC, the agency performs public health assessments of waste sites; maintains health surveillance systems and registries for hazardous substances; provides consultation to governments and corporations regarding the use, transport, and storage of hazardous substances; responds to emergency releases of hazardous substances; and conducts applied research in hazardous substance assessment and containment. The agency also maintains a series of education and training initiatives concerning hazardous substances.
- The *Substance Abuse and Mental Health Services Administration* administers programs for the prevention, treatment, and rehabilitation of substance abuse and mental illness. The agency manages two large federal block grant programs that provide states with funds to implement an array of prevention and treatment programs: the Mental Health Services Block Grant and the Substance Abuse Prevention and Treatment Block Grant. The agency also maintains an extensive surveillance and research portfolio concerning the quality, cost, accessibility, and outcomes of mental health and substance abuse services for prevention, treatment, and rehabilitation. Finally, the agency is actively involved in providing technical assistance and consultation to mental health and substance abuse service providers.

Other Health and Human Services Agencies

Several other agencies within the DHHS play important roles in public health activities although their primary area of operation lies outside the functional domain of the U.S. Public Health Service. Prime among these agencies is the Health Care Financing Administration (HCFA), which administers medical care financing programs that include the Medicare program for disabled and elderly individuals, the Medicaid program for low-income families and children, and the newly developed S-CHIP, which covers low- and moderate-income uninsured children. As discussed previously, the Medicaid and S-CHIP programs are important financing systems not only for medical care, but also for public health services needed by vulnerable and underserved populations. HCFA exercises only partial control over the design and operation of these programs because individual states have flexibility to modify eligibility standards, program benefits, and delivery and payment mechanisms under these programs. Moreover, many states have secured federal waivers in order to institute Medicaid managed care programs that deviate from federal program requirements—such as those programs that restrict a beneficiary's freedom of choice in provider selection.

Because it controls a substantial proportion of the nation's health care financing resources through the Medicare and Medicaid programs, HCFA often uses its influence and its purchasing power to effect changes in clinical and administrative practice across the entire U.S. health system. For example, HCFA creates incentives for managed care plans to participate in the quality measurement initiatives that are maintained by the National Committee for Quality Assurance, and to field periodic consumer satisfaction surveys using a common measurement instrument developed by the AHRQ. HCFA also carries out periodic inspections and surveys of health care facilities that participate in the Medicare and Medicaid programs in order to ensure quality of care in these facilities. These activities are likely to affect the quality of care not just for beneficiaries of federal health programs, but also for the millions of other health care consumers who are served by these providers.

Other agencies within the DHHS that contribute to public health activities include the Administration on Aging, which administers social and health services programs for older Americans, and the Administration for Children and Families, which operates programs for the social and economic support of children and families. The

Administration on Aging's programs that are relevant to public health include those that address the health information and health education needs of the elderly; the nutritional, social support, and long-term care needs of the elderly; the health and social support needs of formal and informal caregivers for the elderly; and the safety, injury prevention, and violence prevention needs of the elderly. By comparison, the Administration for Children and Families' programs that are relevant to public health include the federal Head Start program that provides early educational opportunities and nutritional support to young impoverished children; the Family and Youth Services program that, among other activities, provides health education and counseling services to homeless and runaway youth; programs to prevent and treat sexual abuse among children; and programs that provide health and support services to children and adults with developmental disabilities and mental retardation.

Finally, the DHHS maintains several offices at the departmental level that are designed to coordinate public health activities across the major agencies and units within the department. These offices help the department as a whole to realize opportunities for cross-agency collaboration in addressing major public health issues that span multiple areas of operation and expertise. These offices also help the department to achieve a unified voice in communicating public health issues to the public and other major constituencies in health. The Office of the Surgeon General, perhaps the most widely known departmental office, serves as the nation's leading spokesperson for public health issues. The surgeon general also oversees the Commissioned Corps of the U.S. Public Health Service, a collection of more than 6,000 federal health professionals who provide first-response intervention in the event of national public health emergencies. The Office of Disease Prevention and Health Promotion works to coordinate federal preventive health programs across the department, including the effort to develop and monitor national health promotion and disease prevention objectives for the nation through the *Healthy People 2000* and *Healthy People 2010* programs.[16,17] The Office of Emergency Preparedness coordinates health-related disaster preparedness and response activities for the department, and the Office of International and Refugee Health serves as the department's coordinating agency for global health initiatives. Several other department-level offices develop policy, public awareness strategies, and research initiatives for major national health priorities, including the Office of HIV/AIDS Policy, the Office of Minority Health, the Office on Women's Health, the Office of Family Planning, the Office of Adolescent Pregnancy Programs, and the President's Council on Physical Fitness and Sports.

Nonhealth Agencies with Public Health Responsibilities

A number of other federal agencies are not a part of the DHHS but nonetheless contribute to public health activities on a national level. These agencies include the following:

- The *Department of Agriculture* sponsors an array of health-related programs involving nutritional support, migrant health, food safety, and the prevention of occupational exposure to pesticides. Among the best-known public health programs administered by this department is WIC.
- The *EPA* develops and enforces a wide array of environmental health and safety programs.
- The *Department of Housing and Urban Development* administers programs to address the health and social problems of populations residing in public housing facilities, homeless shelters, and economically disadvantaged communities.
- The *Department of Education* maintains programs to address the health education and health services needs of students.
- The *Department of Labor* administers programs to promote health and safety in the workplace.

These agencies make important contributions to public health activities through programs and services they administer independently and in cooperation with other federal agencies.

Federal Oversight, Governance, and Advisory Organizations

To understand the organization and operation of federal agencies in the domain of public health, it is necessary to examine the intricate systems for governance, oversight, and advice under which these agencies function. These oversight systems help to shape the policy and programmatic agendas of federal agencies while also ensuring that the agencies remain accountable to the executive and legislative branches of federal government and responsive to the needs of constituents and the public at large. Among agencies organized within the DHHS, all programs and services fall under the jurisdiction of the Office of the Inspector General (OIG) for investigations of potential fraud and abuse cases. Recent enforcement efforts of the OIG in the Medicare and Medicaid programs have resulted in substantial resource recoveries and several cases of criminal prosecution for inappropriate billing practices among providers. The OIG also reviews for inappropriate and inadequate financial management practices among state agencies and other recipients of federal public health and health services grant funds.

Programs and services maintained by the DHHS agencies also fall under the purview of the Office of Civil Rights for ensuring equal access to programs and services for all eligible population groups. In recent cases, this office's review and inspection authority has extended to the domain of patient enrollment and provider contracting with managed care plans that participate in the Medicare and Medicaid programs. This office is also involved in ensuring that health facilities funded under the federal Hill-Burton Act provide adequate access to free and reduced-fee health services for uninsured and underinsured individuals and families. Agencies outside the DHHS are not subject to these specific oversight mechanisms, but many of these agencies fall under similar review processes maintained by other cabinet-level executive departments.

All agencies in the executive branch of federal government are subject to the oversight responsibilities of the president. The Office of Management and Budget serves as the president's lead agency for overseeing the programs and activities of the executive branch and for evaluating the effectiveness of agency programs, policies, and administrative procedures. This office is also the lead agency for making funding allocation decisions within the executive branch and for preparing the president's federal budget requests to Congress. In reviewing agency programs and operations, a key area of interest for this office lies in the reduction of unnecessary burdens placed on members of the public. All federal public health research studies and surveillance systems involving human subjects therefore come under the scrutiny of this office, including a review of data collection instruments. The Office of Management and Budget is also the lead agency for the administration of the Government Performance and Results Act of 1993. In compliance with this program, all federal agencies must submit periodic performance plans, program performance measures, and progress reports to demonstrate the effectiveness and efficiency of federal programs and services. This office reviews performance measures, approves performance plans, and assists federal agencies in identifying strategies for performance improvement. In addition to the oversight provided in the executive branch, federal public health agencies are also subject to legislative oversight carried out by the GAO. This office, which has already been described, carries out a broad set of activities in performance measurement, policy analysis, and financial auditing at the behest of Congress.

Federal agencies also make use of a wide array of external advisory committees to help shape their programs and policies in public health as well as in other spheres of activity. Scientific advisory committees consisting of leading researchers and scholars are maintained by agencies such as NIH, the AHRQ, and the CDC, and carry out a broad mission in public health research and surveillance. Similarly, scientific review committees are assembled by these agencies to review and evaluate specific proposals for research funding. Review committees are often empowered to go beyond simple advisory activities and play a substantial role in making decisions concerning awards of funding.

Advisory committees made up of health care industry representatives and health care consumer groups are often empanelled to oversee the regulatory and rule-making activities carried out by federal health agencies. Appointments to these committees are most commonly made by senior officials within the agencies themselves. Although often invisible to external observers, these types of committees can have substantial influence over the organization and operation of federal agencies. These committees may function as catalysts for interorganizational coordination and collaboration because federal agencies often appoint representatives from organizations that currently or potentially act in partnership with the agencies. Advisory committees may also reflect political relationships within the executive branch or between the executive and legislative branches of federal government. For these reasons, knowledge concerning the structure and composition of external governance and advisory committees may be relevant for understanding the roles that federal health agencies play in public health activities.

One final advisory body that provides important assistance in formulating and evaluating federal public health policy is the Institute of Medicine (IOM) within the National Academy of Sciences. Congress established the National Academy of Sciences in 1863 to serve as an external source of research, investigation, and advice for any federal agency requesting assistance. The IOM, which joined the National Academy of Sciences in 1970, conducts health policy studies and reviews on a wide variety of topics in response to federal government requests and in pursuit of information needs identified by the institute's own members. The institute is an independent nonprofit organization that empanels committees of the nation's top scholars and practitioners to study health policy issues and to report findings and recommendations to policy makers, health professionals, and the public at large. The institute has produced many influential studies of public health issues on topics such as emerging infectious diseases, vaccine safety, bioterrorism, medical care quality assurance, community health assessment, and public health performance measurement. The institute's landmark 1988 report on the U.S. public health system, *The Future of Public Health*, sparked nationwide efforts to measure, reorganize, and improve the practice of public health not only within federal agencies, but also at state and local levels.[18] The work that Congress and numerous federal agencies perform in the domain of public health is aided immeasurably by the independent analysis and expertise contributed by the IOM.

State Agencies Contributing to Public Health

Whereas federal roles in public health consist primarily of national policy development and resource allocation activities, state public health agencies are responsible for administering specific public health programs and services on a statewide basis. Part of this responsibility requires agencies to carry out the regulatory and policy objectives outlined in federal public health policies, and part of this responsibility requires the development and implementation of new policies and programs tailored to the specific health needs, resources, and priorities within the state governments. State public health agencies are operational in all 50 states, the District of Columbia, and eight U.S. territories. Federal agencies and the programs they administer have a substantial influence on the structure and function of state health agencies; nonetheless, state agencies exhibit marked diversity in their organization and operation due to the historical and contemporary effects of state-specific political, economic, social, and environmental forces. Understanding this variation is requisite for understanding the larger architecture of public health practice in the United States because state agencies play a pivotal role in shaping the public health activities of local health departments as well as nongovernmental organizations.

State Health Agencies

The organization of state health agencies generally follows one of two basic models: a *free-*

standing agency structure headed by an administrator who reports directly to the state's governor, or an organizational unit within a larger *superagency structure* that includes other functions such as medical care and social services programs.[19] Approximately two-thirds of the states in the United States employ the free-standing agency model for their health agency, in which the state health agency is a cabinet-level unit within the executive branch of state government. For example, Washington State employs the free-standing structural model for its health agency (Figure 3–3). This agency contains administrative units for core public health functions such as epidemiology, health facilities licensing, infectious disease control, MCH services, preventive health care, and environmental health programs. This agency is distinct, however, from the state departments that administer medical assistance (Medicaid) and social services programs.

In the remaining one-third of states, the health agency is organized within a superagency structure that also includes agencies that administer nonhealth-related activities such as social services and environmental programs.[20] In these states, the health agency does not occupy a cabinet-level position within the executive branch of government, but rather the superagency provides cabinet-level representation for public health issues along with other issues within its purview. An example of this organizational model is found in North Carolina's Department of Health and Human Services (Figure 3–4). In addition to its public health division, this agency contains administrative divisions for aging ser-

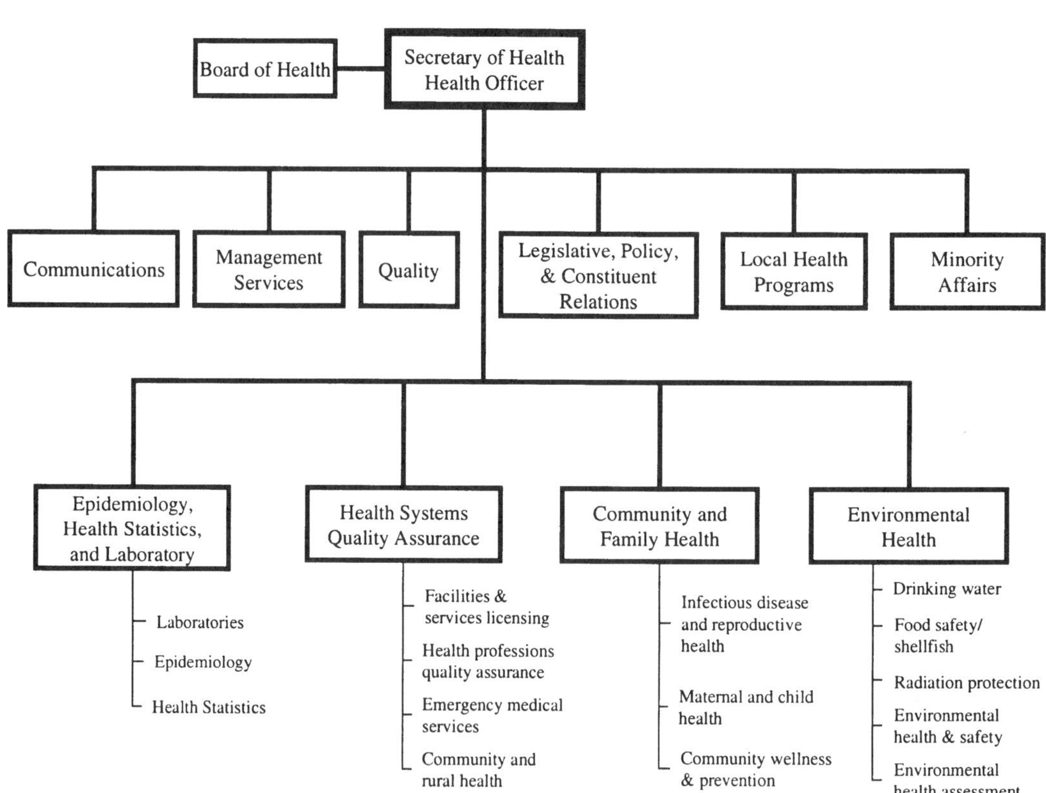

Figure 3–3 Organizational Structure of a Free-Standing State Health Agency: Washington State Department of Health.

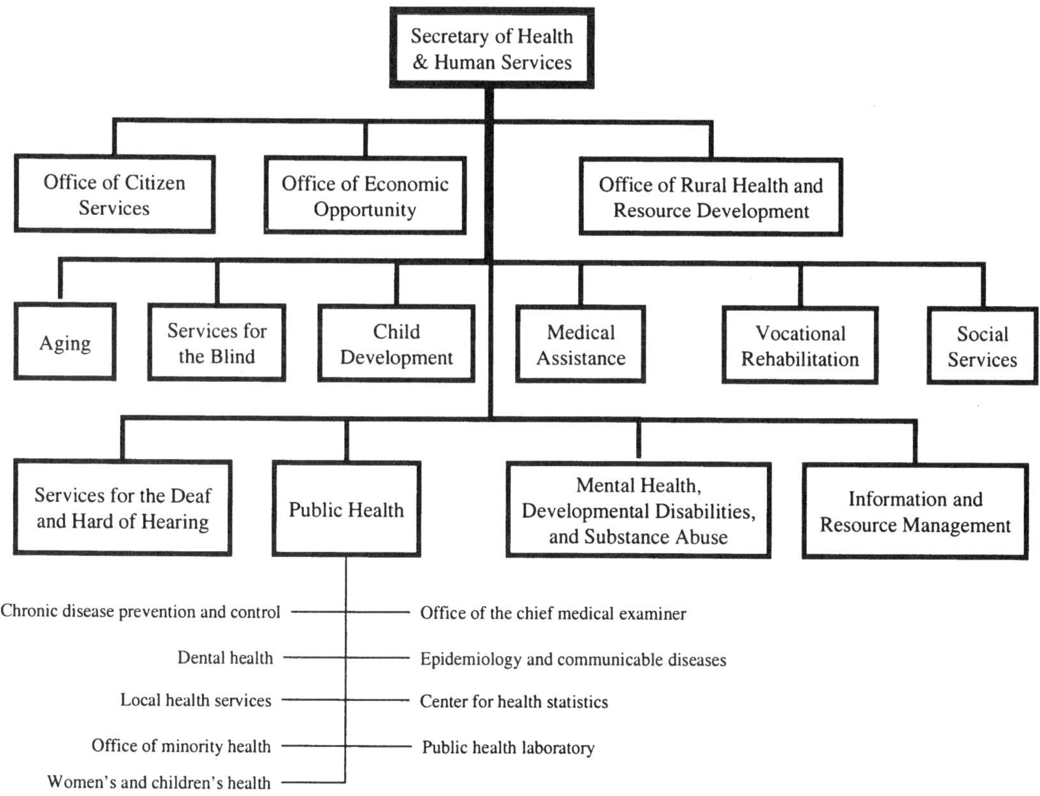

Figure 3–4 Organizational Structure of a State Health Agency within a Super-Agency: North Carolina Department of Health and Human Services. *Source:* Data from North Carolina Department of Health and Human Services.

vices, blind and disabled services, medical assistance (Medicaid), mental health and substance abuse services, and other social services. A cabinet-level secretary of health administers the entire department, and the state's public health director reports directly to the secretary. These two alternative models of state health agency organization offer clear trade-offs in terms of institutional complexity, governmental authority and power, and visibility within the state government bureaucracy.

Regardless of the organizational model used, most states do not consolidate all public health responsibilities within a single governmental agency. Rather, these functions are typically distributed across an array of separate departments and agencies. For example, state health agencies function as the lead environmental agency in only 15 states; in the remaining 35 states, a separate environmental agency carries out this authority.[19,20] Such organizational arrangements run counter to the recommendations of the IOM, which argued in its 1988 review of public health services that states should organize all health-related functions within a single agency, including environmental health services, Medicaid and other medical care programs, mental health and substance abuse services, and health professions and facilities licensing.[18] Nevertheless, political and managerial realities often lead state officials to adopt organizational structures that appear less than optimal from an operational perspective. Interagency and interorganizational mechanisms, therefore, are required to achieve operational objectives that cannot be maintained through structural design alone.[21]

Consensus has yet to be reached concerning the optimal organizational structure for a state health agency, as states aggregate and disaggregate their state health agencies continually—usually in response to leadership changes at the governor or cabinet levels. For example, in 1996, North Carolina extracted its state public health agency from a superagency framework that also contained agencies for environmental protection and natural resources and combined it with the state human services agency to form a new superagency encompassing health and human services. At approximately the same time, Michigan separated its former superagency of public health, environmental protection, and human services into three separate agencies. State public health agencies serve as the designated state Medicaid agency in only five states, and as the state mental health authority in only four states.[19,20] Most state health agencies are empowered with the authority for health professions and health facilities licensing, and for maintaining programs for children with special health care needs.

In nearly half (23) of the states, state health agencies are statutorily required to have a physician as their senior administrator.[19,20] This administrator is appointed by the governor in most states, although a state board of health appoints this official in 4 states and a superagency administrator appoints this official in 14 states. State boards of health enable citizens to participate in the governance of their state health agencies in 40 states. These boards have policy-making authority in 23 states, and in the remaining 17 states, they function in an advisory capacity only.

A key feature in the organization and operation of state health agencies is the administrative relationship between the state agency and the local public health agencies that operate within the state.[22] This relationship varies substantially from state to state, depending largely on the governmental powers that are delegated to local governments under state constitutions and state legislation. State health agencies rely heavily on local public health agencies to implement health policies and programs at the local level, but all state agencies do not have strong and direct administrative authority over the operation of these local agencies. Two-thirds of the states extend home rule authority to local governments or grant these governments the option of assuming this authority.[19] With home rule authority, local governments can adopt their own local constitutions and exercise a broad range of governmental powers usually reserved for states, such as the levying and collection of taxes to support local programs and services.

State health agencies may have much less administrative control over the operations of local health agencies that function under home rule authority; therefore, in many of these cases, states must rely on other means such as resource allocation and regulatory authority to influence the operations of local agencies. In these cases, state agencies maintain *decentralized administrative relationships* with the local agencies, which operate under the direct control and authority of local government.[22] Decentralized administrative relationships between state and local health agencies exist in 16 of the states.[19] In other states and localities where home rule authority does not exist, state health agencies may directly control and operate local health agencies as centralized administrative units of the state. State agencies may establish operating rules for the local agencies and make key decisions regarding agency staffing, financing, and organization.[22] Such *centralized administrative relationships* exist in 10 states. Three of these states (Delaware, Rhode Island, and Alaska) do not contain any local public health agencies and are therefore served only by the state health agency. In two other states (Vermont and Hawaii), the state agency operates regional offices that function as local public health agencies.[19]

Other states operate with a third type of administrative relationship in which local health agencies are subject to the shared authority of both the state agency and the local government.[22] This *shared authority model* exists in 7 states.[19] Finally, in the remaining 16 states, state health agencies maintain decentralized relationships with local health agencies in some jurisdictions within the state while exercising centralized administrative control over agencies in other jurisdictions.[19] This *mixed authority model* predominates among states that include some local governments with home rule authority and other local governments without such authority.

More than half of the nation's state health agencies organize their jurisdiction into subunits such as districts or regions for the purposes of program administration.[19,20] In these states, district offices often maintain close working relationships with the local public health agencies that fall within their catchment area. In states without such districts, public health programs are administered centrally, as are relationships with local public health agencies. In all but two states, a county system of government operates at the local level, with state governments relying heavily on this system for the implementation of state programs and services.[19,20] Even in the presence of county government systems, many state health agencies must interact not only with county public health agencies, but also with public health agencies organized by other forms of local government.

Other State Agencies Contributing to Public Health

Because of the diversity of ways in which the official public health agency is organized and empowered at the state level, many state agencies other than this official agency may contribute substantially to public health activities. These contributions may be carried out in concert with the official state agency through an array of interagency relationships, or they may be produced quite independently of the official agency. The predominant public health contributors include the following types of agencies:

- *Environmental protection:* These state agencies are often charged with enforcing federal environmental health regulations as well as state-specific policies. Jurisdiction over water, air, soil, and waste disposal issues are commonly granted to these agencies, whereas food protection enforcement authority may be retained within the state public health agency. In some states, the environmental protection agency is organized within a larger department of natural resources management.
- *Human services:* In states without superagencies, the human services department often serves as the single-point-of-contact state Medicaid agency. The administrative separation between Medicaid authority and public health authority is disconcerting to some observers because Medicaid programs and public health programs serve many of the same population groups, and because of the powerful effects that Medicaid financing policies have on public health programs and services. State Medicaid agencies also maintain jurisdiction for monitoring the quality and accessibility of services delivered by managed care plans that participate in state Medicaid and S-CHIP programs. In states without superagencies, the need for coordination between state Medicaid programs and state public health programs is often addressed through interagency coordinating councils and steering committees consisting of representatives from both agencies. State human services agencies also often administer state programs for mental health, substance abuse, and developmental disabilities services.
- *Labor:* State departments of labor often administer programs for work force safety and wellness. These departments may also have jurisdiction over workers' compensation insurance funds.
- *Insurance:* State departments of insurance maintain regulatory authority over managed care plans and other types of health-insuring organizations. Increasingly, these agencies are called on to establish systems for monitoring the quality, cost, and accessibility of care provided by these types of organizations. These activities are widely regarded as within the purview of public health agencies.
- *Transportation:* State transportation agencies are substantively involved in traffic safety campaigns as well as policy initia-

tives designed to reduce mortality and morbidity due to automobile crashes.

- *Housing:* State housing departments often contribute to public health activities that address the health needs of public housing clients and homeless individuals. For example, programs to detect and control the incidence of TB and other communicable diseases among homeless shelter residents have become important state agency functions.
- *Agriculture:* Agriculture agencies are increasingly involved in public health activities including health interventions for migrant and seasonal farm workers, programs to ensure the safety of agricultural products, and programs to provide nutritional assistance and support to vulnerable populations.
- *Governor's office:* In addition to cabinet-level state agencies, a variety of state offices focusing on public health issues are often organized within state governors' offices. These offices typically serve to attract public and legislative attention to high-priority health issues, to develop state policies and plans for addressing these issues, and to attract external resources to the state for use in addressing these issues. Examples include executive offices for aging, child abuse and neglect, substance abuse, and violence prevention.

State Intergovernmental Relationships

A diverse collection of governmental agencies forms the public health infrastructure at the state level. State agency involvement in public health activities tends to focus on statewide program administration and policy development; nevertheless, these agencies are also substantively involved in program implementation at the community level. A 1998 survey of the nation's largest local public health jurisdictions found that state agencies were involved in direct program implementation at the community level in 98 percent of all local jurisdictions containing at least 100,000 residents.[7] In these jurisdictions, local public health administrators reported that state agencies were directly involved in performing more than one-third of the core public health services undertaken within the jurisdictions. The official state public health agency provides leadership and direction for many of these activities, but other state agencies are often key contributors as well.

One increasingly important vehicle of interaction between state and local public health agencies exists in the form of performance measurement activities. State health agencies face both internal and external pressures to measure the products and outcomes of public health activities undertaken within their jurisdictions. Increasingly, state legislatures are demanding greater accountability for funds spent on public health and other publicly funded services. A growing number of state health agencies are developing performance measurement systems to meet these legislative mandates.[23,24] Similarly, the federal effort to develop "performance partnerships" with state health agencies as a condition of continued grant funding places additional emphasis on the ability of state health agencies to measure the performance of public health activities at state and local levels and to demonstrate accountability for federal funds. State agencies also use performance measurement activities to monitor progress toward their own internal objectives for organizational effectiveness and efficiency.

A recent survey of state health agency administrators indicates that these agencies are responding to the incentives for performance measurement, as 22 state health agencies had developed systems to measure the performance of local public health organizations as of mid-year 1998, and another 12 states had developed plans for such systems.[25] Most state agencies report using the information produced by these systems for state-level planning and decision making, but nine agencies also report providing the information to local public health agencies for their own use in performance improvement activities. At least two states, Illinois and Michigan, report using performance measurement activities as part of a state-level accreditation and certification process for local public health agencies.[26] Most recently, the federal government has begun involvement in performance measurement activities through the National Public Health Performance Standards Program under development by the CDC.[27] This initiative brings together governmental agencies from federal, state, and local levels to form a standardized national approach for measuring the performance of public health organizations and for instituting a voluntary accreditation program. This initiative represents an increasingly important vehicle for intergovernmental interaction and information sharing in public health.

An additional and perhaps more traditional forum for state and federal intergovernmental relations is the professional organization for state health officials, the Association of State and Territorial Health Officials. Consisting of senior administrators from each state and territorial public health agency, this organization serves not only as a forum for professional exchange among the state health agencies, but also as a powerful voice for state public health issues in Washington. The association develops consensus statements and policy positions on a broad array of state and national public health issues, as well as model state legislation to assist members in the policy development process within their home states. The association also serves as a vehicle for developing and implementing multistate responses to specific public health issues having a regional impact. Examples of such issues include water and air quality concerns, population migration and development patterns, hazardous waste transport and disposal, natural disaster response and recovery, and socioeconomic trends. Through forums such as this association, state agencies obtain a voice in national public health policy development and maintain mechanisms for intergovernmental communication and coordination.

Local Governmental Agencies in Public Health

Local governmental public health agencies retain the most direct and immediate responsibility for performing public health activities at the community level. Their prevalence across the nation varies with the definition used to describe them, but recent studies estimate that more than 2,800 agencies are operational as of 1997 when defined as "an administrative or service unit of local or state government, concerned with health, and carrying some responsibility for the health of a jurisdiction smaller than a state."[28(p.2)] The organizational structures and operational characteristics found among local public health agencies are more diverse even than those observed at state and federal levels. Several explanations for this variation are readily apparent. First, the local governmental entities that sponsor these agencies vary widely in their political authority and jurisdiction—including counties, cities, rural townships, special districts, and state governments. Second, local public health agencies vary widely in the size and composition of the populations they serve. Finally, these agencies show marked diversity in the political, economic, social, and intergovernmental environments in which they operate. Any statistician can confirm that the relative variation in any measure is generally greater across small units of aggregation than across larger units of aggregation. Likewise, public health needs, resources, values, and priorities appear to vary more across local public health jurisdictions than across state jurisdictions. The structure and function of local public health agencies are in many ways tailored to these community-specific parameters.

Organizational Structure

Most local public health agencies are units of county government. A 1997 survey of these agencies indicates that nearly two-thirds are county departments and another 10 percent are units of combined city–county government entities (Exhibit 3–1).[28] Eight percent of the departments are organized as district or multicounty departments—a strategy used by some small and rural local governments to realize economies of scale by combining their health operations. Most of the remaining departments are operated by cities (8 percent) and towns (10 percent).

The vast majority of local public health agencies (81 percent) operate in tandem with a local board of health.[28] These boards vary widely in

Exhibit 3–1 Characteristics of U.S. Local Health Departments, 1997

Governmental Structure	
County departments (%)	61
City/town departments (%)	18
Multicounty/district departments (%)	8
Joint city–county departments (%)	10
Other (%)	2
Local Board of Health	
Board exists (%)	81
Board has policy-making authority (%)	51
Jurisdiction Served	
Less than 50,000 residents (%)	66
50,000 to 500,000 residents (%)	31
More than 500,000 residents (%)	4
Average population size of jurisdiction	99,354
Median population size of jurisdiction	30,000
Financial Resources	
Average annual expenditures ($1,000s, 1996–97)	5,508
Median annual expenditures ($1,000s, 1996–97)	690
Average expenditures per capita ($)	41
Staffing	
Average full-time equivalent (FTE) staff	71
Median FTE staff	16
Average FTE staff per 100,000 residents	151

Source: Data from National Association of County and City Health Officials (NACCHO), *1997 National Profile of Local Health Departments*, NACCHO.

their structure and function. Most boards contain appointed members only, but nearly one-third include elected officials as members.[29] In some cases, a preexisting elected body such as a board of county commissioners or a city council serves as the local board of health. Local boards of health predominate among departments serving small jurisdictions of less than 50,000 residents. Approximately half of the local boards perform both advisory and policy-making functions for their local public health agency, according to a 1996 survey of board representatives.[29] Policy-making functions may include responsibilities such as reviewing and approving the departmental budget, establishing broad departmental policies and objectives, appointing the department's senior administrative and clinical officials, and evaluating the performance of the department and its leadership. In the remainder of cases, boards provide advice to local health departments but wield no policy-making authority. For this reason, most of the nation's local health departments operate without a true governing board that carries out responsibilities beyond advisory activities.

Nearly two-thirds of the nation's local health departments serve jurisdictions of less than 50,000 residents.[28] By comparison, departments serving the nation's largest jurisdictions—those with more than 500,000 residents—make up only 4 percent of the national population of local health departments. The remaining 31 percent of departments serve jurisdictions of between 50,000 and 500,000 residents. Interestingly, departments serving jurisdictions of at least 100,000 residents cover more than 70 percent of the total U.S. population, but they comprise only 20 percent of all U.S. local public health agencies.

Scope of Public Health Services

The scope of public health services performed by local public health agencies varies markedly across regions and states. These agencies typically adapt their service offerings in order to complement the breadth and accessibility of public health services delivered by other community providers. Nearly all local agencies are involved in communicable disease control activities. A 1997 survey of the nation's local health departments revealed that 93 percent offer childhood immunizations and 92 percent offer adult immunizations.[28] More than two-thirds of the departments offer testing for STDs, and 64 percent provide treatment services for these diseases.

The delivery of primary care services by local public health agencies continues to be an issue of much discussion and debate. In some communities, these agencies provide comprehensive primary care services because there are no alternative sources of care for individuals who cannot access private medical providers due to insurance status, financial need, or language and cultural barriers.[1,4] Still, some observers argue that obligations for delivering personal health services detract local public health agencies from their primary mission in performing population-based public health services such as surveillance, health education, and policy development.[18] Despite this unresolved debate, 84 percent of local health departments are actively involved in delivering well-child care and/or sick-child care—either directly or by contract with other community providers.[4,28] More than two-thirds of the departments are engaged in providing early childhood developmental testing and screening services through the federal Early and Periodic Screening, Diagnosis, and Treatment (EPSDT) program. Nearly one-third of local public health agencies offer obstetrical services—most commonly routine prenatal care.[28]

In the area of health promotion and disease prevention activities, 68 percent of the nation's local health departments are engaged in tobacco prevention programs, and 45 percent offer tobacco use cessation services.[4,28] Nearly half of the local departments provide injury prevention and control services such as bicycle helmet and child safety seat distribution programs, and 87 percent report operating health education and behavioral risk reduction programs such as those that focus on nutrition and physical activity.[4,28]

Nearly all local health departments are involved in some type of environmental health activity.[4] (See Chapter 26 for a detailed discussion of the environmental health programs of public health organizations.) The most frequently performed environmental activities among the nation's local departments include food safety inspections (84 percent), lead screening and abatement (82 percent), sewage disposal monitoring (78 percent), and drinking water monitoring (77 percent).[28] Among other types of population health services, 83 percent of local departments indicate performing epidemiologic surveillance and assessment activities.

A growing trend among local public health agencies in some areas of the nation involves the privatization of certain types of public health functions—most often the delivery of personal health services.[30] A growing proportion of local agencies report providing some types of services through contracts with other organizations rather than directly providing the service.[4] Contracting appears increasingly prevalent for services such as immunization delivery, prenatal care, and child health and developmental screening services. The growth of Medicaid managed care initiatives and S-CHIP programs has encouraged this activity in some states because these initiatives have induced larger numbers of private health care providers to serve Medicaid recipients and other population groups who traditionally seek care from public health agencies.[31]

Staffing and Financing

Local public health agencies are sparsely staffed in comparison to many other types of organizations having a comparable scope and scale of activity.[4,32] Half of the nation's local health departments employ fewer than 20 full-time equivalent staff, and one-quarter of these departments employ fewer than 8 staff members.[4,28] The average local health department manages approximately 150 staff per 100,000 individuals residing within the jurisdiction. Correspondingly, local health departments operate with relatively modest levels of financial resources. The average annual local department budget totaled $5.5 million in 1997, but the median department operated with less than $700,000, and nearly one-quarter of the nation's departments managed less than $250,000 during that year.[4,28] On a per capita basis, the average local health department spent $41 per resident per year. (See Chapter 17 for a detailed discussion of financing in public health organizations.)

The largest share of revenue for local public health agency activities derives from state government, including federal pass-through funds. State-derived funds accounted for 40 percent of the average local health department's revenue in 1992–93, with local government sources accounting for another 34 percent of this revenue.[33] Local health departments obtain the remaining funds from private grants and from fee-based revenue in serving Medicaid recipients (7%), Medicare recipients (3%), and privately insured and uninsured clients, and from assessing permitting and licensing fees. Existing evidence suggests that local health agencies have become increasingly reliant on fee-based revenue over the past several decades.[31,34] A 15-year longitudinal study of a diverse group of local health departments indicated that fee-based revenue sources have become increasingly important components of local public health financing, whereas direct federal grants have declined precipitously over the period between 1981–97.[35] State and local funding sources for local public health activities appear to have remained relatively stable over this time period.

The mechanisms through which local health departments obtain state and local revenue vary considerably.[1,35] In some states, local health departments receive a dedicated share of revenue from a specific financing vehicle collected within their jurisdiction, such as a motor vehicle registration tax or a gasoline tax. In other states, most of the state revenue is transferred to local agencies via contracts and grants that are subject to periodic reauthorizations and renegotiations. At the local level, departments may also receive dedicated shares of revenue streams such as property taxes or sales taxes, or they may receive funds through the annual legislative budgeting and appropriations processes. Dedicated revenue streams are often preferred by local public health administrators because these funding mechanisms allow administrators to engage in long-range planning and development activities with accurate projections of future revenues. These mechanisms, however, reduce legislative control over resource allocation decisions and are therefore used sparingly if at all in many states and localities.

Other Local Governmental Agencies Contributing to Public Health

The official local health department is by far not the only unit of local government that contributes to public health agencies in a given jurisdiction. A 1998 study of public health activities in the nation's largest local jurisdictions (those with 100,000 or more residents) indicated that the official local public health agency contributes only approximately two-thirds of the total volume of public health activities performed within the average jurisdiction (Figure 3–5).[7] Other units of local government participate in public health activities in 92 percent of these large jurisdictions, and these other agencies are involved in an average of 32 percent of all essential public health activities performed within these jurisdictions (Table 3–1).

Frequent contributors to public health activities include local social service agencies, elementary and secondary public schools, housing departments, fire and police departments, planning offices, parks and recreation departments, public libraries, public transit authorities, waste management agencies, and water and sewer authorities.[35] These organizations often maintain valuable resources for developing and implementing communitywide public health initiatives such as support staff, specialized expertise, building space and equipment, information and communications infrastructure, and public outreach mechanisms. In any given jurisdiction, these organizations are not necessarily units of the same governmental entity. Many local public health jurisdictions fall within multiple, overlapping spheres of local governmental authority, such as those of counties, cities, townships, school districts, transportation authorities, and water and sewer authorities. The extent to which these types of agencies are involved in public health activities varies widely across communities.[7,35] Mechanisms for interagency communication and coordination are likely to influence such involvement. Structures such as intergovernmental coordinating councils and interagency planning committees may serve as forums for developing multisectoral responses to local public health issues.

NONGOVERNMENTAL PUBLIC HEALTH ORGANIZATIONS

Governmental public health organizations are in many cases the dominant institutions within public health delivery systems. These organizations control most of the human and capital resources that are dedicated specifically for public health activities within the United States. Nonetheless, nongovernmental organizations play instrumental roles in the production of public

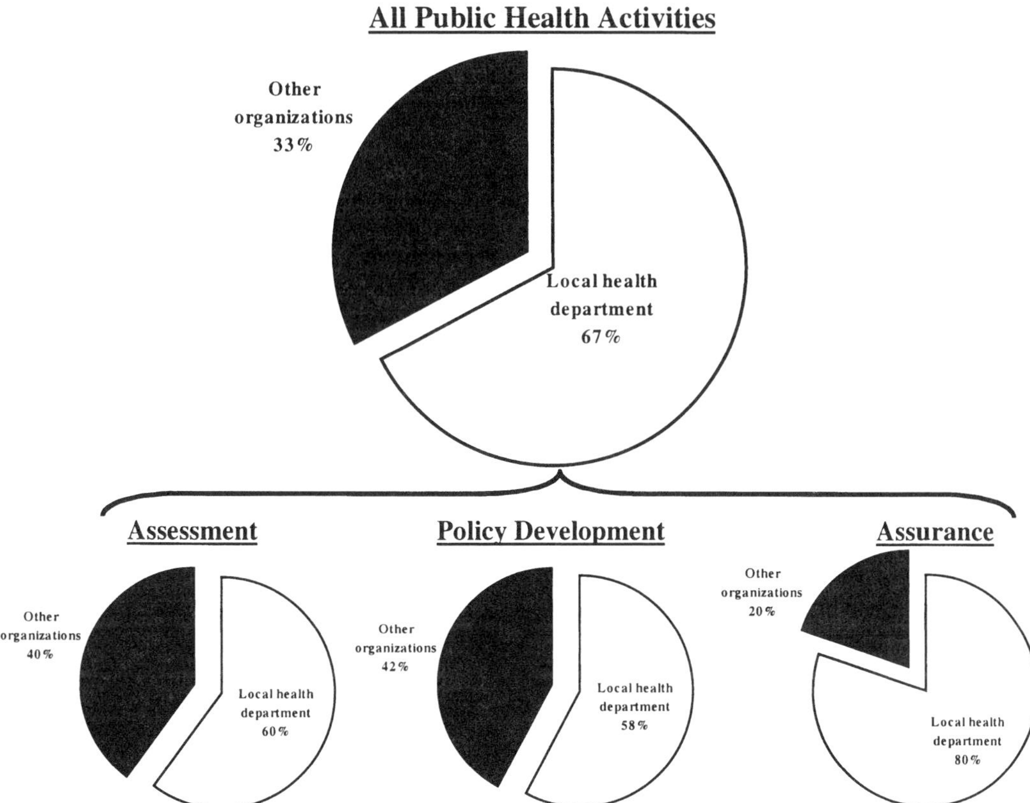

Figure 3–5 Local Health Department Contributions to Local Public Health Activities. *Source:* Unpublished data from G.P. Mays, C.A. Miller, and P.K. Halverson, *Performing Essential Public Health Services in the Nation's Most Populous Communities,* © 1998, University of North Carolina at Chapel Hill School of Public Health.

health services, both independently and in concert with governmental health agencies. Nongovernmental efforts in public health delivery include aspects of medical practice that contribute to public health practices and outcomes. Collaborative activities in medical practice and public health practice have become more visible and more prevalent in recent years as the growth of managed health care has begun to encourage medical care providers to manage the health care needs of defined populations rather than those of individual patients.[36] Other types of nongovernmental organizations maintain a long history of involvement in public health activities such as voluntary associations, philanthropic institutions, and some health professions schools. Some of the most frequent nongovernmental contributors to public health activities are described in the following paragraphs.

Community Hospitals and Health Systems

Community hospitals have long been important contributors to local public health activities. The federal Hill-Burton program, which financed many hospital construction and capital improvement projects over the past half-century, required hospitals that used this funding to provide charitable services. Begun in the mid-1940s, this program established a strong tradition of charity care among community hospitals. As providers of uncompensated acute care services, hospitals continue to play invaluable roles in ensuring access to health care for vulnerable

Table 3–1 Organizational Contributions to Public Health Activities in U.S. Local Public Health Jurisdictions with at Least 100,000 Residents

	*Percentage of Jurisdictions In Which Selected Organizations Participate in Public Health Activities**								
Public Health Activity	*State Agency*	*Hospital*	*Nonprofit Agency*	*Local Agency*	*Private Physician/Grp.*	*University*	*Health Center*	*Managed Care Plan*	*Federal Agency*
Any public health activity	97.7	96.6	95.2	91.7	85.2	65.5	46.7	45.3	44.2
Specific types of activities									
1. Community health needs assessment	42.6	58.2[b]	55.4	49.1	23.3	31.8[a]	19.9	14.5	6.8
2. Behavioral risk factor surveillance	24.5[b]	22.1	19.8	17.9	5.8	15.6	5.2	5.8	4.6
3. Adverse health events investigation	82.1[ab]	56.3	13.1	43.8	48.0[a]	12.5	11.4	7.1	21.9[a]
4. Access to laboratory services	79.5[b]	49.0	4.3	17.9	25.4	9.7	4.3	5.1	15.7
5. Analysis of health determinants	36.7	46.7[b]	45.0	38.1	21.2	24.1	13.8	11.2	5.2
6. Analysis of preventive services use	15.5[b]	13.5	11.7	10.0	7.2	7.2	4.6	4.6	2.6
7. Support and communication networks	47.6	66.5[a,b]	64.2[a]	62.2[a]	37.8	29.8	24.4	18.3	10.6
8. Information provision for elected officials	31.9	26.8	32.5[b]	32.2	14.8	10.5	8.0	4.0	3.4
9. Prioritization of health needs	33.3	49.6[b]	47.9	45.9	25.6	25.4	15.1	11.4	5.7
10. Implementation of public health initiatives	46.7	60.7	63.9[b]	51.0	35.5	25.8	21.5	14.0	9.7
11. Community action planning	20.6	34.7[b]	33.8	31.2	19.8	16.0	10.3	9.5	4.6
12. Planning for resource allocation	14.0	16.2	14.5	17.4[b]	8.0	6.6	6.0	2.8	2.3
13. Resource deployment for priority needs	27.9	35.3[b]	33.6	32.2	15.8	12.6	8.9	7.5	5.7
14. Self-assessment of local health dept.	12.6[b]	3.4	4.3	12.1	1.4	4.9	1.1	1.7	0.6
15. Provision of & linkage to health services	44.5	57.8	59.8[b]	47.1	44.0	17.8	25.6[a]	20.4[a]	8.3
16. Evaluation of public health services	21.5[b]	13.8	14.0	14.3	4.9	7.4	3.4	2.9	4.3
17. Use of process/outcome measures	27.4[b]	11.5	15.0	17.0	6.1	5.5	4.0	2.3	4.0
18. Public information dissemination	47.4	48.9[b]	46.6	34.6	23.7	21.4	14.0	14.6	10.0
19. Media information dissemination	37.6[b]	33.0	25.9	27.9	12.0	8.8	5.7	6.3	5.4
Average: Assessment Activities (#1–#6)	46.6[b]	40.8	24.8	29.4	21.7	16.7	9.8	8.0	9.4
Average: Policy Development Activities (#7–#12)	32.1	42.1	42.5[b]	39.7	23.4	18.9	14.1	9.9	6.0
Average: Assurance Activities (#13–#19)	31.1[b]	28.9	28.3	26.3	15.3	11.2	8.9	7.9	5.5
Average: All Activities	36.6	37.3[b]	31.9	31.8	20.2	15.6	11.0	8.6	7.0

[a]Largest participation measure in the column (activity most frequently performed by the type of organization listed in the column heading)
[b]Largest participation measure in the row (type of organization most frequently reported to perform the activity listed in the row heading)
*As reported by the local health department director
Source: Unpublished data from G.P. Mays, C.A. Miller, and P.K. Halverson, *Performing Essential Public Health Services in the Nation's Most Populous Communities,* © 1998, University of North Carolina at Chapel Hill School of Public Health.

and underserved populations. The charitable missions of many public and nonprofit hospitals motivate these organizations to engage in community health activities that extend beyond the realm of acute care.[37] More recently, hospitals face pressures from policy makers and regulators to demonstrate the production of community benefits in order to retain their tax-exempt status and their accreditation status. Additionally, the growth of managed care and capitated financing arrangements in many communities creates financial incentives for hospitals to engage in public health activities as strategies for reducing costs and encouraging greater efficiency in hospital utilization. For example, hospitals in some areas with low rates of insurance coverage have become involved in operating ambulatory care clinics for uninsured populations in order to reduce the costly utilization of emergency department services.[35] Similarly, hospitals are expanding their involvement in health promotion and disease prevention initiatives in order to attract the growing numbers of health care consumers and purchasers who value these activities.

Hospitals contribute to local public health activities in a variety of ways. In some communities, hospitals participate in directly providing community health services through efforts such as operating primary care clinics for underserved populations, sponsoring community health education programs, and conducting health screening fairs. Hospitals are also major contributors to community health assessment efforts. These contributions appear to be motivated in part by the Joint Commission on Accreditation of Health Care Organizations' recent decision to require its accredited hospitals to engage in community health assessment.[37] Hospitals are important contributors to these efforts because of their unique positions within communities to observe disease effects and identify intervention areas. Finally, hospitals make important contributions to local efforts in public health planning and policy development. In many communities, hospitals wield significant political power through the substantial human and capital resources that they control. Consequently, hospitals can be powerful agents for mobilizing communities around public health issues and for organizing collaborative efforts to address these issues. Hospitals also maintain large administrative data systems that can offer important insight into public health problems within the community, through information such as age- and diagnosis-specific reasons for hospital admissions and emergency department visits.

Ambulatory Care Providers

Ambulatory care providers also make important contributions to public health in many communities. These providers include private physician practices as well as nonprofit health centers supported by federal, state, and local government subsidies. Private physicians often engage in public health activities through local and state medical societies.[35] Medical societies vary widely in the extent of their involvement in public health activities. Some societies maintain only minimal involvement through participation in community health planning and policy development activities. Other medical societies are actively involved in designing and operating community health interventions such as free medical clinics, health fairs, and community health assessments. Private physicians may also contribute to public health activities independently, through such diverse efforts as volunteering in community health clinics, serving on local boards of health, or developing service agreements with local health departments for providing reduced-fee care to the uninsured. Additionally, ambulatory care providers participate passively in an important, nationwide public health surveillance system for infectious diseases, the National Notifiable Disease Reporting System. Physicians who diagnose a patient with one or more of the 50 diseases included in this system are required to notify the state or local public health agency that is locally responsible for this surveillance system so that this agency can initiate appropriate disease control activities and transmit the appropriate information to the CDC.

In addition to private practice physicians, nonprofit health centers also play important roles in public health practice in the communities in which they operate.[38] These centers include those that receive grants through one of the five federal health center programs administered by the HRSA (community health centers, migrant health centers, homeless health centers, public housing health centers, and school-based health centers), as well as those that are supported through state, local, or private funding. Some of these clinics offer comprehensive primary care services; others specialize in areas such as family planning (i.e., Planned Parenthood clinics), pediatrics, or STD services. In addition to ensuring access to primary care services for vulnerable and underserved populations, these health centers serve as important sources for health education, counseling, and social support services. Often, health centers and local health departments develop reciprocal referral agreements and other collaborative arrangements for targeting health services to vulnerable populations.[37] In some cases, health centers are operated directly by local health departments.

Managed Care Plans

Managed care plans are achieving a growing presence in many local communities, and some of these plans make important contributions to local public health practice in the communities in which they operate. For some plans, these contributions are motivated by altruistic missions of community service; other plans seek to achieve financial gains through these contributions by lowering overall medical care use and increasing market share.[39] Many plans are able to communicate with large numbers of community residents and health care providers through extensive networks of enrollees and affiliated providers. Some plans use this capacity to encourage health promotion and disease prevention practices among their enrollees, and to create incentives for affiliated providers to deliver appropriate clinical preventive services to their patients. Plans may also contribute to community health initiatives that target broad segments of the community population, as strategies for improving general population health and for promoting awareness of their organization among consumers, providers, and purchasers. For example, programs that distribute bicycle helmets to children or child safety seats to new parents have become popular methods for managed care plans to achieve heightened visibility in their service areas.[39]

Managed care plans also participate in public health activities as strategies for obtaining information about community health risks and disease patterns.[40] Plans use this type of information to anticipate health risks among their current and potential enrollees. In order to obtain this information, some managed care plans participate with other community organizations in community health assessment and surveillance efforts. Other plans conduct surveillance activities within their own enrollee populations and contribute this information to public health assessment efforts maintained by other community organizations.

Nonprofit Agencies

A range of other nonprofit organizations engage in public health activities at local, state, and national levels. Prime among these agencies are the local, state, and national chapters of voluntary health associations such as the American Heart Association, American Cancer Society, American Diabetes Association, and American Lung Association. These organizations implement public awareness campaigns and health education initiatives concerning disease risks and advocate for the public and private support of prevention, treatment, and control interventions. Similarly, social service organizations such as the United Way, the Urban League, and Rotary International are often active in sustaining community-level efforts to identify health risks and to implement community health interventions. Through their active fund-raising efforts, these organizations often serve as important sources of local, nongovernmental revenues to fund public health interventions carried out through a variety of organizations.

In addition to these national affiliates, many communities are served by locally developed organizations that have formed around community-specific needs and resources. These organizations include neighborhood associations, parent–teacher associations, church groups, and local environmental coalitions. These groups often participate in policy development activities such as community health planning activities and political lobbying efforts. In many communities, these groups also play important roles in implementing community health interventions, such as church-based and school-based health education programs and local environmental restoration projects.

Philanthropic Foundations

Important public health functions are also supported by an expanding array of philanthropic foundations and charities. Several large and well-established health foundations maintain a distinguished history of supporting research and demonstration initiatives in public health. These initiatives have helped to develop the public health infrastructure at state and local levels, while also building the public knowledge base concerning how best to organize, deliver, and finance public health activities at state and local levels. Two of the largest and most active national foundations in public health are the Robert Wood Johnson Foundation in Princeton, New Jersey and the W.K. Kellogg Foundation in Battle Creek, Michigan. The Kellogg Foundation's Community-Based Public Health Demonstration Initiative, which operated during the early and mid-1990s, sponsored a series of pilot programs across the nation that brought local public health agencies, community-based organizations, and academic institutions together for joint planning and program development activities. The initiative produced several successful models of community-oriented public health delivery that have begun to be replicated in other areas. Currently, the Kellogg Foundation maintains several large-scale public health initiatives in collaboration with other organizations, including the following:

- The *Turning Point Program* focuses on improving public health infrastructure through enhanced relationships and shared resources among state health agencies, local public health agencies, and community organizations. The Robert Wood Johnson Foundation is another major sponsor of this initiative.
- The *Community Care Networks Demonstration Program* explores interorganizational models for integrated health and human services delivery among public health agencies, hospitals, social service organizations, ambulatory care providers, and community organizations. The American Hospital Association is another major sponsor of this initiative.

Another type of foundation, which has seen marked growth over the last decade, is the community foundation. Acquisitions, mergers, and ownership conversions among local hospitals and health plans are generating substantial revenues that are being used to launch numerous new local health foundations.[41] In some communities, these foundations play important roles in developing and financing community health interventions. For example, some foundations sponsor extensive community health assessment activities designed to identify health risks and gaps in the health service delivery systems. Other foundations support the delivery of uncompensated health care to uninsured and underinsured community residents. For example, several large health foundations have been created in California as a result of managed care plan conversions, including the California Endowment and the California Health Foundation.

Universities

Universities and other institutions of higher education also make important contributions to local public health practice in many communities. Health professions schools such as schools of public health, medicine, and nursing are perhaps the most common contributors. Faculty from schools of public health often provide technical assistance to local health departments and other community organizations for activities such as conducting disease investigations, community health assessments, and community health planning activities. Additionally, health professions schools often collaborate with community health agencies in developing sites for internships and residencies for health professions students. These types of arrangements provide communities with additional clinical and administrative manpower that can be used to implement new community health interventions. Finally, universities may contribute to local public health practice by developing specialized training and continuing education opportunities for local health professionals. Recent advances in information and communication technology are facilitating the development of these opportunities through distance learning modalities. Increasingly, university consortia such as the Association of Schools of Public Health and the Association of Academic Medical Colleges are actively encouraging and supporting university involvement in public health practice activities.

It is important to note that health professions schools are not the only institutions of higher education that contribute to local public health practice. Other types of institutions—including liberal arts colleges, community colleges, and technical schools—also play important roles in contributing technical assistance, training, and educational expertise to community health interventions.

Other Organizations

A range of other organizations may contribute to public health activities in local communities. In some localities, employers are becoming active in promoting health within their work forces. Employer activities include efforts to reduce work site health risks, promote healthy lifestyles and behaviors among employees and their families, and assist in the early identification and treatment of diseases. For example, employers may contribute to community health education campaigns in areas such as smoking cessation, physical activity, and nutrition.[35] Similarly, employers may sponsor community health fairs and other initiatives designed to identify and address health risks within the community. Employers may undertake these activities independently or through associations such as business coalitions, local chambers of commerce, and economic development councils. Employers face compelling incentives for engaging in these types of activities given their potential effects on employee productivity and costs incurred for health insurance and workers' compensation benefits.

Other organizations contributing to public health activities include elementary and secondary schools, religious organizations, professional associations, labor unions, and other community-based organizations. These organizations vary widely in their involvement in public health issues and in their motivations for doing so. Nonetheless, their potential for making meaningful contributions should not be overlooked within individual communities.

INTERORGANIZATIONAL EFFORTS IN PUBLIC HEALTH

Interorganizational relationships have become a widely prevalent approach for improving quality, efficiency, and accessibility in public health as in other fields of practice.[42] Much of the collaborative activity occurring to date among health-related organizations has focused on enhancing performance within individual organizations. More recently, health organizations have begun to expand the scope of their collaborative efforts to address health issues that exist beyond the boundaries of individual organizations.[43] These collective efforts strive for health improvement within broad segments of the community population, although they also may offer opportunities for individual organizational gain as well. Examples range from coordinated efforts to increase childhood immunization rates within a neighborhood to jointly sponsored programs that provide health care to uninsured populations.[37] These initiatives, termed public health partnerships because of their loose and flexible structures, are defined here as coordinated efforts among public health organizations to address health problems and risks faced by broad segments of a community's population.

The term *partnership* indicates that coordination is achieved through loosely structured agreements between organizations that fall somewhere between the two extremes of ad hoc exchange and a single-firm bureaucracy.[44,45] The public health partnerships examined in this chapter are conceptually and operationally equivalent to the phenomenon of *strategic alliances* that has been identified and studied extensively in the business and health care fields for more than a decade.[28,44,46] Consequently, this chapter draws heavily on the existing body of information concerning strategic alliances to identify opportunities for public health organizations.

The organizational motivations for engaging in public health partnerships are varied and range from economic gain to community health improvement.[47] Consequently, a broad array of organizations—both public and private, proprietary and nonprofit—participate in these arrangements. For organizations with an overriding mission of public service and community benefit, partnerships offer strategies for achieving an enhanced impact on community health through pooled resources and expertise. Organizations may also face individual economic incentives for participating in public health partnerships. Partnerships may offer opportunities for addressing community health issues that impose substantial financial or administrative burdens on health care organizations—such as uncompensated care costs faced by hospitals or preventable diseases faced by managed care plans. The financial incentives for collaboration may be particularly powerful for organizations that operate under capitated payment systems and other managed care arrangements that reward efficiency in health services utilization.

A number of recent initiatives offer evidence of the broad and growing appeal of public health partnerships. A national collection of hospital associations led by the Hospital Research and Educational Trust recently implemented the Community Care Network Demonstration program.[48] This initiative provides funding to 25 community partnerships—consisting of hospitals, physician clinics, public health agencies, and human service providers—for the purpose of creating coordinated service delivery networks designed to improve community health status. A nationally recognized health policy organization, the Institute for Healthcare Improvement, launched a similar effort in 1993 to support the development of community-based partnerships based on the principles of continuous quality improvement. These partnerships addressed health issues such as infant mortality, teen violence, child abuse, chronic diseases, and injury prevention. A subsequent effort begun by the institute in 1996 facilitated the development of public health partnerships focused on the prevention of motor vehicle injuries.[49,50] The Healthcare Forum, another health policy organization, has arranged conferences and training sessions on the subject of community health partnerships since 1993. This organization, in partnership with several other contributors, is currently supporting the development of six partnerships designed to serve as national models of collaboration.[51]

Support for public health partnerships extends beyond these focused demonstration initiatives. Federal health officials have identified these arrangements as essential elements of national health care reform.[52] Similarly, the IOM's Public Health Committee concluded in its influential 1996 report that partnerships between public health agencies and private health care organizations were one of the key prerequisites for sustainable community health improvement.[53] Moreover, a broad range of professional associations have endorsed the concept of public health partnerships—including the American Hospital Association, the American Association of Health Plans, the NACCHO, and the National Association of Community Health Centers. Several recent community health assessment and planning guides have emphasized the importance of developing collaborative relationships among health-related organizations, including those produced by the CDC and others.[54,55] Many state and local associations have also joined the chorus for communitywide collaboration, including hospital associations, medical societies, and managed care trade groups.

Despite growing interest and involvement in public health partnerships, until recently, there has been very little systematic examination of these arrangements. In the absence of clear evidence regarding optimal structural and operational characteristics, health care organizations are pursuing these arrangements through a diversity of strategies. These strategies are likely to vary substantially in the costs imposed on and benefits accrued to organizations and communities.[21] The following paragraphs present some of the major structural and operational characteristics of interorganizational partnerships in public health that have developed to date. To illustrate these interorganizational structures, results from a recent study of 60 diverse local public health jurisdictions located in 15 U.S. states are described, examining the structures that exist (and fail to exist) within these jurisdictions.[37]

Table 3–2 Proportion of Selected Organizations That Participate in Public Health Partnerships

Type of Organization	*N*	*% Participating in Partnerships*
Local health departments	61	97
Hospitals	263	55
Managed care plans	385	22
Community health centers	85	71

Source: © Joint Commission Journal on Quality Improvement, Vol. 24, No. 10. Oakbrook Terrace, IL: Joint Commission on Accreditation of Healthcare Organizations, 1998, p. 522. Reprinted with permission.

Partnership Participants and Their Motivations

A broad range of health-related organizations participate in public health partnerships. These organizations include health care providers, payers, purchasers, professional and trade associations, advocacy groups, social service agencies, and neighborhood associations. Some of these organizations maintain broadly defined missions of public service and community benefit, such as public health departments and other governmental and nonprofit agencies. Other organizations have more narrowly defined organizational interests that are nonetheless compatible with the objectives of public health partnerships. Some of the most common types of partnership participants are described in the following paragraphs.

Public Health Organizations

Local public health departments are among the most frequent participants in public health partnerships. As governmental agencies charged with the mission of promoting health and preventing disease within their jurisdictions, these departments often have much to contribute and much to gain from these arrangements. Health departments are engaged in some form of partnership activity in virtually all (97 percent) of the study communities (Table 3–2).

A detailed study of the partnerships maintained by health departments in eight case study communities reveals a variety of reasons for engaging in these activities.[37] Prime among them is the ability to share the costs of implementing new public health interventions. Through public health partnerships, many health departments secure the participation of other community organizations in financing and operating public health activities that might not be achievable by the health department alone. Some health departments report using this strategy to expand local public health activities in the face of stagnant or declining public funding. Other departments report using public health partnerships as vehicles to secure external funding for new public health activities through grants and contracts. Health departments also indicate using public health partnerships as strategies for transferring existing public health responsibilities to other community organizations.[28,30]

Hospitals

Hospitals are also frequent participants in public health partnerships. Of 263 hospitals operating within the study communities, more than half (55%) participate in some form of public health partnership.[37] Government-owned hospitals appear significantly more likely to engage in these partnerships as compared with privately owned hospitals.[56] However, for-profit hospitals appear no less likely than nonprofit hospitals to participate in partnerships.

A case study analysis of partnerships in eight communities revealed that these arrangements often involve multiple separately owned hospitals, and therefore entail cooperation among competing organizations.[57] Several participants in these multihospital efforts indicated that they offer opportunities for enhanced community health impact by securing large resource contributions and achieving broad community coverage. However, participants also reported that competitive pressures within the partnerships can limit the scope of activities to be achieved and slow the pace of decision making and action.

The case study analysis of local public health partnerships uncovered a variety of reasons for hospital participation in public health partnerships.[57] These include

- creating demonstrable community benefits, particularly for nonprofit hospitals that often face political or regulatory obligations to provide these benefits as justification for their tax-exempt status
- providing new health services outside of the acute care domain, particularly health promotion, disease prevention, and health education services in high demand by consumers and purchasers
- sharing the costs of community interventions that can reduce utilization of resource-intensive services such as inpatient care, emergency department utilization, and uncompensated care delivery
- promoting awareness of hospital services and capacities among local health care consumers, providers, and purchasers

Managed Care Plans

Managed care plans appear somewhat less likely than hospitals to engage in public health partnerships. Only 22 percent of the 385 plans operating within the study communities participate in some type of partnership with the local health department.[37] For-profit plans appear significantly less likely to engage in partnerships as compared with nonprofit plans.[58] Nonetheless, managed care plans appear to make substantial contributions to partnership activities in the communities in which they participate. (See Chapter 30 for a detailed discussion of interactions between managed care plans and public health organizations.)

Managed care plans operating in the case study communities reported many of the same reasons as hospitals for participating in public health partnerships. Several plans added the following reasons:

- obtaining patient-level health information for use in care management processes, particularly information concerning out-of-network health care services received by their members, such as immunizations received through local health departments or laboratory tests received through community screening programs
- obtaining community-level information concerning health risks and disease prevalence that can be used to anticipate the health service needs of members or to project the costs of serving new population groups within the community
- meeting the requirements of state Medicaid agencies and other purchasers for working collaboratively with other community organizations

Community Health Centers

Community health centers are also important partnership participants in the communities in which they operate. These centers provide primary care services to vulnerable and underserved populations and include some organizations that receive federal funding for this purpose and others that operate on state, local, and private funding. More than two-thirds of the 85 health centers operating within the study communities participate in some type of public health partnership.[37] Of 33 partnerships involving health centers, two-thirds involve participation by all health centers operating within the community. However, because many communities are served by a single health center, only a minority of these partnerships (27%) involve participation by multiple health centers.

Community health centers operating within the eight case study communities reported two primary reasons for participating in partnerships.

- securing continued roles in providing health services to the beneficiaries of Medicaid, Medicare, and other public programs that are rapidly moving to managed care
- securing the funding and resources necessary to serve growing numbers of uninsured and underinsured individuals within their communities

Other Partnership Participants

Observations in the case study communities reveal that a broad array of other organizations participate in public health partnerships.[37] In some communities, private physicians and physician groups are important contributors to these activities—often through the mobilizing forces of local medical societies. Voluntary associations and advocacy groups are also important participants in many public health partnerships. These organizations include local chapters of national associations—such as the American Heart Association, American Lung Association, and American Cancer Society—as well as independent grassroots organizations that organize around local health issues. These organizations often play critical roles in promoting community awareness of partnership activities and in mobilizing citizen participation in these activities.

A variety of other health and human service organizations participate in public health partnerships. These organizations include mental health agencies, long-term care facilities, family planning agencies, public assistance programs, child welfare organizations, educational institutions, and government regulatory agencies. In a small but growing number of communities, employers maintain substantial leadership and development roles in public health partnerships. In most of these communities, participating employers are large businesses (more than 1,000 employees) or are part of employer associations such as local chambers of commerce or health care purchasing groups.

Partnership Models

Public health partnerships assume a variety of forms. This variation occurs along three important dimensions. First and perhaps most importantly, partnerships vary in their strategic orientation, which involves the types of organizational objectives pursued through collaborative efforts.[44] Second, partnerships vary in their functional characteristics, which involve the range of activities implemented through the partnership. Finally, partnerships vary in their structural characteristics, which involve the array of organizational tools that are used to establish and maintain relationships between multiple organizations.[44] Within each of these dimensions, a number of alternative models exist that offer both advantages and disadvantages to public health organizations and the communities they serve.

Strategic Orientation of Partnerships

Organizations pursue a wide range of interests through public health partnerships. Conceptually, these interests can be distilled into three basic strategic orientations that summarize the organizational motivations behind most collaborative activity (Figure 3–6).[44] Understanding the strategic orientation of a given public health partnership can assist participating organizations in anticipating and responding to the behavior of their partners.

Some partnerships are developed primarily to allow participating organizations to gain knowledge and expertise in a new field of operation. These types of collaborative arrangements, often termed *opportunistic* partnerships, typically last only long enough for the participating organizations to gain sufficient knowledge to assist them in pursuing their own individual interests.[44] The limited duration and restricted focus of these types of partnerships may cause the arrangement to yield relatively small community-level benefits, although the organization-level benefits may be substantial. However, the community-level benefits that flow from these arrangements may still be substantial if, for example, durable public goods such as service accessibility and

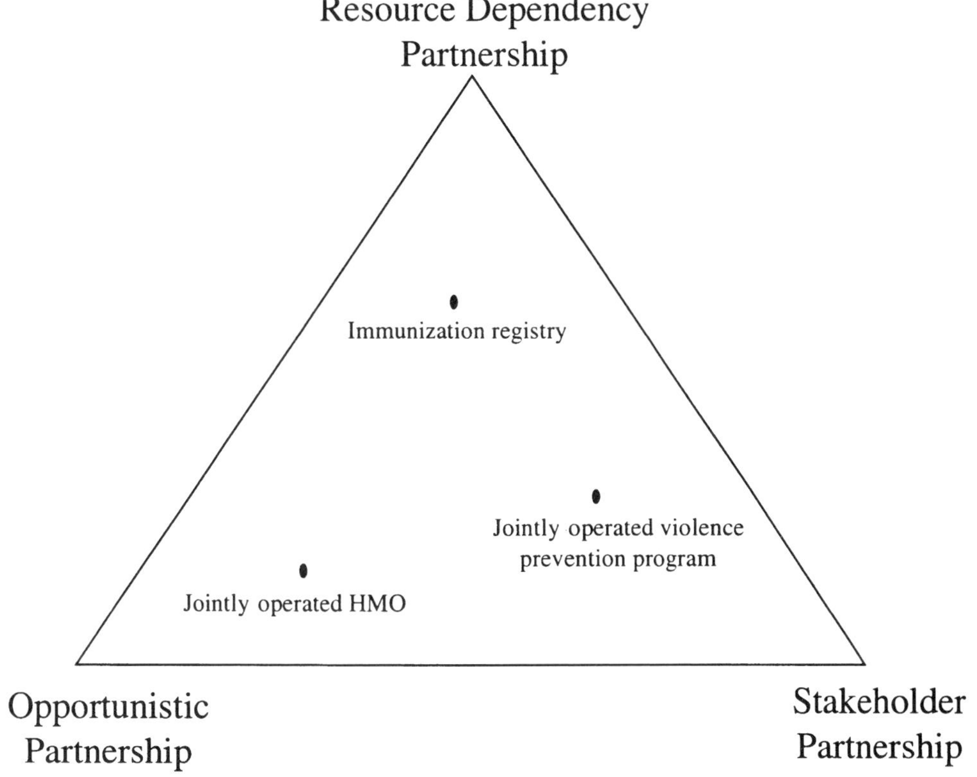

Figure 3–6 Three Strategic Orientations for Public Health Partnerships. *Source:* © Joint Commission Journal on Quality Improvement, Vol. 24, No. 10. Oakbrook Terrace, IL: Joint Commission on Accreditation of Healthcare Organizations, 1998, p. 524. Reprinted with permission.

quality are expanded as a result of the relatively brief information exchange that takes place between partnership participants.

For example, in one community, a local public health agency and a commercial health maintenance organization (HMO) formed a partnership to develop the community's first managed care plan for serving Medicaid beneficiaries.[35] Through this partnership, the public health agency gained expertise in managed care skills such as prospective budgeting, utilization review, and provider profiling. At the same time, the HMO gained expertise in serving Medicaid beneficiaries—who differed considerably from the HMO's commercial enrollees in their health and social service needs. After several years of operation, the two organizations ended their partnership and developed competing Medicaid managed care plans using the information and experience they gained through collaboration.

Other public health partnerships are formed to provide a resource or service needed by multiple health care organizations. These *resource dependency* partnerships are similar to opportunistic partnerships in that the participants use the partnership primarily to pursue individual organizational interests.[39] Organizations form these partnerships to share the costs of a product or service that is needed by different organizations for different purposes. In doing so, public goods are created that contribute to the process of community health improvement. The public goods created by these partnerships range from population-based disease surveillance and health information systems to communitywide efforts in clinical practice guideline development and dissemination. Because these partnerships are formed to address ongoing resource needs, the community benefits produced by them are often less transitory than those produced through opportunistic partnerships. As a consequence, these partnerships often require longer and larger resource commitments by participating organizations.

An example underway in several study communities involves the construction of communitywide immunization registries.[37] These registries are designed to store and retrieve the immunization histories of age-appropriate community residents so that underimmunized children can be readily identified and addressed with appropriate interventions. In several communities, partnerships consisting of hospitals, physician practices, managed care plans, and public health agencies have formed to develop, finance, and implement these registries. These partnerships offer public health agencies enhanced opportunities for preventing outbreaks of communicable diseases within their jurisdictions. At the same time, these partnerships offer managed care plans and other private providers the opportunity to track the immunization histories of their individual patient populations. In doing so, these private organizations can avoid the delivery of unnecessary vaccinations, identify alternative sources of immunization services used by their patients, develop targeted interventions for chronically underimmunized patients, and report more accurate measures of patient immunization status to payers, regulators, and accreditation bodies.

A third type of public health partnership involves organizations that pursue a shared mission or set of interests through collective action. In contrast to opportunistic and resource dependency partnerships, these *stakeholder* partnerships are formed by organizations that seek to achieve a common outcome from their collective efforts.[39] This outcome typically involves improvement in one or more areas of community health. To achieve this improvement, stakeholder partnerships often seek participation from the widest possible array of organizations that may contribute to the outcome of interest. Because participating organizations share a common mission rather than simply a common resource need, stakeholder partnerships typically achieve greater levels of organizational commitment and support than other types of partnerships. As a result, these types of partnerships may hold the greatest potential for achieving sustained community health improvement. They also may be the most difficult type of partnership to develop and maintain due to the need to achieve consensus concerning the partnership's core mission and goals.

Most of the stakeholder partnerships observed to date have involved highly visible community health issues.[35,37] For example, one community's high rate of domestic violence motivated a collaborative effort among two hospital systems, a local health department, several social service agencies, and the local law enforcement agency. Each of the participating organizations reported a shared interest in and responsibility for reducing the substantial health and social services costs associated with domestic violence on a communitywide basis. In response, the organizations developed a jointly financed and jointly operated violence prevention program to provide education, case management, and counseling to families exhibiting signs of domestic violence. In contrast to the resource dependency partnership model, these organizations were motivated by a common mission of reducing community violence rather than by a common need for a particular resource or service.

Many public health partnerships do not perfectly fit one of the three strategic orientations described here. Partnerships often derive from a combination of these orientations, with any given partnership occurring closer or further away from a given strategic orientation (Figure 3–6). For example, organizations may form a jointly operated HMO primarily for opportunistic reasons, but they may also seek to address shared resource needs through the partnership. Therefore, opportunistic motivations may have the strongest influence on this partnership, followed by resource dependencies. By comparison, a partnership to develop an immunization registry may be motivated primarily by resource dependencies (i.e., the mutual need for immunization information), while opportunistic and stakeholder considerations play lesser roles in shaping the partnership. Partnerships may also evolve over time from one strategic orientation toward another. Through the process of partnership participation, organizations gain information about their partners that may motivate them to modify their strategic relationships—for example, to capitalize on newly discovered resources or to limit the risk of loss from newly discovered liabilities in their partners. Despite these complexities, knowledge about a partnership's strategic orientation can assist organizations in anticipating and managing the behavior of their partners.

Functional Characteristics of Partnerships

Through public health partnerships, organizations engage in a broad array of activities designed to achieve strategic objectives and enhance community health. Most partnerships can be classified into one of four functional categories: service delivery, planning and policy development, surveillance and assessment, and education and outreach. These categories are described in the following paragraphs.[37]

Service Delivery. Collaborative efforts in service delivery appear to be a common type of functional activity performed through public health partnerships (Table 3–3). In a recent study of partnerships in 60 diverse public health jurisdictions, more than 40 percent of hospitals and community health centers participate in these types of activities, compared with 21 percent of managed care plans and 87 percent of local health departments.[37] Most of these service delivery partnerships involve joint referral arrangements designed to enhance service accessibility and service coordination at the community level. For example, in one study community, the local hospitals, community health center, and medical society participate in an agreement to refer patients who are at risk for diabetes to a screening and case management program operated by the local health department. Other service delivery partnerships involve joint efforts to finance and deliver community services. Organizations may contribute funding or in-kind resources to these efforts—such as staff time, equipment, supplies, and office space. For example, of the 45 study hospitals involved in the joint production of community services, 75 percent contribute funding, 42 percent contribute staff time, and 49 percent contribute equipment and supplies to these efforts.[37]

Table 3–3 Percentage of Selected Organizations That Participate in Public Health Partnerships, by Functional Type of Partnership

	Type of Organization[a]			
Functional Type	*Health Departments (N = 61)*	*Hospitals (N = 263)*	*Managed Care Plans (N = 385)*	*Health Centers (N = 85)*
Service delivery	87%	53%	21%	46%
Planning and policy development	33%	16%	4%	18%
Surveillance and assessment	23%	6%	1%	16%
Education and outreach	18%	11%	5%	19%
No partnership participation	3%	45%	78%	29%

[a]Columns do not sum to 100% because some organizations engage in multiple partnerships and some partnerships accomplish multiple functions.

Source: © Joint Commission Journal on Quality Improvement, Vol. 24, No. 10. Oakbrook Terrace, IL: Joint Commission on Accreditation of Healthcare Organizations, 1998, p. 526. Reprinted with permission.

Planning and Policy Development. A second functional area commonly addressed by public health partnerships involves the development of coordinated plans and policies for responding to health issues. Through these partnerships, organizations engage in activities such as conducting joint strategic planning and priority-setting sessions to delineate the respective roles of alternative community organizations in addressing health issues; adopting mutually developed service delivery standards, guidelines, and policies; and formulating public health policies and lobbying for their adoption by local, state, and federal legislative bodies. For example, in one study community, a coalition consisting of hospitals, managed care plans, physicians, and a local health department developed restrictive standards for tobacco sales and tobacco use that were successfully adopted by the local board of county commissioners following an extensive lobbying effort.[35] In another community, a partnership consisting of local managed care plans, hospitals, and the local health department developed a standardized form for monitoring and reporting the delivery of developmental screening services to Medicaid beneficiaries.[39] The partnership successfully secured the adoption of this form by all primary care physicians who served beneficiaries enrolled in the community's 10 Medicaid managed care plans.

Surveillance and Assessment. A third group of public health partnerships involves collective efforts to identify health risks and diseases within the community and to assess the performance of health organizations and interventions in addressing community health needs.[37] These partnerships include activities such as sponsoring communitywide surveillance efforts to identify behavioral risk factors within the community, conducting community health needs assessments to identify perceived needs for new programs and services, and sponsoring research efforts to assess the effects of health policies, programs, and services on health status within the community. In one community, a managed care plan and local health department sponsored a telephone survey of community residents and health plan enrollees regarding their health behaviors and risks.[39] The organizations used information from the surveillance effort to design both communitywide and organization-specific interventions to address public health issues such as smoking cessation, diet, and physical activity. In another community, a coalition of hospitals, managed care plans, and physicians sponsored a study of community residents who had recently sought care for digestive disorders to determine the appropriateness of treating these residents for the bacteria *H. Pylori.*

Education and Outreach. A final group of public health partnerships focuses on educating community residents and health care providers about health promotion and disease prevention practices. These efforts include disseminating information on beneficial health behaviors and clinical practices as well as providing outreach to encourage participation in health programs and services. In one of these communities, for example, a coalition of managed care plans and the local health department sponsored an on-site training program in childhood immunization practices that was conducted with all of the pediatricians and family practice physicians operating within the community.[37] In another community, a coalition of hospitals and managed care plans sponsored a breast cancer awareness campaign that included targeted health education messages in the local media and a telephone information and referral line.

Public health partnerships often support activities in several of the functional areas described here. For example, a partnership may include a health education component as well as a service delivery component, as in one community's diabetes awareness and management program.[37] Partnerships may also evolve over time from one functional area to another. Community assessment efforts, for example, often progress into planning and policy development activities. The organizational membership of a partnership may change during this evolution, as may its strategic orientation. These trend effects are described further in the section on partnership life cycles.

Structural Characteristics of Partnerships

Public health partnerships are maintained through an array of interorganizational relationships that structure the ways in which participating organizations interact. Four basic types of structural relationships are observed among the partnerships identified in this study: informal collaboration, contractual agreements, shared governance, and shared ownership. Each of these alternative relationships offers advantages as well as disadvantages in areas such as development and maintenance costs, organizational flexibility, enforceability, and reversibility. Each of these structural relationships is described in detail in the following paragraphs.

Informal Collaboration. The most informal types of relationships are based on loosely structured agreements between organizations that are maintained by mutual expectations and patterns of behavior. Organizations participating in these informal collaborative groups typically maintain a long history of operating within the same community or market and depend on reputation and peer pressure to enforce the expected behavior of their partners. Shared experiences and repeated interaction enable participating organizations to predict with confidence their partners' actions, thereby eliminating the need for more formal mechanisms of enforcing agreements. Most often, these partnerships focus on collaborative activities that entail relatively little risk to the participating organizations. For activities involving higher levels of risk or resource commitment, participating organizations are likely to demand stronger ways of enforcing the provisions of the partnership.

In one recent study of public health partnerships in 60 public health jurisdictions, local health departments and hospitals were found to participate in informal collaborative groups more commonly than in other types of partnership structures (Table 3–4).[37] These types of organizations maintain long histories of operation within their communities compared with other types of health care organizations—allowing them to use their reputation as an assurance of behavior rather than using more formalized and costly assurance methods. Only a minority of the managed care plans and health centers that engage in community health partnerships do so through informal structures.

Contractual Agreements. A second, more formalized structural arrangement used in public health partnerships is the contractual agreement. Contracts are used to specify organizational roles and performance expectations within multi-institutional ventures, and to create legal mechanisms for enforcing these expectations. Contracts are particularly important for partnerships involving organizations that lack a shared mission or set of incentives—such as opportunistic and resource dependency partnerships. Moreover, contractual partnerships are often used for collaborative activities requiring substantial financial risk. In these cases, the addi-

Table 3–4 Percentage of Selected Organizations That Participate in Public Health Partnerships, by Structural Type of Partnership

	Type of Organization[a]			
Structural Type	*Health Departments (N = 61)*	*Hospitals (N = 263)*	*Managed Care Plans (N = 385)*	*Health Centers (N = 85)*
Informal collaboration	67%	34%	7%	19%
Contractual agreements	23%	21%	14%	42%
Shared governance/shared ownership	7%	1%	1%	9%
No partnership participation	3%	45%	78%	29%

[a]Columns do not sum to 100% because some organizations engage in multiple partnerships.

Source: © Joint Commission Journal on Quality Improvement, Vol. 24, No. 10. Oakbrook Terrace, IL: Joint Commission on Accreditation of Healthcare Organizations, 1998, p. 528. Reprinted with permission.

tional costs entailed in establishing and enforcing contracts are justified by the risk that is avoided or limited through contract provisions.

Managed care plans and health centers appear to rely on contractual partnerships more frequently than other types of structural arrangements (Table 3–4).[37] Although most managed care plans do not participate in any type of partnership, nearly two-thirds of the plans that do participate rely on contractual agreements. By comparison, 59 percent of participating health centers rely on contracts, as do 38 percent of participating hospitals and 24 percent of participating local health departments.[37] Most managed care plan partnerships involve service delivery functions, which are more likely than other types of partnerships to be carried out through contractual agreements. Partnerships involving service delivery functions often entail substantial risks—including the risk of failing to recover the costs of providing services and the risk of being held responsible for the outcomes of service delivery. Contractual agreements are used in service delivery partnerships to share these risks equitably among participating organizations.

Shared Governance. A third structural model used in public health partnerships involves arrangements for shared governance among participating organizations. Rather than formalizing the content of interaction through contractual agreements, this approach formalizes the decision-making process to be used in developing and implementing collective action. In doing so, shared governance arrangements add flexibility to the partnership structure by avoiding the need to specify fully the nature of collective action and the contingencies for every foreseeable outcome of this action.

Two basic arrangements for shared governance are commonly observed among public health partnerships. In the first arrangement, each participating organization grants membership on its governing board to representatives from partnering organizations. As an alternative to reciprocal board membership, some organizations choose to establish a separate corporate entity to conduct partnership activities, along with a separate governing board for the new entity. Under either model, an organization's degree of power and representation on the governing board is typically commensurate with the organization's resource commitment to partnership activities.

The shared governance arrangement is used in one study community to organize collaborative activities in community health assessment, planning, and health education.[37] A large employer serves as the founding organization for the partnership by establishing a wholly owned subsidiary to house partnership activities. Ten other organizations participate in the governance of the new corporation, including employers, hospitals, medical practices, managed care plans, a community health center, and the local health department. Three organizations—the founding employer, a hospital, and a managed care plan—contribute the majority of financial resources to sustain the effort, and therefore maintain greater representation on the governing board. Community health activities conducted through the partnership include a communitywide survey of resident health status and behavioral risk factors, a comparative study of surgical rates and outcomes at local hospitals, a collaborative effort to develop and disseminate clinical practice guidelines on a communitywide basis to local physicians, and a community-level health education effort to increase age-appropriate mammography utilization.

Shared Ownership. A fourth and final structural arrangement for public health partnerships closely parallels the shared governance model but involves the added dimension of mutual ownership. Under this arrangement, each of the organizations participating in the partnership maintains equity ownership in a separate corporate entity that is formed to administer partnership activities. As a result, each organization shares in the financial liabilities and assets accrued by the new entity. This structural arrangement helps to align the incentives faced by participating organizations and create a single, shared mission for the jointly owned venture.

The shared ownership arrangement is used in one study community by a group of three hospitals and a network of community health centers to sustain a coordinated care program for serving vulnerable and underserved populations within a 15-county region.[35,37] The hospitals—which include a county-owned facility, an academic medical center, and a nonprofit children's hospital—each maintain one-quarter ownership in the corporation, and the network of health centers owns the remaining one-quarter share. The shared nonprofit corporation is licensed as an HMO and serves uninsured residents as well as Medicaid beneficiaries.

Taken together, shared governance and shared ownership arrangements are relatively rare within the communities examined in this study (Table 3–4).[37] Nonetheless, these arrangements are notable for their ability to sustain multiorganizational, multifaceted community efforts. They appear to accommodate more organizational participants and more functional activities than less-formalized arrangements, suggesting a superior ability to manage operational complexity. At the same time, these arrangements are likely to incur larger development costs and necessitate greater sacrifices of individual organizational control than less formalized and less integrated structural models.

The Ecology of Public Health Partnerships

Like most other institutional innovations, public health partnerships appear sensitive to both organizational and environmental characteristics.[46] An organization's decision to participate in a partnership is likely to be shaped by factors such as community health needs and resources, market structure, and organization-specific attributes such as mission, capacity, expertise, and organizational structure (Figure 3–7).

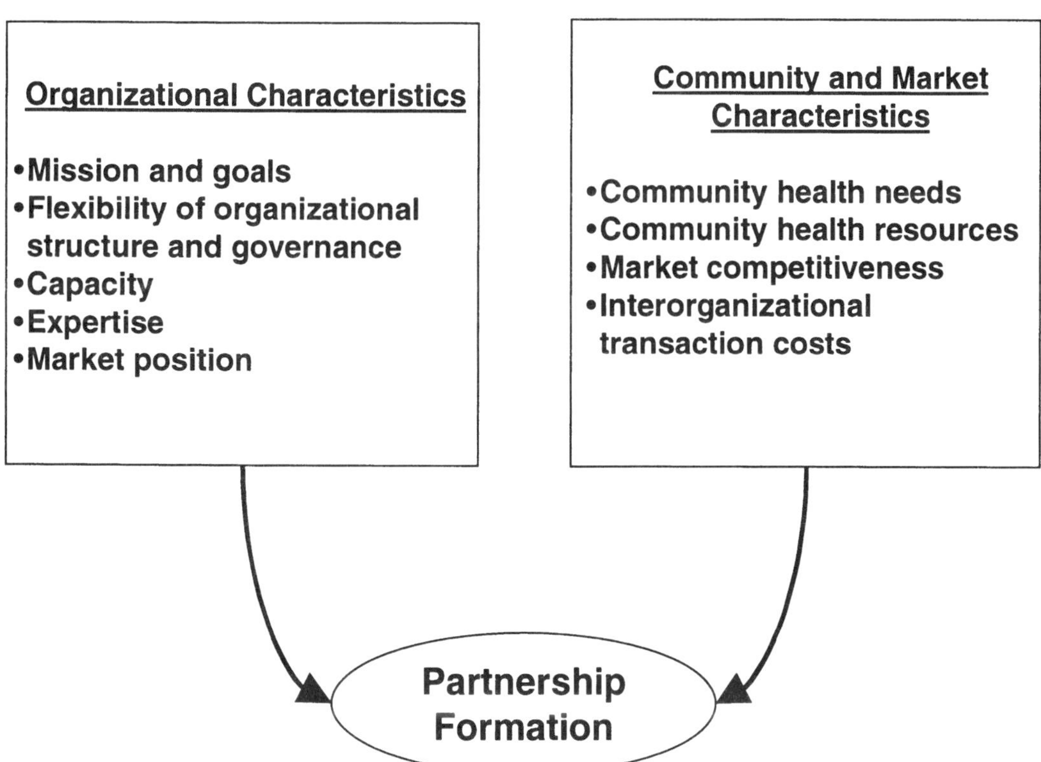

Figure 3–7 Organizational and Environmental Factors Affecting the Development of Public Health Partnerships. *Source:* © Joint Commission Journal on Quality Improvement, Vol. 24, No. 10. Oakbrook Terrace, IL: Joint Commission on Accreditation of Healthcare Organizations, 1998, p. 530. Reprinted with permission.

To explore the effects of these types of characteristics on partnership formation, several specific classes of public health partnerships are examined: (1) partnerships between hospitals and local public health departments, (2) partnerships between managed care plans and public health departments, and (3) partnerships between community health centers and public health departments. These types of partnerships are of particular interest because they involve participation from both medical care and public health organizations—the two types of organizations most frequently involved in community health improvement efforts. This analysis uses data on the 263 hospitals, 385 managed care plans, 85 community health centers, and 61 health departments that operate within 60 study communities.[37] For each partnership class, multivariate ordered logistic regression models are used to estimate the effects of various organizational, community, and market characteristics on the probability of partnership formation. The dependent variable used in each model takes on one of three ordered values corresponding to the outcomes of no partnership, informal partnership, and formal partnership (contractual, shared governance, or shared ownership). Highlights from each model are described in the following paragraphs.

Results from the multivariate models suggest that ownership status is one of the strongest predictors of both hospital and managed care plan partnerships with local health departments. Government-owned hospitals are significantly more likely than their private sector counterparts to participate in partnerships with local health departments, after controlling for other organizational, community, and market characteristics ($p < 0.01$). Similarly, nonprofit managed care plans are significantly more likely than for-profit plans to engage in health department partnerships ($p < 0.05$). These relationships may stem from the fact that public and nonprofit organizations are more likely than for-profit entities to share a mission of community service with local health departments.[37] Additionally, these organizations are more likely to serve the vulnerable and underserved population groups that are also targeted by local health departments. Ownership (public vs. private) is not found to be a significant predictor of partnerships between community health centers and local health departments.

Organizational proximity also emerges as a strong and significant predictor of both hospital and managed care plan partnerships with local health departments ($p < 0.01$). Organizations that maintain corporate offices within the jurisdiction served by the local health department are substantially more likely to partner with the department, compared with those organizations that maintain their corporate offices elsewhere. Locally managed organizations are likely to be more visible and more geographically accessible to health departments, thereby allowing for stronger reputation effects and lower transaction costs. Interestingly, proximity is not found to be a significant predictor of partnerships between health centers and local health departments.

Several additional organizational characteristics affect the development of public health partnerships. Hospitals with larger market shares show a higher propensity for engaging in partnerships with health departments ($p < 0.01$), as do managed care plans with larger geographic service areas ($p < 0.10$). Partnerships with these types of organizations offer opportunities for health departments to reach large segments of the community population. Moreover, organizations with larger market shares often have more to gain from these partnerships—which typically see improvements in populationwide health status.

Community and market characteristics also appear influential in the development of public health partnerships. Community poverty rates positively affect the development of both managed care plan and health center partnerships with local health departments ($p < 0.10$ and $p < 0.01$, respectively). This finding suggests that the demand for uncompensated care and publicly subsidized care may motivate the formation of public health partnerships. Physician availability within the community appears to affect hospital and managed care plan partnerships with health departments negatively ($p < 0.05$ and $p < 0.10$, respectively), indicating that health manpower shortages may provide motivation for these arrangements. HMO market penetration also emerges as a significant positive predictor of hospital, managed care plan, and health center partnerships with health departments ($p < 0.10$, $p < 0.01$, and $p < 0.10$ respectively), suggesting that market incentives for efficiency provide some motivation for community health improvement initiatives. The existence of a Medicaid managed care program within the community has an independent, positive effect on health center partnerships with health departments ($p < 0.10$), suggesting that such programs encourage closer integration among safety-net providers. Finally, market consolidation (as measured by the number of competitors in each market) appears to facilitate hospital and managed care plan partnerships with health departments ($p < 0.10$ and $p < 0.01$, respectively). This finding suggests that the incentives for community collaboration are greater when a relatively small number of organizations control the market and share responsibilities for community health. This finding may also indicate that in less competitive markets, organizations have more slack resources available to contribute to public health partnerships.

These estimates from multivariate models reveal that several organizational and market-level characteristics had significant effects on partnership formation within a sample of 60 local communities. The magnitude of these effects was substantial, as illustrated in Figure 3–8 using estimates from the multivariate models. These results suggest that current organizational and marketplace trends taking shape in the health care industry offer mixed implications for public health partnerships. For-profit conversions and privatization initiatives may have an inhibiting effect on partnerships because of the observed relationships between ownership status and partnership formation. Similarly, the rise of regional and national health care conglomerates—and the resulting demise of locally managed organizations—may pose challenges for partnership development. At the same time, growing managed care penetration and market consolidation appear likely to encourage additional partnership activity. The net effects of these trends on public health partnerships remain far from clear. To develop partnerships within this climate, organizations must be willing to capitalize on emerging market incentives while seeking creative solutions to organizational barriers.

The Life Cycle of Public Health Partnerships

The public health partnerships observed within eight case study communities demonstrate how these relationships evolve over time in response to organizational and environmental changes.[37] Based on interviews with partnership participants in 1995 and again in 1997, a flowchart that profiles the alternative life cycle paths for partnerships was developed, as reported by the participants (Figure 3–9). All of the organizations that participate in partnerships reported engaging in either formal or informal processes for evaluating the arrangement on a periodic basis. Through these evaluation processes, organizations assess whether the arrangement is meeting organizational and community expectations regarding its operation and its outcomes. Most partnership participants reported engaging in informal, internal evaluation activities in order to assess the partnership's performance relative to their individual organization's objectives. Most often these evaluations involved simple, qualitative comparisons of costs incurred and benefits accrued through the partnership, or periodic meetings of key organizational stakeholders to discuss the perceived performance of the partnership in meeting goals. For example, a children's hospital in one community used periodic measures of evening emergency room utilization to evaluate the success of an after-hours community pediatric clinic that was jointly administered with the local health department.[37] The observed declines in utilization that occurred after implementation of the clinic were interpreted as evidence of partnership success in meeting one of the hospital's key internal goals.

Some partnership participants also reported that a formal, interorganizational evaluation process is part of their partnership activities. Such processes are carried out through collaborative efforts among the partnership participants and are focused on assessing performance in meeting shared objectives. These evaluations range from quantitative outcome and process studies to qualitative methods involving group opinion and consensus. In one community, a hospital and a local health department rely on a quantitative

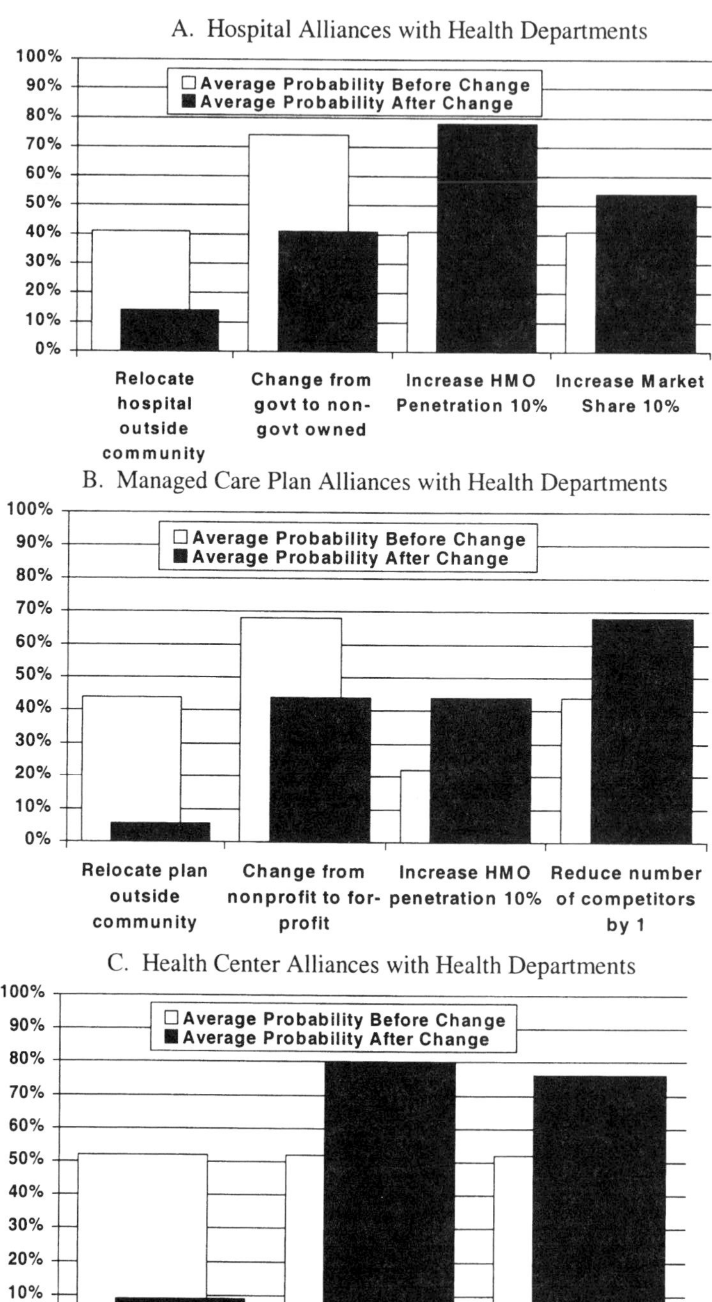

Note: Probabilities are computed using regression coefficients from the ordered logit models together with average values for the explanatory variables included in the models. Modal values are used for dichotomous explanatory variables.

Figure 3–8 Effects of Changes in Selected Organizational and Environmental Characteristics on Average Probability of Partnership Formation. *Source:* © Joint Commission Journal on Quality Improvement, Vol. 24, No. 10. Oakbrook Terrace, IL: Joint Commission on Accreditation of Healthcare Organizations, 1998, p. 532. Reprinted with permission.

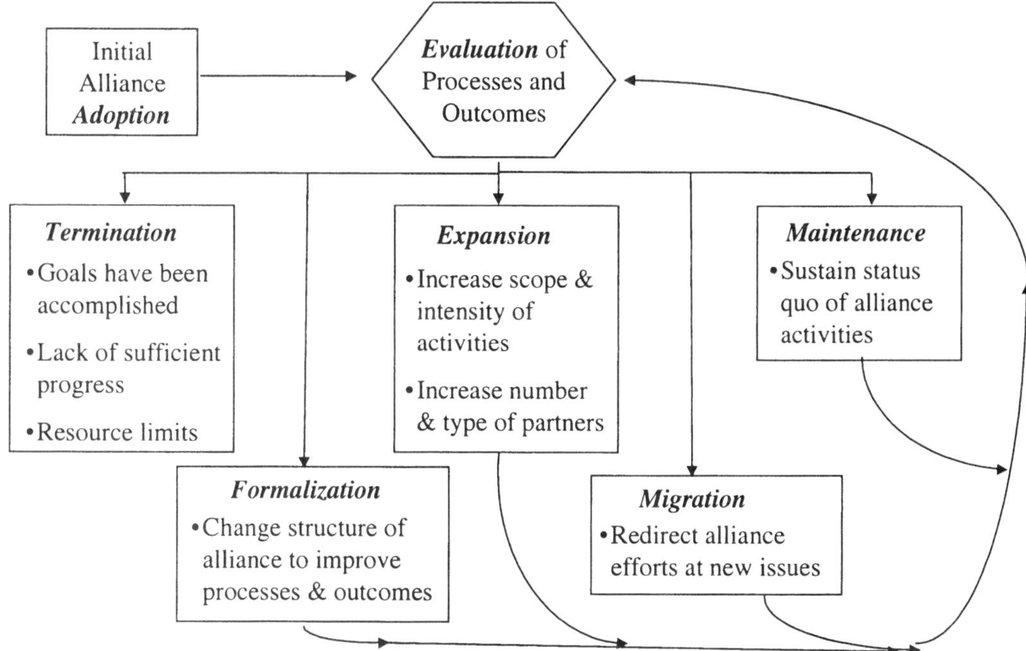

Figure 3–9 The Life Cycle of Public Health Partnerships. *Source:* © Joint Commission Journal on Quality Improvement, Vol. 24, No. 10. Oakbrook Terrace, IL: Joint Commission on Accreditation of Healthcare Organizations, 1998, p. 533. Reprinted with permission.

evaluation strategy to track the effects of a jointly administered public health program that transfers responsibility for operating public health clinics to the hospital.[59] As part of this strategy, the organizations work together with a university-based research center in analyzing measures of service quality and efficiency that are both process based (e.g., marginal product of labor, service utilization rates, referral rates) and outcome based (e.g., vaccination coverage rates, prenatal care uptake rates, low birth weight rates, adolescent pregnancy rates).

In response to both formal and informal evaluations, partnership participants may adopt an array of possible actions (Figure 3–9). Organizations often choose simply to *maintain* existing partnership arrangements in order to sustain current performance levels or allow additional time for objectives to be met. A two-year follow-up of public health partnerships operating in eight case study communities suggests that maintenance approaches are used only for relatively brief periods of time.[37] Most partnerships underway within these communities appear to have used one or more active strategies for adapting the partnership during this period in order to meet new or unfulfilled expectations.

Several of the public health partnerships observed in this study appeared to undergo a *migration* strategy in which the partnership was redirected at new tasks and goals that were identified by the participants. This is often used once original partnership objectives have been met, or when participants are faced with changes in organizational or community needs. In one community, for example, a partnership that was originally formed to conduct provider education activities regarding childhood immunization practices redirected its efforts to focus on supporting appropriate lead poisoning screening practices among community providers.[37] Partnership participants indicated that this migration occurred because the group's immunization objectives had largely been met and because lead poisoning had become an issue of heightened community concern.

Another possible strategy for partnership adaptation is one of *expansion*, in which participants extend the scale or scope of activities addressed through collective action. With this strategy, partnership participants maintain their original objectives and activities, but they may also adopt new areas of operation. Partnerships may expand the volume or range of services delivered, the geographic areas served, or the population groups targeted by their collective actions. In doing so, some partnerships also expand their membership to include a greater number or a wider diversity of participating organizations. Expansion activities appear to be used by organizations after smaller successes have been achieved through the partnership.[37] For example, in one case study community, a partnership that initially focused on encouraging age-appropriate women to seek mammography services was expanded to include a component that encouraged community providers to offer appropriate mammography counseling and recommendations to their patients.

As a fourth strategy, some organizations attempt to enhance the performance of their partnership by changing its structure through a process of *formalization*. This process may entail developing new contract language, governance arrangements, or ownership arrangements in an effort to enforce expected levels of performance. Organizations in one community, for example, chose to move from an informal collaborative structure to the development of a jointly owned nonprofit corporation in order to enhance the operation of jointly administered health education initiatives.[37] Participants hoped that this formalization would facilitate their efforts at coordination and joint management of educational programs. Participants also expected that their new structure would enhance their visibility and credibility with external stakeholders, thereby assisting them in such efforts as securing outside funding and providing outreach to community members.

Finally, some partnership participants choose to *terminate* their initiatives for reasons including goal fulfillment, insufficient performance, or excessive cost. Partnership termination is not automatically regarded as a sign of partnership failure, however. In fact, most of the terminated partnerships observed in this study resulted from goal fulfillment rather than problems with performance or cost.[37] Partnership termination appears particularly common among opportunistic partnerships and resource dependency partnerships, where shared interests may be narrowly defined and rapidly achieved.

Developing and Managing Public Health Partnerships

In reviewing the experience of public health partnerships across a variety of organizations and communities, several common themes emerge regarding the successful development and management of these arrangements. Drawing on these themes, a set of recommendations is identified to help organizations pursue optimal partnership strategies.

1. Identify a boundary spanner.

Perhaps most importantly, partnerships appear to require an organization or individual who is able to span the boundaries of multiple organizations and develop a shared vision for collective action. As other studies of interorganizational partnerships have noted, the role of the boundary spanner is critical in motivating awareness of and interest in collaboration.[28,42,46] Among the partnerships examined in this study, a wide variety of organizations and individuals were observed to fill this role. Local health departments served this role in many of these efforts—in several cases assuming the role of a neutral third party in fostering collaborative activity among competing health care organizations. In other communities, private organizations appeared better suited to boundary-spanning roles because of their existing interorganizational relationships or their freedom from cumbersome government regulations in areas such as contracting and purchasing.

In a dramatic example of the former arrangement, the local health department in one study community serves as the lead agency in an effort to develop a comparative, communitywide report card of health care quality among health plans, hospitals, and other local medical care providers.[35,37] Health plans report that they recruited the health department to serve in this boundary-spanning role because of the agency's scientific expertise and its reputation for neutrality and objectivity.

2. *Secure buy-in from key stakeholders and opinion leaders.*

The successful adoption of any innovation requires the awareness and support of key decision makers. Because the partnerships described here target community-level issues and outcomes, the pool of relevant stakeholders is likely to be large and extend well beyond the set of potential partnership participants. Support from key opinion leaders may be required to ensure the partnership sufficient visibility and acceptance within the community. Furthermore, support from relevant policy and regulatory officials may give the partnership added legitimacy while helping partnership members to identify and anticipate potential legal and regulatory issues. Partnership developers should therefore invest time early in the development process in informing and soliciting feedback from these types of community stakeholders, especially where these stakeholders are not formal partnership participants.

3. *Recognize and respond to participation constraints.*

It appears critical that individuals responsible for developing partnerships have the ability to recognize the participation constraints faced by potential partnership participants and to devise explicit strategies for addressing these constraints. Organizations face financial, legal, political, administrative, and cultural barriers to participating in partnerships that may or may not be tractable. Some organizations find it useful to devise an explicit participation strategy early on in the partnership development process—one that includes contingencies for key organizations that may abstain from partnership membership. In developing this strategy, it appears important to recognize the opportunity costs faced by potential partnership members and to identify participation incentives that are tailored to these costs. In this way, the participation strategy can be used to secure the sustained involvement of essential partnership participants.

In one study community, a partnership formed by a group of health plans, hospitals, employers, and physician groups failed to include the participation of a local health plan that specialized in serving Medicaid beneficiaries.[35] This lack of participation appeared notable given that the partnership was formed to conduct a community health assessment and improvement process—an effort with substantial implications for Medicaid beneficiaries and other traditionally vulnerable and underserved populations. The nonparticipating health plan cited the partnership's focus on employed, commercial populations as a reason for its disengagement, whereas participating organizations reported that the noncooperative behavior stemmed from competitive pressures created by the recent entrance of new organizations into the Medicaid managed care market. Regardless of whether cultural or competitive factors explain the lack of participation, it appears possible that targeted incentives—such as access to Medicaid-specific health data—could have been used effectively to ensure full community participation. Administrators at the nonparticipating health plan indicated a willingness to join the partnership if membership were offered and if access to relevant community health data were assured.

4. *Keep the structure simple.*

This study reveals a variety of possible structural arrangements, both formal and informal, for sustaining public health partnerships. As with many other managerial decisions, simplicity should be a powerful criterion when choosing an appropriate partnership structure.[28] Many of the public health partnerships observed in this study are based on informal agreements and relatively simple contractual agreements. These structures require relatively little development, management, and maintenance costs when compared to the more formalized shared ownership and shared governance models. Where possible, partnership managers should take advantage of natural participation incentives and shared interests to guide and enforce behavior among organizations, rather than resorting to more formalized and complex interorganizational structures. Ultimately, in making structural decisions, managers must balance the risks entailed in the partnership with the costs of alternative partnership structures. Larger risks justify more costly and complex structural safeguards.

5. Ensure incentive compatibility among participants.

Ensuring incentive compatibility emerges as another critical managerial task in developing and sustaining public health partnerships.[28] Organizations report participating in public health partnerships for a variety of reasons—some of which may not be compatible with overall partnership objectives or with the individual interests of other participants. Successful partnership managers appear able to choose structural arrangements that mediate potential incentive conflicts among partnership participants. In some cases, explicit contractual agreements and risk-sharing provisions are required to counteract underlying incentives for noncooperative behavior among partnership members.

For example, several managed care plans and a local health department jointly sponsored a community-based family planning education campaign that initially entailed incompatible incentives.[37] Health plans faced a clear incentive to refer low-income patients with family planning needs to health department clinics where they could receive free services. Such incentives placed excessive financial burdens on the health department and undermined the continuity of care received by health plan members. To address this incentive compatibility problem, the health department successfully negotiated reimbursement arrangements for family planning services with most of the managed care plans—thereby creating financial incentives for plans to deliver these services themselves. For cases where health plan members continued to use health department family planning services, the agreements included provisions for the health department to share with the health plans information concerning services delivered to their members. As this example illustrates, the ability to address issues of incentive incompatibility effectively appears to hinge on: (1) recognizing the nature of the incompatibility, (2) clearly defining the areas of shared interest, and (3) developing interorganizational arrangements that counteract the incentives for noncooperative behavior without eliminating the incentives for collaboration.[28]

6. Ensure effective communication and information flows among participants.

The task of managing communication and information flows among partnership members also appears as an essential element of successful public health partnerships. Many partnership participants reported that the efficient flow of information among organizations was often critical for enabling service coordination and integration to occur. Achieving this flow requires the development of effective protocols for interorganizational communication, explicit policies for information sharing, and reliable systems for data exchange. Adding to the challenge, partnership participants reported that information protocols and policies must be sufficiently flexible to address individual concerns about: (1) the proprietary nature of some types of organizational information and (2) the need for confidentiality in patient-specific health information. Achieving interorganizational consensus about these issues appears far from automatic in many cases.

Partnerships observed in several communities addressed both confidentiality and proprietary concerns by establishing a separate, private corporate entity to collect, process, and manage shared information among participating organizations.[37] This approach was used in the development of a communitywide immunization registry in one community and in the development of a community health information and assessment system in another community. Partnership participants indicated that the corporate entity shields proprietary information from being disseminated inadvertently or in response to public sector information requests under the federal Freedom of Information Act statutes. The entity also enforces confidentiality requirements and ensures the compatibility and quality of data from multiple institutions.

7. Develop an explicit evaluation strategy.

Partnership managers face the important task of developing appropriate processes for monitoring organizational and community performance. Many of the partnerships examined in this review appeared to fall short in this task, relying primarily on informal evaluation processes maintained by individual organizational participants. Clearly, an effective evaluation process hinges on the existence of adequate communication and information flows across participating organizations. Partnership managers must take the additional step of establishing processes for developing and disseminating appropriate measures of performance from this information. These processes ensure that optimal decision making can occur among partnership participants at all stages of the partnership life cycle. In doing this, performance measurement activities must keep pace with changes in partnership structures, processes, and outcomes.

An ideal evaluation strategy focuses both on organization-specific outcomes and on community-level outcomes.[25] Measuring organization-specific outcomes is likely to be essential for the ongoing support and assistance of key internal stakeholders. However, from a public health perspective, the effects on community health outcomes are of primary importance. The ability to demonstrate these community-level effects to key external stakeholders may prove essential in securing ongoing community support and assistance and in recruiting an expanded pool of partnership participants.

8. *Maintain momentum through staged successes.*

Finally, public health partnerships, like other organizational innovations, can maintain and build momentum through periodic, staged successes.[60] Small successes early on in the partnership process can build confidence among partnership participants and provide motivation for subsequent accomplishments. As participants gain experience in working successfully within the partnership structure, increasingly complex and difficult objectives can be undertaken. Managers should therefore follow an explicit plan for staged successes that begins with small and easily accomplished tasks and progresses to more complex and far-reaching objectives. In turn, the partnership evaluation strategy should be designed to provide timely feedback concerning each of these staged objectives.

Public health partnerships vary markedly in their objectives, structures, and functions. On the whole, this variation appears healthy rather than problematic. Public health administrators require many degrees of freedom in designing multi-institutional arrangements to fit specific community needs and organizational capacities. Administrators must also ensure that these arrangements remain flexible and adaptive to changing needs and priorities over time. The challenges entailed in forming and maintaining public health partnerships should not be underestimated; administrators must strike a balance among diverse organizational interests and complex community needs. It is equally important, however, not to undervalue the opportunities for public health improvement created by collaboration.

• • •

This study of the public health delivery system in the United States reveals the complexity of the constellation of organizations participating in public health activities across the United States. No clear division of labor emerges among different types of organizations involved; nonetheless, the scale and scope of activity that is produced rivals many organized national health systems. Governmental health agencies factor prominently in this mix of institutions, reflecting the federalist system of government from which they derive. Nongovernmental organizations are also active participants and often leaders in public health delivery at local, state, and national levels. Many public health activities are now carried out not within institutions but between them, through interorganizational and intergovernmental partnerships. The number and variety of health care organizations that participate in these relationships is impressive and encouraging. Evidence from a growing number of communities suggests that partnerships are addressing complex public health issues that cannot be managed effectively by any one organization acting alone. By pooling the resources and skills of multiple organizations within the community, these efforts offer promising strategies for improving the public health delivery system in the United States.

CHAPTER REVIEW

1. Government authority in public health is generally distributed in the following way:
   - Federal authority is carried out primarily through policy development, public health financing, and broad regulatory enforcement.
   - State authority extends to specific public health regulatory functions, as well as responsibilities in public health resource allocation and program administration.
   - Local government responsibilities focus on implementing public health policies and interventions within communities.
2. Many of the federal agencies with public health responsibilities are organized within the U.S. DHHS. Most of these agencies form the U.S. Public Health Service, including the CDC, the HRSA, NIH, the AHRQ, the FDA, the Indian Health Service, the Substance Abuse and Mental Health Services Administration, and the ATSDR.
3. Wide variation exists in how public health responsibilities are organized within state health agencies. State agencies typically follow one of two general structural models:
   - the free-standing agency model
   - the superagency model
4. Administrative relationships between state and local public health agencies assume one of four basic forms:
   - decentralized relationships
   - centralized relationships
   - shared authority relationships
   - mixed authority relationships
5. An increasing amount of public health activity occurs through interorganizational relationships, often termed partnerships. Key elements of these relationships include their strategic orientation, their structural design, and their functional characteristics.

REFERENCES

1. C.A. Miller and M-K. Moos, *Local Health Departments: Fifteen Case Studies* (Washington, DC: American Public Health Association, 1981).
2. K.J. Arrow, "The Organization of Economic Activity: Issues Pertinent to the Choice of Market Versus Non-Market Allocation," in *Collected Papers of K.J. Arrow,* Vol. 2, ed. K.J. Arrow (Cambridge, MA: Harvard University Press, 1969), 147–185.
3. B.J. Turnock, *Public Health: What It Is and How It Works* (Gaithersburg, MD: Aspen Publishers, 1996).
4. N. Rawding and C. Brown, "An Overview of Local Health Departments," in *Local Public Health Practice: Trends and Models*, eds. G.P. Mays et al. (Washington, DC: American Public Health Association, 2000).
5. P.R. Lee and A.E. Benjamin, "Health Policy and the Politics of Health Care," in *The Nation's Health,* 4th ed., eds. P.R. Lee and C.L. Estes (Boston, MA: Jones and Bartlett, 1994), 121–137.
6. T.J. Litman, "The Politics of Health: Establishing Policies and Setting Priorities," in *The Nation's Health,* 4th ed., eds. P.R. Lee and C.L. Estes (Boston, MA: Jones and Bartlett, 1994), 107–120.
7. G.P. Mays et al., "Performing Essential Public Health Services in the Nation's Most Populous Communities: Who Contributes?" *Journal of the American Medical Association* (Under review).
8. W.L. Roper, "Regulating Quality and Clinical Practice," in *Regulating Managed Care: Theory, Practice, and Future Options*, eds. S.H. Altman et al. (San Francisco: Jossey-Bass, 1999), 145–159.
9. D.W. Moran, "Federal Regulation of Managed Care: An Impulse in Search of a Theory," *Health Affairs 16,* no. 6 (1997): 7–33.
10. B.C. Fuchs, *Managed Health Care: Federal and State Regulation* (Washington, DC: Congressional Research Service, 1997).

11. U.S. General Accounting Office, *Performance Budgeting: Past Initiatives Offer Insights for GPRA* (Washington, DC: 1997).
12. U.S. Department of Health and Human Services, Panel on Performance Measures and Data for Public Health Performance Partnership Grants, *Assessment of Performance Measures for Public Health, Substance Abuse, and Mental Health* (Washington, DC: National Academy Press, 1997).
13. D.A. Rochefort and R.W. Cobb, *The Politics of Problem Definition: Shaping the Policy Agenda* (Lawrence, KS: University of Kansas Press, 1997).
14. U.S. General Accounting Office, *Vaccines for Children: Reexamination of Program Goals and Implementation Needed to Ensure Vaccination* [PEMD-95–22] (Washington, DC: 1995).
15. U.S. General Accounting Office, *Lead Poisoning: Federal Health Care Programs Are Not Effectively Reaching At-Risk Children* [HEHS-99–18] (Washington, DC: 1998).
16. U.S. Department of Health and Human Services, *Healthy People 2000: National Health Promotion and Disease Prevention Objectives* (Washington, DC: U.S. Government Printing Office, 1991).
17. U.S. Department of Health and Human Services, *Healthy People 2010,* Conf. ed. (Washington, DC: U.S. Government Printing Office, 2000).
18. Institute of Medicine, *The Future of Public Health* (Washington, DC: National Academy Press, 1988).
19. U.S. Centers for Disease Control and Prevention, Public Health Practice Program Office, *Profile of State and Territorial Public Health Systems: United States, 1990* (Atlanta, GA: 1991).
20. M. Maralit et al., *Transforming State Health Agencies To Meet Current and Future Challenges* (Washington, DC: National Governors Association, 1997).
21. A.D. Kaluzny et al., *Partners for the Dance: Forming Strategic Alliances in Health Care* (Ann Arbor, MI: Health Administration Press, 1995).
22. G.H. DeFriese et al., "The Program Implications of Administrative Relationships between Local Health Departments and State and Local Government," *American Journal of Public Health 71,* no. 10 (1981): 1,109–1,115.
23. D.E. Nelson et al., "Outcome-Based Management and Public Health: The Oregon Benchmarks Experience," *Journal of Public Health Management and Practice 1,* no. 2 (1995): 8–17.
24. S.R. Griffin and P. Welch, "Performance-Based Public Health in Texas," *Journal of Public Health Management and Practice 1,* no. 3 (1995): 44–49.
25. G.P. Mays et al., "Assessing the Performance of Local Public Health Systems: A Survey of State Health Agency Efforts," *Journal of Public Health Management and Practice 4,* no. 4 (1998): 63–78.
26. B.J. Turnock and A. Handler, "Is Public Health Ready for Reform? The Case for Accrediting Local Health Departments," *Journal of Public Health Management and Practice 2,* no. 3 (1996): 41–45.
27. P.K. Halverson et al., "Performance Measurement and Accreditation of Public Health Organizations: A Call to Action," *Journal of Public Health Management and Practice 4,* no. 4 (1998): 5–7.
28. National Association of County and City Health Officials, *National Profile of Local Health Departments* (Washington, DC: NACCHO, 1998).
29. National Association of Local Boards of Health, *National Profile of Local Boards of Health, Centers for Disease Control and Prevention* (Washington, DC: NALBOH, 1997).
30. P.K. Halverson et al., "Privatizing Health Services: Alternative Models and Emerging Issues for Public Health and Quality Management," *Quality Management in Health Care 5,* no. 2 (1997): 1–18.
31. S. Wall, "Transformation in Public Health Systems," *Health Affairs 17,* no. 3 (1998): 64–80.
32. R.B. Gerzoff et al., "Full-Time Employees of the U.S. Local Health Departments 1992–1993," *Journal of Public Health Management and Practice 5,* no. 3 (1999): 1–9.
33. National Association of County and City Health Officials, *1992–93 National Profile of Local Health Departments* (Washington, DC: NACCHO, 1995).
34. J.S. Koeze, "Paying for Public Health Services in North Carolina," *Popular Government* 60 (1994): 11–20.
35. G.P. Mays et al., *Local Public Health Practice: Trends and Models* (Washington, DC: American Public Health Association, 1999).
36. W.L. Roper and G.P. Mays, "The Changing Managed Care–Public Health Interface, *Journal of the American Medical Association 280,* no. 20 (1998): 1,739–1,740.
37. H. Nelson, *Nonprofit and For-Profit HMOs: Converging Practices but Different Goals?* (New York: Milbank Memorial Fund, 1996).
38. D.J. Lipson and N. Naierman, "Snapshots of Change in Fifteen Communities: Safety-Net Providers," *Health Affairs 15,* no. 2 (1996): 33–48.
39. P.K. Halverson et al., "Not-So-Strange Bedfellows: Models of Interaction between Managed Care Plans and Public Health Agencies," *Milbank Quarterly 75,* no. 1 (1997): 1–26.
40. G.P. Mays et al., "The Contributions of Managed Care Plans to Public Health Practice" A National Survey of Local Public Health Jurisdictions, *American Public Health Association 127th Annual Meeting Abstracts* (Washington, DC: American Public Health Association, 1999).
41. T. Lewin and M. Gottlieb, "In Hospital Sales, an Overlooked Side Effect," *New York Times,* 27 April 1997, 1.

42. R.M. Kanter, "Collaborative Advantage: The Art of Alliances," *Harvard Business Review* 72 (1994): 96–108.
43. R.M. Kanter, "Becoming PALs: Pooling, Allying, and Linking across Companies," *Academy of Management Executives 3,* August (1989): 183–193.
44. G.P. Mays et al., "Managed Care, Public Health, and Privatization: A Typology of Interorganizational Arrangements," in *Managed Care and Public Health,* eds., P.K. Halverson and C.P. McLaughlin (Gaithersburg, MD: Aspen Publishers, 1997), 185–200.
45. W.R. Scott, "Innovation in Medical Care Organizations: A Synthetic Review," *Medical Care Review 47,* no. 2 (1990): 165–192.
46. G.P. Mays et al., "Collaboration To Improve Community Health: Trends and Alternative Models," *Joint Commission Journal on Quality Improvement in Health Care 24,* no. 10 (1998): 518–540.
47. U.S. Centers for Disease Control and Prevention, Committee on Community Engagement, *Principles of Community Engagement* (Atlanta, GA: Public Health Practice Program Office, Centers for Disease Control and Prevention, 1997).
48. G.J. Bazzoli et al., "Public–Private Collaboration in Health and Human Services Delivery: Evidence from Community Partnerships," *Milbank Quarterly 75,* no. 4 (1997): 533–561.
49. M.L. Knapp and T. Reiley, "Community-Based Improvement: Preventing Motor Vehicle Injuries," *Quality Connection 6,* no. 3 (1997): 1–4.
50. L.A. Headrick et al., "Working from Upstream To Improve Health Care: The IHI Interdisciplinary Professional Education Collaborative," *Joint Commission Journal on Quality Improvement* 22 (1996): 149–164.
51. L. Cavaluzzo, "Creating Healthier Communities: A Compendium of Models," *Healthcare Forum Journal 40,* no. 3 (1997): 35–50.
52. E.L. Baker et al., "Health Reform and the Health of the Public," *Journal of the American Medical Association* 272 (1994): 1,276–1,282.
53. Institute of Medicine, Public Health Committee, *Healthy Communities: A New Look at the Future of Public Health* (Washington, DC: National Academy of Sciences, 1996).
54. National Association of County and City Health Officials, *Assessment Protocol for Excellence in Public Health* (Washington, DC: NACCHO, 1991).
55. L.W. Greene, "PATCH: CDC's Planned Approach to Community Health, an Application of PRECEED and an Inspiration for PROCEED," *Journal of Health Education 23,* no. 3 (1992): 140–147.
56. P.K. Halverson et al., "Working Together? Organizational and Market Determininants of Collaboration between Public Health and Medical Care Providers," *American Journal of Public Health* (under review), 1998.
57. P. Lorange and J. Roos, *Strategic Alliances: Formation, Implementation, and Evolution* (Cambridge, MA: Blackwell, 1993).
58. G.P. Mays et al., "The Effect of Ownership on Interorganizational Relationships between Managed Care Plans and Public Health Agencies," (under review), 1998.
59. S.R. Keener et al., "Providing Public Health Services through an Integrated Delivery System," *Quality Management in Health Care 5,* no. 2 (1997): 27–34.
60. P.K. Halverson et al., "Strategies for Managing the Public's Health: Implications and Next Steps," in *Managed Care and Public Health,* eds. P.K. Halverson et al. (Gaithersburg, MD: Aspen Publishers, 1998), 350–363.

CHAPTER 4

The Public Health Work Force

Robert B. Gerzoff
Kristine M. Gebbie

The public health system's most essential resource is its work force. The U.S. public health work force consists of individuals from a wide variety of professions, technical disciplines, and educational backgrounds. This diversity both challenges and motivates efforts to define and assess the composition of the work force. By understanding work force skills, training needs, and practice settings, public health decision makers can design programs and policies that make optimal use of this essential and powerful resource.

The public health work force includes individuals from almost every discipline and profession associated with health services. It also encompasses numerous professions both within and outside the health arena. Each profession and individual brings to public health a special combination of knowledge, skills, abilities, and, perhaps most importantly, world view. This diversity is essential to the vitality and success of public health efforts. Those persons who effectively administer public health services, programs, and agencies blend this rich array of resources into teams that serve the needs of their communities. This chapter identifies and describes the public health work force and examines strategies for educating and training workers that can effectively provide essential public health services to the nation's communities.

DEFINING THE PUBLIC HEALTH WORK FORCE

Intuition suggests that it should be possible to define the public health work force using one or a combination of four classification schemes commonly used in other labor data-gathering efforts: educational preparation, professional discipline (licensed or certified profession), work responsibility/activity, and site of employment. Unfortunately these classification schemes break down when applied to public health workers. Public health is practiced in an extremely wide range of settings and by individuals with diverse backgrounds that confound the usual methods of categorization.

Although most public health workers have attained educational levels of at least an associate or bachelor's degree, there is no single public health degree. The Master of Public Health (MPH) is often regarded as the standard entry to the field, but public health careers begin with numerous other degrees in areas such as engineering, environmental science, education, or the social or behavioral sciences. In fact, the majority of the members of the American Public Health Association do not hold an MPH, and only one-quarter to one-third are reported to have graduate public health training.[1]

Many of the disciplines that contribute to public health have licenses monitored by the states, such as nurses, physicians, dentists, psychologists, and veterinarians. Sanitarians, health educators, nurses, and many other occupations also have official credentials that attest to the capabilities of the professionals within their chosen specialty. For public health, however, there is no single credential a professional can show to demonstrate proficiency in public health practice. The problem is even more basic: the public health community has not defined a common body of knowledge with which all public health practitioners should be familiar. Movement toward such a definition underlies some of the objectives in the public health infrastructure portion of *Healthy People 2010: Objectives for the Nation.*[2]

Any attempt to define the public health work force based on the qualifications of the individuals practicing public health is further complicated by the fact that public health efforts are often the result of a mix of volunteers, paid individuals, professionals, and lay persons. This is in no way a detriment and is, in fact, one of public health's major strengths. Particularly as public health efforts become more focused on the socioeconomic and behavioral determinants of health, this blending becomes vitally important to the success of public health. It does, however, confound attempts to define the work force.

Attempts to enumerate the work force by work setting or employment locale are equally problematic (Figure 4–1). For example, a typical definition focuses on those individuals who work in official local, state, and federal health agencies. Except for its utility in very targeted research, attempts to apply this official definition to address current policy and administrative issues are quickly met with a storm of criticism. Because contemporary public health practice emphasizes collaboration and inclusion, most applications require looser definitions that enable more people, rather than fewer, to be counted as part of the public health effort.

In many official settings, much public health work is carried out in nonhealth governmental offices. Public health programs exist in departments of environment, agriculture, labor, educa-

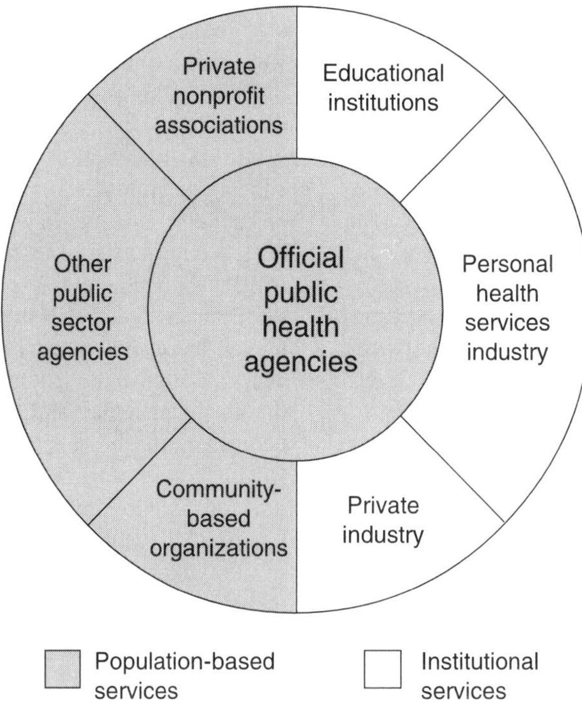

Figure 4–1 The Professional Public Health Work Force: Major Work Settings. *Source:* Reprinted from V.C. Kennedy, W.D. Spears, H.D. Loe, and F.I. Moore, Public Health Workforce Information: A State-Level Study, *Journal of Public Health Management and Practice,* Vol. 5, No. 9, pp. 10–19, © 1999, Aspen Publishers, Inc.

tion, natural resources, social welfare, transportation, and policy—in other words, nearly every branch of government. For example, there is no question that occupational safety and health are public health programs and that occupational health workers, including governmental industrial hygienists, occupational health nurses and physicians, and laboratorians, should be considered public health workers. Yet at the federal level and in most state governments, these persons work not in a health department, but more typically in a department of labor.

Public health workers are also employed in numerous settings outside the government. Many corporations, because they recognize the impact on their productivity and profitability, have undertaken public health efforts. Though often focused on employee populations, some businesses have reached out to entire communities. Workers in labor unions often monitor health impacts or threats to health and inform their members about health issues. Voluntary health organizations such as the American Cancer Society, American Diabetes Association, and American Heart Association have sizable work forces. They provide essential public health services—often in active collaboration with one or more governmental health agencies. By any definition and regardless of their place of employment, these individuals are public health workers. An important and sizable nongovernmental segment of the public health work force consists of individuals who work in the personal health care system. Despite being employed in personal health care, these individuals provide community health promotion, gather health statistics, track nosocomial infections, or undertake community health planning.

Thus, the traditional methods of defining a work force do not appear to have much utility for public health. In recent years however, a working definition has emerged that seems to serve the dual purposes of clearly identifying the central characteristics of the work force and of specifically including the less traditional participants: "The public health workforce is composed of those individuals whose major work focus is delivery of one or more of the essential services of public health, whether or not those individuals are on the payroll of an official, voluntary or not-for-profit public health agency."[3(p.4)]

This definition is more functional than structural, that is, it is focused on what the workers do, as opposed to their job titles, professional education, or who writes their paychecks. It specifically refers to those individuals who work in what are considered to be the traditional public health settings: "official" is generally thought to include state and local health departments and health units of the U.S. Department of Health and Human Services (DHHS). At the same time it acknowledges settings that may be neither traditional nor obvious.

For any practical application, this approach of defining the public health work force by being inclusive and encompassing eventually must be limited. There are many individuals whose work only contributes incidentally to the public's health. These might include the intensive care nurse who appropriately reenforces reduction in tobacco use by limiting smoking on the part of a patient's family, or the highway patrol member who reduces injuries by enforcing speed limits on interstate highways. Although these persons do contribute to public health, their contribution is secondary to the main objectives of their employment. Rarely are public goals considered in planning their day-to-day work.

Defining the public work force in this interdisciplinary and inclusive fashion highlights a major challenge facing public health today. For every public health problem, one must specify the particular combination of skills needed to address the problem and exactly which professions and individuals possess those skills. This is not an easy task. Traditional views on project staffing can lead to missing valuable contributions that individuals can make. For example, in some agencies, physicians are seen as essential because they are able to oversee clinical services, write prescriptions, and authorize immunizations. Yet under the laws of most states, advanced practice nurses can provide many of these same services. Thinking of the public health physician as primarily a special set of letters on a prescription pad fails to acknowledge the need for a medical perspective in planning and interpreting epidemiologic studies, or the special role the public health physician can play in communicating public health priorities to the community. Likewise, thinking of "inspection and enforcement" as the reason one needs sanitarians and environmentalists may cause one to overlook important contributions they can make to community health planning or emergency response activities. It also obscures the fact that other public health workers can and do conduct a variety of inspections and on-site consultations (e.g., in child care facilities and nursing homes).

A broadened perspective is applicable at all staff levels. If the relationship between a public health organization and the community it serves is to be healthy and helpful, it is important that the person who answers the phone, the one who opens the door, the one delivering specimens to a laboratory—in other words, everyone—has a sense of the mission of public health and of the way his or her tasks and the tasks of others contribute. A mishandled phone call alerting health officials to a possible case of food poisoning may be just as much a contributor to an unnecessarily large outbreak as a misdiagnosis under the microscope or poor epidemiologic analysis. A rude janitor can do more to drive a tuberculosis (TB) patient away from completing therapy than the overly insistent disease control specialist or poorly prepared visiting nurse. Clerks in the vital records office, outreach workers, drivers, volunteers—all can contribute to a healthier public. Work force improvement plans must not overlook training for these support and administrative staff. Although their needs may not be elaborate, they and ultimately the community will benefit from the regular receipt of information on priorities and issues, on the way their work contributes, and on ways that their own behavior serves as a model for public health in the community.

This definition of the public health work force, although meeting many political and policy needs, does not allow for a reliable enumeration of the work force. To that end, more rigorous definitions are needed. Most if not all research or evaluation efforts will need to develop a project-specific definition. Regardless, investigators, managers, and policy makers should be cognizant of a framework developed by the U.S. government.

The government agency responsible for tracking the entire U.S. work force is the Department of Labor, Bureau of Labor Statistics. The bureau classifies job occupations using a numerical coding scheme called the Standard Occupational Classification (SOC) system. In creating the SOC, the federal government intended that all major occupational data gatherers would use this classification as the basic framework for their information collections so that it could serve as the nation's comprehensive occupational classification framework. The latest version of the SOC (1998 revision)[4] classifies workers at four levels of aggregation: (1) major group, (2) minor group, (3) broad occupation, and (4) detailed occupation. All occupations are clustered into one of 23 major groups. Within these major groups are 98 minor groups, 452 broad occupations, and 820 detailed occupations.

It is important to realize that none of the SOC detailed categories are specific to public health. One might expect that the majority of those individuals in some detailed occupational categories such as epidemiologist would be in public health, but there is no way to know for certain. An epidemiologist might be tracking hospital infections or doing pure epidemiologic research. Whether such individuals should be counted as part of the public health work force will depend on the particular question being asked. Thus, the SOC is only the beginning framework for public health work force investigations. Useful work force studies will need to gather more detailed information, including job responsibilities, work location, and daily activities.

HISTORICAL PERSPECTIVES ON THE PUBLIC HEALTH WORK FORCE

Work Force Structure

The diversity and basic structure of the U.S. public health work force was established with the founding of public health. Lemuel Shattuck's 1850 *Report of the Massachusetts Sanitary Commission* recognized that public health needed a variety of workers with a variety of skills.[5] He called for state and local boards of health whose members were to be qualified physicians. Presaging the current work of epidemiologists and registrars, each physician was also expected to keep records of vital statistics and patient contacts. Shattuck made a point to emphasize the importance to public health efforts of nurses and those with sanitary science backgrounds. These two positions still constitute the core of today's local public health work force.[6] Echoing contemporary calls for broader collaborative efforts with religious institutions, he suggested that public health matters be discussed by clergymen at least once a year. And paralleling what we do today, he recommended that measures be taken to ensure safe food and control smoke and other nuisances. After nearly 150 years, the broad basis that first determined the structure of the public health work force is essentially unchanged.

The work force pattern that evolved from the foundation that existed in Shattuck's era was one of ever-increasing diversification, specialization, and professionalization. In 1922, the Committee on Municipal Health Department Practice published an article that prescribed the work force needed to staff a city health department serving a population of 100,000.[7] At the head of each department would be a health officer supported by a clerk and two stenographers. The health officer would oversee eight bureaus with nine divisions. The divisions of epidemiology and communicable diseases were to be headed by physicians. Nurses featured prominently; 30 were recommended to carry out the preventive functions of public health. Additional nurses, specifically for clinical settings, were also suggested. Overall, the committee recommended a ratio of one nurse to each 2,000–2,500 persons in the population served. Sanitary and nuisance inspectors were expected to serve districts with approximately 25,000 people. These were lofty goals, and few departments ever came close to having the prescribed numbers. Still, the vision shows the direction in which public health was headed.

The bacteriologic revolution and an increased acknowledgment of the depth of knowledge needed to effectively protect the public's health brought further breadth and specialization to the public health work force. By 1945, the list of recommended personnel included health educators and differentiated statistical clerks from other clerks, health officers from other administrative medical personnel, and engineers from sanitarians.[8]

Surveys of today's public health work force commonly include more than two dozen occupational categories. Some, such as toxicologist, industrial hygienist, or environmental health specialist, are the product of life in our modern industrial age. Others, such as social worker, public health information specialist, or dietician, are the result of increased attention to the social and behavioral determinants of health. Careful consideration reveals, however, that these jobs are just specializations of work that was already described in the late 1800s. This is not unexpected. Despite a century of changes, the basic functions and purposes of public health remain the same.

Work Force Assessments

Until recently, the government had made a substantial effort to track the number of official public health workers, particularly those who were employed locally and working in the nation's largest cities. From 1923 to 1946, the U.S. Public Health Service bulletins regularly included reports that summarized the public health work force. The authors of these reports were some of public health's legends, including C.-E.A. Winslow and Joseph W. Mountin.[9,10] In 1945, Haven Emerson used these data to create a plan for structuring and administering public health for the entire nation.[8]

From 1946 until the mid-1960s, the Public Health Service continued to gather and report data on local health units and their employees using a standardized report of public health personnel.[11]* Local jurisdictions wishing to receive state or federal monies were required to provide the data requested on those forms. Under a variety of titles, survey results were reported nearly every year. Recognizing their importance to the public health system, government officials conducted a separate census of public health nurses nearly every year between 1940 and 1960.[12] The data contained in all of these reports were amazingly detailed, especially when one realizes that the data were compiled without the aid of computers. They provide a rich comparative time series on all aspects of local public health, not just personnel, and show how public health coverage grew in the United States.

Legislative changes brought an end to those surveys sometime in the late 1960s. No consistent, longitudinal assessments of the public health work force have been conducted since that time. The motivation for collecting work force information in the 1920s until the mid-1960s had been to track the nation's progress in establishing local public health jurisdictions for the entire nation. By the 1960s that goal had, for all practical purposes, been attained. The focus and legislative mandate for work force tracking then changed to supporting health manpower training efforts. This focus included all health personnel, of which public health manpower was only one small portion.

The result of this switch in focus was a series of reports to Congress on the status of health personnel in the United States. In the first of that series (and using data from the late 1970s), the Bureau of Health Professions conducted a study summarizing the status of the entire public health work force.[13] That report found that there were approximately 500,000 public health workers—250,000 public health workers in the primary public health work force and another 250,000 ancillary workers. The data from the report continued to be cited in later reports to Congress throughout the 1980s and early 1990s. Amazingly, the same numbers are cited to this day. That report was the last detailed national accounting of the public health work force.

Recent efforts to assess the public work force originate within states. There are few examples, but the motivation for these assessments usually involves specific legislative or policy initiatives. In the state of Washington, for example, training needs of the work force needed to be assessed.[14] In Texas, the state health department had a general need for information so they could conduct work force planning.[15] The Texas study was noteworthy because it took a statistical survey sampling approach and examined not just the official public health agencies, but also numerous other agencies that provide public health services. A federal desire to understand rural local health systems led to a detailed investigation that compared the local public work force in Wyoming and Idaho. Despite both states being rural and in the same region of the country, the authors reported large differences in both work force structure and organization.[16] These three reports set the standard for most future work force studies—state based, multiorganizational, and policy motivated.

DETERMINANTS OF THE SIZE AND STRUCTURE OF THE PUBLIC HEALTH WORK FORCE

The roles, size, and structure of the public health work force are determined not only by the public health problems it faces, but also by the broader social, political, and economic environment in which it operates. Of these factors, perhaps the largest influence on public health today is the economic environment. The major factors currently influencing the public health work force are outlined in the following paragraphs, and the underlying economic agents within each factor are highlighted.

Evolving Health Care Environment and Systems of Care

Public health practice is tied inextricably to the systems of personal health care delivery and

*Similar reports with other titles can be found going back to 1946. Many were authored by Cliford Greves and Josephine Cambell.

financing. Examples abound. One of the essential services of public health is ensuring that individuals are linked to needed care, including direct service provision. The ability of the personal care system to provide effective perinatal services is a key part of health improvement. Efforts to limit nosocomial infections and reduce the use of antibiotics can only succeed with the active partnership of the personal care system. Despite attempts to increase attention to population health, the huge proportion of health-related dollars spent on personal health care (approximately 98 percent of the total) ensures that concern about personal care dominates health discussions. Thus, effective public health practice and an effective public health work force are highly dependent on a clear understanding of the current structure and future direction of the medical care system.

During the past three decades, health care costs have risen dramatically. The pressures to limit these costs have given rise to a panoply of health care purchasing and insurance arrangements generally referred to as managed care. (See Chapter 30 for a detailed discussion.) Government agencies, whether federal, state, or local, have also felt the financial pinch and turned to managed care arrangements to provide personal care services for their clients. The result is that many functions that traditionally have been performed by the government are now in the hands of nonprofit and, frequently, for-profit private providers.

Much of the worry associated with the move to private providers stems from concerns that individuals will have fewer personal choices regarding the source and content of their health care. Although limiting an individual's freedom to decide his or her health is of some interest, public health's main concern is when these systems fail to provide persons with the care they need. If managed care or other private providers are to be the personal care providers in a community, then the local public health work force must take steps to ensure that all individuals within the community have access to them.

Another concern for public health is the limited population perspective that managed providers may bring with their business. The larger systems of care such as health maintenance organizations (HMOs), prepaid practices, and multihospital systems can and do employ individuals with public health perspectives and training; smaller groups are less likely to do so. Regardless of their size, managed care organizations must be encouraged to either begin, continue, or expand their community-based public health efforts.

Many public health workers are suspicious when managed care reaches out to the larger community. Some view these programs as a threat to their jobs; others are dubious that the efforts of a private entity will reach out to the whole community. From a careful look at managed care's potential role and contribution, it is apparent that although managed care entities may become vigorous and helpful partners, they cannot replace traditional public health or the traditional public health worker. For example, although it may be of clear benefit to a managed care plan to be actively involved in seeing that enrollees with a sexually transmitted disease (STD) are diagnosed and treated, for legal and practical reasons, most plans will not be in a position to do the community-based case finding that should follow. Likewise, although a hospital might well conduct some health promotion programs (at least partially to increase visibility in the community), financial considerations make sustaining a long-term, comprehensive program in support of behavior change throughout the population unlikely.

With these limitations in mind, however, medical care systems should be sought actively as partners for public health organizations. Their increasingly sophisticated health care data systems contain valuable information that can be coupled with traditional public health data sources for early alerts to problems or improved planning and evaluation. The leadership of medical care systems, if appropriately informed and committed, can be effective advocates for good public health programs and systems in the community.

Privatization of Government Functions

The move to private providers goes beyond just providing personal care services. It is part of a widely held perspective that views government's appropriate role as one of steering activities rather than performing them. This concept, popularized in the book *Reinventing Government*, has led many public decision makers to reshape and shrink the public work force by seeking private organizations to perform what previously had been performed by those on the public payroll.[17]

Although public health has not been a primary target of the privatization movement, neither has it been entirely ignored. Workers who provide personal care services (e.g., nurses, physicians, and social workers) are most often the target of privatization efforts. In many areas, visiting nurse associations and home health and maternal/child health services are now contracted by local governments rather than being part of the governmental system. Health clinics are often outsourced to area hospitals or private practice groups. In some areas, entire local health departments have been turned over to local hospital corporations.[18–22]

A major implication of this move to private providers is a need for public health workers with new skills. Workers need experience in contract writing, management, and supervision. They must also be able to foster collaborations and resolve conflicts between organizations with diverse and often conflicting missions. In the language of the Institute of Medicine, they must also be able to ensure that quality services are provided in a timely, cost-effective manner.[23]

When a public health program is privatized, managers and policy makers need to remember that although there is a reduction in the directly managed public health work force, the employees of the new organization (who might well have just left the public payroll) remain in the public health work force. These individuals should be included as resources and partners in community health improvement efforts. And the public entity paying for the service needs to retain at least some public health skills in order to write and monitor effective contracts.

A further work force concern brought about by the privatization of services and the focus on population in private organizations is that the public sector is now competing with the private sector for the same skilled work force. The slow pace with which public personnel systems move to improve salary and grade levels leaves traditional public health agencies at a distinct disadvantage. More than one public health manager has been heard to describe the governmental public health agency as an on-the-job training site for other institutions. Workers who come to the public sector directly out of school quickly master governmental programs and approaches. Just as quickly they move to more flexible and better-paying positions in the private sector.

Funding for Public Health

If saying that funding is a major determinant of the size and structure of the public health work force is a truism, so too is saying that there are never sufficient funds. Since the birth of contemporary public health practice in the late 1800s, discussions concerning how many and what types of workers are needed have always resulted in a call for more workers and more money to hire those workers. Perhaps the easiest way to understand, justify, and communicate a request for increased work force funds is not to focus on the absolute level of funding desired, but to compare the dollars dedicated to public health versus those spent on medical care.

As a proportion of all U.S. medical care dollars, the proportion of dollars spent on public health efforts has been remarkably constant, between one to three percent.[24–26] Recent figures include much funding for public health-provided clinical care. Looking at strictly population-based prevention efforts, the proportion appears to be less than one percent.[27] Requests for funding and more public health workers become more meaningful when placed in this context and juxtaposed with a need for a greater emphasis on prevention.

Despite national trends, year-to-year funding for individual public health programs rises and falls, and funding by individual states and localities fluctuates widely. These fluctuations have a number of causes. Given that much of public health is funded from general tax revenue (local, state, or national), the condition of the general economy obviously will have a large influence. Funding is also affected by the general attitude the body politic has concerning government. During periods when government is seen as a necessary evil rather than as a positive force for improving society, funds for public health programs will be more difficult to gather than when the reverse is true. Funding for public health is also affected by the degree to which the services that have been funded are seen as necessary and effective and are widely communicated not only to the direct recipients, but also to the general public and policy makers.

Public health's role in providing clinical services (both those associated with specific disease control programs and those provided as a safety net) is another source of funding instability. (See Chapter 17 for a detailed discussion.) In recent years, the substantial shift of Medicaid-funded personal health services into private programs of managed care plans has led to a marked reduction in clinical services and associated revenues to public health agencies. From a work force perspective, this shift has two important impacts. First, it may free up staff, allowing them to focus on population-focused activities such as health promotion. Frequently this requires that staff receive training and updates in new skills. Second, staff of the agencies that currently are providing the clinical services become critical partners with public health, and thus need to be informed regularly about how their clinical services mesh with other public health services and priorities. They also must receive training in pertinent content areas with an emphasis on community perspectives.

The economic pressures from limited funding, privatization, and managed care all act to constrain the growth of the public health work force. To be sure these are only three of many factors that could be mentioned as determinants of the public health work force. The result of these pressures is that public health administrators must plan carefully and look to deploy workers in the most efficient manner possible. A major impediment to providing public health services, particularly at the local level, has and continues to be the inability of small districts and programs to gather the resources needed to staff public health initiatives adequately. To gain the needed economies of scale, administrators must abandon "turf wars" mentality and be open to cross-jurisdictional contracting, sharing of employees, private sector collaboration, and other forms of mutual assistance. Such arrangements need to be considered both within and between governmental levels.

Behavioral Interventions

From a social perspective, the largest influence on the public health work force of the future may be the public's perception of the public health problems it faces. When infectious diseases ravaged a city, there was little dissent that swift action was needed. However, when the origin of many public health problems are rooted in individual behaviors, as they are now, the perceptions are different. Many people perceive such problems not as public health problems, but rather as problems of individual responsibility and individual choice. If one chooses to drink, smoke, or partake in any unhealthy behavior, many people believe that it is not only their choice, but their right to do so. Viewed from this perspective, public health interventions designed to alter behaviors are not just intrusive, but threatening and possibly unconstitutional.

The increasing use of behavioral interventions in public health has added a special dimension to the relationship of public health agencies and organizations to communities, one meriting special attention. Despite a growing body of science on behavior and behavior change, as a society, we appear to remain suspicious of the application of this knowledge. This becomes evident in the public response to efforts to support behavior change in areas that traditionally were held as very private, or associated with deeply imbedded social attitudes. For example, the response of many people to efforts limiting the intended and unintended injuries associated with handguns is that this is not a public health concern. Likewise, many community members believe that education about sexuality, reproduction, and STDs, at least at ages up to 15 or 16, is strictly a matter for family and should not involve the educational system or other community groups. Difficulty responding responsibly to substance abuse, and the intersection of substance abuse with bloodborne diseases such as hepatitis B, hepatitis C, or human immunodeficiency virus (HIV), provides another illustration. The challenge for public health administrators is to find the resources to employ experts in behavior change and then be able to use them within a collaborative community framework.

THE STRUCTURE OF THE CURRENT WORK FORCE

No inventory of public health workers could ever claim to be exhaustive. Still, there are some occupations that are present throughout the public health system and essential to its effectiveness (Figure 4–2 and Table 4–1). The characteristics of those jobs are worth noting, and in the following paragraphs, some of those characteristics and occupations are summarized.

Generalists versus Specialists

Current dialogue in public health often begins with an affirmation of a view of health as the product of a complex interaction among multiple forces rather than the linear result of the treatment of individual diseases with singular causes.[28] If that is the case, then the public health work force must include individuals who understand

- the immediate and global physical environment
- the social environment (family, community, social strata, geopolitics)
- genetics
- human behavior and its development and modification
- functional status of individuals, families, and communities

Public health leadership in a community should make every effort to assemble a staff who collectively encompass this rich mix of knowledge. Not all of the resources may be on the full- or part-time employed staff. Some of those individuals with the required backgrounds may be available from a partner agency, nearby college, state or large local health department, or federal agency. Effective administrators will have a plan for tapping the necessary resources when appropriate. This plan will include regular input from all perspectives in program planning, development, implementation, and evaluation. It will also detail links needed for emergency situations.

Many public health workers are generalists. Particularly in small communities or neighborhoods, generalist public health workers—often public health nurses or sanitarians—are the only visible component of the public health work force. For their communities, these individuals are able to manage day-to-day public health services and provide first-line public health response in emergencies appropriately. Considering the range of concerns to be handled in a given week or month, their contributions are limited by their inability to become deeply immersed in any one problem. The lone local public health nurse, for example, may have to move from immunizations to elder health to prenatal education to directly observed TB therapy to HIV counseling and testing to interpretation of the monthly state vital records/reportable disease summary. Thus, generalists need ready access to specialist consultation in all program areas and need to be supported by a system of regular updates and refreshers on public health priorities and programs. Perhaps most importantly, generalists need a system that will provide continued general support and encouragement!

Especially when dealing with larger populations, most programs benefit from specialized staff who are able to devote their knowledge and skills full time to single areas of public health concern. Such areas can be defined as a single kind of threat to health (vector control), a single disease area (STDs), a single health resource (outreach and access to care), or a single public health skill (epidemiology, microbiology, or health education). Finding the right number of specialists, providing them with the resources necessary to fulfill their potential, and linking them appropriately with each other and with

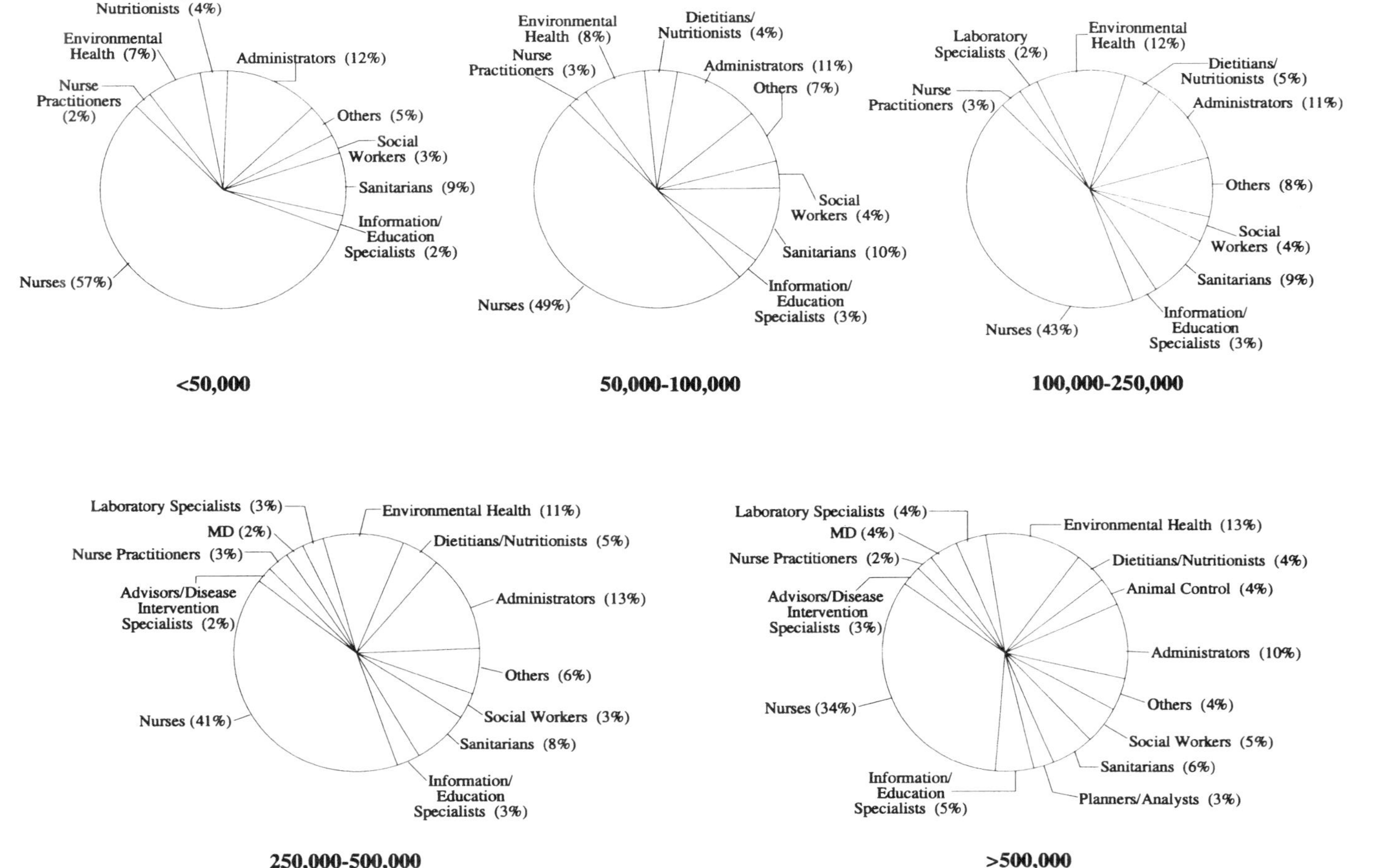

Figure 4–2 Local Health Department Staff Composition (in Percent) for Five Jurisdiction Sizes: United States, 1992–1993. Each circle represents 100% of the responding staff for local health departments in the population category noted below the circle. *Source:* Reprinted from R.B. Gerzoff, C.K. Brown, and E.L. Baker, Full-Time Employees of U.S. Local Health Departments 1992–1993, *Journal of Public Health Management and Practice,* Vol. 5, No. 3, pp. 1–9, © 1999, Aspen Publishers, Inc.

Table 4–1 Percentage of Local Health Departments (LHDs) Having at Least One Full-Time Employee in the Listed Job Classification: United States, 1992–1993

	Population Category (in Thousands)					
	<50	*50 to 100*	*100 to 250*	*250 to 500*	*>500*	*All*
Number of LHDs	1,209	334	203	80	66	1,892
Percent of LHDs	64	18	11	4.2	3.5	100
Nurses	86	91	95	96	97	89
Administrators	57	77	84	90	88	66
Sanitarians	36	56	49	51	53	42
Environmental health specialists	27	43	60	68	64	36
Dieticians/nutritionists	17	41	67	76	89	32
Public information specialists/ health educators	12	42	62	66	94	27
Nurse practitioners/physician assistants	12	34	57	64	85	26
Social workers	11	27	42	61	73	21
Physicians	4	16	37	54	77	14
Laboratory specialists	2	15	37	51	73	12
Animal control specialists (non-DVM)	5	12	18	20	41	10
Dental assistants/hygienists	2	12	25	39	68	10
Public health advisors/disease intervention specialists	3	8	21	39	53	9
Epidemiologists	3	3	18	28	67	8
Dentists	1	5	14	23	52	6
Planners/analysts	0	3	11	19	67	5
Toxicologists	0	0	0	3	6	0.3
Industrial hygienists	0.2	0.3	3	4	20	1
Veterinarians	0.3	0.9	0	6	17	1
Other	56	61	61	69	55	58

Source: Reprinted from R.B. Gerzoff, C.K. Brown, and E.L. Baker, Full-Time Employees of U.S. Local Health Departments 1992–1993, *Journal of Public Health Management and Practice,* Vol. 5, No. 3, pp. 1–9, © 1999, Aspen Publishers, Inc.

generalists is one of the enduring challenges for public health leaders and managers. With the growth of new knowledge concerning health and the determinants of health, it is likely that the need for specialists will continue to grow and that their numbers will increase throughout the public health work force.

Epidemiologists and Biostatisticians

Epidemiology is the study of the distribution and determinants of health-related states or events in specified populations, and the application of this study to the control of health problems. By this definition, nearly all of those people who work in public health are epidemiologists in one sense or another. Those individuals considered to be epidemiologists, however, generally have a degree in epidemiology, and the major focus of their work is the surveillance of health problems in a community and the study of the effectiveness of different interventions. Epidemiology can be the primary speciality for a graduate or postgraduate degree, generally an MS, MPH, or PhD. It can also be a graduate specialization added to initial preparation in medicine, nursing, or other health field. Preparation in epidemiology can come as a primary degree earned from a school of public health or as a graduate specialization added to initial preparation in medicine, nursing, or another health field. While epidemiologists previously were concerned exclusively with infectious and vectorborne diseases, some now specialize in understanding and analyzing the distribution and occurrence of conditions resulting from occupational and environmental exposure. They study the complete range of health threats, including pesticides, toxic chemicals, and radioactivity.

Most epidemiologists work in federal or state agencies. Epidemiologists are employed only by the largest local agencies. Looking to improve their prevention efforts and minimize costs, epidemiologists are increasingly employed by private health agencies such as HMOs and managed care organizations. Epidemiologists are also employed by individual hospitals, medical centers, and hospital systems in programs to control nosocomial infections. A small portion is employed in the private sector in consulting firms and other corporations. These positions may be in conducting research, consulting, or providing oversight on scientific investigations.

The work of epidemiologists frequently overlaps with that of biostatisticians, whose primary focus is using statistical theory, techniques, and methods to identify and analyze health problems and the effectiveness of health services. They may also use their statistical skills to provide measurements needed for public health plans and public health policy. Much of a biostatistician's work revolves around the compiling, processing, and analyzing of data.

Educators and Behavioral Scientists

The public health work force also needs to include an adequate number of individuals with skills in education and behavioral sciences. (See Chapter 12 for a detailed discussion.) The origin of public health in the physical sciences and the laboratory, and its primary attention to conditions that can be alleviated with a physical intervention, has caused today's work force to lack social scientists. The more we know about humans and human behavior, however, the more obvious it becomes that even diseases that are seen as strictly "physical" can only be ameliorated effectively using behavioral science. For example, our efforts to control STDs are severely limited without advanced knowledge of human sexual behavior and sexual decision making. In other areas such as promoting increased exercise, changing individual eating patterns, or reducing stress, behavioral science is the main driver of program planning. There is an immediate need for public health agencies to recruit and retain behavioral and social scientists to complement the more traditional mix of public health expertise.

Environmental Health Specialists

Environmental health specialists manage a multiplicity of population-based health issues addressed by the control and management of environmental factors. (See Chapter 26 for a detailed discussion.) Their day-to-day concerns include air and water quality, toxic substance management, solid waste management, and industrial hygiene. Job titles for individuals working in environmental health are extremely varied, but include scientist, engineer, geologist, hydrologist, toxicologist, risk assessor, industrial hygienist, and sanitarian.

The lead national agency that employs environmental health specialists is the Environmental Protection Agency. However, environmental specialists are found in almost all federal offices. Within state governments, environmental workers are frequently employed not in a health department, but in a separate department of environmental quality, health, or protection. Locally, environmental specialists will most often be employed in a local health department. As in the states, environmental specialists in large cities are often found in a separate environmental agency.

Of course, not all environmental workers are government employees. A large portion of the environmental health work force is employed by the private sector in consulting and engineering firms. These firms are hired by clients to help them assess environmental risks and comply with government environmental regulations. All organizations associated with the preparation of food products—from mills and bakeries to meat-packing houses and restaurants—use a variety of sanitarians and environmental health specialists.

Nurses

Public health nursing in the United States originated with the work of Lillian Wald at the Henry Street Settlement House in New York City. Wald and her colleagues were actively involved in a wide range of disease prevention and health promotion efforts targeted at vulnerable and visible urban immigrant population.[29]

Public health nurses are distinguished from other nursing specialty areas by their focus on populations rather than individuals, and by their interest in disease prevention. Although public health agencies often employ nurses with a diploma or associate degree, a public health nurse generally has a bachelor's degree. In larger agencies, nurses with public health preparation work in community-based programs or hold leadership positions. Other nurses are limited to clinical or more support positions. Public health nursing covers most aspects of public health but is most visible in infectious disease control programs such as directly observed therapy for TB, maternal and child health (MCH) programs, and immunizations. Newer programs in which nurses have been active include lead poisoning identification and abatement, tobacco control, injury prevention, and mental health services.

Preventive Medicine Workers

Preventive medicine is the specialty area providing postgraduate medical preparation for work in public health. The American College of Preventive Medicine is the related specialty organization. Over the past three decades, the number of preventive medicine physicians has been declining. The decrease has been particularly large for preventive medicine physicians in public health. In 1970, 3,029 identified themselves as public health preventive medicine physicians. By 1997 that number was cut nearly in half to 1,670.[30]

Despite the existence of the specialty, physicians practicing in public health come from almost every field of medicine. Given the range of public health interests, it is not unusual for a public health agency to employ someone with expertise in pediatrics, obstetrics, infectious diseases, emergency medicine, or pathology. On the job, physicians from these specialties learn a great deal about public health, community- and population-focused medicine, and health promotion, and frequently are quite successful with their public health efforts. The reasons for the diverse backgrounds are varied, but perhaps the primary one is the failure of medicine to acknowledge public health fully as an area requiring advanced preparation. Although it would be unacceptable for someone without a surgical residency to be placed in charge of an operating room, it is often the case that physicians without preventive medicine training and without a graduate public health degree are placed in leadership positions in public health. Indeed, one study found that 78 percent of local health department directors had no formal public health training.[31] In the past and to a certain degree still today, some organizations believed that physicians were the natural leaders of any health-related activity. Physicians were sought to lead public health efforts, even if other individuals from other professions were better prepared for the particular challenge.

There has been some movement away from this point of view. In some sectors, it seems that physicians have become an unnecessary luxury, to be employed in public health only for their ability to sign prescriptions and oversee clinical services. In 1945 all of the directors of local health departments were physicians. By 1995 only 32 percent were physicians.[31] The interdisciplinary nature of public health requires that the knowledge of human health brought by physicians be available in many specific programs and at the leadership level. The inclusion of medical expertise, however, should be done with a careful evaluation of the public health perspective of the physician(s) available and not in a manner that either over- or undervalues the knowledge, skills, and abilities of the other members of the public health team.

Nutritionists

Given the influence that diet and eating have on health outcomes, it is no surprise that nutritionists are part of the public health work force. Nutritionists plan nutrition programs and supervise the preparing and serving of meals. They help prevent and treat illnesses by promoting healthy eating habits, scientifically evaluating clients' diets, and suggesting diet modifications, such as less salt for those with high blood pressure or reduced fat and sugar intake for those who are overweight. They run food service systems for institutions such as hospitals and schools, promote sound eating habits through education, and conduct research. Major areas of practice are clinical, community, management, and consultancies.[32] The advent of the U.S. Department of Agriculture–funded Special Supplemental Food Program for Women, Infants, and Children, commonly known as WIC, has raised awareness of the value of nutritional interventions and is documented as one of the most successful public health programs. A substantial proportion of the *Healthy People 2010* goals for the nation will only be met if nutritionists' skills are tapped in program design and development.[2]

Cultural competence plays a unique role in public health nutrition. Although cultural competence is an asset and requirement of any public health program, the need for culturally competent nutritionists is perhaps greater than for any other public health specialty. The continued flow of immigrants from around the globe means that most communities must regularly update food-related activities and information to accommodate the habits and preferences of those from other cultures.

MCH Workers

Rather than being a single occupation, the category of MCH worker encompasses a number of professions and skills. MCH programs are often staffed by physicians, nurses, health educators, nutritionists, social workers, and others interested in the health of mothers and children. Physicians may be specialists in family medicine, pediatrics, or obstetrics and gynecology. Similarly, MCH nurses may specialize as midwives, women's health care practitioners, or pediatric nurse practitioners.

MCH is also an area of specialization within many schools of public health. Some offer an MPH with this area as the degree focus. Training can cover a wide variety of topics, including family planning, comprehensive maternity care, growth and development, comprehensive pediatric care, genetics, and inborn errors of metabolism (e.g., phenylketonuria).

Maternal child health is one of the many areas within public health in which individuals hired for a specific programmatic skill with little public health preparation (such as an obstetrician employed to provide prenatal care, or a nurse practitioner employed to provide family planning services, or a social worker employed to counsel families with a high-risk newborn) may move over time into more generalized roles or programs. Absent good on-the-job training in general public health, or time and interest in obtaining additional formal preparation, these MCH specialists are at a distinct disadvantage when they need to respond to the demands of broader public health work. Although their employment should not be discouraged, the employing agency would be wise to have a career development plan in place to assist those who wish to move from a specialty area to public health.

Health Services Administrators

Managing public health programs is a unique challenge; funding streams are usually complex, and the programs are not easily analyzed using the tools appropriate for the private sector. With every resident of the service community as client, analysis of cost/benefit and investment payoffs do not fit a sales or customer model. Many of those served by public health may not know that they have been served, or may not be happy about the experience (for example, a restaurant forced to close temporarily due to a food-handling problem).

Because public health recruits managers not only from public health training programs but also from business settings and public administration training programs, public health leaders need to ensure that the new recruits are adequately oriented to a public health perspective. That said, it is also important for public health managers to listen to and learn from those trained in settings such as industrial administration, business management, human resource management, information technology, and other business management specialties. To cross-fertilize managerial perspectives and expertise, public health organizations can exchange staff with other national, state, and local agencies and institute a variety of training strategies.

Dental Health Workers

Public health agencies employ dentists and dental hygienists in both preventive and restorative roles. In addition to supporting the fluoridation of public water supplies, public health agencies promote children's dental health through education, the application of sealants, and the application of topical fluoride in areas without fluoridated drinking water. Those agencies with clinical services may also provide dental examinations and restorative dentistry as a part of ensuring care for those individuals without other sources of care.

EMPLOYMENT SETTINGS

Although public health workers are found in both private and public settings, the largest portion of the primary public health work force is employed in the three government sectors. Regardless of where public health employees work, they are likely to interact with government officials at some level. The next few paragraphs describe the "official" public health work force.

Because such a large proportion of public health workers is employed in the public sector, their job titles, qualifications, and duties are generally defined by a public personnel system. (See Chapter 16 for a detailed discussion.) These personnel systems are affected by various governmental policies, including fair employment practices, equal employment opportunity, career advancement, and demonstration of capacity through work experience in lieu of education—all of which have pushed toward less specific job requirements. This and the sometimes slow pace of change in such systems has made it difficult to update job requirements as public health has evolved. Therefore, those managing the "public" public health work force must be flexible when matching needed skills to job titles and positions that have appropriate pay and status and be cautious in interpreting numbers that describe the size of some groups within the work force.

The governmental presence at the local level is almost universally the local health department (LHD)—whether it is a unit of local government or a branch of the state health agency. These departments are "where the rubber meets the road," where services are delivered and monies are spent. Thus, the number and types of employees who are employed locally depend on the particular services being provided and the available funding. Funding and service depend in turn on the size of the jurisdiction that is being served, its proximity to major urban centers, and the area's unique problems. Regardless, the largest portion of the work force in almost all local health departments are nurses, administrators, and some form of environmental employee, typically a sanitarian. Those positions make up at least 50 percent of the local work force. Informally, the total work force in local health departments across the nation is estimated to be approximately 145,000 full-time and 47,000 part-time employees.[6]

Local public health workers are supported by workers from a vast array of community-based organizations (CBOs), voluntary health organizations (i.e., local chapters of the American Cancer Society or American Heart Association), or personal health care providers. Often, these community efforts match or exceed that of the official governmental local public health work force. Some CBOs have regular full-time staff; others operate on a strictly volunteer basis. Often, CBOs are affiliated with a local charity, religious, or political institution. Some CBOs address a specific health or other community problem; others are more concerned with the general health and well-being of the community. Regardless, it is important for all public health workers to be aware of the CBOs operating in their area and, most importantly, look to them as partners. The most fruitful public health endeavors are those that involve the community through its CBOs.

State public health agencies provide three kinds of public health services: broad administrative and policy setting for the whole state, supervisory and support services for local public health efforts, and direct services to citizens. This latter role arises either where there is no other local governmental public health presence or when the state and local body politic have determined that it is most effective for the state to be the provider. In addition, states historically have been the recipient of most federal public health funds and have the responsibility for overseeing those expenditures. The states in turn provide money to the local health departments, where it is spent on programs and services. Lately this pattern has changed as the federal government sought to fund local programs directly. Recent efforts for states' rights, a move toward block grants rather than categorical grants, and federal cutbacks suggest that states will once again be the major public health budget overseers. State health departments are estimated to provide approximately $1.8 billion per year to local authorities.[33]

The state public health work force is estimated at approximately 130,000 full-time equivalent positions.[34] Although recent data on the state public health work force are lacking, it can be assumed that the staffing patterns in state health departments very much depend on the particular services and functions for which the state is responsible, the health priorities it seeks to address, and the programs it conducts. This is not unlike the situation for LHDs. Compared with local districts, however, states, because of their fiscal, regulatory, and policy-setting responsibilities, have a larger proportion of their employees in managerial and oversight positions and fewer providing direct services.

With the advent of the Environmental Protection Agency, states began creating separate environmental agencies, moving programs to protect waterways, air, and soil out of the general public health agency. States have also made various decisions for the organizational location of programs of worker health and safety and supervision of the food and dairy industries. Because of this diversity, it has been even more difficult to estimate the size of the state public health work force.

To some extent, federal public health agencies carry out all public health functions, even directly providing some personal health services. (See Chapter 3 for a detailed discussion.) The major federal focus, however, is setting policy for the nation, conducting research and health-related investigations, and administering grants and funds. Of necessity, these activities are carried out in cooperation with states and local authorities.

The major federal employer is the DHHS. The DHHS employs nearly 60,000 individuals. These workers are employed in eight operating divisions within the DHHS, including the Agency for Healthcare Research and Quality, Agency for Toxic Substances and Disease Registry, Centers for Disease Control and Prevention, Food and Drug Administration, Health Care Financing Administration, Health Resources and Services Administration, Indian Health Service, National Institutes of Health, and Substance Abuse and Mental Health Services Administration. The two largest employers are the Indian Health Service and the National Institutes of Health. They account for just more than half of the employees. Most DHHS employees are employed in either clinical research or clinical service settings. The Health Care Financing Administration is not always included on the list of public health agencies within the DHHS but is clearly concerned with issues of access to care for two populations: the elderly (through Medicare) and the poor (through Medicaid). The remaining employees are more likely to be employed in settings where the focus is population-based prevention. Approximately one-third of all DHHS employees are in medical or health-related occupations, and another 11 percent are biologists or chemists.[35]

TRAINING FOR PUBLIC HEALTH WORKERS

Public health workers arrive on the job with diverse educations and experience. Much of this educational preparation will have been specific to a single professional practice area and may or may not include specific public health content. Thus, many workers need not only on-the-job and technical/vocational training for a specific task, but also general orientation to public health. Even with an appropriate public health background, staff development and continued learning opportunities are a necessity. To provide appropriate training, administrators need to understand the diversity of educational backgrounds a public health worker may bring to his or her job.

Formal public health degree preparation may begin at the associate level and can continue through doctoral study. A number of college and university programs offer a bachelor's degree in public health. These programs prepare students in community development, health promotion, or environmental health. Graduates are eligible for entry positions in almost any aspect of public health, providing they receive adequate supervision and support. An individual with only a bachelor's or associate's degree and no or very limited work experience would not be prepared to work independently or to assume leadership in a program area.

The MPH degree is the most widely accepted and recognized preparation for public health practice, especially for a position of program responsibility. The capacity of the nation's schools and programs in public health, however, is such that only a small fraction of those in the work force have attained this degree.[36] These programs ensure that all graduates have at least a basic introduction to epidemiology, biostatistics, environmental health, behavioral science, and management. Graduates can also specialize in one of these fields, or in a program area such as MCH, international health, or public health laboratory science. A large proportion of those seeking the MPH have had some work experience in a public health organization and expect to return to a position of greater responsibility. Others follow the MPH with study for the DrPh or PhD in public health—training that provides an opportunity for deeper specialization and development of research skills. Most schools describe the role of the PhD as preparing students for academic careers; the DPh is perceived as a practice degree, supporting a higher level of leadership or innovation in service organizations.

The preparation of the majority of the public health work force with postsecondary education is in a discipline other than public health, such as medicine, nursing, dentistry, nutrition, social work, biology, chemistry, engineering, or education (the list is almost endless). Although accrediting bodies expect that both medicine and baccalaureate nursing curricula will include content on prevention and public health, actual student experience varies widely. These other disciplines, while preparing students in an area that is very relevant to public health, have little specific content on the perspectives, values, and skills necessary to deliver essential public health services. Once recruited and employed in public health, however, these individuals often seek out continuing education opportunities or return to school for the MPH.

Nursing and public health nursing professions are often confusing because of the multiple routes of entry. Individuals may sit for the registered nurse (RN) licensing examination after completing an educational program that may range from 24 months to 5 years, and having earned an associate degree, a bachelor's degree, a master's degree, or (in rare instances) a doctorate. In many parts of the country, the nursing work force is such that public health agencies routinely fill vacancies with nurses who have less than a bachelor's degree. Without a bachelor's degree, these nurses will have had little, if any, exposure to public health content in their studies. These nurses do a very effective job in clinic-based practice, and many have learned on the job to fill other community-based roles. However, they are at a disadvantage similar to that of the environmental health employee who has a bachelor's degree in biology and has learned public health sanitation on the job. Although they have learned the specific job responsibilities and technical knowledge, they have not had the opportunity to develop an understanding of the population perspective necessary for effective public health work. Consequently, their program management and development skills, as well as their future growth, are limited.

Nursing schools also offer graduate degrees in public health nursing and community health nursing. These programs include much content that is similar to that offered in the MPH, but they may omit key topics such as environmental health. Nonetheless, graduates are well prepared for many leadership roles in public health organizations.

Other disciplines such as environmental engineering, social work, and nutrition offer graduate degrees that are extremely relevant to public health. However, the amount of general public health information included in these programs varies widely. The graduates of these programs are well equipped to fill specialized positions in public health, and will learn on the job about public health. Many of those seeking graduate degrees may have begun work in public health with less training, and use formal education as a strategy for career advancement. The employing agency must assess the amount of on-the-job or continuing education training needed to ensure that these specialists have sufficient public health orientation to collaborate effectively with all partners.

Certification and licensure programs in public health make work force training backgrounds even more complex. Some public health professions (medicine, nursing, dentistry) require licensure to practice in every state. Other professionals, such as sanitarians, are licensed in some states, certified or registered in others, or left to voluntary standards in still others. In medicine, in addition to a license to practice, there is an expectation that individuals will seek certification in a specialty area. Most pertinent to public health is the previously mentioned one in preventive medicine from the American College of Preventive Medicine. The limited number of physicians certified in this area means that most physicians working in public health are certified in another area, with pediatrics, obstetrics, infectious disease, and family medicine being the most common. Nurses who have advanced practice preparation (midwives, pediatric nurse practitioners, family nurse practitioners, women's health nurse practitioners) and work in public health settings are required by all states to have additional certification beyond the basic registered nurse license. Public health educators may be certified by the Society for Public Health Education, though in most areas, this is not required by state law.

Public health organizations must be attentive to position descriptions and recruitment requirements, if they hope to recruit individuals with appropriate levels of public health knowledge. Given the range of preparation possible, organizations must also recognize that some of the most effective individuals have acquired the necessary competencies through unusual routes. Although laws on licensure, for example, must be followed, there should be flexibility in matching the person to the job, remembering that with the exception of particular tasks associated with particular licenses (e.g., prescribing by a physician, dentist, nurse, or physician's assistant), individuals with widely varied educational preparation may have the combination of competencies sought. There is movement toward some form of general certification in basic public health skills that would be offered to all public health workers, which might make it easier for the employer or manager to assess readiness for various positions.

Future Directions in Training

Public health organizations have begun to explore strategies for developing a readily available core of public health knowledge that could be tapped as a part of new employee orientation or existing work force updates. Based on a number of recent efforts, it appears possible to identify a core content that could make up this preparation.[37] Basic content could include an orientation to the values, history, and world view of public health. The other key content areas include assessment and epidemiology, analytic thinking, effective communication skills, community development, policy development, politics, and organizational effectiveness. Although some individual public health organizations have developed programs encompassing all or part of this content, there is increasing interest in making it available through regional consortia and using distance-based technologies such as the Internet or satellite downlinks. Such methods allow the use of master teachers and avoid duplication. Regional or national distance learning also allows for improved quality control of the training and can be extremely cost effective.

Providing public health continuing education through distance learning approaches can benefit all forms of public health training programs, and all public health practitioners need regular updates in their areas of responsibility. As new threats to health are understood or new interventions are developed, public health workers need to master the new material.

Although many public health workers are in urban areas with extensive resources and short distances to educational centers, a large proportion work in small and isolated agencies. There may be no one to take a worker's place when training is at another site. One day of training may be a three-day trip. Managers must be sure that workers have both the money and the time needed to attend these training opportunities. Job responsibilities must be covered and adequate resources provided. Distance learning technologies may help to relax these constraints.

Administrators must also ensure that professionals who for reasons of licensure or certification need continuing education credits can get credit for public health training. This may take some effort on the part of public health organizations that may have routinely made one- or two-day "update" conferences available, but have not gone through the often tedious paperwork needed to offer official credit. Another increasingly available option is converting continuing education credits into academic credit with some additional work (and fees). This approach, if more widely developed, would allow staff who may not have originally understood the need for a graduate degree in public health to get a head start on formal preparation through the conversion of credit for knowledge already gained through agency-supported continuing education.

Finally, managers must personally hold and foster the attitude that education is not simply a series of time-limited classes leading to a specific set of letters to insert after one's name, or a single set of skills to be employed indefinitely. Learning is a lifelong process, and learning about work should be continuous and stimulating. Although there may be specific times to gain skills, or to earn a degree, there is always something to be learned that will make the current job better, more rewarding, more interesting, more challenging, and more successful. Every new thing that is learned becomes a building block toward some new opportunity that should be even more interesting and rewarding.

THE FUTURE OF THE PUBLIC HEALTH WORK FORCE

Any attempt to predict the future size and structure of the public health work force must be made with extreme caution. The diversity of the work force in terms of both its occupations and its tasks, coupled with the lack of up-to-date information, makes firm conclusions extremely difficult. Another complicating factor is the role of government. Governments fund schools of public health, public health training, and community public health programs. It is thus a large, if not the largest, influence on the structure of the public health work force. Whether they are federal, state, or local, governments determine the budgets that ultimately determine the numbers and types of individuals hired. Thus, all those factors that influence politics will also influence the public health work force.

Although it cannot be argued with authority, it can be reasonably asserted that the demand for public health workers is likely to continue to grow for at least the next decade. U.S. local health departments reported 6 percent of their budgeted positions to be unfilled.[6] Growth rates for the number of nurses employed in a variety of community settings have been more than 20 percent for the past several years.[38] Demands for behavioral and social scientists are expanding and adding a whole new sector to the public work force. The public's concern with the risks associated with technologies such as genetically modified crops or electromagnetic fields will undoubtedly continue for the foreseeable future and thus continue to expand the breadth of public health and its work force.

The individuals needed to fill these positions will come from a variety of sources. The primary source for the core public health professional will continue to be the nation's schools of public health. The number of graduates has increased more than 50 percent from 1985 to 1995.[39] Although such a large increase would seem to be sufficient to meet the demand for new public health workers, firm conclusions are impossible because of several limitations.

The first is that nearly 17 percent of the graduates are foreign nationals. What percentage of them continue to work in the U.S. public health work force is unknown. Of those who choose to remain in the United States, little data is known about the sectors where they ultimately find work. Increasingly, graduates from schools of public health are finding employment in areas outside the bounds of traditional public health, particularly in HMOs and other private health care institutions. The focus of their work in these employment settings may or may not be population-based public health.[39]

To the public health community, the need for more public health workers and enhanced training is self-evident and unquestionable. To those in government who make and pay for resource allocation decisions, the needs are not so obvious. Compelling arguments for public health work force development can be made, but the evidence must first be gathered in research directed toward establishing the current size and structure of the public health work force.

CHAPTER REVIEW

1. The public health work force consists of individuals whose major work focus is the delivery of one or more of the essential services of public health, whether or not those individuals are on the payroll of an official, voluntary, or nonprofit public health agency.
2. The size and structure of the public health work force is highly sensitive to health policy and marketplace trends that affect the scope of activity carried out by public health organizations. These trends include evolving systems of health care delivery and financing, privatization initiatives in government health programs, changes in federal and state public health funding, and innovations in public health technologies and interventions.
3. The optimal distribution of public health workers between generalists and specialists depends on the size and complexity of the populations served. This distribution is likely to shift toward specialist training as public health knowledge and technology becomes broader and more complex.
4. Core disciplines represented within the public health work force include epidemiologists, biostatisticians, health educators and behavioral scientists, environmental health specialists, preventive medicine specialists, nutritionists, MCH specialists, public health nurses, public health social workers, and dentists.
5. Government health agencies are a dominant employment setting for public health workers, as are nonprofit and community-based organizations. Private sector employment is growing rapidly among many types of public health professionals, particularly as health plans and medical care providers begin to acquire capacities for population-based health care management.
6. Educational and training programs for public health workers include formal bachelor's and master's level degree programs in public health (BSPH and MPH), medical degree programs with residencies in preventive medicine and public health, nursing degree programs with specialties in public health and community health, and nondegree certificate programs in specific public health disciplines. A majority of current public health workers completed postsecondary education in a discipline other than public health.

REFERENCES

1. E.S. Carpenter, *Proposed Credentialing System for Public Health Professionals: What Would It Mean for Schools of Public Health* (Ann Arbor, MI: Association of Schools of Public Health, 1990).
2. U.S. Department of Health and Human Services, Public Health Service, *Healthy People 2010: Objectives for the Nation* (Washington, DC: U.S. Government Printing Office, 2000).
3. Public Health Functions Project, *The Public Health Workforce: An Agenda for the 21st Century* (Washington, DC: U.S. Department of Health and Human Services, 1997).
4. Department of Labor, Bureau of Labor Statistics, *Standard Occupational Classification,* rev. ed. (Washington, DC: 2000).
5. L. Shattuck, *Report of the Sanitary Commission of Massachusetts, 1850* (Cambridge, MA: Harvard University Press, 1948).
6. R.B. Gerzoff et al., "Full-Time Employees of U.S. Local Health Departments 1992–1993," *Journal of Public Health Management Practice 5,* no. 3 (1999): 1–9.
7. C.-E.A. Winslow and H.L. Harris, "An Ideal Health Department for a City of 100,000 Population," *American Journal of Public Health 12,* no. 11 (1922): 891–907.

8. H. Emerson and M. Luginbuhl, *Local Health Units for the Nation* (New York: The Commonwealth Fund, 1945).
9. J.W. Mountin et al., *Ten Years of Federal Grants in Aid for Public Health: 1936–1946* [Public Health Bulletin No. 300] (Washington, DC: Superintendent of Documents, 1949).
10. Treasury Department, U.S. Public Health Service, *Report of the Committee on Municipal Health Department Practice* (Washington, DC: U.S. Government Printing Office, 1923).
11. U.S. Department of Health, Education, and Welfare, Public Health Service, *Public Health Personnel in Local Health Units,* rev. ed. [Publication No. 682] (Washington, DC: U.S. Government Printing Office, 1967).
12. U.S. Department of Health and Human Services, Public Health Service, *Nurses in Public Health* (Washington, DC: U.S. Government Printing Office, 1960).
13. U.S. Department of Health and Human Services, Public Health Service, Health Resources Administration, *Public Health Personnel in the United States, 1980* [HRP-0904085] (Washington, DC: U.S. Government Printing Office, 1992).
14. Northwest Center for Public Health Practice, *A Profile and Training Needs Assessment of Community/Public Health Professionals in Washington State* (Seattle, WA: 1998).
15. V.C. Kennedy et al., "Public Health Workforce Information: A State-Level Study," *Journal of Public Health Management and Practice 5,* no. 9 (1999): 10–19.
16. M. Richardson et al., *Local Health Districts and the Public Health Workforce: A Case Study of Wyoming and Idaho* [Working paper 56] (Seattle, WA: Center for Work Studies, University of Washington, 1999).
17. D. Osborne and T. Gaebler, *Reinventing Government* (New York: Plume Books, 1992).
18. L. Kertesz, "Public Facilities Going Private," *Modern Healthcare,* 9 September, 1996, 32–41.
19. S.R. Keener et al., "Providing Public Health Services through an Integrated Delivery System," *Quality Management in Health Care 5,* no. 2 (1997): 27–34.
20. S.H. Lopez et al., *The Quiet Dismantling of Public Health: The Impact of Pennsylvania State Health Center Privatization and Staff Cutbacks* (Harrisburg, PA: Keystone Research Center, 1998).
21. J.R. Pierce, "Transformation of a Local Health Department from Primary Care to Core Public Health," *Public Health Reports* 113 (1998): 152–159.
22. S. Wall, "Transformations in Public Health Systems," *Health Affairs 17,* no. 3 (1998): 64–80.
23. Institute of Medicine, *The Future of Public Health* (Washington, DC: National Academy Press, 1988).
24. "Only Three Cents for Health," *American Journal of Public Health 23,* no. 2 (1933): 139.
25. Health Care Financing Administration, *1998 National Healthcare Expenditures* (Washington, DC: 1999).
26. R.E. Brown, *National Expenditures for Health Promotion and Disease Prevention Activities in the United States* [BHARC-013/91/019] (Washington, DC: Battelle Human Affairs Research Centers, Medical Technology and Policy Research Center, 1991).
27. Centers for Disease Control and Prevention. "Estimated Expenditures for Essential Public Health Services—Selected States, Fiscal Year 1995," *Morbidity and Mortality Weekly Report 46,* no. 7 (1997): 150–152.
28. B.C. Amick et al., *Society and Health* (New York: Oxford University Press, 1995).
29. D.J. Mason and J.K. Leavitt, *Policy and Politics in Nursing and Health Care,* 3rd ed. (Philadelphia: W.B. Saunders, 1998).
30. D.S. Lane, "A Threat to the Public Health Workforce: Evidence from Trends," *American Journal of Preventive Medicine 18,* no. 1 (2000): 87–96.
31. R.B. Gerzoff and T.B. Richards, "The Education of Local Health Department Top Executives," *Journal of Public Health Management and Practice 3,* no. 4 (1997): 50–56.
32. Bureau of Labor Statistics, *1998–1999 Occupation Outlook Handbook* (Washington, DC: U.S. Government Printing Office, 1999).
33. Public Health Foundation, *Public Health Agencies 1991: An Inventory of Programs and Block Grant Expenditures* (Washington, DC: Public Health Foundation, 1991).
34. Public Health Foundation, State Health Agency Staffs, *1991 Final Report of a Contract with DHHS-PHS-HRSA.* (Washington, DC: Public Health Foundation, 1992).
35. U.S. Department of Health and Human Services, *HHS Employment Profile and HHS: What We Do* (Washington, DC: 1999).
36. F. Moore, *Analysis of the Public Health Workforce, Final Report from Contract No. HRSA 85–266P* (Washington, DC: HRSA, 1985).
37. K.M. Gebbie and I. Hwang, *Preparing Currently Employed Public Health Workers for Changes in the Health System* (New York: Columbia University School of Nursing, 1998).
38. Division of Nursing, Bureau of Health Professions, Health Resources and Services Administration, U.S. Department of Health and Human Services, *The Registered Nursing Population,* March 1996 (Washington, DC: Division of Nursing, 1997).
39. Association of Schools of Public Health, *Annual Data Report, 1995* (Washington, DC: 1997).

CHAPTER 5

Public Health Law

Lawrence O. Gostin

Laws are enacted to influence healthy behavior, respond to health threats, and enforce health and safety standards. Public health law is principally concerned with government's assurance of the conditions for the population's health—what government may, and must, do to safeguard human health. Federal, state, and local governments exercise public health powers derived from the complex legal relationships among these levels of government. Protecting and preserving community health is not possible without an effective legal framework to guide a wide range of private endeavors.

Preservation of the public's health is among the most important goals of government. The enactment and enforcement of law, moreover, is a primary means by which government creates the conditions for people to lead healthier and safer lives. Law creates a mission for public health authorities, assigns their functions, and specifies the manner in which they may exercise their authority. The law is a tool for public health practice, which is used to influence norms for healthy behavior, identify and respond to health threats, and set and enforce health and safety standards. The most important social debates concerning public health take place in legal fora—legislatures, courts, and administrative agencies—and in the law's language of rights, duties, and justice.[1] It is no exaggeration to say that "the field of public health...could not long exist in the manner in which we know it today except for its sound legal basis."[2(p.4)]

The Institute of Medicine (IOM), in its foundational 1988 report, *The Future of Public Health*, acknowledged that law was essential to public health, but cast serious doubt on the soundness of public health's legal basis. Concluding that "this nation has lost sight of its public health goals and has allowed the system of public health activities to fall into disarray," the IOM placed some of the blame on an obsolete and inadequate body of enabling laws and regulations.[3(p.19)] The IOM recommended that

> states review their public health statutes and make revisions necessary to accomplish the following two objectives: [i] clearly delineate the basic authority and responsibility entrusted to public health agencies, boards, and officials at the state and local levels and the relationship between them; and [ii] support a set of modern disease control measures that address contemporary health problems such as AIDS, cancer, and heart disease, and incorporate due process safeguards (notice, hearings, ad-

---

This chapter is based on a more substantial examination and analysis of American public health law contained in Lawrence O. Gostin, *Public Health Law: Power, Duty, Restraint* (Berkeley, CA, and New York, NY: University of California Press and Milbank Memorial Fund, 2000).

ministrative review, right to counsel, standards of evidence).[3(p.10)]

This chapter reviews the state of public health law in the United States. First, a theory and definition of public health law is offered. Second, public health powers within the constitutional design are explained. Third, the current structure of federal, state, and local health agencies is examined. Finally, the future of public health law is considered, explaining the deficiencies in state public health statutes and proposing guidelines for law reform.

A THEORY AND DEFINITION OF PUBLIC HEALTH LAW

Public health law is often used interchangeably with other terms that signify a connection between law and health, such as health law, law and medicine, and forensic medicine. Despite the similarity of these names, public health law is a distinct discipline capable of definition. I define public health law as the study of the legal powers and duties of the state to ensure the conditions for people to be healthy (e.g., to identify, prevent, and ameliorate risks to health in the population), and the limitations on the power of the state to constrain the autonomy, privacy, liberty, proprietary, or other legally protected interests of individuals for the protection or promotion of community health.

Public health law has at least five characteristics that help separate it from other fields at the intersection of law and health: government, populations, relationships, services, and coercion.

Government's Essential Role in Public Health Law

Public health activities are the primary (but not exclusive) responsibility of government. The importance of government in ensuring the conditions for the population's health is demonstrated by its constitutional powers and its role in a democracy. The Preamble to the Constitution reveals the ideals of government as the wellspring of communal life and mutual security: "We the People of the United States, in Order to form a more perfect Union, establish Justice, insure domestic Tranquility, provide for the common defence, promote the general Welfare, and secure the Blessings of Liberty to ourselves and our Posterity, do ordain and establish this Constitution…." The constitutional design reveals a plain intent to vest power in government at every level to protect community health and safety. Government is empowered to collect taxes and expend public resources, and only government can require members of the community to submit to regulation.

The role of government in a democracy also helps explain its importance in advancing the public's health. People form governments precisely to provide a means of communal support and security. Acting alone, individuals cannot ensure even minimum levels of health. Individuals may procure personal medical services and many of the necessities of life; any person of means can purchase a home, clothing, food, and the services of a physician or hospital. Yet, no single individual, or group of individuals, can ensure his or her health. Meaningful protection and assurance of the population's health requires communal effort. The community as a whole has a stake in environmental protection, hygiene and sanitation, clean air and surface water, uncontaminated food and drinking water, safe roads and products, and the control of infectious disease. Each of these collective goods, and many more, are essential conditions for health. Yet, these goods can be secured only through organized action on behalf of the population.

This discussion does not suggest that the private and voluntary sectors are not important in public health. Manifestly, private (e.g., managed care), charitable (e.g., the Red Cross), and community (e.g., human immunodeficiency virus [HIV] support) organizations play roles that are critical to public health. Nevertheless, communal efforts to protect and promote the population's health are primarily a responsibility of government, which is why government action represents a central theoretical tenet of what we call public health law.

Serving the Health Needs of Populations

Public health focuses on the health of populations rather than on the clinical improvement of individual patients. Generally, public health focuses on communal health, whereas medicine focuses on the health of individuals. Classic definitions of public health emphasize this population-based perspective: "As one of the objects of the police power of the state, the 'public health' means the prevailingly healthful or sanitary condition of the general body of people or the community in mass, and the absence of any general or widespread disease or cause of mortality."[4(p.721)] Public health services are those that are shared by all members of the community and are organized and supported by, and for, the benefit of the people as a whole. Thus, whereas the art or science of medicine seeks to identify and ameliorate ill health in the individual patient, public health seeks to improve the health of the population.

Relationships between Government and the Public

Public health contemplates the relationship between the state and the population (or between the state and individuals who place themselves or the community at risk) rather than the relationship between the physician and the patient. Public health practitioners and scholars are interested in organized community efforts to improve the health of populations. Accordingly, public health law observes collective action—principally through government—and its effects on various populations. The field of public health law similarly examines the benefits and burdens placed by government on legally protected interests. This is in direct contrast to the field of health care law, which concerns the microrelationships between health care providers and patients as well as the organization, finance, and provision of personal medical services.

Population-Based Services

Public health deals primarily with the provision of population-based health services rather than personal medical services. The core functions of public health agencies are those fundamental activities that are carried out to protect the population's health:

- *assessment:* the collection, assembly, and analysis of community health needs
- *policy development:* the development of public health policies informed through scientific knowledge
- *assurance:* assurance of the services necessary for community health

Activities regarded as essential public health services include efforts to monitor community health status and investigate health risks; inform, educate, and empower people about health; mobilize community partnerships; regulate individual and organizational behavior; evaluate effectiveness, accessibility, and quality of personal health services; and pursue innovative solutions to health problems.[5] Moreover, the public health community is increasingly interested in scientific methodologies to monitor the efficacy of services.[6]

Demand Conformance with Health and Safety Standards

Public health possesses the power to coerce individuals for the protection of the community and thus does not rely on a near-universal ethic of voluntarism. Although government can do much to promote public health that does not require the exercise of compulsory powers, it alone is authorized to require conformance with publicly established standards of behavior. The degree of compulsory measures necessary to safeguard the public health is, of course, subject to political and judicial resolution. Yet, protecting and preserving community health is not possible without the constraint of a wide range of private activities. Absent an inherent governmental authority and ability to coerce individual and community behaviors, threats to public health and safety could not be reduced easily.

Having defined public health law and distinguished it from other fields, it will be helpful to examine the public health law in our constitutional system of government.

PUBLIC HEALTH IN THE CONSTITUTIONAL DESIGN

No inquiry is more important to public health law than understanding the role of government in the constitutional design. If public health law is principally about government's assurance of the conditions necessary for the population's health, what must government do to safeguard human health? Analyzing this question requires an assessment of duty (what government must do), authority (what government can, but is not required to, do), limits (what government cannot do), and responsibility (which government—whether federal, state, or local—is to act).

The U.S. Constitution is the starting point for any analysis concerning the distribution of governmental powers. Although the Constitution is said to impose no affirmative obligation on governments to act, provide services, or protect individuals and populations, it does serve three primary functions: (1) it allocates power among the federal government and the states (federalism), (2) it divides power among the three branches of government (separation of powers), and (3) it limits government power (to protect individual liberties).[7] In the realm of public health, then, the Constitution acts as both a fountain and a levee; it originates the flow of power—to preserve the public health—and it curbs that power—to protect individual freedoms.[8]

If the Constitution is a fountain from which government powers flow, federalism represents a partition in the fountain that separates federal and state powers.[9] By separating the pool of legislative authority into these two tiers of government, federalism preserves the balance of power among national and state authorities. Theoretically, the division of government powers is distinct and clear. The federal government is a government of limited power whose acts must be authorized by the Constitution. The states, by contrast, retain the powers they possessed as sovereign governments before ratification of the Constitution.[10] The most important state authority is the power to protect the health, safety, morals, and general welfare of the population. In practice, however, the powers of the federal and state governments intersect in innumerable areas, particularly in areas of traditional state concern, like public health.

Federalism functions as a sorting device for determining which government (federal, state, or local) may respond legitimately to a public health threat. Often, federal, state, and local governments exercise public health powers concurrently. Where conflicts among the various levels of government arise, however, federal laws likely preempt state or local actions pursuant to the supremacy clause: the "Constitution, and the Laws of the United States...and all Treaties made...shall be the supreme law of the Land."[11]

In addition to establishing a federalist system, the Constitution separates governmental powers into three branches: (1) the *legislative* branch, which has the power to create laws; (2) the *executive* branch, which has the power to enforce the laws; and (3) the *judicial* branch, which has the power to interpret the laws. States have similar schemes of governance pursuant to their own constitutions. By separating the powers of government, the Constitution provides a system of checks and balances that is thought to reduce the possibility of governmental oppression.

The separation of powers doctrine is essential to public health. Each branch of government possesses a unique constitutional authority to create, enforce, or interpret health policy. The *legislative branch* creates health policy and allocates the necessary resources to effectuate that policy. Some believe that legislators are ill-equipped to make complex public health decisions. (See Chapter 23 for a detailed discussion.) Yet, as the only "purely" elected branch of government, members of federal or state legislatures ultimately are politically accountable to the people.

The *executive branch,* which enforces health policy, has an equally significant role in public health. Most public health agencies reside in the executive branch and are responsible for implementing legislation that may often require establishing and enforcing complex health regulations. The executive branch and its agencies are uniquely positioned to govern public health. Public health agencies are designed and created for the purpose of advancing community health. They have sufficient expertise and resources to focus on health problems for extended periods of time. Agencies, however, may occasionally suffer from stale thinking, complicity with the subjects of regulation, and the inability to balance competing values and claims for resources.

The *judicial branch,* which interprets the law and resolves legal disputes, also has an important role concerning public health. Courts can exert substantial control over public health policy by determining the boundaries of government power and the zone of autonomy, privacy, and liberty to be afforded individuals. Courts decide whether a public health statute or policy is constitutional, whether agency action is authorized legislatively, whether agency officials have sufficient evidence to support their actions, and whether governmental officials or private parties have acted negligently. Although the exercise of judicial power may serve public health, courts may fail to review the substance of health policy choices critically. Federal judges, once appointed, are politically less accountable (though state judges may be elected). Courts are bound by the facts of a particular case or controversy, may be overly influenced by disfavored expert opinions, and may focus too intently on individual rights at the expense of public health protections.

The separation of powers doctrine is not a model of efficiency. Dividing broad powers among branches of governments significantly burdens governmental operations, which may actually thwart public health. The constitutional design appears to value restraint in policy making: legislative representatives reconcile demands for public health funding with competing claims for societal resources; the executive branch straddles the line between congressional authorization and judicial restrictions on that authority; and the judiciary tempers public health measures with individual rights. As a result, the possibility of strong public health governance by any given branch is compromised in exchange for constitutional checks and balances that prevent overreaching and foster political accountability.

A third constitutional function is to limit governmental power to protect individual liberties. Governmental actions to promote the communal good often infringe on individual freedoms. Public health regulation and individual rights may directly conflict. Resolving the tension between population-based regulations and individual rights requires a trade-off. Thus, although the Constitution grants extensive powers to governments, it also limits that power by protecting individual rights and freedoms. The Bill of Rights (the first 10 amendments to the Constitution), together with the Reconstruction Amendments (13th, 14th, and 15th Amendments) and other constitutional provisions, create a zone of individual liberty, autonomy, privacy, and economic freedom that exists beyond the reach of the government.* Public health law struggles to determine the point at which governmental authority to promote the population's health must yield to individual rights and freedoms.

Understanding and defining the limits of public health powers by the federal, state, and local governments is an integral part of our constitutional system of government. In the following sections, the constitutional authority and exercise of public health powers by each of these levels of government are explored.

Federal Public Health Powers

The federal government must draw its authority to act from specific, enumerated powers. Before an act of Congress is deemed constitutional, two questions must be asked: (1) does the Constitution affirmatively authorize Congress to act, and (2) does the exercise of that power improperly interfere with any constitutionally protected interest?

In theory, the United States is a government of limited, defined powers. In reality, political and judicial expansion of federal powers through the doctrine of implied powers allows the federal government considerable authority to act in the interests of public health and safety. Under the doctrine of implied powers, the federal govern-

*See, for example, Article I, § 9 (federal and state government may not criminally punish conduct that was lawful when committed); Article I, § 10 (no state shall impair the obligation of contracts); and Article IV ("Citizens of each State shall be entitled to all Privileges and Immunities of Citizens in the several States") of the Constitution.

ment may employ all means "necessary and proper" to achieve the objectives of constitutionally enumerated national powers.[12] For public health purposes, the chief powers are the powers to tax, to spend, and to regulate interstate commerce. These powers provide Congress with independent authority to raise revenue for public health services and to regulate, both directly and indirectly, private activities that endanger human health. The taxing power is a primary means for achieving public health objectives by influencing, directly and indirectly, health-related behavior through tax relief and tax burdens. Tax relief encourages private, health-promoting activity; tax burdens discourage risk behavior. Through various forms of tax relief, government provides incentives for private activities that it views as advantageous to community health (e.g., tax benefits for self-insured health care plans).

Public health taxation also regulates private behavior by economically penalizing risk-taking activities. Tax policy discourages a number of activities that the government regards as unhealthy, dangerous, immoral, or adverse to human health. Thus, the government imposes significant excise or manufacturing taxes on tobacco, alcoholic beverages, and firearms; penalizes certain behaviors such as gambling; and influences individual and business decisions through taxes on gasoline or ozone-depleting chemicals that contribute to environmental degradation.

The spending power provides Congress with independent authority to allocate resources for the public good or general welfare without the need to justify its spending by reference to a specific enumerated power.[13] Closely connected to the power to tax, the spending power authorizes expenditures expressly for the public's health. The grant of such expenditures can be conditioned on a number of terms or requirements. The conditional spending power is thus like a private contract: in return for federal funds, the states agree to comply with federally imposed conditions. Such conditions are constitutionally allowed provided the conditions are clearly authorized by statute and a reasonable relationship exists between the condition imposed and the program's purposes.[14,15]

The need for federal public health funds effectively induces state conformance with federal regulatory standards. Congress and federal agencies use conditional spending to induce states to conform to federal standards in numerous public health contexts, including direct health care, prevention services, biomedical and health services research, public health regulation and safety inspection, and workplace safety and health.

The commerce power, more than any other enumerated power, affords Congress potent regulatory authority. Congress has the power to regulate: (1) all commerce among foreign nations and Indian tribes and (2) interstate commerce among the states.[16] Although the scope of the interstate commerce power has been judicially limited during the course of our constitutional history, the current conception of Congress' commerce powers is extensive.

The Court's modern construction of the interstate commerce power has been described as "plenary" or all-embracing, and has been exerted to affect virtually every aspect of social life.[17,18] The expansive interpretation of the commerce clause has enabled the national government to invade traditional realms of state public health power, including the fields of environmental protection, food and drug purity, occupational health and safety, and other public health matters. Thus, the commerce clause gives national authorities the power to regulate throughout the public health spectrum.

Any legitimate exercise of federal taxing, spending, or commerce power in the interests of public health may be determined to trump state public health regulation. By authority of the supremacy clause, Congress may preempt state public health regulation, even if the state is acting squarely within its police powers. Federal preemption occurs in many areas of public health law, such as with cigarette labeling and advertising regulations and occupational health and safety.

The federal government, however, sometimes does not preempt state laws. Congress may offer states the choice of either establishing regulatory schemes that reflect federal standards or having federal regulation preempt state law. This model, known as "cooperative federalism," is found in federal public health statutes concerning water quality, occupational health and safety, and conservation, and is the predominant approach to federal–state relations in environmental law.

As a result of broad interpretations of its supreme, enumerated powers, the federal government has a vast presence in public health. It is nearly impossible to find a field of public health that is not heavily influenced by U.S. governmental policy. Public health functions, including public funding for health care, safe food, effective drugs, clean water, a beneficial environment, and prevention services, can be found in an array of federal agencies. The bulk of all federal health responsibilities lies with the Department of Health and Human Services (DHHS) and its many subagencies, including the Centers for Disease Control and Prevention (CDC), the National Institutes of Health (NIH), and the Food and Drug Administration (FDA). The Department of Agriculture, the Department of Labor (DOL), and the Environmental Protection Agency (EPA), to name a few, also have important public health functions.

State Police Powers

Despite the broad federal presence in modern public health regulation, historically, states have had a predominant role in providing population-based health services. States still account for the majority of traditional public health spending for public health services (not including personal medical services or the environment). The 10th Amendment of the Constitution reserves to the states all powers that are neither given to the federal government nor prohibited by the Constitution. These reserved powers, known as the police powers, support a dominant role in protecting the public's health.[19]

The police powers represent the state's authority to further the goal of all government, which is to promote the general welfare of society. Police powers can be defined as

> the inherent authority of the state (and, through delegation, local government) to enact laws and promulgate regulations to protect, preserve and promote the health, safety, morals, and general welfare of the people. To achieve these communal benefits, the state retains the power to restrict, within federal and state constitutional limits, private interests—personal interests in liberty, autonomy, privacy, and association, as well as economic interests in freedom of contract and uses of property.[20]

This definition of "police power" reflects three principal characteristics: (1) the government purpose is to promote the public good, (2) the state authority to act permits the restriction of private interests, and (3) the scope of state powers is pervasive. States exercise police powers for the common good, that is, to ensure that communities live in safety and security, in conditions that are conducive to good health, with moral standards, and, generally speaking, without unreasonable interference with human well-being.

Government, in order to achieve common goods, is empowered to enact legislation, regulate, and adjudicate in ways that necessarily limit, or even eliminate, private interests. Thus, government has inherent power to interfere with personal interests in autonomy, liberty, privacy, and association, as well as economic interests in ownership and uses of private property. The police power affords state government the authority to keep society free from noxious exercises of private rights. The state retains discretion to determine what is considered injurious or unhealthful and the manner in which to regulate, consistent with constitutional protections of personal interests.

Police powers in the context of public health include all laws and regulations directly or indirectly intended to reduce morbidity and premature mortality in the population. The police powers have enabled states and local governments to promote and preserve the public health in areas ranging from injury and disease prevention to sanitation, waste disposal, and water and air pollution. Police powers exercised by the states include vaccination, isolation and quarantine, inspection of commercial and residential premises, abatement of unsanitary conditions or other nuisances, and regulation of air and surface water contaminants, as well as restriction on the public's access to polluted areas, standards for pure food and drinking water, extermination of vermin, fluoridization of municipal water supplies, and licensure of physicians and other health care professionals.

Local Public Health Powers

In addition to the significant roles that federal and state governments have concerning public health law in the constitutional system, local governments also have important public health powers. Public health officials in local governments, including counties, cities, municipalities, and special districts, are often on the front line of public health. They may be directly responsible for assembling public health surveillance data, implementing federal and state programs, administering federal or state public health laws, operating public health clinics, and setting public health policies for their specific populations.

Although states have inherent powers as sovereign governments, localities have delegated power. Local governments in the constitutional system are subsidiaries of their states. As a result, any powers that local governments have to enact public health law or policies must be granted either in the state constitution or in state statutes. Sometimes state grants of power are so broad and generic that they afford cities home rule. For example, if the state constitution expressly affords a city the power to protect the health, safety, and welfare of local inhabitants, this is an important guarantee of home rule. Absent constitutionally protected delegations of power to local governments, however, states may modify, clarify, preempt, or remove "home rule" powers of local government.

New Federalism

Since the founding of the United States, the division of federal and state governmental powers has been an important and highly controversial part of our federalist system of government. The Supreme Court, at least since Franklin Delano Roosevelt's New Deal, has liberally interpreted the federal government's enumerated powers, leading to an unprecedented expansion of national public health authority. More recently, however, the Rehnquist Court has emphasized that there exist enforceable limits on Congress' powers. Known as new federalism, federal courts have begun to hold that federal police powers should be circumscribed, with more authority returned to the states.

The Supreme Court has narrowed the scope of the commerce power, holding that the federal government cannot regulate purely intrastate police power matters. In *United States v. Lopez,* the Court held that Congress exceeded its commerce clause authority by making gun possession within a school zone a federal offense. Concluding that possessing a gun within a school zone did not "substantially affect" interstate commerce, the Court declared the statute unconstitutional.[21]

In addition to *Lopez*, the Court has held in a series of recent cases that Congress, even if empowered to act for the public good, must exert its authority in ways that do not excessively intrude on state sovereignty. In *New York v. the United States*, the Supreme Court struck down a federal statute providing for the disposal of radioactive waste as violating the 10th Amendment.[22] The Constitution, stated the Court, does not confer upon Congress the ability to "commandeer the legislative processes of the States by directly compelling them to enact and enforce a federal regulatory program."[22(p.175)] The Supreme Court used the same reasoning to overturn provisions in the Brady Handgun Violence Prevention Act, which directed state and local law enforcement officers to conduct background checks on prospective handgun purchasers.[23]

In this era of new federalism, some federal public health laws may be vulnerable to state challenges. National environmental regulations are particularly at risk because they invade core state concerns and are being challenged in the court system.

In summary, a highly complex, politically charged relationship exists between various levels of government regulating for the public's health—federal, state, and local. The Constitution ostensibly grants the federal government limited powers, but these powers have been construed in ways that have facilitated an enormous growth of national public health authority. The Constitution does not grant states any power because, as sovereign governments that predated the Republic, the states already had broad powers. Known as the police powers, states may act to protect the health, safety, and well-being of the population. Local governments, as subsidiary entities of states, possess only those public health powers delegated by the state. In an era of new federalism, the Supreme Court has gradually limited federal public health powers and returned them to the states. Even so, the vast majority of public health functions currently exercised by the federal government are likely to survive constitutional scrutiny.

THE MODERN PUBLIC HEALTH AGENCY

The deep-seated problems of modern society caused by industrialization and urbanization pose complex, highly technical challenges that require expertise, flexibility, and deliberative study over the long term. Solutions cannot be found within traditional governmental structures such as representative assemblies or governors' offices. As a result, governments have formed specialized entities within the executive branch to pursue the goals of population health and safety. These administrative agencies form the bulwark for public health activities in the United States. Public health agencies are found at all levels of government—federal, state, and local.

Federal Public Health Agencies

The modern role of the federal government in public health is broad and complex. Public health functions, which include public funding for health care, safe food, effective drugs, clean water, a beneficial environment, and prevention services, can be found in an array of agencies. The bulk of all health responsibilities lies with the DHHS and its many subparts. (See Chapter 3 for a more detailed discussion.) However, the Department of Agriculture, the DOL, and the EPA, to name a few, also have important public health functions.

The DHHS is the umbrella agency under which most public health functions are located. Under the aegis of the DHHS, various programs promote and protect health. The Health Care Financing Administration was created in 1977 to administer the Medicare and Medicaid programs. The CDC provides technical and financial support to states in monitoring, controlling, and preventing disease. The CDC's efforts include initiatives such as childhood vaccination and emergency response to infectious disease outbreaks. NIH conducts and supports research, trains investigators, and disseminates scientific information. The FDA ensures that food is pure and safe, and that drugs, biologicals, medical devices, cosmetics, and products that emit radiation are safe and effective.

The DOL administers a variety of federal labor laws, some of which pertain to workers' rights to safe and healthy working conditions. Specifically, the Occupational Safety and Health Administration (OSHA) develops occupational safety and health standards and monitors compliance. In 1970, the EPA was created to control and reduce pollution in the air, water, and ground. The EPA develops national standards, provides technical assistance, and enforces environmental regulations.

State Public Health Agencies

The state's plenary power to safeguard citizens' health includes the authority to create administrative agencies devoted to that task. State legislation determines the administrative organization, mission, and functions of public health agencies. Contemporary state public health agencies take many different forms that defy simple classification. (See Chapter 3 for a more detailed discussion.) Before 1960, state public health functions were located in health departments with policy-making functions residing in a board of health (e.g., issuing and enforcing regulations). As programs expanded (e.g, increased federal funding for categorical programs and block grants), certain public health functions were assigned to other state agencies (e.g., mental health, medical care financing for the indigent, and environmental protection). Currently, 55 state-level health agencies (including the District of Columbia, American Samoa, Guam, Puerto Rico, and the U.S. Virgin Islands) exist, each of which may be a free-standing, independent department or a component of a larger state agency.

The trend since the 1960s has been to merge state health departments with other departments—often social services, Medicaid, mental health, and/or substance abuse—to form superagencies. Under this framework, the public health unit is often called a *division* of health or public health. Another common framework is to assign public health functions to a cabinet-level agency. Under this framework, the public health unit is often called a *department* of health or public health.[24–26]

The trend has also been to eliminate or reduce the influence of boards of health. These boards, once ubiquitous and highly influential, are now often replaced or supplemented with specialized boards or committees established by state statute to oversee technical or politically controversial programs (e.g., genetics, rural health, expansion of health care facilities).[27] The chief executive officer of the public health agency—the commissioner or, less often, the secretary—is usually politically appointed by the governor, but may be appointed by the head of a superagency or, rarely, the board of health. Qualification standards may include medical and public health expertise, but increasingly, chief executives with political or administrative experience are appointed.

Local Public Health Agencies

Local government exercises voluminous public health functions derived from the state, such as air, water, and noise pollution; sanitation and sewage; cigarette sales and smoking in public accommodations; drinking water fluoridation; drug paraphernalia sales; firearm registration and prohibition; infectious diseases; rodents and infestations; housing codes; sanitary food and beverages; trash disposal; and animal control. Local government also often regulates (or owns and operates) hospitals or nursing homes.

Municipalities, like the states, have created public health agencies to carry out their functions.[28] Local public health agencies have varied forms and structures: centralized (directly operated by the state), decentralized (formed and managed by local government), or mixed.[29,30] Local boards of health, or less often, governmental councils, still exist in most local public health agencies with responsibility for health regulation and policy. The courts usually permit local agencies to exercise broad discretion in matters of public health, sometimes even beyond the geographic area if necessary to protect the city's inhabitants (e.g., during a waterborne disease outbreak).

Local public health agencies serve a political subdivision of the state such as a city (a municipality or municipal corporation), town, township, county, or borough. Some local public health functions are undertaken by special districts that are limited governmental structures that serve special purposes (e.g., drinking water, sewerage, sanitation, or mosquito abatement).

Rule Making, Enforcement, and Quasi-Judicial Powers

Public health agencies are part of the executive branch of government but wield considerable authority to make rules to control private behavior, interpret statutes and regulations, and adjudicate disputes about whether an individual or company has conformed with health and safety standards. Under the separation of powers doctrine, the executive branch is supposed to enforce law, but not enact or interpret it. Nevertheless, the lines between law making, enforcement, and adjudication have become blurred with the rise of the administrative state.

The courts, at least theoretically, can carefully scrutinize legislative grants of power to public health agencies. Conventionally, representative assemblies may not delegate legislative or judicial functions to the executive branch. Known as "nondelegation," this doctrine holds that policy-making functions should be undertaken by the legislative branch of government (because assemblies are politically accountable), whereas adjudicative functions should be undertaken by the judicial branch (because courts are independent).

The nondelegation doctrine is rarely used by federal courts to limit agency powers.* The doctrine, however, has received varying interpretations at the state level—some jurisdictions liberally permit delegations whereas others are more restrictive. New York State's highest court, for example, found unconstitutional a health department prohibition on smoking in public places because the legislature, not the health department, should make the "trade-offs" between health and freedom. "Manifestly," the court said, "it is the province of the people's elected representatives, rather than appointed administrators, to resolve difficult social problems by making choices among competing ends."[31(p.1356)]

Rule Making

Although public health agencies possess considerable power to issue detailed rules, they must do so fairly and publicly. Federal and state administrative procedure acts (as well as agency-enabling acts) govern the deliberative processes that agencies must undertake in issuing rules. (Unless specified by statute, state administrative procedure acts generally have been held not to apply to local governmental agencies). Administrative procedure acts often require two different forms: (1) *informal*, simple and flexible procedures often consisting of prior notice (e.g., publication in federal or state register), written comments by interested persons, and a statement of basis and purpose for the rule; and (2) *formal*, more elaborate procedures often requiring a hearing.

Enforcement

Health departments do not possess only legislative power. They also have the executive power to enforce the regulations that they have promulgated. Enforcement of laws and regulations is squarely within the constitutional powers of executive agencies. Although legislatures set the penalty for violations of health and safety standards, the executive branch monitors compliance and seeks redress against those who fail to conform. Pursuant to their enforcement power, health departments may inspect premises and businesses, investigate complaints, and generally monitor the activities of those who come within the orbit of health and safety statutes and administrative rules.

Quasi-Judicial

Modern administrative agencies do not simply issue and enforce health and safety standards. They also interpret statutes and rules as well as adjudicate disputes about whether standards are violated. Federal and state administrative procedure acts and agency-enabling legislation often enumerate the procedures that agencies must follow in adjudicating disputes. Rarely, these laws require *formal adjudications*. Formal adjudications typically are conducted by an administrative law judge (ALJ), followed by an appeal to the agency head. Formal adjudications usually include notice, the right to present evidence, and agency findings of fact and law as well as reasons for the decision. Even in the absence of statutory requirements, federal and state constitutions require procedural due process if the regulation deprives an individual of "property" or "liberty" interests.

In summary, modern administrative agencies exercise *legislative power* to issue rules that carry heavy penalties, *executive power* to investigate potential violations of health and safety standards and prosecute offenders, and *judicial power* to interpret law and adjudicate disputes over violations of governing standards. Agency powers have developed for reasons of expediency (because of agency expertise) and politics (because "specialists" are presumed to act according to disinterested scientific judgments).

Although ample agency power is critically important for achieving public health purposes, it is also troubling and perplexing in a constitu-

*Since 1935, the Supreme Court has rarely invalidated health and safety regulation as an impermissible delegation of law-making power to the executive. *See, e.g., Touby v. United States,* 500 U.S. 160 (1991).

tional democracy. One important problem is that commercial regulation may simply transfer wealth from one private interest group to another rather than promote a public good. For example, licenses can exclude competitors from the market, or regulation of one industry may benefit another providing comparable services (e.g., coal, electrical, or nuclear energy). A related problem is that agencies may be unduly influenced, or "captured," by powerful constituencies or interest groups. Agencies, over the long term, may come to defend the economic interests of regulatory subjects. Finally, agencies may operate in ways that appear unfair or arbitrary, inefficient or bureaucratic, or unacceptable to the public. The very strengths of public health authorities (e.g., neutrality, expertise, and broad powers) can become liabilities if they appear politically unaccountable and aloof from the real concerns and needs of the governed. This is why governors' offices, representative assemblies, and courts struggle over the political and constitutional limits that should be placed on agency action that is nominally intended for the public's health and safety.

PUBLIC HEALTH LAW REFORM*

Effective public health protection is technically and politically difficult. Law cannot solve all, or even most, of the challenges facing public health authorities. Yet, law can become an important part of the ongoing work of creating the conditions necessary for people to live healthier and safer lives. A public health law that contributes to health will, of course, be up-to-date in the methods of assessment and intervention it authorizes. It should also conform to modern standards of law and prevailing social norms. It should be designed to enhance the reality and the public perception of the health department's rationality, fairness, and responsibility. It should help health agencies overcome the defects of their limited jurisdiction over health threats facing the population. Finally, both a new law and the process of its enactment should provide an opportunity for the health department to challenge the apathy about public health that is all too common within both the government and the population at large.

The law relating to public health is scattered across countless statutes and regulations at the state and local level. Problems of antiquity, inconsistency, redundancy, and ambiguity render these laws ineffective, or even counterproductive, in advancing the population's health. In particular, health codes frequently are outdated, built up in layers over different periods of time, and highly fragmented among the 50 states and territories.

Problem of Antiquity

The most striking characteristic of state public health law and the one that underlies many of its defects is its overall antiquity. Certainly, some statutes are relatively recent in origin, such as those relating to health threats that became salient in the latter part of the twentieth century (e.g., environmental law). However, a great deal of public health law was framed in the late nineteenth and early to mid-twentieth century and contains elements that are 40–100 years old (e.g., infectious disease law). Certainly, old laws are not necessarily bad laws. A well-written statute may remain useful, effective, and constitutional for many decades.

Nevertheless, old public health statutes that have not been altered substantially since their enactment are often outmoded in ways that directly reduce both their effectiveness and their conformity with modern standards. These laws often do not reflect contemporary scientific understandings of injury and disease (e.g., surveillance, prevention, and response) or legal norms for the protection of individual rights. Rather, public health laws use scientific and legal standards that prevailed at the time they were enacted. Society faces different sorts of risks today and deploys different methods of assessment and intervention. When many of these statutes were written, public health (e.g., epidemiology

**Source:* This section originally appeared at 99 Colum. L. Rev. 59 (1999). Reprinted by permission.

and biostatistics) and behavioral (e.g., client-centered counselling) sciences were in their infancy. Modern prevention and treatment methods did not exist.

At the same time, many public health laws predate the vast changes in constitutional (e.g., tighter scrutiny and procedural safeguards) and statutory (e.g., disability discrimination) law that have transformed social and legal conceptions of individual rights. Failure to reform these laws may leave public health authorities vulnerable to legal challenge on grounds that they are unconstitutional or that they are preempted by modern federal statutes such as the Americans with Disabilities Act. Even if state public health law is not challenged in court, public health authorities may feel unsure about applying old legal remedies to new health problems within a very different social milieu.

Problem of Multiple Layers of Law

Related to the problem of antiquity is the problem of multiple layers of law. The law in most states consists of successive layers of statutes and amendments—built up in some cases over 100 years or more in response to existing or perceived health threats. This is particularly troublesome in the area of infectious diseases, which forms a substantial part of state health codes. Because communicable disease laws have been passed piecemeal in response to specific epidemics, they tell the history of disease control in the United States—for example, smallpox, yellow fever, cholera, tuberculosis, venereal diseases, polio, and acquired immune deficiency syndrome (AIDS). Through a process of accretion, the majority of states have come to have several classes of communicable disease law, each with different powers and protections of individual rights: those aimed at traditional sexually transmitted diseases (or venereal diseases), including gonorrhea, syphilis, chlamydia, herpes; those targeted at specific currently or historically pressing diseases, such as tuberculosis and HIV; and those applicable to "communicable" or "contagious" diseases, a residual class of conditions ranging from measles to malaria whose control does not usually seem to raise problematic political or social issues. There are, of course, legitimate reasons to treat some diseases separately. Nevertheless, affording health officials substantially different powers, under different criteria and procedures, for different diseases is more an accident of history than a rational approach to prevention and control.

The disparate legal structure of state public health laws can significantly undermine their effectiveness. Laws enacted piecemeal over time are inconsistent, redundant, and ambiguous. Even the most astute lawyers in departments of health or offices of the attorneys general have difficulty understanding these arcane laws and applying them to contemporary health threats.

Problem of Inconsistency among the States and Territories

Public health laws remain fragmented not only within states but also among them. Health codes within the 50 states and the U.S. territories have evolved independently, leading to profound variation in the structure, substance, and procedures for detecting, controlling, and preventing injury and disease. In fact, statutes and regulations among American jurisdictions vary so significantly in definitions, methods, age, and scope that they defy orderly categorization. Ordinarily, a different approach among the states is not a problem and is often perceived as a virtue; an important value of federalism is that states can become laboratories for innovative solutions to challenging health problems. Nevertheless, there may be good reason for greater uniformity among the states in matters of public health. Health threats are rarely confined to single jurisdictions, but pose risks within whole regions or the nation itself. For example, geographic boundaries are largely irrelevant to issues of air or water pollution, disposal of toxic waste, or the spread of infectious diseases.

Public health law, therefore, should be reformed so that it conforms with modern scientific and legal standards, is more consistent within and among states, and is more uniform in its approach to different health threats. Rather than making artificial distinctions among diseases, public health interventions should be based primarily on the degree of risk, the cost and efficacy of the response, and the burdens on human rights. A single set of standards and procedures would add needed clarity and coherence to legal regulation and would reduce the opportunity for politically motivated disputes about how to classify newly emergent health threats.

Guidelines for Public Health Law Reform

Public health law reform efforts should include the following elements:

1. *Define a mission and essential functions. Take responsibility for ensuring the conditions of health.*

State public health statutes should define a cogent mission for the health department and identify a full set of essential public health functions that it should, or must, perform. Broad, and well-considered, mission statements in state public health statutes are important because they establish the purposes or goals of public health agencies.[32] By doing so, they inform and influence the activities of government and, perhaps ultimately, the expectations of society about the scope of public health.

2. *Provide a full range of public health powers.*

Voluntary cooperation is the primary way to obtain compliance with public health measures. However, where voluntary strategies fail, public health officials need a full range of powers to ensure compliance with health and safety standards. At present, public health officials in many states have a sterile choice of either exercising draconian authority, such as deprivation of liberty, or refraining from coercion at all. The temptation is either to exercise no statutory power or to reach for measures that are too restrictive of individual liberty to be acceptable in a modern democratic society. As a result, authorities may make wrong choices in two opposite directions: failing to react in the face of a real threat to health or overreacting by exercising powers that are more intrusive than necessary. Public health authorities need a more *flexible* set of tools, ranging from incentives and minimally coercive interventions to highly restrictive measures.

3. *Impose substantive limits on powers (a demonstrated threat of significant risk).*

Whereas public health authorities should have all the powers they need to safeguard the public's health, statutes should place substantive limits on the exercise of those powers. The legislature should clearly state the circumstances under which authorities may curtail liberty, autonomy, privacy, and property interests. At present, a few state statutes articulate clear criteria for the exercise of public health powers; others provide vague or incomplete standards; still others leave their use partly or wholly within the discretion of public health officials. Although public health authorities may prefer an unfettered decision-making process, the lack of criteria does not serve their interests or the interests of regulatory subjects. Effective and constitutionally sound public health statutes should set out a rational and reliable way to assess risk to ensure that the health measure is necessary for public protection. Most importantly, public health authorities should be empowered to employ a compulsory intervention only to avert a significant risk based on objective and reliable scientific evidence and made on an individualized (case-by-case) basis.

4. *Impose procedural limits on powers (procedural due process).*

There are good reasons, both constitutional and normative, for legislatures to require health authorities to use a fair process whenever their decisions seriously infringe on liberty, autonomy, proprietary, or other important interests. For example, if health authorities seek to close a restaurant, withdraw a professional (e.g., physician) or institutional (e.g., restaurant) license, or restrict personal freedom (e.g., civil confinement), they should provide procedural due process. Procedural protections help to ensure that health officials make fair and impartial decisions and to reduce community perceptions that public health agencies arbitrarily employ coercive measures. Where few formal procedures exist, public health officials risk rendering biased or inconsistent decisions and erroneously depriving persons and businesses of their rights and freedoms. Although public health authorities may feel that procedural due process is burdensome and an impediment to expeditious action, it can actually facilitate deliberative and accurate decision making.

5. *Provide strong protection against discrimination.*

Throughout the modern history of disease control, the stigma associated with serious diseases and the social hostility that is often directed at those with, or at risk of, disease has interfered with the effective operation of public health programs. The field of public health has always had to consider issues of race, gender, sexual orientation, and socioeconomic status carefully. Persons who fear social repercussions may resist testing or fail to seek needed services. As part of any effort to safeguard the public's health, legislators must find ways to address both the reality and the perception of social risk. Public health statutes should have strong nondiscrimination provisions.

6. *Provide strong protection for the privacy and security of public health information.*

Privacy and security of public health data are highly important from the perspective of both the individual and the public at large. Individuals seek protection of privacy so that they can control intimate health information. They have an interest in avoiding the embarrassment and stigma of unauthorized disclosures to family or friends. They similarly have an interest in avoiding discrimination that could result from unauthorized disclosures to employers, insurers, or landlords. At the same time, privacy and security protection can advance the public's health. Privacy assurances can facilitate individual participation in public health programs and promote trust between health authorities and the community. Public health laws, therefore, should have strong safeguards of privacy to protect these individual and societal interests.

THE FUTURE OF PUBLIC HEALTH LAW

This chapter explores the varied roles of law in advancing the public's health. The field of public health is purposive and interventionist. It does not settle for existing conditions of health, but actively seeks effective techniques for identifying and reducing health threats. Law is a critically important but perennially neglected tool in furthering the public's health. To achieve improvements in public health, law must not be seen as an arcane, indecipherable set of technical rules buried deep within state health codes. Rather, public health law must be seen broadly as the authority and responsibility of government to ensure the conditions for the population's health. As such, public health law has transcending importance in how we think about government, politics, and health policy in America.

CHAPTER REVIEW

1. Public health law has at least five characteristics that help separate it from other fields at the intersection of law and health:
   - government
   - populations
   - relationships
   - services
   - coercion
2. Political and judicial expansion of federal powers through the doctrine of implied powers allows the federal government considerable authority to act in the interests of public health and safety. For public health purposes, the chief federal powers are the powers to tax, to spend, and to regulate interstate commerce.
3. Police powers provide a dominant role for the states by affording authority to promote the general welfare of society. The state and, through delegation, the local government enact laws and promulgate regulations to protect and promote health.

4. The Supreme Court has narrowed the scope of the commerce power, holding that the federal government cannot regulate purely intrastate police power matters. Some federal public health laws may be vulnerable to state challenges.
5. Public health agencies are part of the executive branch of government but wield considerable authority to make rules to control private behavior, interpret statutes and regulations, and adjudicate disputes. Health departments also have the executive power to enforce the regulations they have promulgated.
6. The most striking characteristic of state public health law is its *antiquity*. Public health laws use scientific and legal standards that prevailed at the time they were enacted.
7. Public health law should be reformed so that it conforms with modern scientific and legal standards, is more consistent within and among states, and is more uniform in its approach to different health threats.

REFERENCES

1. L.O. Gostin et al., "The Law and the Public's Health: A Study of Infectious Disease Law in the United States," *Columbia Law Review 99,* no. 1 (1999): 59–128.
2. F.P. Grad, *Public Health Law Manual,* 2d ed. (Washington, DC: American Public Health Association, 1990).
3. Institute of Medicine, *The Future of Public Health* (Washington, DC: National Academy Press, 1988).
4. *Black's Law Dictionary,* 7th ed. (New York: West, 1999).
5. Department of Health and Human Services, *Vision of 2010: Healthy People in Healthy Communities* <http://odphp.osophs.dhhs.gov/pubs/hp2000>; *see* Kristine M. Gebbie, *Identification of Health Paradigms in Use in State Public Health Agencies* (New York: Columbia University, School of Nursing, 1997).
6. J.S. Durch et al., eds., *Improving Health in the Community: A Role for Performance Monitoring* (Washington, DC: Institute of Medicine, 1997).
7. E. Chemerinsky, *Constitutional Law: Principles and Policies* (New York: Aspen Law & Business, 1997), 1–6.
8. J. Areen et al., *Law, Science and Medicine,* 2d ed. (New York: Foundation Press, 1996), 520.
9. J.G. Hodge, Jr., "Implementing Modern Public Health Goals through Government: An Examination of New Federalism and Public Health Law," *Journal of Contemporary Health Law & Policy* 14 (1997): 93–126.
10. *Gibbons v. Ogden,* 22 U.S. 1 (1824).
11. U.S. Constitution, art. 6, cl. 2.
12. *McCulloch v. Maryland,* 17 U.S. (4 Wheat.) 316 (1819).
13. *United States v. Butler,* 297 U.S. 1 (1936).
14. *Pennhurst State School and Hospital v. Halderman,* 451 U.S. 1 (1981).
15. *South Dakota v. Dole,* 483 U.S. 203 (1987).
16. U.S. Constitution, art 1, sec. 8, cl. 3.
17. *NLRB v. Jones & Laughlin Steel Corp.,* 301 U.S. 1 (1937).
18. *United States v. Darby,* 312 U.S. 100 (1941).
19. *Jacobson v. Massachusetts,* 197 U.S. 11 (1905).
20. L. Gostin, *Public Health Law: Power, Duty, Restraint* (Berkeley, CA: University of California Press, 2000).
21. *United States v. Lopez,* 115 Sup. Ct. 1624 (1995).
22. *New York v. the United States,* 505 U.S. 144 (1992).
23. *Printz v. United States,* 117 Sup. Ct. 2365 (1997).
24. S. Dandoy, "The State Public Health Department," in *Principles of Public Health Practice,* eds. D. Scutchfield and W. Keck (Albany, NY: Delmar Publishers, 1997).
25. B. Turnock, *Public Health: What It Is and How It Works* (Gaithersburg, MD: Aspen Publishers, 1997), 145–156.
26. K.M. Gebbie, "Steps to Changing State Public Health Structures," *Journal of Public Health Management and Practice 4,* no. 5 (1998): 33–41.
27. D.J. Gossert and C. Arden Miller, "State Boards of Health, Their Members and Commitments," *American Journal of Public Health 63,* no. 6 (1973): 486–493.
28. C. Arden Miller et al., "Statutory Authorization for the Work of Local Health Departments," *American Journal of Public Health 67,* no. 10 (1977): 940–945.
29. National Association of County and City Health Officials, *Profile of Local Health Departments, 1992–1993* (1995).
30. G.P. Mays, P.K. Halverson, C. Arden Miller, "Assessing the Performance of Local Public Health Systems: A Survey of State Health Agency Efforts," *Journal of Public Health Management and Practice 4,* no.4 (1998): 63–78.
31. *Boreali v. Axelrod,* 517 N.E. 2d 1350 (1987).
32. K.M. Gebbie and I. Hwang, *Identification of Health Paradigms in Use in State Public Health Agencies* (New York: Columbia University School of Nursing, 1997).

CHAPTER 6

Ethics and Public Health

Sholom Glouberman

The major building blocks of public health action include: (1) the implementation of communal measures of sanitation, inspection, and public health nursing; (2) concern with health care coverage; and (3) health promotion. Another, evolving block focuses on inequalities in health. Each of these major elements give rise not only to health policy issues, but also to important ethical questions. An ethical struggle between the sanctity of the individual and the consequences to the larger population is manifest in compulsory vaccination, the detention of contagious individuals, and the mandatory reporting of sexually transmitted diseases (STDs). Similarly, ethical issues arise in debates over expanded health care coverage, including the elements of access and choice. Fostering health promotion raises questions concerning the role of government versus the individual in assuming responsibility for risk behaviors. What is the role of government in reducing health inequalities that are likely related to a variety of social determinants? A recommendation is made for new ways of looking at these traditional ethical issues.

Public health organizations and their managers routinely face ethical issues in developing and applying health resources to improve population health. Whether explicitly considered or implicitly addressed, these issues profoundly shape public health organizations and their relationships with internal and external constituents. Despite substantial changes in both the formulation and the approach to health and social policy, there have been few recent philosophical examinations of the concept of health and its implication for public health practice. In this chapter, a conceptual framework for thinking about health will be described that incorporates current work on health inequalities. This framework facilitates consideration of the fundamental ethical issues in public health.

THE BUILDING BLOCKS OF PUBLIC HEALTH ETHICS

This discussion begins by considering three major building blocks of government involvement in health, which have consequently served as the primary building blocks of public health ethics. These include the early implementation of public health measures such as sanitation, inspection, and public health nursing; the enactment of universal health care coverage; and the introduction of government-sponsored health promotion programs. Governmental health policy initiatives in the United Kingdom and Canada are presented as examples. More recently, research suggests that a fourth block of health policy that is concerned with inequalities in health is emerging. This analysis applies equally to public health systems in the United States and other Western countries.

Block 1: Public Health Measures—How Do We Stop Epidemics and Keep People Healthy?

The recurrent cholera epidemics of the nineteenth century and the discoveries by scientists like John Snow led to the realization that these epidemics were transmitted by contaminated water. A cleaner water supply required some form of governmental intervention if only to regulate and inspect for contaminants. It took a long time for reformers like Edwin Chadwick, a father of public health, to convince government to initiate public health policies for a clean water supply and for other sanitation initiatives such as public health inspection and nursing. This was an important early building block of governmental health policy and ethical views in public health.[1]

For many years public health advocates claimed that the clean water policies of the nineteenth century did more to improve health status than did medical discoveries of the twentieth century, such as penicillin and other antibiotics. More recently there has been some debate concerning the relative impact of these public health measures.[2] It has been argued by some population epidemiologists that improved health owed less to public health measures than to a general increase in prosperity, which afforded better nutrition and housing. Despite this disagreement concerning the extent of their impact on health, it is indisputable that the public health initiatives did contribute considerably to general health improvement and that they continue to answer the question, "How do we keep people healthy?"

Here the efforts were to improve the health of a population by means of interventions that kept people healthy. The focus was on the collective and the environment rather than the individual and the body. It was on prevention rather than treatment.

A major ethical dilemma in health policy and administration involves the struggle between philosophic and analytic frameworks focused on the individual and those frameworks focused on populations. Researchers and practitioners working within frameworks that are focused on individuals see individual human beings as "ends in themselves" and consider each human life as of absolute value. An example of this kind of view is found in the writings of Immanuel Kant and has been called deontological ethics.[3] At its core is the view that one has an ethical obligation to do the right thing regardless of cost or consequences. According to this series of views, the autonomy of individuals takes precedence over the consequences of actions to a population.

A second series of views calculates the well-being of the population as a whole against its individual members, and considers that overall well-being may force the sacrifice of the well-being of some individuals. According to proponents of these views, the consequences of one's actions are critical. Jeremy Bentham was the leading figure in the nineteenth-century reform movement that dealt with public problems on a scientific basis. He argued along with John Stuart Mill for developing ways of calculating the overall consequences of our actions. Their consequentialist position became known as utilitarianism. The objective of this view is best characterized by the motto "the greatest good for the greatest number."[4]

The public health movement grew out of the utilitarian tradition. A major founder of public health was Edwin Chadwick, a follower of Jeremy Bentham and a reformer who was firmly on the side of consequentialist health policy directed at the population. He argued for improved sanitation and better housing. He collected data on the health of the population, and his statistical work was an early forerunner of more recent work on inequalities in health and the need to provide an evidence base for policy decisions.[1]

The individual and population-based frameworks can support dramatically different policy and administrative decisions in public health. In recent times, the issues that surround this building block of policy and ethics include compulsory vaccination, the detention of contagious individuals, and mandatory reporting of STDs. Current practices and positions concerning compulsory vaccination vary quite a lot between jurisdictions. Attempts to increase the number of people vaccinated against a variety of diseases range from incentives to individuals and their physicians to the requirement that all children present a vaccination certificate upon school entry. There are similar ranges of policy and practice over the other public health issues mentioned above. In all of these cases, there is an ethical struggle between the sanctity of the individual and the consequences to a larger population. If individual autonomy is given the highest value, then responsibility for decisions about everything from vaccination to reporting of STDs must remain with the individual. If societal consequences are paramount, then individual rights must be subservient to them. These two value sets appear to be incompatible.

Block 2: Universal Health Care Coverage—How Do We Diagnose and Treat People with Ill Health?

A second building block of health policy and public health ethics was the introduction of government-funded health services. The poor health of recruits for the Boer War in the United Kingdom led people to think about how to ensure the diagnosis and treatment of those who suffered from ill health. There was an emerging role for government in the provision of health care to an entire population. But it was not until after the Second World War that the National Health Service was created in the United Kingdom. It was believed that universal medical coverage would completely "cure" the population of ill health so that, in time, there would be a reduction in the need for it. In Canada, widespread ill health from the time of the Depression and World War II led to the enactment of Medicare in 1968.[5]

Once more there was a delay between the ideas associated with this second building block of policy and ethics and its final implementation. And there is also some dispute regarding the extent of the contribution of universal health care coverage to the health of the population. Some researchers claim that improvements in health status after the initiation of universal health care coverage were less a result of these governmental policies than a result of similar increases in prosperity and other changes. Despite these debates, there is little disagreement with the view that universal medical coverage has contributed to the treatment of ill health.[5]

Medical services focus primarily on the individual and the body rather than on the collective and the environment. They provide diagnosis and treatment, which together with the existing and expanding prevention programs would seem to provide complete health coverage to the population.

Debates concerning universal health care coverage are instructive from an ethical point of view. In most countries, the medical profession as a whole has been initially opposed to the introduction of universal insurance for health care coverage. Public health movements have advocated universal coverage. But the debates in different countries have a great deal to do with how health care is viewed by the population at large. It is possible to distinguish between such views in Canada, Great Britain, and the United States. In Canada, health care is seen as part of the infrastructure of the country. It is like the road system or the electrical grid or the regulatory mechanisms of the banking system. As such, it is a responsibility of government to ensure full coverage because it is one of the things that keeps the country together and allows it to function. Therefore, it must be somewhat transparent and perform reasonably well. In Great Britain, the National Health Service is seen as a governmental service: it is part of a welfare state that provides support and services to all of its citizens. Like many governmental services, it carries some opportunity cost but provides services for those who want it. One can also access medical services privately so that one can avoid the waits that seem to be an inevitable cost of access to public services. In the United States, health care is often treated as a commodity—an item that can be bought and sold. In fact, consumerism and choice are seen to be essential features of health care systems. It is therefore not surprising that there has been some resistance in the United States to paying for other people's health care.

It is commonplace these days that values stand behind policies and actions. Hence the interest in ethics. However, this case suggests that "facts" have an impact on value decisions. It is a factual matter that health care is part of the infrastructure or a governmental service or a commodity. Each case presents a different perspective on the place of government and the role of universal health care coverage. If health care is infrastructural, then there is a clear role for government. In the United States, it is broadly accepted that the monetary and banking systems are infrastructural to a free market society. Government plays a critical role in regulating these systems and had no choice but to involve itself when there was a crisis in the savings and loan sector. In Canada, because the blood supply is part of the country's infrastructure, the government had no choice but to involve itself heavily when there were problems with the purity of the blood supply. A major inquiry and large payments to patients followed.

Block 3: Health Promotion—How Do We Improve People's Health?

In the 1960s and 1970s, Thomas McKeown argued that "in order of importance the major contributions to improvement in health in England and Wales were from limitations of family size (a behavioural change), increase in food supplies and a healthier physical environment (environmental influences), and specific preventive and therapeutic measures."[6]

His idea that there are more important influences on health than traditional public health measures and medical care had a strong effect on thinking about health. McKeown's ideas shaped the content and direction of the Lalonde report, arguably the most significant Canadian health policy document in the last 25 years. The Lalonde report articulated the health field concept that recognizes four elements "affecting the level of health in Canada": human biology, environment, lifestyle, and health care organization. These four major influences on health can be used as a "tool for analyzing health problems, determining health needs of Canadians and choosing the means by which those needs can be met."[7(p.32)]

The Lalonde report recommended that governmental policy be extended to encourage people to assume more responsibility for their own health through improvements in their lifestyles and to create healthier social environments, which would also contribute to the health of individuals and populations. The report marks a transition in governmental policy to place increasing emphasis on health promotion. The ideas in it were expanded on in the Epp report *Achieving Health for All: A Framework for Health Promotion* and in the Ottawa Charter.[8] These later reports emphasized the importance of the social environment, power and control, coping skills, social justice, housing, education, and civil society in promoting health. They also specified action: the need for health workers to advocate and act to improve health. They set in motion major changes at the federal and provincial levels. As a result of these reports, Health Canada reorganized itself and many provinces also adjusted institutional structures to facilitate health promotion.

Between 1974 and today, the health promotion literature has reported on an increasing number of influences on health, which interact in complex ways. A recent document considers that there are at least 12 critical determinants of health, including social support networks, education, employment and working conditions, social environments, physical environments, personal health practices, healthy child development, biology and genetic endowment, health service, gender, and culture.

This third building block of health policy and ethics, like the first two, took some time to implement. Some health promotion advocates argue that it has not been fully implemented yet. And just as there were debates concerning the impact of traditional public health and universal health insurance, there are disagreements concerning the efficacy of health promotion, which made more explicit the differences in beliefs and values of different groups.

The role of government and the extent to which it is paternalistic is at the core of ethical discussions concerning many health promotion initiatives. Should individuals be allowed knowingly to assume risks that harm only themselves?

Does the government have the right to interfere in the lives of its citizens and force them to engage in risk-reducing behaviors? The debate over seat belt legislation is a good example. The consequences of not wearing seat belts are injuries to the person who does not wear them in case of an accident. There are few or no consequences to the health of others. This makes it more difficult to mount a consequentialist argument for the mandatory use of seat belts. (When the argument becomes one based on cost to the system, it results in discussions about whether the risk taker should bear those costs.) Debates over reducing lifestyle risks by making mandatory the use of bicycle helmets, or controlling cigarette smoking and alcohol consumption, tend to follow similar patterns.

The sets of facts and values that stand behind such issues can be taken together. How much of health behavior is the responsibility of individuals and how much is the responsibility of government and hence beyond individual responsibility? What are appropriate interventions in each case? The array of answers for these questions can be traced to incompatible views concerning the role of government in general, and conflicts about where individuals can in fact assume responsibility. It is especially interesting to compare views about addictive behavior with respect to alcohol, tobacco, and mind-altering drugs and then to consider government's role in reducing risk in each case. It may also be useful to consider the struggle between autonomy of individuals and professional paternalism, which has had a significant part to play in recent discussions regarding the doctor–patient relationship.

The Emerging Building Block: Inequalities in Health—Why Are Some People Healthy and Others Not?

It has been known for a very long time that the level of health of a population is closely associated with a number of nonhealth factors. Edwin Chadwick presented mortality tables as early as 1842, which indicated that gradients of child mortality correlate with the level of the child's father's occupation.[1] Gradients of a wide variety of health indicators along social class lines have been an ongoing feature of epidemiologic studies. They became even more apparent when statistical data began to be gathered using formal class definitions in Great Britain early in this century. A 1957 epidemiology text is a good example. "Cancer of the stomach, myocardial degeneration, pneumonia and ulcer of the stomach have a definite rising gradient from Social Class I to V."[9] Infant mortality followed the gradients in 1932, and continued to follow them in 1950.[9]

"The Black Report" of 1980 was a landmark study of health inequalities in the United Kingdom.[10] It provided clear and more complete evidence of gradients of socioeconomic status following differences in health. Richard Wilkinson's *Unhealthy Societies: The Afflictions of Inequality* continued in this tradition by using gradients to present the socioeconomic correlations with health disparities.[11] His sources were epidemiologic studies in the United Kingdom and other developed countries. Similar studies in Canada and the United States have shown that mortality, various kinds of morbidity, self-reporting of health, and similar health measures seem to follow gradients of education, social status, income, and other socioeconomic circumstances.

"Why are some people healthy and others not?" This is the question that forms the title of a prominent publication by Canadian researchers on inequalities in health. They have amassed population-based evidence in a systematic and integrated way in an attempt to understand how different factors influence health. The result has been to demonstrate that social environments have a far stronger impact on health than individual behaviors. Trying to understand these social–structural dimensions has become a central focus of their research. Health promotion researchers recognized these impacts but did not engage in detailed empirical research needed to identify the correlation between social gradients and health status and to explain their interaction.

Researchers studying inequalities in health have attempted to integrate evidence of what is known about identifiable factors that influence health over the life course from large-scale population health studies. Along the way, evidence regarding the relative contribution of health care, the physical environment, and genetics has been assessed, and the conclusion has been that these factors are far less critical than the social environment over the course of a person's life. A range of measures of health status, including mortality, morbidity, and self-assessment of health, all vary according to such socioeconomic measures as education, social class, occupation, income, and economic status.

Researchers in health inequalities have "drilled down" into various social determinants and assessed the significance of more particular factors. After showing that the rank of civil servants was a good indicator of morbidity and mortality, British researchers began to look more carefully at the nature of work and how it is performed. Recent Whitehall studies indicate that lack of control over work contributes significantly to ill health. In fact, after correcting for smoking, alcohol consumption, and nutrition, it is the most significant contributor to heart disease in the population studied.[12]

Other studies look more carefully at particular components of people's lives. Correcting for other differences such as smoking, nutrition, and other health-related behaviors, studies have shown that hopelessness is tied to cardiac disease. A study of 2,500 Finnish males used measurements of the blood flow in their carotid arteries to show that hopelessness is closely correlated with the onset of atherosclerosis.[13]

POLICY IMPLICATIONS

Despite the clear conclusions of recent research concerning health inequalities, there has been some difficulty in framing and adopting the policy consequences of this work. In the foreword to *Tackling Inequalities in Health,* Sir Donald Acheson stated, "Today the question is not whether these facts are valid but who cares and what can be done about them."[14(p.ix)] Similar complaints have been heard in Canada from researchers in health inequalities.

After the publication of "The Black Report," there was a political division on interpreting its results. "The House of Commons debate of 6 December 1982...developed on strict party lines and reached its forgone conclusion by 10 PM."[15] This division of perspectives on the results of research remains. Sir Donald Acheson concluded, "In the circumstances it is particularly unfortunate that the issue has become a party political football."[14(p.ix)]

One set of arguments focuses on individuals. With this argument, everyone must have the relatively untrammelled freedom to accumulate wealth. This will result in the greatest increase in the wealth of the population as a whole and will also improve the wealth of the most socioeconomically deprived. There is an explicit recognition in this belief that health and well-being follow wealth. Improvements in wealth therefore will increase the health of the whole population—the least well off as well as everyone else. Although inequalities may persist, general improvements will affect everyone. At the same time, it may be necessary to provide a safety net for the worst off.

In support of this belief, there are those researchers who argue that improvement in health in industrialized countries over the last 150 years is mainly due to an increase in general prosperity. There has also been a narrowing of longevity differences so that everyone lives longer and the gradients of disparity along class lines are shallower. As mentioned earlier, higher incomes and improved diet, housing, and working conditions are more significant factors than either sanitation or medical advances. An example of this kind of change is the reduction of infant mortality, which has been to the benefit of all classes. Even though inequalities remain, there is evidence that in the long term, except for occasional blips, the differences between the best off and worst off have been reduced.[16]

The other side argues that reducing inequalities not only improves the health of the least favored but also results in an improvement of health of the whole population. Wilkinson is a good example of someone who holds this view. Using examples that compare the United Kingdom with Sweden, Wilkinson argues that in countries like Sweden where there is less disparity between classes, not only is the health of the least well off improved, but so is the health of the best off. Sir Douglas Black concluded, "A radical cure demands nothing less than a renewed dedication to the welfare state."[15(p.9)]

The epidemiologic studies do not provide direct causal accounts of illness; instead, they indicate risk factors. A significant risk of a condition does not constitute a causal explanation. The gradients of health indicate varying degrees of risk of illness at different socioeconomic levels of the population. It remains true that at each level, some people are sick and others are healthy. However, the presence of proven risk factors cannot predict individual outcomes of disease. There is still no way to ascertain whether a particular person will get lung cancer or not. Jill who is poor and smokes like a chimney can remain healthy and live a long life, whereas Jack who is a rich, nonsmoking vegetarian jogger can die early of lung cancer.

Socioeconomic risk factors cannot, and should not, be identified with direct causes. It remains true that even though someone may be at higher risk because of his or her social and economic situation, the luck of the draw remains of prime importance in the risk of most illnesses. This is reflected in population-based data like the Whitehall studies, which indicate that of the known factors that affect heart disease among British civil servants, the most significant known ones may be job status, or control over work, but even larger components remain unknown.[12]

Even if it were accepted that reducing inequalities would improve the health of the population, the question remains, "Equality of what?" There is widespread disagreement among egalitarians about what should be equalized in order to improve general well-being (and by implication, the health of the population). This is true on a number of fronts, including health, education, welfare, and so forth. (See NY Review article on Black disagreement and Cohen's article in *The Quality of Life*.)[17]

Tackling Inequalities in Health suggests four levels of policy initiative to this end.

1. strengthening individuals
2. strengthening communities
3. improving access to essential facilities and services
4. encouraging macroeconomic and cultural change

It quickly points out that "despite some successes, efforts to strengthen individuals and communities have had a minimal impact on reducing inequalities in health. Greatest gains in health in the past have resulted from improvements in living and working conditions."[14(p.xviii–xix)]

It concludes that "a worthwhile agenda for tackling inequalities in health must therefore include a strong focus on reducing poverty and a commitment to the careful monitoring of the impact of major public policies on health, particularly among the most vulnerable groups."[14(p.xix)]

This kind of conclusion leaves government departments of health with a particular dilemma: if their mission is to improve the health of the population, or even if they adopt a mission of reducing inequalities in health, the policy tools available to them are limited. They cannot themselves develop policies for "macroeconomic or cultural change." Nor can they develop policies that will increase access to essential facilities outside of the health portfolio, such as housing, or circumstances such as control over work.

This frustration of purpose is apparent in many departments of health. Governmental officials in health recognize their inability to develop policies that will change socioeconomic circumstances. Officials in other governmental departments, when faced with the declared desire by the Ministry of Health to develop such policies, often consider their efforts to result from a kind of health imperialism. Must health be the focus of all governmental policy? What is the relationship between the health of the population and other governmental objectives?

IDEAS RELEVANT TO AN UNDERSTANDING OF HEALTH

Changes in three big ideas have had a substantial impact on the current concept of health. The state of health has moved from a deterministic Newtonian account of the physical world to a post-Einsteinian one with strong consequences to the nature of explanation. People's attitude concerning the natural environment has changed to become far more respectful of it and people's place in it. And finally, people have begun to recognize the importance of interactions between autonomous individuals and their social context. A review of these changing ideas may help unravel some of the puzzles concerning health policy. The changes can be categorized as follows: (1) the extent of uncertainty in individuals' understanding of the physical world, (2) the relationship between individuals and their environment, and (3) individual identity in relation to the social environment.

Uncertainty

For Plato and some other ancient Greek philosophers like Parmenides, the physical world was the world of becoming. According to them, people cannot have knowledge of the physical world but only opinion and uncertainty because the world is constantly changing. For many medieval philosophers, man's uncertainty concerning the physical world was set against divine knowledge: only God can understand the physical world. It is with the rise of modern science that the belief grew that humans can gain a powerful understanding of the physical world. The success of Newtonian physics and science in general resulted in a strongly mechanistic and deterministic picture of the physical universe. Its high point in the early nineteenth century was marked by the work of Pierre Simon Laplace. He envisaged a being, often referred to as "Laplace's Demon," which was capable of complete knowledge of the deterministic universe. Explanation in Laplace's universe required causal links and accurate predictions. There was no room for choice, chance, or uncertainty.[18]

The deterministic picture presented by Laplace is contradicted by the occurrence of a large number of nonpredictable phenomena that occur throughout nature at every level, from the subatomic to the cosmic. Many things like the weather, the stock market, or the next drip of a faucet are not completely predictable. There is now general acceptance of the strong characteristics of uncertainty and indeterminism in the physical world.

In contrast to the Newtonian picture of the world, modern chaos theory speaks of a world in which there is always some uncertainty in any real measurement, which makes it impossible to specify initial conditions to infinite accuracy. Extreme sensitivity to initial conditions (the butterfly effect) makes it impossible to predict the weather accurately over long periods of time. Uncertainty about such phenomena may be the norm rather than a special case. Some people suggest that this uncertainty and the lack of constant stability are important considerations in helping to understand the physical world. Explanation is no longer in terms of prediction and control.

If these ideas are applied to one's understanding of health, they suggest that attempts to consider the human body as the single site for the study of health are insufficient. The Human Genome Project is often presented as a complete explanation of human biology on the Newtonian model. There is no doubt that it will have enormous consequences to one's capacity to understand and control many types of disease. But given that genes set out only some of the initial conditions for health, there will still be a great deal of variation of outcome. An epigenetic perspective on health has already emerged (i.e., that many nongenetic factors will contribute to the initial conditions and hence have strong influence on lifelong health). It is unlikely that there will ever be a complete (causal) account of health (or illness) that considers the body in isolation.

Relation to the Physical Environment

A second big shift in ideas that affects one's understanding of health concerns the relationship between humans and the natural environment. In early animistic cultures, people saw themselves as an element of nature: everything was "ensouled." This close connection to the rest of nature forced a constant focus on the interaction between human affairs and the natural world. In medieval society, although humans were special, the natural world was also a divine creation that demanded consideration and respect. The land needed to rest as did man, and animals were literally *creatures* of God. The Newtonian and especially Cartesian pictures of a mechanical universe increased the distance between humans and the natural world. Scientific advance began to be seen as a solution to problems that occur in nature. This approach grew and reached its peak in the early parts of this century when major engineering and design projects were launched with the view that scientific expertise would always be able to solve any problems that might arise. Rachel Carson's *Silent Spring* marked a renewed realization that humans are part of nature and must learn to respect it rather than attempt to control all aspects of it.[19]

This changing understanding of the connection between humans and nature is mirrored in changes in one's concept of health. A good example of this change occurs in the area of nutrition. It was not so long ago that the scientific future provided a vision of healthy food in the form of pills. The growth of an organic, natural food industry and a growing concern about the possible side effects of genetically engineered produce emerged from a recognition that humans are inseparable from a complex and delicately balanced natural environment. There are two different pictures of what one should ingest. The first is a belief in the magic bullet drug that will deliver health and youth, and the second is the expectation that a more natural organic way of life will maintain health throughout life.

Individuals and the Social Environment

The third "big idea" that has changed today's notion of health has to do with human identity. In primitive societies, individuals identified themselves by means of their relationships with others. A person's network of relationships determined who someone was: for example, daughter of A, sister of B, and cousin of C. The notion of separate personal identity without this kind of reference arose gradually as individuals became responsible for their individual souls in medieval society. Theories of human development from Freud onward continued to recognize the importance of the individual, but there is increasing evidence of the strong impact on identity of the interaction between individuals and their social environment.

THREE WAYS OF THINKING ABOUT HEALTH

There are three main elements in concepts of health: the individual, the social context, and the mode of interaction between them. Three traditional modes of thinking about health can be identified, each comprising one of the three elements.

The first or medical tradition focuses on the individual. Major advances in medical knowledge have resulted from an ever-deepening understanding of the physiology and psychology of the individual person. Interventions on the individual body seek to maintain health and prevent or cure illness. This approach to health is closely tied to the ethics of deontology.

The second tradition, as exemplified by the work of Thomas McKeown, argues that medical intervention is a lesser contributor to the health of an individual than the environment. This emphasis on environmental factors is a strong part of the public health approach, which began with the Sanitarian movements and can be traced through ideas of health promotion and current work on the inequalities in health. Increasingly, this tradition emphasizes the social and economic environment as having the greatest influence on health. This view obviously is associated with consequentialism.

A third view of health that focuses on the nature of interactions between individuals and their environment has begun to be articulated in this century. Talcott Parson's work on the boundary between health and illness relates people's capacities to engage in their social and work environment.[20] His ideas help people to understand health in terms of the relationship between an individual and his or her social context. Antonovsky's discussion of the nature of resiliency identifies the capacity to use the resources one has to respond to misfortune.[21] This echoes Aristotle's description of the fine man as one who can cope with misfortune.

This third way of thinking about health suggests that one might consider ethical imperatives that interact between respect for individuals and one's obligations to them and the social context in which they occur and one's responsibilities to populations. This is the balance that occurs in most areas of public policy. But the balance occurs in different ways in different cultural environments. Thus the degree of involvement of government varies, the responsibility for health care is located differently, and what is considered to be an appropriate balance varies quite widely.

HYPOTHESIS ABOUT HEALTH AND HEALTH IMPROVEMENT

The considerations above have led to the following hypothesis, which can be tested against a number of research results:

> A robust interaction between an individual and his or her social context is a major contributor to health.

Applying this hypothesis to some of the examples described in the earlier parts of the chapter yields some preliminary policy directions.

Health Inequalities: Marmot and Control over Work

When Marmot's results in the Whitehall study declared that control over work was the most critical factor correlated with heart disease, the implication was that control over work is a characteristic of the workplace. However, control over work is not merely an environmental characteristic of the workplace. Some workers feel as if they have little control over their work in circumstances where others feel as if they have a great deal of control. This variance occurs over a broad range of work from policy development to the automobile assembly line. Workers' sense of control over work is a function of the nature of the work environment and also of how the worker interacts with it.

Much of the preventive efforts in the workplace have to do with occupational health and safety issues. A lesson from the Whitehall studies is that there are more opportunities for preventive policies and programs that might be considered. As formulated, health-related policies and programs can be categorized into three groups: ones that target the individual, ones that target the work environment, and ones that focus on the interaction between the two. The hypothesis would then suggest that it is worthwhile to look more carefully at the nature of this interaction for fresh opportunities to improve health in the workplace.

Health Inequalities: The Everson Study

Research efforts are continually discovering finer socioeconomic correlates with health. Everson's study is a good example: it connects self-assessed measures of hopelessness with the onset of atherosclerosis. She defined hopelessness as "negative expectancies about oneself and the future."[13(p.114)] The two items on the questionnaire were, "I feel that it is impossible to reach the goals I would like to strive for;" and "The future seems to me to be hopeless. And I can't believe that things are changing for the better."[13(p.119)] Responses were on a five-point scale from "absolutely agree" to "absolutely disagree."

These statements appear to be less about psychological states of individuals or the nature of the environment than about the interaction between the individual and the environment. In fact, Everson speaks of this in her study: "These notions suggest that individuals in interaction with their environment develop a set of behavioral, social, psychological, and physiological adaptations or adjustments that have a cumulative, generic effect on health."[13(p.120)]

Hopelessness thus is understood to be a result of a deteriorating interaction with one's social context. It is not a mental state but rather a belief about external possibilities and is highly interactive.

Social Marketing: Smoking and HIV Prevention

Social marketing has had very mixed responses in different sectors of the population. Attempts to urge people to stop smoking have worked well in middle-class communities but have been less successful for poor people. Campaigns against acquired immune deficiency syndrome (AIDS) and human immunodeficiency virus (HIV) have had similarly varied results. Campaigns to increase the use of condoms had a strong impact on the organized homosexual community several years ago, but recent attempts to influence intravenous drug users not to reuse needles and to encourage safe sex by a younger and poorer cohort of homosexuals have not been very successful (as evidenced by a new wave of HIV infection in Canada).

One way to understand both the successes and failures of these campaigns is to think about their effect on the community within which individuals are at risk. In middle-class communities, it has become increasingly difficult to maintain a smoking habit and good relations with others. There is increasing community pressure on members to stop smoking. For many people, it is easier to stop smoking than to relieve the strain on relationships that accompanies it. On the other hand, in some poor communities, smoking is a form of cheap entertainment that is encouraged by all, and there is considerable community pressure to take it up. Maintaining good relations with others in these communities requires at least tolerance for smoking and abstention requires a special effort.

A similar case can be made about the varying success of efforts to stop the spread of HIV in different communities. As safe sex became the community norm in the older homosexual community, it became increasingly difficult not to practice safe sex. In the community of intravenous drug users, however, there was no such community uptake. Similarly, younger and poorer members of the gay community spurn the advice of their more respectable elders and their community does not respond well to safe sex campaigns.

Both these cases suggest the special importance of interactions between individuals and their social context. When these interactions are health inducing, social marketing works; when they are not, lack of compliance with health-inducing practices seems to stem less from ignorance than from the nature of one's relationship to a social context. Although much of the focus of social marketing has been the individual, it turns out to be most effective if it impacts on the community to which individuals want to belong.

The Health Care System: How Individuals Relate to It

At meetings with American policy makers, a recurrent theme has been the dramatic difference between Canadian and U.S. health policy issues. An American pointed out that the major issue in the United States is "coverage." There are more than 40 million people in the United States with no health care coverage and, according to some experts, another 20 million are underinsured. In the United States, issues concerning inequalities in health are submerged under the more obvious and painful consequences of inequalities in health care.

This brings up a peculiar role of health care coverage when thinking about health. Far from being measured in terms of its productivity or the outcome of health care interventions, the role of a publicly funded, universally accessible health care system is to provide security that one will be cared for should one become ill. Current public concern in Canada may well be connected to the fear that such care will not be forthcoming given the current state of the health care system.

According to the proposed hypothesis, a universal health care system that provides such security fosters a stronger relationship between individual citizens and the state. This will, if the hypothesis is correct, improve population health status. It would provide one explanation for the differences in health status between those countries with and without universal health care coverage and would identify an interesting preventive aspect of universal coverage.

• • •

The set of ethical issues that confront public health organizations is fluid and expanding; consequently, this work remains preliminary and exploratory. Nonetheless, an expanding body of public health research corroborates the ethical issues identified in this analysis. Research shows, for example, that death rates correspond highly with the nature of social relationships. Death rates for both men and women from coronary disease, stroke, motor vehicle accidents, and some cancers correlate with marriage-related states. The data suggest that people in close relationships are healthier than those who are not, and still healthier than those who have suffered through marriage breakdowns. Further investigation might look for studies that investigate the connection between health and the strength of other relationships such as family, friends, and colleagues. Connecting these studies with other work on inequalities in health may lead to fresh policy and ethical frameworks. Such a framework can be conceptually rigorous and empirically well founded, but, of equal importance, it can guide ethical decision making in public health organizations. Policy and administrative decisions based on such a framework should be easy to articulate, implement, and evaluate. It is also hoped that such a framework can add a new dimension to ethical decision making that goes beyond the historic dichotomy of the individual and the social environment.

Clearly, there are new ways for public health decision makers to view traditional ethical distinctions between individual interests and collective interests. The question yet to be answered concerns how such new perspectives might alter the public's view of contemporary public health decisions and its view of the organizations and professionals that make them.

CHAPTER REVIEW

1. Building blocks of governmental health policy and ethics include
   - basic measures of sanitation, inspection, and public health nursing
   - concern for health care coverage
   - health promotion
   - a current focus on inequalities of health
2. The public health movement grew out of a utilitarian tradition influenced by Jeremy Bentham and his follower Edwin Chadwick, who argued for improved sanitation and housing.
3. Concern for collective health creates ethical conflicts with the autonomy of individuals in areas such as compulsory vaccination, detention of contagious individuals, and mandatory reporting of STDs. These conflicts arise from the incompatible value sets of the individual and society.
4. Debates concerning health care coverage raise ethical issues of unequal access, waiting time, and opportunity to choose health services based on payment.
5. The role and responsibility of government in health promotion initiatives raises questions of paternalism and conflicts with the individual's decision to assume health risks and the attendant consequences.
6. Inequalities of health are closely associated with nonhealth factors, including various social determinants. Higher incomes and improved diet, housing, and working conditions are more significant to health than sanitation or medical care. Official health agencies are unable to change these basic socioeconomic circumstances.
7. Health as a concept is influenced by three views: (1) uncertainty in the understanding of the physical world, (2) relationship of the individual to the physical world, and (3) relationship of the individual to the social environment. The hypothesis explored in this chapter is that a robust interaction between the individual and his or her social context is a major contributor to health.

REFERENCES

1. E. Chadwick, *Report on the Sanitary Condition of the Labouring Population of Great Britain* (London: W. Clowes, for H.M. Stationery Office, 1842).
2. T. McKeown, *The Role of Medicine: Dream, Mirage, or Nemesis?* (Oxford: Basil Blackwell, 1976).
3. I. Kant, *Foundations of the Metaphysics of Morals*, trans. L.W. Beck (Indianapolis, IN: Bobbs-Merrill, 1969).
4. J. Bentham, "Article on Untilitarianism," in *Deontology Together with a Table of the Spring of Action and the Article on Untilitarianism*, ed. A. Goldworth (Oxford: Clarendon Press, 1983).
5. B. Legowski and L. McKay, *The Evolution of Health Policy at the Federal Level* (Ottawa, Canada: Canadian Policy Research Networks, in press).
6. T. McKeown, "The Major Influences of Man'sHealth," quoted in M. Lalonde, *A New Perspective on the Health of Canadians* (Ottawa, Canada: Minister of Supply and Services, 1974).
7. M. Lalonde, *A New Perspective on the Health of Canadians* (Ottawa, Canada: Minister of Supply and Services, 1974).
8. World Health Organization, *Ottawa Charter for Health Promotion* (Ottawa, Canada: Canadian Public Health Association, 1986).
9. I. Taylor and J. Knoweldon, *Principles of Epidemiology* (London: J & A Churchill, 1957).
10. D. Black et al., "The Black Report," in *Inequalities in Health*, eds. P. Townsend and N. Davidson (London: Penguin, 1980).
11. R.G. Wilkinson, *Unhealthy Societies: The Afflictions of Inequality* (London: Routledge, 1996).
12. M.G. Marmot et al., "Contribution of Job Control and Other Risk Factors to Social Variations in Coronary Heart Disease Incidence," *The Lancet* 350 (1997): 235–231.
13. S.A. Everson et al., "Hopelessness and Risk of Mortality and Incidence of Myocardial Infarction and Cancer," *Psychosomatic Medicine 58*, no. 113 (1996): 113–121.
14. D. Acheson, *Tackling Inequalities in Health* (London: The King's Fund, 1995).
15. D. Black, "Inequitable variation," *Journal of Royal College of Physicians London 30*, no. 3 (1996): 8–9.
16. S.R. Johansson, "Food for Thought: Rhetoric and Reality in Modern Mortality History," *Historical Methods 27*, no. 3 (1994): 101–124.
17. G.A. Cohen, "Equality of What?", in *The Quality of Life*, eds. M. Nussbaum and A. Sen (Oxford: Clarendon Press, 1993), 9–29.
18. P.S. Laplace, *Exposition du système du monde* (The System of the World), trans. H.H. Harte (London: Longman, Rees. Orme, Brown, and Green, 1830).
19. R. Carson, *Silent Spring* (New York: Crest Books, 1962).
20. T. Parsons, "Illness and the Role of the Physician: A Sociological Perspective," *American Journal of Orthopsychiatry* 21 (1951): 452–460.
21. A. Antonovsky, *Health, Stress, and Coping*, 1st ed. (San Fransisco, CA: Jossey-Bass Publishers, 1979).

PART II

Operational Issues in Public Health Administration

Despite heterogeneity in both form and function, public health organizations engage in a number of common operational activities considered vital to the task of population-based management and community health improvement. Part II examines the administrative processes and issues involved in carrying out these essential operations. Nine chapters explore issues in data acquisition and surveillance, information systems design and management, processes for public health assessment, health education and health promotion intervention, program evaluation, and public health research. Each chapter describes the relevance and importance of the activity to public health practice and provides an overview of common administrative issues in implementing and managing the activity. Public health professionals in any practice setting require a firm understanding of these operational activities and their associated management issues.

CHAPTER 7

Public Health Data Acquisition

C. Virginia Lee

Data in public health are needed for community health assessment, planning, and evaluation. Attribute data include demographics, socioeconomics, health expenditures, disease prevalence, and mortality. Behavioral risk and environmental information are also key to appraising the health communities. Data are available from federal, state, and local sources. The Centers for Disease Control and Prevention (CDC) is a major source of data for community health planning and measures of preventive effectiveness. State sources of data include vital statistics, disease registries, and Medicaid reports. Local data are available from disease reporting, special surveys, and, increasingly, managed care sources.

HISTORICAL PERSPECTIVE ON DATA COLLECTION

Governments have found it useful to collect statistics on the population, animals, and objects under their jurisdiction since the beginning of civilization. The ancient Babylonians made tabulations of agricultural yields and commodities. Around 600 BC, the ancient Greeks used censuses as a basis for taxation. The Roman Empire was the first government to make extensive documentation of the land it controlled and the populations residing in that land. Registration of deaths and births began in England in the sixteenth century.

Modern public health organizations rely on data to inform all aspects of their operations, ranging from the design and targeting of population-based interventions, to the development of policies and the enforcement of regulations. More specifically, organizations use data to enhance community health assessment and planning activities, which are increasingly carried out with administrative tools that require specific data elements, such as *Assessment Protocol for Excellence in Public Health (APEXPH)*, developed by the National Association of County and City Health Officials (NACCHO). (See Chapter 11 for a detailed discussion.) In this chapter, several categories of data for community assessment and planning are examined, including demographics, socioeconomics, health care expenditures, health care resources and access to primary health care, perinatal indicators, mortality, years of potential life lost, hospitalization, ambulatory medical care, disease prevalence, behavioral risk factors, and environmental hazards. This chapter reviews federal and state sources of data for use in community health planning and the geographic level for which the data are available. Additionally, data acquisition strategies are reviewed, including the use of local health surveys and administrative data from managed care plans. The chapter concludes with a discussion of key data management issues to consider when using data, such as access and confidentiality.

Census of the Population

The first census of the population in the United States was conducted in 1790.[1(p.13)] U.S. marshals collected the data with the help of hired assistants. The first census consisted of six questions.

1. name of head of household
2. number of free white males 16 years of age and older
3. number of free white males under 16 years of age
4. number of free white females
5. number of other free persons
6. number of slaves

The form of the census stayed essentially the same for the next 50 years. In 1840, the government expanded the scope of the census to cover agriculture. By 1860, there were six separate questionnaires with 142 questions total. Among the topics covered in the various questionnaires were population, health, mortality, occupation, income, and agriculture. In 1880, Congress created a temporary civilian census office to handle the data collection. The U.S. Bureau of the Census as a permanent organization within the government was established in 1902. The 1950 decennial census was the first in which computer technology was used to tabulate the data.[1(p.16)]

Vital Statistics

The legal authority to register births, deaths, marriages, divorces, fetal deaths, and abortions lies with the states and territories.[1(p.45)] Virginia first enacted a registration law in 1632, followed by Massachusetts in 1639. Early in the nineteenth century, the decennial census contained questions about births and deaths. However, the results were inconsistent. In 1902, when the Census Bureau was established as a permanent agency, it was authorized to obtain annual copies of records that were kept by state vital statistics offices. In 1880, a national death registration area was established. Later in 1900, a standard certificate of death was recommended. The national birth registration area was established in 1915. By 1933, all states were registering live births and deaths to an extent that national birth and death statistics could be produced.[2] In 1946, responsibility for collecting and publishing national-level vital statistics was transferred to the U.S. Public Health Service.

Reportable Diseases

In the United States, the first collection of data on selected diseases was for diseases in other countries for the purposes of quarantine. In 1878, Congress authorized the U.S. Marine Hospital Service to collect morbidity reports on cholera, smallpox, plague, and yellow fever for U.S. consuls overseas.[3] In 1893, the authority for data collecting and reporting was expanded to include state and municipal data. Legislation enacted in 1902 required that the surgeon general provide forms for the collection of data at a national level in an effort to provide uniformity to the system. The first notifiable diseases annual summary in 1912 had data from 19 states, the District of Columbia, and Hawaii.[4] By 1928, all states, the District of Columbia, Hawaii, and Puerto Rico were participating. Data were reported for 29 specific diseases.[3] In 1961, the CDC assumed responsibility for the collection and publication of data concerning nationally notifiable diseases.[4]

Present Uses of Data

Another nationwide public health planning tool is the *Healthy People* series. This series is a tool that identifies the most significant preventable threats to health and focuses public and private sector efforts to address those threats. *Healthy People* is based on scientific data and is designed to be used for decision making. The first set of national health targets was published in 1979 in *Healthy People: The Surgeon General's Report on Health Promotion and Disease Prevention*.[5] This set of five challenging goals, to reduce mortality among four age groups—infants, children, adolescents and young adults, and adults—and increase independence among older adults, was supported by objectives with 1990 targets that drove action.

Healthy People 2000: The National Health Promotion and Disease Prevention Objectives was released in 1990.[6] It is a comprehensive agenda organized into 22 priority areas, with 319 supporting objectives. Three overarching goals are to increase years of healthy life, reduce disparities in health among different population groups, and achieve access to preventive health services. In the most recent *Healthy People 2000 Review (1998–99)*, some 15 percent of the objectives have reached or surpassed the year 2000 targets.[7] These include child and adolescent death rates. Death rates for children 1–14 years of age have declined by 26 percent from the 1987 baseline to surpass the year 2000 target of 28 deaths per 100,000 population. Preliminary 1997 data indicate a death rate of 25 per 100,000 population for this age group. Progress toward the targets has been made for another 44 percent of the objectives (e.g., prenatal care, child immunizations, and mammography screening). Some 18 percent of the objectives show movement away from the targets (e.g., overweight and diabetes prevalence). Data for 6 percent of the objectives show mixed results, and 2 percent show no change from the baseline. Thirty-five objectives (11 percent) have baseline data but have no additional data with which to evaluate progress. Two new baselines were obtained this year on health promotion programs for older adults and counties with health promotion programs for racial and ethnic groups. Baselines have yet to be attained for nine objectives (3 percent).

Healthy People 2010 began to be developed in 1996 at a meeting of the Healthy People Consortium—an alliance of 350 national membership organizations and 300 state health, mental health, substance abuse, and environmental agencies. At that meeting, consortium members discussed the year 2000 framework, goals, objectives, and improvements needed to make the 2010 agenda relevant to the first decade of the twenty-first century. From that meeting and a series of other meetings and forums, a number of focus areas have been identified for *Healthy People 2010.* (See Chapter 2 for a detailed discussion.) Table 7–1 shows those focus areas and the federal agency or office within the U.S. Department of Health and Human Services (DHHS) that is responsible for the lead on each area.

To date, 47 states, the District of Columbia, and Guam have developed their own *Healthy People* plans. Most states have tailored the national objectives to their specific needs. A 1993 NACCHO survey showed that 70 percent of local health departments used *Healthy People 2000* objectives.[8] Building on their successes with *Healthy People 2000,* the state *Healthy People* action contacts, working with community coalitions, are beginning to frame their own versions of *Healthy People 2010.* To encourage groups to integrate *Healthy People* into current programs, special events, publications, and meetings, all *Healthy People* materials are in the public domain.

Leading health indicators, such as those developed from the focus areas shown in Exhibit 7–1, have been selected in a companion process to the development of *Healthy People 2010.* These health indicators reflect the major health concerns in the United States and illuminate behavioral, physical, and social environmental factors important to health. For each of the leading health indicators, specific objectives from *Healthy People 2010* will be used to monitor progress.[9] Overall, *Healthy People 2010* has 476 objectives in 28 focus areas.

For example, one of the 10 indicators is overweight and obesity. Higher body weights are associated with higher death rates, and overweight and obesity is a contributor to many preventable causes of death. Two objectives have been selected to measure progress for this leading health indicator:

- *Reduce the proportion of children and adolescents who are overweight or obese.*
- *Reduce the proportion of adults who are obese.*

FEDERAL SOURCES OF DATA

The CDC

The mission of the CDC is to promote health and quality of life by preventing and controlling

Table 7–1 *Healthy People 2010* Focus Areas and Their Lead Federal Office or Agency

Focus Area	*Agency/Staff Office Lead/Co-Lead Responsibility*
Access to quality health services	Agency for Healthcare Research and Quality, Health Resources and Services Administration
Disability and secondary conditions	Centers for Disease Control and Prevention, Department of Education/National Institute on Disability and Rehabilitation Research
Educational and community-based programs	Centers for Disease Control and Prevention, Health Resources and Services Administration
Environmental health	Agency for Toxic Substances and Disease Registry, Centers for Disease Control and Prevention, National Institutes of Health
Family planning	Office of Public Health and Science, Office of Population Affairs
Food safety	Food and Drug Administration
Health communication prevention and health promotion	Office of Public Health and Science, Office of Disease, Centers for Disease Control and Prevention
Heart disease and stroke	National Institutes of Health, Centers for Disease Control and Prevention
Injury/violence prevention	Centers for Disease Control and Prevention
Kidney disease	National Institutes of Health
Maternal, infant, and child health	Health Resources and Services Administration, Centers for Disease Control and Prevention
Medical product safety	Food and Drug Administration
Mental health and mental disorders	Substance Abuse and Mental Health Services Administration, Centers for Disease Control and Prevention
Nutrition	Food and Drug Administration, National Institutes of Health
Occupational safety and health	Centers for Disease Control and Prevention
Oral health	Centers for Disease Control and Prevention, National Institutes of Health, Health Resources and Services Administration
Physical activity and fitness	Office of Public Health and Science, President's Council on Physical Fitness and Sports, Centers for Disease Control and Prevention
Public health infrastructure	Centers for Disease Control and Prevention, Health Resources and Services Administration
Respiratory diseases	National Institutes of Health, Centers for Disease Control and Prevention
Sexually transmitted diseases	Centers for Disease Control and Prevention
Substance abuse	Substance Abuse and Mental Health Services Administration, National Institutes of Health
Tobacco use	Centers for Disease Control and Prevention

Source: Reprinted from *Healthy People 2010, Understanding and Improving Health,* Vol. I, 2000, U.S. Department of Health and Human Services.

Exhibit 7–1 *Healthy People 2010* Focus Areas

- Access to quality health services
- Arthritis, osteoporosis, and chronic back conditions
- Cancer
- Chronic kidney disease
- Diabetes
- Disability and secondary conditions
- Educational and community-based programs
- Environmental health
- Family planning
- Food safety
- Health communication
- Heart disease and stroke
- HIV
- Immunization and infectious diseases
- Injury and violence prevention
- Maternal, infant, and child health

Source: Reprinted from *Healthy People 2010: Understanding and Improving Health,* Vol. 1, 2000, U.S. Department of Health and Human Services.

disease, injury, and disability. The CDC is considered the primary prevention agency within the federal government. As such, it is one of the primary sources of data for community health planning and monitoring prevention effectiveness. Table 7–2 shows vital statistics data that are useful for health care planning and selected sources of that information.

The *National Vital Statistics Program* is a major source of national-level vital statistics information that is collected by the National Center for Health Statistics (NCHS). The NCHS collects and publishes data on births, deaths, marriages, and divorces in the United States. Since 1985, all states and the District of Columbia have participated in the Vital Statistics Cooperative Program (VSCP), sending 100 percent of their birth and death records to the NCHS. Data are collected using the U.S. Standard Live Birth and Death Certificates and Fetal Death Reports. The latest revision of these standard certificates was in 1989 when Hispanic ethnicity

Table 7–2 Data for Community Health Planning: Perinatal Indicators, Mortality, and Years of Potential Life Lost (YPLL)

Category	*Source*	*Data Set Name*	*Small Geographic Unit*
Perinatal indicators (e.g., total live births, teenage live births, prenatal care, low body weight live births, live births with mortality or birth defects)	1. National Center for Health Statistics 2. Centers for Disease Control and Prevention 3. State or local registries	1. National Vital Statistics Program (Birth and Fetal Death Certificate) 2. Abortion services statistics 3. Congenital Malformation or Birth Defect Registries	1. County 2. States 3. County Limited local
Mortality (e.g., leading causes of mortality by age and population subgroups)	1. National Center for Health Statistics 2. State vital statistics	1. National Vital Statistics Program (Compressed Mortality File) 2. State vital statistics	1. County 2. Street
Years of potential life lost (YPPL)	1. State vital statistics	1. YPPL statistics are derived from age of death on death certificate	1. County

Source: Adapted from C.V. Lee, *Journal of Public Health Management and Practice,* Vol. 5, No. 4, pp. 7–22, © 1999, Aspen Publishers, Inc.

was added. Among the data on the standard certificates that are collected by some states are maternal education, prenatal care, marital status of mother, Hispanic births, tobacco use, education of the decedent, and Hispanic deaths. Data from the program are available at the county level.

The *Compressed Mortality File* is a county-level national mortality and population database. The mortality database is derived from the detailed mortality files of the National Vital Statistics Program. The population database is derived from intercensal estimates and census counts of the resident population of each U.S. county by five-year age groups, race, and sex. Counties are categorized according to level of urbanization based on the rural–urban continuum codes developed by the Economic Research Service of the U.S. Department of Agriculture.

Abortion services statistics are reported to the CDC from central health agencies, hospitals and other facilities, and the NCHS. The statistics are kept at a statewide level.

The *National Health Interview Survey (NHIS)* is a continuing nationwide sample survey in which data are collected through personal household interviews. Information is collected on personal and demographic characteristics as well as on illnesses, injuries, impairments, chronic conditions, utilization of health resources, and other health topics. The response rate for the survey has been between 95–98 percent over the years. In 1985, the *NHIS* began to include an oversampling of the black population to improve the precision of the statistics.

The National Health and Nutrition Examination Surveys consist of a series of surveys that were undertaken by the NCHS. The purpose of these surveys was to estimate the national prevalence of selected diseases and risk factors, to estimate national population reference distributions of selected health parameters, and to investigate reasons for trends in selected diseases and risk factors. The first *National Health and Nutrition Examination Survey (NHANES I)* was conducted from 1971 to 1974.[10] The purpose was to measure indicators of the nutrition and health status of the American people through dietary intake data, biochemical tests, physical measurements, and clinical assessments for evidence of nutritional deficiency. The target population was the civilian, noninstitutionalized population, 1–74 years of age, living in the coterminous United States. Native Americans residing on reservations were not included. *NHANES II* was conducted from 1976 to 1980 and expanded the nutrition component.[11] The medical components of primary interest were diabetes, kidney and liver functions, allergy, and speech pathology. The target population was expanded to include those persons 6 months to 74 years of age, including people in Alaska and Hawaii. There was oversampling of those persons aged 6 months to 5 years, those aged 60–74 years, and those living in poverty areas. *NHANES III* was conducted from 1988 to 1994 and included those persons 2 to 6 months of age in the target population.[12] There was oversampling of children aged 2 to 35 months, persons over 69 years of age, Black Americans, and Mexican Americans. Table 7–3 includes data from other CDC surveys and from other agencies that related specifically to health care provision.

The *National Health Provider Inventory* (National Master Facility Inventory) is a comprehensive file of inpatient health facilities in the United States. There are three categories of facilities in the inventory: hospitals, nursing and related care facilities, and other custodial or remedial care facilities. To be included in the inventory, hospitals must have at least six inpatient beds, and other facilities must have at least three inpatient beds. The inventory is kept current through reports from state licensing and other agencies for all newly established facilities. In addition, there is a yearly survey of hospitals and periodic surveys of other facilities.

The *National Home and Hospice Care Survey* is an annual national survey of home health agencies and hospices that was begun in 1992. A sample of current and discharged patients is conducted by staff who are familiar with the type of care being received.

The *National Hospital Discharge Survey* is a continuing nationwide sample survey of short-stay hospitals in the United States. Before 1988, lengths of stay greater than 30 days were ex-

Table 7–3 Data for Community Health Planning: Hospitalization, Ambulatory Medical Care, and Estimated Prevalence of Disease

Category (Examples)	*Source*	*Data Set Name*	*Smallest Geographic Unit*
Hospitalization (e.g., leading causes of hospitalization by age and population subgroup)	1. National Center for Health Statistics 2. Health Care Financing Administration 3. Dartmouth Center for Clinical Evaluative Services 4. Medicaid Data System	1. National Hospital Discharge Survey 2. Medicare Statistical System 3. Dartmouth Atlas of Health Care	1. Census regions 2. State 3. Hospital referral region
Ambulatory medical care	1. National Center for Health Statistics	1. National Hospital Ambulatory Medical Care Survey 2. National Ambulatory Medical Care Survey	1. Four national regions 2. Four national regions
Estimated prevalence of disease	1. National Center for Health Statistics	1a. National Health Interview Survey 1b. National Health and Nutrition Examination Survey	1. National
	2. Centers for Disease Control and Prevention	2a. National Notifiable Diseases Surveillance System 2b. AIDS surveillance	2. State
	3. National Institutes of Health	3. Surveillance, Epidemiology, and End Results (SEER) Program	3. County
	4. State cancer registries	4. Cancer and tumor registries	4. County, ZIP code, limited street

Source: Adapted from C.V. Lee, *Journal of Public Health Management and Practice,* Vol. 5, No. 4, pp. 7–22, © 1999, Aspen Publishers, Inc.

cluded. Presently, the only exclusions are discharged newborn infants and discharges from federal hospitals. Abstracts of patient records are prepared from the sample of hospitals selected.

The *National Ambulatory Medical Care Survey* is a continuing national sample survey of ambulatory medical encounters. The survey covers patient–physician encounters with nonfederally employed physicians. Excluded from the survey are telephone contacts; nonoffice visits; visits to hospital-based physicians; visits to anesthesiologists, pathologists, and radiologists; and physicians involved in research, teaching, or administration. A random sample of office visits to nonexcluded physicians is carried out.

The *National Hospital Ambulatory Medical Care Survey* is a continuing annual national sample survey that was initiated in 1992 to examine visits to emergency departments and outpatient departments in nonfederal, short-stay, or general hospitals. Telephone contacts are excluded. Hospital staff are asked to complete patient record forms for a random sample of patient visits during a four-week reporting period.

Acquired Immune Deficiency Syndrome (AIDS) surveillance is conducted by health departments in each state, territory, and the District of Columbia. Reporting sources include hospitals and hospital-based physicians, physicians in nonhospital practice, public and private clinics, and medical records systems. The health departments collect data without personal identifiers using a standard confidential case report form.

The *National Notifiable Diseases Surveillance System* provides weekly provisional information on the occurrence of diseases that are defined as notifiable by the Council of State and Territorial Epidemiologists. The system provides summary data on an annual basis. The reporting of the states and territories to the CDC is voluntary.

The *National Traumatic Occupational Fatalities Surveillance System* is compiled by the National Institute for Occupational Safety and Health (NIOSH) based on information taken from death certificates. The following criteria are used to select the death certificates: age 16 years or older, an external cause of death (ICD-9, E800–E999), and a positive response to the "Injury at work?" item on the death certificate. Guidelines have been completed for filling out the injury at work item so the capture of data should improve. Denominator data come from the Census Bureau's County Business Patterns, supplemented by employment data for agriculture derived from the Census Bureau's 1982 census of agriculture, and public administration employment data taken from the Bureau of Labor Statistics' annual average employment data for 1980–89. Rates are figured for the U.S. civilian labor force.

From a perspective of community health planning, a number of important health problems (e.g., cardiovascular disease, cancer) have a relatively long latency period. In order to plan community interventions, information is needed about behavioral risk factors (e.g., smoking habits, physical activity, diet, and health insurance), as well as morbidity and mortality. At the national level, the CDC collaborates with state health departments on a *Behavioral Risk Factor Surveillance System (BRFSS),* where each state conducts a telephone survey of a sample of state residents using uniform questions. Summary data are made available at the state level. Because behavioral risk factor information is quite useful at the local level, some local health departments are now starting to develop behavioral risk factor surveys specific for their jurisdiction. Table 7–4 shows data sources that can be accessed for information regarding occupation and other activities that may impact health.

National Institutes of Health (NIH)

NIH is one of the world's foremost biomedical research centers and the federal focal point for biomedical research in the United States. NIH's mission is to uncover new knowledge that will lead to better health for everyone. NIH works toward that mission by conducting research in its own laboratories; supporting the research of nonfederal scientists in universities, medical schools, hospitals, and research institutions throughout the country and abroad; helping in the training of research investigators; and fostering communication of biomedical information. The goal of NIH research is to acquire new knowledge to help prevent, detect, diagnose, and treat disease and disability.

NIH has developed the *NIH Information Index* to provide information on: (1) diseases that are currently under investigation by NIH or NIH-supported scientists, (2) major NIH research areas, and (3) important health-related topics. Each listing in the index includes the abbreviated name(s) of the NIH institute, center, division, or other component to call for information, as well as the appropriate phone number(s).

One of the most widely used data sources from NIH is the *Surveillance, Epidemiology, and End Results (SEER) Program.* The National Cancer Institute contracts with selected population-based cancer registries throughout the United States and Puerto Rico to collect data for the SEER Program on residents who have recently been diagnosed with cancer and to collect follow-up data on persons who were previously diagnosed with cancer. The population estimates used to calculate incidence rates are obtained from the Census Bureau. The sample rates from the collecting centers are used to estimate county rates for the entire country.

Table 7–4 Data for Community Health Planning: Occupational Health and Safety, Substance Abuse, Mental Health/Mental Retardation, Behavioral Risk Factors, and Lifestyle Marketing Data

Category	*Source*	*Data Set Name*	*Smallest Geographic Unit*
Occupational health and safety	National Institute for Occupational Safety and Health Bureau of Labor Statistics	National Traumatic Occupational Fatalities Surveillance System	1. State
Substance abuse (e.g., drug-related deaths and emergency room visits, alcohol-related deaths and accidents)	Substance Abuse and Mental Health Services Administration	National Household Surveys on Drug Abuse Drug Abuse Warning Network	1. Four U.S. regions 2. Metropolitan areas
Mental health/mental retardation (e.g., teenage suicides, serious mental retardation in school-age children)	Substance Abuse and Mental Health Services Administration	Monitoring the Future Survey of Mental Health Organizations	1. National
Behavioral risk factors (e.g., current smokers, sedentary lifestyle, not using seat belt)	Centers for Disease Control and Prevention	Behavioral Risk Factor Survey	1. State
Lifestyle marketing data	Commercial sources (e.g., CACI International or Claritas)	Neighborhood or lifestyle segmentation	1. Census tract

Source: Adapted from C.V. Lee, *Journal of Public Health Management and Practice,* Vol. 5, No. 4, pp. 7–22, © 1999, Aspen Publishers, Inc.

The *Monitoring the Future Study* (High School Senior Survey) is a large-scale annual survey of drug use and related attitudes that was begun in 1975. Data are collected using self-administered questionnaires that are given out in classrooms. In 1991, the study was expanded to include eighth and tenth graders in addition to twelfth graders.

Health Care Financing Administration (HCFA)

HCFA is the federal agency that administers the Medicare, Medicaid, and Child Health insurance programs. HCFA provides health insurance for more than 74 million Americans through Medicare, Medicaid, and Child Health. The majority of these individuals receive their benefits through the fee-for-service delivery system; however, an increasing number are choosing managed care plans. In addition to providing health insurance, HCFA also performs a number of quality-focused activities, including the regulation of laboratory testing (Clinical Laboratory Improvements Amendments [CLIA]), surveys and certification of health care facilities (including nursing homes, home health agencies, and intermediate care facilities for the mentally retarded), development of coverage policies, and quality-of-care improvement.

HCFA annually compiles estimates of expenditures for health by type of expenditure and source of funds. Those data are released in the annual reports called *National Health Expenditures.* The American Hospital Association (AHA) data on hospital finances are the primary source for estimates related to hospital care (including expenditures in hospital outpatient clinics, expenses for hospital-based home health agencies, the cost of nursing care provided in a hospital setting, and the salaries of physicians and dentists on hospital staff). Expenditures for home health care and for services of health professionals are estimated using data from the Census Bureau's Service Annual Survey and the quinquennial census of service industries. Estimates for retail spending for prescription drugs are based on industry data on prescription drug transactions. Other estimates in the report are based on a variety of sources.

Estimates of State Health Expenditures are also compiled annually by type of expenditure and source of funds for each state. Data sources for the estimates are the same as noted above for the national estimates.

The *Medicare Statistical System* provides data for examining the program's effectiveness and for tracking the eligibility of enrollees and the benefits they use, the certification of institutional providers, and the payments made for services provided. The system has four major files: the health insurance master file, the service provider file, the hospital insurance claims file, and the supplementary medical insurance payment records file.

The *Medicaid Data System* contains data compiled from forms that are submitted annually by state Medicaid agencies. The user must keep in mind that definitions from the various states may differ, and some states have duplicated counts of recipients. This limits the usefulness of the data to examine areas larger than a state. Comparisons between states should be made with extreme caution.

Health Resources and Services Administration (HRSA)

The HRSA directs national health programs that improve the health of the nation by ensuring quality health care to underserved, vulnerable, and special-need populations and by promoting appropriate health professions work force capacity and practice, particularly in primary care and public health.

The HRSA publishes a report called *Physician Supply Projections.* The projections in this report are based on a model developed by the Bureau of Health Professionals. The model forecasts the supply of physicians by specialty, activity, and state in which they practice. The source of the baseline data for the model is the American Medical Association (AMA) Physician Masterfile for 1986.

The HRSA also publishes *Nurse Supply Estimates,* a report on the supply of nurses in the country. The estimates in this report are based on a model developed by the Bureau of Health Professionals. The model estimates the number of nurses currently licensed to practice, the supply of full- and part-time practicing nurses, and the full-time equivalent supply of nurses for each state. The estimates are divided into levels based on educational attainment: associate degree or diploma, bachelor's degree, master's degree, and doctorate. Data sources for the estimates include the National League for Nursing, the National Council of State Boards of Nursing, and the National Sample Survey of Registered Nurses performed in 1992.

Substance Abuse and Mental Health Services Administration (SAMHSA)

The SAMHSA is the federal agency charged with improving the quality and availability of prevention, treatment, and rehabilitation services in order to reduce illness, death, disability, and cost to society resulting from substance abuse and mental illnesses.

The SAMHSA conducts the *National Household Surveys on Drug Abuse* to collect data on trends in the use of marijuana, cigarettes, alcohol, and cocaine among persons 12 years of age and older. The SAMHSA began collecting the data for the survey in 1971. The survey covers the civilian, noninstitutionalized population 12 years of age and older in the United States. Persons from 12 to 34 years of age, African Americans, Hispanics, and individuals in six selected large metropolitan areas are oversampled.

The *Drug Abuse Warning Network* (DAWN) is a large-scale, ongoing drug abuse data collection system based on information from emergency room and medical examiner facilities. The system collects information about drug abuse occurrences that resulted in a medical crisis or death. The objectives of the system are to monitor drug abuse patterns and identify trends, identify substances associated with drug abuse episodes, and assess the drug-related health consequences. The system was first developed in 1978 and was redesigned in 1988.

The *Survey of Mental Health Organizations* is a biennial inventory of mental health organizations and general hospital mental health services. The purpose of the survey is to determine the sociodemographic, clinical, and treatment characteristics of the patients serviced by these types of facilities.

U.S. Bureau of the Census

The mission of the Census Bureau is to be the preeminent collector and provider of timely, relevant, and quality data about the people and economy of the United States. Its goal is to provide the best mix of timeliness, relevancy, quality, and cost for the data collected and the services provided. The Census Bureau is headed by a director, who is assisted by a deputy director and an executive staff composed of associate directors. The Bureau has 12 regional offices with additional processing centers set up temporarily for the decennial censuses. The sole purpose of the censuses and surveys is to secure general statistical information. Replies are obtained from individuals and establishments only to enable the compilation of such general statistics. The confidentiality of these replies is very important. By law, no one—neither the census takers nor any other Census Bureau employee—is permitted to reveal identifiable information regarding any person, household, or business.

Accurate and current demographic data (e.g., age, sex, race, ethnic group) and projections are critically important for community planning, and also as denominators for the computation of rates. The *decennial census* (e.g., 1990 or 2000) is the "gold standard," and is available from the U.S. Bureau of the Census to the census block group level.[13] Commercial vendors have been able to compact many of the variables from the 1990 census onto one CD-ROM.

Selected socioeconomic variables (e.g., poverty, education level, age of housing) are also available from the Census Bureau to the census block group level. Age of housing is of special interest as part of childhood lead poisoning prevention efforts. In some communities, the tax assessor's office may be able to provide information on age of housing in electronic format. If so, then the local health department's childhood lead poisoning prevention program may find it useful to access and link the electronic housing age data with electronic information about new births. Childhood lead poisoning prevention efforts can then be focused on specific individual houses containing an infant and a high likelihood of the presence of lead-based paint.

The Census Bureau's *mapping program* supports the decennial census through the production of street-level address maps for use by the census enumerators. For the 1990 census, TIGER (Topologically Integrated Geographic Encoding and Referencing) was developed. TIGER uses the street segment to form blocks that are the basis of census geography. TIGER was a collaborative effort between the Census Bureau and the U.S. Geological Survey. An important feature of TIGER data is that each geographic unit has a unique identifier that links it to the population attribute data in the main census files, allowing the collection of a great deal of population information for a wide variety of areas.

The Census Bureau has developed a new online system for data access and dissemination called the *American FactFinder*. Since early 1999, individuals have been able to access data tabulations and maps from the available census data sets. Among the data sets that are presently available in the system are the 1990 Decennial Census Detailed Files, the American Community Survey Summary Tables, the Census 2000 Dress Rehearsal Summary Files, and the 1997 Economic Census Summary Files. Table 7–5 includes data that form the denominators for our analysis such as the demographic and socioeconomic information on a community.

U.S. Bureau of Labor Statistics

The Bureau of Labor Statistics is the major federal agency for collecting information in the fields of labor economics. The bureau is an

Table 7–5 Data for Community Health Planning: Demographic, Socioeconomics, Health Care Expenditures, and Health Care Resources and Access to Primary Care

Category (Examples)	*Source*	*Data Set Name*	*Smallest Geographic Unit*
Demographic data (e.g., age, sex, race, and ethnic distribution)	U.S. Bureau of the Census	1. Decennial and periodic census	1. Census block
Socioeconomic data (e.g., educational level, poverty level, percent unemployed, age of housing, and number of workers by industry)	U.S. Bureau of the Census Bureau of Labor Statistics	1. Decennial and periodic census 2. County Business Patterns	1. Census block group 2. County
Health care expenditures (e.g., number of persons on Medicaid, number of persons in Women, Infants, and Children Program, number of homeless persons, number of food stamp recipients)	Health Care Financing Administration	1. Estimates of National Health Expenditures 2. Estimates of State Health Expenditures	1. National 2. State
Health care resources and access to primary care (e.g., number of primary care physicians, community and migrant health care centers, uninsured/underinsured)	Health Resources and Services Administration	1. Area Resource File 2. Physician Supply Estimates 3. Nurse Supply Estimates 4. National Health Provider Inventory 5. National Home and Hospice Care Survey	1. County 2–5. National

Source: Adapted from C.V. Lee, *Journal of Public Health Management and Practice,* Vol. 5, No. 4, pp. 7–22, © 1999, Aspen Publishers, Inc.

agency within the Department of Labor. The surveys and programs of the Bureau of Labor Statistics include a wide range of subjects under the general categories of employment and unemployment, prices and living conditions, compensation and working conditions, productivity and technology, employment projections, and international programs. One useful survey is the *Non-Farm Payroll Statistics from the Current Employment Statistics,* which includes monthly data on employment, hours, and earnings by industry for selected geographic areas.

U.S. Environmental Protection Agency (EPA)

The EPA was established to protect human health and the natural environment on which human health depends. In 1987, the EPA established a *National Geographic Information Systems Program* to coordinate the use of spatial data. EPA maintains numerous data sets that can be downloaded and used in geographic analysis. Some of the more widely used data sets include the following:

- The *American Indian Lands Environmental Support Project* (AILESP) contains data on current multimedia contaminant releases, recent compliance and enforcement histories for facilities located on or near Indian lands, and other environmental data, such as stream reaches with fish consumption advisories, contaminated fish tissues, and contaminated sediments.
- *Better Assessment Science Integrating Point and Nonpoint Sources* (BASINS) integrates national watershed data and state-of-the-art environmental assessment and modeling tools.
- The *EPA Spatial Data Library System* (ESDLS) is a repository for the agency's new and legacy geospatial data holdings that are accessible through various geographic information systems (GIS) applications.
- The *Geospatial Data Clearinghouse* site provides access to geospatial data used in GIS to identify the location and characteristics of natural or manmade features and boundaries on the earth.
- The Internet-based *Maps on Demand* (MOD) generates maps to display environmental information for the entire United States. MOD accesses data available through the *Envirofacts Data Warehouse.*

Table 7–6 provides sources of environmental data that can have an impact on the health of the population.

Agency for Toxic Substances and Disease Registry (ATSDR)

The ATSDR was established as an agency of the DHHS by the Superfund Act. The agency's *Hazardous Substance Release/Health Effects Database* (HazDat) was developed to provide access to information concerning the release of hazardous substances from Superfund sites or from emergency events and to provide information on the effects of exposure to hazardous substances on the public health. The database includes information on the hazardous waste sites, the contaminants present at the sites, the concentration of the contaminants, the size of the exposed or potentially exposed population, and community health concerns.

The ATSDR has *environmental exposure registries* for several chemicals including benzene, tri-chlor ethylene, and dioxin. The individuals compiling these registries follow persons who have been identified as having environmental exposures to these chemicals and administer questionnaires to identify any health complaints the individuals have noticed. Data are available only for the entire registry population and not for local areas.

STATE SOURCES OF DATA

State Vital Statistics

In the United States, responsibility for the certification of vital events rests with the states. Among the items collected by state vital statistics agencies are information on births, deaths,

Table 7–6 Data for Community Health Planning: Meteorological/Climatological Data and Environmental Hazards

Category	*Source*	*Data Set Name*	*Smallest Geographic Unit*
Environmental hazards (e.g., locations of toxic waste sites)	1. U.S. Environmental Protection Agency	1a. Envirofacts Data Warehouse 1b. EPA Spatial Data Library System 1c. Better Assessment Science Integrating Point and Nonpoint Sources 1d. American Indian Lands Environmental Support Project	1. Local
	2. Agency for Toxic Substances and Disease Registry	2a. Hazardous Substance Release/Health Effects Database 2b. Environmental exposure registries for selected chemicals (e.g., benzene, tri-chlor ethylene, and dioxin)	2a. Local site specific 2b. Registry coverage area

Source: Adapted from C.V. Lee, *Journal of Public Health Management and Practice,* Vol. 5, No. 4, pp. 7–22, © 1999, Aspen Publishers, Inc.

fetal deaths, and induced terminations of pregnancy (abortions). Consistency of the reporting of information is ensured through contracts between the federal government and the states, providing for standardized certification forms that include a standard set of items needed at the federal level.

Birth certificate data can be very useful in health care planning. The registration of births is considered essentially complete, with periodic checks showing registration rates for births at more than 99 percent. Birth registration in this country has been carried out for many years, allowing for time-period analysis of the data. Geographic coverage of births has been complete since 1933. This allows the researcher to use the data for spatial comparisons. Information collected on the certificates can be used for analysis based on maternal age and race. The information is also useful for studying birth weight and some birth defects. Mothers provide demographic information for birth certificates and hospital records provide health information. One major difficulty in using birth certificate data for local analysis is that actual residence data may not be available in electronic form. Data are generally kept in electronic form for county or ZIP code, but not necessarily for street address. Birth certificate information includes residence at the time of birth, which is not necessarily the residence at the time of the exposure of interest. Some studies have indicated that in certain populations, up to 30 percent of women may move during their third trimester. Although certain information such as birth weight is generally considered reliable, problems have been noted with the information on APGAR score, gestational age, and prenatal history. Problems arise from using birth defects information contained on birth certificates because some birth defects do not manifest themselves until the child is older and therefore are not noted when the birth certificate is filled out.

Death certificate information has similar advantages for health care planning as birth certificate information. The registration for deaths is considered essentially complete. And, like birth registration, death registration in this country has been carried out for many years, allowing for time-period analysis of the data. Geographic coverage of deaths has been complete since 1933, allowing the researcher to use the data for spatial comparisons. Information collected on the certificates can be used for analysis based on sex, age, and race. Demographic information on the death certificate is provided by the funeral director. Because certain demographic information (race, ethnicity) for the birth and death certificates is provided by persons with different degrees of closeness to the individual (family member vs. funeral director), the possibility exists that the recorded race of an individual may differ from birth to death. Medical certification of the cause of death is provided by a physician, medical examiner, or coroner. Analysis of death certificate data is useful for rapidly fatal diseases. As with birth certificates, however, a major difficulty in using death certificate data is that the actual residence data may not be available in electronic form. Data are generally kept in electronic form for county or ZIP code, not necessarily for street address. Death certificate information includes the residence at the time of death, which is not necessarily the residence at the time of the exposure of interest. The data are not useful for examining diseases with long latencies or nonfatal conditions.

Fetal death certificates are required by most states for the certification of fetal deaths after 20 weeks' gestation. A problem arises because a fetal death is defined as the death in utero of a fetus that weighs 500 grams or more at birth, irrespective of gestational age. Because the certification requirements do not reflect the definition, the certification of fetal deaths is incomplete. For fetuses born after 28 weeks, certification is nearly complete because most of them weigh greater than 500 grams. However, certification is inconsistent for fetuses born between 20–28 weeks' gestation and incomplete for those born less than 20 weeks' gestation. The problem of data inconsistency and variability of coverage makes the data from fetal death certifications less useful in geographic analysis.

Abortion data are used to provide information on fertility, pregnancy rates, and abortion rates. This information can be used to evaluate the effectiveness of family planning programs and programs aimed at reducing teen pregnancies.

State Disease Registries

Cancers and tumors are the most common groups of diseases for which registries are established. Reporting is generally close to complete for most areas where the registries exist. The data include information on cancer incidence but not mortality. Information from the registries allows for comparisons by age, sex, and race. Residence is considered a personal identifier, and getting such information from the registries at the local level is difficult. The rates of some rare cancers can be very unstable for small areas such as counties. This information is not useful for cancers such as lung cancer, which have a latency period of 20–30 years. Exhibit 7–2 includes those states having cancer registries in 1994.

Congenital malformation or birth defect registries are much less common than cancer registries. Most such registries are passive (do not actively update or confirm information) so the ascertainment rate is not very high for many defects. Residence is considered a personal identifier, and getting information from the registries at the local level is difficult.

Some states, industrial facilities, the NIOSH, and the military have some form of *occupational exposure registries* for selected chemicals. The information contained in these registries is most useful for identifying some health effects reported by persons who have been exposed to occupational levels of those chemicals.

State Medicaid Agency

Created in 1965 under Title XIX of the Social Security Act, Medicaid is a jointly funded, fed-

Exhibit 7–2 Location of U.S. Registries Listed by the National Association of Central Cancer Registries: Cancer in North America, 1990–1994

Arizona	Kentucky	New York
California	Louisiana	North Carolina
CA: Los Angeles	Maryland	Pennsylvania
CA: San Francisco/Oakland	Massachusetts	Rhode Island
CA: San Jose/Monterey	Michigan	Texas
Colorado	MI: Metropolitan Detroit	Utah
Connecticut	Minnesota	Virginia
Delaware	Montana	Washington
Florida	Nebraska	WA: Seattle/Puget Sound
GA: Metropolitan Atlanta	Nevada	West Virginia
Hawaii	New Hampshire	Wisconsin
Idaho	New Jersey	Wyoming
Illinois	New Mexico	Puerto Rico
Iowa		

Source: Data from National Association of Central Cancer Registries.

eral–state health insurance program to provide medical assistance for certain low-income and needy people. In 1996, it covered approximately 36 million individuals, including children; the aged, blind, and/or disabled; and people who are eligible to receive federally assisted income maintenance payments. Federal statutes and regulations provide broad national guidelines for the program. Each state determines its eligibility standards, the scope of services, the rate of payment for services, and how its program will be administered. There are several categorically needy groups that the states must provide services to if they are to receive federal funds. Managed care as an option for Medicaid recipients is increasing rapidly and may soon approach 50 percent. States maintain data on the recipients of services, the scope of services provided, and the cost of the program. In addition to the federal program, several states have "state-only" programs to provide assistance to certain Medicaid-ineligible groups.

State Department of Transportation (DOT)

The DOT and its predecessors often represent one of the longest tenured line agency functions in state government. The DOT generally coordinates the development of transportation with each mode serving its best purpose. Under its auspices fall the entire transportation network, including

- state and local highway system
- a rail network over which tons of equipment, raw materials, manufactured goods, and produce are shipped each year
- public and private aviation facilities
- public transit operators
- major public and private ports

State Planning Agencies

Planning agencies deal with development within their boundaries. Most of planning relates to providing a comprehensive guide to the physical, economic, and social environments of communities. Elements of planning include objectives of land development, zoning controls, transportation, strategies for economic revitalization of depressed areas, and guidelines for environmental protection. Many planning agencies can provide a variety of socioeconomic, demographic, and land use data for use by health care planners.

LOCAL SOURCES OF DATA

Public health agencies can also obtain additional information for their service areas by implementing low-cost telephone surveys. Local public health agencies have information limitations because data from many sources are not applicable to the relatively small geographic areas served by local agencies. Also, vital statistics data and morbidity data collected and available to local health agencies are restricted in scope and may not fulfill a specific information need associated with a health problem or proposed initiative.

Surveys can be designed for these purposes and can take the form of direct questioning, mail, or telephone queries. The advantages of implementing these surveys by a local health agency is that this method works well to obtain information on a particular objective within a defined community. For successful use of this data collection strategy, three requirements must be fulfilled.

1. The design of the survey must ensure that individuals interviewed are representative of the community or group of interest.
2. The survey instrument must be acceptable to respondents in terms of length and content.
3. Implementation cost must be relatively low.

Using a Telephone Survey To Evaluate a Community Folic Acid Intake Campaign

In October 1996, the Onondaga County Health Department (OCHD) launched a campaign to increase folic acid intake among all women of childbearing age in this county of 470,000 people in central New York State. This initiative was based on the U.S. Public Health Service recommendation that all women capable of becoming pregnant consume 0.4 mg of folic acid daily to reduce the risk of having children with spina bifida and other neural tube defects.[14]

Pre- and postcampaign random telephone surveys were conducted to evaluate changes in awareness and use of multivitamins.[15] The first step was to develop a survey tool. This was accomplished through group discussion and a literature review to locate any existing and relevant survey tools. Two instruments were located. One had been created by the Gallup Organization for the March of Dimes and a second was from the Georgia Women's Health Survey.[16,17] With permission of these two organizations, a modified instrument with approximately 20 questions was prepared.

Three criteria can be applied to a survey tool.

1. Does the survey address key questions that derive from the campaign's goal and objectives?
2. Does it provide information that will inform decisions?
3. Does it permit delineation of populations or geographic areas at risk?

The draft survey tool was field tested with 60 women to assess time for completion, unexpected reactions, and flow.

Next, a statistical sample and sampling frame were developed. The overall goal of the sampling methodology was to collect representative, precise information about knowledge and practice regarding folic acid use for women 18–45 years of age. A goal of at least 650 completed surveys was set for each sample, based on a decision to keep the overall margin of error small.

A random sampling design was used with ZIP codes as sampling units. The objective was that the percentage distribution of the completed surveys across ZIP codes would be the same as the percentage distribution of women between the ages of 18–45 years living in these ZIP code areas. However, after meeting these statistical quotas, oversampling was conducted within targeted ZIP codes to increase sample size for racial and ethnic minorities, who make up less than 10 percent of the overall population. Readily available computer software with all telephone listings on CD-ROM was used as the source of local phone numbers for the call lists in each ZIP code. The size of these call lists took into account an expected "hit rate" of 15 dials to 1 completed interview based on the pilot study results.[15]

A volunteer work force was used to staff the 36 calling sessions. The total incremental cost for both the pre- and postsurvey was only $2,500, which was mostly related to telephone charges and food for the volunteers.[15] The survey results are illustrated in Figures 7–1 and 7–2.

A telephone survey using similar methodology was used in 1997 to ascertain the rate of mammography utilization in women over the age of 50 years.[18] Results of this survey, shown in Figures 7–3 and 7–4, were important for communitywide efforts to increase mammography rates.

OTHER SOURCES OF DATA

Managed Care Data

An increasing proportion of individuals are enrolled in managed care organizations. In addition, many states are enrolling increasing numbers of Medicaid recipients into managed care plans for the provision of health services. Data that monitor the receipt of preventive services by managed care organizations are of significant potential importance for public health agencies. Managed care enrollees are a group of individuals who constitute a subpopulation. As enrollment in these plans grows, the aggregate or total of these subpopulations constitutes a substantial proportion of the community population. Data from managed care entities on immunization, blood lead screening, mammography, pap smear screening, and other factors are important to public health agencies for two reasons: (1) information is provided on the performance of individual plans in delivering preventive services and (2) information is available on the status of clinical preventive services in a large proportion of community residents.

The opportunity for using this type of data is now possible because of the development of the *Health Plan Employer Data and Information Set (HEDIS)* by the National Committee for Quality Assurance (NCQA). These measures were initially established by representatives from a variety of health plans and employers to respond to employer need: "How to understand what 'value' the health care dollar is purchasing and

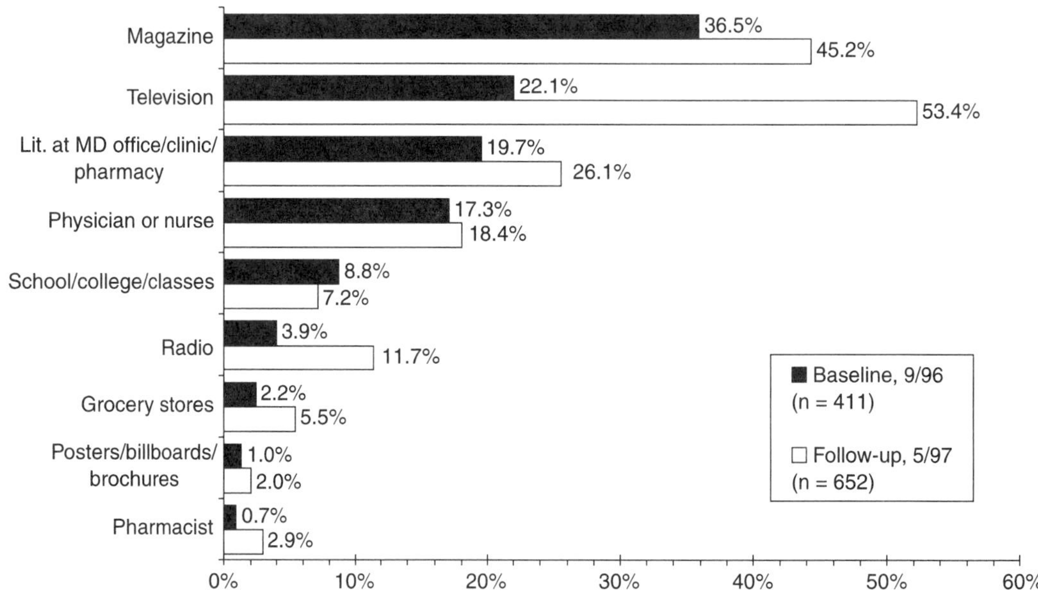

Figure 7–1 Folic Acid Survey, Resident Women 18–45 Years, Onondaga County, NY: Responses to "Where or How Did You Learn about Folic Acid?" *Source:* Onondaga County Department of Health, 1997, Onondaga County, New York.

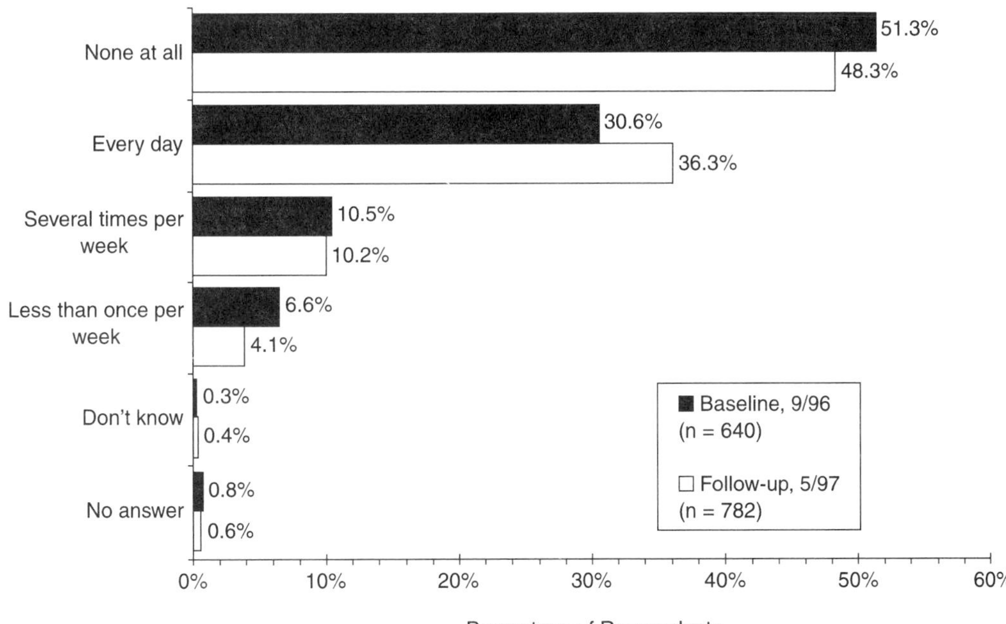

Figure 7–2 Folic Acid Survey, Resident Women 18–45 Years, Onondaga County, NY: Responses to "How Often Have You Taken Multivitamins during the Past 30 Days?" *Source:* Onondaga County Department of Health, 1997, Onondaga County, New York.

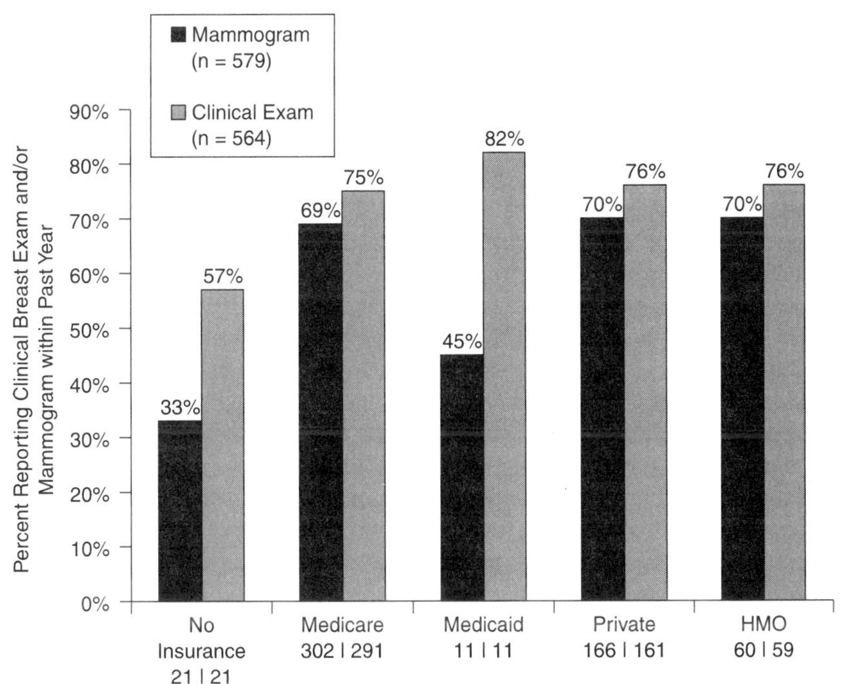

Figure 7–3 Clinical Breast Exam and Mammogram during Past Year by Insurance: Onondaga County, NY, 1997. *Source: Mammography Utilization Survey,* Onondaga County Department of Health, October 1997, Onondaga County, New York.

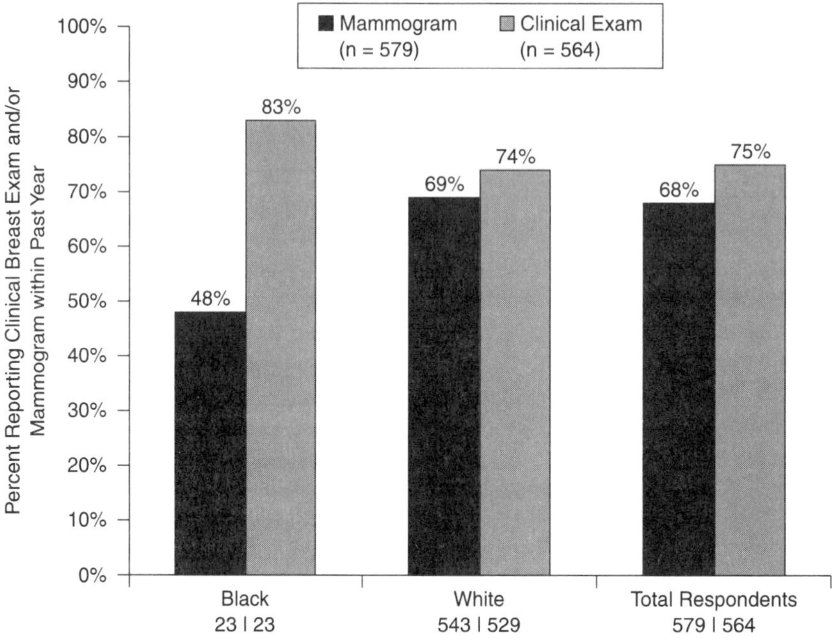

Figure 7–4 Clinical Breast Exam and Mammogram during Past Year by Race: Onondaga County, NY, 1997. *Source: Mammography Utilization Survey,* Onondaga County Department of Health, October 1997, Onondaga County, New York.

how to hold a health plan 'accountable for its performance.'"[19(p.1)] The initial draft document of *HEDIS* measures was completed in 1991 and incorporated into the NCQA evaluation of health plans.[17] Further information on the NCQA accreditation process may be obtained by contacting the NCQA in Washington, DC (www.ncqa.org).

HEDIS 2000, the latest data and information set, is the most widely used set of performance measures in the managed care industry.[20] *HEDIS 2000* contains 56 measures across eight domains of care: effectiveness of care, access/availability of care, satisfaction with the experience of care, health plan stability, use of services, cost of care, informed health care choices, and health plan descriptive information.[20] (See Table 7–7 for *HEDIS 2000* effectiveness of care measures.) Some of the specific areas included in *HEDIS* are preventive measures, including childhood immunization and screening for breast cancer and cervical cancer. These measures are relevant to public health practice and, where available, *HEDIS* uses *Healthy People 2000* goals as benchmarks or standards. For benchmark purposes, NCQA's Quality Compass rates are also available based on 1997 *HEDIS* data from commercial plans nationwide. Quality Compass rates are derived from commercial care plans and therefore are of limited comparability to Medicaid enrollees. The NCQA is currently working with a number of states to develop benchmarks for the Medicaid population.[21]

States may have specific quality assurance reporting requirements (QARRs) designed to examine managed care performance. New York State uses measures largely adopted from the NCQA's *HEDIS* reporting requirements with additional New York State–specific measures needed to address public health issues of particular significance in New York, such as lead screening of children and HIV testing of pregnant women.[21] Commercial and Medicaid immunization rates for New York State managed

Table 7–7 *HEDIS 2000* Effectiveness of Care Measures

HEDIS 2000 *Measures*	*Applicable to:* *Medicaid*	*Commercial*	*Medicare*
Effectiveness of care			
Childhood immunization status	X	X	
Adolescent immunization status	X	X	
Breast cancer screening	X	X	X
Cervical cancer screening	X	X	
Chlamydia screening in women (first year)	X	X	
Prenatal care in the first trimester	X	X	
Check-ups after delivery	X	X	
Controlling high blood pressure (first year)	X	X	X
Beta blocker treatment after a heart attack	X	X	X
Cholesterol management after acute cardiovascular events	X	X	X
Comprehensive diabetes care	X	X	X
Use of appropriate medications for people with asthma (first year)	X	X	
Follow-up after hospitalization for mental illness	X	X	X
Antidepressant medication management	X	X	X
Advising smokers to quit	X	X	X
Flu shots for older adults			X
Medicare health outcomes survey			X

Source: Reprinted with permission from the National Committee for Quality Assurance; *HEDIS® 2000,* Volume 1: What's In It and Why It Matters; page 35; © 2000 by NCQA.

HEDIS® is a registered trademark of the National Committee for Quality Assurance.

care plans in 1977 are shown in Tables 7–8 and 7–9. Only Medicaid lead screening rates are available (Table 7–10).

In interpreting this managed care data for public health purposes, several factors related to the collection and representativeness of the data are important. Two distinct strategies are used for obtaining data on specific performance measures: medical record (or chart review) or administrative or transaction information (claims, encounter data, membership data, pharmacy data).[19] Extracting data from the medical record is expensive, but this data can be more complete than data in administrative databases. Hybrid methods relying on both strategies are often employed. In examining performance measures of plans, adequacy of the data collection is important in establishing whether plan-specific differences in performance are real or are artifacts of the collection processes.

Another issue facing the local public health agency interested in using managed care data is the lack of congruence between the managed care plan service areas with the jurisdiction of the health department. For example, managed care plans may provide services to enrollees in many counties. Therefore, data on performance measures will be collected for all plan enrollees and not specifically for the individual county jurisdiction of the public health agency. Also, because the sample size for medical records or administrative data is limited, adequate data reflecting performance in the individual county may not be available. This is not a problem for public health agencies where boundaries have significant overlap with managed care plans.

However, even where significant overlap does not occur, the performance data of the managed care plan on preventive services is relevant to the public health agency. Poor or questionable performance by the managed care plan throughout its service area is a warning flag that should initiate further inquiry and discussion.

A factor to be considered in interpreting managed care plan performance data is that services provided by the plan are only one of the determi-

Table 7–8 Commercial Immunization Rates, NY State Managed Care Plans, 1997

Plan Name	*Type of Review**	*Number of Records Reviewed*	*Rate*	*Statistical Rating*
CDPHP	H	440	86	✪
CHP/Kaiser	H	418	86	✪
Community Blue	M	411	86	✪
Finger Lakes	H	422	86	✪
Health Care Plan	H	411	88	✪
HMO Blue	H	188	84	✪
HMO-CNY	H	354	83	✪
HSMC	H	288	87	✪
MVP	H	419	79	✪
Oxford Health Plan	H	411	80	✪
Preferred Care	H	411	85	✪
CIGNA Health Care	H	411	67	❍
Empire BC/BS	H	411	68	❍
IHA-Hudson Valley	H	315	75	❍
Prudential Health Care Plan	H	322	69	❍
Vytra	H	411	73	❍
Well Care	H	411	72	❍
Aetna/U.S. Healthcare	H	427	49	●
Healthsource HMO	H	190	53	●
HIP	H	411	50	●
IHA-Buffalo	H	411	65	●
MD:NY	A	157	54	●
NYLCare	H	411	16	●
Physicians Health Services	A	256	52	●
United HealthCare—NYC	A	335	56	●
United HealthCare—Upstate	H	161	58	●
Statewide average			70	
New York City			57	
Rest of state			75	

The following plan had data found to be unreliable: North Medical CHP.

The following plans are included in the statewide average but had sample sizes too small to report individually: Health Now, North American Healthcare, Partner's Health Plans.

*Type of Review: A—Administrative, H—Hybrid, M—Medical Record

Statistical Ratings: ✪ Rate is significantly better than the statewide average.
❍ Rate is not significantly different from the statewide average.
● Rate is significantly worse than the statewide average.

Source: 1999, New York State Department of Health.

Table 7–9 Medicaid Immunization Rates, NY State Managed Care Plans, 1997

Plan Name	*Number of Records Reviewed*	*Rate*	*Statistical Rating*
Bronx Health Plan	411	78	✪
Buffalo Community Health Plan	136	85	✪
CDPHP	295	85	✪
CHP/Kaiser	409	85	✪
Community Blue	202	75	✪
Fidelis Care New York	302	78	✪
Finger Lakes	419	82	✪
Health Plus	308	82	✪
Preferred Care	299	78	✪
Aetna/U.S. Healthcare	427	61	❍
Community Choice	115	61	❍
HealthFirst	411	61	❍
HIP	411	68	❍
IHA-Buffalo	411	61	❍
Neighborhood Health Providers	106	63	❍
St. Barnabas CHP	53	57	❍
Suffolk Health Plan	193	61	❍
Total Care	305	66	❍
WellCare	330	61	❍
CenterCare	411	53	●
Genesis Health Plan	91	38	●
Managed HealthCare System	411	49	●
MetroPlus	411	59	●
NYLCare	86	0	●
Oxford Health Plan	411	52	●
United HealthCare—Upstate	241	36	●
Vytra	276	57	●
Westchester PHSP	357	55	●
Statewide average		64	
New York City		63	
Rest of state		66	

The following plan had data found to be unreliable: ABC Health Plan.

The following plans are included in the statewide average but had sample sizes too small to report individually: CarePlus, Compre-Care, Empire BC/BS, New York Hospital CHP, United HealthCare—NYC.

Statistical Rating: ✪ Rate is significantly better than the statewide average.
❍ Rate is not significantly different from the statewide average.
● Rate is significantly worse than the statewide average.

Source: 1999, New York State Department of Health.

nants of the outcomes measured. Other health determinants such as socioeconomic status and education of the enrollees are also operating. Compliance with recommended visits is influenced by both client and plan factors. For some indicators, severity adjustment has been applied. For example, the New York State Department of Health risk adjusts low birth weight (LBW) rates to take into account differences in the demographic profiles of plans' enrollees. Variables included in the risk adjustment for LBW include education, alcohol use, drug use, smoking, level

Table 7–10 Medicaid Lead Screening Rates, NY State Managed Care Plans, 1997

Plan Name	*Type of Review**	*Number of Records Reviewed*	*Rate*	*Statistical Rating*
Bronx Health Plan	H	196	87	✪
Buffalo Community Health Plan	H	136	94	✪
CDPHP	H	295	78	✪
CHP/Kaiser	H	410	80	✪
Community Blue	H	204	86	✪
Community Choice	M	115	79	✪
Finger Lakes	A	627	76	✪
Health Plus	M	323	80	✪
HIP	H	411	77	✪
Preferred Care	H	299	86	✪
Suffolk Health Plan	M	194	86	✪
Total Care	M	305	74	✪
CenterCare	M	411	72	❍
MetroPlus	M	411	68	❍
Neighborhood Health Providers	M	106	75	❍
Oxford Health Plan	H	411	69	❍
St. Barnabas CHP	M	53	62	❍
Westchester PHSP	H	357	72	❍
Aetna/U.S. Healthcare	H	440	61	●
Fidelis Care New York	H	411	60	●
Genesis Health Plan	M	91	41	●
HealthFirst	M	411	62	●
IHA-Buffalo	M	411	57	●
NYLCare	H	86	42	●
United HealthCare—Upstate	M	241	33	●
Vytra	H	276	55	●
WellCare	H	330	59	●
Statewide average			69	
New York City			69	
Rest of state			68	

The following plans had data found to be unreliable: ABC Health Plan, Managed HealthCare Systems.

The following plans are included in the statewide average but had sample sizes too small to report individually: CarePlus, Compre-Care, Empire BC/BS, New York Hospital CHP, United HealthCare—NYC.

*Type of Review: A—Administrative, H—Hybrid, M—Medical Record

Statistical Ratings: ✪ Rate is significantly better than the statewide average.
❍ Rate is not significantly different from the statewide average.
● Rate is significantly worse than the statewide average.

Source: 1999, New York State Department of Health.

of prenatal care, race/ethnicity, marital status, parity, previous low birth weight, maternal risk factors, and nationality.[21] Similarly, comparing performance rates to a standard such as a year 2000 goal is difficult because of differences between the enrollees of a plan and the *Healthy People 2000* national goal that was developed for the entire U.S. population.

Despite these limitations, managed care data offer significant promise in abetting efforts to improve population health status. In addition to using *HEDIS* measures, public health agencies with registries containing immunization or lead testing data can match these against Medicaid managed care enrollee files to determine compliance with these preventive measures.

Public health staff can use performance data as indicators of potential problems with preventive services. Discussions of performance with managed care entities are warranted and remediation plans are requested. Although the data themselves may not be precise measures of performance, they are an important introduction to a quality assurance process. As these data become increasingly available from organized delivery systems, they will become useful community indicators to measure the provision of preventive services.

Commercial Health Care Databases

A wide array of data sets that can be used in community health planning are available from commercial vendors.

- *CACI International, Inc.* offers data on demographics, businesses, lifestyles, consumer spending, purchase potential, shopping centers, traffic volumes, and crime statistics. The data are available in a variety of formats such as reports, maps, electronic media, software, books, and lists. CACI builds on Census Bureau data to create its collection of databases. In addition to the latest census data, CACI also provides current-year updates and five-year forecasts.
- *Claritas* produces databases related to health care: DRG/ICD-9 Demand; HMOs and Hospitals; Nursing Homes; Physicians; and Senior Life Demographics. In addition to data sets, Claritas offers geocoding and point coding services. The geocoding process appends the following information to the records: block group number, census tract assignments, coordinates (latitude/longitude), lifestyle codes from Claritas' neighborhood segmentation system, and ZIP codes.
- *Healthdemographics* provides health care data and analytic systems. It produces packages of coordinated health care databases called HealthPacs. HealthPacs include demographic data, population-based models of the incidence of diseases by category, and estimates of the demand for services (inpatient, outpatient, physician services, etc.).

Neighborhood Segmentation Data

A neighborhood segmentation system contains neighborhoods that are grouped into clusters, or neighborhood segments, based on demographics and other characteristics (e.g., high proportion of people in the 20–30 age group). This information could be used by public health officials for targeting interventions (e.g., smoking cessation campaigns) or facility siting.

CACI produces a neighborhood segmentation system called ACORN. Similar to CACI, Claritas has a neighborhood segmentation system (PRIZM) based on demographics and "lifestyle" characteristics (e.g., active travelers).

USING THE INTERNET TO ACCESS DATA SOURCES

Government is increasingly recognizing the power of information technology (IT) to provide information to its constituents. In 1994, the National Performance Review strongly endorsed the use of IT to improve the service of government. Under revisions to the Freedom of Information Act, agencies are required to establish electronic records centers to provide more open access to documents and data. Friede and O'Carroll provided an excellent overview of the electronic data resources at the CDC and the ATSDR in their article for the *Journal of Public Health Management Practice.*[22] The article summarized major electronic information resources and provided information on obtaining access, required equipment, cost, and the office responsible for maintaining the data source. The Census Bureau has developed the Integrated Information Solutions Program to improve data access and dissemination.[23] One goal of the program is to integrate the Census Bureau's geographic, demographic, and economic data sets. The system will serve as a data warehouse with an electronic metadata repository. This will allow users to access focused data sets for their use. Some of the national-level sources of data are listed in Exhibit 7–3. In addition to those sources, each state health department maintains an Internet site for data access and querying. In addition, the NCHS provides a link to all state health departments from its Web page (http:www.cdc.gov/nchs/fastats/fastats.htm#S).

ISSUES IN DATA INTERPRETATION

While there are numerous sources of data available for community health planning, several factors influence the ability of health care planners and researchers to use that data. Some of the issues are those of data interpretation such as the rates selected and possible bias. One fac-

Exhibit 7–3 Examples of On-Line Gateways to Data That Can Be Used in Public Health Planning

- American Public Health Association: http://www.doody.com/apha.htm
- Bureau of the Census: http://www.census.gov
  TIGER Home Page: http://www.census.gov/tiger/tiger.html
- CACI: http://www.demographics.com
- Caliper Corporation: http://www.caliper.com
- Centers for Disease Control and Prevention: http://www.cdc.gov
  WONDER System: http://wonder.cdc.gov
  National Center for Health Statistics: http://www.cdc.gov/nchswww
  Behavioral Risk Factor Surveillance System: http://www.cdc.gov/nccdphp/brfss
  STDs or AIDS Surveillance: http://www.cdc.gov/nchstp
- Claritas: http://www.claritas.com
- Dartmouth Atlas of Health Care in the United States: http://www.darthmouth.edu/~atlas/
- Department of Health and Human Services: http://www.healthfinder.org
- Environmental Protection Agency: http://www.epa.gov
  National GIS Program: http://www.epa.gov/ngispr
  EPA Envirofacts: http://www.epa.gov/enviro/index_java.html
- Environmental Systems Research Institute: http://www.esri.com
- Geographic Data Technology: http://www.geographic.com
- Health Care Financing Administration: http://www.hcfa.gov/stats
- Healthdemographics: http://www.healthdemographics.com
- Health Resources and Services Administration: http://www.hrsa.dhhs.gov
- Healthy People 2000: http://odphp.osophs.dhhs.gov/pubs/hp2000/
- Healthy People 2010: http://www.health.gov/healthypeople/
- International Association of Cancer Registries: http://www-dep.iarc.fr
  Cancer Registry Resources: http://www-dep.iarc.fr/resour/manuals.htm
- MapInfo Corporation: http://www.mapinfo.com
- National Association of Central Cancer Registries: http://www.naaccr.org
- National Cancer Registrars Association: http://www.ncra-usa.org
- National Oceanic and Atmospheric Administration Data: http://www.noaa.gov
- National Program of Cancer Registries: http://www.cdc.gov/nccdphp/dcpc/npcr
- National Institutes of Health: http://www.nih.gov
- U.S. Geological Survey: Call: 1-800-USA-MAPS
  Main Home Page: http://www.usgs.gov
  EROS Data Center: http://edcwww.cr.usgs.gov/eros-home.html

tor in data interpretation is that many of the data sets mentioned were not necessarily collected for use in health care planning. Other issues are legal in nature or relate to issues of individual privacy. Those using these data sources must keep in mind all the factors that may influence the outcome of their analysis.

Common Rates Used in Analysis

Data are often presented in the form of a rate. A rate is a type of proportion that includes the element of time. Many of the indicators that are followed attempt to determine the frequency of disease in the population (Where do the cases occur?), the pattern of disease occurrence over time (When do the cases occur?), and the effects of that disease on the health of the population (Who in the population gets the disease?). Common measures used to follow this are the incidence rate, prevalence rate, mortality rate, and relative risk.[24(p.74)]

- The *incidence rate* is the number of new cases of a disease in a population over a specified period of time.
- The *prevalence rate* measures the proportion of people with the disease in the population at a point or period in time.
- The *mortality rate* measures the number of people dying with the disease in a population over a specified period of time.
- The *relative risk* evaluates the rate among those individuals with a selected characteristic (exposed) and compares it to the rate of the unexposed. The relative risk is used to provide an indication of the strength of an association.

Rates for populations can be expressed either as crude rates or as adjusted rates. *Crude rates* are based solely on the number of events in the population over a certain period of time. *Adjusted rates* are statistically transformed to control for the effects of a characteristic that may influence the risk of disease or death.[25] The most common variable that is adjusted for is age because of its profound effects on morbidity and mortality. There are two methods of adjusting rates: direct and indirect. The *direct* method applies the age-specific rates from the study population to a standard population. The *indirect* method uses the age-specific rates of a standard population to get an expected number of events in the study population. A standardized mortality (morbidity) ratio (SMR) is then used to relate the number of events observed to the number expected. The SMR is expressed as the total observed events in the study population over the total expected events in that population. An SMR of greater than 1 indicates that there were more of the events in the population than was expected. Thus, adjusted rates attempt to remove the effects of differences in composition between populations, thereby allowing for the comparison of rates.

Common Biases

Bias is defined as a systematic error in the estimation of an effect. There are three possible sources of bias: selection, information, and confounding. *Selection or sampling bias* occurs when the control group for the study is not representative of the population. *Information, observation, or misclassification bias* occurs during the collection phase of a study. Misclassification bias is a problem for environmental and other studies that use surrogates of exposure such as distance to a facility. Observation bias can also arise when either the subjects or the investigators are not blinded to exposure status of the subject. A very important source of bias is that of *confounding*, which is a mixing of two or more effects. This occurs when the estimate of the effect of an exposure under study is changed because of the effect of an extraneous factor. For a factor to be a confounder, it must have an effect on the occurrence of disease. A confounding factor must be associated with both the exposure and the disease under study. All types of bias must be considered and steps must be taken to deal with them in any study that is undertaken.

Ecologic Fallacy Issue

The ecologic fallacy problem occurs when it is assumed that results based on grouped data can be applied to individuals who make up the groups under study. The ecologic fallacy occurs because ecologic studies cannot distinguish between associations that are created by the selection of groups or associations that are in the individual data before they are grouped. Ecologic studies are based on measurements from population samples and the data from such studies are averaged over the population. The studies often use proxy measures for both exposure and disease. In addition, it is usually not possible to control for confounding in the analysis.[24] All of these factors make the associations seen in ecologic studies uncertain; therefore, it is difficult to make inferences based on the data.

Modifiable Units Problem

The modifiable units problem was identified back in the 1930s when it was shown that different results could be obtained by using different areal units for analysis. Correlation between variables is generally higher when areas are aggregated together.[26] When examining the degree of spatial association, one must keep in mind that the association depends on the size and nature of the areal units that are used. The selection of areal units used in many spatial studies is arbitrary and often subject to change. There are no standard guidelines for aggregating data for analysis. The modifiable units problem has two components: a scale problem and an aggregation problem.[27] The scale problem occurs when data that are collected for one scale are aggregated together for analysis at a different scale (one covering a larger area). The aggregation problem occurs when examining the data at the same scale (e.g., counties) but combining the counties together into a different number of zones. Thus, it is important to examine the data using a variety of groupings in order to understand fully the associations that are seen.

Standardization of Data from Various Sources

When using data from a variety of sources, steps need to be taken to standardize the variables for comparison. Various agencies have different needs for the data that are collected and may define the variables in different ways to meet their needs. The user needs to examine the criteria used to define the variables in the data set, the time period covered by the data, and the quality assurance steps taken in data collection. Certain variables such as race and ethnicity have standard collection requirements for the federal agencies that are established by the Office of Management and Budget. There are also national standards for the collection of spatial data. There are no over-riding national standards for the collection of health data, so the user must be mindful that the data may have been collected in a manner that would affect the overall interpretation of combined results.

LEGAL ISSUES REGARDING DATA RELEASE AND SECURITY

Government agencies are creatures of statute or of constitutions that were written before the electronic age. Therefore, the present laws lack guidance for establishing a uniform public policy regarding the ownership of intangible information assets. In 1985, there were more than 400 "information service organizations" in the private sector that repackage raw government information and resell it.

Public access to government information is a fundamental right that operates to check and balance the actions of elected and appointed officials. The Office of Technology Assessment (OTA) reported in 1988 that the federal government spends $6 billion each year on information dissemination (not including the cost of collection, processing, or agency automation).[28] The OTA said at that time that congressional action was urgently needed to resolve federal information dissemination issues and set policy direction for future federal agency activities.

Legal precedent directs custodial agencies to release or withhold records in consideration of the balance between the privacy of individuals and the public's right to know. In a Freedom of Information Act (FOIA) case heard before the Supreme Court in 1989, the court ruled that "FOIA's central purpose is to insure that the Federal Government's activities be opened for public scrutiny, not that information about private citizens that happens to be in the Federal Government's warehouse be so disclosed."[29] The court recognized the difference between a computerized databank and the source records. Unfortunately, the burden for making the distinction between products and records falls on the custodial agencies. The case discussed the possibility that departing from the original purposes of the FOIA could threaten to convert that federal government into a clearinghouse for personal information that had been collected concerning millions of persons under a variety of different situations. The previous interpretations may change because there have been changes in the FOIA that expand it to cover electronic records. The amendment to the FOIA that was passed in September of 1996 requires that computer-based information kept by federal agencies be subject to disclosure and that agencies must comply, if they can, to requests for records in electronic form. This may have a future impact on the type of information kept in computer databases.

Limitations to protect information that fits under Open Records Act privacy exceptions must be established before the development of the databases. Some courts, in looking at the balance between privacy and right-to-know, have reached a compromise that can result in a tremendous burden of resources for some agencies. "When an academic researcher wants information about test scores and income levels, courts have required the custodial agency to perform a statistical analysis of the 'private' data, and provide this analysis in response to an open-records request for otherwise private information. This so-called 'redaction' requirement places a burden on the agency to produce information that did not exist, and was not necessary for agency purposes, to meet the outside request."[28(p.256)] It was simpler in the pre-electronic age to review a specific request and determine whether a privacy issue was involved. When an agency is offering a computer database for public application, the issues become much broader and more obscure. The custodial agency should anticipate what can be done through different forms of access, and any privacy invasion that may result. GIS systems are particularly vulnerable to use that results in an invasion of privacy.

In the related issue of the liability of government agencies for effects from the use of provided goods and services, the use of disclaimer language must be considered. The government has the right not to engage in discretionary functions such as the marketing and selling of GIS and other computer products. Once the decision to engage in a discretionary activity or function has been made, a government agency may be held liable for the negligence of its employees' and agents' actions in the performance of the discretionary activity. Negligence may take the form of incorrect information that is entered into a database that results in the production of an incorrect product. If that leads to damaging results and the information provided by the agency led the injured party to justifiably rely on the information or product, then liability is likely. By issuing and selling information products, the custodial agency assumes a duty to invest sufficient resources that are necessary to achieve what the government and the courts will agree to be proper care in maintaining the database.

There is also a question of whether the Uniform Commercial Code applies. As a general rule, Article 2 of the Uniform Commercial Code applies only to the sale of goods and not to the provision of services. However, courts have found that electricity transmitted over wires and natural gas pumped through pipes are "moveable goods" and therefore subject to the code. It is yet to be seen if electronically transmitted data will be considered similarly.

• • •

Public health officials and health administrators can incorporate a wide variety of types of data as part of community assessment and planning efforts. An increasing amount of data is now becoming available on-line over the Web. In addition, planners can incorporate data from federal programs and from local and state sources. The key to successful data acquisition is the development of effective and mutually beneficial data partnerships among the organizations that produce and use health-related data. These partnerships must protect data confidentially and privacy, and ensure that data are collected to support a wide variety of community health planning needs. Public health administrators must carefully consider the questions that need to be answered from a community planning perspective and the data that will be most advantageous in answering those questions.

CHAPTER REVIEW

1. Collecting data is necessary for the assessment and monitoring of community health and for evaluating the effectiveness of preventive programs.
2. Sources of health data are available at federal, state, and local levels. For each source, a critical parameter is determining the population size and the smallest geographic unit for which the information is applicable.
3. Within the federal government, a broad range of data sets are available from multiple agencies, including the CDC, NCHS, NIOSH, Bureau of Labor Statistics, HCFA, HRSA, and others.
4. At the state level, sources of data include
   - vital statistics
   - disease reporting
   - disease registries
   - Medicaid information
5. At the local level, additional information can be gathered by surveys for special purposes. Other sources of data can be sought, such as from managed care entities.
6. The Internet is now a readily available method for accessing data sources. Multiple federal data sets are now available electronically, and each state health department maintains an Internet site for data access and querying.
7. To be successful in working with data, queries or hypotheses are structured first, a plan or design to answer these questions is then constructed, and finally, data are sought recognizing potential biases including reporting, measurement, and selection.

REFERENCES

1. H.S. Shryrock et al., *The Methods and Materials of Demography* (New York: Academic Press, 1976).
2. J.A. Weed, "Vital Statistics in the United States: Preparing for the Next Century," *Population Index 61,* no. 4 (1995): 527–539.
3. F. Mullan, *Plaques and Politics: The Story of the United States Public Health Service* (New York: Basic Books, Inc., 1989).
4. Centers for Disease Control and Prevention, "Summary of Notifiable Diseases, United States, 1997," *Morbidity and Mortality Weekly Report 46,* no. 54 (1998).
5. U.S. Department of Health, Education, and Welfare, *Healthy People: The Surgeon General's Report on Health Promotion and Disease Prevention* (DHEW [PHS] Publication No. 79–55071) (Washington, DC: Public Health Service, 1979).
6. U.S. Department of Health and Human Services, *Healthy People 2000: The National Health Promotion and Disease Prevention Objectives* (DHHS Publication [PHS] No. 91–50213) (Washington, DC: Public Health Service, 1990).
7. National Center for Health Statistics, *Healthy People Review 2000 Review, 1998–99* (Hyattsville, MD: Public Health Service, 1999).
8. Office of Disease Prevention and Health Promotion, Department of Health and Human Services, "Healthy

People 2000 Fact Sheet." http://odphp.osophs.dhhs.gov/pubs/hp2000/hp2kfact.htm. Accessed 25 April 2000.

9. U.S. Department of Health and Human Services, *Healthy People 2010: Understanding and Improving Health, Vol. 1* (Washington, DC: Public Health Service, 2000).
10. National Center for Health Statistics, Centers for Disease Control and Prevention, "National Health and Nutrition Examination Survey." http://www.cdc.gov/nchs/nhanes.htm. Accessed 25 April 2000.
11. C.M. Loria et al., "Plan and Operation of the NHANES II Mortality Study, 1992," *Vital Health Statistics 1,* no. 38 (1999).
12. National Center for Health Statistics, "Plan and Operation of the Third National Health and Nutrition Examination Survey, 1988–94," *Vital Health Statistics 1,* no. 32 (1994).
13. U.S. Department of Commerce, U.S. Census Bureau Home Page. http://www.census.gov/index.html. Accessed 25 April 2000.
14. U.S. Centers for Disease Control and Prevention, "Recommendations for the Use of Folic Acid To Reduce the Number of Cases of Spina Bifida and Other Neural Tube Defects," *Morbidity and Mortality Weekly Report 41,* no. RR-14 (1992).
15. D. Cibula et al., *Obtaining Quality Information on a Shoe-String Budget: A Low-Cost Evaluation of a County-Wide Campaign Promoting Folic Acid* (Syracuse, NY: Onondaga County Department of Health, 1997).
16. March of Dimes Foundation, *Preparing for Pregnancy: A National Survey of Women's Behavior and Knowledge Relating to the Consumption of Folic Acid and Other Vitamins and Pre-Pregnancy Care* (White Plains, NY: 1995).
17. F. Serbanescu and R. Rochat, *Georgia Women's Health Survey—1995: Preliminary Report* (Atlanta, GA: Georgia Department of Human Resources, Division of Public Health, 1996).
18. Onondaga County Health Department, *Breast Cancer and Mammography Utilization in Onondaga County, New York* (Syracuse, NY: 1997).
19. National Committee for Quality Assurance. *Health Plan Employer Data and Information Set* (Washington, DC: 1993).
20. National Committee for Quality Assurance. *HEDIS 2000 Technical Specifications.* Vol. 2. (Washington, DC: 1999).
21. New York State Department of Health. *Quality Assurance Reporting Requirements, 1997: A Report on Managed Care Performance* (Albany, NY: 1999).
22. A. Friede and P.W. O'Carroll, "CDC and ATSDR Electronic Information Resources for Health Officers," *Journal of Public Health Management and Practice 2,* no. 3 (1996): 10–24.
23. M. Wallace et al., Integrated Information Solutions: The Future of Census Bureau Data Access and Dissemination (Presentation at the National Conference on Health Statistics, Washington, DC, August 2, 1999).
24. K.J. Rothman, *Modern Epidemiology* (Boston: Little, Brown and Co., 1986).
25. J.S. Mausner and S. Kramer, *Epidemiology—An Introductory Text* (Philadelphia: W.B. Saunders Co., 1985).
26. M. Green and R. Flowerdew, "New Evidence on the Modifiable Areal Unit Problem," in *Spatial Analysis in a GIS Environment,* eds. P. Longley and M. Batty (New York: John Wiley & Sons, 1997).
27. S. Openshaw, "The Modifiable Areal Unit Problem," in *Concepts and Techniques in Modern Geography* No. 38 (Norwich, England: Geo Books, 1984).
28. J.C. Antenucci et al., *Geographic Information Systems: A Guide to the Technology* (New York: Van Nostrand Reinhold, 1991).
29. *U.S. Department of Justice v. Reporters Committee for Freedom of the Press,* 489 U.S., 103 L Ed 2d 774; 109 Sup. Ct. (1989).

CHAPTER 8

Public Health Surveillance

Theresa Hatzell
Tim E. Aldrich
Willard Cates, Jr.
Euichul Shin

Surveillance is the primary mechanism through which public health organizations acquire information concerning population health. Surveillance systems vary widely in both structure and function; consequently, the optimal system design is contingent on an organization's specific information needs and resources as well as the characteristics of the populations and health issues under study. In developing and maintaining surveillance systems, public health administrators must use current epidemiologic knowledge in tandem with effective managerial strategies.

Effective public health management requires an iterative cycle of formulating public health objectives, designing and implementing interventions, measuring the population-level impact of programs, and using that information to revise program targets and interventions. An essential input for this cycle is continuously updated information reflecting the current health status of the population. Public health surveillance is the primary mechanism through which public health organizations generate and process this information for use in management, policy, and practice.[1] Described as an essential step in the "systematic and ongoing assessment of the health of a community,"[2(p.18)] surveillance permits public health agencies to assess trends in disease and other health conditions, measure the prevalence of risk factors and health behaviors, and monitor the utilization of health services. Conclusions drawn from this information can then be used for decision making and action at multiple levels of the public health system.

This chapter provides an overview of surveillance systems and strategies that are relevant to the public health administrator. The first section describes the various functions that surveillance serves in public health and the corresponding configurations of surveillance systems. This is followed by an overview of basic epidemiologic techniques used in conducting surveillance activities. This overview is not intended to be a comprehensive "how to" guide to surveillance. Rather, the section presents fundamental information relevant to public health managers, whether they have ultimate oversight responsibility for a surveillance system within a public health agency, or they wish to capitalize fully on the program-enriching capacity of surveillance data. Readers seeking more detailed discussion of surveillance techniques are directed to other texts written for epidemiologists and other technicians directly responsible for surveillance operations.[3–6] The final section of this chapter describes administrative and managerial activities that support surveillance system operations.

FUNCTION AND FORM OF PUBLIC HEALTH SURVEILLANCE SYSTEMS

Functions: What Purpose Does Surveillance Serve?

Surveillance activities support public health management at many levels, beginning with the establishment of health objectives. Surveillance systems provide information about the leading causes of sickness, injury, and disability (collectively referred to as morbidity) as well as death (mortality) within the population served by the public health agency. Although surveillance was originally focused on communicable diseases, surveillance systems now monitor the occurrence of a broad range of health events. These include infectious and chronic disease, injury, disability, occupational health events, environmental exposures, personal behavior, and the use of health services. Health officers rely on this information as they select targets for public health action. Surveillance also provides the public health officer with information on the occurrence of risk factors that are already known to be immediate precursors to disease or injury, such as obesity, smoking, illicit drug use, or exposure to harmful agents. Further, public health officers can rely on the surveillance of health service utilization to assess whether the population is taking full advantage of preventive and curative services. Documented underutilization of available health services may point to the need for public health intervention to reduce barriers to care.

Once officials establish priorities for public health interventions, they can rely further on surveillance data to design and target specific programs. Surveillance provides information about the characteristics of people most affected by health conditions and where these people reside. Programs can then be formulated to reach targeted populations and respond to their specific needs. Once services are designed and implemented, surveillance data can be further used to measure program impact. By analyzing trends in the specific health condition, policy makers can determine whether their program achieved its desired effect. Surveillance data can then be used to support programmatic decision making about whether interventions should be continued, modified, expanded, or terminated.

Aside from supporting routine public health program management, surveillance activities are essential for timely response to immediate public health needs. Surveillance is used to detect disease outbreaks and epidemics, and to identify newly emerging diseases. Of primary concern are diseases with high severity and strong infectivity that can be controlled by prompt action. A 1999 outbreak of salmonella infection in the northwest United States serves as an example.[7] Salmonella infection typically causes diarrhea, abdominal cramping, fever, and dehydration; in a small proportion of cases, severe complications can lead to death. State health officials in Washington State were notified of 85 cases of salmonella infection that occurred between June 10 and July 9, 1999. An investigation revealed that 67 of these people had consumed a particular brand of unpasteurized orange juice. Meanwhile, in neighboring Oregon, 57 cases of salmonella infection were identified by state health officials, all occurring in the latter half of June. Thirty-nine of these people drank the same brand of orange juice. After collaborative investigations by the two states and discussions with the U.S. Food and Drug Administration (FDA), the manufacturer voluntarily issued a recall of the juice. Further investigations identified salmonella in samples of the juice, dispensers in restaurants, and the juice factory. Smaller outbreaks were reported in 13 other states among individuals who drank the juice during the same period. In response to this outbreak, the FDA proposed regulations to improve the safety of juices through pasteurization, or at a minimum, labeling that warns consumers of possible risks associated with the product.

Public health surveillance is also able to reveal issues warranting in-depth investigation through formal epidemiologic studies. Surveillance systems can monitor large cohorts of individuals over time, producing databases that contain longitudinal information on disease occurrence and risk factors. The American Cancer Society (ACS), for example, compiles data from central cancer registries in 21 states and the National Vital Statistics Program. Combining interview data with surveillance data on cancer incidence and mortality, ACS has published research findings on chronic disease and lifestyle risk factors drawn from an immense cohort developed through its volunteer networks.[8]

Regional studies in the United States can be conducted by linking epidemiologic surveillance systems from neighboring states with databases from hospital discharge systems and insurance organizations. A prototype of this application has been completed for the three southeastern states that comprise the "stroke belt"—Georgia, South Carolina, and North Carolina. Through their collaborative use of hospital discharge databases, the three state health departments have achieved large sample sizes that offer the statistical power needed to perform valuable analyses for extremely high-risk subgroups such as African American Medicare beneficiaries in rural areas. Collaboration between federal agencies in defining consistent variable coding systems at the national level facilitates such surveillance linkages to support research developments.

A final function served by surveillance is to support comprehensive public health policy formulation, such as the development of disease control plans.[9] Policy makers can then use surveillance to evaluate disease control programs and to assess the impact of specific policy decisions. In the United States, the Centers for Disease Control and Prevention (CDC) has urged all states to develop strategic, statewide disease control plans. As a part of that recommendation, close collaboration with the appropriate surveillance systems is explicitly urged. For example, the CDC's recent initiative to eliminate syphilis draws heavily on the syphilis surveillance infrastructure established during the past half-century.

Surveillance System Forms

Surveillance systems take on a variety of forms depending on the health events being monitored and the purposes the system is intended to serve. Chapter 7 provided a comprehensive discussion of sources of health data, many of which are obtained through surveillance activities. Major types of surveillance activities are highlighted in the following paragraphs.

Notifiable Disease Reporting

The CDC defines notifiable diseases as those for which regular, frequent, and timely information regarding individual cases is considered necessary for the prevention and control of disease. The Association of State and Territorial Health Officials (ASTHO) has defined the national notifiable diseases since 1948. The ASTHO's Council of State and Territorial Epidemiologists (CSTE), in consultation with the CDC, makes recommendations every three years about diseases that should be reported by states and territories. In 1997, the CSTE recommended the reporting of 52 infectious diseases and 4 health conditions (acute pesticide poisoning, silicosis, elevated blood lead levels, and tobacco use).[10] Each year, the CDC publishes the national recommendations for disease reporting in *Morbidity and Mortality Weekly Report, Summary of Notifiable Diseases.*

State legislatures hold final authority to determine which of the nationally recommended conditions to include on the local list of notifiable diseases. The majority of states and territories require reporting of most of the health conditions recommended nationally by the CSTE, but variation does exist based on local public health priorities. Reporting requirements are mandated either through statutes, health department regulations, or a combination of both.[11] States have an obligation to keep systems updated to ensure that notifiable disease information is relevant to public health concerns. Moreover, information requirements should be as streamlined as possible to encourage compliance by those persons responsible for collecting and submitting surveillance data.

Health care providers are responsible for reporting notifiable diseases upon case detection. Public health laboratories are also assigned responsibility for reporting notifiable diseases, particularly for diagnoses that are aided by laboratory confirmation. Both clinicians and laboratories typically report to local or state public health agencies. The state epidemiologist is responsible for collection, analysis, interpretation, and data dissemination regarding notifiable diseases within the state. Surveillance findings on notifiable diseases from the state are forwarded to the CDC for compilation, analysis, and dissemination at the national level. The CDC manages weekly transfer of data on notifiable diseases from state health departments through the National Electronic Telecommunications System for Surveillance (NETSS). The NETSS was developed by the CDC and the CSTE for electronically collecting, transmitting, analyzing, and publishing weekly reports of notifiable diseases and injuries from 50 states and major metropolitan areas and territories.[12] The NETSS relies on standard case definitions and reporting procedures to heighten data accuracy and comparability. The CDC has also established the Public Health Laboratory Information System (PHLIS), which permits the compilation and transmission of data on laboratory-confirmed disease incidence from public health laboratories to the CDC.

Vital Statistics Surveillance

Mandatory data recorded at the time of birth and death are known as vital statistics. Birth and death certification and the tracking of infant mortality and occupational deaths are examples of vital statistics surveillance. This form of surveillance is useful for monitoring long-term trends in causes of death and identifying differences by subpopulation (e.g., racial or age groups) or geographic location.[13] Advantages offered by vital records data are that they provide near complete coverage of the population, and the specific data items are frequently confirmed by medical data. One possible disadvantage of relying on vital records for surveillance, however, is that extensive time may be needed for the compilation of population-based data and its subsequent release.[14]

Sentinel Surveillance

Sentinel surveillance most commonly refers to targeted reporting by a specially designated sample of providers. In this type of surveillance, a network of clinicians routinely reports information on a specified set of health events. The CDC's national influenza surveillance effort provides an example. The CDC receives weekly reports from 122 cities and metropolitan areas summarizing the total number of deaths occurring in these cities/areas, as well as the number of deaths due to pneumonia and influenza. Epidemiologists from the CDC then combine information from these sentinel sites with data from the 121 Cities Mortality Reporting System to evaluate patterns of influenza mortality in the United States and the severity of the currently circulating virus strains.

The generalizability of the sentinel surveillance results depends on how closely the populations served by the sentinel providers represent the general population. What is sacrificed in the precision of population estimates may be made up for in the timeliness of the data and the consistency of the reporting. In fact, sentinel surveillance may be considered a cost-effective alternative to universal reporting because resource requirements are lower for a smaller set of reporters, and the providers who voluntarily participate in the system may be more motivated to report accurate, complete, and timely data.

The term sentinel surveillance has two other applications. First, disease occurrence can be monitored in special "sentinel groups" with a particular risk profile for disease occurrence. For example, human immunodeficiency virus (HIV) infection has been monitored in blood donors, pregnant women, military recruits, and prisoners, among other groups.[2] Sentinel surveillance can be conducted without establishing the disease status of individuals within a sentinel population, for example, among all patients seeking care at a particular clinic. Anonymous screening uses blood specimens collected for other purposes, with identifying information removed from the specimens.[15] Based on the screening results, estimates of disease prevalence can be made for the general population of which the sentinel population is representative. For example, in some developing nations, the prevalence of HIV infection among women of childbearing age is estimated by screening women seeking prenatal care services.

Finally, the term "sentinel health event" refers to conditions for which even a single case serves as a warning signal that improvements in preventive measures are warranted.[16] Sentinel health events include illnesses and injuries described as avoidable, and deaths deemed as "untimely." In the United States, a single case of maternal mortality is an example of a sentinel event warranting closer scrutiny. The CDC's National Institute of

Occupational Safety and Health (NIOSH) uses sentinel surveillance to monitor the occurrence of selected serious injuries, exposures, illnesses, and deaths in the workplace.[17]

Registries

Registries are used to compile information on health events from multiple sources, linking data to a particular individual over time.[13] They are particularly useful for monitoring the incidence, prevalence, and economic burden of chronic diseases such as cancer.[18] Registries can be used for surveillance of the incidence of a health event in a population when the intention is to collect information on all cases occurring within that population. For example, the National Cancer Institute's Surveillance, Epidemiology, and End Results (SEER) Program compiles data from 11 population-based cancer registries and 3 supplemental registries covering approximately 14 percent of the U.S. population. Since 1970, this SEER database has been the "gold standard" for cancer incidence in the United States. However, because it was suspected that regional variation was not described adequately, 1992 federal legislation stipulated that all states will operate central cancer registries. This national program of central cancer registries produces an annual publication of cancer incidence and mortality for the United States and Canada.[19]

Health Surveys

Surveys can serve as a surveillance mechanism when they are used periodically to collect a set of information on health conditions, risk factors, or health-related knowledge, attitudes, or practices. Surveys are used to estimate the prevalence of conditions within a population based on information provided by a representative sample. In the United States, for example, the National Center for Health Statistics (NCHS) sponsors the *National Health and Nutrition Examination Survey (NHANES),* collecting clinical and biologic data on a random sample of Americans.[20] The NCHS also conducts the *Hospital Discharge Survey,* collecting data on health conditions requiring hospitalization from 7,500 randomly selected inpatient facilities. The *National Health Interview Survey* is an example of a national telephone survey conducted annually in the United States to ask a sample of adults about their experiences with specific illnesses, injuries, and disabilities, as well as their use of health services. The *Behavioral Risk Factor Surveillance Survey* is another telephone survey used to monitor adult health behaviors and the use of preventive services.[13]

Internationally, behavioral surveillance surveys are playing an important role in HIV control programs due to the important role that individual behaviors play in determining future trends in the epidemic (Exhibit 8–1).[21]

Combined Approaches

A combination of surveillance methods may be required to obtain a complete and accurate picture of health conditions. New initiatives in chronic disease surveillance, for example, rely on a combination of data collection approaches. In 1996, the ASTHO, the organization that advises the federal government and state health departments on notifiable diseases, recommended that information on the prevalence of avoidable risk factors be collected. As a result of this recommendation, states are now expected to conduct surveillance for more than 70 chronic disease indicators.[22] States are encouraged to monitor these indicators as a means of evaluating disease control programs and measuring progress toward national health priorities. The suggested indicators are drawn from the entire range of surveillance data sources, such as death certification systems, cancer registries, and surveys of lifestyle factors such as the Behavioral Risk Factor Surveillance System. Eventually, the surveillance system will include community-level indicators reflecting environmental and policy changes associated with chronic disease control, such as the number of miles of walking trails, sales volumes for fruits and vegetables, and proportion of restaurants with nonsmoking areas.[22,23]

SURVEILLANCE SYSTEM DESIGN AND OPERATIONS

Within most public health organizations, direct responsibility for surveillance operations lies in the hands of epidemiologists, biostatisticians, and other data management specialists.

Exhibit 8–1 Application of Behavioral Surveillance Surveys for HIV/Acquired Immune Deficiency Syndrome (AIDS) Control

Since 1986, Family Health International (FHI) has pioneered ways to curtail the spread of HIV/AIDS internationally. With support from the U.S. Agency for International Development, FHI has developed behavioral surveillance surveys (BSS) as one methodology for predicting the course of HIV/AIDS epidemics in developing countries and evaluating the impact of AIDS control interventions. BSS consist of systematic and repeated cross-sectional surveys that measure the prevalence of unsafe behaviors. They are typically administered to a few key target groups at high risk for HIV infection.[a] Beginning with rapport-building questions to encourage respondents to share sensitive information honestly, surveys pose a small but carefully chosen set of questions about risk behaviors and characteristics that help to predict the course of the epidemic, such as those listed below.

- age at first intercourse
- type of sex partners (e.g., casual, commercial)
- number of sex partners by type
- condom use
- needle sharing (for injection drug user surveys)
- other factors affecting risk taking, such as alcohol and substance use

Since launching the methodology in 1993, FHI has supported implementation of BSS in more than 25 AIDS control initiatives in Asia, Africa, and the Caribbean. The National AIDS Control Program of Ivory Coast in West Africa provides one case example. A first round of BSS was carried out in 1998. Six municipalities from throughout the country were selected for inclusion in the study along with four subpopulations of interest: female commercial sex workers, youth ages 15–19, male migrant workers, and long-distance drivers. The sample size for each of these groups was based on expected levels of selected indicators, desired confidence levels, feasibility, and time constraints. Results were disseminated in a series of reports that were widely distributed and publicized through the National AIDS Control Program. Since their publication, BSS findings have been used to focus the national HIV prevention strategy as well as for the development and implementation of a variety of HIV-oriented interventions. Ivory Coast will continue to conduct additional rounds of BSS to measure the impact of its HIV control initiative.

Thailand has already conducted repeated rounds of BSS to assess the impact of its national HIV control program. Between round 1 and round 3 of the BSS, specific public health interventions led to marked increases in condom use with sex workers, as illustrated below.

Percent of males reporting condom use during last sex with a female sex worker: Thailand, 1991–1995

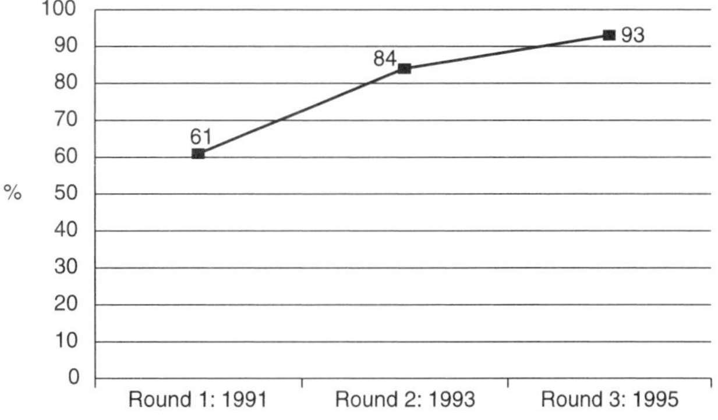

[a]S. Mills et al., "HIV Risk Behavior Surveillance: A Methodology for Monitoring Behavioral Trends," *AIDS* 12 (Suppl 2, 1998): S37–S46.

Source: Data from K.E. Nelson, D.D. Celentano, S. Eiumtrakol, D.R. Hoover et al., Changes in Sexual Behavior and a Decline in HIV Infection among Young Men in Thailand, *New England Journal of Medicine,* 335, pp. 297–303, © 1996, Massachusetts Medical Society.

Public health managers must be able to communicate with these technicians about system operations in order to carry out general oversight responsibilities and to make management-related decisions that affect surveillance activities. This section presents an overview of key technical aspects of surveillance operations, including mechanisms for the timely collection, analysis, interpretation, dissemination, and subsequent use of data.

Establish System Objectives

Surveillance system design begins with the specification of system objectives. In the United States, surveillance policy is established through intergovernmental alliances between the federal, state, and local levels. The CDC coordinates the development of national disease control strategies that include the collection and use of specific forms of surveillance data. State health departments then receive financial support from federal grants to establish surveillance mechanisms in compliance with the CDC guidelines. As a part of establishing a surveillance system, it is recommended that one engage its stakeholders, that is, the data suppliers and eventual data users. A common approach is to form an advisory committee to guide the implementation and operation of the surveillance system. Close collaboration is required among the different tiers for this system to be successful in achieving national disease control objectives. Surveillance requirements need to be sufficiently systematized across jurisdictions for data to be comparable and meaningful at the national level. At the same time, reporting requirements should be flexible enough to permit adaptation to local public health priorities.

Within this context, state- and local-level planners must delineate the purpose they expect the system to serve. Typically, surveillance data will serve one or more of the following objectives:

- Measure the prevalence of a health problem in the community.
- Examine the source causes of diseases.
- Evaluate the success of disease control interventions.
- Detect changes in individuals' behaviors that impact their health.
- Generate and evaluate hypotheses concerning disease origins.
- Serve as a springboard for focused research.

Because surveillance systems are intended to produce information to support public health action, the process of delineating system objectives must include careful consideration of the expected follow-up activities. Intended consumers of information, particularly those represented on the advisory committee, should be consulted when surveillance system objectives are first being established to help ensure that surveillance data will be used appropriately and optimally. The public health manager can play an important role in ensuring that the agencies or individuals expected to use surveillance data will actually exploit them in public health planning and programming.

Establish the Population under Surveillance

Although public health surveillance relies on records of individuals, the unit of watchfulness is the population of which the individuals are constituents. Therefore, the population targeted for surveillance must be explicitly defined. Surveillance activities may focus on populations at levels ranging from a neighborhood to a nation to the entire world. Within the domain of interest, surveillance may focus on the entire population, or on special subgroups delineated by such factors as age, race, or sex.

Select and Define Health Events To Be Monitored

Each step of surveillance activities—reporting, analysis, interpretation, and dissemination—requires substantial resources, and the total cost of surveillance rises incrementally with each additional health event that is monitored. Consequently, the selection of health events to be tracked by the surveillance system must involve prioritization in order to arrive at surveillance targets of primary public health interest. Various criteria have been proposed for assessing the relative importance of health events to be included in the system.[2,24]

- disease prevalence
- disease severity

- most frequent causes of premature death or disability
- leading causes for hospitalization or use of ambulatory services
- leading causes for health care expenditures
- potential for prevention
- strength of risk factor for leading causes of morbidity and mortality
- feasibility of collecting data

Prioritization of health events often requires more than just objective comparisons based on quantifiable measures. The selection process is improved through the use of qualitative techniques aimed at building consensus. Professional and community opinion must be sought to reflect local health concerns and the priorities of the public health agency.

Once a health event is selected for surveillance, a case definition must be developed based on the disease outcome of interest and the potential exposures under study. Classification systems such as the *International Classification for Diseases*, originated by the World Health Organization in 1979, help to define disease states.[13] Cases can be classified as confirmed, probable, and suspect according to their conformity with the disease classification criteria. Laboratory confirmation is often necessary when the clinical presentation of a disease may be indeterminate, such as in the case of hepatitis or many forms of cancer.

The precision of surveillance data is influenced by case definitions, which may vary over time or according to local diagnostic capability or practices. For example, when acquired immune deficiency syndrome (AIDS) surveillance was initiated in 1982, a set of opportunistic infections was used as an indicator of the underlying immunodeficiency. In 1987, the World Health Organization established new diagnostic criteria, emphasizing HIV infection status. At that time, however, many developing nations had to continue relying on the clinical diagnosis of AIDS because limited laboratory facilities precluded confirmation of HIV status and cultural or histologic diagnosis of characteristic infections.[15] An experience from a southeastern coastal city in the United States further illustrates the influence of diagnostic requirements on the accuracy of surveillance data. A series of deaths from the late 1990s was recorded in the mortality files, each classified as chronic obstructive pulmonary disease in the absence of postmortem pathologic evaluations. The state's central cancer registry, by contrast, requires pathologic diagnosis for classification. Analysis of cancer registry data subsequently revealed that those deaths represented a statistically significant cluster of rare pleural cancer that previously had been obscured by the standard mortality surveillance system.[25]

Establish Reporting Procedures

Once health events have been selected for surveillance and case definitions have been formulated, systems and procedures must be established for obtaining data. Surveillance managers must delineate what type of information is to be collected and how. Data collection instruments are then formulated to obtain needed information. Forms typically use a coding system to standardize data collection and entry. The instrument may be quite simple or rather complex, depending on the application. For example, the national infectious disease reporting format has minimal requirements; only the diagnosis, personal identifying information to avoid double counting, and a few additional data items are collected, with all information fitting onto a short card. For cancer registries, the data set includes information on diagnosis, pathology, and treatment, generally requiring a multipage form. Two samples of data collection forms are presented in Exhibits 8–2 and 8–3. Exhibit 8–2 is a standard, brief reporting card for nationally notifiable diseases. Exhibit 8–3 illustrates the complexity of the coding procedures used in longer forms, such as those used to collect cancer registry data. Electronic reporting is generally the standard procedure used in both types of data collection.

Exhibit 8–2 Standard Reporting Card for Nationally Notifiable Diseases

2000 SCDHEC DISEASE REPORTING CARD

Disease reporting is required by SC Code of Laws Section 44-29-10, Regulation 61-20. **For Urgent Reporting See Back**

Patient's Name (Last) (First) (Middle) | Date of Birth Month/Day/Year | Race: White ☐ Asian ☐ Black ☐ Hisp. ☐ Am.Ind. ☐ Unk. ☐ | Sex: Male ☐ Female ☐ Not Stated ☐ | Hospital ID or Social Security #

Patient's Address / Telephone Number | City and Zip Code | County

Disease (Include Stage, if appropriate) | Criteria for Diagnosis: Clinical ☐ Laboratory ☐ Both ☐ | Day Care Center Child / Staff ☐Yes ☐No ☐Unknown | For DHEC Use Only — (Initial and date) County review date______ State review date______ C P S

Date of Onset ☐of Diagnosis, or ☐of Symptoms | Food Service Worker ☐Yes ☐No ☐Unknown

Specific Laboratory Test / Date / Results | For STD: Pregnant? ☐ Yes ☐ No; Treated ☐ Yes ☐ No; Treatment Planned ☐ Yes ☐ No; Treatment Unk ☐ Yes | Number of Cases Diagnosed Last Month (report by # only) Mumps ______ Varicella ______ Influenza-Like Illness ______ Herpes simplex, primary genital ______

Hepatitis Serology Results	**Pos**	**Neg**	**Not Tested/Unk**
IgM Hepatitis A antibody (IgM anti-HAV)	☐	☐	☐
Hepatitis B Surface antigen (HBsAg)	☐	☐	☐
IgM Hepatitis B core antibody (HBcAb-IgM)	☐	☐	☐
Antibody to Hepatitis C - EIA	☐	☐	☐
Antibody to Hepatitis C - RIBA	☐	☐	☐

Report Acute Viral Hepatitis only unless patient is a pregnant chronic carrier

Diagnosis: Hepatitis A ☐ Hepatitis B ☐ Hepatitis C ☐ Other ☐ ______; Acute ☐ Chronic ☐ Unknown ☐

Clinical/Epidemiology	**Yes**	**No**	**Unk**
Jaundice	☐	☐	☐
Elevated LFTs	☐	☐	☐
Pregnant	☐	☐	☐
Hx of IV drug use	☐	☐	☐

Date DHEC 1129 Card Completed | Responsible Physician & Telephone # for follow-up information | Reporting Laboratory Person & Telephone #

Case reported to local County Health Department Yes☐ No☐ ☐ SEND MORE CARDS TO: Address

MAIL OR CALL NON-URGENT REPORTS TO YOUR COUNTY HEALTH DEPARTMENT OR CALL 803-898-0861 (M–F, 9–5) OR 1-800-616-SICK (7425) 24 hrs/day.

DHEC 1129 (12/1999)

Source: South Carolina Department of Health and Environmental Control.

Surveillance system managers must establish who will report the case, when, and to whom. A major issue is whether the surveillance system will be passive or active. In the case of *passive* surveillance, public health officials rely on health care providers to report the occurrence of a health event voluntarily, as mandated by state law. With *active* surveillance, health officials routinely contact clinicians to inquire about notifiable diseases, or they review appropriate documents such as medical records and laboratory reports to locate notifiable diagnoses. Active surveillance generally achieves more complete and accurate reporting than passive surveillance, but the former approach is far more labor intensive and costly for the public health agency.

A major challenge for any surveillance system manager is to maintain a consistent flow of data and to achieve maximally complete reporting. A multifaceted approach is needed to keep health care professionals motivated to contribute to surveillance activities. First, the surveillance system manager must provide clinicians with the support they need to conduct their reporting responsibilities. Clinicians may be greatly aided by procedural manuals that specify the list of notifiable conditions, case definitions, information recording requirements, and reporting schedules. Other ideas for encouraging physicians' compliance with reporting requirements include keeping reporting procedures as simple as possible, establishing 24-hour toll-free numbers for reporting, and providing addressed, postage-paid envelopes or postcards to facilitate data transfer.[26]

Surveillance system managers must create incentives to maintain clinicians' continuous participation in surveillance activities. Continuous feedback is an essential factor in sustaining clinicians' interest. Clinicians are motivated by information on local health conditions, particularly in forms of use in caring for their patients. The experience of Korea illustrates how its communicable disease surveillance system was greatly enhanced through innovative reporting and dissemination procedures (Exhibit 8–4).

Analyze and Interpret Surveillance Data

Epidemiologists can apply a variety of analytic techniques to meet specific objectives of surveillance activities. These objectives can be

Exhibit 8–3 Data Collection Form for Cancer Registry

Cancer Identification

Topography Code: __ __ __. __ Text: ____________________

Sequence Number: __ __

Histology/Behavior-Grade: __ __ __ __/ __ __ Text: ____________________

Type of Patient: __ 1 = Inpatient 2 = Outpatient 3 = IP and OP 8 = Other, including physician's office 9 = Unknown

Diagnostic Confirmation: __

1 = Positive Histology
2 = Positive Exfoliative Cytology, no positive histology
4 = Pos. Microscopic confirmation, method not specified
5 = Positive laboratory test/ marker study
6 = Direct visualization, without microscopic confirmation
7 = Radiography and other imaging techniques, without microscopic confirmation
8 = Clinical diagnosis only (other than 5, 6, or 7)
9 = Unknown whether or not microscopically confirmed

Laterality: __

0 = Not a paired site
1 = Right
2 = Left
3 = One side, R or L not specified
4 = Bilateral, origin unknown
9 = Paired site, laterality unknown, midline tumor
*Unknown Primary = 0

Class of Case: __

0 = Dx here, all 1st Rx elsewhere
1 = Dx and all/part 1st Rx here
2 = Dx elsewhere, all/part 1st Rx here
3 = Dx and all 1st Rx elsewhere
4 = Dx and 1st Rx here before ref. date
5 = Dx at autopsy
6 = Dx and all 1st Rx only in staff physician's office
8 = By death certificate only
9 = Unknown

TM 1: __ TM 2: __

0 = Not done, not ordered, not performed
1 = POSITIVE
2 = NEGATIVE
3 = Borderline, undetermined Pos or Neg
8 = Ordered, but results not on chart
9 = Unknown or Not Applicable (all sites other than those listed in *ROADS* Table pages 116–117)

Extent of Disease:

Date of Admission __ __ - __ __ - __ __ __ __

Date of Initial Diagnosis: __ __ - __ __ - __ __ __ __

Date of Discharge __ __ - __ __ - __ __ __ __

SEER Summary Stage: __

0 = In situ
1 = Localized
2 = Regional by Direct Extension
3 = Regional to Lymph Nodes
4 = Regional (both 2 and 3)
5 = Regional, NOS
7 = Distant mets/systemic disease (Leukemia, Multiple Myeloma, Reticuloendotheliosis, Letterer-Siwe's disease)
9 = Unstaged, unspecified, Unknown (*Unknown primary) Class 3 or 4 when stage at initial Dx unknown

Size of Tumor: __ __ __ mm (ie: 02.1 cm = 021 mm)

Refer to *ROADS* for detailed instruction (pages 121–122)

Size of tumor is the largest dimension, or the diameter of the PRIMARY tumor.

Record EXCISED tumor size as stated by Pathologist, NOT incisional biopsy or resected tumor size. Do NOT add tumor sizes

If no pathology excised tumor size, may use size as stated on: (listed in preference order) Operative report, Scans, X-rays, or Physical Examins

Malignant Melanoma—Record Depth of Invasion

998 = Esophagus—Entire circumference
Stomach—Diffuse; widespread, 3/4 or more, linitis plastica
Colorectal—Familial polyposis (histology 8220 or 8221 with behav. code 2 or 3)
Lung—Diffuse, entire lobe or lung
Breast—Diffuse; widespread, 3/4 or more; inflammatory carcinoma

999 = Not recorded, Not available
If no size other than tissue chips from prostate or bladder (Do Not Add)
If any of following: Hematopoetic neoplasms, Hodgkin's/Non-Hodgkin's Lymphoma, Mycosis Fungoides of skin, Kaposi's Sarcoma, Letterer-Siwe's Leukemia, Multiple Myeloma, Reticuloendotheliosis, Unknown primary

continues

Exhibit 8–3 continued

Regional Nodes Positive: __ __

00 = All nodes examined negative
01 = One positive lymph node
02 = Two positive lymph nodes
etc
96 = 96 or more positive lymph nodes
97 = positive nodes but # not specified (LN aspiration when cytology or histology pos)
98 = No nodes examined
99 = Unknown if nodes are positive or negative, NA, patient Rx prior to Surg., Brain, Leukemia, Lymphoma, Multiple Myeloma, Reticuloendotheliosis, Letterer-Siwe, Unknown Primary

Regional Nodes Examined: __ __

00 = No nodes examined, no nodes surgically removed
01 = One node examined
02 = Two nodes examined
etc
97 = 97 or more lymph nodes examined
98 = Nodes examined, but # not specified (LN aspiration when cytology or histology pos)
99 = Unknown if nodes were examined, NA, patient Rx prior to Surg., Brain, Leukemia, Lymphoma, Multiple Myeloma, Reticuloendotheliosis, Letterer-Siwe, Unknown Primary

Source: South Carolina Central Cancer Registry.

Exhibit 8–4 Improving Surveillance through Technological Innovation: Korean Communicable Diseases Surveillance System

Based on the Communicable Disease Prevention law first enacted in 1954, a surveillance system was designed to monitor communicable disease occurrence, detect epidemics, and introduce disease control measures as promptly as possible. For 40 years, physicians were expected to follow the same set of procedures for reporting any occurrence of 29 notifiable diseases. For category I diseases, which are acute and rapidly spreading infectious diseases like cholera, physicians were expected to report an individual patient's epidemiologic information immediately after onset. In the case of category II and III diseases, which are less severe, chronic infectious diseases, physicians had to report only the number of cases either weekly or monthly, depending on the condition. Physicians sent surveillance information to the local community health center (CHC). Each CHC had its own communicable disease control work force for the investigation of epidemics, conducting control activities when needed. CHCs then reported the frequencies of the notifiable diseases to the provincial health department, which compiled data on disease frequency in their areas (city or province) and reported the frequencies to the Ministry of Health and Welfare (MOHW). The Communicable Diseases Surveillance Office at the National Institute of Health received the nationwide data from the MOHW and conducted an analysis. The results were edited and published in the *Communicable Diseases Monthly Report* and distributed to public and several private medical facilities free of charge.

Studies of Korea's surveillance system documented several opportunities for improvement.[a] First, notifiable disease reporting rates were very low in general. Investigators documented an overall disease reporting rate of only 27 percent in 1994, on par with rates determined by other studies.[b] The reporting rate for typhoid fever was estimated to be only 20 percent in Korea in the latter part of the 1990s.[c] The poor reporting was attributed to a variety of factors. Physicians were unaware of their notification duty, they found the process of notification too complicated or burdensome, they lacked immediate access to reporting forms, and they felt uncertain about the disease diagnosis.

The surveillance system had other serious problems. Delays in reporting were common. Surveillance data passed through three major tiers, with each step requiring substantial time because the individuals responsible for collecting and reporting notifiable disease data had other responsibilities besides surveillance. The surveillance system also relied on outdated data analysis techniques. The most sophisticated analysis was mere calculation of disease frequency by geographic region and month. Results were published in a monthly newsletter that was distributed on a limited basis. Finally, coordination between data analysts and

continues

Exhibit 8–4 continued

public health authorities was inadequate, in part due to the nature of the notifiable diseases. For public health administrators at the CHC level, evidence of disease outbreaks could lead to blame about failure to meet responsibilities. A serious disincentive to support efficient surveillance operations thus existed on the part of an important partner in the system.

These defects eventually prompted an outcry from academia and government to improve Korea's national surveillance system. In 1993, the Korean National Institute of Health decided to improve the system by piloting the National Computerization of Communicable Diseases Surveillance Network in Kyong-gi province.[d] The system was modeled after the French Communicable Diseases Network (FCDN).[e,f] Improvement efforts are now in the pilot stage of development. Sentinel physicians have started to report certain kinds of non-notifiable diseases such as influenza-like illness. Health authorities at the provincial level are now sending electronic information about the notifiable disease cases through the computerized network. Surveillance data are collected and analyzed by the National Institute of Health using analytic software developed by computer programmers in collaboration with epidemiologists, statisticians, and geographic information systems specialists. Surveillance findings are then rapidly distributed through the Internet (http://dis.mohw.go.kr/). This system eliminates delays in data processing that had previously been incurred by letter, fax, and manual calculation. The whole surveillance feedback loop—from disease reporting to analysis to results dissemination—can be completed as quickly as one week.

Physicians and public health authorities are motivated to participate in surveillance activities now that they can obtain useful forms of epidemiologic information very quickly and easily. Preliminary evidence of high participation rates in surveillance activities by sentinel physicians is a testimony to the system's success. An attitudinal change has also occurred now that the utility of surveillance activities has become more apparent. Documented evidence of a disease outbreak in a specific county is no longer a source of shame for health officials. Rather, problems detected through surveillance indicate that officials are being vigilant toward the local community's health. Interviews with some clinicians have revealed their satisfaction in participating at the "cutting edge" sentinel surveillance. The MOHW is now in the process of expanding the information network to the nation's 244 counties and to a broader range of diseases.

[a]J.S. Kim, "The Improvement of Statistics and Reporting in Notifiable Communicable Disease Surveillance in Korea," *Journal of Korean Medical Association 37,* no. 1 (1984): 24–31.

[b]E. Shin et al., "Estimation of Reporting Rates of Notifiable Acute Communicable Disease and Characteristics Related to Reporting in Korea," *The Journal of Catholic Medical College 49,* no. 4: 1197–1209.

[c]K. Meng, "Comparison of Communicable Diseases Occurrence between Korea and Japan," *Korean Journal of Epidemiology* 9 (1987): 165–167.

[d]E. Shin, "Communicable Diseases Surveillance System, Version 1.0," *Communicable Diseases Monthly Report 5,* no. 8 (1994): 85–88.

[e]P. Garnerin et al., "The French Communicable Diseases Computer Network: A Seven-Year Experiment," *The Annals of the New York Academy of Sciences* 670 (1992): 29–42.

[f]A. Valleron et al., "A Computer Network for the Surveillance of Communicable Diseases: The French Experiment," *American Journal of Public Health* 76 (1986): 1289–1292.

to detect epidemics, monitor long-term trends or seasonal variation, project future occurrence of disease or injury, or plan and evaluate public health programs. With surveillance, the occurrence of health events is measured in terms of the basic epidemiologic parameters of time, place, and person. Relative to time, data analysis addresses questions about how trends in health events at one point in time compare to those of another period. Comparisons of health events in different geographic locations—ranging from neighborhoods to cities to nations—constitute the comparisons by place. Concerning person, descriptions of the health event are organized by various characteristics of the population, such as age, sex, and racial and ethnic groups.

These analyses should transform surveillance data into useful information concerning the distribution of health events in a population. Table 8–1 presents a sample of the most common techniques used for analyzing and presenting surveillance data.

In all cases, the analysis of surveillance data is descriptive, meaning that statistical techniques are used to describe patterns in health events. Using strict definitions for establishing etiology, surveillance data should not be used to test hypotheses about health events because the essentials of sampling theory have not been satisfied.[27] Rather, surveillance data frequently generate hypotheses to be tested through more formal study.

The analysis of surveillance data must take into consideration unintended reporting inaccuracies or inconsistencies that can introduce bias. Consistency and completeness of reporting are known to vary based on the health care setting.[20] Data on the incidence of sexually transmitted disease, for example, tend to be more accurate in states with laws requiring that positive tests be reported. Additionally, cases detected in public sector facilities are more likely to be reported to health authorities than cases diagnosed by private clinicians, leading to higher reported disease rates among individuals more likely to seek care in public clinics. Even at a single time and place, surveillance data can be biased. For example, respondents' faulty recall or reluctance to admit to stigmatic conditions can lead to underreporting in surveillance surveys that rely on self-reporting of health events.[28]

Surveillance system managers have two major strategies for reducing the effect of bias. First, they must strive to base analyses on data sets that are as complete, comparable, and representative as possible. National programs often define minimally acceptable standards for data collection and processing.[29] Funds for the field work associated with the operation of an active surveillance system (e.g., for quality control reviews, case-finding audits, etc.) are sound investments for a reliable surveillance database. Second, surveillance system managers should be keenly aware of the potential for bias and should explore its possible influence on patterns in health events. (Chapter 14 on public health research further discusses approaches for minimizing the effect of measurement error in data collection and analysis.)

The ultimate objective of public health surveillance is to collect information for action. Accordingly, once surveillance data are analyzed, public health officials must determine the implications of the findings. Typically, the health officer or epidemiologist is charged with evaluating trends in notifiable diseases on a regular basis. A committee composed of academic epidemiologists and agency consultants can be formed to supplement the epidemiologic review of a complex data analysis, and to assist with the formulation and support for recommendations for public health action. Thresholds for public health action should be set in advance so that any unusual events in the distribution of health will be identified and appropriate interventions can be implemented.

Just as surveillance activities have expanded to include varied public health domains, the needs for interpretation of surveillance data have diversified as well. The CDC's National Program of Cancer Registries, for example, recommends that states should allocate resources for epidemiologic guidance, especially for the interpretation and translation into action of the cancer registry data. Since the mid-1990s, chronic disease epidemiology posts and programs have been recommended by the National Chronic Disease Center as a part of the expected state's capacity for chronic disease control. Similarly, in recent years, greater attention has been placed on the interpretation and use of maternal and child health data derived from vital records for monitoring interventions aimed at reducing infant mortality and ensuring children's access to health care.

Disseminate and Apply Surveillance Findings

A critical component of surveillance activities is the reporting of surveillance findings to appropriate stakeholders, including health authorities,

Table 8–1 Common Techniques Used for Analyzing Surveillance Data

Technique	*Description*	*Insight Derived from Technique*	*Examples*
Crude rate	$\frac{\text{Number of health events}}{\text{Population}}$	Allows comparisons between populations and across time	Infant mortality rate (IMR), expressed as deaths among children under age one per 1,000 live births
Standardized rate	Crude rates are adjusted to minimize the effect of confounding variables within a population.	Permits comparisons of the incidence of a health event across populations that may not be comparable with respect to a factor associated with that health event, such as age, race, or socioeconomic status	Annual mortality rates standardized to the U.S. population as estimated by the 1940 Census
Graph	Visual display of quantitative information	Visually illustrates patterns, trends, changes, similarities, and outliers in data	**Bar Graph**
Table	Direct presentation of quantitative data, organized in rows and columns	Organizes data to reveal patterns and relationships among variables	**Table**
Mapping	Graphic representation of data using location and geographic coordinates	Provides a quick, clear illustration of variation in health events within a geographic area	**Map**

policy makers, clinicians, and the general public. Individuals and agencies that contribute data to the surveillance system will be most compliant with reporting requirements when they see products from the system.

A variety of mechanisms exist for publicizing surveillance findings. At the national level, the CDC publishes the *Morbidity and Mortality Weekly Report* as a means of rapidly disseminating surveillance data submitted by state health departments. Individual state agencies may produce weekly or monthly newsletters, electronic bulletins, press releases, news conferences, and public meetings. Visual displays such as graphs, tables, and maps help the audience to understand the data and appreciate their significance. Many disease registries publish a concise report annually and make their database available for interested researchers; then, periodically, such as every three to five years, these registries publish a detailed report with extensive analyses and narratives.

The dissemination strategy must correspond to the purpose of the surveillance activities. Particular attention should be focused on establishing a message that is comprehensible, relevant, and readily interpreted by the intended audience. Effective communication may be accomplished via public hearings or small group discussions with key individuals. The media can be an ally for information distribution by judicious use of prepared statements and carefully planned content. Wherever possible, system managers should target informed reporters (e.g., scientific writers) for such directed information releases. Cultivating credibility is also a sound policy; public health managers are urged to keep lines of communication to the media open in times of "no news" in order to prepare them for broader, less sensational themes such as screening for cancer.

Exhibit 8–5 illustrates how surveillance methods can be combined and results subsequently disseminated to achieve remedial intervention for a priority public health issue.

Exhibit 8–5 Managing a Population-Based Surveillance System: A Sentinel Health Event Study

The Chronic Disease Epidemiology Branch (CDEB) of the state department of health implemented a sentinel health event surveillance system to assess avoidable diabetes mortality in South Carolina. A sentinel health event is defined as a relatively uncommon health event, readily diagnosed, with a manageable course. CDEB chose diabetic ketoacidosis (DKA) as the sentinel health event to evaluate diabetes mortality risks. This choice was based on data from North Carolina suggesting that persons dying of DKA represented to be unmanaged diabetes cases.[a]

The investigation began with compilation of population-based data from a variety of surveillance systems. Collaborative data access agreements facilitated the process. The Bureau of Vital Records furnished data on deaths from DKA (ICD Code 250.3) for the calendar years 1996 and 1997. Two years of data were chosen to provide a level of temporal consistency, so that a single year fluctuation in deaths could be distinguished from a more compelling, recurring pattern. The investigators compiled data on hospital discharges and emergency room admissions related to cases of DKA. Finally, data were obtained from the Behavioral Risk Factor Surveillance System (BRFSS) on patterns of risk relevant to diabetes, such as obesity and use of preventive services. Each form of data included identifiers for age group, race, and sex.

The goal of the investigation was to identify population subgroups with excessive rates of DKA. Initially, statisticians assessed the distribution of DKA cases at the county level, stratified by sex and race. It was not appropriate, however, to compare the number of DKA cases directly because the total number of people in each subgroup differed. The statisticians therefore standardized the number of DKA deaths by dividing the data by the total number of "all diabetes" deaths for each subgroup. Epidemiologists then used these more comparable figures in analyses to determine which risk factors were most strongly associated with DKA deaths.

Preliminary analyses revealed that the number of cases was most elevated for African American

continues

Exhibit 8–5 continued

females, who became the focus of further analyses. The investigators applied geographic clustering methods to assess the adjacency of counties in which African American females were at greatest risk for DKA deaths. The hospital discharge and emergency room patterns were consistent with the mortality data, indicating a concentration of DKA cases among African American females in a specific series of counties in the coastal region of the state. Although BRFSS data were not statistically reliable at the county level, risk patterns were consistent with the rest of the findings. Specifically, African American females in that region of the state were less likely to see a physician regularly and had higher frequencies of related risk factors such as obesity.

Epidemiologists selected eleven "sentinel" deaths from a single county for in-depth investigation to assess missed opportunities for prevention of the DKA death. Trained medical record reviewers examined medical records in the hospitals where the DKA deaths had occurred to determine the extent to which they were under medical surveillance. Contacts with surviving family members were arranged through local health officials and attending physicians when the medical records were insufficient for determination of clinical details. This investigation revealed two primary risk factors for DKA death: (1) personal isolation and (2) inadequate follow-up for established clinical studies (e.g., blood sugar monitoring).

A report focusing attention on avoidable circumstances leading to death from DKA was prepared for the Diabetes Initiative of South Carolina and for the health director in the county in which these deaths occurred. The findings were also disseminated through a state health department newsletter and through presentations before audiences who were specifically concerned with diabetes care within the state. The study findings led to recommendations for diabetes case management, including more intensive involvement of family members and local health care providers. Continuing medical education and family member education materials were disseminated by local voluntary agencies and health departments. In some medical clinics, specialized software was acquired to remind clinicians of the overdue visits for their patients with diabetes.

[a]R.A. Bell et al., "Medical Examiner Cases Associated with Previously Undiagnosed Diabetes Mellitus, North Carolina, 1994," *Southern Medical Journal 91,* no. 2 (1999): 151–154.

MAINTAINING SURVEILLANCE SYSTEM OPERATIONS

The previous sections described surveillance system components and techniques. Once the system is designed and implemented, the public health manager must provide support to ensure consistent and effective execution of surveillance operations. This section describes public health management issues of particular relevance to surveillance activities.

Human Resource Needs for Effective Surveillance

Public health administrators must ensure effective communication and collaboration across the diverse disciplines that contribute to the surveillance system. Key among these disciplines is the surveillance system manager, who often holds a graduate degree in public health, most frequently specializing in epidemiology or biostatistics. Other important professionals include database specialists and technicians trained in data file design, linkage, maintenance, and editing. Some larger surveillance systems also employ full-time computer systems programmers. Statisticians work to compile, analyze, and report results from surveillance systems, as well as to assist in designing surveillance systems that support valid, reliable, and relevant results. In addition, epidemiologists are frequently involved in designing systems and interpreting surveillance data.

Maintaining a qualified staff is an important consideration for good surveillance. Specialized training exists for many surveillance system functions. Degree programs exist for those persons responsible for medical record coding, known as accredited record technicians. Many technical colleges and trade schools offer this associate-level degree through a two-year curriculum. Bachelor's programs are present in most states for medical record administrators. Some graduate programs also offer advanced-level training. The National Cancer Registrars Association is one professional organization that many surveillance staff join for their high-quality training and informative annual meeting. The CDC's NCHS offers training opportunities and career development programs. More generally, funds for continuing education and professional organization memberships for professional development are crucial budget considerations with surveillance systems.

Meeting Federal Data Standards

The 1996 Health Insurance Portability and Accountability Act (HIPAA) included provisions for creating national standards for administrative health data management that have important implications for public health surveillance. Several major sources of surveillance data are likely to be affected by this legislation, including hospital discharge databases, disease registries, trauma registries, and vital statistics.[30] It will therefore be in the interest of public health managers to be aware of evolving federal standards and to take necessary measures for compliance.

Another likely consequence of HIPAA is increased scrutiny of public health systems' data use policies and the treatment of patient identifiable information. According to NCHS's Public Health Data Standards Consortium,[30]

> Public health agencies are now being asked to explicitly justify the need for such data and are charged with demonstrating how the benefits of this information outweigh privacy encroachments. Public health agencies have historically had a difficult time convincing policy makers that health data collection is a valuable activity and the growing concerns regarding the confidentiality of patient records will only exacerbate this reluctance. In the absence of pressing financial or communicable disease crises, policy makers are hesitant to fund abstract, seemingly academic, data gathering exercises. The specter of data misuse and confidentiality concerns will only further alarm and mobilize an already wary public.

Public health agencies have always recognized that the sensitive nature of surveillance data necessitates that measures be taken to ensure confidentiality.[31] To balance the principles of access to data and patient confidentiality, surveillance systems must establish protocols and procedures to make determinations on requests for information for scientific research.[32] The data release protocol should include a clearly defined classification scheme to promote equal treatment of data requestors and data providers, expedite the release process, and encourage the release of a broad spectrum of data elements without compromising confidentiality.[29]

At the national level, the CDC and the CSTE have created a policy for the release of data from the National Notifiable Diseases Surveillance System for research purposes. Many individual states have also legislated mandates to establish advisory boards or scientific review committees to oversee the release of confidential surveillance data. Committee membership should include experts from appropriate disciplines who are experienced in the analysis of health data, disease coding, registry operations, and bioethics. Depending on whether the surveillance system is part of the state health department or university, additional criteria may be required by the review committees.

Surveillance System Evaluation

All public health surveillance systems require periodic evaluation to ensure that the system remains focused on its ultimate public health objectives and operates as efficiently and effectively as possible.[9] Evaluation should assess whether the information produced by the surveillance system is theoretically and functionally useful for public health programming and policy making. The CDC advocates for including those persons responsible for promoting health in the population—the surveillance system's stakeholders—in the design and execution of the evaluation. This approach helps to ensure that evaluation results are most useful and credible to those who need the information most.

The CDC has played a leading role in establishing and updating guidelines for surveillance system evaluation, which are posted on its Internet site (http://www.cdc.gov). These guidelines describe the evaluation process, beginning with a review of the surveillance system's purpose and objectives. The process continues with a thorough examination of system operations, taking into consideration six key qualitative attributes of surveillance systems: simplicity, flexibility, acceptability, sensitivity, predictive value positive, and representativeness. Evaluation culminates in the formulation of recommendations for system-strengthening intervention. To assess the utility of surveillance functions, evaluators are encouraged to verify that surveillance activities are integrated into the overall public health system, and that their results are routinely received, understood, and applied by appropriate policy makers.[9]

CHAPTER REVIEW

1. Surveillance systems produce data that support
   - public health planning and priority setting
   - intervention design and targeting
   - detection and response to emergent public health needs such as disease outbreaks
   - epidemiologic investigation of health issues, including disease etiology, risk factors, and prevention and control opportunities
   - public health policy development and resource allocation
   - program and policy evaluation
2. Primary surveillance system design formats include
   - notifiable disease reporting
   - vital statistics surveillance
   - sentinel event surveillance
   - registries
   - health surveys
3. Major operational activities to be accomplished in surveillance systems include
   - establishing system objectives
   - defining the population under surveillance
   - defining the health events to be monitored
   - formulating reporting procedures
   - specifying analytic strategies for use with surveillance data
   - disseminating and applying information from surveillance systems
4. Key managerial strategies for sustaining surveillance systems within and across public health organizations include
   - attracting and retaining appropriate human resources and monitoring their performance
   - ensuring the performance of the surveillance system as a whole, including meeting federal data standards and privacy protections
   - implementing effective internal evaluation processes to enable continual improvements in the quality and efficiency of surveillance systems

REFERENCES

1. S.B. Thacker and R.L. Berkelman, "Public Health Surveillance in the United States," *Epidemiologic Reviews* 10 (1988): 164–190.
2. S.M. Teutsch, "Considerations in Planning a Surveillance System," in *Principles and Practice of Public Health Surveillance*, eds. S.M. Teutsch and R.E. Churchill (New York: Oxford University Press, 1994), 18–30.
3. S.M. Teutsch and R.E. Churchill, eds., *Principles and Practice of Public Health Surveillance* (New York: Oxford University Press, 1994).
4. W. Halperin and E. Baker, eds., *Public Health Surveillance* (New York: Van Nostrand Reinhold, 1992).
5. H. Menck and C. Smart, eds., *Central Cancer Registries—Design, Management and Uses* (Switzerland: Harwood Academic Publishers, 1994).
6. C.L. Hutchison et al., eds., *Cancer Registry Management: Principles and Practice* (Dubuque, IA: Kendall/Hunt Publishing Co., 1997).
7. "Outbreak of Salmonella Serotype Muenchen Infections associated with Unpasteurized Orange Juice—United States and Canada, June 1999," *Morbidity and Mortality Weekly Report (MMWR)* 48 (1999): 582–585.
8. M.J. Thun et al., "Aspirin Use and Reduced Risk of Fatal Colon Cancer," *New England Journal of Medicine* 325 (1991): 1,593–1,596.
9. U.S. Centers for Disease Control and Prevention, Guidelines Working Group, "Draft Updated Guidelines for Evaluating Surveillance Systems," *Morbidity and Mortality Weekly Report* January 19, 2000.
10. S. Roush et al., "Mandatory Reporting of Diseases and Conditions by Health Care Professionals and Laboratories," *Journal of the American Medical Association* 282 (1994): 164–170.
11. S.B. Thacker, "Historical Development," in *Principles and Practice of Public Health Surveillance,* eds. S.M. Teutsch and R.E. Churchill (New York: Oxford University Press, 1994), 3–17.
12. T.D. Vacalis et al., "Electronic Communication and the Future of International Public Health Surveillance," *Emerging Infectious Diseases* 1 (1995): 34–35.
13. N.E. Stroup et al., "Sources of Routinely Collected Data for Surveillance," in *Principles and Practice of Public Health Surveillance,* eds. S.M. Teutsch and R.E. Churchill (New York: Oxford University Press, 1994), 31–85.
14. M.C. Lynberg and L.D. Edmonds, "Surveillance of Birth Defects," in *Public Health Surveillance,* eds. W. Halperin and E. Baker (New York: Van Nostrand Reinhold, 1992), 157–177.
15. J. Chin, "Public Health Surveillance of AIDS and HIV Infections," *Bulletin of the World Health Organization* 68 (1990): 529–536.
16. D.D. Rustein et al., "Measuring the Quality of Medical Care: A Clinical Method," *New England Journal of Medicine* 294 (1976): 582–588.
17. P.J. Seligman and T.M. Frazier, "Surveillance: The Sentinel Health Event Approach," in *Public Health Surveillance,* eds. W. Halperin and E. Baker (New York: Van Nostrand Reinhold, 1992), 16–25.
18. P.L. Garbe and S.B. Blount, "Chronic Disease Surveillance," in *Public Health Surveillance,* eds. W. Halperin and E. Baker (New York: Van Nostrand Reinhold, 1992), 130–141.
19. V.W. Chen and X.C. Wu, eds., *Cancer in North America, 1991–95. Volume One: Incidence, Volume Two: Mortality* (Sacramento, CA: North American Association of Central Cancer Registries, 1999).
20. W. Cates, "Estimates of the Incidence and Prevalence of Sexually Transmitted Diseases in the United States," *Sexually Transmitted Diseases* 26 (1999): S2–S7.
21. E. Pisani, T. Brown, T. Saidel, T. Rehle, and M. Carael. *Meeting the Behavioral Data Collection Needs of National HIV/AIDS and STD Programmes.* A joint IMPACT/FHI/UNAIDS Workshop: Report and Conclusions May 1998.
22. E.J. Lengerich, ed., *Indicators for Chronic Disease Surveillance: Consensus of CSTE, ASTCDPD, and CDC* (Atlanta, GA: Council of State and Territorial Epidemiologists, 1999).
23. R. Meriwether, "Blueprint for a National Public Health Surveillance System," *Journal of Public Health Management and Practice* 2 (1996): 16–23.
24. D.N. Klaucke, "Evaluating Public Health Surveillance," in *Principles and Practice of Public Health Surveillance,* eds. S.M. Teutsch and R.E. Churchill (New York: Oxford University Press, 1994), 158–174.
25. T.E. Aldrich, S.W. Bolick, and L.A. Cave. *A Report of Cancer in ZIP Code 29405* (Columbia, SC: Department of Health and Environmental Control, 1999).
26. M. Wharton and R.L. Vogt, "State and Local Issues in Surveillance," in *Principles and Practice of Public Health Surveillance,* eds. S.M. Teutsch and R.E. Churchill (New York: Oxford University Press, 1994), 218–234.
27. W. Cates and G.D. Williamson, "Descriptive Epidemiology: Analyzing and Interpreting Surveillance Data," in *Principles and Practice of Public Health Surveillance,* eds. S.M. Teutsch and R.E. Churchill (New York: Oxford University Press, 1994), 96–135.

28. J.E. Anderson et al., "Factors Associated with Self-Reported STDs: Data from a National Survey," *Sexually Transmitted Diseases* 21 (1994): 303–308.
29. J. Seifert, ed., *Standards for Cancer Registries.* Vol. III. Standards for Completeness, Quality, Analysis, and Management of Data (Springfield, IL: North American Association of Central Cancer Registries, 1994).
30. Public Health Data Standards Consortium, "Issue Brief 1999," National Center for Health Statistics. http://www.cdc.gov/nchs/otheract/phdsc/issue_group.htm. Accessed 13 April 2000.
31. R.A. Hahn, "Ethical Issues," in *Principles and Practice of Public Health Surveillance,* eds. S.M. Teutsch and R.E. Churchill (New York: Oxford University Press, 1994), 175–189.
32. D.M. Parkin, *Guidelines on Confidentiality in the Cancer Registry* (Lyon, France: International Association of Cancer Registries [IARC Internal Report No. 92/003], 1992).

CHAPTER 9

Using Information Systems for Public Health Administration

Stephen Parente

Public health organizations require well-designed information systems in order to make optimal use of the mounting supply of health-related data. Organizations rely on these systems to inform managerial decision making and improve operations in areas such as epidemiologic surveillance, health outcomes assessment, program and clinic administration, program evaluation and performance measurement, public health planning, and policy analysis. Key design considerations in developing information systems include service-based and population-based application objectives, units of analysis, data sources, data linkage methods, technology selection and integration strategies, and information privacy protections. A growing collection of models and resources now exists for developing effective information systems for public health organizations.

Information systems have emerged as an essential public health tool. Today, information systems provide real-time data to guide public health decisions. The rise in importance of health information systems (HISs) has three fundamental sources: (1) the expanding breadth of data available from multiple public and private sources, (2) advances in information technology (IT), and (3) the growing recognition of the power of information in public health decision making. Administrative data from public and private health service providers as well as insurers contain an electronic history of health care cost and use. Government surveys provide an unprecedented level of detailed information on health status, functional status, medical care use and expenditure, nutrition, sociodemographics, and health behaviors.

HISs support a wide variety of public health system objectives, including

- epidemiologic disease and risk factor surveillance
- medical and public health outcomes assessment
- facility and clinic administration (billing, inventory, clinical records, utilization review)
- cost-effectiveness and productivity analysis
- utilization analysis and demand estimation
- program planning and evaluation
- quality assurance and performance measurement
- public health policy analysis
- clinical research
- health education and health information dissemination

IT has now advanced to the point that one year of the Medicare program's entire claims history—roughly 200 million observations—can be analyzed on a high-end personal computer (PC) workstation. Advances in IT are dramatically influencing public health organizations and their historical roles in collecting and disseminating data. Vital statistics and disease registries—critical functions of public health departments at both the local and national level—are being transformed by IT and its emphasis on evidence-based decision making. Yet, HIS resources remain difficult to develop and manage in addressing current public health challenges. Data sets are located in a balkanized array of separate computing platforms with little interconnectivity. For HISs to be effective, public health administrators must assess available data sources, design blueprints for extracting information and knowledge, and evaluate the benefits derived from these systems.

This chapter examines concepts, resources, and examples of HISs for public health organizations. Issues and implications for public health management are explored in the following five areas.

1. contemporary concepts and applications of HISs in public health
2. systems and technology building
3. available databases
4. operational models
5. privacy and security

CONTEMPORARY CONCEPTS AND APPLICATIONS

What is public health information? A more telling question may be what is not public health information because the scope of data required to examine scientifically the multiple and overlapping health, social, and environmental factors that affect a population can be enormous. Traditionally, public health or epidemiologic data consist of vital statistics, disease registries, and other surveillance-based resources. However, these resources are often limited in scope because they only record natality, morbidity, mortality, and perhaps some measure of environmental and behavioral influences. Managing health resources effectively at the population level requires a much broader scope of data resources to measure the effectiveness and cost of health interventions and policies.

An examination of public health applications of HISs is facilitated by an understanding of the two most common applications of these systems in practice. First, information systems are used to store and make available service data that reflect activities performed by public health organizations and other health-related entities. Second, information systems store and make available population-based data that are important for surveillance, program evaluation, policy making, and priority setting in public health. These two common applications are not separate but interact extensively.

For example, routinely collected service data by local public health agencies often include the results of blood lead screening of children under five years of age, immunization status, and encounter data recording the results of client visits for tuberculosis (TB) and sexually transmitted diseases (STDs). Other routinely collected service data include records of individual client encounters in the federal Special Supplemental Food Program for Women, Infants, and Children (WIC) and other early intervention programs. These service data are important for the effective management of individual care by public health and ambulatory care providers. Importantly, these data reflect individual transactions and can be used to monitor program performance and to describe a group of users at a particular facility—but they do not necessarily offer information about an entire community or population.

An important practical distinction exists between the service-based application of HISs and the population-based application, which offers information about defined communities and population groups of interest. To support this latter application, information systems must integrate data from major populationwide sources such as vital statistics registries and disease surveillance systems. In some cases, service data may also contribute to population-based information.

For example, the National Notifiable Diseases Surveillance System (NNDSS), formed more than a century ago, serves as a major source of populationwide data. This system captures information on disease incidence for approximately 50 diseases, which require accurate and timely information for effective prevention and control. The Centers for Disease Control and

Prevention (CDC) receives reports of disease from the 50 states, 2 cities (New York City and the District of Columbia), and 5 territories.[1] This database is most useful to public health agencies because of its ability to analyze trends and conduct comparisons of disease incidence among communities.

Population-based information systems may also be constructed from service-level data. The immunization registries recently implemented by many state and local public health agencies provide an excellent example of this use. These registries record immunization status and vaccinations provided to all children residing within a defined geographic area so that this information is available not only to the initial provider, but also to other providers, health plans, and schools. Many of these registries incorporate birth certificate data for children born in the community, adding a population denominator. This is an example of an information system that provides service-level information that is helpful to individual providers and their patients, while also providing population-level information that is helpful to public health organizations for surveillance, program evaluation, and policy making. A key qualification, however, is that a large proportion of the children in the community must be captured by such information systems in order for population-based information to have validity and reliability.

Drawing on the successes of immunization registries, a growing number of local public health organizations are developing computerized information systems for other purposes. For example, some local systems track the results of blood lead screenings performed at public health clinics, thereby producing important service information regarding the number of children screened, those with elevated blood lead levels, and those receiving follow-up treatment and lead abatement services. This information is based on service data, but if the systems can capture data on all children in a defined community, then valuable population-based information can become available.

The relatively recent availability of state-of-the art computing technology has enabled public health organizations to collect health data rapidly and extract meaningful information about community health status.[2] The major challenge is to integrate data sources and develop networks that make this information optimally available to public health organizations at all levels of government as well as to appropriate entities in the private sector. The current impetus to have a surveillance capability supported by a national network of public health HISs is fueled by concerns about bioterrorism and emerging infectious diseases, resulting in sizeable investments by the CDC for constructing linked information systems. (See Chapter 28 for more information on the use of public health information in managing disasters.)

Major practical goals for the future development of HISs for public health organizations include the following:

- Integrate the multiple data sources available for public health purpose.
- Network information systems to make interaction and information flow between different entities feasible.
- Use health care delivery information systems to produce public health information regarding preventive services, preventable diseases, and quality of care.

Integration

Government public health agencies have historically designed computer-based information systems for single programs. For years, the same data were entered and maintained in many different, often incompatible, systems that supported different public health programs.[3] This duplicative and fragmented information infrastructure hindered the ability of public health managers to know what data existed and how to access them. For example, most local public health agencies maintain multiple programs for children, including lead toxicity prevention, immunization, WIC, and early intervention services. Meanwhile, the local departments of social services enroll families in Medicaid. Despite the fact that Medicaid and public health programs serve client populations that overlap substantially in most communities, the databases used to manage these programs are entirely separate in most cases, reflecting the categorical mechanisms that support these programs. Information systems integration can offer opportunities for improved service delivery and enhanced population-based decision making and management.

Linkage of data sets is often an effective method to obtain information across programs. For example, linkage of WIC records with Medicaid, birth and death, and hospital discharge files has enabled program analysts to document the effectiveness of the WIC program in reducing infant death and costly neonatal hospitalizations. Similarly, linking lead screening registries, Medicaid eligibility files, and managed care plan enrollment files can enable public health organizations to monitor compliance with lead screening by health plans. Apart from such special-purpose studies, HISs are needed to integrate information concerning the various health services provided to a population in order to facilitate improved service delivery and to enable population-based management by public health organizations. A growing number of models now exist for integrating public health information, many of which are described later in this chapter.

Public health agencies are also beginning to innovate by using unconventional data sources such as market research databases. For example, electronic information compiled from grocery and drug store sales can be used as part of an HIS to identify the purchase of cigarettes concomitantly with products associated with pregnancy or infants, such as diapers. This information by ZIP code can help target or evaluate public health intervention programs, such as efforts to prevent tobacco use in the perinatal period.

Networks

Another major function of HISs in public health is to create linked networks of information that can strengthen public health operations by: (1) facilitating communication among public health practitioners throughout the United States, (2) enhancing the accessibility of information, and (3) allowing swift and secure exchange of public health data.[4] As a prominent example, the CDC initiated the Information Network for Public Health Officials (INPHO) in 1992. The CDC has been the major supporter of efforts to create networks that link public health information from localities and states with that of federal agencies. Information networks of this type are increasingly indispensable for disease surveillance activities, particularly in cases of local disease outbreaks that have the potential to spread regionally and nationally. In this way, HISs can help to create and sustain effective interorganizational relationships among public health organizations.

Utilization of Health Care Delivery Systems

Public health organizations can also benefit from timely access to health care services information from providers of personal health care services.[4] For example, immunization registries must acquire information on immunization status from multiple community providers who deliver vaccinations. In a growing number of communities, public health organizations are able to obtain relevant and timely information from the systems that are maintained by health care delivery organizations. Large delivery systems can offer information on the delivery and utilization of preventive services (including missed opportunities for prevention), the incidence of preventable diagnoses and comorbidities, and the quality of health care facilities and providers (such as rates of medical errors, mortality, and hospital infections).

These types of resources drive the contemporary development of HISs among public health organizations, and they reflect a basic change of thought regarding the delivery of medical and public health services subsequent to the 1993 federal health reform initiative. This initiative accentuated the need for informed decision making by consumers, providers, employers, and governments. For example, the Clinton Administration reform plan relied solely on analyses of the 1987 *National Medical Expenditure Survey*

(NMES) to draw conclusions about the future demand for and cost of health care in the United States. Between the time the *NMES* was fielded and 1993, the dominance of fee-for-service gave way to managed care as the primary health financing mechanism for the private and public insurance market. As a result, the 1987 *NMES* could not reliably estimate the impact of the administration's health care reform proposal without significant and possibly questionable assumptions. The limitations of the data increased the administration's interest in an annual survey, which could provide better estimates of a rapidly changing market. In 1996, the Agency for Health Care Policy and Research fielded the *Medical Expenditure Panel Survey (MEPS),* providing a national annual survey instrument to track changes in health care use and cost as well as health status and insurance coverage. A similar demand for information came from employers, who wanted health plans to provide standardized information on the value of their products. The result was a cooperative effort between employers and health insurers to develop a common set of health plan performance measures known formally as the *Health Plan Employers Information Data Set (HEDIS),* developed by the National Committee for Quality Assurance. Some of the *HEDIS* measures were prevention oriented (e.g., immunization) and thus illustrated the principle of obtaining public health information from a health care delivery information system.[4] (See Chapter 11 for more information on the evaluation of public health information.)

Building new databases for multiple purposes such as *MEPS* and *HEDIS* required a clear identification of HIS objectives as well as knowledge of the strengths and weaknesses of established data structures. This knowledge is essential in determining which structures can be recycled in building a new database, such as using existing health insurer records for *HEDIS,* and which structures need to be newly constructed, such as designing medical record abstraction protocols for obtaining disease and outcomes data for *HEDIS.* With appropriate design, medical encounter data (service data) can be used for several population-based purposes, including community health assessment, surveillance, and evaluation.

BUILDING SYSTEMS AND TECHNOLOGY

A common misperception in developing HISs for public health applications is the expectation that such systems are analogous to their counterparts in IT-intensive industries such as banking or manufacturing. Health is a combination of many uncertain inputs. These inputs range from the unique biologic and behavioral characteristics of the individual patient or population under study to health insurance characteristics and the accessibility of health resources to the practice styles of physicians and other health professionals, as well as to thousands of possible diagnoses, comorbidities, risk factors, and interventions. In combination, these inputs generate millions of possible outcomes for a given health episode. Consequently, the HISs used to support public health applications and decision-making may need to be more complex and costly than the systems supporting applications in other industries and professions.

In building an HIS, the field of health informatics constitutes a multidisciplinary core of expertise including specialists from the fields of

- computer science
- electrical engineering
- medicine, nursing, and allied health
- management, finance, and accounting
- operations research
- economics
- sociology
- survey design
- epidemiology
- statistics

These disciplines work in combination to produce HISs to serve the public health system objectives described above. In designing and managing HISs, public health administrators require the ability to: (1) distinguish between data, information, and knowledge; (2) define units of analysis for the level of data aggregation; and (3) understand the health IT architecture of system(s) to be used.

Data versus Information versus Knowledge

Data are raw facts and statistics that are collected as part of the normal functioning of a business, clinical encounter, or research experiment. *Information* is data that has been processed in a structured, intelligent way to obtain results that are directly useful to managers and analysts. *Knowledge* is obtained by using information to explain the context of a problem or situation. To illustrate all three concepts, consider the operation of a car. During driving, a driver generates data on the speed of the vehicle by tracking the revolutions of the wheel in a defined time period. The speedometer converts this data on wheel revolutions and time to information on the current miles per hour traveled. The driver uses this information to generate the knowledge that he or she is over the speed limit and needs to slow down. The blue and red lights in the rear view window provide knowledge to the driver that he or she will not arrive at his or her destination on time.

In public health, data are obtained from a variety of sources ranging from patient history at a clinical visit to health insurance claims to bacteriology laboratory reports. To be valuable for generating information and knowledge, data must be readily accessible and reliable. Generally, electronic data in standardized formats are most efficient. However, data that are easy to obtain may not be the most accurate or precise. For example, electronic health insurance claims data will identify a specific immunization on a particular date but not indicate the child's overall immunization status. For that information, medical records or reports from a computerized immunization registry are needed. Thus, the cost of obtaining accurate and precise knowledge concerning a child's immunization status may be outside the scope of existing data collection processes. Ethical questions also arise if immunization data had to be transferred from another source and parental consent had not been given.

In developing a database, the manager needs to consider (1) the information objective, (2) cost and feasibility, and (3) whether threats to personal privacy are an issue.

Defining a Unit of Analysis in an Information System

To turn data into information, a manager must choose a unit of analysis. The unit of analysis determines a level at which data will be aggregated and analyzed in order to generate information. The four most common units of analysis in public health are

1. person/patient
2. vendor/supplier
3. program
4. region/population

For example, an average diabetic patient is associated with 200 billing records in a year. The information can be bundled at the person/patient level by building a set of counts for the frequency of a certain service that is vital to recommended diabetic care, such as the number of Hemoglobin A1c or diabetic retinopathy screening tests. Once completed, a database with one observation per diabetic patient is created to compare patient-level variation in quality of care. This type of bundled procedure can be completed for a variety of different levels of analysis.

Generally, the unit of analysis should correlate to the population of interest for a management decision. For example, if the principal focus of an evaluation is patient compliance with a disease management program, then the correct unit of analysis is the patient. If, however, the goal of the analysis is to compare how different disease management programs perform to improve the health of the population, the appropriate unit of analysis is the program. Vendors or suppliers in health care can be physicians, hospitals, group practices, public health clinics, health insurers, or any other health-related organization. Regions can be defined in a variety of ways, including state, interstate regions (e.g., the Midwest), metropolitan statistical area, county, and ZIP code. Populations can be defined by residence within a given geopolitical subdivision, by sociodemographic characteristics such as age and ethnicity, or by health conditions such as diagnoses or behavioral risk factors. Other health-related units of analysis are defined by diseases, medical procedures, or other health interventions.

Health IT Pyramid

The physical component of an HIS is a computer or network containing software applications to collect and analyze data. From a manager's perspective, the health IT pyramid is a useful conceptual model for building and enhancing an HIS. As seen in Figure 9–1, the base of the pyramid is the computer hardware that will form the foundation of an HIS. The second level is software needed to operate the hardware and collect information needed to conduct business. The third layer are software applications that provide the financial and administrative "life support" for an organization such as billing systems, provider scheduling systems, and communication applications such as e-mail and file transfer protocols to the Internet using the World Wide Web interface. The fourth and top level of the pyramid includes decision support software applications to guide management decisions.

- The pyramid's foundation should be wide and adaptable enough to support the structures above it. For IT, the base of the pyramid constitutes the mainframe or large server with adequate storage capacity, processing speed, and workstation links to complete the business of health care. A mainframe platform offers the ability to perform a large sheer volume of transactions and reliability of the equipment. Increasingly, the PC platform has the speed and data storage capabilities needed to handle mainframe-sized analysis, but it does not have the mainframe's contingency components for failed disk drives and memory. Such failures can cost a 1,000-person health care organization tens of thousands of dollars per hour in wasted productivity. Although advanced PC-based servers and minicomputers, such as Sun Microsystems's workstations, can be configured to have equivalent reliability to mainframes, the cost of transferring platforms can be larger than the savings achieved from using technology that is less expensive than a mainframe.

Other important pieces of hardware include the input and output devices used to enter and report electronic data. Common input devices include the keyboard, mouse, and scanner. For medical care, other input devices include specialized machines to obtain clinical data, including imaging devices (such as computerized tomography [CT] scans and magnetic resonance imaging [MRI]), and biomedical probes to

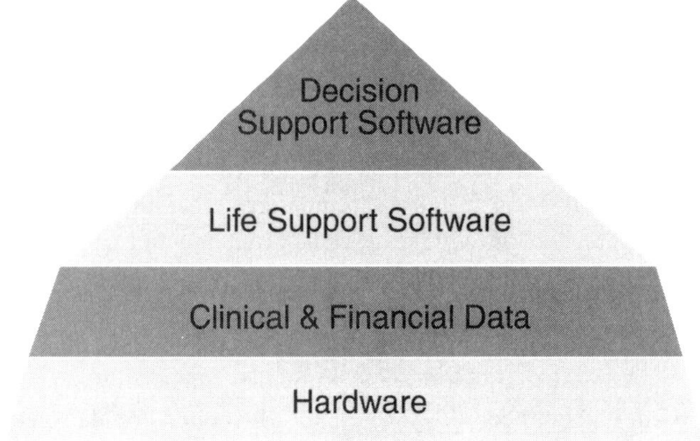

Figure 9–1 The Health Information Technology Pyramid

monitor heart, lung, and brain capacity. Common output devices include monitors, printers, and audio speakers.

- The operating system and basic data collection software constitute the second level of the pyramid. Mainframes use the IBM MVS system; microcomputers and PC servers use UNIX and Microsoft server products such as Microsoft Windows NT Server or Microsoft Windows 2000 Server. These systems provide instructions to the hardware to process data and run advanced software applications. This second tier includes the software needed to collect data for the operation of the organization. For example, the second tier includes software applications that allow a pathologist to enter data on a clinical specimen to a hospital's computer. It also includes the software to read data from other organizations or state agencies. For a county health department, the second tier would contain a data entry software application to record vital statistics information.
- The third tier of the pyramid represents "life support" software applications. These computer applications process the data collected in the second tier of the pyramid and use it for operational purposes. For example, a hospital billing department would take the pathologist's data entry in the previous example and price it based on the supplies and time resources used for cost accounting. Depending on the hospital's financial arrangement with the patient's insurer, the billing department will either submit a claim to the insurer for services rendered or record the resources internally as part of a negotiated fixed fee for pathology services. In this case, the billing department processed the data regarding a health service and converted it to another form of data regarding information resource use for internal and external purposes. In this tier, information may be generated for clinicians, but not for managers. For example, a software application can be used to take the data inputs from an intensive care unit (ICU) and convert them into information for a treating provider. However, a fourth tier application would use the results of the ICU inputs as well as the data on the treating provider's resource use to compare the effectiveness of all ICU providers.
- Decision support software applications are the fourth and final tier of the health IT pyramid. These applications are used for decision support. For example, statistical analysis of cost and use patterns among a series of cost centers for strategic planning purposes would be completed using decision support software such as Structured Query Language (SQL), Microsoft Access or Microsoft Excel, SPSS, or SAS. Increasingly, custom-designed software applications are built to meet very specific needs of health managers.

For example, the migration of a hospital billing system from a mainframe to a PC server environment should be undertaken so as to not adversely impact the pyramid's upper tiers. Likewise, new decision support applications can be used without affecting hardware or basic data of the system. This framework should allow a manager to identify which tier is affected by a proposed change in an HIS and the impact on other tiers.

Technical Considerations

For most public health analyses, the abilities of a PC workstation (circa 2000) are adequate. With processing speeds on most of the major technology platforms in excess of 500 to 600 megahertz, and the ability to link processors together, specifying technical requirements is not very meaningful. Larger information systems are required if data collection is to be ongoing and collected at different sites of a network. This involves the creation of a client–server platform managed over the Internet with appropriate security protocols in place. The use of claims data would require a large workstation or server depending on the size of the database being used.

Although technology has advanced, knowledge of using computing resources to process data efficiently can be more valuable than the capital expense of IT. Three key issues are discussed in the following paragraphs.

1. *Data storage requirements:* Computer data storage management is a valuable skill. It is learned from experience and knowledge of the capacities of different data platforms such as CD-ROMs, digital versatile disks (DVDs), and mainframe computer tape. Although there are few substitutes for experience, there are several rules to follow.
   - Know the size of the data you are working with in terms of bytes, not just observations. This will tell you whether you need to have 100 megabytes of storage versus 100 gigabytes (or 100,000 megabytes) of storage. The easiest way to know the size of your database is to multiply the number of observations by the record length. Thus, a claims file with a record length of 450 bytes and approximately 6 million observations will need approximately 2.7 gigabytes (or 2.7 billion bytes) of storage space.
   - Plan on having at least three times as much computer space as the size of your database on the computer. This amount of space is needed to sort the data and to combine and create new files that will be the analytic files.
   - Work toward creating a small analytic file that you need to run your analyses.
   - Once you have created your ideal file, use it for several weeks to make sure it is the ideal file and then carefully back up and remove the source data and secure it in a safe environment.

   As a practical matter, most public health databases are distributed on CD-ROM. As such, they are no larger than 650 megabytes and can be accommodated on modern PCs where hard drives in excess of 10 gigabytes (or 10,000 megabytes) are commonly found. When data start being distributed on DVD, the range in storage capacity is presently between 3 gigabytes and 15 gigabytes, depending on which data storage format wins out.
2. *Data processing performance:* When working with very large databases, the time to pass through millions of observations can be measured in hours if not days unless the appropriate equipment is being used. For large database management, the key issue is input/output (I/O) speed of the hard drives. Hard drives for these tasks must be fast (at least 10,000 revolutions per second) and contain suitable cache. A computer must read and store every piece of information on the hard drive on a given file. High-end workstations and servers use redundant arrays of inexpensive disks (RAID) controllers with cached memory to speed this process up. If resources are not an issue, one can also build a random access memory (RAM) disk made of memory chips alone to bypass the use of hard drives, although this is yet to be a conventional method of data management and can lead to greater data loss in the event of a power failure.
3. *Software packages to build and use analytic files:* Depending on your analysis, different software packages may be used to develop the analytic file and perform statistical analysis. Software packages such as SAS can do almost anything from data management to statistical manipulation. However, other data management packages such as Microsoft FoxPro, PowerBuilder, and Oracle provide faster access times, particularly if the data can be structured in a relational database format. For most analyses, calculations from common spreadsheet programs such as Microsoft Excel may be sufficient. For more advanced statistical analysis, SPSS, STATA, and SAS are commonly used. STATA has a user-friendly interface that converts just about any database to a STATA database as well as to other non-STATA formats (e.g., from Microsoft

FoxPro to SAS). For budgeting purposes, the software that best suits the analysis should be chosen. The learning curve costs on different software package may exceed the saving in price.

SOURCES OF DATA FOR INFORMATION SYSTEMS

Common Data Structures in Public Health

Electronic databases are one of the great resources for public health organizations in building information systems. National databases such as the *National Health Interview Survey (NHIS)* and the *National Death Index* provide public health professionals with valuable resources to gauge the health of the population. However, databases come in many shapes and sizes. The shape of a database can be characterized by whether it is wide, deep, or multidimensional. A *wide* database is one with many variables—one per observation in the database. A *deep* database contains many observations. A *multidimensional* database has variables that can be linked across different time periods or different databases. These databases are generally thought of as relational databases.

Information systems must be designed to accommodate the various forms of electronic data they use. Although there are many forms of electronic data to be encountered by the public health professional, the most common are described in the following paragraphs.

- *Transaction data:* This is the most prevalent form of data in health insurance and provider transaction data. A good example of transaction data is a checking account. Each month, a person receives a statement of debits and credits. If a debit was voided or changed, an identical observation with a negative debit amount (also thought of as a credit) will follow to cancel the debit. If the record is to be changed, a third observation will follow that is identical except a different positive debit amount will appear to reflect the appropriate debit now that the original debit has been cancelled. Generally, health transaction data will record the date of medical services, the procedure performed, and the diagnosis of the patient. For a given patient, there could be many observations in a given year reflecting the extent of medical services provided. A programmer/analyst must know how to "clean" the administrative data of extraneous "adjudication" observations in place to yield the correct debit to an insurer. Once cleaned, a programmer/analyst can read the data and count services and resources used in a variety of different statistical and database software applications. When using transaction data for health services or outcomes research, it is important to remember that the database was built for the purpose of accounting, not research. As a result, the analyst must be prepared for the incompatibility of transaction data for a research project focused on health status or improvement measurement.[5]
- *Registry data:* Registry databases are common in public health. Most registries are organized at the person level. Examples include state tumor registries or the national mortality database. Data are usually collected through a questionnaire completed by a medical provider at a key point in an individual's life. Often, these registries provide the only national inventory of all persons with a disease or persons who have reached a critical event in their lives such as birth, marriage, parenthood, or death. Registries are found at the provider level as well. These files are primarily used for membership in organizations such as the American Medical Association (AMA) or for payment information for medical care delivery reimbursed by a public or private health insurer. These databases are often ready for analysis once the analyst is familiar with their structure and history. Multiple records per person may occur if repeated events are recorded with different data entry dates. Thus, an analyst must use caution to develop nonduplicative data files if a person-level unit of analysis is desired.

- *Survey data:* Health surveys are completed when transaction or registry data are insufficient. The data are usually structured to be ready for analysis at either the person or the organization level. Survey data can be gathered primarily through mail, telephone, or personal interview. There are two major types of person-level surveys found in public health: those completed at the national level (e.g., the *National Health Interview Survey*) and those completed to represent a smaller geographic or organizational population (e.g., a managed care organization's risk assessment of the personal behavior of their members). Public health managers hoping to use national survey data to assess the wellness of their community must recognize that the samples are designed to generalize the nation, not a state or region of the country. To be generalizable, a national survey will have person-level weights used to multiply an individual's response so as to create a national summary statistic. For example, a 40,000-person survey will have weights averaging 6,750 to generalize to the U.S. population of 270 million. The weights will vary in size depending on whether certain geographic or sociodemographic features in the population will be under- or overcounted to achieve national representation. If survey data are unavailable, one could think about "building" rather than "buying" a survey. However, the cost of designing and deploying an adequate survey device that will yield a response rate sample participants (e.g., the number of respondents divided by the number of eligible sample participants) is not trivial and often is the most expensive component of a formal program evaluation.
- *Relational data:* Relational database structures were designed with economy in mind. Identifying key variables for file linkage is the key attribute of relational database structure. All types of data described above could be structured as a relational database. The value of a relational database is that linkages are made between files that permit faster and more efficient summation than conventional databases. Assume that a wide database with a transaction format contains 10 five-digit diagnosis code variables and an associated 70-character diagnosis description variable for each patient. Assume further that there are 10 possible diagnosis codes. This is an enormously wasteful use of data storage because not all of the diagnosis code and description variables (with a total length of 75 characters each) are filled. If the transaction file is five million observations, there will be a significant amount of empty space on the data file if, on average, 2 of the 10 possible diagnosis segments are filled. The diagnosis descriptions could be moved to a relational database format where each observation is a unique diagnosis code. The linking variable would be the five-digit diagnosis code. This one design change would reduce the size of the transaction file by approximately 18 200-megabyte mainframe data tapes. Although relational database structures are not necessary to complete an analysis, the size and scope of the data involved may require changes in data structure in order to achieve sufficient data economy to proceed with an analysis.

Common Databases Available for Public Health

A solid understanding of health IT and data structure is required for the optimal design of public HISs. Fortunately for public health managers, there are rich data resources available at federal and state levels. This section provides a brief overview of the most common databases available to health managers and researchers in developing HISs. (A more detailed review of data sources available to support a variety of public health activities is found in Chapter 7.) Most of the databases described here are federal- or state-specific in their focus. Although a federal focus may be too broad for local and regional health policy issues, federal surveys can still provide two significant benefits. First, national databases provide field-tested survey instruments or data abstraction tools that can be applied to a more focused information system. Second, federal surveys can provide a comparison database for information systems that also use state and local data sources in order to gauge the effectiveness of local initiatives.

Government Survey Data

The federal government collects a broad array of data that may be used by public HISs. The U.S. Department of Health and Human Services (DHHS) has the largest health data collection responsibility. However, other federal government departments such as defense, labor, and commerce also collect critical health data.

The phrase "national probability sample" describes a survey instrument that has been deliberately designed to reflect the U.S. national population's sociodemographic variation in age, gender, race, income, and education. If a state-level analysis was attempted, the survey could produce misleading estimates if survey respondents were over- or underweighted to reflect their proportional representation within the nation.

Another important concept is the panel survey. In this design, a panel or cohort of survey participants is followed during several rounds of the questionnaire. For example, some surveys such as the *MEPS* and the *Medicare Current Beneficiary Survey (MCBS)* follow participants for at least two years to track health status and cost. Panel surveys are valuable to assess long-term impacts in health care, such as a lack of health insurance or follow-up from a massive heart attack.

Most federal surveys are collected on an annual basis and are generally available as public use files one to two years following the completion of the data collection period. These data are available for a small fee to cover the cost of producing the databases. A list of nearly all of the government surveys used for health is available on the Internet at http://www.census.gov/publication/www/dbna/dbn-sum-tab.html.

Several examples of government-sponsored survey data are provided in the following paragraphs.

- *Current Population Survey (CPS):* This survey is completed annually and contains basic information in health care use. It is collected by the Department of Labor and can be purchased as a public use file. It is often available before any other federal survey with health data. The sample consists of approximately 52,000 housing units and the persons in them. The survey's primary goals are to provide estimates of employment, unemployment, and other socioeconomic characteristics of the general labor force, of the population as a whole, and of various subgroups of the population.
- *NHIS:* This survey, collected by the National Center for Health Statistics (NCHS) within the DHHS, is a national probability sample of the health status of the population. A two-part questionnaire is used with a sample size of approximately 49,000 households yielding 127,000 persons. The NHIS has had continuous data collection since 1957 for national estimates through household interviews by U.S. Census Bureau interviewers. The *NHIS* provides the sampling frame for other NCHS surveys and is linked to the *National Death Index* (discussed later). Both a core survey of demographic and general health information and a supplement focusing on different populations are deployed.
- *MEPS:* The Agency for Healthcare Research and Quality (AHRQ), as part of the DHHS, fields an annual national probability sample that focuses on health care expenditures of an individual. This survey also collects information on a survey responder's employer (if appropriate), insurer (if appropriate), and provider. The survey has been in use since 1996 and is seen as an ongoing continuation of the *National Health Expenditure Surveys* completed in 1977 and 1987.
- *National Health and Nutrition Examination Survey III (NHANES):* The *NHANES* is sponsored jointly by the CDC and the NCHS as part of the DHHS. This third version of *NHANES* represents a sample of

40,000 people who were interviewed between the period of 1988–94.The primary goal of the *NHANES III* was to estimate the national prevalence of selected diseases and risk factors. Target diseases and areas of special interest include (but are not limited to) cardiovascular disease, chronic obstructive pulmonary disease, diabetes, kidney disease, gallbladder disease, osteoporosis, arthritis, infectious diseases, substance abuse, tobacco use, child health, mental health, environmental health, and occupation health. Public use files from the *NHANES* are currently available.

- *NCHS Medical Care Use Surveys:* The NCHS has several annual surveys of health care services designed to profile the use of services regardless of public or private payer. The surveys are specific to inpatient, ambulatory care, home care, and other types of services. These are excellent surveys for national comparisons of changes in the use of ambulatory and inpatient care. However, they are not able to generalize to any area smaller than a multistate sample (e.g., the northeast United States).
- *MCBS:* The Health Care Financing Administration (HCFA) started the *MCBS* as an annual panel survey in 1992.[1] The *MCBS* has one of the most innovative database designs. Approximately 14,000 Medicare beneficiaries receive three rounds of a household survey each year. For those beneficiaries not in a Medicare health maintenance organization (approximately 90 percent of the over age 65 population), Medicare claims data (described in greater detail below) are extracted and linked to the survey data. As a result, analysts can identify health and functional status indicators from the survey and correlate them to medical care use patterns. The *MCBS* has been used to look at the expansion of the Medicare prescription drug program, near-poor Medicare benefits expansion through the Qualified Medicare Beneficiary Program, and changes in the Medicare home health use and expenditure. Each survey respondent is in the survey for three years to develop a longer term database for outcomes and policy research.

Administrative/Claims Data

The use of administrative data in public HISs has dramatically increased as the cost to work with the data has been reduced and the quality of data, relative to its past quality, has improved significantly. Administrative data are defined as the data elements that are generated as part of a health care organization's operations. For example, health insurers generate claims data to record the services that are reimbursed by the insurer. There are three significant advantages to using administrative data. First, the data cover a large breadth of services ranging from inpatient services to prescription drug use and immunizations. Second, administrative data are an inexpensive source of data when contrasted to other forms of health service data such as medical records. The third advantage is the timeliness of availability when compared with government surveys and other data sources. The most commonly used administrative databases are described to illustrate the range of data available for use in information systems.

- *Medicare National Claims History File (NCHF):* The NCHF is more of a database architecture than a single file. Generally, it includes two file types. One file type is an annual 5 percent sample of the roughly 40 million Medicare beneficiary population. This file is sold as a public use file by HCFA. The second file type includes specialized data extracts of the NCHF across the Medicare population. An example of this type of file is any patient who received either a coronary artery bypass graft procedure (CABG) or angioplasty in 1990 and their claims for the next five years. Within these data, one can track health outcomes, such as repeat hospitalizations for cardiac conditions as well as mortality. Reimbursed services included in the claims file are inpatient, outpatient, hospice, medical equipment, provider services (e.g., physician), home health care, and skilled nursing care. The key identifying variables for the NCHF data extracts are inpatient diagnosis-related groups (DRGs), physician procedure codes, and diagnosis codes. Unlike survey data, the NCHF can be used to develop state-, county-, and possibly even ZIP code–level analysis, depending on the prevalence of the condition or treatment under investigation.

- *State Hospital Discharge Records:* Nearly half of all states maintain annual hospital discharge summary records. These data are valuable for examining changes in inpatient service use and cost. For example, changes in the use of CABGs and angioplasty over several years can be assessed by different age, gender, and health insurance payer categories. The principal advantage of using hospital discharge records for health policy purposes is that they contain data on all payers, whereas the NCHF only provides data on Medicare. Hospital discharge data can be obtained directly from a state's government or from the AHRQ Healthcare Cost and Utilization Profile (HCUP) standardized databases. Specifically, the State Inpatient Database (SID) involves 22 states. The advantage of the SID is that it allows an analyst to obtain data from 11 of the 22 states in a standardized format from AHRQ. For more information on the SID database, refer to http://www.ahrq.gov.
- *State Medicaid Claims Data:* Most states maintain claims data for reimbursements from their Medicaid programs. The states with more advanced Medicaid systems include (but are not limited to) California, Maryland, Pennsylvania, and Wisconsin. As with the Medicare claims data, Medicaid claims include data on inpatient, outpatient, physician, pharmacy, and skilled nursing services. Also available are provider data and Medicaid-eligible beneficiary data. It is vital to secure the eligibility file to properly account for truncated beneficiary enrollment periods. For example, one Medicaid recipient may have been enrolled for one month, whereas another may have been enrolled for one year. If both recipients received an equal number of physician services during a calendar year, the absence of applying the denominator of enrolled months will lead to faulty conclusions on service use. The quality of these data varies widely. For example, managed care capitation contracts may not require the collection of encounter information. Therefore, an analyst seeking to complete a multistate Medicaid study will be faced with the task of understanding each state's claims data idiosyncrasies.

Regional Data

Although survey and claims data provide person-specific information on health status, socioeconomic status, and medical care received, these data lack information on the environment in which the person resides. Regional databases providing county and other geographic data can be merged with administrative and survey data to develop a useful information system. Two of the most common databases used for this purpose are discussed in the following paragraphs.

- *Area Resource File (ARF):* The Health Resources and Services Administration (HRSA) within the DHHS generates the ARF. The ARF is an annual summary of county-specific data on health facilities, health professions, measures of resource scarcity, health status, economic activity, health training programs, and socioeconomic and environmental characteristics. When an administrative database provides a county identifier, the ARF is one of the most effective resources of supplemental regional data. The file also contains geographic codes and descriptors that enable it to be linked to many other files and to aggregate counties into various geographic groupings (e.g., metropolitan statistical areas, state, or region). The ARF contains data from more than 50 different source files including NCHS detail mortality and natality records, American Hospital Association (AHA) facilities, and AMA physician specialty data. All information contained on the file is derived from existing data sources. For more information on the ARF, visit the following Internet site: http://www.arfsys.com/overview.htm.

- *Hospital Wage Index File:* HCFA produces a Hospital Wage Index File that provides detailed data of hospital staff hours and wages used within the Medicare program's prospective payment system. The wage indexes are county specific and can be used to generate input price measures for economic analyses. The data file can be downloaded directly from HCFA as a public use file. The Internet location for these public use files is http://www.hcfa.gov/stats/pufiles.htm.

Program Data

Public health and social services programs often develop client-tracking databases, a specialized type of administrative database that provides valuable information for program management and evaluation. For example, program data might include a case history for a client enrolled in a diabetes management program sponsored by a local public health agency or managed care plan. The database provides dates of services that may be linked with other administrative data to determine if services are delivered and used appropriately and if the program improves the health behavior and health status of a patient or population.

The best way for a manager to obtain program data is to build its collection into a new public health initiative. The value of data collection for the management and evaluation of new programs is considerable if the program has yet to demonstrate its cost-effectiveness. If a manager needs program data for an existing initiative, the best strategy is to make a sweeping inventory of all possible data that could be recorded. Sometimes, the data may need to be extracted from a "live" system. For example, if a social services department has a data collection system for tracking clients, but has never used the file for analysis, it may be possible to "extract" relevant analytic information and conduct a retrospective analysis.

Vital Statistics Data

Tracking vital statistics, including the collection of birth and death records, is one of the nation's oldest public health activities. However, the development of a national death index for mortality data and a national natality database are fairly recent developments. Prior to the 1970s, states, cities, and towns may have recorded such data but did not forward the data to a national database. These data are used largely for epidemiologic surveillance, but they are also important resources for developing public HISs. The three most common forms of the data are discussed in the following paragraphs.

- *National Natality Data:* In the United States, state laws require birth certificates for all births, and federal law mandates the national collection and publication of births and other vital statistics data. The National Vital Statistics System, the federal compilation of these data, results from cooperation between the NCHS and the states to provide access to statistical information from birth certificates. An annual, national natality database is available from the NCHS as a public use file.
- *National Death Index:* The states and the NCHS cooperate to develop a database of mortality data. This unique database provides valuable information on the cause of death by ICD-9-CM diagnosis code. The current file contains data for 1979 through 1997. This database is only available by special request.
- *Disease registries, including state and federal notifiable disease reporting systems:* The disease registries maintained by federal and state governments are also key ingredients for use as part of public HISs. Tumor registries are one of the most common databases of this type. These databases are critical to track the morbidity of major diseases over time and by geographic re-

gion. Infectious disease registries with links to federal and state governments are essential to provide public health managers with vital information on the geographic dispersion and rate of morbidity associated with a disease outbreak in near real time.

Private Industry Data

Private industry data can be used when no other data are publicly available to address a public health issue. Often the price of obtaining these data may give an analyst pause. However, the price may be worth paying if the net societal benefit is positive after accounting for the cost of the data.

Private industry data can be useful to understand private sector developments in health care financing that impact public health. For example, accounting and consulting firms may have completed state- and region-specific estimates of managed care prices that would be useful for developing Medicaid managed care programs.

There are several types of organizations selling private industry data. For some organizations, the sale of the data is a source of supplemental income if the database construction and maintenance is financed by another core line of business. For other groups, it is their primary source of income. Two of the most common types of organizations selling data are described below.

- *Proprietary data organizations:* These organizations buy administrative data from insurers, employers, and state agencies to build a health care market surveillance system for activities ranging from risk adjustment of new managed care markets to pharmaceutical pricing. The data can either be purchased outright with actual patient identifier information removed or be processed by the firm to provide a customized report for a given diagnosis, treatment, geographic location, or type of provider. Most of these organizations operate on a for-profit basis and expect to be well compensated for data purchases. The most common examples of these types of firms are HCIA and the MEDSTAT group.
- *Pharmaceutical companies:* Pharmaceutical companies finance their own clinical trial studies involving the collection of detailed medical record abstractions as well as administrative data. These studies have the advantage of being population based. However, they focus on a small subset of individuals and may not be generalizable to a larger group unless the disease in question has a high prevalence (e.g., asthma). Buying the data used by these organizations is not a customary practice. However, a public health manager may partner with a pharmaceutical company to secure access to the data in exchange for programmatic information assisting the pharmaceutical firm with their marketing strategy. If the incentives of the pharmaceutical firm and public health manager are aligned, both will benefit from such collaboration. An example of collaboration is a city's public health agency working in conjunction with a company producing a new TB drug to slow the rate of infection.

Using and Enhancing Public Health Databases

Few established databases provide the precise information needed for the management and evaluation of public health programs. For example, the *MCBS* describes the number of nursing home admissions for elderly persons over 85 years of age. To compare the number of admissions with the number of county nursing home beds, an analyst must link the *MCBS* to the ARF in order to obtain a variable for the number of nursing home beds. If an analyst needs further information on unmet needs for nursing home beds and quality of care in nursing facilities, the *MCBS* may need to be supplemented with other data sources or a new surveillance activity. Supplementing a database with new data is often a very expensive and timely proposition. The next section shows how to use databases as well as tailor existing databases to increase their value for an analysis.

Using Secondary Data Systems for Population-Based Surveillance

Public health data managers distinguish between primary and secondary database collection activities. Collecting new data from survey instruments or medical record abstraction creates a *primary database.* A *secondary database* consists of existing data systems such as administrative data and ongoing federal surveys. The primary advantage of using secondary data is their cost economy. For population-based surveillance, secondary data are a cost-effective instrument for answering public health questions. Three specific examples of using secondary data for public health analyses are presented to illustrate their value.

1. *Measuring period prevalence of a disease or treatment:* Ideally, public health managers would like to have real-time information of disease incidence and prevalence. Nationally, the CDC has such systems in place, with the capacity to narrow an investigation to the local level in case of public health emergencies such as rapid transmission of infectious and communicable diseases. As part of a public health surveillance activity, secondary data can provide information on the period prevalence of a disease or treatment. A period prevalence statistic is the number of unique individuals with a given diagnosis or receipt of a treatment in a specified period of time. For example, one can use the five-percent sample of the Medicare claims database to identify the period prevalence of diabetes within the United States. To generate this estimate, an analyst would write a computer program to scan 10 million claims records and record instances where a diagnosis code of 250.xx is recorded. With this subset of claims data, the analyst would count unique beneficiary identifiers, dividing by the total number of beneficiaries (i.e., 5 percent of the Medicare population or 40 million ÷ 5 percent = 2 million) to create a period prevalence estimate. A similar analysis could identify the number of patients who received a CABG in a given year.
2. *Variation in diagnosis or treatment as an early warning system:* Secondary data can be used to develop an "early warning system" of a population-based trend. In this case, early warning means finding patterns in health care diagnosis and treatment that suggest more serious public health concerns, such as a rise in TB-related hospitalizations in the Medicaid population. Variation in the period prevalence or use rate of a medical procedure can be identified across geographic regions or across time periods. One common method used to assess the extent of variation is the coefficient of variation, which equals standard deviation divided by the mean. The higher the standard deviation, relative to mean, results in higher variation. A more intuitive way of assessing variation is to use a graphic representation for geographic areas or time trends. If a long period of time is assessed (e.g., 10 or more years), one could animate geographic and temporal patterns.
3. *Deviation from best practice indicators:* A best practice indicator involves two elements: (1) a statistic by which to gauge medical care quality or access and (2) a threshold value for the statistic to identify a best practice. For example, if a primary care physician has a childhood immunization rate of 95 percent, and the best practice threshold identified by a managed care plan is 90 percent, the physician has a best practice indication. Using secondary data, one can simply extend the use of analyses identifying variations in period prevalence and treatment use by establishing a threshold for when a best practice has been achieved. Mathematically, one can replace the coefficient of variation calculation with a measure of the mean variance of prevalence or treatment use from the best practice threshold and divide it by the best practice threshold value. However, this constructed "coefficient of best practice" should be used care-

fully in managerial application to avoid providing incentives for seeking the best practice threshold and no higher.

Identifying a Population

Populations can be identified from administrative and survey data. Several approaches to identifying these populations are described.

- *Administrative data:* The primary advantage of administrative data is that it contains data on a broad range of health conditions and services. However, these data are not designed for health services research, although this may change as insurance companies and providers reengineer their databases for quality improvement and the production of value-added services. Currently, administrative data have huge breadth, but little depth. Still, the range of possible variables to identify a population is good, and population identification is seen as a key strength of administrative data as a precursor to more in-depth clinical and outcomes research that may involve primary data collection activities. Populations can be identified with claims data using the following variables:
  1. disease (identified by ICD-9-CM diagnosis code[s])
  2. procedure (identified by DRGs for inpatient services, revenue center codes for hospital outpatient services, and the AMA's Current Procedural Terminology [CPT] code system for physician and other ambulatory care. HCFA uses a variant of the CPT system called the Health Care Procedure System [HCPC], which includes additional codes for supplies and covered Medicare expenses.)
  3. pharmaceutical agent received (identified by the National Drug Code [NDC] System)
  4. demographics (including age, gender, and sometimes race)
- *Survey data:* Survey data can easily identify populations because they are designed for population-based research. The most common variables used in surveys are
  1. disease (e.g., asthma)
  2. demographics (including age, gender, race, income, education)
  3. health behaviors (e.g., smoking and alcohol consumption)
  4. program received (e.g., participation in a welfare to work program)
  5. outcome generated (e.g., improvement in health status following a treatment)

Measuring the Impact of Programmatic Intervention

In addition to surveillance, public health data evaluate interventions. The most straightforward assessments measure the health of a person before and after a health intervention, whether a medical procedure or a social services program. However, this type of analysis needs additional scientific rigor to state conclusively that the intervention resulted in the monitored impact. To do so requires a controlled study where another "identical" population does not receive the intervention or treatment. Operationally, this is a difficult prospect in health care because of liability issues for the people receiving the "placebo." From a public health management perspective, the path of least resistance is to look for a natural experiment where only one of two similar groups received the intervention. If a natural experiment is not an option, one can try to generate one's own variable to control for other factors that might bias the results of an uncontrolled intervention.

File Linkage

The primary prerequisite for linking files is a common unit of analysis. In the case of the *MCBS,* the common unit of analysis is the beneficiary identifier to link survey and claims information. However, if one supplemented the *MCBS* with county-specific data on provider supply using the ARF, the common unit of analysis would be the county identification number. Regardless of whether the analyst will use an existing data source or generate a new one, a linking variable must always be present. In addition, the presence of a set of linking variables for different data files enables the development of a relational database structure.

Issues for Supplementing Databases with New Data

Supplementing a database with new data can be a costly and time-consuming proposition. Unless all other avenues to obtain additional data are exhausted, one should not try to originate a supplemental database. If no other option exists for obtaining the precise data needed, then the survey method should fit the scope of the project.

The three basic methods to survey a population are (in order of increasing cost per survey) mail, telephone, and in-person interviews. The main advantage of the in-person interview is a higher response rate and better quality information that is less prone to misinterpretation by the survey respondent. To achieve a high response rate using a mail survey may require many subsequent mailings and, possibly, follow-up by telephone. In these instances, the low projected cost of obtaining the data by mail will be countered by additional costs for more surveys as well as the time spent waiting for the information. If one needs to survey a population, it is best to work with an established contract survey organization that is knowledgeable in avoiding common errors in the development of a survey instrument. Also, a public health organization can solicit competitive bids for a contract from survey research firms where an achieved response rate of at least 55–60 percent can be negotiated as part of a fixed price agreement.

The cost of repeating a new data collection activity should also be taken into consideration. If the project demands an annually updated database, an expensive data collection initiative will be a significant burden. One alternative approach is to survey a special population once to assess the extent of a public health problem and report the findings in a monograph focusing on one issue. For example, HCFA uses the *MCBS* in this fashion to create specialized survey supplements to examine different issues affecting the elderly in more detail. If the information gathered is found to be critical for continued analysis, then a separate case can be made for integrating an ongoing data collection strategy for a select group of data elements. A further option may be to modify the existing "core" survey instrument or administrative data system used to collect the data of interest presently on a continual basis.

HIS APPLICATIONS IN PUBLIC HEALTH ADMINISTRATION

There are several operating public HISs of note. These initiatives range in scope from federal to local sponsorship. Some provide a general database for a full range of public health issues, while others are designed for specific disease tracking or program evaluation.

- *The CDC's INPHO:* The INPHO system was developed as a framework for public health information and practice based on a state-of-the-art telecommunications network.[4] The INPHO is part of a strategy to strengthen public health infrastructure. The three concepts of the INPHO are linkage, information access, and data exchange (Exhibit 9–1). The CDC works with state and local area health agencies to build local- and wide-area networks. Second, the CDC has expanded "virtual networks" through the use of CDC WONDER. This is a software system that provides access to data in the CDC's public health databases. Third, the CDC has encouraged each state to connect with the Internet to have access to information.

  Georgia (discussed in more detail below) pioneered the program in early 1993. By 1997, 14 more states made the INPHO vision integral to their public health information strategies: California, Florida, Illinois, Indiana, Kansas, Michigan, Missouri, New Jersey, New York, North Carolina, Oregon, Rhode Island, Washington, and West Virginia. A second round of INPHO projects was funded through a cooperative agreement program, with awards made in the

Exhibit 9–1 INPHO: The Vision, the Need, the Basic Concepts

The Vision
- an integrated telecommunications network linking the public health community and providing exchange of data and information

The Need
- connecting a fragmented system
- linking public health professionals
- empowering communities with information
- leading and responding to health reform

The Basic Concepts
- linkage
- information access
- data exchange

Source: Reprinted from E.L. Baker, A. Freide, A.D. Moulton, and D.A. Ross, CDC's Information Network for Public Health Officials (INPHO): A Framework for Integrated Public Health Information and Practice, *Journal of Public Health Management and Practice,* Vol. 1, No. 1, p. 45, © 1995, Aspen Publishers, Inc.

spring of 1998. The program promotes the integration of information systems, with special emphasis on immunization registries. The cooperative agreements were funded as either implementation projects (Florida, Georgia, Missouri, and New York) or demonstration projects (Iowa, Maryland, Montana, Nevada, and Texas). In 1998, the INPHO, in partnership with the University of Washington School of Public Health, established a public health informatics training program for public health advisors and state health officers, and initiated a resident informatics fellowship position. Throughout the 1990s, the program has functioned as a federation of states and organizations with shared interests. More information on the initiative is available at http://www.phppo.cdc.gov/INPHO/about_inpho.htm.

- *CDC WONDER:* CDC WONDER was designed by the CDC to put critical information into the hands of public health managers quickly and easily. Originally a PC-based system, it is now available from any computer with an Internet connection, solving the problem of dedicating workstations to a specific database. As such, it is one of the few truly national public health data resources available with real-time access to anyone in the world. With CDC WONDER, one can
  1. Search for and retrieve *Morbidity and Mortality Weekly Review* articles and prevention guidelines published by the CDC.
  2. Query dozens of numeric data sets on the CDC's mainframe and other computers via "fill-in-the blank" request screens. Public use data sets about mortality, cancer incidence, hospital discharges, AIDS, behavioral risk factors, diabetes, and many other topics are available for query, and the requested data can be readily summarized and analyzed.
  3. Locate the name and e-mail addresses of the CDC staff and registered CDC WONDER users.
  4. Post notices, general announcements, data files, or software programs of interest to public health professionals in an electronic forum for use by CDC staff and other CDC WONDER users.

  For more information on CDC WONDER, refer to http://wonder.cdc.gov/#aboutWonder.
- *State public HISs:* States have multiple public HISs mirroring the complicated array of categorical programs with different funding sources. Commonly maintained information systems can include computerized immunization registries, lead toxicity tracking, early intervention databases for children with a disability, congenital disease registries in addition to vital statistics data, Medicaid utilization, and disease reports. The need for integrated information systems and the support of the INPHO project has spurred models in a number of states. Efforts will be described in Missouri, Georgia, Illinois, and New York.

1. *Missouri:* The Missouri Department of Health had a problem with 67 information systems that ran on different platforms and could not communicate with one another.[3] To solve this problem, the Missouri Health Strategic Architectures and Information System (MOHSAIC) was developed. An integrated client service record was an important component of this initiative. From the client's perspective, it was irrelevant if the services were labeled WIC, prenatal care, diabetes, Maternal and Child Health Services Block Grant, or local funding. Considerable effort and staff resources were committed to develop this system. Also, integrated systems magnify concerns about confidentiality. Benefits included increased capability for community health assessment, coordination of services, outreach, and linkages to primary care delivered by larger networks.[3]
2. *Georgia:* Georgia was the first site of the CDC INPHO initiative. Georgia was able to develop quickly as a demonstration site through a unique consortium of state agencies with academic health partners and IT partners. For example, members of the consortium included the Medical College of Georgia as well as the Georgia Center for Advanced Telecommunications Technology and the Emory University School of Public Health. The program also had initial funding from the Robert Wood John Foundation.[2] The infrastructure includes 81 clinics and 59 county health departments.

   The Georgia INPHO system includes local- and wide-area computer networks, office automation and e-mail, a public health calendar, an executive HIS, and electronic notification of public health emergencies. Before the project began, the state public health office operated 13 small unlinked local-area networks. With the INPHO project, hardware and software were consolidated into one integrated network system.
3. *Illinois:* Cornerstone is a management information system developed in Illinois to integrate maternal and child health services. The design expands on the existing WIC program PC-based computer system.[6] This system is an example of a state information system integrating several related programs as compared with wide integration pursued by Missouri, Georgia, and New York State.

   Risk assessment and demographic information are captured once and used for multiple programs. Exchange of information, risk assessment, assurance of follow-up, and referral are assisted by this information system.
4. *New York:* New York State is implementing an ambitious far-reaching plan for the integration of public health information. Development of this information system was assisted by funding from the CDC. The New York State Department of Health has developed an enterprisewide infrastructure for electronic health commerce. This effort has three major components.
   - a public Web site (www.health.state.ny.us) of health information serving as an Internet portal with an average of 850,000 hits per week and provider of data to consumers, researchers, and providers on health issues and data
   - the Health Information Network (HIN), a public and private health data interchange that can receive 440,000 connections with a system of 1,300 local health user accounts spread across all New York counties (Exhibit 9–2)
   - the Health Provider Network (HPN) targeted at private data information interchange between state and health care providers including clinical laboratories, managed care plans, pharmacies, hospitals, and continuing care facilities

The New York health e-commerce initiative is using the Internet and Web page interface to connect users and databases in a secure environ-

Exhibit 9–2 The New York State Health Information Network (HIN) Web System

- News and information of general interest to local health: Examples include grant awards, contracts, meeting minutes, and calendar of events.
- Data queries: Access interactive data queries for generating statistical reports for births, deaths, communicable diseases, and inpatient hospital stays. These data queries enable the counties to dynamically generate frequencies, cross-tabulations, charts, maps, and rates from these databases.
- Health emergency alerts: Specialized Web programs allow the state health department to post and broadcast epidemiologic problem alerts and other health notices instantaneously to specific local health staff over HIN.
- Health program information: Examples include emerging infections, immunization, communicable disease, chronic disease, lead poisoning and prevention, and child health.
- Electronic reporting systems: The HIN has a highly sophisticated system for electronic reporting and tracking of diseases. The system provides a series of electronic forms that enable designated local health staff to submit and track case-level reports for communicable diseases, sexually transmitted diseases, and TB. The forms post the case records in a central integrated database that is accessible by appropriate state and local health staff. The system uses sophisticated business rules for editing and quality assurance of the data. Provisions are also available to allow local health staff to download case report data as well as upload data from local systems in predefined format. Statistical and case-level queries and reports are also available to designated local health infection control practitioners. The New York State Department of Health is currently working with clinical labs to establish an electronic lab reporting system whereby positive lab reports for notifiable conditions will be electronically submitted over the Health Provider Network (HPN) in HL7 format, where they will be processed, edited, and distributed electronically to appropriate local health departments. Another emerging surveillance system on the HIN is lead in a child's blood. In this system, clinical laboratories submit blood lead results to the state department of health via the HPN. The reports are processed and electronically distributed to the appropriate local health departments, where they may be queried and downloaded. An HIN Web system for tracking child lead case histories is currently under development.
- General utilities: The HIN provides general utilities to facilitate data exchange between state and local health. An example is the secure file transfer utility, which allows any state or local health users to exchange files securely without encryption software. The intended recipient receives notice by e-mail that the sender has posted a file for him or her. The sender receives notice by e-mail when the intended recipient has picked up the file. All files are scanned for viruses prior to posting.
- Directory services: HIN users may query for e-mail addresses and phone numbers of state and local health staff as well as health providers connected to the HPN. Other services enable the HIN user to look up his or her individual access permissions to applications and data on the HIN.
- Health provider network access: HIN users are also given default access to the HPN Web system.

Source: New York State Integrated Child Health Information System, August 9, 1999, New York State Department of Health.

ment. For the HIN, the Web-based interface functions as a closed intranet where Web encryption of secure socket layers is established transparently to the user to protect the security and confidentiality of data.[7]

A large effort has been undertaken to ensure information security on the HIN due to the confidential nature of data transactions between state and local public health departments. Organizational and individual security agreements are required for HIN access.[8] Very narrow access is provided for highly confidential items such as case reports for notifiable disease. Particular restrictions and security arrangements will be in place for HIV reporting. More broadly defined access exists for statistical data queries.

New York State is currently developing an Integrated Child Health Information System (ICHIS) that will be accessible through the HIN. This will meet county health department needs that are linked across a number of department of health databases (Figure 9–2).

Future Public Health Information Systems

The broad range of public HIS applications developed over the past 10 years demonstrates how managers are seeking to improve the scope and quality of their data systems. HIS experts consistently state that the future lies in building an infrastructure that is both easy to use and able to demonstrate value for its investment.[9,10] To build such an infrastructure requires data standards as well as translators for different standards to help bridge the transition from the current system.[11]

One of the most promising developments is the use of the Internet as the platform to collect data, turn data into information, and monitor the health of the population. The development of Internet-based software that is not dependent on operating systems or statistical computing software represents one less barrier to building an infrastructure. (The Internet's ease of software deployment through the use of a simple connection and a Web browser will lead to faster dissemination of standard data translation tools.) Even more powerful is the transition of the medical profession from an arcane paper-based data collection world toward e-commerce for business-to-business applications where new standards can be applied from the beginning of data collection and management activity, not retrofitted. Public concerns about the privacy of health-related information in this new environment are motivating new policies for information use that hopefully will build the public's trust in emerging health information applications while preserving the ability of public health organizations to use health data for essential surveillance, research, and management activities.

Amid the opportunities for developing HISs, substantial barriers remain, but these barriers are becoming less technical and more political. Pub-

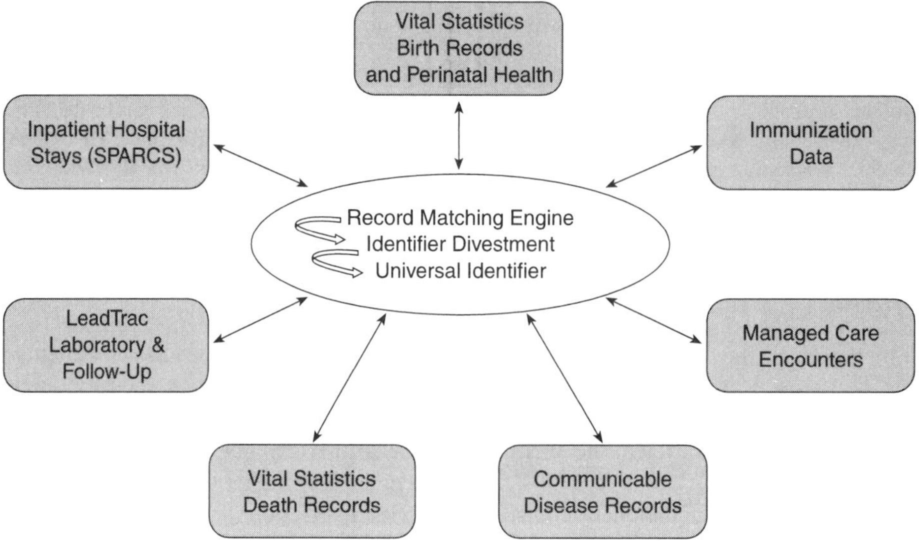

Figure 9–2 Creating a Profile of a Child's Health. *Source:* Reprinted from *ICHIS Technical Paper No. 2,* March 8, 1999, New York State Department of Health.

lic health managers seeking to develop and use the IT infrastructure must be prepared to demonstrate its value to society constantly.

PRIVACY ISSUES

The public's concern for the privacy of personal health information has become a major policy issue. Unfortunately, this concern is not easily addressed. At the heart of this issue is the paradox that health data must be identifiable if they are to be valuable for public health interventions. Complicating the issue is that an encrypted personal identifier still yields a personal identifier. HISs must remain responsive to these evolving data privacy and confidentiality issues.

The public's desire for health data privacy appears to exceed its desire for public health and biomedical research. In a 1993 Lou Harris survey on the public's attitudes on health data privacy, 64 percent of the sample responded that they did not want medical records data used for biomedical research unless the researchers obtained the patient's consent. When asked if they favor the creation of a "national medical privacy board" to hold meetings, issue regulations, and enforce standards for protecting medical information privacy, 86 percent responded favorably.[12]

Two recent developments advanced the privacy debate. The first development was the passage of the Health Insurance Portability and Accountability Act (HIPAA) in 1996, which created a timetable for the adoption of national medical privacy legislation by the year 2000. The combination of HIPAA and privacy laws creates the first national policy to prosecute those persons who breach the medical privacy of an individual. The penalties can range from fines to prison.

For public health research, it is unclear how this legislation will affect the use of administrative data and medical records. Currently, major biomedical research studies involving the use of medical records obtain approval of their research protocol through an Institutional Review Board (IRB). (See Chapter 15 on "Human Subjects Protection" for more information.) The IRBs decide whether the research will safeguard the privacy of study participants' health data. Uncertainty surrounds the use of electronic medical records. Electronic medical records are seen as the future of medical chart data collection, though they are not in widespread use. Current proposals state that only "operational activities" may be permitted to use electronic medical records. Other uses must be cleared by the IRBs, which could require patient consent.

This proposed legislation, if fully implemented, may ultimately compromise the ability of researchers to obtain a representative sample for research purposes. For example, consider past studies linking lung cancer to smoking. These studies involved the use of medical records where patients did not provide their consent although the research protocol was approved by an organization's IRB. If patient consent was required to use the data, a disproportionate share of lung cancer patients who were smokers may have decided not to participate.

In the case of administrative data, there is an exemption in the HIPAA legislation permitting the use of claims data for public health purposes. Other uses of administrative data, such as the sale of health insurance claims to consulting firms or pharmaceutical companies, are not discussed in the legislation and could be construed as a proprietary public health activity. However, this activity is unlikely to be viewed as a public health exemption as originally formulated by the legislation. Another possible exemption is the release of encrypted data instead of a social security number or other individually identifiable information (III). Here as well, the definition of individually identifiable is not clearly specified in the HIPAA legislation. The proposed medical privacy rule by the DHHS offers more clarity on the definition of III, but not an operational definition. To some organizations, the operating definition of III is social security number or last and first name. To other organizations, it is a large list of variables including any combination of name, social security number, date of birth, gender, date of service, procedure code, diagnosis code, or patient ZIP code; that is, any data useful for public health research.

In the wake of these federal policy deliberations, several states have adopted their own privacy legislation. It is likely that these initiatives will be secondary to the federal legislation unless they contain more restrictive regulations than federal law.

Ultimately, data are provided to public health managers and researchers as an act of trust. If one individual or organization violates that trust, the public's confidence may erode immediately. The Harris poll results show consistently that health data confidentiality and security issues are an important public concern.[12] In developing and using HISs, public health administrators and researchers must demonstrate that the public's trust is deserved. To do so, contemporary HISs must ensure that society receives an optimal return on its public investments in data resources—a return that ultimately must be realized through more effective public health interventions and improved community health status.

CHAPTER REVIEW

1. Public health organizations rely on information systems to support a number of key operations, including
   - epidemiologic disease and risk factor surveillance
   - medical and public health outcomes assessment
   - program and clinic administration (billing, inventory, client tracking, clinical records, utilization)
   - cost-effectiveness and productivity analysis
   - utilization analysis and demand estimation
   - program planning and evaluation
   - quality assurance and performance measurement
   - public health policy analysis
   - clinical research
   - health education and health information dissemination
2. Two of the most common types of applications for information systems in public health organizations are
   - *service-based applications* that track encounter-level information on the users and providers of specific services (These applications are useful for program administration and management of services for individual clients.)
   - *population-based applications* that track information on defined populations of interest (These applications are useful for surveillance, program evaluation, planning, and policy development.)
3. Well-designed information systems consist of a "pyramid" of technology that includes: (1) necessary hardware for data storage, computing, and exchange; (2) software for operating hardware and for collecting and managing core data sources; (3) administrative software for use in activities such as billing, financial management, communications, and scheduling; and (4) decision support software to produce information needed for managerial and clinical decision making.
4. Technical considerations in developing an information system include *data storage requirements*; *data processing performance requirements*, including data linkage capabilities; and *software requirements* for building and using analytic files.
5. A variety of data sources can be integrated within a public HIS. Common data sources include survey data, administrative claims data, program administration data, regional/geographic data, registry data, and private industry data. Common data structures include transactional data, cross-sectional data, time series and panel data, and relational databases.

6. Well-designed public HISs must provide strong protections for the privacy and confidentiality of information derived from person-specific health-related data. These protections must cover data acquisition, storage, and linkage and retrieval activities, as well as analytic and reporting activities. Information systems must be responsive to the privacy provisions of recent federal and state legislation.

REFERENCES

1. D. Koo and S.F. Wetterhall, "History and Current Status of the National Notifiable Diseases Surveillance System," *Journal of Public Health Management and Practice 2,* no. 4 (1996): 4–10.
2. K.A. Chapman and A.D. Moulton, "The Georgia Information Network for Public Health Officials (INPHO): A Demonstration of the CDC INPHO Concept," *Journal of Public Health Management and Practice 1,* no. 2 (1995): 39–43.
3. G.H. Land et al., "Developing an Integrated Public Health Information System for Missouri," *Journal of Public Health Management and Practice 1,* no. 1 (1995): 48–56.
4. J.M. Corrigan and D.M. Nielsen, "Toward the Development of Uniform Reporting Standards for Managed Care Organizations: The Health Plan Employer Data and Information Set," *Journal of the Joint Commission on Quality Improvement 19,* no. 12 (1993): 566–575.
5. S.T. Parente, J.P. Weiner, D. Garnick, et al., "Developing a Quality Improvement Database Using Health Insurance Data: A Guided Tour with Application to Medicare's Claims History File," *American Journal of Medical Quality,* Winter 1995, 162–176.
6. J.R. Nelson, "Cornerstone: Illinois' Approach to Service Integration," *Journal of Public Health Management and Practice 2,* no. 1 (1996): 71–74.
7. I. Gotham, personal communication, NYS Department of Health August, 1999.
8. E.L. Baker et al., "CDC's Information Network for Public Health Officials (INPHO): A Framework for Integrated Public Health Information and Practice," *Journal of Public Health Management and Practice 1,* no. 1 (1995): 43–47.
9. E.L. Baker, Jr. and D. Ross, "Information and Surveillance Systems and Community Health: Building the Public Health Information Infrastructure," *Journal of Public Health Management and Practice 2,* no. 4 (1996): 58–60.
10. N. Milio, "Beyond Informatics: An Electronic Community Infrastructure for Public Health," *Journal of Public Health Management and Practice 1,* no. 4 (1999): 84–94.
11. J. Lumpkin et al., "The Development of Integrated Public Health Information Systems: A Statement by the Joint Council of Governmental Public Health Agencies," *Journal of Public Health Management and Practice 1,* no. 4 (1995): 55–59.
12. Lou Harris and Associates. Health Information Privacy Survey, 1993 (New York: Harris, 1993).

CHAPTER 10

Geographic Information Systems for Public Health

Alan L. Melnick

The ability to access and use geographically based data is now essential for designing and managing population-based public health initiatives. Geographic information systems (GIS) allow for the integration, storage, retrieval, analysis, and communication of data with a spatial or geographic component. Analysis and display of the data on maps provide public health administrators with powerful tools to promote better understanding about population health needs and disease risks among community members, health care providers, policy makers, and other important leaders.

HISTORY OF GIS IN PUBLIC HEALTH

As early as 1854, John Snow, the father of modern epidemiology, plotted the geographic distribution of cholera deaths in London, demonstrating the association between the deaths and contaminated water supplies.[1] In doing so, he forever linked the new science of epidemiology with the use of geographic information to reveal relationships between environment and disease.[2]

Of the three core epidemiologic variables of time, place, and person, place has always been the most difficult and time consuming to analyze and depict.[2] In the past, when public health practitioners focused mainly on communicable disease control, push pins or dots drawn on maps usually proved effective in helping to analyze and control disease outbreaks. The modern public health practitioner, however, is responsible for analyzing and responding to more complex health issues in a rapidly changing, diverse environment. The social, environmental, and behavioral determinants of health have a strong geographic component. To work effectively with communities in improving health status, modern public health practitioners and their community partners will need easy, immediate access to accurate, geographically based data.[3] New developments in GIS technology are making this possible.

Limitations of Pre-GIS Analysis

For several reasons, local health consumers and health planners have rarely used the health data that are collected routinely by local and state governments. First, the data are not timely. For example, up to two years can elapse before states report vital statistics data. Then, the data arrive in hard copy form, containing limited analysis at the county level. Such hard copy data are not amenable to further analysis, leaving local planners asking the responsible state agency to make specific data runs, which requires additional time and staff support.[4] Second, many different agencies at the local, state, and federal levels collect and maintain health-related data in different formats in different locations, making the data less accessible for consumers, health planners, and local health departments. Third, data that were analyzed and reported at the county level and above are not useful for assessing the health of diverse communities within large- or even medium-sized counties. Such macrolevel data fail to capture the unique essential characteristics of the individual communities, leaving little opportunity for local public health professionals to seek dialogue and strengthen relationships with populations within their counties. By providing easy access to a variety of data that are analyzable at the community level, modern GIS promise to address these problems, enabling public health practitioners to engage diverse communities in a partnership to improve community health.[4]

Emergence of Modern GIS

Several factors contributed to the development of GIS. Computers became smaller, faster, more accessible, and less expensive. Software became easier to use. Landscape and census data became available in digital format, allowing the linkage of health-related data sets to a geographic map.[5]

FEATURES OF GIS

Definition

GIS are automated computer packages that are defined more by their functions than by what they are.[5] GIS integrate several functions, including the capture and incorporation of data sets, the storage of data, the retrieval of data, the statistical manipulation of data, data analysis, data modeling, and the display of the data on maps.[5,6] The incorporated data must have a spatial or geographic component. Because much of the data collected today have some geographic reference, such as a street address, GIS have the potential to revolutionize public health practice. With GIS, public health practitioners can map health-related issues such as mortality and birth rates at the neighborhood or even street level.[7] In addition, GIS are tools for understanding and displaying disease or disease risks related to environmental exposures or social demographic data.[2] For example, studies have used GIS to demonstrate the relationship between childhood lead poisoning cases by census block with older housing stock.[8] The public health uses of GIS will be described later in this chapter.

Data Acquisition and Storage: Creating Spatial Databases

To perform geographic analyses, GIS require a foundation of spatial, or geographic, data. The creation of the U.S. Bureau of the Census' Topologically Integrated Geographic Encoding and Referencing (TIGER) files as a foundation database contributed to the development of modern GIS.[9] Updated, easily obtainable versions of the TIGER geographic data files include detailed street and address range information, along with political and administrative boundaries such as counties, ZIP codes, census tracts, and census block groups.[10] TIGER/Line files are available to order at the Census Bureau TIGER home page at http://www.census.gov/geo/www/tiger/index.html. Updated geographic data files are also available from commercial vendors, but may be expensive.[7]

The next step in a GIS analysis is to obtain the attribute data and link them to the geographic database.[10] Attribute data relate to any public health issue of interest, and can include health, social, and environmental data. Examples of attribute data include the Census Bureau's extensive demographic, economic, and social data sets; state and local vital statistics (perinatal and mortality data); and law enforcement data (reported arrests). To link to the geographic foundation, the attribute data must include a geographic reference, such as an address field. For example, to analyze birth rates by geography, each record in the birth database must include a field with the mother's street address. GIS can analyze any attribute database, such as arrest data, that includes a field with a location.

Geocoding is the process by which GIS software matches each record in an attribute database with the geographic files. The GIS software converts each address in the attribute file to a point on a map. The software then compares each address with the corresponding information in the foundation spatial database. A match occurs when the two agree.[10]

Map Making and Data Analysis

Once stored and geocoded, the data are ready for analysis and display. The power of GIS technology stems from its ability to allow users to analyze and display health-related data in new and effective ways.[5] The simplest form of display would be analogous to a push pin depiction—events, such as reported cholera cases, displayed as dots on a map. In one study, local public health planners created a map showing the home locations of children who had high blood lead levels (Figure 10–1).[10] Areas with larger numbers of children with reported high lead levels show up as clusters of triangular-shaped black dots. Like other epidemiologic studies, this map raised an additional question. Was clustering a reflection of high blood lead prevalence or a reflection of greater screening efforts? A second map, in which circular clear dots displayed all children screened, answered the question, revealing the varying patterns of children with high and low blood lead levels (Figure 10–2).[10]

Of course, GIS can perform much more complex tasks than a simple mapping of events.[5] The overlay capability of GIS allows the user to display more than one attribute on a map at a time. For example, the Centers for Disease Control and Prevention (CDC) has identified older housing as the most significant risk factor for lead exposure in young children. Local public health planners might be interested, then, in identifying the location of older housing in targeting lead exposure prevention efforts. If the data were available, a map could overlay the triangular black dots of reported childhood lead cases with the location of houses built before 1960. In this

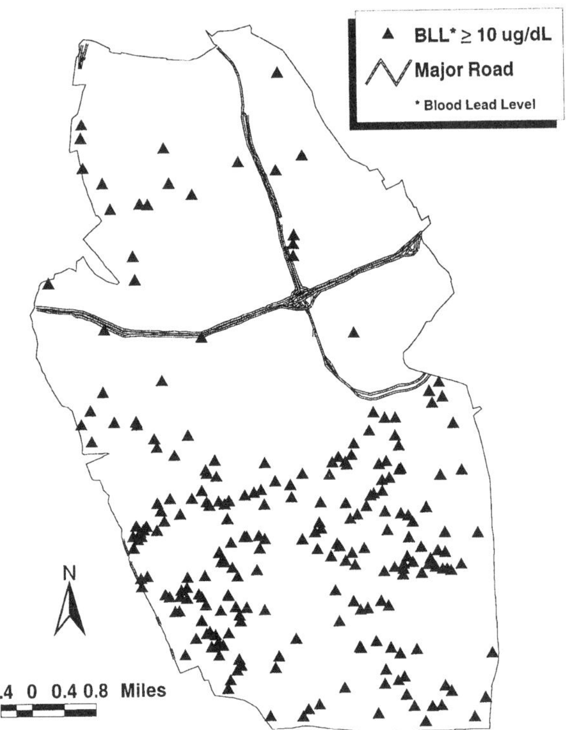

Figure 10–1 Children with Elevated Blood Lead. *Source:* Reprinted from S. McLafferty and E. Cromley, Your First Mapping Project on Your Own: From A to Z, *Journal of Public Health Management and Practice,* Vol. 5, No. 2, p. 79, © 1999, Aspen Publishers, Inc.

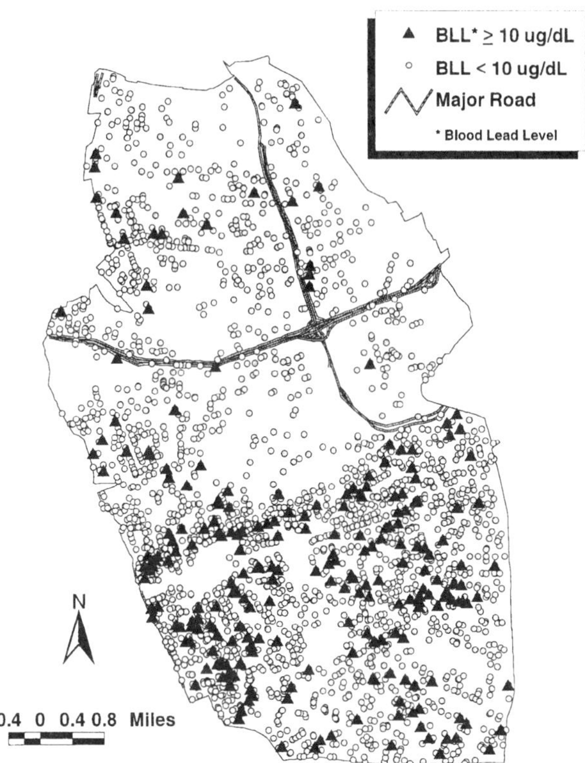

Figure 10–2 Children Screened for Lead. *Source:* Reprinted from S. McLafferty and E. Cromley, Your First Mapping Project on Your Own: From A to Z, *Journal of Public Health Management and Practice,* Vol. 5, No. 2, p. 80, © 1999, Aspen Publishers, Inc.

case, dots of different colors and shapes could represent older housing. Alternatively, the user could overlay the reported lead cases with a map showing the percentage of homes built before 1960 by census tract or census block group.[10] Each census block group could be colored or shaded based on its range of percentage of housing built before 1960. This type of map, in which a given area, or polygon, is shaded with different colors to depict variations of features such as the percentage of older housing stock, is called a *choropleth* map. Public health planners in Duval County, Florida, used overlays to create such a map. Census block groups were shaded based on the percentage of older housing, with reported childhood lead poisoning cases displayed as black dots (Figure 10–3).[11] This map was quite useful in focusing blood lead screening efforts.

Buffering is another powerful feature of GIS analysis. Using this feature, GIS can create polygons based on the distance from a target object.[7] Buffers are particularly useful in identifying people at risk of exposure to environmental hazards. A GIS study of childhood lead risk could define a 25-meter zone around main roads to identify areas with potentially high levels of lead-contaminated soil from past use of leaded gasoline (Figure 10–4).[12] The same study could then identify and locate children living within these areas who would benefit from lead screening. Another study used buffering to evaluate potential health risks and health risk perceptions of minority populations living within 0.2 miles of businesses that store hazardous chemicals (Figure 10–5).[13]

PUBLIC HEALTH GIS APPLICATIONS

Because the numerous determinants of health have strong geographic components, GIS tech-

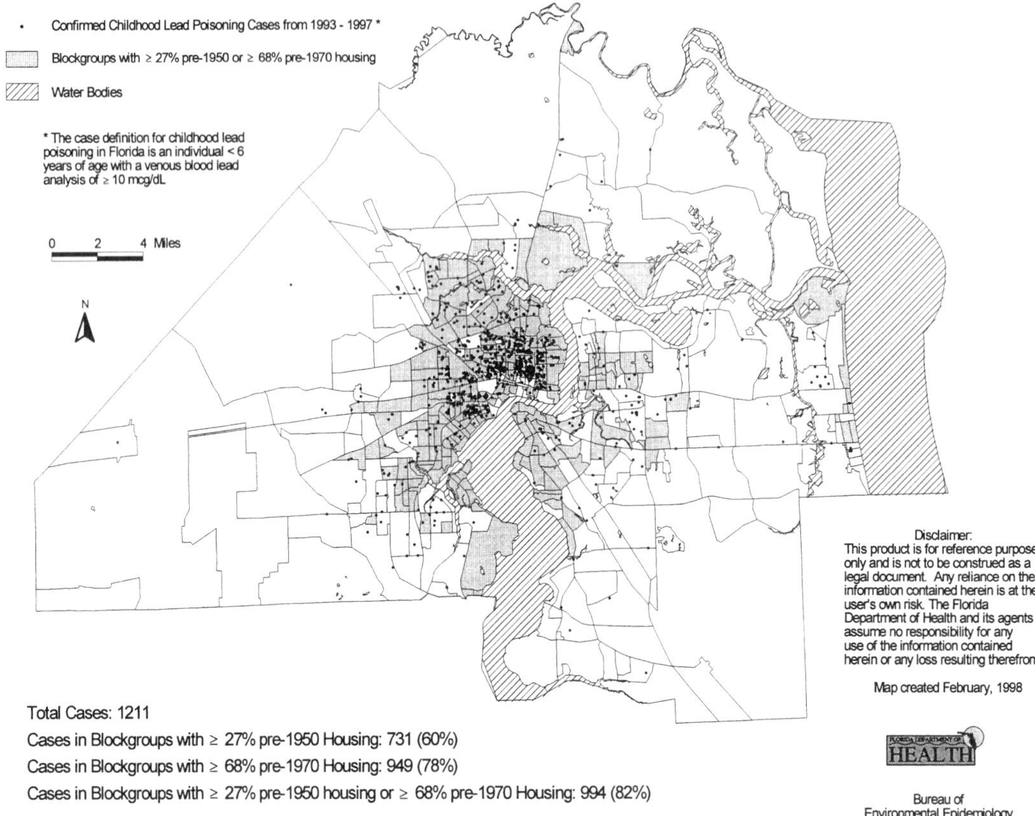
Confirmed Childhood Lead Poisoning Cases from 1993 - 1997 *
Blockgroups with ≥ 27% pre-1950 or ≥ 68% pre-1970 housing
Water Bodies
* The case definition for childhood lead poisoning in Florida is an individual < 6 years of age with a venous blood lead analysis of ≥ 10 mcg/dL
0 2 4 Miles
N
Disclaimer:
This product is for reference purposes only and is not to be construed as a legal document. Any reliance on the information contained herein is at the user's own risk. The Florida Department of Health and its agents assume no responsibility for any use of the information contained herein or any loss resulting therefrom.
Map created February, 1998
Total Cases: 1211
Cases in Blockgroups with ≥ 27% pre-1950 Housing: 731 (60%)
Cases in Blockgroups with ≥ 68% pre-1970 Housing: 949 (78%)
Cases in Blockgroups with ≥ 27% pre-1950 housing or ≥ 68% pre-1970 Housing: 994 (82%)
HEALTH
Bureau of Environmental Epidemiology

Figure 10–3 Development of Childhood Blood Lead Screening Guidelines: Duval County, FL, 1998. *Source:* Bureau of Environmental Epidemiology, Duval County, Florida.

nology has many public health applications. These applications range from epidemiology, including research, to community health assessment and community health planning.

Epidemiology

Perhaps the most direct use of GIS technology is as a tool for understanding and displaying disease or disease risks that are related directly to environmental exposures.[2] For example, GIS have depicted nitrate levels in water, Iodine-131 releases from the Hanford Nuclear Reservation, and childhood lead poisoning cases by census block with older housing stock.[8,11,14,15] Cohort studies have used GIS to identify populations with risk of exposure to magnetic fields from high-powered electrical lines.[12] By integrating GIS with statistical methods, epidemiologists can use GIS for modeling, a spatial analysis process that can identify disease risk factors. A study of Lyme disease in Baltimore County, Maryland, obtained data for 53 environmental variables at the residences of Lyme disease patients. Combining GIS with a logistic regression analysis, researchers rapidly identified Lyme disease risk factors over a large area (Figure 10–6).[16]

Many diseases cluster geographically whether or not they are related to environmental exposure.[2] One of the most useful features of GIS is their ability to identify and analyze space–time clusters or "hot spots" of disease.[5] An early GIS application called the Geographical Analysis Machine (GAM) was used to evaluate whether spatial clusters of childhood leukemia were located near nuclear facilities in Britain.[5,17]

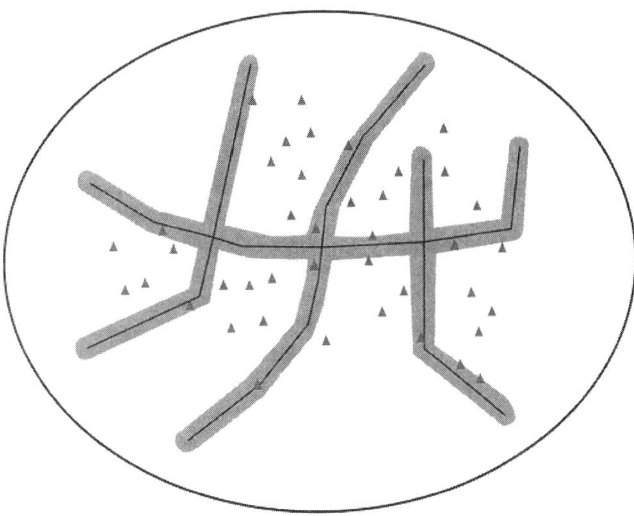

Figure 10–4 25-m Zones around Main Roads. *Source:* Reprinted from M.F. Vine, D. Degnan, and C. Hanchette, Geographic Information Systems: Their Use in Environmental Epidemiological Research, *Environmental Health Perspectives,* Vol. 105, No. 6, pp. 598–605, 1997, Environment Health Information Services, published by National Institute of Environmental Health Sciences, National Institutes of Health.

Community Health Assessment and Planning

For public health administrators and practitioners, the most exciting aspect of GIS technology is its potential to revolutionize the process of community health improvement by improving access to health-related data. Every community or neighborhood has assets and capacities in addition to needs.[18] GIS will enable communities to assess many of these factors, strengths, and weaknesses related to community well-being and allow them to evaluate actions they take to improve their health status.[4] This potential is a consequence of several features inherent in GIS.

The relational and overlay features of GIS encourage the rapid incorporation of multiple attribute data sets, including data sets not traditionally viewed as related to public health. Attribute data are available from many sources, both government and commercial.[19] (See Chapter 7 for a more detailed discussion.) Census data, available from the Census Bureau, includes demographic and socioeconomic data at the census block group level. Demographic data, useful as denominator data in calculating rates, contain information on age, gender, race, and ethnicity. Socioeconomic data include educational level, poverty level, employment, and age of housing.[19]

Depending on the state and locality, many data sets are easily obtainable, such as vital statistics data (perinatal and mortality), health care expenditures, access to primary care data, hospital discharge data, and behavioral risk factor data.[19] Table 10–1 lists a few examples of commonly available data sets.

One vision for community health assessment suggests other data such as high school dropout rates, commuting time, and domestic abuse.[4] Communities can add data on neighborhood assets, such as local business, religious, and cultural organizations.[18] Software "data wizards" make it easy for partners to incorporate additional data sets into the system, further encouraging multiple agencies to share data.[4]

The feature of unlimited scale of analysis is particularly helpful when performing community health assessments and program evaluations in densely populated counties. Large counties often contain many diverse and sizable communities

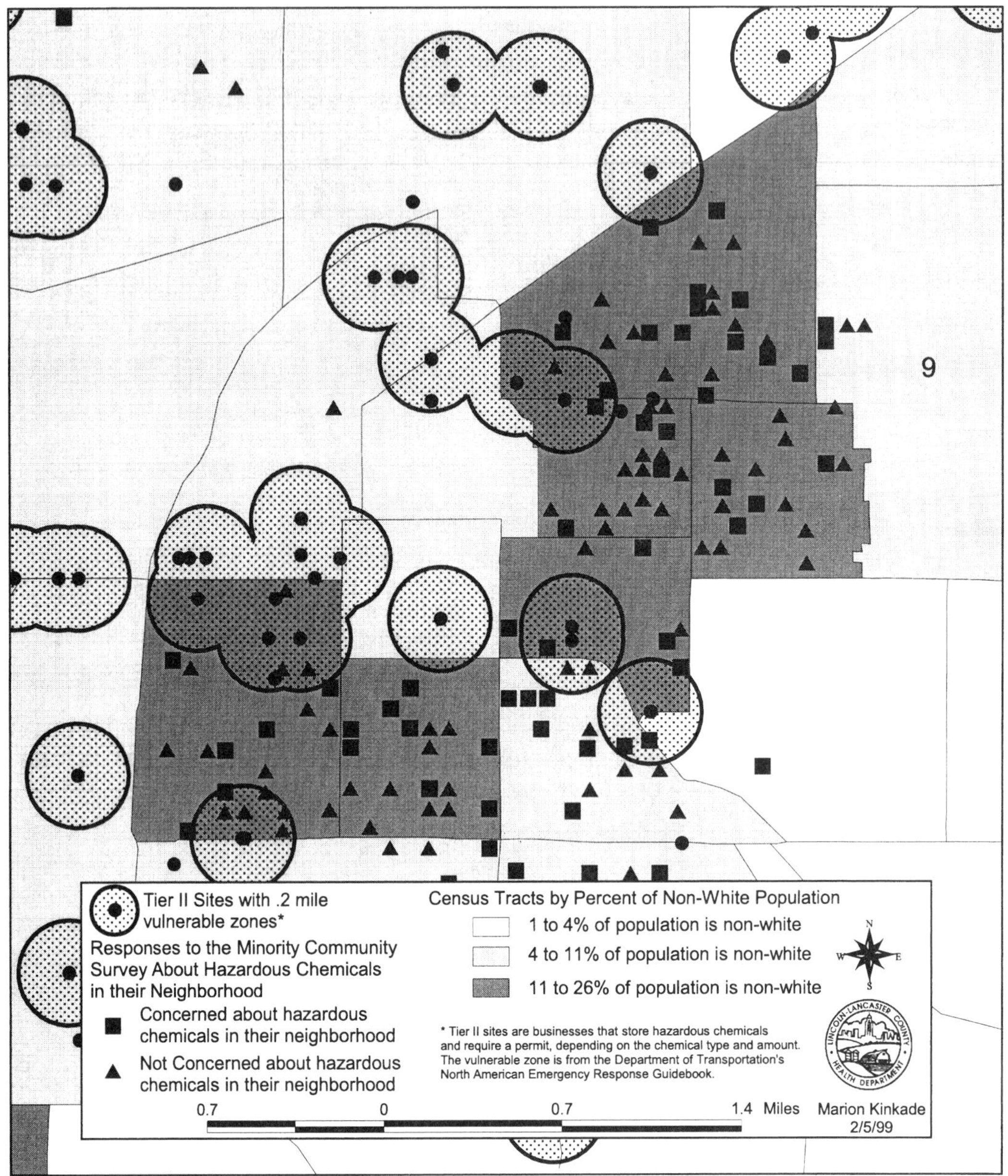

Figure 10–5 Responses to the Survey of Environmental Health Hazard Risks in the Minority Community, in Relation to the Primary Minority Census Tracts and the Evacuation Zones for Tier II Sites in Lincoln, NE, February 1999. *Source:* Lincoln-Lancaster County Health Department, Lincoln, Nebraska.

whose borders do not necessarily coincide with county boundaries. As a result, summaries based on these boundaries may not accurately capture community characteristics. For example, a large county may have low teen birth rates compared to the state, whereas several communities within the county may have markedly elevated rates. In this instance, county-level data are not useful in target-

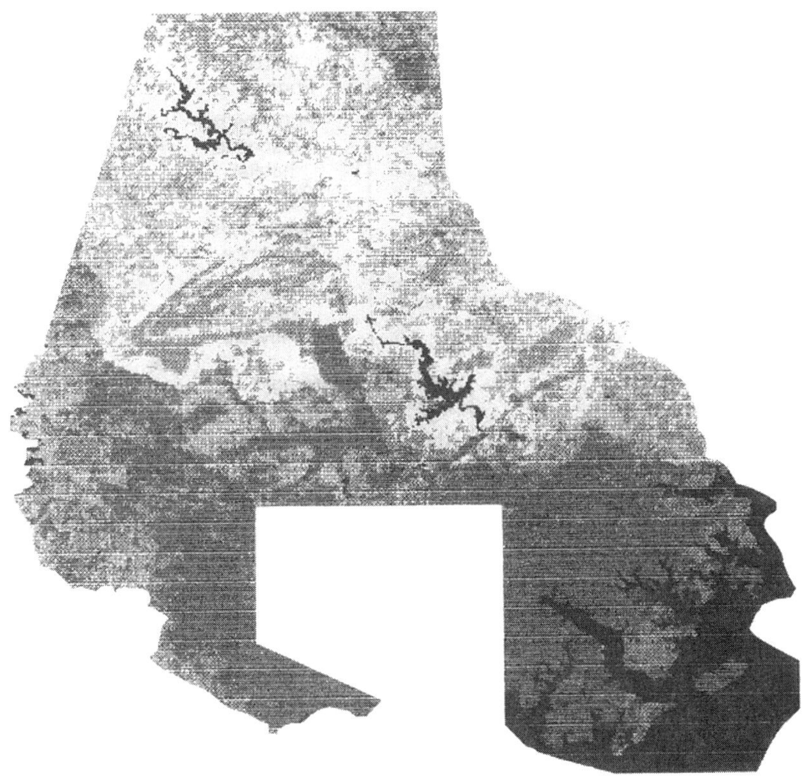

Note. Lighter shading indicates increased risk.

Figure 10–6 Lyme Disease—Risk Density Map from Logistic Regression Model That Used Environmental Variables in Baltimore County, MD, 1989–90. *Source:* Reprinted with permission from G.E. Glass et al., Environmental Risk Factors for Lyme Disease Identified with Geographic Information Systems, *American Journal of Public Health,* Vol. 85, No. 7, pp. 944–948, © 1995, American Public Health Association.

ing teen pregnancy prevention efforts. Using GIS, public health practitioners and their community partners can analyze and display the data at the local, subcounty, community level. They can compare their teen birth rate measures statistically with state data, national data, and benchmarks. They can also display available resources for teen pregnancy prevention by overlaying physical features such as health and social work facilities, roads, public transit routes, and travel time.[4,20] Over time, they can use the analytic features of GIS to evaluate the outcomes of pregnancy prevention or other public health efforts within their communities.[4]

The flexibility to define community geographically is invaluable in community health planning. GIS software can aggregate census block groups into a variety of community definitions, such as high school attendance areas or legislative districts. Likewise, GIS software can aggregate attribute data, such as vital statistics data, into the same areas for analysis. For example, a GIS prototype application analyzed teen birth rates, teen male arrest rates, and adequacy of prenatal care by high school attendance area, and compared these rates with overall county rates, state rates, and benchmarks.[4] Overlays allow users to look at two variables simultaneously so they can visualize spatial patterns and relationships. For example, GIS could depict teen birth rates with *Youth Risk Behavior Survey (YRBS)* results for high school attendance areas. Alternatively, those persons inter-

Table 10–1 Types and Potential Sources of Attribute Data

Category (Examples)	*Source (Varies by State)*	*Level of Analysis (Varies by State and Locality)*
Demographic data (e.g., age, sex, race, and ethnic distribution)	U.S. Bureau of the Census	Census block group, county, state
Perinatal indicators by age and population subgroups (e.g., births, repeat births, prenatal care, low birth weight)	State vital statistics	Census block group (if address included on birth certificate), county, state
Pregnancies; abortions	State vital statistics	County (abortion data do not contain street address), state
Mortality (by age and population subgroups) including years of potential life lost	State vital statistics	Census block group if address included on death certificate; otherwise county and state
Hospitalization (causes by age and population subgroup)	Depends on state—may be Medicaid agency	Varies (census block group, ZIP code, county, state depending on how residence is reported)
Ambulatory encounter data (by diagnosis age and population subgroup) for Medicaid population	State Medicaid agency	Census block group, county, state
Reportable disease (communicable disease, including sexually transmitted disease, lead poisoning, pesticide exposure)	Local health department, state epidemiologist	Census block group, county, state
Immunization of two-year-olds	Depends on state—may be state health department	Varies
Cancer incidence (by age and population subgroup)	State cancer registry	Census block group, county, state
Behavioral risk factors	Centers for Disease Control and Prevention	ZIP code, state
Youth risk behaviors (Youth Risk Behavior Survey)	CDC, state health department	High school, state
Synar reports (reports of tobacco outlet inspections)	Depends on state—agency responsible for alcohol and drug treatment planning	Census block group, county, state
Arrests by residence (causes by age and population subgroup)	County law enforcement (e.g., Sheriff's office), state justice department	Census block group, county, state

Source: Data from A. Melnick, S. Seigal, J. Hildner, and T. Troxel, Clackamas County Department of Human Services Community Health Mapping Engine (CHiME) Geographic Information Systems Project, *Journal of Public Health Management and Practice,* Vol. 5, No. 2, pp. 64–69, © 1999, Aspen Publishers, Inc.; and C.V. Lee and J.L. Irving, Sources of Spatial Data for Community Health Planning, *Journal of Public Health Management and Practice,* Vol. 5, No. 4, pp. 7–22, © 1999, Aspen Publishers, Inc.

ested in improving prenatal care could evaluate the percentage of first trimester care and income level by legislative district.

GIS programs can be Internet compatible, making them easily accessible. Most communities have access to Internet-capable libraries, where they could create customized maps to meet their needs.[4] GIS Internet packages can be designed for users without formal epidemiologic skills, and tutorials can be added. For example, tutorials can provide explanations of concepts such as incidence rates, prevalence, confidence intervals, and the need for age adjustment when evaluating mortality rates.[4,21]

Perhaps the greatest strength of GIS technology is that its product is a picture.[2] Epidemiologists often present analyses in formats that are only comprehensible by other epidemiologists. Program managers, policy makers, and others who must act on results need these results in a way they can digest and therefore believe. GIS take complex data and translate them into easily understandable information. This feature promises to enhance collaboration between all partners involved in community health improvement.

LESSONS LEARNED AND CHALLENGES

Like any other new technology, GIS comes with limitations and a potential for problems. Limitations include limited availability of data, inconsistent data quality, lack of a trained work force, and costs. Potential problems include community definitions, confidentiality, and misinterpretation of results.

Data Availability and Quality

As with any analysis, useful GIS output is dependent on useful input. Many commonly used databases, such as mortality data or hospital discharge data, frequently lack an address. Public health professionals will have to encourage their data-sharing partners to include address fields to make their data useful for community health planning. Encouraging data producers to geocode the data before release will further facilitate incorporation of the data set into effective GIS applications.

Many important data sets are not available, and when they are, users must be careful to evaluate their quality.[2,12] Quantitative information regarding the measured factor, such as environmental hazard exposure, must be present and accurate. Numerator address data may be missing, wrong, or (particularly in rural areas) impossible to match.[2,12] Inaccuracies may exist in denominator data and in the geographic data file, especially if they are outdated. The match rate between geospatial and attribute databases is directly dependent on their quality. Misspellings, empty address fields, and geographic files that are not up-to-date with the latest road maps lead to low match rates. For example, new housing developments often create new roads that may not be present on an old file. Low match rates, in turn, lead to selection bias in subsequent analyses. Public health professionals need to ensure that GIS users carefully assess and account for these limitations in their analyses. Depending on the quality of the data, unmatched records often need to be evaluated one at a time, which is a potentially cumbersome process. To solve these problems, standards for currency, quality, and completeness of data incorporated into GIS will need to be developed and adhered to. Government and commercial suppliers will have to provide metadata—data about the data—allowing users to evaluate data quality in relation to these standards.[7,13]

Trained Work Force and Costs

Many public health organizations will have to invest in hardware, software, and trained staff to apply GIS successfully. In a small study conducted by the National Association of County and City Health Officials (NACCHO), the cost to do relatively small projects was $10,000–$15,000, which is beyond the reach of small, rural health departments.[13] Staff time is required to acquire data sets, geocode the data, check the quality of the data, perform the analyses, and answer questions concerning the data. Increasing the availability of geocoded data would help cut this time.[7] For example, if state health departments released geocoded vital statistics data, they would encourage the use of GIS. At the local level, public health departments can reduce costs and improve collaboration by sharing data sets, trained staff, software, and hardware with other community partners.

Defining Community

When using GIS for community health improvement, public health officials and their partners will need to be both careful and flexible in defining community. How to portray a community will be constrained by the quality of the data and the perceptions of those within the depicted community. Although GIS projects can define communities in many geographic ways—ZIP codes, census tracts, census block groups, high school attendance areas, legislative districts, cities, and counties—in any given situation, all are not equally appropriate.[2] On a case-by-case basis, public health officials can share their community maps with community partners to obtain comments. Then, using GIS, they can easily redraw the community boundaries, selecting the most appropriate mapping strategy.[2]

Confidentiality

Confidentiality issues pose a significant limitation for public health officials intending to share health-related data with community partners or place data on the Internet. Data containing personal addresses can be as identifying as data with names. Without appropriate, clear laws, guidelines, and standards regarding confidentiality and data release, health agencies and consumers may be unwilling to provide needed information.[9] Those persons responsible for maintaining the data files should ensure appropriate precautions in order to prevent unauthorized access. Great care and thought must precede the depiction of address data linked to confidential information.

One possible solution is to remove identifiers such as name or address, presenting aggregated data only. State and federal agencies have traditionally reported data aggregated at the county, state, and federal levels. Public health officials can do the same for geocoded community-level data by aggregating it into any selected community definition. For example, public health officials could share GIS data wizard software with hospitals unwilling to release discharge data. Local hospitals could then use the wizard to geocode the personal health data and aggregate it by legislative district boundaries. Then, they could remove the personal identifiers such as name and address and release the aggregated data to the public health officials for incorporation into the Web-based GIS. In this way, public users would only view data that was aggregated at the legislative district level.

When small numbers (numerator or denominator) are involved, the possibility exists that aggregated data could still be ascribed to individuals. This is particularly true when GIS users stratify their community health analyses by multiple demographic variables, such as gender and ethnicity. To avoid this, public health officials must develop safeguards, built into the software, that restrict the analysis, reporting, and depiction of very small numbers.[4] For example, standards could prohibit the release of a health statistic, such as teen birth rate, if the population denominator (teenage females) were less than 50. If the denominator were a cohort defined by an event, such as all births, a standard could prohibit release of percentage of outcomes (e.g., first trimester care) for a community with fewer than 10 events (births). Alternatively, GIS applications can allow users to analyze data aggregated over two or more years when rates for a single year are unstable due to small numbers.

Even if GIS studies do not identify individuals, group disclosure, especially in studies of environmental exposure, can lead to financial risk for individuals in an exposed community, including decreased property values and increased insurance cost.[22] GIS technology is just one more reason to develop a nationally uniform framework of information sharing that protects privacy while permitting public health practice.[2]

Misinterpretation of Results

Ironically, the strength of GIS technology may be its biggest shortfall. The elegance of GIS is that they integrate many complex data sets into an easily understandable picture—a map. Because of this, GIS technology is becoming available to a diversity of users, many with little understanding of public health and epidemiologic principles. Many determinants of health, including age, ethnicity, socioeconomic status, and education, cluster geographically. Consequently, most GIS analyses will find an association between geography and health outcomes. Usually, however, these outcomes will cluster geographically because of underlying population characteristics, not because of the geography itself. Users without epidemiologic training may be tempted to misinterpret why geographic clustering is occurring, often as proof of a pet theory.[2]

The conflicting analyses of the London 1854 cholera epidemic provide a perfect example. For John Snow, geographic analysis of cholera death clustering implicated the Broad Street pump. However, using the same data, the England General Board of Health was convinced that nocturnal vapors from the Thames River were responsible.

As GIS technology becomes more widely available, inexperienced users, including those in policy-making positions, may be tempted to make individual-level inferences from ecologic data and make false assumptions concerning the nature of associations between exposure and health.[2,12] The job of public health officials is to ensure that any interpretation of geographically referenced health data looks beyond maps to a wider range of analytic tools. For example, a superficial analysis of the geographic variation in childhood asthma hospitalization rates could have led to the conclusion that different populations have different burdens of illness. Closer study revealed that geographic variation in hospital bed supply and hospital proximity, not asthma itself, were independent predictors of admission.[23]

Public health professionals can help prevent these mistakes by building safeguards into Internet-based GIS applications. For example, pop-up help screens could contain messages discussing the concept of ecologic fallacy and the need for caution about drawing conclusions when cause-and-effect relationships have not been established previously.[4,21] In addition, built-in links to appropriate county health officials would allow inexperienced users to obtain consultation.

GETTING STARTED WITH GIS

Before a public health organization invests in a GIS application, it should determine whether it really needs the application or if other, cheaper alternatives might suffice.[24] For example, a small organization with limited resources serving small numbers of residents may not benefit from a detailed geographic analysis. In many cases, other government or private organizations may have already developed a GIS application and would welcome partnership with the public health organization.

The basic components of GIS include appropriate hardware and software. Hardware recommendations change rapidly but should at least include the basic components listed in Table 10–2.[24] Over the past few years, the variety of GIS software products has markedly increased. Each easily obtainable product has its own advantages and disadvantages, as shown in Table 10–3.[24]

FUTURE OF GIS AND THE ROLE OF PUBLIC HEALTH OFFICIALS

As GIS technology evolves and becomes more widely available, the role of public health officials will undoubtedly evolve with it. Many more data

Table 10–2 Recommended Hardware Configuration for a Local Health Department That Wants To Get Started with GIS

- Windows 95 or above; Windows NT for network systems
- 266 MHZ Pentium II processor (or faster) with graphics refresh capability
- 64 MB of RAM
- Video card with 4 MB RAM
- 4 GB or greater hard drive
- 24x or faster CD-ROM
- 17-inch monitor or bigger
- Color printer (laser or inkjet) with at least 300x300 dots per inch resolution
- Back-up capability (e.g., Iomega Zip drive, tape backup, CD-ROM writer, or LAN backup)
- Ability to connect to Internet
- *Optional:* Color scanner with OCR capability

Source: Reprinted from S.E. Thrall, Geographic Information System (GIS) Hardware and Software, *Journal of Public Health Management and Practice,* Vol. 5, No. 2, p. 83, © 1999, Aspen Publishers, Inc.

Table 10–3 Selected GIS Software Products: Advantages and Disadvantages

GIS Software	*Advantages*	*Disadvantages*
ArcView GIS	• Works with ARC/INFO • Excellent tutorials and documentation	• Modules priced separately
Autodesk World	• Reads/writes popular GIS and database formats • Scripting language is Visual BASIC	• Very limited documentation • No geographic or demographic data included
Community 2020	• Links with HUD data • Web forum for users	• Based on older *Maptitude 3.0* rather than more recent, enhanced *Maptitude 4.0* • Data templates limited to HUD data
EpiMap	• Public domain • Simple to use • Written by the CDC	• Very limited GIS features • DOS based but work is underway on a Windows-based version
Geomedia	• Open GIS • Enterprise solution • Scripting language is Visual BASIC	• Open GIS functionality does not support all popular GIS formats • Very limited documentation • No geographic or demographic data included
MapInfo	• Excellent documentation • Many established users • Much after-market data	• Few branch offices • Quality of resellers may vary greatly
Maptitude	• Excellent price • Bundled with abundance of data • Exports data in variety of GIS formats	• Small user base • Limited sources of documentation

Source: Reprinted from S.E. Thrall, Geographic Information System (GIS) Hardware and Software, *Journal of Public Health Management and Practice,* Vol. 5, No. 2, p. 87, 1999, Aspen Publishers, Inc.

sets—containing information on a broad range of social, demographic, and health-related data—will be available on the Web. The same information now available only to public health organizations will be available to the public.[25]

Rather than posing a threat, the new technology poses incredible opportunities for public health officials and their communities. GIS technology is eminently compatible with the core public functions of assessment, policy development, and assurance.[26] Public health managers will have many important roles to play, such as building data systems, mobilizing community partnerships, serving as resources, inserting (and teaching) science, and ultimately facilitating community health improvement.

Building Data Systems and Mobilizing Community Partnerships

GIS can encourage public health organizations and communities to form partnerships to assess community health status. Through dialogue with their public health partners, communities can decide what data are relevant for community health improvement. Public health organizations can then help obtain the data sets and incorporate them into an effective assessment system. They can es-

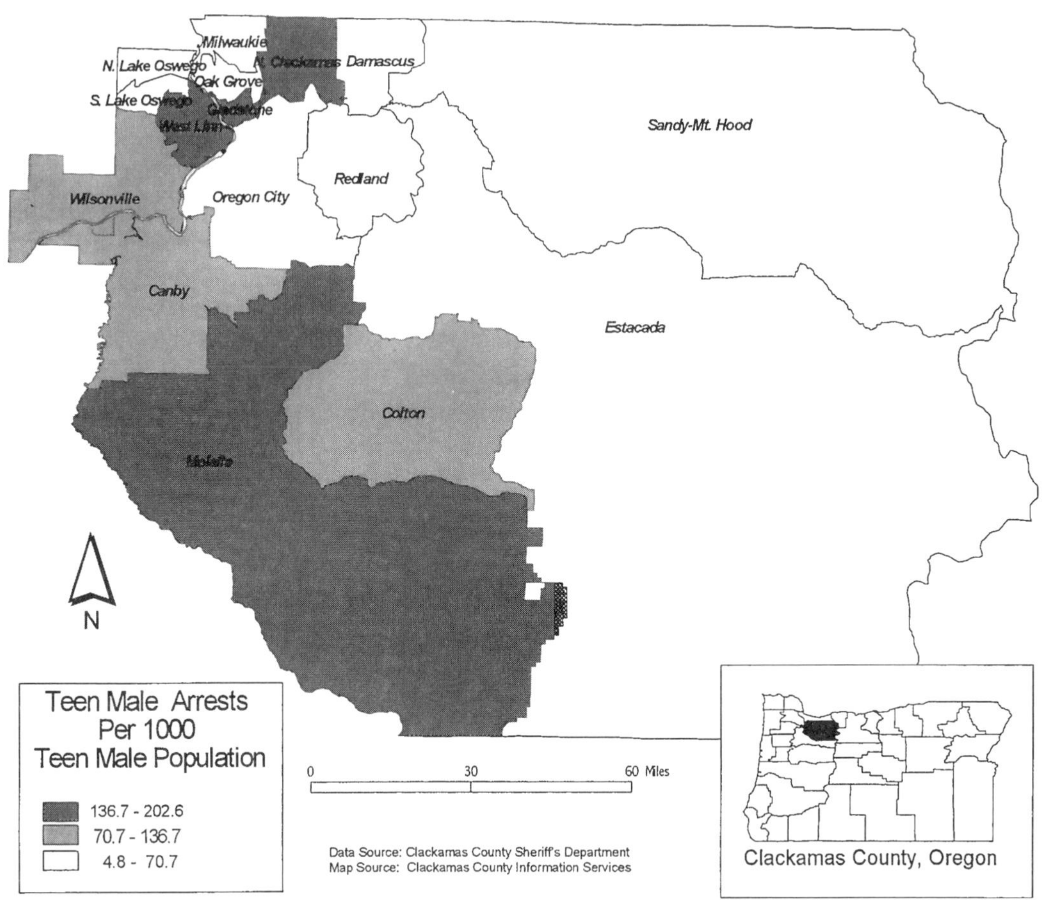

Figure 10–7 Teen Male Arrest Rates, Ages 10–17, by High School Attendance Area: Clackamas County, OR, 1995. *Source:* Clackamas County Information Services, Clackamas County, Oregon.

sentially create a "one-stop" shopping data system, eliminating the need for users to search for data from multiple sources.

An early prototype GIS application is one example of how this may work. Figure 10–7 is a map of teen male arrest rates by high school attendance areas in Clackamas County, Oregon.[4] Juvenile arrests are one of Oregon's benchmarks—measurable indicators for which data are reliably, regularly, and economically available. Through a public process, Oregon established a set of benchmarks related to three community goals: (1) quality jobs for all; (2) safe, caring, and engaged communities; and (3) healthy, sustainable surroundings.[27,28]

Ten of the current Oregon benchmarks have focused on traditional public health indicators such as infant mortality and percentage of adequately immunized two-year-olds. However, connections exist between all three of the community goals and most benchmarks. The Clackamas County Public Health Division has viewed the teen arrest rate as a benchmark with public health implications and as one for which GIS could play an important role in developing community partnerships.

Historically, local law enforcement agencies had used the location of crime and arrest events rather than incident rates in determining where to deploy resources. With public health input, the Juvenile Crime Subcommittee of the Local Public Safety Coordinating Council became interested in looking at juvenile arrest rates as a measure of community health and safety. Their interest increased when they found that they could use GIS to map and analyze juvenile arrest rates, and associated risk factors, at the subcounty, community level.

On the sample map, the case definition for a teen male arrest is age (10–17), male gender, and an arrest report by law enforcement agencies. The GIS application calculated rates based on the residence of the arrested teen (Table 10–4). Public health officials selected high school attendance areas as a community definition because of the potential to design interventions and educational messages targeted at high school teachers, students, and parents. Public input through several focus groups confirmed high school attendance area as a reasonable definition of community. Using census block group aggregations, local health officials and their partners analyzed and mapped (on choropleth maps) juvenile arrest rates for each high school attendance area in the county. The application enabled communities to calculate confidence intervals around these rates to determine whether community juvenile arrest rates were significantly above or below benchmark rates.

As the system is developed, it could help community members visualize patterns of juvenile arrests in relationship to demographic factors, specific crimes committed, and community health indicators, such as the poverty rate.[4] In addition, by obtaining other data sets such as the *YRBS* data, health officials could help communities examine relationships between juvenile arrest rates and behavioral risk factors. With a time trend statistical analysis feature, future applications could enable community partners to evaluate the effectiveness of neighborhood-level juvenile crime prevention initiatives over time.

Diffusing the Technology, Serving as Resources, and Inserting the Science

Public health organizations wanting dialogue and strengthened relationships with local com-

Table 10–4 Teen Male Arrest Rates, Ages 10–17, per 1,000 Teen Male Population, by High School Attendance Area, Clackamas County, OR, 1995

High School Attendance Area	*Number of Teen Male Arrests*	*Teen Male Population*	*Rate per 1,000*
Canby	171	1,325	129.1
N. Clackamas	207	1,091	189.7
Damascus	7	843	8.3
Estacada	47	1,835	25.6
Gladstone	140	691	202.6
Milwaukie	82	1,904	43.1
Molalla	196	1,218	160.9
N. Lake Oswego	39	1,137	34.3
Oak Grove	79	1,858	42.5
Oregon City	118	2,566	46.0
Redland	20	447	44.7
S. Lake Oswego	6	1,249	4.8
Sandy–Mt. Hood	110	1,823	60.3
West Linn	212	1,486	142.7
Wilsonville	77	707	108.9
Colton	34	430	79.1

Source: Clackamas County Information Services, Clackamas County, Oregon.

munities, and wanting to develop policy through collaboration, will have to make health information readily available. The information will have to be of high quality and adequately referenced. Health officials at all levels—local, state, and federal—will have to work with their public and private partners to develop guidelines for metadata. These guidelines should include standards for geocoding and data quality. In addition, health officials at all levels will have a responsibility, with their public and private partners, to develop guidelines on data sharing and confidentiality. Adequate guidelines should lead to the development of new and improved data sets, such as morbidity data, that will be relevant to every community.

Once data become readily available, public health organizations will have an additional responsibility to work with their partners in teaching them basic concepts in epidemiology and ensuring that they use the data appropriately. Fortunately, GIS are compatible with existing community planning tools, such as the *Assessment Protocol for Excellence in Public Health (APEXPH)*.[29] (See Chapter 11 for a more detailed discussion.) In many communities, a major issue has been how to assess community health given the chaotic location of health-related data. *APEXPH98* software integrated with GIS will provide communities with a tool to organize the process of health assessment at the subcounty level.[4] The next iteration of planning tools, such as *Assessment and Planning Excellence through Community Partners for Health (APEXCPH)* and the *Protocol for Assessing Community Excellence in Environmental Health (PACE-EH),* will be compatible with GIS.[30,31]

Facilitating Community Health Improvement

Like other analytic tools, the greatest promise of GIS technology lies in raising additional questions rather than in coming up with answers. The map will begin or advance, but not end, the process of community health improvement. In this way, the development of GIS and other new technologies may change the fundamental roles of public health organizations. The public health professional of the twenty-first century will work closely with his or her community partners to ask questions about community health at the neighborhood level. Together, they will use the new technology to develop neighborhood-based programs that rely on community strengths and meet community needs. Public health organizations will serve as resources and facilitators in gathering data, ensuring data quality, and inviting their partners to the community health improvement table. As the technology and information become more available, public health organizations will lead the way in promoting assessment, policy development, and assurance as community responsibilities rather than government responsibilities.

CHAPTER REVIEW

1. GIS require a foundation of spatial or geographic data. Easily obtainable geographic data files are available from the Census Bureau with detailed street and address information and administrative boundaries including census tract, ZIP codes, and county boundaries.
2. The next step is to obtain attribute data and link them to the geographic database. Examples include vital statistics and law enforcement data. GIS can analyze any attribute database, such as arrest or birth data, that includes a field with a location.
3. *Geocoding* is the process by which GIS software matches each record in an attribute database with the geographic file. The GIS software converts each address in the attribute file to a point on the map. The data are ready for analysis and display.
4. The overlay capability of GIS allows the user to display more than one attribute on a map at a time.

5. Confidentiality issues pose a significant limitation because data with personal addresses can identify individuals. One possible solution is to present aggregated data.
6. Misinterpretation of results can occur if the GIS user regards associations between geography and health outcomes as causally related. Usually, outcomes will cluster geographically because of underlying population characteristics and not because of the geography itself.
7. GIS encourage public health officials and communities to form partnerships to assess community health status.

REFERENCES

1. J. Snow, *On the Mode of Communication of Cholera,* 2d ed. (New York: Commonwealth Fund, 1936).
2. A.L. Melnick and D.W. Fleming, "Modern Geographic Information Systems—Promise and Pitfalls," *Journal of Public Health Management and Practice 5,* no. 2 (1999): viii–x.
3. W.L. Roper and G.P. Mays, "GIS in Public Health Policy: A New Frontier for Improving Community Health," *Journal of Public Health Management and Practice 5,* no. 2 (1999): vi–vii.
4. A. Melnick et al., "County Department of Human Services Community Health Mapping Engine (CHiME) Geographic Information Systems Project," *Journal of Public Health Management and Practice 5,* no. 2 (1999): 64–69.
5. K.C. Clarke et al., "On Epidemiology and Geographic Information Systems: A Review and Discussion of Future Directions," *Emerging Infectious Diseases 2,* no. 2 (1996): 85–92.
6. U.S. Tim, "The Application of GIS in Environmental Health Sciences: Opportunities and Limitations," *Environmental Research* 71 (1995): 75–88.
7. M.Y. Rogers, "Getting Started with Geographic Information Systems (GIS): A Local Health Department Perspective," *Journal of Public Health Management and Practice 5,* no. 4 (1999): 22–33.
8. S. Wilkinson et al., "Lead Hot Zones and Childhood Lead Poisoning Cases, Santa Clara County, California, 1995," *Journal of Public Health Management and Practice 5,* no. 2 (1999): 11–12.
9. C.M. Croner et al., "Geographic Information Systems (GIS): New Perspectives in Understanding Human Health and Environmental Relationships," *Statistics in Medicine* 15 (1996): 1,961–1,977.
10. S. McLafferty and E. Cromley, "Your First Mapping Project on Your Own: From A to Z," *Journal of Public Health Management and Practice 5,* no. 2 (1999): 76–82.
11. C. Duclos et al., "Development of Childhood Blood Lead Screening Guidelines, Duval County, Florida, 1998," *Journal of Public Health Management and Practice 5,* no. 2 (1999): 9–10.
12. M.F. Vine et al., "Geographic Information Systems: Their Use in Environmental Epidemiologic Research," *Environmental Health Perspectives 105,* no. 6 (1997): 598–605.
13. P.H. Bouton and M. Fraser, "Local Health Departments and GIS: The Perspective of the National Association of County and City Health Officials," *Journal of Public Health Management and Practice 5,* no. 4 (1999): 33–41.
14. M. Ralston, "Elevated Nitrate Levels in Relation to Bedrock Depth, Linn County, Iowa, 1991–1996," *Journal of Public Health Management and Practice 5,* no. 2 (1999): 39–40.
15. W.D. Henriques and R.F. Spengler, "Locations Around the Hanford Nuclear Facility Where Average Milk Consumption by Children in 1945 Would Have Resulted in an Estimated Median Iodine-131 Dose to the Thyroid of 10 Rad or Higher, Washington," *Journal of Public Health Management and Practice 5,* no. 2 (1999): 35–36.
16. G.E. Glass et al., "Environmental Risk Factors for Lyme Disease Identified with Geographic Information Systems," *American Journal of Public Health 85,* no. 7 (1995): 944–948.
17. S. Openshaw et al., "A Mark 1 Geographical Analysis Machine for the Automated Analysis of Point Data Sets," *International Journal of Geographic Information Systems* 1 (1987): 335–358.
18. J.L. McKnight and J.P. Kretzman, *Mapping Community Capacity* (Evanston, IL: Northwestern University, Institute of Policy Research, 1996).
19. C.V. Lee and J.L. Irving, "Sources of Spatial Data for Community Health Planning," *Journal of Public Health Management and Practice 5,* no. 4 (1999): 7–22.
20. A. Gordon and J. Womersley, "The Use of Mapping in Public Health and Planning Health Services," *Journal of Public Health Medicine 19,* no. 2 (1997): 139–147.
21. H. Morgenstern, "Ecologic Studies," in *Modern Epidemiology,* 2d ed., eds. K.J. Rothman and S. Greenland (Philadelphia: Lippincott-Raven Publishers, 1998), 459–480.
22. L.H. Cox, "Protecting Confidentiality in Small Population Health and Environmental Statistics," *Statistics in Medicine* 15 (1996): 1,895–1,905.

23. D.C. Goodman and J.E. Wennberg, "Maps and Health: The Challenges of Interpretation," *Journal of Public Health Management and Practice 5,* no. 4 (1999): xiii–xvii.
24. S.E. Thrall, "Geographic Information System (GIS) Hardware and Software," *Journal of Public Health Management and Practice 5,* no. 2 (1999): 82–90.
25. G.I. Thrall, "The Future of GIS in Public Health Management and Practice," *Journal of Public Health Management and Practice 5,* no. 4 (1999): 75–82.
26. Committee for the Study of the Future of Public Health. Institute of Medicine, Division of Health Care Services, *The Future of Public Health* (Washington, DC: National Academy Press, 1988).
27. Oregon Progress Board, *Oregon Benchmarks. Standards for Measuring Statewide Progress and Institutional Performance. Report to the 1995 Legislature* (Salem, OR: 1994).
28. Oregon Progress Board, *Oregon Shines II. Updating Oregon's Strategic Plan. Highlights. A Report to the People of Oregon from the Oregon Progress Board and the Governor's Oregon Shines Task Force* (Salem, OR: 1997).
29. National Association of County and City Health Officials. *Assessment Protocol for Excellence in Public Health (APEXPH)* (Washington, DC: 1991).
30. National Association of County and City Health Officials, *Assessing and Planning Excellence through Community Partners for Health (APEXCPH)* (Washington, DC: 1998).
31. National Association of County and City Health Officials. *Protocol for Assessing Community Excellence in Environmental Health (PACE-EH)* (Washington, DC: 1998).

Chapter 11

Public Health Assessment

Paul K. Halverson
Glen P. Mays

Public health organizations use assessment processes to transform empirical and practical information into knowledge that guides administrative and policy decision making. The assessment process involves a comparative analysis and interpretation of health information from many different sources in order to determine priorities and strategies for addressing the health needs of a defined population. Managing an effective assessment process requires skills in empirical data analysis, group process facilitation, negotiation, interorganizational relations, and consensus development.

Public health organizations require a thorough understanding of current and potential health needs within the populations they serve. Through the activity of assessment, public health organizations transform information into practical knowledge about population health needs. The processes involved in public health assessment are heavily dependent on, yet distinct from, the activities involved in producing and managing population health, including public health surveillance and health information systems development. Assessment involves a critical, comparative analysis and interpretation of health information in order to determine the relative importance and priority of multiple public health issues facing a defined population. Both quantitative and qualitative analytic skills are used to carry out this function.

Institutional perspective plays a powerful role in shaping the processes and outcomes of public health assessment. Public health organizations, therefore, face a key responsibility in determining the extent to which various organizations and individuals have a voice in the assessment process. Managing an effective assessment process requires a diverse set of skills not only for the analysis and interpretation of health information, but also for group process facilitation, negotiation, interorganizational decision making, and consensus development. This chapter reviews the administrative processes used by public health organizations and professionals to assess health needs in the population so that policies and interventions can be tailored to address these needs.

Assessment is widely recognized as a core public health function to be carried out by organizations at all levels of the public health delivery system. (See Chapter 2 for more information.) Despite broad consensus about the importance of this function, the successful implementation and institutionalization of assessment processes within public health organizations is rarely automatic. For example, a 1998

Source: This material, except where otherwise noted, is published in the public domain. No copyright applies. Material on pp. 267–272 (see footnote on p. 272) and sections entitled "Assessment and Tools for Public Health Organizations" and "Implementation and Management Strategies" adapted from G.P. Mays et al., Continuous Quality Improvement in Public Health Organizations, pp. 360–403, in *Continuous Improvement in Health Care: Theory, Implementation, and Applications,* 2nd ed., C.D. McLaughlin and A.D. Kaluzny, eds., © 1999, Aspen Publishers, Inc.

survey of the nation's largest local public health agencies found that, on average, only two-thirds of the activities regarded as essential components of a public health assessment process were performed by these agencies.[1] Less than one-third of the agencies maintained a process for prioritizing health needs within their jurisdictions. Additionally, a longitudinal case study of 15 diverse local public health agencies located in eight different states found that most of these departments reduced their involvement in assessment activities during the five-year period between 1992–97—a period when most of these departments experienced substantial health system change created by the implementation of Medicaid managed care programs.[2]

These findings call attention to the difficulties encountered by public health organizations in carrying out the assessment function effectively while simultaneously addressing other organizational responsibilities. Paradoxically, public health organizations require an effective assessment process in order to make informed decisions regarding other responsibilities in public health service delivery and policy development. For this reason, gaps in the assessment process can cause a downward spiral in organizational performance, as poor policy and program decisions result in fewer organizational resources being available to support assessment activities. The challenge for public health managers lies in investing sufficient intellectual and institutional resources in the assessment process, even though these activities are rarely supported by dedicated funding streams or required by explicit legislative mandates.

This chapter examines both opportunities and challenges faced by public health organizations in implementing an assessment process. First, we examine several important attributes of public health assessment activities that public health organizations must consider either explicitly or implicitly when designing and managing assessment activities. Second, the chapter explores an array of organizational tools and protocols that have been developed over the past decade to facilitate public health assessment activities. These tools, together with the processes developed internally by public health organizations, offer valuable strategies for initiating and sustaining assessment activities within communities. Finally, this chapter examines a set of implementation and management issues that public health organizations encounter while carrying out public health assessment activities. Alternative strategies for addressing these issues are considered. Throughout this chapter, examples of public health assessment efforts involving both governmental and nongovernmental organizations are examined in order to illustrate the benefits and challenges of assessment in the diverse multi-institutional environments that characterize modern public health practice.

KEY CHARACTERISTICS OF PUBLIC HEALTH ASSESSMENT INITIATIVES

Public health organizations exhibit substantial variation in the design and management of assessment activities. There is no single tool or method that is universally used for assessing population health needs. Nevertheless, it is possible to identify a core set of attributes across which public health assessment activities vary. These attributes reflect the objectives of the assessment activity, the organizations and individuals involved, and the specific measurement and decision-making strategies used. Each of the attributes examined in the following paragraphs are considered by public health organizations involved in assessment activities. Successful public health managers actively consider these characteristics in designing an assessment process to fit the needs of their organizations and the populations they serve.

Defining and Delineating the Assessment Process

There continues to be substantial variation in how public health organizations define the scope of public health assessment. In 1988, the Institute of Medicine (IOM) devised a simple definition of public health assessment that has served as the basis for many recent initiatives.[3] The

IOM framework defines assessment as one of three core public health functions to be performed by organizations at all levels of the public health system. Assessment is defined as "the regular and systematic collection, analysis, and dissemination of information on the health of the community, which enables community health needs to be identified." [3(p.44)]

Subsequent work by the Centers for Disease Control and Prevention (CDC) led to the delineation of three specific practices that comprise the assessment function as defined by the IOM.[4] These practices, which were identified by a working group of public health experts convened by the CDC during 1991–92, include the following:

- *Assess* the health needs of the community.
- *Investigate* the occurrence of health effects and health hazards of the community.
- *Analyze* the determinants of identified health needs.

Under sponsorship by the CDC, several groups of researchers have used these definitions of public health practice to develop systems for measuring the performance of public health activities within states and communities.[5,6] Each of the three assessment practices was linked to a set of measurable public health performance indicators for this purpose. Using results from these studies, researchers identified a subset of six public health indicators that appear to reflect the core public health activities that organizations undertake as part of an assessment process. These six indicators include the following:

1. A formal community needs assessment process exists in the jurisdiction that systematically describes the prevailing health status in the community.
2. The local public health agency surveys the population for behavioral risk factors at least every three years.
3. Timely investigations of adverse health events are conducted within the jurisdiction on an ongoing basis—including communicable disease outbreaks and environmental health hazards.
4. Necessary laboratory services are available to the local public health agency to support investigations of adverse health events and meet routine diagnostic and surveillance needs.
5. An analysis is conducted regularly of the determinants of, and contributing factors to, priority health needs in the jurisdiction, the adequacy of existing health resources, and the population groups most affected.
6. The local public health agency conducts an analysis of age-specific participation in preventive and screening services at least every three years.

Another federal effort to define the scope of public health practice was undertaken during the national policy debate over health care reform that took place throughout 1993–94. An expert committee convened by the U.S. Department of Health and Human Services (DHHS) identified a set of 10 essential public health services that are ostensibly independent of the IOM and CDC formulations, but conceptually similar to these earlier efforts.[7] Four of these essential public health services relate to the assessment process and include the following:

1. Monitor health status to identify and solve community health problems.
2. Diagnose and investigate health problems and health hazards in the community.
3. Evaluate the effectiveness, accessibility, and quality of personal and population-based health services.
4. Conduct research for new insights and innovative solutions to health problems.

The federal government has tested this framework in evaluations of state public health agency expenditures and in assessments of state programs funded through the federal Maternal and Child Health Services Grant.[8] The essential services framework has achieved broad support at the federal level, but as yet it appears to be used sparsely within state and local public health organizations.[9]

The frameworks developed by the IOM, CDC, and DHHS are conceptually similar, but it is unlikely that any one of them represents the last word for defining the complex task of public health assessment. A recent survey of state public health organizations revealed that few of these organizations use any single framework in an unaltered form.[9] Many organizations develop their own approaches to public health assessment that are based only loosely on existing definitions and frameworks.

Although the means are still imperfect, the need to define the public health assessment function in terms that can be easily translated to practice has become widely accepted. Considering the great variability in the structure and function of public health organizations, it is not surprising that a variety of approaches now exist for defining the scope of public health assessment. To be successful, the definition that is used must provide a good fit with the public health resources, capacities, and priorities existing in a given setting.

Assessment Focus: Internal versus External Processes

A basic distinction can be made between assessment efforts that focus on the internal operations of a public health organization (often called a self-assessment) and those that focus on processes and outcomes that depend on the actions of multiple organizations and individuals (often called an environmental or community assessment). For example, an *internal* assessment effort conducted by a local health department may focus on the delivery and uptake of immunizations provided through the department's public health clinics. By contrast, an *external* assessment effort may focus on immunization uptake among all physician practices and clinics that operate within the local health department's jurisdiction. Both types of activities potentially contribute to a local health department's need for information on how to improve community immunization rates and reduce the incidence of vaccine-preventable diseases. Internal and external assessment activities, however, may address markedly different facets of the public health problem under study, and may require vastly different allocations of resources, skills, legal authority, and political clout.

In choosing the appropriate focus for an assessment activity, public health organizations need to consider a variety of factors, including

- the nature of the public health problem being targeted
- the internal strengths and weaknesses of the organization
- the current and potential roles played by external organizations and individuals in the problem under study
- the public health organization's current and potential relationships with these external entities

In some cases, an external focus may be infeasible due to insufficient resources and skills, or a lack of political will in the external environment. In other cases, an internal focus may be inappropriate because of the limited effects that internal processes have on the public health problem under study. For example, improving immunization rates only among health department clients may be insufficient to achieve meaningful improvements in community immunization coverage. Therefore, an external assessment effort that targets the immunization practices of all community providers may be needed. In still other cases, an internal assessment may provide initial information needed to generate support for subsequent external efforts.

The Role of Public Health Organizations in the Assessment Process

A third attribute of assessment activities delineates the roles that public health organizations play in implementing and managing these processes. These roles reflect the growing body of evidence in organizational sociology suggesting that organizations follow a staged process in adopting new technologies and operations. Organizations progress from awareness of a problem to identification of a potential solution to implementation of the solution and, finally, to institutionalization of the solution. Public health organizations may assume roles in any or all of these stages in adopting assessment activities. For internally focused assessment activities, these stages may all occur within the public health organization. For externally focused assessment activities, however, other organizations may play critical roles in the adoption process. Public health organizations may play an *initiating* role for assessment efforts by raising awareness about a public health problem, only to let other organizations assume responsibility for implementing and institutionalizing an assessment process around the problem. Public health organizations may play a *convening* role in assessment efforts by bringing organizations and individuals together for the purpose of designing and implementing an assessment process.

During the stage of assessment implementation, public health organizations may choose among several alternative levels of involvement, including

- a *governing* role, wherein the public health organization assumes primary responsibility for directing and managing the assessment process
- a *participatory* role, which entails shared responsibility for managing the assessment process with other organizations
- a *contributing* role, which involves providing information, resources, and expertise to an assessment process that is actively managed by other organizations

The public health organization's role in assessment activities will depend on its own mission, skills, and resources—and those of other organizations having an interest in the public health problems being examined. By encouraging other organizations to assume key responsibilities in public health assessment efforts, public health organizations sacrifice some measure of control over these efforts. In return, however, public health organizations benefit from the additional expertise and resources contributed by these other organizations. Collaborative assessment processes also offer public health organizations opportunities for gaining new knowledge about assessment methods and tools from organizations already skilled in these approaches, including hospitals, managed care plans, medical practices, and laboratories. For example, in one community examined in a recent case study analysis of local public health systems, a private hospital assumed primary responsibility for implementing a process aimed at assessing barriers to routine health care for community members.[2] In this case, the local public health agency participated extensively in the assessment process, but the hospital assumed primary responsibility for the core activities of conducting surveys and focus groups with community residents, and convening local providers to assess their perceptions on access to care.

Levels of Analysis and Authority in the Assessment Process

A fourth critical attribute of the public health assessment process concerns the levels of analysis that are used in conducting assessment activities. Government public health functions are carried out at federal, state, and local levels, with overlapping jurisdictions of authority existing for many public health activities. Assessment efforts reflect these different levels of authority. An important task for public health organizations, therefore, entails identifying the most appropriate level for implementing an assessment effort and encouraging assessment activities to be performed at that level. Some public health problems are addressed most effectively through interventions at state or national levels rather than at the local level. Enhanced legal authority or political will may exist at these higher levels, and superior resources may be available to address the problem. Many public health problems extend beyond the boundaries of a single local community, and therefore require broader governmental authority to carry out effective assessment activities. Moreover, the problem under study may stem from a characteristic of a state or federal program, rather than from local activities. For example, environmental health problems such as water quality and hazardous waste disposal often fall into this category because many state governments exercise regulatory authority over these issues. Rather than attempting to lead an assessment effort at the local level, local public health agencies may achieve better results by contributing to state-level or federal-level assessment initiatives.

Conversely, other public health issues involve primarily local populations, resources, and health needs. Often, these issues can be addressed most effectively through community-level efforts rather than large-scale state or national interventions. For example, the task of improving the accessibility of family planning services within a community is likely to be best informed by a local assessment effort. In this case, the processes of service delivery, outreach, and education are implemented primarily by local community organizations and are therefore amenable to local information about community health needs. In other cases, local assessment efforts may be implemented because larger-scale state or national efforts are not feasible due to a lack of political will. For example, some local communities have initiated assessment efforts around the task of improving health insurance coverage for the uninsured, in part because state and federal initiatives to address this problem have failed to be implemented.[10]

Assessment activities may also involve public health organizations at multiple levels of authority. Local assessment efforts may be implemented as components of larger state or national assessment efforts, with linkages maintained through communication and information flows among the various levels of public health authority. These approaches are designed to inform public health activities simultaneously at these multiple levels of authority, and are particularly relevant in cases where performance at one level of the public health system has substantial influence on performance at another level. For example, Florida's state health agency maintains a state-level assessment process designed to improve public health outcomes in areas such as infant mortality, adolescent pregnancy, and the incidence of communicable diseases.[11] As part of this effort, individual assessment processes are implemented at each local public health unit within the state. These local assessment efforts identify strategies designed to improve the delivery of public health services at the community level. These efforts also generate information about local resource needs and priorities that inform the state-level assessment process. The state assessment effort uses this local information to improve decision making regarding state budget allocations, policy making, and program development.

The administrative relationships that exist among local, state, and federal public health organizations play important roles in assessment implementation. In states such as Florida, local public health agencies are organized as centralized administrative units of the state public health agency. The state agency maintains direct authority for all public health activities within the state. In other states, local public health organizations are decentralized and operate under the direct authority of local governments and local boards of health. In still other states, local public health agencies operate under state authority for some public health functions (e.g., communicable disease control and environmental health protection) and under local authority for other functions (e.g., health promotion and disease prevention activities and community health assessment). *Centralized* public health jurisdictions may offer state agencies enhanced authority for organizing and coordinating assessment processes at the local level, whereas *decentralized* jurisdictions may offer greater opportunities for incorporating local needs, priorities, and values in the assessment process. Public health organizations therefore face the need to tailor their assessment activities to the specific interorganizational and intergovernmental context in which they operate.

Federal public health agency relationships with state and local public health organizations also help shape assessment efforts. Federal agencies interact with state and local organizations primarily through the provision of public health funding, technical assistance, and regulatory oversight. Much federal public health funding is now disbursed through block grants and similar "pass through" arrangements to state health agencies, rather than through categorical grants made directly to local public health organizations. Increasingly, federal agencies use these funding vehicles to encourage assessment activities at state and local levels. For example, the Maternal and Child Health Services Block Grant administered by the U.S. Health Resources and Services Administration (HRSA) requires state grantees to conduct formal needs assessment processes and to develop performance objectives and measures for their programs based on this assessment.

Other federal agencies are developing similar performance measurement criteria for their public health funding programs, pursuant to requirements of the federal Government Performance and Results Act of 1993. These federal efforts, many of which are described in Chapter 3, provide additional motivation for public health organizations to implement assessment processes.

Federal agencies may also encourage assessment implementation through their regulatory authority. Agencies such as the U.S. Environmental Protection Agency (EPA) use their regulatory authority to enforce compliance with federal public health standards such as those concerning air quality, water quality, and solid waste disposal. State and local public health organizations that do not meet these standards are required to adopt remediation processes, which offer opportunities for the application of assessment methods. Since 1995, the EPA's Reinventing Environmental Protection initiative requires the use of assessment methods as part of community-based strategies to achieve and exceed federal environmental health standards.[12]

Federal public health agencies also encourage the implementation of assessment methods by providing technical assistance to state and local public health organizations. Organizations such as the CDC's Public Health Practice Program Office provide information and support to state and local public health agencies seeking to implement assessment methods. The CDC carries out its technical assistance role in partnership with professional associations such as the National Association of County and City Health Officials (NACCHO) and the Association of State and Territorial Health Officials. Through these partnerships, the CDC has been instrumental in developing several resources to support assessment processes, which are discussed in the following sections. Other federal agencies such as the HRSA provide similar types of technical assistance to public health organizations for assessment activities.*

Public Participation in Assessment

Another important attribute of the public health assessment process concerns the extent of public participation. Organizations at all levels of the public health delivery system face the need to remain responsive to community needs, values, and priorities. Some public health organizations ensure this responsiveness through the direct involvement of community representatives in public health decision making and governance. These organizations may operate under governing boards consisting of community representatives, or they may appoint community members to serve on public health task forces empowered to address specific community health issues. Other public health organizations rely on indirect approaches for ensuring responsiveness and accountability to the public, such as governing boards consisting of publicly elected officials that are accountable to public interests through the electoral process.

These same levels of public participation are often extended to assessment activities conducted by public health organizations. Some organizations directly involve community representatives in their assessment processes. For example, organizations may field community surveys and focus groups designed to elicit community perceptions concerning public health issues. The community health assessment process maintained by a local health department and local United Way chapter in California uses this strategy for identifying priority health issues within this community.[13] Another approach involves the appointment of community representatives to working committees that are charged with analyzing, interpreting, and prioritizing health information collected through the assess-

---

*From heading "Key Characteristics of Public Health Initiatives" to here, adapted from G.P. Mays et al., 1999. See note on p. 266.

ment process. This approach was used recently in a series of community demonstration projects supported through the W.K. Kellogg Foundation's Community-Based Public Health Initiative.[2] Each of the seven demonstration projects brought together public health organizations, academic institutions, and community-based organizations to form collaborative processes for identifying community health needs, developing and implementing interventions, and evaluating outcomes. Representatives from community-based organizations—including churches, neighborhood associations, and other local groups—shared responsibility for problem identification, intervention, and evaluation with the governmental public health organizations and academic institutions. Steering committees made up of representatives from each participating organization used consensus-driven processes to make decisions about how to evaluate and prioritize public health issues within the community. This approach was designed to ensure that improvement processes were focused on issues of high importance to community members, and that they involved organizations and individuals with substantial knowledge of and experience with community health problems. Although foundation support for these projects officially ended in 1996, most of the projects continued to operate successfully. A new demonstration effort launched jointly by Kellogg and the Robert Wood Johnson Foundation, entitled "Turning Point: Collaborating for a New Century in Public Health," retains the emphasis on direct community participation in public health assessment and improvement processes.

Other public health organizations employ assessment processes that involve more indirect mechanisms for community participation. These processes rely on community representatives to identify community health needs; however, they often do not directly involve these representatives in the decision-making processes that determine the prioritization, implementation, and evaluation of public health improvement efforts. For example, many public health organizations invite community participation and comment in the early phases of a community health assessment process. During the early phases, organizations assess community perceptions regarding the most pressing public health issues and elicit opinions about the most promising strategies for addressing these issues. In many of these efforts, direct community participation is limited to the task of problem identification. Decisions regarding which issues should receive priority, which interventions should be implemented, and how interventions should be evaluated remain the direct responsibility of public health organizations.

The degree of community participation may have important implications for the success of public health assessment efforts. Direct forms of community participation may help to ensure that the assessment process maintains a high degree of visibility and responsiveness to public health problems as experienced by community members. Direct participation may also add substantial time and resource commitments to the assessment process because community members must learn about assessment concepts and build trust and familiarity with other participants in the process. Furthermore, assessment processes involving direct community participation may experience difficulties in reaching consensus about key public health issues and potential interventions, given the diversity of opinion and perspective that is likely to exist among participants. In choosing among alternative strategies for community participation, public health managers must balance the trade-offs among responsiveness, feasibility, and efficiency.

Evaluative Methods Used for Assessment

Public health assessment efforts vary widely in the methods used to measure and evaluate public health issues. This variation results, in part, from the alternative ways that public health organizations define the scope of public health practice. This variation also stems from the alternative types of information that are available for a given public health issue in a given population, and the alternative analytic techniques that are available for evaluating this information. Public health assessment activities may rely on information concerning the structural dimensions of public health practice, the clinical and administrative processes used in practice, and the health outcomes that result from practice. Moreover, assessment activities may use measures that reflect elements of public health need as well as attributes of public health practice, including its technical quality, effectiveness, appropriateness, comprehensiveness, accessibility, and efficiency.

Methods for evaluating health information also vary substantially, but they uniformly entail comparisons.[14] Some public health assessment initiatives rely on comparisons with a priori standards and goals identified by experts, such as the *Healthy People 2010* national goals for health promotion and disease prevention identified by the U.S. Public Health Service.[15] Comparisons with these types of goals have the advantage of being relatively simple to carry out once data are available, and of being widely recognizable and understandable. These comparisons, however, have the disadvantage of focusing on only a single level of performance, so that continued improvement is de-emphasized once the standard is met (a phenomenon known as a *ceiling effect*). Some assessment initiatives use comparisons over time—also called trend analysis—so that changes in performance can be detected and measured for a given indicator. This method addresses the problem with ceiling effects, but it is limited in its ability to evaluate how much improvement is adequate and desirable over a given period of time. Finally, some improvement initiatives rely on benchmark comparisons with other public health organizations so that performance can be evaluated in relation to similar organizations and/or exemplary organizations in the field. Combining methods based on a priori standards, trend analysis, and benchmarking can be particularly powerful for assessing public health needs and motivating continuous improvement in public health performance.

ASSESSMENT METHODS AND TOOLS FOR PUBLIC HEALTH ORGANIZATIONS

Over the past decade, many different public health assessment and improvement activities have been implemented within the field of public health at local, state, and national levels. These efforts reflect the concepts and methods of assessment in varying ways and with varying degrees of success. More importantly, these activities provide models, tools, and insight for public health organizations to use in designing and managing their own assessment efforts. Six general types of activities have relevance for assessment activities undertaken by public health organizations.

1. community assessment and planning tools
2. public health guidelines
3. community health report cards
4. public health information networks
5. performance-based contracting systems
6. public health performance measurement systems

Each of these activities is examined in the following paragraphs for the advantages and disadvantages they may offer public health organizations in implementing and managing assessment activities.

Community Assessment and Planning Tools

A number of tools and protocols have been developed to assist public health organizations in identifying and assessing community health problems within their jurisdictions and in planning strategies to address these problems. These tools may serve as important foundations and frameworks for implementing assessment activities within specific institutional contexts.

National Health Objectives

Perhaps the most prominent public health planning tools of the past two decades have been those developed by the U.S. Public Health Service to identify measurable national health objectives. These efforts identified a set of high-priority health issues, formulated national improvement goals for each issue, and specified measurement criteria and data sources to be used in assessing improvement. Objectives were identified for the years from 1980 to 1990 in the document entitled *Healthy People*, and from 1990 to 2000 in the document entitled *Healthy*

People 2000.[16,17] Objectives are now available for the *Healthy People 2010* document that will cover the period from 2000 to 2010.[15] *Healthy People 2000* includes objectives in 22 general areas of health (see Exhibit 2–7). In each area, three types of health objectives are identified: those that target *health status outcomes* for the health issue, those that target *health services and interventions*, and those that target *health risk factors*. For example, a health outcome objective in the area of child health states: "Reduce the infant mortality rate to no more than 7 per 1,000 live births."

These national objectives have assisted many public health organizations in their assessment processes by identifying a set of priority health issues in need of attention and by offering measurable goals against which performance may be judged. As a tool for public health improvement, however, these objectives are limited in that they are not sensitive to public health problems of local and regional interest that may not be reflected in broad national trends and priorities. Additionally, these national objectives identify specific performance levels to be achieved rather than establish a process for continuous improvement. To complement the national objectives and address some of their limitations, several additional community health planning tools have been developed in conjunction with the U.S. Public Health Service's efforts.

Health Planning Tools

One of the most prominent health planning tools, the *Planned Approach to Community Health* (PATCH), was developed by the CDC in 1985.[18] The PATCH protocol outlines a standard process that public health organizations can follow for analyzing a few selected health issues, determining their root causes and key intervention points, and planning effective strategies for addressing the issues. Expanding on this effort, the American Public Health Association developed a protocol to assist public health organizations in creating community health planning and monitoring systems that address a comprehensive range of health-related problems. This protocol, named *Healthy Communities 2000: Model Standards*, was developed in 1991 and was explicitly designed to link with the *Healthy People 2000* national objectives.[19,20] Using this protocol, public health organizations develop a plan based on measurable public health objectives that target specific public health outcomes, processes, and population groups. Both process and outcome objectives are emphasized in the protocol. The Texas Department of Health, for example, used this protocol in developing performance-based objectives for local public health departments within the state.[21] Objectives were constructed so that the time frame and quantity of improvement could be specified by each local agency, as in the following outcome and process examples:

- The rate of bicycle-related injuries in children ages 5–14 in *[name]* County will be reduced from *[number]* per 100,000 in FY *[year]* to *[number]* per 100,000 in FY *[year]*.
- By end of FY *[year]*, secure passage of a local ordinance requiring mandatory use of bicycle helmets.

Another assessment and planning tool, the *Assessment Protocol for Excellence in Public Health* (APEXPH), was developed by the NACCHO with sponsorship from the CDC in 1991 to serve as a self-assessment workbook for public health officials.[22] The workbook includes components for assessing the internal capacity of public health organizations as well as the external capacity of other organizations serving the community. The workbook relies on an array of process indicators, including those addressing public health authority, community relations, community health assessment, policy development, financial management, personnel management, program management, and governing board procedures. An expanded version of this protocol, the *Assessment and Planning Excellence through Community Partners for Health* (APEXCPH), is currently under development.[23] This new protocol aligns the indicators in APEXPH with the 10 essential public health services identified by the DHHS, and expands the community capacity indicators to include a broader array of community organizations and activities.

Drawing on these efforts, the U.S. Agency for Health Care Policy and Research (now the Agency for Healthcare Research and Quality) developed a planning tool designed specifically to assist local health departments in responding to managed health care systems. This workbook, entitled *Assessing Roles, Responsibilities, and Activities in a Managed Care Environment: A Workbook for Local Health Officials*, provides guidelines for health departments to use in areas such as assessing budgets, staffing, and service delivery activities; developing managed care contracts and affiliations; assessing community health needs; and monitoring policy and marketplace trends.[24]

Health Assessment and Improvement Tools

Other assessment tools formally integrate the tasks of collecting and analyzing community health data with the processes of community health planning, priority setting, and intervention. In many communities, the hospital industry has become actively involved in developing and applying these tools. Pioneered by efforts in Pennsylvania, Vermont, and Wisconsin, growing numbers of state hospital associations actively encourage their members to conduct community health assessment and improvement initiatives within their service areas.[25] The Pennsylvania association's assessment process, which has served as a model for many assessment initiatives across the country, involves a five-step sequence involving

1. compiling a community health profile
2. identifying priorities for community health needs
3. developing an action plan
4. implementing community health interventions
5. evaluating the interventions[26]

The assessment initiative adopted by the Wisconsin association draws heavily on the Pennsylvania model as well as the APEXPH protocol that was originally developed for public health agencies.[9] Hospitals in California are now required by state law to conduct periodic community health assessments using an established protocol in order to maintain their nonprofit status. Hospitals must also demonstrate involvement in community health assessment as part of the accreditation process conducted by the Joint Commission on Accreditation of Healthcare Organizations.

The IOM Model

The proliferation of community health assessment and improvement efforts in the public and private sectors led the IOM to convene an expert panel to review the many existing processes and recommend a consensus approach for undertaking these efforts. The IOM's work identified several essential characteristics of an effective community health assessment and improvement effort.[27] These characteristics include

- use of an iterative process that cycles continuously through the tasks of assessment, action, and evaluation
- use of a team approach, through which decisions are made largely by consensus among community representatives
- use of an incremental strategy for improvement, whereby progress is accomplished through a series of small steps rather than through major breakthroughs

The IOM proposed a model for community health improvement processes consisting of two related cycles of implementation (Figure 11–1).[27] The first cycle consists of five main activities: forming a community health coalition, collecting and analyzing data for a community health profile, and identifying and prioritizing important community health issues. As part of activities in this first cycle, the IOM proposed a set of 25 indicators for use in assessing community health status (Exhibit 11–1).[28] These indicators are an expanded version of a consensus set of 18 indicators that were recommended in 1991 by the CDC to track progress toward achieving *Healthy People 2000* objectives.[29] Of course, for any specific community, these general indicators may need to be supplemented with additional measures corresponding to the specific

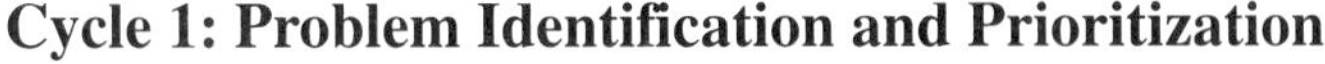

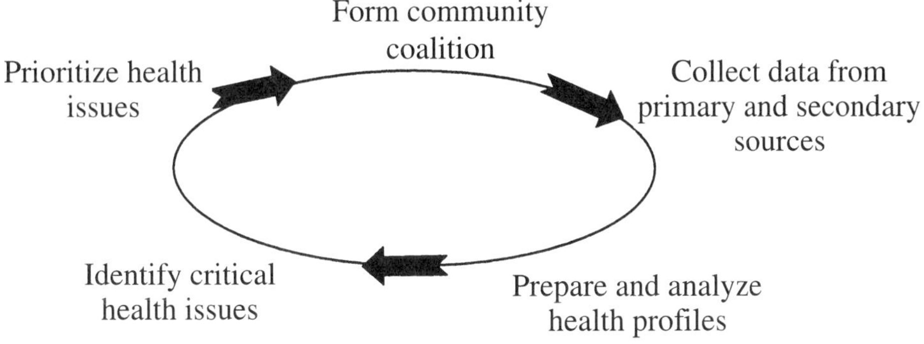

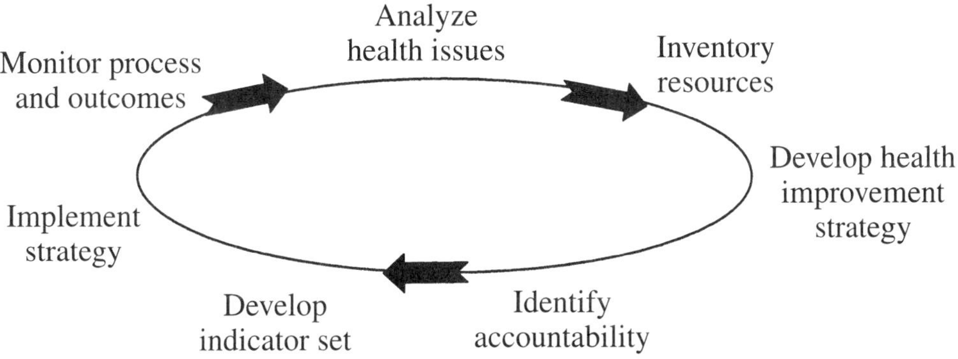

Figure 11–1 The Community Health Improvement Process. *Source:* Adapted with permission from *Improving Health in the Community: A Role for Performance Monitoring,* © 1997 by the Committee on Using Performance Monitoring to Improve Community Health, Institute of Medicine. Courtesy of National Academy Press, Washington, D.C.

problems and needs of that community. Community improvement strategies may be broad based, simultaneously exploring a number of health issues, as in the APEXPH model. Alternatively, strategies may focus on a small number of specific issues, as in the PATCH model.

Once a specific health issue has been targeted by a community, the IOM health improvement process moves on to the analysis and implementation cycle (Figure 11–1). The steps in this second cycle include analysis of the health issue, an inventory of health resources, development of a health improvement strategy, discussion and negotiation to establish where accountability lies, development of a set of performance indicators for accountable entities, implementation of the health improvement strategy, and measurement to monitor the outcome of efforts by community organizations.

To help identify risk factors for problematic health outcomes, organizations can use the process for cause and effect analysis identified in the APEXPH model.[22] The State of Florida Department of Public Health and Rehabilitative Services has successfully used this type of analysis to help communities identify promising public health interventions.

A critical step in the community health improvement process is to formulate appropriate action based on the results of a community health

Exhibit 11–1 Community Health Indicators Proposed by the Institute of Medicine

Sociodemographic Characteristics

1. Distribution of the population by age and race/ethnicity
2. Number and proportion of persons in groups such as migrants, homeless, and the non-English speaking, for whom access to community services and resources may be of concern
3. Number and proportion of persons aged 25 and older with less than a high school education
4. Ratio of the number of students graduating from high school to the total number of students who entered 9th grade three years previously
5. Median household income
6. Proportion of children less than 15 years of age living in families at or below the poverty level
7. Unemployment rate
8. Number and proportion of single-parent families
9. Number and proportion of persons without health insurance

Health Status

10. Infant mortality rate by race/ethnicity
11. Number of deaths or age-adjusted death rates for motor vehicle crashes, work-related injuries, suicide, homicide, lung cancer, breast cancer, cardiovascular diseases, and all causes, by age, race, and gender
12. Reported incidence of acquired immune deficiency syndrome, measles, tuberculosis, and primary and secondary syphilis, by age, race, and gender as appropriate
13. Births to adolescents (ages 10–17) as a proportion of total live births
14. Number and rate of confirmed abuse and neglect cases among children

Health Risk Factors

15. Proportion of 2-year-old children who have received all age-appropriate vaccines, as recommended by the Advisory Committee on Immunization Practices
16. Proportion of adults aged 65 and older who have ever been immunized for pneumococcal pneumonia, and the proportion who have been immunized in the past 12 months for influenza
17. Proportion of the population who smoke, by age, race, and gender
18. Proportion of the population age 18 and older who are obese
19. Number and type of U.S. Environmental Protection Agency air quality standards not met
20. Proportion of assessed rivers, lakes, and estuaries that support beneficial uses (e.g., fishing and swimming approved)

Health Care Resource Consumption

21. Per capita health care spending for Medicare beneficiaries

Functional Status

22. Proportion of adults reporting that their general health is good to excellent
23. During the past 30 days, average number of days for which adults report that their physical or mental health was not good

Quality of Life

24. Proportion of adults satisfied with the health care system in the community
25. Proportion of persons satisfied with the quality of life in the community

Source: Adapted with permission from *Improving Health in the Community: A Role for Performance Monitoring,* © 1997 by the Committee on Using Performance Monitoring to Improve Community Health, Institute of Medicine. Courtesy of National Academy Press, Washington, D.C.

assessment. The IOM uses the term *accountable entities* to refer to stakeholders that are expected to achieve specific results as part of the community's strategy for addressing a health issue. Traditionally, communities have viewed the local public health agency as the primary accountable entity. As described earlier, however, solutions to public health problems require action by multiple groups within a community, and accountability should be recognized as an issue of shared responsibility. An important part of the community health improvement process is to designate accountable entities and to establish agreements among entities that specify areas of responsibility, measures of performance, and rewards for successful performance. Performance gaps should trigger problem analysis and a reformulation of each stakeholder's approach to the health issue.

Public Health Practice Guidelines

Practice guidelines are another management tool for public health organizations that hold much potential for facilitating the conduct of public health assessment processes. Like their counterparts in medical care, public health practice guidelines provide scientifically based, tailored information regarding optimal methods for implementing public health interventions for specific population groups. Like health objectives and standards, practice guidelines can be powerful tools in public health assessment processes by creating a metric for evaluation and comparison. Guidelines can be used to detect and eventually reduce unnecessary variation in the implementation of public health interventions, thereby enhancing the effectiveness and efficiency of these interventions.

The development of practice guidelines has occurred slowly in the field of public health, principally because of the limited availability of scientifically valid information regarding the outcomes and costs of public health interventions. For many of these interventions, the outcomes accrue over long periods of time, making scientific evaluation methodologically difficult and financially costly. Nonetheless, several important sources of public health guidelines exist for assisting organizations in implementing public health quality improvement initiatives. First, organizations may use externally developed guidelines such as those issued by the U.S. Preventive Services Task Force and the Public Health Service Task Force developing the *Guide to Community Preventive Services*. Additionally, a growing number of organizations implement internally developed guidelines based on evidence that has been collected and analyzed within the organization.

Externally Developed Guidelines

One of the most widely recognized external sources for public health practice guidelines is the *Guide to Clinical Preventive Services: An Assessment of the Effectiveness of 169 Interventions*, issued by the U.S. Preventive Services Task Force.[30] Based on an extensive review of scientific evidence, the task force constructed guidelines for the provision of more than 100 primary and secondary prevention services designed to address more than 70 illnesses and health conditions. The evidence used to develop these guidelines included randomized controlled trials, controlled trials, cohort and case-control studies, multiple time series studies, uncontrolled experiments, and expert opinion. For each intervention, guidelines specify the sociodemographic characteristics of the target population, the timing and sequence of component processes, the contraindications associated with each intervention, and the health risks and benefits of each intervention. Originally produced in 1989, the guide was updated in 1996 to reflect new scientific evidence and newly developed interventions. Evidence from randomized controlled trials serves as the gold standard for guideline development, but the guide continues to be heavily dependent on expert opinion and nonrandomized studies due to the limited clinical research in many areas of prevention practice.

Expanding on the process for clinical preventive services, the CDC appointed a Task Force on Community Preventive Services to develop similar guidelines for population-based public health interventions that target communities, schools, and work sites rather than individual patients. Although still under development, the *Guide to Community Preventive Services* is expected to offer guidelines in the following areas:[31]

- preventing community health problems
- changing risk behaviors
- changing ecosystems, including environmental concerns
- cross-cutting public health activities

Additional sources for externally developed public health practice guidelines exist, although most address clinical rather than population-based prevention. These include specialized task forces and advisory panels convened by the National Institutes of Health and the CDC, such as the Advisory Council for the Elimination of Tuberculosis, which developed guidelines for the implementation of tuberculosis prevention and control programs.[32] Professional associations such as the American College of Preventive Medicine are also active in developing and disseminating prevention practice guidelines.[33,34]

Internally Developed Guidelines

Increasingly, public health organizations are engaging in efforts to develop their own practice guidelines—either alone or in combination with other health organizations. These tools are based on evidence and experience amassed by individual organizations in serving specific population groups. One approach to creating local guidelines is to begin with a nationally developed guideline and tailor its specifications to the individual needs and capacities of the organization and the community it serves. The Texas Department of Health used this approach in developing its performance measurement process for district health departments, drawing heavily on guidelines established in the American Public Health Association's *Healthy Communities: Model Standards* and the NACCHO's APEXPH. Texas went beyond the generic practices described in these resources by developing specific process objectives tailored to the capacities and policy priorities of its local health agencies.[21]

Similarly, the Denver Health Authority in Colorado developed an internal quality assessment process based on guidelines established for managed care plans in the National Committee for Quality Assurance's *Health Plan Employer Data and Information Set (HEDIS)*. Denver added performance elements that were not included in *HEDIS* but that were perceived as important by key stakeholders, including staff, local and state policy officials, and consumers.[35] The agency also eliminated *HEDIS* elements that did not appear relevant to the organization or that proved to be too difficult to measure accurately. Denver used the resulting process to demonstrate accountability for contract funds received from local and state governmental agencies.

Some public health agencies adopt practice guidelines developed by other organizations with which they interact. Managed care plans are key among those organizations helping to disseminate practice guidelines among public health agencies. Public health agencies that contract with plans for the delivery of personal health services adopt many of the same health plan guidelines used by medical care providers. These may include practices for assessing patient health status, delivering clinical preventive services, and making referrals to other health care providers. Agencies participating in health plan provider networks often benefit from the quality improvement processes maintained by these plans, which may allow agencies to compare their own performance in a guideline area with that of other providers. The Memphis and Shelby County Health Department, for example, uses the information it receives from health plans to compare its performance with private providers in areas such as childhood and adult immunization, cervical and breast cancer screening, and asthma and diabetes management.[2] The agency uses documentation of its performance to negotiate favorable contracts with health plans and to demonstrate accountability to local government officials and the public.

Public health agencies play important roles in disseminating public health practice guidelines to managed care plans and other health care organizations. For example, following a large measles outbreak, the City of Milwaukee Health Department conducted on-site provider education seminars with community physicians—including those in managed care plans—regarding optimal strategies for childhood immunization delivery. More recently, the health department has sponsored workshops on TB diagnosis and treatment strategies for physicians practicing in managed care plans.[36] Health plan executives in Milwaukee identify the local health department as an important source of information concerning effective prevention practices. In Vancouver, Washington, the Southwest Washington Health District conducts periodic on-site workshops with community physicians concerning optimal ways for storing vaccines—an effort motivated by an earlier health department study that showed widespread use of inappropriate storage techniques.[2]

In some communities, public health agencies have begun to work jointly with other health care organizations to develop communitywide practice guidelines.[37] These efforts represent potentially powerful strategies for improving community health through the coordinated actions of multiple stakeholders—including health care providers, purchasers, insurers, and consumers. In one such initiative in Genesee County, Michigan, a local public health agency is working in partnership with a group of hospitals, health plans, employers, community-based organizations, unions, and the local medical society.[2] This coalition has formed working groups to develop a broad range of community practice guidelines in areas such as primary care, clinical preventive services, chronic disease treatment and control, and violence prevention. Once guidelines are developed, each participant works to encourage adoption and implementation within his or her organization as well as among peer organizations.

Community Health Report Cards

Report card systems are becoming popular strategies for monitoring and improving performance in many areas of health care. Although they vary widely in their structure and content, report card systems typically consist of a set of standardized performance measures that are collected consistently across a group of organizations, individuals, or other entities under study. Using these measures, report card systems employ a metric for comparing and profiling the performance of each entity against its peers on a periodic basis. These systems are distinct from other types of assessment approaches that rely primarily on trend analysis or on comparisons against a priori performance standards and goals.

Report cards are being used in other sectors of the health care field to monitor performance and encourage improvement through comparison.[38–44] Recent evidence suggests that report card methodologies are also being used to assess community-level health issues in some localities.[45] These existing approaches appear to vary widely in their purpose, scope, and methodology.

Report cards offer several distinct advantages over other assessment approaches, including: (1) encouraging continuous improvement in performance rather than establishing specific floors or ceilings for performance; (2) motivating performance improvement through benchmarking and comparisons with peers; (3) enabling aggregate measures of performance across a group of organizations, individuals, or communities using standardized measures; and (4) creating a framework for identifying best practices among the entities under study. In the medical care field, report card systems are thought to be particularly effective in improving performance among organizations that compete for patients, revenue, or other resources—such as hospitals, physician practices, and managed care plans. In these settings, report cards are used as tools for marketing services to patients, payers, and purchasers. Some evidence suggests that these systems motivate substantial improvements in medical care practice.[38–44]

Report card systems are used at the community level to promote collaboration and information-sharing rather than competition. By facilitating comparisons of community-level health measures across local areas, report card systems can serve as tools for mobilizing collaborative, interorganizational efforts in community health improvement. Report card systems can be used to profile the aggregate effects of multiple health organizations and interventions within a community, thereby exposing gaps in performance that need remedy. To be sure, local public health agencies and other community health organizations already have an extensive battery of tools, protocols, and planning guides for conducting community health assessment.[18,20,22,46] Nonetheless, by enabling comparisons among peer groups of local communities, report card systems may offer local public health agencies more meaningful and relevant measures of community health performance than other assessment approaches.[14]

Community health report card systems are attractive tools for organizations other than local public health agencies.[47] If broadly implemented, these systems may assist state and federal health agencies in targeting health resources and services to areas of greatest need, and in evaluating the community-level effects of health-related interventions. These systems may be used to integrate the reporting requirements and accountability systems of multiple federal and state health programs, thereby reducing reporting duplication and respondent burden while enhancing program assessment and evaluation activities. Similarly, report card systems may help to inform the progress toward performance-based contracting initiatives in public health, which are currently taking shape at both federal and state levels.[21,48–50] Under these initiatives, state and local governments may use report card systems to obtain improved measures of public health performance at the community level and thereby demonstrate accountability for funds that are appropriated to support public health activities. Finally, report card systems may prove to be valuable tools in the movement toward national performance standards and accreditation programs for local public health agencies.[51] An appropriately structured report card system may provide an ideal framework for establishing performance standards and measuring performance levels among participating agencies.

A frequent criticism of standardized assessment tools and reporting systems in public health is that they fail to account for the unique ways in which public health is organized and administered at local levels.[52] Local public health officials have raised this issue in relation to community health report cards, questioning the local relevance and utility of a standardized system designed for broad implementation. Recent studies have begun to explore the extent to which there exists a degree of commonality in the assessment needs and capacities of local public health agencies that might support a standardized report card system.[47,53] These efforts examine whether a core set of community health indicators can be identified that are scientifically sound, locally available, and widely regarded as relevant and useful for measuring community health status. Early results from these efforts suggest that such indicators may be identifiable and useful. A representative survey of the nation's local health agencies during 1997 uncovered that a strong majority of agencies would find comparative assessment data from a national report card initiative to be useful, and that a core set of community health indicators are available at the local level to form the basis of such an initiative.[47]

Additional research and development efforts are needed to identify relevant, reliable, and feasible indicators of community health that can be used to monitor outcomes and practices at the community level.[54] The set of 25 indicators proposed by the IOM provides an appropriate starting point for this work (Exhibit 11–1). Ultimately, consensus needs to be reached on a minimum data set that will permit valid comparisons to be made across local and state jurisdictions, and that will facilitate progress toward achieving state and national health objectives. The measures included in this set must be readily and uniformly acceptable and understandable, be measurable using easily available data, and indicate specific interventions for public health action as well as broad general measures of community health and program effectiveness. Additionally, strategies are needed for measuring outcomes and practices in small geographic areas, where statistics may not be stable because of small denominators. Valid methods are needed for adjusting community outcomes for the severity of health problems being addressed and the underlying risks that are present in individual communities. Finally, methods must be developed for identifying groups of communities appropriate for comparison and benchmarking purposes, such as groups based on population size, sociodemographic composition, and/or health resources availability.

Public Health Information Networks

Public health assessment strategies often face the challenge of acquiring and integrating community health information from multiple sources in order to monitor practices and outcomes adequately at the community level. A number of computerized information management systems have been developed to assist community efforts to collect and display data from multiple sources. (For a full review, see Chapter 9.) These systems hold great potential for facilitating the conduct of public health assessment processes. Two recent examples are the Michigan and CDC APEXPH Information Manager, and the Seattle-King County Department of Public Health VISTA PH computer software.[55,56] These computer programs facilitate the display of data such as demographics, adult death rates, infant death rates, hospitalization rates, and infectious disease rates.

Many other public health information systems are currently under development at state and local levels to facilitate public health assessment and decision making. A number of these efforts have been supported by the CDC's Information Network for Public Health Officials (INPHO) program. These efforts are working to establish integrated information networks that can support information sharing and communication across public health organizations within the states. Other efforts are carried out through state health data organizations, hospital associations, managed care plans, and health care purchasing coalitions.[57] These state and local resources complement the information systems available at the national level through such resources as the CDC WONDER on-line warehouse of public health data and information and the National Library of Medicine's on-line databases of health sciences literature. Public health managers at state and local levels need to be able to identify and understand the array of information resources and systems that can be used for assessing public health needs within the populations they serve.

Performance-Based Contracting Systems

Performance-based contracting mechanisms represent yet another management tool for public health organizations that may facilitate the conduct of public health assessment efforts. By making contract awards and financial payments contingent on measurable attributes of performance, these mechanisms can create powerful incentives for organizations to assess public health problems and demonstrate the impact of programs and services. In the domain of medical care, managed care plans have pioneered numerous strategies for performance-based contracting, including risk-adjusted capitation payment rates, payment withholds and bonuses based on provider performance, and payment formulas based on performance in specific clinical areas (such as immunization rates). In the field of public health, performance-based contracts are currently being applied on at least two levels. First, federal grant-making agencies are beginning to use performance-based contracting principles as part of the grants they issue to state and local public health agencies. Much of this activity is occurring in response to the Government Performance and Results Act of 1993, which requires federal agencies to track outcomes associated with the public funds they administer. The DHHS is rapidly moving toward implementation of "performance partnerships" grants with state health agencies, which would require these agencies to establish action plans and measurable performance objectives as part of their contracts with the DHHS for federal public health funding.[48]

Second, many state and local health agencies have begun to use performance-based contracting principles in their relationships with other health organizations. Many of these efforts are being adopted as part of public health privatization efforts that transfer responsibility for certain public health functions from public agencies to private (or quasi-private) contractors.[58] For example, the local health department in Milwaukee, Wisconsin, contracts with a network of community health centers to provide specified clinical services to health department clients. Similarly, in Mecklenburg County, North Carolina, the county health department contracts with a hospital-based integrated delivery system for the provision of most personal health services that are traditionally provided by the health department.[59] Performance-based contracting mechanisms offer public health agencies promising strategies for assessing the quality of services and activities that are purchased from contractors such as private health care providers.

Several implementation characteristics of performance-based contracting activities warrant close attention. First, these activities require a clear definition of the public health functions and services to be carried out under the contract and a clear delineation of responsibilities to be assumed by each party. Without these elements, contract provisions can be difficult if not impossible to enforce. Second, performance-based contracting requires accurate, reliable methods for assessing public health impact and performance. Performance measures that are self-reported by the contractor introduce a clear moral hazard for "upcoding" these measures in order to receive higher payments. Therefore, effective performance-based contracting strategies require substantial investments in assessment methods that are resistant to these types of gaming. Third, performance-based contracting initiatives must be supported by effective plans for enforcing contract provisions and payment rates. Barriers to effective contract enforcement are due to the lack of alternative contractors, the risk of reducing the financial viability of contractors, and the political influence maintained by contractors. Public health agencies must anticipate these barriers and incorporate contract mechanisms that offer alternative methods of enforcement.

Several state health agencies have initiated performance-based contracting efforts as part of their public health quality improvement efforts. Rhode Island's Department of Health delivers personal health services and community health services exclusively through contracts with private providers such as community health centers and voluntary health associations because the state is not served by a system of local health departments.[9,60] Currently, the state relies primarily on process-based measures of performance in developing and enforcing contracts with private providers. These measures include such elements as waiting times, appointment availability, service volume, and consumer-initiated complaints. The state is in the process of developing strategies to link contracts with measurable public health outcomes—particularly those that are emphasized in the *Healthy People 2000* national health objectives. Similarly, Washington State's Department of Health is exploring the feasibility of developing performance-based contracting mechanisms linked to an 84-indicator performance measurement system for local health departments, based on the IOM's 1988 framework.[9,60] The Utah Department of Health is phasing in performance-based contracting mechanisms in four core areas: services provided under the federal Preventive Health Services Block Grant, services provided through the federally supported Children with Special Health Care Needs Program, services provided through the federal Special Supplemental Food Program for Women, Infants, and Children (WIC) program, and services provided through state human immunodeficiency virus (HIV) and TB prevention and control programs.[9,60] Utah develops individually tailored action plans with each contractor, specifying both short-term process objectives and long-term outcome objectives. Objectives are developed through a process that includes input from contractors as well as consumers, and that links with the national *Healthy People 2000* objectives.

Public Health Performance Measurement Systems

Public health researchers and policy makers have begun to develop and implement approaches for measuring the performance of public health organizations. Increasingly, these approaches are being used at local, state, and national levels to monitor the overall adequacy of the public health delivery system and to ensure accountability for public health spending. (For a full description of these approaches, see Chapter 18.) Performance measurement systems can also facilitate in the conduct of public health assessment activities. Two frequently used performance measurement instruments are those developed by researchers at the University of North Carolina at Chapel Hill and the University of Illinois—both of which are based on the three core public health functions identified by the IOM and an associated list of 10 public health practices identified by a work group convened by the CDC.[4,6,61] Other performance measurement approaches have developed around a set of 10 essential public health services identified by the DHHS and the Essential Public Health Services Work Group.[7,8,62,63] Additionally, many public health organizations have developed their own approaches for monitoring performance.[9]

The performance measurement system developed by Miller and colleagues has received considerable attention because it focuses on the contributions made to public health practice by all providers serving the community—both public and private—rather than limiting the focus to the roles of governmental agencies.[9] This approach is particularly useful for public health assessment activities designed to evaluate the extent to which the local public health infrastructure meets existing community health needs. The organizing framework for this measurement system is the three core public health functions identified by the IOM, linked with the 10 public health practices subsequently delineated. A group of indicators was developed for each practice drawing on materials from many sources, including *Healthy People 2000* and the APEXPH process. Eight to 10 indicators were selected for each of the 10 public health practices, yielding a total of 84 indicators. Responses to the survey were obtained from local health department directors. These indicators are combined to compute performance measures for each surveyed public health jurisdiction, indicating the adequacy of performance for each practice, the proportional contribution to performance by the local health department, and the other types of organizations that contribute to each practice within the jurisdiction. Schematic representation of the results can be presented in graphic form, as illustrated in Figure 11–2. Note that the top graph line for each public health jurisdiction indicates the extent to which core public health activities are performed within the jurisdiction in each of the 10 practice areas. The bottom graph line illustrates the contribution to each of the practices by the local health department. Codes at the bottom of the graphic indicate the other types of providers that contribute to each practice.

Most recently, several popular performance measurement protocols were combined and condensed into a set of 20 public health performance indicators, each one linked to the three core public health functions identified by the IOM.[64] During 1998, these 20 indicators, shown in Exhibit 11–2, were used in a national survey of all local health departments serving jurisdictions of at least 100,000 residents ($N = 496$). Results confirmed that wide variation in performance persists despite many public health improvement efforts implemented at national, state, and local levels during the 1990s (Table 11–1). On average, 64 percent of the 20 public health indicators were performed in local public health jurisdictions. The average local health department performed 24 percent of these services directly, accounting for 67 percent of the total community effort devoted to public health activities in the areas studies.

Public health agencies use a variety of other approaches for measuring organizational performance. A survey of the nation's state health agencies during 1997 revealed that 88 percent of public health agencies surveyed had some level of involvement in local public health performance measurement systems.[9] Of these departments, 50 percent maintained an ongoing performance assessment process that was currently active, 30 percent were engaged in developing a new or revised performance assessment process that was not yet active, and 20 percent reported past involvement in a performance assessment process that was no longer active.

Building on many of these existing efforts, the CDC has initiated a collaborative effort to develop and implement a national performance measurement system for state and local public health organizations. Although still under development, the National Public Health Performance Standards Program will include performance standards and measures designed to facilitate quality improvement efforts, practice-based research initiatives, and accountability systems for state and local public health organizations. An example of the draft performance standard and measures for the activity of *monitoring health status to identify community problems* is shown in Exhibit 11–3. This example illustrates the elements that the CDC has found to comprise an

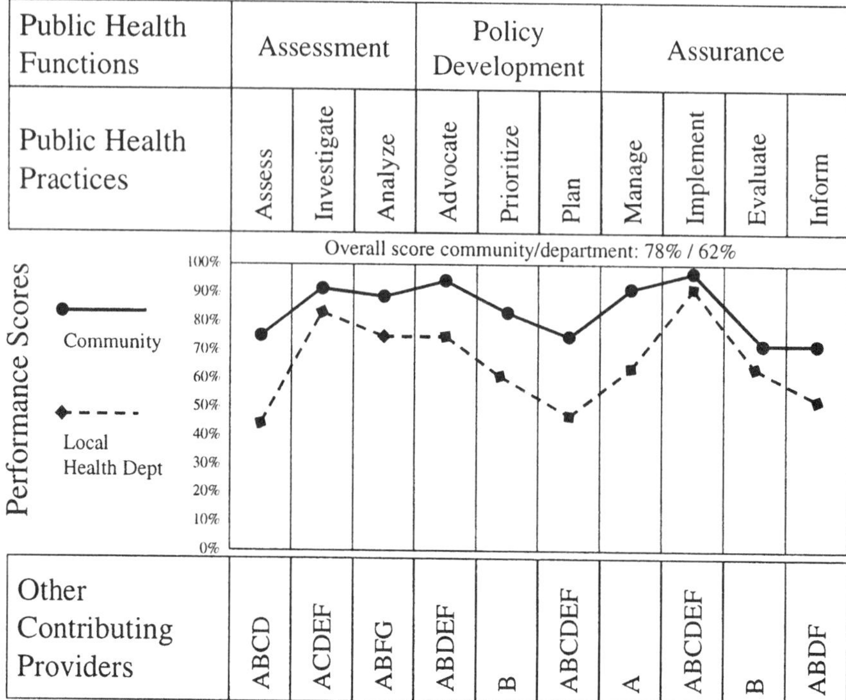

Other provider codes: A=state agencies; B=local agencies; C=nonprofit agencies; D=hospitals; E=community health centers; F=universities; G=other.

Figure 11–2 Public Health Performance Profile for a Sample Community and Local Health Department. *Source:* Reprinted with permission from C.A. Miller, K.S. Moore, T.B. Richards, and J.D. Monk, A Proposed Method for Assessing the Performance of Local Public Health Functions and Practices, *American Journal of Public Health,* Vol. 84, No. 11, pp. 1743–1749, © 1994, American Public Health Association.

optimal public health assessment process carried out at the local level. These definitions and standards are likely to change over time as the CDC refines its measurement system to keep pace with changes in standards of practice. Once fully operational, the National Public Health Performance Standards Program promises to be an important information resource for public health organizations to use in designing and implementing public health assessment activities.

IMPLEMENTATION AND MANAGEMENT STRATEGIES

A variety of tools and methods are now available to assist public health organizations in implementing assessment and improvement efforts at local, state, national, and even international levels. Nonetheless, public health organizations have generally not been as quick to adopt and apply these methods as have organizations in other sectors of the health care field.[65] Public health organizations face several unique challenges in implementing and managing assessment processes that must be anticipated, recognized, and addressed to ensure success. Some of the most common challenges are examined in the following sections.

Securing Start-Up and Maintenance Resources

Public health organizations frequently operate in an environment of constrained resources that

Exhibit 11–2 Twenty Indicators of Local Public Health Performance

1. In your jurisdiction, is there a community needs assessment process that systematically describes the prevailing health status in the community?
2. In the past three years in your jurisdiction, has the local public health agency surveyed the population for behavioral risk factors?
3. In your jurisdiction, are timely investigations of adverse health events conducted on an ongoing basis—including communicable disease outbreaks and environmental health hazards?
4. Are the necessary laboratory services available to the local public health agency to support investigations of adverse health events and meet routine diagnostic and surveillance needs?
5. In your jurisdiction, has an analysis been completed of the determinants of and contributing factors to priority health needs, the adequacy of existing health resources, and the population groups most effected?
6. In the past three years in your jurisdiction, has the local public health agency conducted an analysis of age-specific participation in preventive and screening services?
7. In your jurisdiction, is there a network of support and communication relationships that includes health-related organizations, the media, and the general public?
8. In the past year in your jurisdiction, has there been a formal attempt by the local public health agency to inform officials about the potential public health impact of decisions under their consideration?
9. In your local public health agency, has there been a prioritization of the community health needs that have been identified from a community needs assessment?
10. In the past three years in your jurisdiction, has the local public health agency implemented community health initiatives consistent with established priorities?
11. In your jurisdiction, has a community health action plan been developed with community participation to address priority community health needs?
12. In the past three years in your jurisdiction, has the local public health agency developed plans to allocate resources in a manner consistent with community health action plans?
13. In your jurisdiction, have resources been deployed as necessary to address priority health needs identified in a community health needs assessment?
14. In the past three years in your jurisdiction, has the local public health agency conducted an organizational self-assessment?
15. In your jurisdiction, are age-specific priority health needs effectively addressed through the provision of or linkage to appropriate services?
16. In your jurisdiction, have there been regular evaluations of the effects of public health services on community health status?
17. In the past three years in your jurisdiction, has the local public health agency used professionally recognized process and outcome measures to monitor programs and to redirect resources as appropriate?
18. In your jurisdiction, is the public regularly provided with information about current health status, health care needs, positive health behaviors, and health care policy issues?
19. In the past year in your jurisdiction, has the local public health agency provided reports to the media on a regular basis?
20. In the past three years in your jurisdiction, has there been an instance in which the local public health agency has failed to implement a mandated program or service?

Source: Reprinted from B.J. Turnock, A.S. Handler, and C.A. Miller, Core Function-Related Local Public Health Practice Effectiveness, *Journal of Public Health Management and Practice,* Vol. 4, No. 5, pp. 26–32, © 1998, Aspen Publishers, Inc.

limits their ability to allocate scarce human and financial capital to assessment initiatives. Funding streams for public health organizations are often limited and inflexible—particularly when they consist primarily of governmental appropriations, categorical grant programs, and charitable contributions. Nonetheless, public health organizations must secure an initial supply of human and financial resources that is sufficient to launch the assessment effort. A large and per-

Table 11–1 Average Public Health Performance Scores for Local Public Health Jurisdictions Serving Populations of at Least 100,000 Residents: United States, 1998

		Performance Scores			
Indicator	*N*	*Community Performance*	*Adequacy of Community Performance**	*Health Dept. Contribution*†*	*Health Dept. Contribution as % of Community Performance*†*
1 Needs assessment	335	73%	36%	21%	58
2 Behavioral risk factor survey	331	47%	22%	11%	52
3 Adverse health events investig.	336	99%	75%	57%	76
4 Laboratory services	336	96%	73%	37%	50
5 Analysis of health determinants	333	63%	30%	16%	54
6 Participation in preventive serv.	333	29%	13%	8%	61
7 Support and communication	333	79%	43%	21%	48
8 Inform elected officials	335	82%	38%	29%	77
9 Prioritization of health needs	335	67%	35%	21%	61
10 Implementation of initiatives	333	83%	35%	21%	61
11 Community action plan	333	42%	16%	9%	54
12 Plans to allocate resources	335	27%	11%	7%	63
13 Resources for priority needs	333	50%	19%	10%	54
14 Self-assessment	333	57%	32%	29%	89
15 Provision/linkage of services	332	76%	36%	19%	51
16 Evaluation of services	333	35%	16%	12%	71
17 Process/outcome measures	331	47%	22%	16%	75
18 Public information	334	76%	33%	20%	61
19 Media information	335	76%	40%	31%	78
20 Mandated program/services	323	92%	92%	92%	100
Assessment (#1–#6)	336	67%	41%	25%	60
Policy development (#7–#12)	336	63%	29%	18%	61
Assurance (#13–#20)	336	63%	36%	28%	78
Total score	335	64%	35%	24%	67

Note: Performance scores represent the proportion of communities/departments that perform the selected public health activity.
*Scores adjusted for perceived adequacy of performance (five-point scale)
†Scores adjusted for proportion of effort contributed by the local health department (five-point scale)

manent funding stream is not essential because successful assessment efforts often become self-sustaining once early successes lead to resource reallocation and an expanding base of support from core organizational resources. Start-up resources, however, are essential, and may need to be pieced together from multiple sources such as demonstration grants issued by local foundations, volunteer labor, and in-kind donations from local health care organizations.

Achieving Institutional Flexibility and Control

Second, governmental public health agencies often function under stringent operational re-

Exhibit 11–3 National Public Health Performance Standards Program Criteria for Local Community Health Assessment Profiling

Definition:

A community health profile (CHP) is a comprehensive compilation of measures within multiple categories, or domains, that describe health status at a community level and the resources available to address health needs.

Model Community Standard:

The local public health system (LPHS) compiles and maintains a comprehensive community health profile (CHP). The CHP includes measures within multiple domains that research has suggested are related to health status at both the individual and community levels. These domains include: Community assets and quality of life; Environmental health characteristics; Demographic characteristics; Socioeconomic characteristics; Community health status; Maternal and child health measures; Behavioral risk factors; Sentinel events; Social and mental health measures; Infectious disease measures; and Health resource measures.

The CHP is the vehicle by which trends in health status, along with correlated risk factors and resource consumption, are tracked over time and compared with local peers and referenced to PHS levels and/or benchmarks. Such data and information are displayed in formats that can be readily understood by diverse audiences, such as the media and community-based organizations. The LPHS promotes the communitywide use of the CHP and ensures that the CHP (both the total profile and any "fact sheet" summaries) can be easily accessed in a timely manner by the community.

The CHP provides a common set of measures to drive the prioritization of community health issues and resource allocation decisions by LPHS partners and to monitor population-based health status improvement over time.

Source: Public Health Practice Program Office, *National Public Health Performance Standards Program, Local Instrument,* 1999, Centers for Disease Control and Prevention.

quirements concerning such activities as personnel management, purchasing, and contracting. As a result, these organizations seldom have full and immediate control over their own operational processes. Launching an effective public health assessment effort, then, may require more administrative flexibility than is typically available to governmental public health organizations. Several managerial strategies may be effective in addressing this constraint. For example, public health agencies may collaborate with private organizations that have fewer administrative constraints, and allow these private partners to assume responsibility for those assessment activities that are difficult for a public agency to initiate and maintain. Alternatively, public health agencies may cultivate sufficient political support for their assessment efforts in order to secure exemptions from administrative requirements—at least on a temporary demonstration basis. Finally, public health agencies may seek changes in their organizational structures in order to facilitate the conduct of assessment activities. As an extreme example, the public health agency and hospital system in Denver, Colorado, successfully achieved local and state approval to convert from a county agency to an independent health care authority chartered by the state government.[2] This change substantially enhanced the agency's ability to undertake a variety of assessment and quality improvement efforts.

Managing Activities across Organizational Boundaries

Implementation of public health assessment processes may be complicated by the fact that public health processes and outcomes are inherently multiorganizational in nature, with no single institution within the community able to monitor and respond to population health needs and outcomes. To be effective in improving health at the population level, assessment methods and improvement strategies often must be implemented across organizational boundaries—a daunting task for many public health organizations. Nonetheless, multiorganizational efforts for public health assessment and improvement have become increasingly common in recent years, fueled in part by marketplace and policy developments that have created shared incentives for improving health at the population level.[64,66] These developments have also created new opportunities for using assessment methods as part of multiorganizational public health partnerships. To capitalize on these opportunities, public health organizations must actively pursue strategies for building effective interorganizational relationships around assessment processes. Key elements of such a strategy include

- identifying major internal and external stakeholders that have influence over the public health issues to be addressed through the assessment process
- facilitating shared interests in assessment among multiple community organizations
- anticipating the participation constraints faced by key stakeholders and designing appropriate incentives to ensure full participation in the assessment process
- implementing effective mechanisms of communication and information sharing across organizations
- developing multi-institutional consensus about the design and operation of the assessment process, including measurement strategies and decision-making and priority-setting mechanisms
- ensuring appropriate collection and analysis of objective and subjective data measured from multiple institutional perspectives
- communicating data effectively to all stakeholders using language and concepts understandable to all
- ensuring an adequate voice for all stakeholders in priority-setting activities
- developing effective mechanisms for addressing dissenting views and perspectives
- developing consensus around collective actions that can be taken to address shared assessment interests

Responding to External Pressures for Assessment

A final reason for the limited uptake of assessment and improvement processes by public health organizations has been the lack of sufficient external pressure to do so. Public health organizations historically have not faced significant external pressures from competitors, consumers, purchasers, and regulators to improve quality and efficiency in service delivery. Increasingly, public health organizations are no longer protected from these market and policy forces. Many agencies now face an environment in which they must actively compete for patients, negotiate relationships with managed care plans and other private health care organizations, and demonstrate accountability for the public funds they receive from local, state, and federal sources. In this environment, growing numbers of public health organizations turn to assessment and improvement processes for insight on how best to reposition their institutions within an evolving health system.

Case Study: Public Health Assessment Efforts in North Carolina[67]

Several recent public health assessment efforts conducted in North Carolina offer insight regarding implementation and management strategies. Comprehensive community health assessment efforts were launched in four North Carolina counties during the 1994–97 period, each one initiated by a multiorganizational coalition consisting of the local health department, local hospitals and health care professionals, and various community organizations. All four of the counties were located in the central region of the state, and most contained a mix of rural and urbanized areas (Table 11–2). In each case, faculty and staff from a university-based school of public health served as consultants to the assessment process, providing expertise with assessment planning, data collection and analysis, and data interpretation and priority setting. Each of the assessment efforts used the same basic process of implementation, which closely mirrored the IOM model and the hospital association models described earlier.[26,27,67] The university faculty refined the assessment model in response to specific needs and concerns identified by the participants in each community. Specifically, the model was designed to

- Involve the broadest possible range of organizations and individuals in each community that have an interest in health.
- Ensure that the assessment is driven by decisions made by community members themselves, rather than by influences from outside of the community (including consultants).
- Ensure that the assessment process is highly sensitive to local issues and priorities.
- Focus on the goal of health improvement through intervention planning.

The assessment process used in each community consisted of five phases. The first phase focused on assessment planning and leadership development (Figure 11–3). During this phase, the initial assessment participants identified the range of organizations and individuals within the community that maintained interest and/or expertise in health issues, and actively recruited these stakeholders to provide leadership and guidance for the assessment process. In most communities, these stakeholders included recognized community and governmental leaders, public health officials, hospital administrators, prominent health professionals, and other key opinion leaders. A steering committee consisting of these representatives then engaged in initial planning activities for the assessment effort. Key issues addressed in the planning process included funding and fund-raising, budgeting, staffing, decision-making and management processes, and scheduling for the assessment effort.

The second phase of the assessment process was devoted to data collection and analysis. During this phase, the university consultants worked under the guidance of the steering committee to obtain a broad range of health-related data about the community, using both primary data collection strategies and secondary data acquisition (Exhibit 11–4). In each community, a sample of community residents was surveyed via telephone using random-digit dialing techniques, which produced information on self-reported health status, behavioral risk factors, use of preventive health services, and access to health care. Qualitative health data were collected by conducting interviews and focus groups with members of important professional and sociodemographic groups within the community, such as health care providers, business owners, education and social service professionals, public health clinic clients, senior citizens, teenagers, nursing home residents, emergency room patients, church members, and residents of minority and low-income neighborhoods. These primary data were supplemented by acquiring existing data from sources including national and state vital statistics systems, national and state notifiable disease reporting systems, local and

Table 11–2 Characteristics of the Communities That Implemented a Public Health Assessment Process

	County			
Characteristic	*Alamance*	*Chatham*	*Davidson*	*Orange*
Setting	Urban/rural	Rural	Urban/rural	Urban/rural
Population	113,000	39,000	133,000	106,000
Poverty rate	8.9%	9.7%	9.8%	13.9%
Percentage of high school graduates	67.9	70.0	69.2	83.6
Percentage of age 65+ years	15	15	12	9
Hospital beds	340	68	221	592
Physicians/100,000 population	122	101	62	1,254
Infant mortality rate	10.5	12.0	8.5	10.6
Employment base	Manufacturing	Government	Manufacturing	University
Year of assessment	1996–97	1996–97	1994–95	1996–97

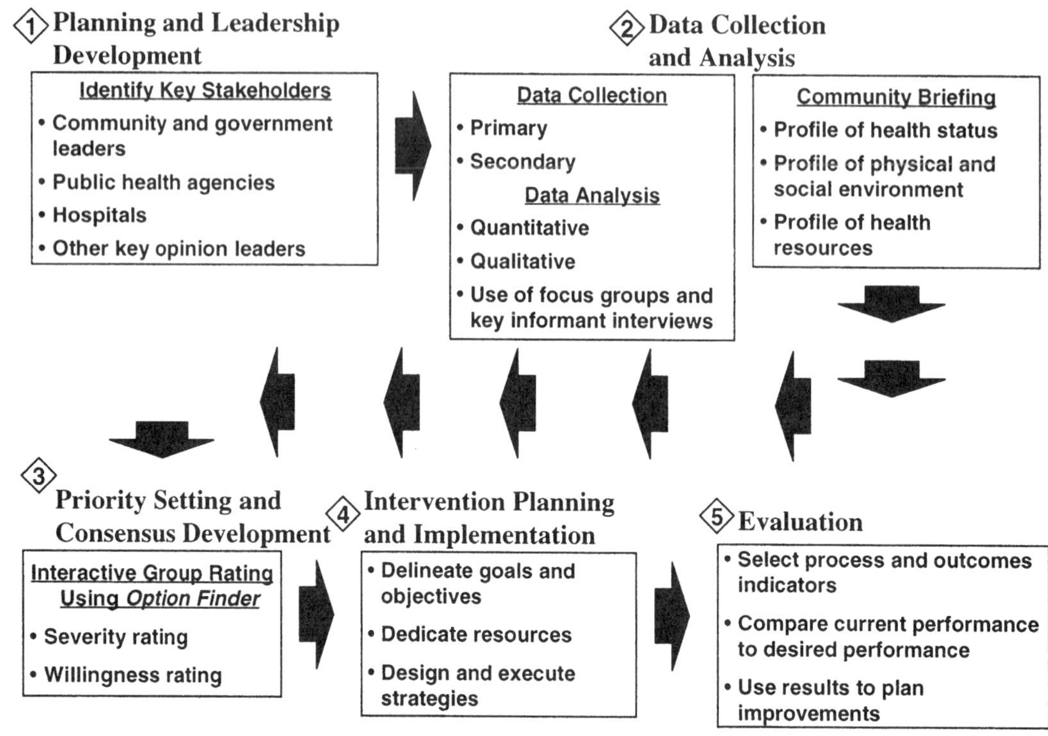

Figure 11–3 Community Health Assessment and Improvement Process Example

state public health agency surveillance systems, local hospital administrative records, and service records and annual reports from local health and social service organizations.

Data from all of these sources were analyzed and profiled in a community health status report developed by the consultants and the steering committee. Where possible, community health measures were compared with data from similar communities, state and national norms, and state and national health objectives such as the *Healthy People 2000* objectives. The report was disseminated and publicized widely within each community through the local media and community organizations. A public briefing was held in each community, during which key findings from the report were reviewed and discussed, and community opinions regarding the findings were elicited.

The third phase of the assessment process involved priority setting and consensus development around identified community health issues. During a widely publicized public forum, community members were asked to express their opinions about each of the community health issues identified in the report. A computerized polling device linked to handheld keypads was used to elicit individual, anonymous community perceptions about the relative impact and importance of each health issue, and about the willingness of community members to address the health issue through available community resources.[68] A subset of priority health issues was then identified by plotting each issue on a priority-setting grid based on average community ratings of perceived impact and perceived willingness to act (Figure 11–4). The issues that rated highly in both attributes fell within the top quadrant of the grid and were selected for further consideration. This subset of issues was then prioritized further by community members using the polling device.

Exhibit 11–5 shows the community health issues that were rated highest on impact and willingness in each community (in rank order), along with the issues that were given the highest priority for action in each community. Both similarities

Exhibit 11–4 Example Data Sources Used in a Community Health Assessment and Improvement Process

Quantitative Data		Qualitative Data
Secondary Data	***Primary Data***	***Primary Data***
• National health statistics (NCHS) • State health statistics (DEHNR) • Vital records information • Annual filings with state and federal agencies • Annual reports of major health organizations • State and local inspection reports • Strategic plans • Service records • Governing board meeting minutes • Other reports	• Survey representative sample of community residents by telephone and mail • Survey gathers data on behavioral risk factors (BRFS), access to health services, and health status	• Focus groups with key community segments: – providers – business – education – health dept. clinic patients – single mothers – seniors – nursing home residents – teenagers – churches – special populations • Key informant interviews: – physicians – dentists – emergency services – social services – mental health – health administrators

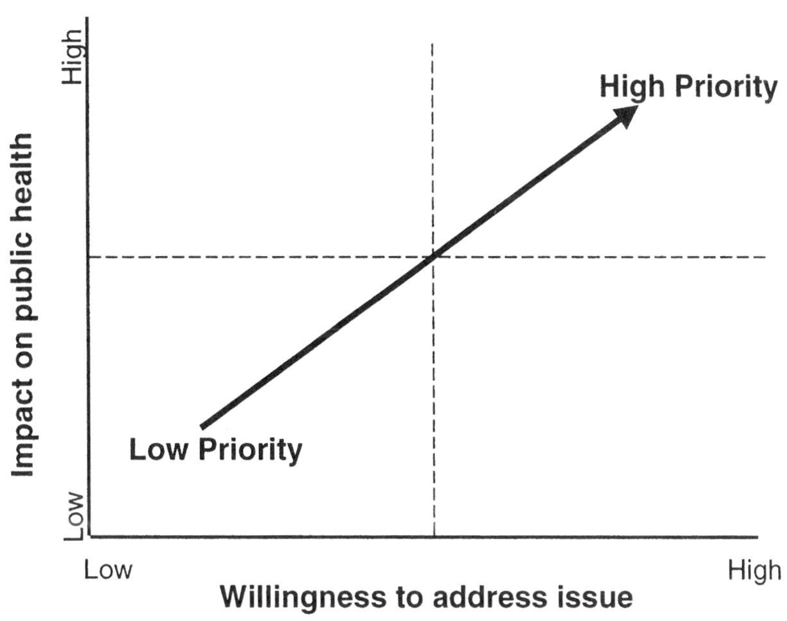

Figure 11–4 Priority-Setting Grid Example for a Community Health Assessment and Improvement Process

Exhibit 11–5 Highest-Ranking Community Health Issues in Four Community Assessment Processes

Alamance	*Chatham*	*Davidson*	*Orange*
1. Substance abuse*	1. Substance abuse*	1. Teen pregnancy*	1. Teen pregnancy*
2. Child abuse/ neglect*	2. STDs*	2. Substance abuse*	2. Preventive services*
3. Medical care cost*	3. Housing*	3. Preventive services*	3. Child abuse/ neglect*
4. Cigarette smoking*	4. Rabies	4. Infant mortality	4. Child services*
5. Awareness of services*	5. Social & recreation opportunities	5. Motor vehicle crashes	5. Substance abuse
6. AIDS education	6. Education	6. Violence	6. Health insurance
7. Mental health		7. Suicide	7. Dentist availability
		8. Transportation	8. AIDS education
		9. Health insurance	9. Parenting skills
		10. Health manpower	10. Poverty disparities
			11. Prenatal care

*Issue received priority for community action

and differences are evident in the set of issues chosen by each community forum, reflecting common health needs as well as unique priorities and values. The notable variation in community health priorities underscores the importance of using assessment methods that are responsive to community-specific needs and perceptions. The priorities identified in the four communities are not entirely consistent with objective measures of local disease burden and severity—precisely because these priorities are subject to community perceptions and willingness to act. The prioritization methods used in the communities ensure that the identified health issues are not only important from a public health perspective, but also tractable given local priorities and values. The success that is achieved in addressing priority issues can subsequently be used to mobilize community efforts around important but less tractable health problems.

The issue of tobacco use provides an interesting example of the prioritization process used in the communities. In all four counties, tobacco use was rated highly in terms of impact/importance, but only one county rated this issue highly in terms of willingness to address the issue (see Exhibit 11–5). By contrast, all four counties rated the issue of substance abuse (other than tobacco) highly in terms of both impact and willingness to act. This result may be explained by the fact that tobacco farming and/or manufacturing are key components of the local economy in the three counties that indicated a low willingness to address tobacco issues. Consequently, community members appeared reluctant to address the issue of tobacco use at the time of the assessments, given the impact it might have on local residents and given the community reactions it might engender. By focusing initially on substance abuse, however, the communities are likely to develop knowledge, skills, and relationships that will facilitate the subsequent implementation of an effective and publicly acceptable campaign against tobacco use. In this way, the assessment methods employed in these communities incorporate local capacities and priorities—both tangible and intangible—in evaluating public health needs.

The final phases of the assessment process involved planning, implementing, and evaluating community interventions to address the priority health issues. In each of the communities, these improvement-oriented activities were carried out by task forces that formed around each of the priority health issues. The task forces developed goals and objectives for improvement, researched and designed interventions based on these goals, and sought the resources necessary to implement the interventions. The task forces also designed and implemented evaluation strategies for the interventions, using both process and outcome measures of intervention performance. The interventions that were implemented varied widely both within and between communities, ranging from public education campaigns about health risks, to expanded public health clinic hours and services, to new community programs for adolescents. In all four communities, tangible public health interventions were implemented in response to the assessment process. In most cases, these interventions and their evaluation strategies were integrated with existing organizations and programs in the community in order to ensure the long-term stability and survival of the interventions. In one community, however, a new community organization was formed to oversee and coordinate ongoing activities in assessment, intervention, and evaluation. These alternative strategies target the most difficult task of the public health assessment process—that of responding effectively to identified public health needs and priorities.

Public health assessment and improvement efforts ideally become ongoing processes in which achievements in one area motivate new initiatives in other areas. The communities examined here all experienced early successes in their assessment efforts, but the long-term viability and effectiveness of these efforts remains to be seen. The obstacles encountered in implementing the assessment efforts were numerous and varied—many of which were specific to local organizational and community contexts. Nonetheless, several tasks involved in the assessment process posed challenges that were common across the four communities, and therefore warrant special attention. These tasks include the following:

- ensuring the participation of community leaders and stakeholders who are often overly committed to other tasks
- securing representation from disadvantaged and vulnerable population groups
- processing and prioritizing large volumes of diverse health information
- developing action plans to address issues that are not fully within the control of the public health system

In overcoming these challenges, participants involved in the assessment efforts attributed their successes to a number of factors, including

- innovative presentation of data in reports and public forums
- rigorous recruitment efforts for securing participants in priority-setting process
- strong linkages between data analysis and the priority-setting process
- careful consensus development processes for identifying priorities, including a mix of high-technology methods and practical, low-technology approaches

• • •

The assessment model examined in this chapter by no means represents a gold standard approach for identifying and responding to population health needs. Many different tools and models exist for carrying out this vital activity, each offering unique benefits and limitations. The challenge for public health administrators lies in developing and managing an assessment process that fits the unique capacities and needs within the communities served. An ideal assessment process, therefore, must be tailored to the specific organizations and populations involved. Only through such a process can public health organizations acquire the information and insight necessary for achieving meaningful improvements in population health.

CHAPTER REVIEW

1. Assessment is typically defined as the regular and systematic collection, analysis, and dissemination of information on the health of a community, which enables community health needs to be identified. Assessment processes may involve a variety of specific activities, including
   - *identifying* health needs in the community and among important population groups
   - *investigating* the occurrence of health effects and health hazards in the community
   - *analyzing* the determinants of identified health needs in a community or population group
2. Some assessment activities are carried out internally within public health organizations, whereas others are designed to include participation and decision making from multiple organizations serving a population of interest. In choosing the appropriate focus for an assessment effort, public health organizations must consider
   - the nature of the public health problem being targeted
   - the internal strengths and weaknesses of their organization
   - the current and potential roles played by external organizations and individuals in the problem under study
   - the public health organization's current and potential relationships with these external entities
3. Public health organizations may play various roles in an assessment process, including those of *initiating* the process, *convening* major stakeholders, *governing* and managing the process, *participating* in joint management and oversight, and/or *contributing* resources and expertise to an externally managed process.
4. A variety of administrative tools and processes may facilitate the conduct of public health assessment activities. These elements include
   - community planning and priority-setting tools
   - community health report cards
   - public health practice guidelines and standards
   - public health information networks
   - performance-based contracting systems
   - public health performance measurement systems
5. Several factors have been found to be important to the successful development and management of public health assessment activities, including
   - involving the broadest possible range of organizations and individuals in each community that have an interest in the problem under study
   - ensuring that the assessment process is driven by decisions made by community members themselves, rather than by influences from outside the community (including consultants)
   - ensuring that the assessment process is highly sensitive to local issues and priorities
   - focusing the assessment effort on the goal health improvement through intervention planning

REFERENCES

1. G.P. Mays et al., "Performing Essential Public Health Services in the Nation's Most Populous Communities: Who Contributes?" (Center for Public Health Practice Working Paper, School of Public Health, The University of North Carolina at Chapel Hill, 1999).
2. G.P. Mays et al., *Local Public Health Practice: Trends and Models* (Washington, DC: American Public Health Association, 2000).
3. Institute of Medicine, *The Future of Public Health* (Washington, DC: National Academy Press, 1988).
4. W.W. Dyall, "Ten Organizational Practices of Public Health: A Historical Perspective," *American Journal of Preventive Medicine* 11 (1995): 6–8.
5. C.A. Miller et al., "A Proposed Method for Assessing Public Health Functions and Practices," *American Journal of Public Health 84,* no. 1 (1994): 1,743–1,749.

6. B.J. Turnock et al., "Local Health Department Effectiveness in Addressing the Core Functions of Public Health," *Public Health Reports 109,* no. 5 (1994): 653–658.
7. E.L. Baker et al., "Health Reform and the Health of the Public: Forging Community Health Partnerships," *Journal of the American Medical Association* 272 (1994): 1,276–1,282.
8. K.W. Eilbert et al., "Public Health Expenditures: Developing Estimates for Improved Policy-Making," *Journal of Public Health Management and Practice 3,* no. 3 (1997): 1–9.
9. G.P. Mays et al., "Assessing the Performance of Local Public Health Systems: A Survey of State Health Agency Efforts," *Journal of Public Health Management and Practice 4,* no. 4 (1998): 63–78.
10. D.J. Lipson and N. Naierman, "Snapshots of Change in Fifteen Communities: Safety-Net Providers," *Health Affairs 15,* no. 2 (1996): 33–48.
11. D.L. Speake et al., "Integrating Indicators into a Public Health Quality Improvement System," *American Journal of Public Health 85,* no. 10 (1995): 1,448–1,449.
12. U.S. Environmental Protection Agency, *The Changing Nature of Environmental and Public Health Protection: An Annual Report on Reinvention* (Washington, DC: U.S. Government Printing Office, 1998).
13. J.E. Fielding et al., "Community Health Report Cards: Results of a National Survey," *American Journal of Preventive Medicine 17,* no. 1 (1999): 79–86.
14. R.B. Gerzoff, "Comparisons: The Basis for Measuring Public Health Performance," *Journal of Public Health Management and Practice 3,* no. 5 (1997): 11–21.
15. U.S. Department of Health and Human Services, *Healthy People 2010: Conference Edition* (Washington, DC: U.S. Government Printing Office, 2000).
16. U.S. Department of Health, Education, and Welfare, *Healthy People: The Surgeon General's Report on Health Promotion and Disease Prevention* (Washington, DC: U.S. Government Printing Office, 1977).
17. U.S. Department of Health and Human Services, *Healthy People 2000: National Health Promotion and Disease Prevention Objectives* (Washington, DC: U.S. Government Printing Office, 1991).
18. L.W. Greene, "PATCH: CDC's Planned Approach to Community Health, an Application of PRECEED and an Inspiration for PROCEED," *Journal of Health Education 23,* no. 3 (1992): 140–147.
19. American Public Health Association, *Healthy Communities 2000: Model Standards* (Washington, DC: 1991).
20. American Public Health Association, *The Guide to Implementing Model Standards: Eleven Steps Toward a Healthy Community* (Washington, DC: 1993).
21. S.R. Griffin and P. Welch, "Performance-Based Public Health in Texas," *Journal of Public Health Management and Practice 1,* no. 3 (1995): 44–49.
22. National Association of County and City Health Officials, *Assessment Protocol for Excellence in Public Health (APEXPH)* (Washington, DC: 1991).
23. National Association of County and City Health Officials, "Assessment and Planning Excellence through Community Partners for Health." http://www.naccho.org/project49.htm. Accessed 22 March 2000.
24. L. Bartlett et al., *Assessing Roles, Responsibilities, and Activities in a Managed Care Environment: A Workbook for Local Health Officials* (Washington, DC: U.S. Department of Health and Human Services, 1997).
25. R.L. Gordon et al., "Prevention and the Reforming U.S. Health System: Changing Roles and Responsibilities for Public Health," *Annual Review of Public Health* 17 (1996): 489–509.
26. The Hospital Association of Pennsylvania, *A Guide for Assessing and Improving Health Status* (Harrisburg, PA: 1993).
27. Committee on Using Performance Monitoring To Improve Community Health, Institute of Medicine, *Improving Health in the Community: A Role for Performance Monitoring* (Washington, DC: National Academy Press, 1997).
28. E.B. Perrin and J.J. Koshel, eds., *Assessment of Performance Measures for Public Health, Substance Abuse, and Mental Health* (Washington, DC: National Academy Press, 1997).
29. National Center for Health Statistics, "Consensus Set of Health Status Indicators for the General Assessment of Community Health Status—United States," *Morbidity and Mortality Weekly Report 40,* no. 27 (1991): 449–451.
30. U.S. Preventive Services Task Force, *Guide to Clinical Preventive Services: An Assessment of the Effectiveness of 169 Interventions* (Baltimore, MD: Williams & Wilkins, 1989).
31. M. Pappaioanou and C. Evans, "Development of the *Guide to Community Preventive Services:* A U.S. Public Health Service Initiative," *Journal of Public Health Management and Practice 4,* no. 2 (1998): 48–54.
32. P.M. Simone, "Essential Components of a Tuberculosis Prevention and Control Program: Recommendations of the Advisory Council for the Elimination of Tuberculosis," *Morbidity and Mortality Weekly Report 44,* no. RR-11 (1995): 1–16.
33. R. Patel and L. Kinginger, "Childhood Immunizations: American College of Preventive Medicine Practice Policy," *American Journal of Preventive Medicine 13,* no. 2 (1997): 74–77.
34. R. Ferrini, "Screening Asymptomatic Women for Ovarian Cancer: American College of Preventive Medicine Practice Policy," *American Journal of Preventive Medicine 13,* no. 6 (1997): 444–446.
35. P.K. Halverson et al., *Managed Care and Public Health* (Gaithersburg, MD: Aspen Publishers, Inc., 1997).

36. P.K. Halverson et al., "Managed Care and the Public Health Challenge of TB," *Public Health Reports 112,* no. 1 (1997): 22–28.
37. G.P. Mays et al., "Collaboration To Improve Community Health: Trends and Alternative Models," *Joint Commission Journal on Quality Improvement in Health Care 24,* no. 10 (1998): 518–540.
38. S. Auerbach, "Report Cards Found To Improve Health Care," *Washington Post*, 6 January 1998, A08.
39. D.R. Longo et al., "Consumer Reports in Health Care: Do They Make a Difference in Patient Care?" *Journal of the American Medical Association* 278 (1997): 1,579–1,584.
40. M.R. Chassin et al., "Benefits and Hazards of Reporting Medical Outcomes Publicly," *New England Journal of Medicine 334,* no. 6 (1996): 394–398.
41. "Health Care Report Cards," *New York Times,* 10 July 1995, A12.
42. National Committee on Quality Assurance, *Report Card Pilot Project* (Washington, DC: 1995).
43. U.S. General Accounting Office, *Report Cards Are Useful but Significant Issues Need To Be Addressed* (Washington, DC: 1994).
44. Pennsylvania Health Care Cost Containment Council, *A Consumer Guide to Coronary Artery Bypass Graft Surgery: Pennsylvania's Declaration of Health Care Information* (Harrisburg, PA: 1991).
45. J.E. Fielding and N. Halfon, "Characteristics of Community Report Cards—United States, 1996," *Morbidity and Mortality Weekly Report 46,* no. 28 (1997): 647–655.
46. U.S. Agency for Toxic Substances and Disease Registry, *ATSDR Public Health Assessment Guidance Manual* (Boca Raton, FL: Lewis Publishers, 1992).
47. G.P. Mays et al., "Developing a Model Report Card of Community Health: A Proposed Methodology?" (Center for Public Health Practice Working Paper, School of Public Health, The University of North Carolina at Chapel Hill, 1999).
48. U.S. General Accounting Office, *Performance Budgeting: Past Initiatives Offer Insights for GPRA* (Washington, DC: 1997).
49. D.E. Nelson et al., "Outcome-Based Management and Public Health: The Oregon Benchmarks Experience," *Journal of Public Health Management and Practice 1,* no. 2 (1995): 8–17.
50. Washington State Department of Health, *Public Health Improvement Plan: A Blueprint for Action* (Olympia, WA: 1996).
51. B.J. Turnock and A. Handler, "Is Public Health Ready for Reform? The Case for Accrediting Local Health Departments," *Journal of Public Health Management and Practice 2,* no. 3 (1996): 41–45.
52. C.A. Miller et al., "Flexibility in Measurement of Public Health Performance [editorial]," *Journal of Public Health Management and Practice 3*, no. 5 (1997): 1–2.
53. G.P. Mays et al., "Identifying Indicators for a National Community Health Report Card," *Prevention 98 Meeting Abstracts* (Washington, DC: American College of Preventive Medicine, 1998), 75.
54. P.K. Halverson and G.P. Mays, "Disease Management: A Public Health Perspective," in *A Health Care Professional's Guide to Disease Management*, ed. J.B. Couch (Gaithersburg, MD: Aspen Publishers, Inc., 1998), 29–51.
55. E.H. Vaughn et al., "An Information Manager for the *Assessment Protocol for Excellence in Public Health,*" *Public Health Nursing 11,* no. 6 (1994): 399–405.
56. Epidemiology, Planning, and Evaluation Unit, Seattle-King County Department of Public Health, *Vista/PH Software for Public Health Assessment: User's Guide* (Seattle, WA: Seattle-King County Department of Public Health, 1995).
57. D.N. Mendelson and E.M. Salinsky, "Health Information Systems and the Role of State Government," *Health Affairs 16,* no. 3 (1997): 106–119.
58. P.K. Halverson et al., "Privatizing Health Services: Alternative Models and Emerging Issues for Public Health and Quality Management," *Quality Management in Health Care 5,* no. 2 (1997): 1–18.
59. S.R. Keener et al., "Providing Public Health Services through an Integrated Delivery System," *Quality Management in Health Care 5,* no. 2 (1997): 27–34.
60. G.P. Mays et al., "Continuous Quality Improvement in Public Health Organizations," in *Continuous Quality Improvement in Health Care: Theory, Implementation, and Applications,* 2nd ed., eds. C.P. McLaughlin and A.D. Kaluzny (Gaithersburg, MD: Aspen Publishers, Inc., 1999), 360–403.
61. C.A. Miller et al., "A Screening Survey To Assess Local Public Health Performance," *Public Health Reports* 109 (1994): 659–664.
62. K. Eilbert et al., *Measuring Expenditures for Core Public Health Functions* (Washington, DC: Public Health Foundation, 1996).
63. H.A. Grason and B. Guyer, *Public MCH Program Functions: Essential Public Health Services To Promote Maternal and Child Health in America* (Baltimore, MD: The Johns Hopkins University School of Hygiene and Public Health, 1995).
64. Institute of Medicine, *Healthy Communities: New Partnerships for the Future of Public Health* (Washington, DC: National Academy Press, 1996).
65. F.D. Scutchfield et al., "The Presence of Total Quality Management and Continuous Quality Improvement Processes in California Public Health Clinics," *Journal*

of Public Health Management and Practice 3, no. 3 (1997): 57–60.

66. R. Lasker, *Medicine and Public Health: The Power of Collaboration* (New York: New York Academy of Medicine, 1997).
67. T.A. Hatzell et al., "Beyond Assessment: Achieving Community Health Improvement through Local Partnerships [abstract]." *Proceedings of the 1997 Joint Meeting of the Public Health Conference on Records and Statistics and the NCHS Data Users Conference* (Washington, DC: U.S. Government Printing Office, 1997), P27.
68. Option Technologies Interactive, *The OptionFinder* (Ogden, UT: Option Technologies, 1997).

Chapter 12

Public Health Education and Health Promotion

Judith M. Ottoson
Lawrence W. Green

Public health organizations use health education strategies to facilitate voluntary adaptations of behavior that are conducive to health. Health education influences current behavior such as participation in health-promoting activities, appropriate use of health services, health supervision of children, and adherence to appropriate medical and nutritional regimens. *Health promotion* encompasses a broader set of educational, organizational, environmental, and economic interventions to support behavior and conditions of living that are conducive to health. Designing and managing successful health education and health promotion interventions require strong institutional capacities in applied behavioral science, community assessment, and program administration.

Behavior, environment, human biology, and community organization interact to shape the health of populations. Various scientific and professional subspecialties have emerged within the core disciplines of public health to address these complex interactions. These subspecialties include environmental epidemiology, behavioral ecology, behavioral medicine, health psychology, social medicine, medical geography, and social epidemiology. Application of the scientific knowledge and technologies developed within these public health subspecialties falls largely to community health workers, especially through the vehicle of health education. Public health education employs a combination of methods designed to facilitate voluntary adaptations of behavior that are conducive to health. It too has subspecialties such as patient education, school health education, population education, environmental education, sex education, nutri-

---

Acknowledgment: The health education planning model presented in the first part of this chapter is referred to as PRECEDE (predisposing, reinforcing, and enabling constructs in educational diagnosis and evaluation), based on L.W. Green, "Toward Cost–Benefit Evaluations of Health Education: Some Concepts, Methods, and Examples," *Health Education Quarterly* 2 (suppl. 1) (1974): 34. The health promotion model described in the second part is an elaboration called PRECEDE-PROCEED, combining health education with policy, regulation, and organization for educational and environmental development (PROCEED). See L.W. Green and M.W. Kreuter, *Health Promotion Planning: An Educational and Ecological Approach*, 3d ed. (Mountain View, CA: Mayfield, 1999). Much of this chapter's rendition of the model and the fields of health education and health promotion is based on L.W. Green and J.M. Ottoson, *Community and Population Health,* 8th ed. (NY: McGraw-Hill, 1999), Chapters 4 and 12, with permission of the publisher. Most of the references in the bibliography are applications of the model, among the 850 or so published applications that can be found in the periodically updated bibliography at http://www.lgreen.net. The two textbooks provide examples of applications to other health problems in clinical, school, workplace, and other community settings.

tion education, dental health education, mental health education, and occupational health education.[1] The broader efforts of community or population health promotion may go beyond voluntary changes in behavior. These efforts may include regulatory and environmental control strategies designed to channel, restrain, or support behavior that is conducive to health or quality of life for the person, the community, or a population.[2] Nonetheless, health education strategies are a core element of most health promotion efforts that target communities and population groups.

This chapter examines the health education and health promotion strategies used by public health organizations to improve community health. The first part of this chapter focuses specifically on the design and management of health education approaches directed at voluntary changes in behavior. The second part of the chapter examines linkages between health education strategies and the larger field of health promotion, with attention given to policy, regulatory, organizational, and environmental factors that enable health education strategies to achieve health promotion goals.

PUBLIC HEALTH EDUCATION

Community and population health education interventions are designed to elicit, facilitate, and maintain positive health practices in large numbers of people. The practices in question may be those of individuals whose health is at risk, or those whose behavior influences the health risks faced by other individuals and populations, such as through exposures to environmental threats. *Elicit, facilitate,* and *maintain* refer to the processes of change supported by increasing the understanding, skills, and support that motivate individuals to undertake voluntary actions conducive to their health. They reflect the efforts of health education to affect factors that predispose, enable, or reinforce behavior that is related to health. For purposes of this chapter, health education is defined as any combination of learning opportunities that are designed to facilitate voluntary adaptations of behavior that are conducive to health.

Health education addresses current behavior such as the participation in health-promoting activites, appropriate use of health services, health supervision of children, and adherence to appropriate medical and nutritional regimens. Health education also addresses issues in child and youth development that create the cognitive and behavioral foundation for future health. Within their families and with peers at school, children form predispositions—knowledge, attitudes, and values—that can prevent or promote many of the health problems associated with later adult life. Good planning in health education ensures that programs combine these channels of influence appropriately to support voluntary patterns of behavior that are conducive to health.

A Focus on Health Behavior

Human behavior relates to health in both direct and indirect ways, as shown in Figure 12–1. The direct effect of personal and social behavior on health (arrow *a*) occurs when behavior exposes an individual, group, or population to more or less risk of injury, disease, or death. Sometimes, the exposure is subtle, as with small but repeated doses of a substance that may become addictive or cumulative in their effect. Drugs and fatty food are examples of this type of exposure. At other times, behavior may pose an immediate and excessive risk, such as eating a poisonous or infected food. Acute risks to health in food production, distribution, advertising, and

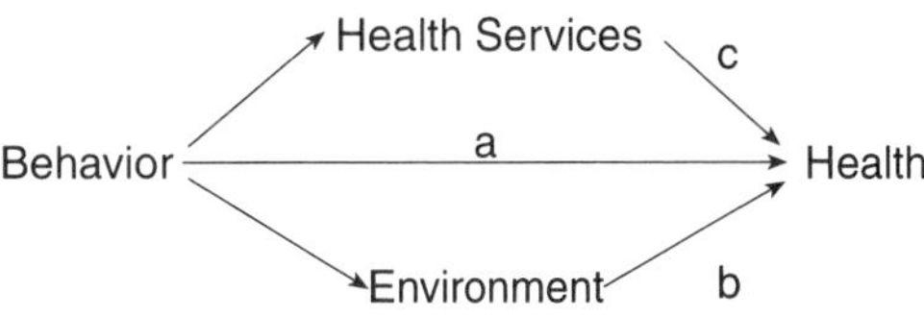

Figure 12–1 Behavior of lifestyle can have a direct effect (**a**) on health or an indirect effect on health through exposure to the environment (**b**) or on the use of health services (**c**). *Source:* Reprinted with permission from L.W. Green and M.W. Kreuter, *Health Promotion Planning: An Educational and Ecological Approach,* 3rd ed., p. 116, © 1999, Mayfield Publishing Co.

consumption have been minimized in the social history of health by the environmental and regulatory controls that are administered by public health agencies.

Behavior influences health indirectly through the environment (arrow *b*) to the degree that people will plan individual or community actions to bring about changes in the environment. Examples of behavioral influences on health through environment include

- participating in efforts to control toxic waste disposal
- organizing a lead paint removal program in the neighborhood
- voting on referenda or for elected officials in support of community water fluoridation
- advocating drunk driving laws or other automobile safety provisions
- writing letters to the editor concerning food and drug labeling
- signing a petition on air and water pollution controls
- boycotting stores that sell cigarettes to minors

Behavior also influences health indirectly through health services (arrow *c*). This can happen in at least three ways. Individuals, groups, or organizations can

- Influence the distribution and delivery of services through action in the legislative and health planning process.
- Use (or not use) available services in a timely and appropriate way.
- Follow (or fail to follow) the medical or preventive regimens prescribed by their health service providers.

Voluntary Behavior

Health education assumes that beneficial, voluntary health behavior in both children and adults results from a combination of planned, consistent, integrated learning opportunities. To achieve these ends, community or population health education systematically applies theories and methods from the social and behavioral sciences, epidemiology, ecology, administrative science, and communications. These approaches are informed by scientific evaluations of health education programs in schools, at worksites, in medical settings, and through the mass media. Further, indirect evidence is borrowed from experiences outside of the fields of health and education. Community development, agricultural extension, social work, marketing, and other enterprises in human services and behavior change all contribute to the understanding of planned change at the community level and in other populations.

Planned learning experiences to influence voluntary changes in behavior, as distinct from *incidental* learning experiences, link the educational approach to community and population health. Health education is also distinguished from other change strategies that may be excessively permissive, regulatory, or coercive. Behavioral changes resulting from education are by definition voluntary and freely adopted by people, with their knowledge of alternatives and probable consequences. Some behavioral change strategies may have unethical components. Behavior modification techniques, for example, qualify as health education only when people freely request them to achieve a specific behavioral result, such as controlling eating or smoking habits, that they desire. Principles of planning for community health education call for the participation of consumers, patients, or citizens in the planning process.

Mass media qualify as educational channels for community or population health up to the point that commercial or political interests control the media strictly for profit or propaganda. The regulation of advertisers and the media may be necessary as a more coercive, economic, or legalistic strategy to protect consumers from, for example, deceptive advertising claims concerning the health value of food products. Such was the case when communities took action to restrict the advertising of certain foods and toys on Saturday morning television programs directed at young children. Several countries restrict the advertising of tobacco and alcohol in the mass media. Third World nations took action to restrict the marketing of powdered milk formula for bottle feeding of babies because it was leading the public to use unsanitary water and bottles in place of breast feeding.

Planning for Public Health Education Programs

To achieve sound health education programming and effectiveness, public health organizations required an informed and comprehensive planning process.[3] An understanding of the stages and components of health education planning is therefore requisite for public health administrators. The PRECEDE model on which planning phases discussed here are based has been applied in more than 850 published applications. These include, for example, applications in community diabetes and arthritis self-management in native populations; breast and cervical cancer screening in low-income populations and in rural populations; encouraging bicycle helmet use among children; reaching mothers of preschool-aged children with a smoking cessation program; prevention of diarrhea infant mortality in rural Mexico; prevention of heart disease in Fabreville and Montreal, Quebec; parent education for self-management of cystic fibrosis and asthma; a nutrition program for low-income mothers of preschool children, and for Vietnamese mothers; and increasing Medicaid child health screenings.[4–18]

Phases of Planning for Public Health Education

An educational plan for community health or population health ideally begins with an analysis of social issues or quality-of-life concerns.

- Phase 1 begins with a social assessment (Figure 12–2, *bottom*) of the ultimate community concerns or outcomes and the social assets they have or need, rather than with an administrative assessment to choose educational interventions (Figure 12–2, *top*).
- Phase 2 is an epidemiologic assessment to identify the incidence, prevalence, and cause of the health problems associated with the quality-of-life concerns in a given population.
- Phase 3 is a behavioral analysis of the priority health problem to determine specific behaviors causing it.
- Phase 4 is a further analysis of the factors influencing each behavior implicated in the cause of each health problem. Health education based more on favorite techniques than on systematic analysis of behavior and of the learning problems influencing the behavior will tend to be inefficient if not ineffective.
- Phase 5 involves matching behavioral priorities with adequate methods. Indeed, administrative decisions concerning the best match of behavioral priorities and adequate methods and materials depend on the accuracy of the preceding phases in problem assessment.

Social Assessment. The ideal starting point in planning is an assessment of the social concerns and assets of the community or population. Starting with social or quality-of-life issues rather than with health problems ensures that the health planners appreciate the broader context of issues that are paramount in the community. This step requires an understanding of the subjective concerns and values of the community, as well as objective data on social indicators such as unemployment, housing problems, teenage pregnancy, violence, and poverty. Consideration of varying community perceptions should take place early in program development. Health programs are not likely to be successful without community support and participation in the planning process.

Epidemiologic Assessment. The social concern or quality-of-life issues in the community or population can be analyzed for priority health problems embedded within them. Once the priority health problem is analyzed, addressing and solving that problem becomes the overall program goal for a community health or population health program. The agency sponsoring the program should use the most recent available demographic, vital, and sociocultural statistics to define the characteristics of the subpopulations experiencing the health problem. Planners can review the problem from the perspective of related agencies, a review of previously published reports, and the U.S. Health and Human Services objectives for the nation.[19] They can gain

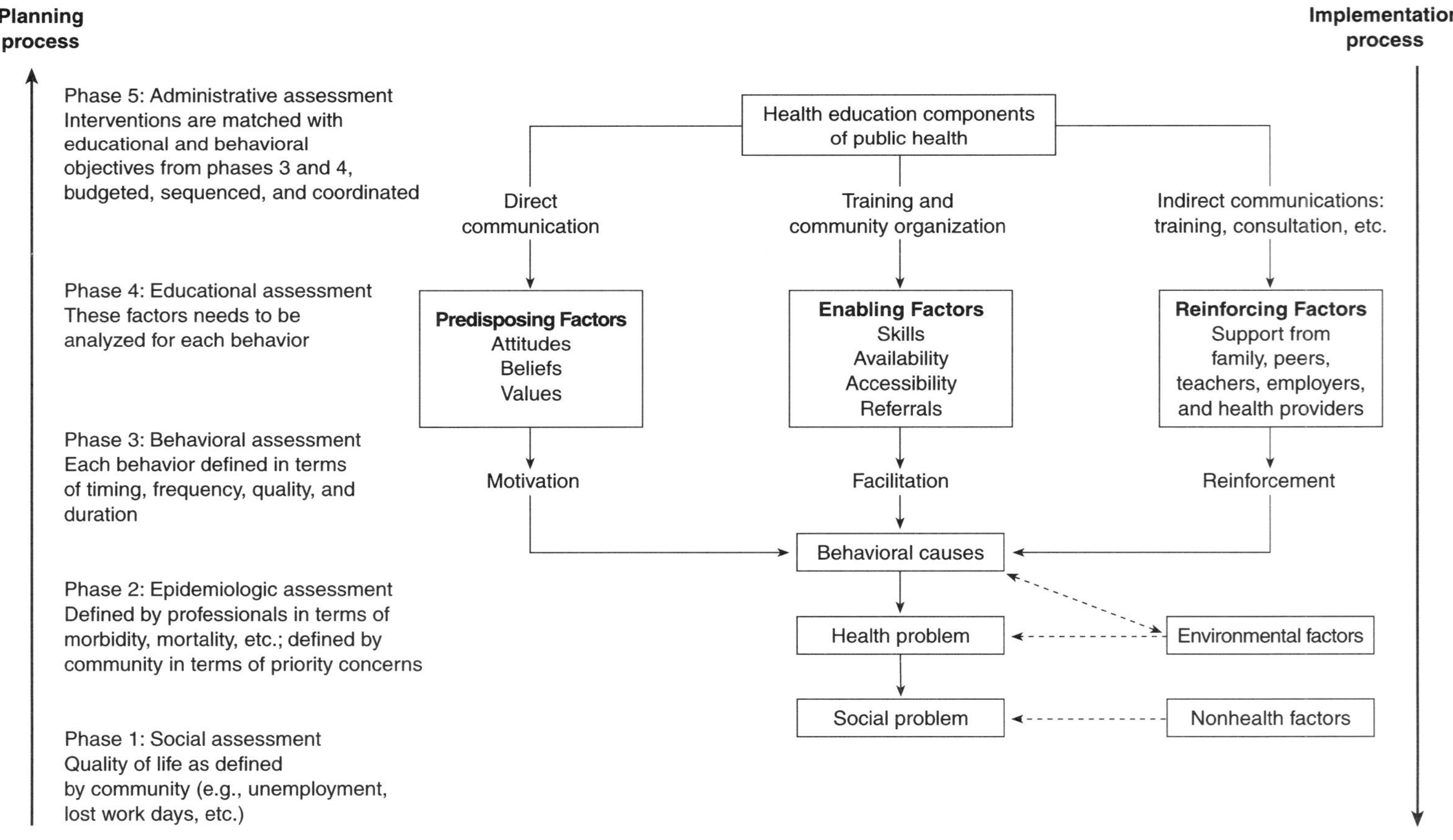

Figure 12–2 The PRECEDE model for health education begins the planning process at the end of a presumed causal chain (bottom left) with social assessment. Subsequent phases work "backward" through the causal links to the development of a health intervention. Evaluation criteria are embedded in each of these phases as objectives. The implementation process reverses the planning process by working from the educational program toward amelioration of the health problem and toward quality-of-life concerns. *Source:* Reprinted with permission from L.W. Green and M.W. Kreuter, *Health Promotion Planning: An Educational and Ecological Approach,* 3rd ed., p. 35, © 1999, Mayfield Publishing Co.

perspective on the experience of the community with the health problem by reviewing similar data from other cities, states, or regions.

Citizens or lay participants in the planning process at this stage can help identify population subgroups within the community, such as adolescent mothers and preschool youth, who may have special problems and needs.[20] Information on these subpopulations can include geographic distribution; occupational, economic, and educational status; age and sex composition; ethnicity; health indicators, including age-specific morbidity; and service utilization patterns.

Behavioral Assessment. Once the health problem has been defined and the program goal and high-risk subpopulations have been identified, the behavioral problems or barriers to the community solution of the problem can be specified (Figure 12–2, phase 3). The following guidelines should be considered when performing the behavioral assessment.

- Specify the behaviors that are presumably contributing to the health problem as concretely as possible. Make an inventory of as many possible behavioral determinants as one can imagine.
- Identify the nonbehavioral factors (environmental, biologic, and technological factors) contributing to the problem as determinants for which strategies other than health education must be developed.
- Review research evidence that shows that the behaviors identified as possible causes are amenable to change through educational interventions and that such change will improve the health problem in question.
- For each health problem, identify one or more of the relevant dimensions of health behavior. For example, in prenatal care, one behavioral dimension is the timing or promptness of the care, which should begin with the first trimester of pregnancy.

An assessment should lead to the selection of specific behaviors that will be the target of the educational interventions. Rarely, if ever, does an agency have the resources necessary to influence all the behaviors contributing to a health problem. Therefore, an initial selection of some of the behaviors should be made. The selection often must be influenced by policies governing required services of the agency. Priorities might also consider legal and economic factors affecting the desired behaviors, agency resources and expertise available, political viability of the educational interventions, the possibility of continued funding, and the probability of quick program success. The reasons for selecting specific behaviors as the priority focus of the educational interventions should be justified.

The two most important objective criteria for the selection of priority behavioral targets for health education are: (1) evidence that the behavioral change will make a difference in the reduction of the health problem and (2) evidence that the behavior is amenable to voluntary change.

Educational Assessment. Once the behaviors have been selected, they can be subjected to further analysis for assessment of their causes (Figure 12–2, phase 4). The following sets of factors should be considered as *causes* of each behavior:

- *predisposing factors:* knowledge, attitudes, beliefs, and values that motivate people to take appropriate health actions
- *enabling factors:* skills and the accessibility of resources that make it possible for a motivated person to take action
- *reinforcing factors:* the attitudes and climate of support from providers of services, families, and community groups who reinforce the health behavior of an individual who is motivated and able to adopt the behavior but who will discontinue the behavior if it is not rewarded

Planners should consult representatives of the various segments within the agency and community who are potentially affected by the program. Failure to assess some of these factors and to develop a community health education program addressed to all three sets of these factors would seriously limit the impact of the program. Selecting the health education methods for a community health program follows almost automatically from a thorough identification and ranking of predisposing, enabling, and reinforcing factors influencing the health behaviors.

Administrative Assessment. The final phase of the process includes the assessment of available resources to support the selected educational methods. Resources can be identified through survey information obtained from organizations and agencies at national, state or provincial, and local levels. Some examples of resources include citizens' groups, industry, labor organizations, religious groups, colleges, advertising agencies, drama groups, pharmacies, local facilities (e.g., libraries, health centers, hospitals, training centers, town halls, gathering places), personnel (e.g., volunteers, agency staff, social workers), communications resources (e.g., numbers of telephones and use of radios, billboards, local television and radio stations, newspapers, newsletters, organization bulletins, Internet and World Wide Web sites), and funding sources available for the educational program through the health service agency itself and related organizations. This identification and assessment of available resources should lead to the further refinement of objectives, strategies, and methods. Advocacy for the reallocation of resources or the changes in policy required to support the program may be necessary at this phase of the planning process.

The coordination and budgeting of resources into a timetable that corresponds to the community health program is the next step. Both require constructive participation by staff, other organizations, and area residents. By including other organizations and community members in the planning, one obtains their personal commitment to realizing program success, which can help eliminate duplication of services. Most importantly, their participation enables program planners to incorporate the interests, perspectives, and values of various stakeholders into the educational activities of the program. The principle of participation usually applies to representatives of related agencies, institutions, and organizations in the community, to the agency staff who will implement the program activities, and to community residents in the target.

It should be noted that the assessment process used as part of health education planning is analogous to assessment processes that public health organizations may undertake for other purposes (see Chapter 11 for a discussion of these purposes and processes). Consequently, public health organizations may wish to undertake health education assessment efforts as part of larger public health assessment processes.

Components of Planning for Public Health Education

The following discussion concerning assessment in health education planning contains a number of cross-cutting concerns at issue in all phases of planning, including the identification of the target population, writing of clear objectives, and the use of health education methods and theories. These issues weave through the preceding assessment phases and continue through organizational implementation and program evaluation in an iterative way, requiring the planner and practitioner to back and fill with new knowledge and understanding as experience with the community or population grows. This process makes planning both a technical and a socially negotiated process.

Priority Target Populations. An early program planning task is the identification of the populations who are at risk, or those who are most affected by the health problem. These populations are the target for, and the intended beneficiaries of, most of the educational interventions, and thus constitute the primary target group that planners should consult. It is the understanding of this group that focuses the social assessment and is deepened in subsequent rounds of epidemiologic, behavioral, educational, and administrative assessments. An iterative and deep understanding of the target population sidelines an ineffective "one size fits all" approach to educational interventions.

The primary target population should receive direct communication designed to influence members' predisposition to accept the recommended health practices. Planners need to describe the primary target population by their geographic, occupational, economic, educational, age, sex, and ethnic distributions. Planners should consult or collaborate with representative persons from the described population and cooperating agencies in the further development of the educational plans. The characteristics of the target population that provide the basic analysis for the specification of community health programs are also the basis for the development of educational interventions.

In addition, education must also be directed toward populations who are not affected by the health problem, but who are in a direct position to influence those who are. These "gatekeepers" and social reinforcers, such as parents, spouses, teachers, peers, employers, and opinion leaders, are often an intermediate or additional target population for educational programs. To develop the enabling factors for health education programs, planners can direct educational interventions toward these intermediate target groups. For example, one intermediate target group for community organization efforts would be directors of other agencies who control resources that would enable or facilitate the health behavior. Another intermediate target group might be employers, friends, or family members who would receive training, consultation, or supervision in reinforcing the recommended health behavior.

Objectives as Planning Tools. At each of the assessment phases previously discussed, clear statements of objectives serve as a guiding tool not only for the planning, but also for the eventual evaluation of public health education programs. To exemplify the components of objectives, we focus here on the development of behavioral objectives (Figure 12–2, phase 3).

The objectives for behavior change derive from the findings of the behavioral assessment. The proper statement of the objectives should lend purpose to the program plan and direction to its implementation.

Because education appears to be more abstract and difficult to define or measure than some of the other activities of community health programs, time spent on the formulation of objectives in educational planning is especially important. Objectives should be expressed as intended outcomes. They may apply to providers and to the organization or system, as well as to the consumers. Each objective should answer the following question: *Who* is expected to achieve or become *how much* of *what* by *when* and *where*?

The desired behaviors (what) should describe what the participants will do or not do as a result of the program that they could not or did not do (to the same extent) before the program. The conditions of the action should be stated in the following way:

- *who:* some logical portion (percentage) of the target group who is expected to change
- *how much* or *to what extent:* an amount of behavioral change that will depend on available resources
- *what:* the action, change in behavior, or health practice to be obtained
- *when,* or *how soon,* or *within what time period:* will be determined by the urgency of the health problem in the population and by the rate of change that can be expected from the amount and type of effort that is devoted to the program
- *where:* geographic, political, or institutional boundaries derived in part from the original description of the health problem

In most community health or population-based programs, "how much" refers to the number of people or percentage of the population expected to change their behavior as a result of the program. For individuals, "how much" would refer to the level of accomplishment (e.g., number of monthly prenatal visits). Planners should word their objectives in such a way as to imply their assessment criteria. They should state the objectives in concrete terms with at least an implied if not stated scale of measurement that can be used to evaluate progress and achievement of the objective.

The test of good objectives is their ability to communicate expected results. Lucidity and precision in their formulation should accomplish several things. First, these objectives should provide limits to expenditure of time and effort on specific educational interventions. Second, they should identify criteria for measurement of program achievement. Third, they should lead to task analyses for selection, training, and supervision of staff. Finally, these objectives, like others, should provide orientation to cooperating agencies and to the general community.

Health Education Methods and Theories. Having set priorities and selected strategies, the next step is to plan for the appropriate educational tools, tactics, and methods. Regardless of the setting in which the community health promotion program occurs, there are three basic types of educational strategies at its core.

1. direct communications with the target population to *predispose* behaviors that are conducive to health: These include lecture/discussion, individual counseling or instruction, mass media campaigns, audiovisual aids, educational television, and programmed learning. Interpersonal or two-way communication and demonstration processes provide the most favorable environment for learning, and generally have greater long-term behavioral effects. One-way communication, such as the use of pamphlets, may be appropriate in the early phases of a program or when other methods with more lasting outcomes are not feasible, and when the audience is literate.
2. training methods to *enable* or *reinforce* behaviors that are conducive to health: These include skills development, simulations and games, inquiry learning, small group discussion, modeling, and behavior modification.
3. organizational methods to *support* behaviors that are conducive to health: These include community development, social action, social planning, and economic and organizational development. Such methods usually go beyond health education in supporting behavior.

A single educational intervention cannot be relied on to have a significant, lasting impact on an individual's health behavior. Only through repeated educational reinforcement by health staff, aides, community leaders, friends, and family, can health education affect human behavior in the context of today's complex community health problems.

One of the most noticeable changes in prevention programs in community health in recent years has been the increasing integration of behavioral theory into health education and other phases of program development.[21] Insofar as health behavior is only partially understood (the level of understanding varies with the complexity of the health behavior), multiple theories have been used in planning for prevention programs. The most successful programs consult relevant behavioral theory in their planning to clarify the assumptions about the causes of behavior on the basis of which strategies are selected or developed.[22]

Implementing Public Health Education Programs

Once the planning operations have been developed and refined, the educational components of the community health program can move toward implementation. At this phase, if involvement of concerned persons has been obtained and detailed written plans are available to staff, volunteers, and cooperating agencies, all will be aware and (ideally) agreed on the program's aims and general strategies. Planning participants should be committed to assuming their roles in the educational efforts. To initiate the program will require more specific logistical planning and resource identification, equipment and materials assembly, design of procedures, and training and orientation of staff, volunteers, and cooperating agencies.

Putting the Educational Plan in Reverse

Planning for health education programs works "backward" in the causal chain from the social assessment of ultimate outcomes to the administrative assessment of immediate targets of change, as seen in Figure 12–2. The implementation of plans reverses the flow to work "forward" from the administrative assessment toward educational interventions that influence behavioral changes that resolve health problems and ultimately meet the social concerns of the population. If the planning process has carefully paved the way from social concerns to educational programs—with adequate assessment, information, and social support—the road back should be a visible and viable one. The health educator or administrator approaches implementation with a well-documented and supported plan in hand. If not, the usual bumps and twists in any implementation path may turn into impassable gaps and crevices.

Assessing Barriers and Facilitators to Implementation

To implement the educational plan, an assessment of factors that may impede or facilitate program activities must be conducted. Both the barriers and facilitators to the program should be assessed.

Barriers. Barriers to the achievement of educational objectives can assume several forms. Some examples of social, psychological, and cultural barriers include citizen and staff bias, prejudice, misunderstanding, taboos, unfavorable past experiences, values, norms, social relationships, official disapproval, or rumors. Communication obstacles include illiteracy and local vernacular. Economic and physical barriers include low income and inability to pay for prescribed drugs or the means of transportation to medical services, and long distances over difficult terrain to medical or health education facilities. Legal and administrative barriers include residence requirements to be eligible for services, legal requirements that the program operate within defined geographical boundaries, and policies or regulations that restrict program implementation.

Facilitators. Facilitators to the achievement of program objectives go beyond the mere absence of barriers. The predispositions of area residents who are favorable to the implementation of the program may include past and favorable experience with similar programs, and high credibility of the program's sponsoring agency. Other capabilities facilitating the program might be high education levels of consumers, dynamic and supportive local leaders and organizations, skilled staff with experience, open channels of communication with consumers, and support from other agencies. In addition, some geographic and physical enabling factors may serve as program assets, such as population distribution, density, and access to facilities.

The introduction of new or unfamiliar schemes for promoting awareness and health behavior has its greatest opportunity for success when it is integrated into existing systems of knowledge transfer and influence within the community. Schools, local media, clubs, churches, neighborhoods, and ethnic associations are the most effective channels of communication. In addition, planners should identify barriers in additional objectives that indicate how much and when the program will surmount each of the barriers.

Priorities for Implementation

Resources are often scarce in relation to the great needs in public health. When budgets are reduced, the first line item to get cut is often the health education component. To ensure the most economical use of the resources available, priorities among alternative educational activities must be considered. Related to this pressing need for efficiency is the need for effectiveness. For an activity to be effective, the most effective combination of educational interventions and activities available must be selected. The first step is to determine which procedures are feasible, given limited staff, services, money, and time, and then to combine these resources to achieve the best support of program objectives.

The following guidelines can be used to set priorities:

- Obtain opinions and contributions from community members on priorities for educational services.

- Delineate the areas that will provide the greatest benefits to the most recipients.
- Phase program activities with a gradual beginning.
- Limit the number and range of activities, with initial emphasis on areas that are most amenable to quick and early success and activities requiring minimum staff training.
- Review the most recent scientific literature on the evaluation of health education methods relevant to the local program to guide these decisions on priorities.
- Develop a contingency plan to aid program survival in the event of future reduction of resources.

Beyond these general principles, the selection of educational efforts in strategic patterns or combinations depends on the particular circumstances of each site, the specific objectives, and the expectations for sustaining or institutionalizing the program.

Using Educational Methods and Media

Methods, media, and materials can be pretested in the intended target audience to determine their acceptability to the particular group and their convenience (e.g., time demands, personnel requirements, and situational concerns such as light and sound). They should also be selected based on their efficiency and effectiveness. Efficiency relates to fixed costs, continuing costs, space and maintenance requirements, and staff and time needs to convey a message. Presumed effectiveness is based on confidence in the ability to communicate messages, arouse attention and interest, promote interaction, use suitable repetition and message retention techniques, and encourage desired attitudes and the adoption of practices.

Managing Human Resources for Health Education

Some health workers and allied personnel may be uninformed concerning methods of health education; others may feel that educational efforts are too slow, complex, and of dubious efficacy. Training or continuing education for these workers can provide them with time to discuss their concerns and develop their competence and confidence. Training in health education should be differentiated from technical training related to health and medical content. Health education training underscores the attitudinal and behavioral factors essential to long-term health maintenance, the cultural perceptions of the target population, and the necessity of well-planned and properly sustained action. Knowledge of these factors can help health workers achieve the health behavior changes required by the objectives of the community health.

Although many health professionals are involved in various forms of health education, one group of professionals, the certified health education specialist (CHES), has specialized training in the planning, implementation, and evaluation of public health education. CHES professionals are typically assigned the responsibility for planning, implementing, and evaluating community health education programs because they have specialized training in public health or community health education and experience in a community health agency or institution. Competencies tested for the CHES include the following:

- planning at the community level, including epidemiologic and sociological research methods, community organization, and health services administration
- assessment and adaptation of communications to attitudinal, cultural, economic, and ethnic determinants of health behaviors
- educational evaluation within the context of community health (as distinct from formal curriculum evaluation), including biostatistics, demography, and behavioral research methods

When these skills are not available within the staff of a community health agency, consultation for the planning and preparation stages of health education programs may be obtained from other organizations employing CHES professionals. Continuing education and inservice training are important to maintaining up-to-date knowledge and skills in all community health staff.

The CHES may work in a variety of different settings, such as public health departments, hospitals, voluntary agencies, educational institutions, or for-profit organizations. What links educators in these various settings is their training and intent of facilitating voluntary actions by the public with regard to health. In some organizations, health educators work as part of a team with other health professionals to achieve intended outcomes. For example, a health educator may work as a team member with a physician, nurse, nutritionist, and social worker to develop and implement programs for maternal and child health. In other organizations, health educators may all work in the same department and be loaned to other departments, such as nursing or nutrition, to help plan and implement health education programs. Both models of organization have their advantages and disadvantages; the former promotes collaboration among health professionals and the latter may allow health educators to better support each other, but isolate them from other health professionals. Careful consideration needs to be given to the placement of health education specialists.

Staff training may include orientation aimed at sensitizing staff members to their educational function and to the general objectives of the education program. It may also include preparation in recognizing educational opportunities, communication skills, and reinforcement techniques; training priorities for those staff members in contact with consumers; and continuing education.

Volunteers are not free of cost. Proper use of volunteers requires continuous, careful supervision and training. These items should be budgeted in the educational plan. A thorough plan for training volunteers might include a content designed to foster their interest in health education and in the program's need for their insight into the attitudes, reactions, and daily lives of the target population. It can also include training in communications skills, teamwork roles, and limits of volunteers' responsibility and authority.

Data Collection and Records

Documenting the implementation process not only provides guidance for present action, but also provides statistics and financial accounts that are useful for evaluation and future planning. Good records and documentation, supervisor reports on quality control, and other process evaluations can provide immediate feedback on whether things are working satisfactorily. *Records* provide for continuous monitoring of program impact; for supervision, training, and staff development; and for evaluation of program process and outcome. *Peer review* among health professionals helps to maintain quality control, but it must be based on standards and documentation of practice. *Feedback* on patients' or clients' utilization and satisfaction with health services should provide data for program adjustment and redirection. *Population surveillance* will aid in continuous health education planning and evaluation.

Information collection can be integrated into daily routines and may require coordination among various units and sites in order to provide meaningful data for future planning. Information collection that requires additional paperwork must always be weighed against other demands for time. Small additions and checklists may be integrated into existing records with little effort and with staff acceptance. For more intensive narrative reporting and recording, special efforts during limited time periods may be acceptable and may provide sufficient data without generating staff resistance and unmanageable amounts of paperwork. The educational plan should clearly identify the use and purpose of new forms and records.

Scheduling Implementation

Timing is crucial to the success of the educational plan of action. It requires an analysis of when, where, and who is responsible for implementation. This analysis will provide the starting and completion date required for each activity in relation to the total program. Consideration of the training required, production schedules for material, and staff loads guide the development of timetables. A task analysis and time sequence of activities should integrate the educational implementation with the total program plan. Planners should consider external events when scheduling to avoid conflict with community happenings, school openings, holidays, and related community schedules. The implementation stage is a logical progression from the previous stages of assessment, planning, and organizing.

Evaluating Public Health Education Programs

Evaluation is the comparison of an object of interest against a standard of acceptability (see Chapter 13 for a detailed discussion of evaluation in public health organizations).[23] The evaluation of a health education program, then, is the systematic assessment of the operations or outcomes of a program against standards for the purposes of improving the program. The evaluation of a program needs to be guided by the standards of program evaluation: accuracy, feasibility, propriety, and utility. That is, evaluation needs to be not only technically well done and ethically conducted, but also feasible in cost and effort and directed toward program improvement.

The various levels of objectives developed in the assessment phases of planning—epidemiologic, behavioral, educational, and administrative—shape the dimensions and standards that are used during evaluation to determine the value (success or failure) of the program or its components. If the objectives were well developed during the planning stage, evaluation can proceed with ease, as compared with programs that have no developed standards for judging their success or failure. The involvement of various stakeholders in determining the dimensions and standards used to judge program value is essential in the highly political context of program evaluation. If stakeholders do not accept the dimensions and standards as those they would use in judging value, they are not likely to accept or use the results of the evaluation.

Program evaluation, at the very least, is an assessment of the worth or merit of a program, a method, or some other object of interest. It may provide an estimate of the degree to which spent resources result in intended activity, and the degree to which performed activities attain goals. The determination of whether the program has met its goals is based on criteria indicated by precise statements of objectives along with subjective impressions and reporting. Evaluation can suggest which of several alternative educational strategies is the most efficient and which steps have an effect on the behavior specified. Evaluation provides accountability for time spent. Results usually offer a sense of accomplishment to staff and consumers or sponsors of the program.

Formative and Process Evaluation

Formative evaluation is the earliest phase of process evaluation. Formative evaluation refers to preliminary assessments of the appropriateness of materials and procedures before beginning the program. Sources of data for formative evaluation include pretesting of materials, access to planning by relevant stakeholders, and adequate resources. *Process evaluation* refers to continuous observation and checking to see whether the program activities are taking place with the quality and at the time and rate necessary to achieve the stated objective. Process evaluation requires ongoing sources of data that often include budget reports on monthly expenditures in specific categories where rate of expenditures would indicate the amount of program activity relevant to the achievement of objectives.

Professional consensus usually provides the source of the standards of acceptability in formative and process evaluation. The data for process evaluation often come from routine records kept on encounters with consumers, patients, or clients. These might include, for example, clinic attendance records tabulated weekly or monthly for total numbers of patients. Staff can tabulate systematic samples of the records in more detail to estimate progress on such variables as broken appointment rates, sources of referral, and trimester of first visit for pregnant women. Another type of data available for process evaluation is administrative records. Administrators can tabulate personnel records to assess the number of home visits attempted, the number completed, the number of group sessions conducted, and the time allotted for various educational functions.

Supervisors should conduct periodic reviews of personnel to assess staff performance. Time should be set aside on the agenda of staff and community meetings for consideration of strengths, weaknesses, and adaptation of ongoing programs. There should be a plan for charting records over time or comparing progress statistics with other programs or standards.

Outcome Evaluation

Outcome evaluation, sometimes referred to as summative or impact evaluation, assesses the achievement of program effects. Intended program effects are contained in objectives that were developed during the planning phase. The more precisely stated the objectives, the more meaningful the evaluation. Outcome evaluation asks the following questions: What are the results of program efforts in the promotion of health behavior? Has there been any change in the attitudes of the clients toward recommended actions, or change in their ability to carry out the recommended actions, or change in the resources and social support for such actions in the community? An outcome evaluation may also assess unintended program effects that may be either beneficial or harmful to intended recipients.

Data concerning program outcomes can be assessed with quantitative or qualitative approaches. *Quantitative* approaches attempt to measure intended outcomes; *qualitative* approaches are more concerned with explaining why and how outcomes occurred, whether or not they were intended. For quantitative measurement, planners or evaluators should obtain baseline information on a period prior to the program's inception for comparison with similarly gathered data during the program or following the program. The evaluation of a specific educational component (e.g., a pamphlet or a group discussion) should not depend on the comparison of people who receive only that method with people who receive nothing. The comparison should be between a group receiving a comprehensive health education program and another group receiving everything *except* the component to be evaluated. The outcome statistics (knowledge, attitude, and behavioral outcomes) should be better for subgroups who were exposed to the entire program than for those who were exposed to everything except for specific methods or materials of interest. If the evaluation finds no significant difference, it would suggest ways to reduce costs and increase efficiency by eliminating those methods or procedures from the program.

Evaluators should report on outcomes to the affiliated organizations, agencies, and institutions participating in the program and to the clients and general public. Reports can encourage their continued participation by noting their contribution to, or influence on, the program. Finally, practitioners should seek to publish case histories and reports in professional journals and newsletters for use by other departments, programs, or projects and to contribute to the advancement of professional knowledge, practice, and policies.

Limits of Health Education

People may not truly have the resources or support necessary to make independent decisions and to take voluntary actions when some of the determinants of health are factors beyond their control. Whether they were born in a democratic country to loving parents with access to resources sets some limits on their ability and will to act independently or to control the determinants of their health. These limits must be recognized by public health organizations in designing and managing health education programs.

Such considerations also set limits on how much health education alone can achieve health objectives without placing undue responsibility for change on people who are relatively powerless to make such change. This excessive reliance on health education has been referred to as "victim blaming." Combining health education with policy and regulatory actions that empower the relatively powerless and restrain the more powerful who might exploit them overcomes this risk of victim blaming.

Health education is necessary even when the changes in health risks require regulatory or environmental controls on behavior. For example, health education in a democratic society must precede such controls as drunk driving or seat belt enforcement to gain the public's understanding and support required to pass legislation. It also helps to gain the public's cooperation in abiding by the new regulations. Community health promotion, then, is the combination of health education with related organizational, environmental, and economic supports to foster behavior that is conducive to health.

Linking Health Education and Health Promotion

Population health and community health promotion require an understanding of health behavior that goes beyond the specific actions of individuals and includes more than educational interventions alone to change behavior. Lifestyle, a broader concept than behavior, describes value-laden, socially conditioned behavioral patterns. This concept has a rich history of study in anthropology and sociology. Only recently has it taken on special significance in epidemiology, population health, and community health promotion. It is a concept that public health administrators need to understand in managing the broad-ranging, complex, and often politically charged interventions of health promotion. This section examines how health education strategies fit within the larger set of health promotion approaches that may be used by public health organizations to improve community health.

Lifestyle

The mid-century shift from acute infectious diseases to chronic, degenerative diseases as the leading causes of death in Western societies brought a new perspective to epidemiology. No longer could isolation and suppression of a single germ or agent control the predominant diseases. Now, the causes of most chronic diseases tend to be multiple and elusive. These causes defy simple environmental control measures because they involve people's pleasures and rewards, their social relationships and physical needs, and, ultimately for some, their habits and addictions. They involve lifestyle.

Lalonde identified lifestyle as one of the four elements of his health field concept; the other elements include health services, environment, and human biology.[24] Of these, lifestyle is responsible for more than half of the years of life that are prematurely lost in the more developed nations (Figure 12–3). Tobacco use, diet (in combination with physical activity), and alcohol use are the three leading determinants of the leading causes of death in North America. Together, they account for some 38 percent of premature deaths. To put these revealing statistics in more positive terms, the greatest gains in preventing premature death and disability can be achieved today through community supports or policies for more healthy lifestyles. Reducing risk means that chances of developing a disease are lowered. It does not guarantee that a disease will be prevented. Because several factors are involved in the development of disease, risk reduction usually involves several strategies or approaches.

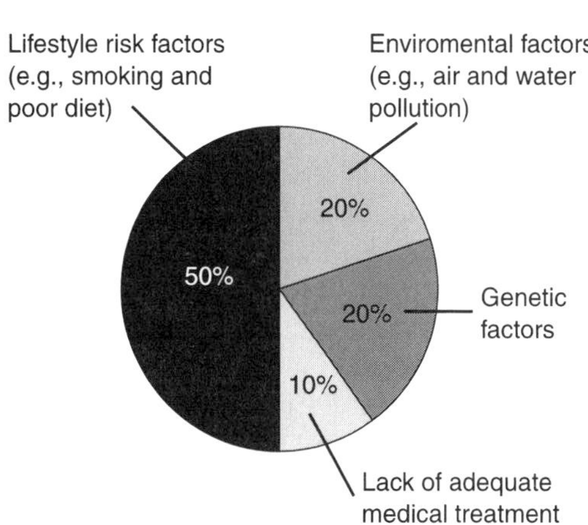

Figure 12–3 Lifestyle risk factors contribute as much as the combination of health care, environment, and human biology to the years of life lost prematurely (before age 75). *Source:* Centers for Disease Control and Prevention, U.S. Department of Health and Human Services.

Broad Supports for Lifestyle Change

Health education typically has been called on to alert the public to complex community health problems, but health education by itself can hardly be expected to solve such problems. The lifestyles in question are too embedded in organizational, socioeconomic, and environmental circumstances for people to be able to change their own behavior without concomitant changes in these circumstances. Health promotion combines health education with organizational, economic, and environmental supports for behavior and conditions of living that are conducive to health.

The entire burden for improved health or risk reduction must not be placed on the individual alone. The responsibility must be shared between individuals and their families; between families and their communities; and between communities and their state, provincial, and national governments. Each level of organizational influence on behavior must assume some responsibility for setting the economic and environmental conditions that will support healthy lifestyles. Families, for example, must set examples for children. Communities must provide facilities and pass local ordinances to encourage, enable, and reinforce healthy behavior. State and national governments and private organizations must assume responsibility for the production, sale, and advertising of foods and other substances that can be either helpful or harmful to health.

HEALTH PROMOTION

Any program that has to deal with such complex problems related to lifestyle must address the social, environmental, economic, psychological, cultural, and physiological factors encompassed by the lifestyle in question. In the first part of this chapter, the PRECEDE model of health *education* was introduced. That model will now be expanded to include the additional elements of economic, organizational, and environmental supports for behavior that are conducive to health and applied as the PRECEDE-PROCEED model of health *promotion*.[2] Note that this health promotion model, as shown in Figure 12–4, includes health education at its core along with other types of organizational and regulatory interventions. The combined model has been applied to health promotion programs at international, national, and local levels for planning and evaluating such complex interventions for such complex lifestyle problems.

This section of the chapter begins with a review of the different levels of prevention and different types of prevention strategies. These levels and strategies are used to compare and contrast health education and health promotion approaches. This understanding paves the way for application of the PRECEDE-PROCEED model.

Levels of Prevention

Health professionals sometimes employ a taxonomy of three levels of prevention: primary, secondary, and tertiary. *Primary* prevention is accomplished by activities that promote optimum health and provide specific protection against the onset or incidence of a health problem (e.g., proper nutrition, genetic counseling, fluoridation, and disease inoculation). *Secondary* prevention refers to activities concerned with the early assessment and prompt treatment of health problems (e.g., the Papanicolaou [Pap] smear, regular physical examination, referral programs for troubled employees, neonatal metabolic screening). *Tertiary* prevention refers to minimizing the disability from existing illness through treatment and rehabilitation efforts (e.g., treatment for persons with lung cancer, alcoholism rehabilitation, treatment of sexually transmitted diseases). Whereas primary prevention may reduce the *incidence* of a health problem, secondary and tertiary prevention can reduce its *prevalence*.

Prevention Strategies

Three types of strategies can be used in each of the three prevention levels to accomplish health promotion goals.

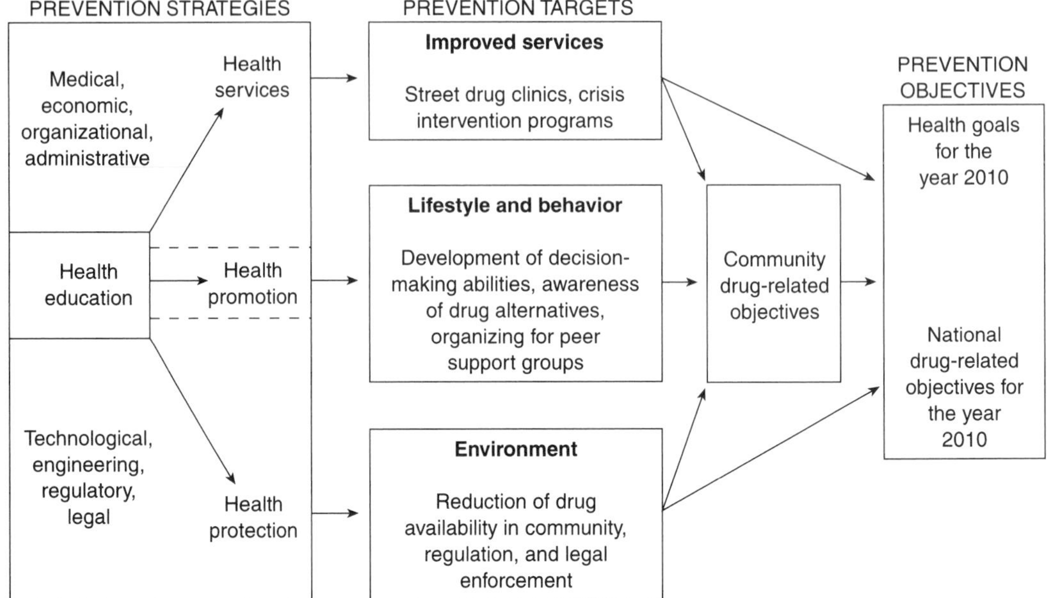

Figure 12–4 The structure of the objectives for the nation in health promotion are seen here as applied to drug abuse prevention. The relationship of community health education and health promotion also is shown as part of the prevention strategies box to the left. Health promotion, however, can serve community development needs other than the prevention of specific diseases or lifestyle problems. *Source:* Reprinted with permission from L.W. Green and M.W. Kreuter, *Health Promotion Planning: An Educational and Ecological Approach,* 3rd ed., p. 226, © 1999, Mayfield Publishing Co.

- *Educational strategies* inform and educate the public about issues of concern, such as the dangers of drug misuse, the benefits of automobile restraints, or the relationship of maternal alcohol consumption to fetal alcohol syndrome.
- *Automatic-protective strategies* are directed at controlling environmental variables, such as public health measures providing for milk pasteurization, fluoridation, infant immunizations, and the burning or chemical killing of marijuana crops.
- *Coercive strategies* employ legal and other formal sanctions to control individual behavior, such as required immunizations for school entry, mandatory tuberculosis testing of hospital employees, compulsory use of automobile restraints, and arrests for drug possession or use.

Table 12–1 provides examples of community health programs and measures classified by level of prevention and category of prevention strategy. The examples illustrate traditional public health strategies and new strategies in community health promotion and drug misuse prevention.

Planning for Health Promotion Programs

Planning for health promotion programs follows the same phases as those involved in planning for health education programs. One of the differences in planning for health promotion, though, is a broader look at the ecologic influences on health behavior and outcomes and a willingness to consider measures beyond those aimed at voluntary changes in health behavior. To illustrate the use of a health promotion planning and evaluation framework, the following section applies the PRECEDE-PROCEED model to the complex issues of substance abuse. Tobacco, alcohol, and other drug abuse prevention programs incorporating the integrated

Table 12–1 Examples of Intervention Strategies for Each Level of Prevention of Health Problems, Including Those Associated with Drug Misuse

	Levels of Prevention		
Type of Strategy	*Primary*	*Secondary*	*Tertiary*
Educational	Genetic counseling School health education Public education about drugs	Community hypertension screening education programs Teacher training in recognition of drug problems	Drug education programs for patients in coronary care
Automatic-protective	Fluoridation of community drinking water systems Legal control of prescription drugs	Neonatal metabolic screening Requiring medical prescription for drug refills	Referral to community mental health center for counseling following discharge from drug treatment center
Coercive	Immunization requirements for schoolchildren Arrests of drug traffickers	Mandatory classes for persons convicted of driving while intoxicated or using illicit drugs	Mandatory treatment for persons having an addiction or a sexually transmitted disease

Source: Reprinted with permission from L.W. Green and J. Ottoson, *Community and Population Health,* 8th ed., © 1999, McGraw-Hill Companies.

health promotion approach of educational, organizational, and economic supports for lifestyle conducive to health have a much greater chance of success than programs directed at only one of these categories.

When using the health promotion framework in Figure 12–4 to plan community drug prevention programs, one starts with the final consequences—namely, social problems that are usually defined as community drug-related problems but not necessarily as health concerns. One works back from there to the original causes—that is, the causes of the behavior that influenced the health problem or community drug-related social problem.

Social Assessment

The first phase involves a consideration of the quality of life in a community by assessing the assets and social problems of concern to the various segments of the population. This phase of the model has the same purpose and process as that previously discussed in application of the model for health education. It has the effect of forcing planners to consider the desirable social outcomes of a program before setting priorities on health or selecting program approaches.

It also helps justify a program to the community. This is especially important in the planning of community drug prevention programs because of the relationship between drug-related health problems and the social problems of a community. For example, when a community has a large number of drug-dependent persons, it is likely that there will be high rates of violent and nonviolent crime, school truancy, early dropouts from school, juvenile delinquency, and unemployment (all social problems). Conversely, when a community is experiencing such social problems as high unemployment, inadequate housing, inadequate private and public school programs, or discrimination, a serious drug dependence problem will be present because the use of drugs for some will be a method of coping with the social problems.

By identifying the major social problems of concern to the community, one can select potential outcome evaluation measures and gain an understanding of the community's concerns as they relate to the particular health problem that is the target of the prevention program. A community's social problems can be diagnosed from analyses of existing records, files, publications, and informal interviews and discussions with leaders, key informants, and representatives of various community populations. This is an important first step that should not be undertaken too hastily because its outcome may well affect program scope and quality as well as the extent of community support.

Epidemiologic Assessment

The objective of the epidemiologic assessment phase is to identify the specific health problems that appear to be contributing to the social problems noted in the preceding phase. Using data from community surveys, hospital admissions, city and county health departments, health systems agencies, and selected state or provincial and national agencies, trends in the drug-related morbidity, mortality, and disability information can be identified.

The incidence, prevalence, distribution, intensity, and duration of each identified health problem should be described. These data can be analyzed to determine the populations that are most affected by the health problem. This process will often reveal and locate a variety of existing health problems such as drug dependence, drug-related psychoses, drug-related depression or anxiety, injuries, and other drug-related problems such as acquired immune deficiency syndrome, serum hepatitis, and endocarditis. The use of spatial maps to depict the distribution of the identified health problems within the city or county is an effective way of presenting data if there is reason to believe that the problems vary by geographic location.

The results of epidemiologic analyses should be used to develop program objectives. The objectives should be stated in epidemiologic terms and answer the following questions: Who will be the recipients of the program? What benefit should they receive? How much of that benefit should they receive? By when or for how long? For example, it has been estimated that in a 6-month period, approximately 1,000 persons die of drug overdose in New York City. Therefore, a program objective for a drug prevention program in New York City could be stated as follows: "To reduce the number of drug overdose deaths in New York City by 25 percent within 1 year and an additional 25 percent within the next year, until the national average is reached." The major drug-related health problem for most communities would not be death or drug overdose; rather, it would be physiological or psychological dependence.

Behavioral and Environmental Assessment

This phase of the planning process is where the health education model previously discussed is expanded beyond a behavioral assessment to an environmental assessment, in keeping with the broader health promotion focus. The behavioral and environmental assessment requires the systematic identification of health behaviors that appear to be causally linked to each of the health problems identified in the epidemiologic assessment. The outcome of the behavioral assessment is the generation of a ranked list of specific behaviors to be used as the basis for specifying the behavioral objectives of the program.

The process of identifying the health behaviors linked to the health problems usually relies on the professional literature. The review of the literature can be combined with structured and unstructured interviews of persons who are familiar with the health problem (such as drug treatment personnel), data from observations, and intuition based on personal experiences. In the case of drug dependence, the behavioral causes leading to the health problem are drug use and drug misuse. These should be perceived not as distinct behaviors but, rather, as a continuum of drug use to drug misuse with varying types and amounts of drugs used. Distinct behaviors within the continuum could be specified, such as misuse of prescription medications, use of illicit drugs such as marijuana and cocaine, and use of illicit drugs in a manner that predisposes the user to health problems.

A second part of this phase is the identification of environmental factors that contribute to the health problem. These are the organizational and environmental conditions that influence the health problem and the behavior but that are not controlled directly by the behavior of the target population. Nonbehavioral causes of drug dependence include such factors as the housing situation in the community, the school environment, and the law enforcement activity in the community. Identification of these factors is important because it provides the planners with direction for health promotion activity other than educational measures, such as organizational and economic interventions directed at the regulation of the environment and the availability of services.

Educational and Ecologic Assessment

The educational and ecologic assessment identifies factors that require change to initiate and sustain the process of behavioral and environmental change. The determinants of health and social conditions identified in this phase will become the immediate targets or objectives of a program.

In this phase, the planner assesses the relative influence of various predisposing, enabling, and reinforcing factors on each of the identified behavioral and environmental causes of the health problem. Figure 12–5 focuses attention on the order of causation of behavior, as indicated by the numbered arrows. People first have an initial motivation to act (predisposing factors). They then deploy their resources and skills to enable the action, or acquire them through training and organizational arrangements in the community. Third comes a reaction to the behavior from someone else (or in the case of drug use, the drug effects themselves), which reinforces or discourages the behavior. The reinforcement and strengthening or the punishment and discouragement of the behavior, in turn, affect the predisposing factors by strengthening or extinguishing the motivation to act. Finally, the person has an increased ability to take certain actions, which tends to increase the predisposition or motivation to take such actions.

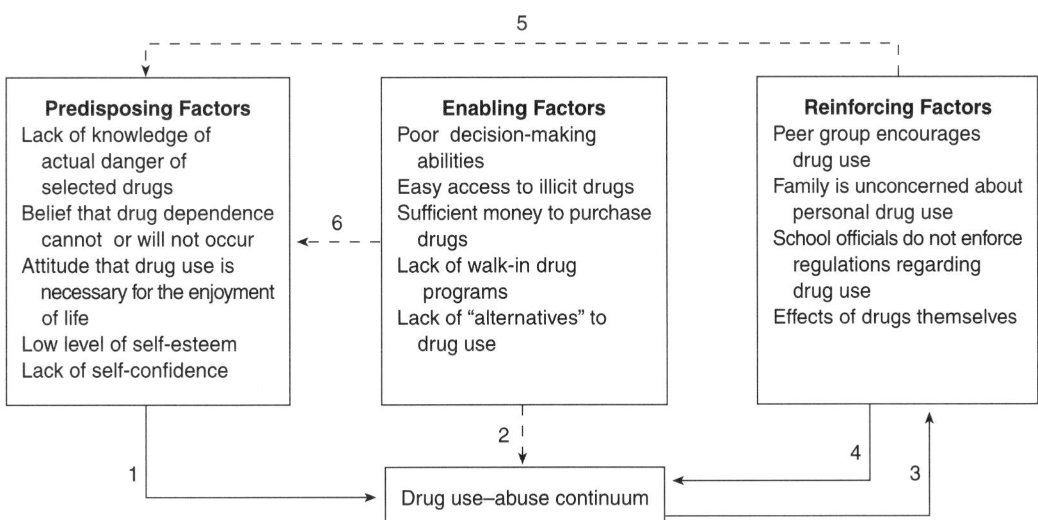

Figure 12–5 The three categories of factors influencing lifestyle are shown here as related to drug use and abuse. The numbered arrows indicate the appropriate expected order of cause and effect. *Source:* Reprinted with permission from L.W. Green and M.W. Kreuter, *Health Promotion Planning: An Educational and Ecological Approach,* 3rd ed., p. 155, © 1999, Mayfield Publishing Co.

In the process of identifying and listing factors in the three areas, one may include factors that seem to encourage the behavior as well as those that seem to discourage the behavior.

After completing the list of predisposing, enabling, and reinforcing factors, the next step is to select those factors that will be most likely to bring about the desired behavior. The factors that should be selected as targets for the program are those that are most changeable and most important. Changeability is assessed from data (evidence-based) or professional judgments. The factors determined to be both important and changeable form the basis of the prevention program. This level of specificity helps to use scarce resources in the most appropriate manner as well as to increase the chances of the program being successful. Difficult choices will be made in this phase of the planning process, but in the decision-making process, the level of understanding of the nature of the problem usually increases.

Administrative Assessment

The administrative assessment phase assesses the resources that are available and the organizational problems that are likely to be encountered as the program becomes operational. Factors such as interagency cooperation, staffing patterns, and budgeting should be thoroughly discussed. This phase of planning analyzes the potential problems within programs, within organizations, and between organizations. A well-conceived program is seldom effective without an implementation plan.

In this phase, the right combination of strategies is selected to affect the priority predisposing, enabling, and reinforcing factors. As a general rule, selected communication methods are effective in altering predisposing factors; organizing resources and training are effective in altering enabling factors; and strategies such as consultation, training, feedback, and group development are effective in altering reinforcing factors. Refer to Table 12–1 for an example of considerations in selecting appropriate educational and other strategies according to the level of prevention.

HEALTH EDUCATION VERSUS HEALTH PROMOTION

For purposes of this chapter, health promotion is defined as any combination of educational, organizational, environmental, and economic supports for behavior and conditions of living that are conducive to health. With health education as an integral part of all health promotion interventions, it follows that the interventions should be directed toward voluntary behavior at all levels—individuals, organizations, and communities. At the community, state or provincial, or national level, additional interventions may be legal, regulatory, political, or economic, and therefore potentially coercive. Nevertheless, to be successful, such interventions must be supported by an informed electorate and a consenting public.

Such informed consent requires health education. Ideally, the coercive measures are directed at the behavior of those individuals whose actions may affect the health of others, such as the manufacturers, distributors, and advertisers of hazardous products. Even then, public health education is required to ensure the support of an informed public because taxes, prices, availability of services and products, and jobs may be affected by such regulations of health- or drug-related industries and sources. For example, one part of a health promotion program for drug misuse prevention could target organizational change. Local public leaders could combine health education with various incentives (such as free program consultation services) and persuasion techniques (such as program promotion by local opinion leaders) in an attempt to increase the number of schools offering peer counseling programs for those persons who misuse drugs.

If the program also targeted political change, community organization techniques could be combined with health education activities to develop "concerned parent groups" in neighborhoods and to apply political pressure on local school, law enforcement, and government officials to support drug misuse prevention efforts. If the program directed other efforts toward economic change, health professionals and others could work with representatives of insurance carriers to initiate health insurance reimbursements for counseling and rehabilitation services.

The point is simple: when health education activities are combined with appropriate changes in organizations, political systems, and environmental and economic supports for behavior, the end result is more likely to be favorable than is the result achieved by a series of single, uncoordinated changes. Indeed, uncoordinated changes sometimes make things worse by throwing a community system out of balance and forcing an overreaction or overcompensation by the wrong elements in the community.

The relationships of health education and health promotion activities to the three prevention targets and the relationships of these targets to the health or drug misuse objectives set for the community and the nation are depicted in Figure 12–4. The three prevention targets are not isolated. The human environment and the organization of services continually affect lifestyle. Furthermore, a successful program must effectively integrate and coordinate activities in relation to each of these targets. To facilitate the integration of activities within and between the prevention strategies, a planning framework is needed. The planning framework introduced in the first part of this chapter forces an encompassing and systematic analysis of public health problems in the context of social problems or quality-of-life concerns.

Organization of Health Education and Health Promotion Activities within Public Health Institutions

Placing professional health educators and health promotion specialists within the staffing and organization of public health organizations poses some quandaries. From what has been described here as the tasks of coordinating the necessary components of effective health education and health promotion, it would seem that personnel performing these functions should be distributed to the specific program areas, such as maternal and child health, environmental health, tobacco control, and the like. This would allow each health educator or health promotion personnel to specialize in and learn the content, resources, and community capabilities of the area in which the work is to be done. However, in recent years, many public health organizations have not been able to afford a sufficient number of health education and health promotion specialists to have one assigned to every problem area in which they are needed. The usual, preferred staffing arrangement, then, is to centralize or pool the health education and health promotion staff in a unit that provides planning and organizing services or consultation to the other units within the organization.

The major trap to avoid in centralizing the health education and health promotion staff is turning them into a public relations unit serving the publicity needs of the organization. A separate and distinct public relations officer should serve that purpose and should remain distinct from the health education and health promotion functions described in this chapter.

• • •

There is no simple solution to such health-related lifestyle problems as tobacco use, alcohol misuse, drug misuse, and obesity. Problems as complex as these may defy even well-planned preventive efforts. Nevertheless, the effects of well-planned and systematically implemented preventive efforts are more likely to be successful than the single-focused, uncoordinated efforts that have typified many of the early attempts to address lifestyle, particularly those at the local level.

Specific measurable objectives for the United States have been set in each of the past three decades in the *Healthy People* initiatives of the federal government. If these objectives were met each decade, the scope and intensity of health problems attributable to lifestyle, the environment, and inadequate health services would be appreciably reduced. These objectives can serve to concentrate the limited resources of communities where they can be most productive. To illustrate how community health programs can work toward the objectives, a planning framework encompassing the three areas of lifestyle, environment, and services has been presented.

Health education directed at individuals and decision makers has been demonstrated to influence population changes in simple behaviors such as one-time immunizations and more complex behaviors for those segments of the population that are highly motivated, more affluent, and more educated. Health education can enhance its effect on more complex behaviors (lifestyles) and in poorer, less educated segments of a population by combining the best of educational interventions with advocacy and organizational efforts to effect social environments, including political and economic systems. Applying the latest findings from the rapidly developing research in designing and evaluating prevention programs and ensuring the necessary quality and quantity of resources for programs will not guarantee success, but will increase the probability of reaching the objectives set for a community.

CHAPTER REVIEW

1. Human behavior relates to health in both direct and indirect ways, including
   - the direct effect of personal and social behavior
   - the indirect effect of people planning individual or community actions that result in environmental change
   - the indirect effect through health services related to planned distribution, appropriate utilization, and individual compliance with medical and preventive regimens
2. Behavioral changes resulting from education are by definition *voluntary* and freely adopted by people, with their knowledge of alternatives and probable consequences.
3. The two most important objective criteria for the selection of priority behavioral targets for health education are
   - evidence that the behavioral change will make a difference in the reduction of the health problem
   - evidence that the behavior is amenable to voluntary change
4. Planning sets the foundation for sound health education programming and effectiveness and proceeds through the following stages:
   - social assessment
   - epidemiologic assessment
   - behavioral and environmental assessment
   - educational and ecologic assessment
   - administrative assessment
5. Three types of strategies form the core of health education.
   - direct communication with the target population to predispose behaviors that are conducive to health
   - training methods to enable or reinforce behaviors that are conducive to health
   - organizational methods to support behaviors that are conducive to health
6. Population and community health promotion require an understanding of health behavior that goes beyond the specific actions of individuals and includes more than educational interventions alone to change behavior.
7. Lifestyle, a broader concept than behavior, describes value-laden, socially conditioned behavioral patterns. The greatest changes in preventing premature death and disability can be achieved through community supports or policies for more healthful lifestyles. Planning for health promotion programs follows the same phases as those described for health education.

8. Three types of strategies can be used to accomplish health promotion goals for each of the three levels of primary, secondary, and tertiary prevention.
   - educational: informing and educating the public
   - automatic-protective: controlling environmental factors
   - coercive: employing legal and other formal sanctions to control individual behavior

---

REFERENCES

1. L.W. Green and J.M. Ottoson, *Community and Population Health,* 8th ed. (St. Louis, MO: McGraw-Hill, 1999).
2. L.W. Green and M.W. Kreuter, *Health Promotion Planning: An Educational and Ecological Approach*, 3d ed. (Mountain View, CA: Mayfield, 1999).
3. G. Kok, "Quality of Planning as a Decisive Determinant of Health Education Effectiveness," *Hygiene* 11 (1992): 5–8.
4. M. Daniel and L.W. Green, "Application of the PRECEDE-PROCEED Model in Prevention and Control of Diabetes: A Case Illustration from an Aboriginal Community," *Diabetes Spectrum* 8 (1995): 80–123.
5. P. McGowan and L.W. Green, "Arthritis Self-Management in Native Populations of British Columbia: An Application of Health Promotion and Participatory Research Principles in Chronic Disease Control," *Canadian Journal on Aging* 14 (suppl. 1) (1995): 201–212.
6. C. Morrison, "Using PRECEDE To Predict Breast Self-Examination in Older, Lower-Income Women," *American Journal of Health Behavior* 20 (1996): 3–14.
7. M.B. Dignan et al., "The Forsyth County Cervical Cancer Prevention Project—I: Cervical Cancer Screening for Black Women," *Health Education Research* 9 (1995): 411–420.
8. J.A. Earp et al., "The North Carolina Breast Cancer Screening Program—Foundations and Design of a Model for Reaching Older, Minority, Rural Women," *Breast Cancer Research & Treatment 35,* no. 1 (1995): 7–22.
9. C. Farley et al., "The Effects of a 4-Year Program Promoting Bicycle Helmet Use among Children in Quebec," *American Journal of Public Health 86,* no. 1 (1996): 46–51.
10. M.K. Keintz et al., "Reaching Mothers of Preschool-Aged Children with a Targeted Quit Smoking Intervention," *Journal of Community Health* 19 (1994): 25–40.
11. S.D. Morrison, "PRECEDE Model as a Framework for Using Health Education in the Prevention of Diarrhea Infant Mortality in Rural Mexico," *The Eta Sigma Gamma Monograph Series 12,* no. 1 (1994): 41–49.
12. M.N. Nguyen et al., "Behavioral Diagnosis of 30- to 60-Year-Old Men in the Fabreville Heart Health Program," *Journal of Community Health* 20 (1995): 257–269.
13. G. Paradis et al., "Coeur en Santé St-Henri—A Heart Health Promotion Programme in Montreal, Canada: Design and Methods for Evaluation," *Journal of Epidemiology and Community Health* 49 (1995): 495–502.
14. G.S. Parcel et al., "Self-Management of Cystic-Fibrosis—A Structural Model for Educational and Behavioral Variables," *Social Science and Medicine* 38 (1994): 1,307–1,315.
15. L.W. Green and C.J. Frankish, "Theories and Principles of Health Education Applied to Asthma," *Chest* 106 (suppl. 4) (1994): 219S–230S.
16. D.B. Reed, "Focus Groups Identify Desirable Features of Nutrition Programs for Low-Income Mothers of Preschool Children," *Journal of the American Dietetic Association* 96 (1996): 501–503.
17. D.B. Reed et al., "Assessment of Nutrition Education Needs Related to Increasing Dietary Calcium Intake in Low-Income Vietnamese Mothers Using Focus Group Discussions," *Journal of Nutrition Education 30,* no. 3 (1998): 155–163.
18. M. Selby-Harrington et al., "Increasing Medicaid Child Health Screenings: The Effectiveness of Mailed Pamphlets, Phone Calls, and Home Visits," *American Journal of Public Health* 85 (1995): 1,412–1,417.
19. U.S. Department of Health and Human Services, *Healthy People 2010* (Vol. I and II) (Washington, DC: 2000).
20. G.D. Gilmore and M.D. Campbell, *Needs Assessment Strategies for Health Education and Health Promotion,* 2d ed. (Dubuque, IA: Brown & Benchmark, 1996).
21. K. Glanz and B. Rimer, *Theory at a Glance: A Guide for Health Promotion Practice* (Bethesda, MD: U.S. Department of Health and Human Services, 1995).
22. B.G. Simons Morton et al., *Introduction to Health Education and Health Promotion,* 2d ed. (Prospect Heights, IL: Waveland Press, Inc., 1995).
23. L.W. Green and F.M. Lewis, *Measurement and Evaluation in Health Education and Health Promotion* (Palo Alto, CA: Mayfield, 1986).
24. M. Lalonde, *A New Perspective on the Health of Canadians: A Working Document* (Ottawa: Government of Canada, 1974).

Chapter 13

Evaluation of Public Health Interventions

Michael A. Stoto

Evaluation encompasses the set of tools that are used to measure the effectiveness of public health programs by determining what works. Traditional evaluations in public health have focused on assessing the impact of specific program activities on defined outcomes. Evaluation is also a conceptual approach to the use of data—as part of a quality improvement process—in public health management. Public health organizations must continually improve upon the standards of evidence used in the evaluation of public health so that results can inform managerial and policy decision making. As public health interventions become more integrated within the community, collaboration in evaluation efforts is a growing imperative.

Evaluation concepts and methods are of growing importance to public health organizations, as well as to education and social services programs. Increasingly, public health managers are being held accountable for their actions, and managers, elected officials, and the public are asking whether programs work, for whom, and under what conditions. Public health decision makers need to know which program variants work best, whether the public is getting the best possible value for its investment, and how to increase the impact of existing programs. These evaluation questions are being asked of long-standing programs, new activities, and proposed interventions. These developments parallel today's emphasis on "evidence-based medicine" in clinical areas, and suggest the growing role of "evidence-based management" within public health organizations.

In this context, "evaluation" is, first of all, a set of tools that is used to improve the effectiveness of public health programs and activities by determining which programs work, and also which program variants work most effectively. These tools derive from social science and health services research, and include concepts of study design, a variety of statistical methods, and economic evaluation tools. "Evaluation" is also a conceptual approach to the use of data—as part of a quality improvement process—in public health management.

However defined, evaluation can be useful to managers in public health who need, for example, to do the following activities:

- Judge the effectiveness of new approaches to public health service delivery systems that were developed elsewhere, and judge their potential applicability in one's own jurisdiction. For instance, do the immunization registries being tried in a number of U.S. cities actually result in more children being immunized?
- Judge the effectiveness of new approaches to public health service delivery systems that were developed in one's own jurisdiction. For instance, does the new community-based outreach program actually result in more children being immunized? If not, why not?

- Assess how well an intervention is being implemented in one's own jurisdiction. What fraction of children is being enrolled in the community's new immunization registry at birth? Which children are left out? What can be done to improve coverage?
- Ensure accountability of contractors and other entities with a responsibility to the public health agency. Are the managed care organizations with Medicaid contracts in the community ensuring that the children enrolled in their plans are receiving all of the recommended immunizations? Are some plans doing better than others? Why?
- Demonstrate accountability of internal programs to funders or higher authorities. Are federal funds for immunization being used according to the funders' guidelines? Are they achieving the intended effect?

This chapter begins with a primer on evaluation research methods, used by public health organizations drawing on examples from immunization programs and needle exchange programs to prevent human immunodeficiency virus (HIV) infection. Special issues in the evaluation of community-based interventions are also covered, as are issues of measurement and data. The second section of the chapter deals with practical aspects of program evaluation in public health, drawing on examples from family violence and other areas, and proposes a process for evaluation in public health settings. The final section focuses on performance measurement—in organizations as well as community settings—as a form of evaluation methodology. An extended example dealing with tobacco control illustrates the concept of performance measurement.

EVALUATION METHODS

Terminology

All public health programs can be characterized by their inputs, activities, outputs, and outcomes, as illustrated in terms of a childhood immunization program in Exhibit 13–1. *Inputs* are resources dedicated to or consumed by the program. Inputs can, in some settings, include organizational structures and capacities. *Activities* are what the program does with its inputs to fulfill its mission. *Outputs* are the direct product of program activities. Outputs, sometimes called intermediate outcomes, can sometimes overlap with outcomes, depending on the stage of the intervention. *Outcomes* are benefits for participants during and after program activities.

Within this framework, a number of different types of evaluations are possible.

- *Traditional evaluations* in public health have focused on assessing the impact of specific program activities on defined outcomes. For instance, does the new reminder system increase the number of children immunized? Questions may also be asked concerning the impact of resources on outcomes. For example, do laws requiring complete immunization prior to school entry reduce vaccine-preventable disease?
- *Economic evaluations* include costs and benefits in quantitative terms. Which program, for example, is most effective in terms of dollars per child immunized?
- *Process evaluations* refer to evaluations that are focused on outputs. Such an evaluation might ask, for instance, whether the change in enrollment procedures increases the number of children enrolled in a registry. In these cases, a relationship is assumed between outputs and outcomes (presumably based on research done elsewhere), and evidence of a change in outputs is taken as indirect evidence of an impact on desired outcomes.
- *Formative evaluations* refer to efforts to identify the best uses of available resources, prior to a traditional program evaluation. Formative evaluation often employs qualitative methods such as focus groups or structured interviews to understand a process or system and identify barriers and opportunities for improvement. Project Access in the San Francisco Bay area, for instance, interviewed drug users at

Exhibit 13–1 Examples of Program Inputs, Activities, Outputs, and Outcomes

Inputs	*Activities*	*Outputs*	*Outcomes*
Resources dedicated to or consumed by the program • Money • Staff time • Facilities • Equipment • Laws • Regulations • Funders' requirements	What the program does with inputs to fulfill its mission • Educate consumers. • Educate providers. • Distribute vaccines to providers. • Establish an immunization registry. • Provide technical assistance to providers about reminder systems. • Monitor immunization coverage in the population and health plans.	The direct product of program activities • Number of brochures distributed • Doses of vaccines delivered • Percentage of births enrolled in registry • Number of providers who establish a reminder system • Number of providers who monitor immunization coverage • Program costs	Benefits for participants during and after program activities • Parental awareness of vaccine benefits • Provider awareness • Changed attitudes • Children immunized • Reduced burden of vaccine-preventable disease in immunized children • Reduced prevalence of vaccine-preventable disease in the population • Cost per child immunized

needle exchange programs, shooting galleries, parking lots, and drug treatment centers. Researchers discovered a variety of structural barriers that prevented the users from seeking HIV counseling and testing, such as restricted hours of counseling and testing sites, lack of transportation, complications in drawing blood, and insensitive providers.[1]

- *Empowerment evaluations* involve an approach whereby programs take stock of their existing strengths and weaknesses, focus on key goals and program improvements, develop self-initiated strategies to achieve these goals, and determine the type of evidence that will document credible progress.[2] This approach is discussed in more detail in the following paragraphs.

Efficacy Assessment

Regardless of its ultimate purposes, evaluation is essentially an applied research activity seeking to discover whether a program, in some sense, has beneficial effects for the public's health. The program could be a specific activity in one public health clinic or a comprehensive communitywide activity. The question may be retrospective—Did it work?—before the program is expanded to other venues, or current—Is it working?—to ensure accountability and improve outcomes. The issue may be comparing two or more competing interventions, or assessing whether a particular program is better than nothing. The question may also be whether the program is better in some populations, or under some particular conditions. In every case, however, the central question is one of efficacy: Is some program more effective than some alternative?

Program evaluation thus centers on questions of efficacy, but additional steps are usually necessary in order to make policy decisions about recommendations for individuals and the allocation of resources. Programs shown to be effective in controlled situations, however, may not work in settings where the conditions are different. Effectiveness refers to a program's ability to get results in less than optimal situations. A worksite smoking cessation program developed by highly motivated and skilled health educators for university employees, for instance, may not be as effective when applied by human resources personnel assigned to a large auto manufacturer. Effective programs employ well-developed materials and training so that they can be generalized, that is, transferred from where they were developed to other settings.

The evaluation of public health interventions requires research directed at estimating the unique effects (or net effect) of the intervention, above and beyond any change that may have occurred because of a multitude of other factors. Such research requires study designs that can distinguish the impact of the intervention within a general service population from other changes that occur only in certain groups or that result simply as a passage of time. These designs commonly involve the formation of two or more groups: one composed of individuals who participated in the intervention (the treatment group) and a second group of individuals who are comparable in character and experience to those who participated but who received no services or an intervention that was different from that under study (the control or comparison group).

In order to estimate the net effect of an intervention reliably, the following technical issues must be addressed:[3,4]

- The manner in which the control or comparison groups are formed influences the validity of the inference.
- The number of participants enrolled in each group (the sample size) must be sufficient to permit statistical detection of differences between the groups, if differences exist.
- There should be agreement among interested parties that a selected outcome is important to measure, that it is a valid reflection of the objective of the intervention, and that it can reflect change over time.
- Evidence is needed that the innovative services were actually provided as planned, and that the differences between the innovative services and usual services were large enough to generate meaningful differences in the outcome of interest.

Experimental Designs

Over the last few decades, evaluation researchers have developed a general consensus regarding the relative strength of various study designs, as illustrated in Figure 13–1.[3] The highest level of evidence occurs with *experimental designs* that include randomized controls to restrict a number of important threats to validity. In clinical settings, individual patients are assigned by some random mechanism to a treatment group or a control group, and both groups are observed to see if there is a difference in outcomes of interest. If there is a difference in outcome, it can be assumed to be due to the intervention because the randomization ensures that there are no other differences between the two groups. An additional benefit is that the random allocation per se makes it possible to perform statistical inference, that is, to assess whether the observed differences can be due to chance.

Public health interventions such as immunizations are essentially personal health services, so the randomization model can be used directly. For other programs, the unit of intervention might be social units such as schools, worksites, or even whole communities. In these instances, randomization can still be carried out, but just not on an individual basis.[4,5] Although ethical and political objections are often raised, randomization can be carried out in social settings much more commonly than is currently done. As long as there is equipoise regarding the benefits and harms of the intervention, potential for participants to benefit, and a means of informed consent, randomization is ethically acceptable. Resource constraints that prevent the immediate introduction of a new program to an entire population present an opportunity to randomize which units get the intervention first, and concomitantly evaluate the outcome. Waiting lists can be arranged so that every client eventually receives the service, but those who get it first are chosen at random and compared to those who receive it later.[6]

Quasi-Experimental Designs

In public health, however, random assignment commonly either is not feasible or simply

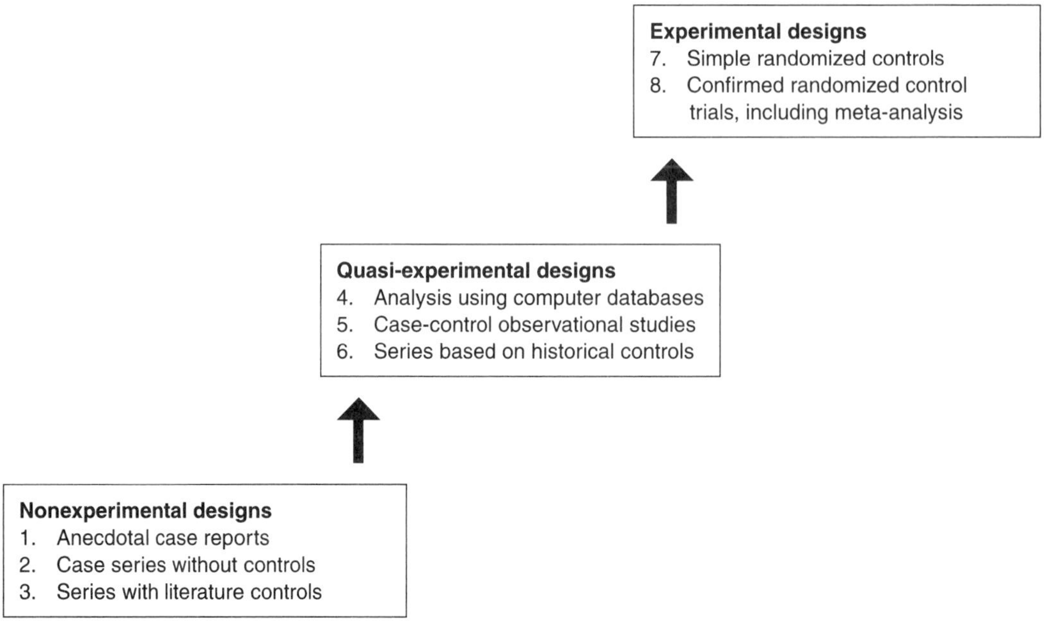

Experimental designs
7. Simple randomized controls
8. Confirmed randomized control trials, including meta-analysis

Quasi-experimental designs
4. Analysis using computer databases
5. Case-control observational studies
6. Series based on historical controls

Nonexperimental designs
1. Anecdotal case reports
2. Case series without controls
3. Series with literature controls

Figure 13–1 Hierarchy of Strength of Evidence in Research Evaluations. *Source:* Adapted with permission from *Violence in Families: Assessing Prevention and Treatment Programs,* © 1998 by the National Academy of Sciences. Courtesy of National Academy Press, Washington, D.C.

is not done. In such instances, *quasi-experimental designs*, the second level of evidence in the hierarchy, can be used to assess the impact of programs. Included in this group are analyses using existing computerized databases, case-control observational studies, and series based on historical controls. Although these designs can improve inferential clarity, they cannot be relied on to yield unbiased estimates of the effects of interventions because the subjects are not assigned randomly. A before–after design, for example, compares some outcome in the same group before and after a program is introduced. Did traffic fatalities go down in the three months after the speed limit was lowered? Designs of this sort, however, are subject to a variety of biases or threats to validity. If fatalities decreased, can it be due to better weather after the speed limit was changed on March 15? Before–after designs can be improved by gathering multiple data points before and after the program is introduced, and by careful examination of other factors, such as weather, that may be responsible for the apparent effect.

Another important quasi-experimental design is to have one or more comparison groups that are thought to be similar to the group receiving the intervention. If immunization coverage rates are higher in a community that has received a special program than in a neighboring community with no such intervention, a prima facie case can be made for the efficacy of the program. A slightly more complex design combines the before–after and control group approaches: teen birth rates are measured in two communities before and after one community attends a special school-based program. In this approach, a larger decrease in teen birth rate in the school that received the intervention than in the control school is interpreted as evidence of efficacy. The major problems with a comparison-group design is that the treatment control groups may differ in some way other than the intervention that explains the outcome. A selection bias, for instance, occurs when more advantaged population groups are more likely to choose or be chosen for a new program. In either of the examples cited, for instance, the differences may reflect a greater social advantage in the intervention group, which explains both the outcome and why they received the program.

When randomization is not possible or is not performed, statistical methods are available to reduce the effect of selection or other biases. If the experimental and comparison groups differ in some respects that may affect the outcomes, multivariate analysis can be used to "adjust" for these differences and isolate the true effect of the intervention. A worksite-based smoking cessation program, for example, may have been tested in two workplaces that differ substantially in the proportion of male and female workers and in the proportion of blue- versus white-collar positions. Because both sex and kind of job could affect smoking cessation success, evaluators might want to adjust for these factors in their analysis. In clinical settings, where patients with more severe illness seek out academic medical centers and are also at higher risk for failure, evaluators "risk adjust" to account for these differences.

Nonexperimental Designs

The lowest level of evidence occurs with *nonexperimental designs,* which consist of case series and anecdotal reports. Although such studies can contain a wealth of useful information, they cannot support inference because they cannot control for factors such as maturation, self-selection, historical influences unrelated to the intervention, and changes in instrumentation.

When a difference is detected between treatment and control groups in a study, the first question an evaluator asks is whether the difference could be due to chance (resulting from sampling individuals to be included). Various statistical techniques, depending on the nature of the research design and data, are available to provide answers to this question. If the analysis suggests that the difference is unlikely to be due to chance, it is said to be *statistically significant.* Statistical significance is sometimes assessed through the examination of *confidence intervals.* A 95 percent confidence interval is a range calculated from the data in such a way that there is a 95 percent chance that the range includes the quantity being estimated. Suppose, for example, an educational program was evaluated in terms of the average difference between the scores of individuals who were in the program and a similar group of controls on a test of knowledge of HIV risk factors. If the average difference was 1.5 points on a 10-point test, and the 95 percent confidence interval was 0.8 to 2.2 (0 is not in the range), the difference can be said to be statistically significant.

Statistical power is the likelihood that an evaluation will detect the effect of an intervention, if there is one. Two factors affect statistical power: sample size and effect size, a quantitative measure of the program's impact, such as a 10 percent improvement in immunization rates. Public health evaluation studies are often based on small samples of individuals, and thus lack sufficient statistical power to detect meaningful effects. Power can be increased by increasing the number of subjects, or by increasing the number of intervention sites, as long as each site adheres to common design elements and applies uniform eligibility criteria. Evaluators planning a study must consider whether the study size and effect size are large enough to ensure a reasonable probability that the program's impact will be statistically significant. Managers considering the results of a negative study should consider whether the study has sufficient power to detect an effect.

A related criterion is the need for careful implementation of the intervention being evaluated. A careful, randomized assessment of an intervention that is poorly implemented is likely to show, with great precision, that the intervention did not work as intended. Such a study will not distinguish between failures of the theory that is being tested and failures of implementation. Program designers need to identify critical elements of programs to explain why effects occurred and to assist others who wish to replicate the intervention model in a new setting.

Economic Analyses

Going beyond efficacy and effectiveness involves a diverse set of techniques sometimes called cost-effectiveness or economic analysis. Consider, for example, mammography for women 40–49 years of age. A group of careful evaluation studies has determined that regular (annual or biannual) mammograms for women in this age group can reduce breast cancer mortality by approximately 0.7 percent.[7] Although there is considerable uncertainty regarding the magnitude of this effect, it is very likely that the effect is positive. Breast cancer mortality, however, is very uncommon for women in their forties. The net effect, on a population level, is a small absolute reduction in mortality levels. Regular mammograms, moreover, are costly to both the women tested and their insurers. Women in their forties who receive 5 to 10 mammograms are likely to have at least one false positive result, causing anxiety, discomfort from biopsies, some unnecessary surgery, and substantial health care costs.

An economic evaluation of a public health recommendation regarding mammography for women aged 40–49 would study at least two perspectives: individuals and society. Individual women should consider the trade-off between a small reduction in mortality and the likelihood of false positives and the costs they entail. Mammography would make more sense, for instance, for women who have a high risk of breast cancer (e.g., because of family history) or who are particularly risk averse. On the societal level, policy makers should consider the clear but relatively small mortality benefits, the financial costs, and the effects of false positive results, as well as other opportunities to promote health and prevent disease that must be forgone if society invests in universal mammography. There are clearly value judgments at both the individual and societal levels that formal evaluation does not address. Evaluation tools, however, can be very useful in informing the personal and political decision-making processes.

Research Synthesis

Because replication is an important part of the scientific process, systematic reviews of existing studies—*research synthesis*—can provide a tool for understanding variations and similarities across studies. It can also uncover robust intervention effects. Before implementing a new program, careful public health managers check the evaluation literature to ensure that the intervention has been shown to be effective in other settings. Because such literature reviews often reveal a confusing range of different findings in evaluation studies of varying quality, techniques such as *meta-analysis* and more generally, research synthesis, are increasingly used in public health.[8,9]

Synthesis of research findings offers the potential to identify areas of agreement and to identify areas needing more research. Synthesis essentially involves a state-of-the-art literature review, presenting and analyzing the available data and framing results so they can be translated into practice and policy. Meta-analysis is a subset of research synthesis that employs special statistical analyses of a collection of results from individual studies for the purpose of integrating the findings. This analysis can increase the statistical precision of the estimates of a program's effect.

In a research synthesis/meta-analysis, the individual study results are the raw data. Thus, in order to avoid bias, an a priori protocol for the selection of studies to be included and their analyses is needed. Search strategies should include bibliographic sources such as the National Library of Medicine (accessible through a medical library or the World Wide Web). Searching the bibliographies of review articles and studies at hand, as well as asking experts in the field for additional references, are also effective methods of research synthesis.

Once the relevant studies are identified, they can be presented through a narrative summary of each article, or an evidence table that lays out key aspects of each study, including the publication date, study population, study design and sample size, definitions of the intervention and of outcome measures, and results. When the available studies are sufficiently similar, statistical summaries can be prepared, as illustrated in the following paragraphs.

As part of the efforts of the Community Preventive Services Task Force, for instance, researchers from the Centers for Disease Control and Prevention (CDC) identified and reviewed the effectiveness of population-based efforts to improve vaccination coverage.[10] The interventions studied included efforts to increase community demand for immunizations such as patient reminder/recall systems; programs to enhance access to immunization services by, say, reducing out-of-pocket costs; immunization mandates at school, child-care, and college entry; and provider-based strategies such as provider reminder/recall systems and the assessment of immunization rates and feedback for vaccination providers. A systematic literature search yielded 126 studies of such interventions. Following a standard approach, the researchers characterized the body of evidence as strong, sufficient, or insufficient based on the numbers of available studies, the strength of their design and execution, and the size and consistency of reported effects. This analysis then formed the basis for the recommendations of the task force.[11]

In another example, researchers evaluated the effectiveness of Bacillus Calmete-Guérin (BCG) vaccine for tuberculosis (TB) by identifying and reviewing 70 articles, 26 of which yielded appropriate quantitative data.[12,13] Figure 13–2 illustrates the analysis of 13 clinical trials in which the relative risk of TB cases was the primary outcome variable.[12] Each line corresponds to one study, labeled by author. The box in the center of each line represents the study's estimate of the vaccine's effectiveness (the size of the box is proportional to sample size); the length of the line represents a 95 percent confidence interval for the estimate. The line identified as "Combined" represents a meta-analysis of the 13 individual studies, summarized as a relative risk of 0.49, with a 95 percent confidence interval of (0.34, 0.70). Thus, although the individual study results vary, as a whole, they represent strong evidence that the BCG vaccine reduces the risk of TB by approximately 50 percent.

In other instances, quantitative combination of results is simply not feasible because the available

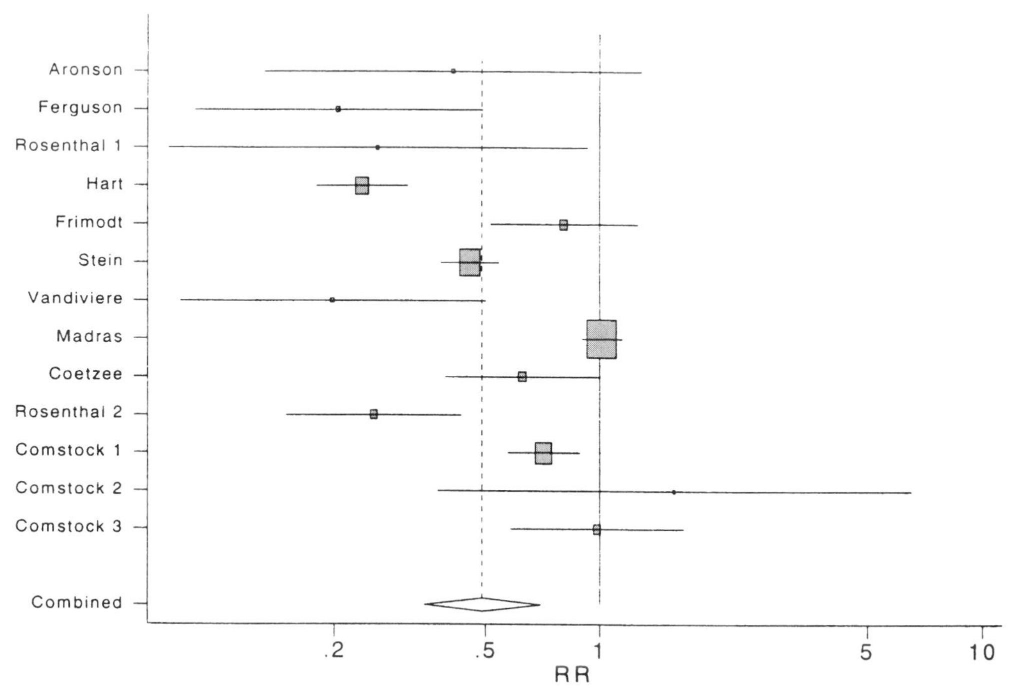

Figure 13–2 Meta-Analysis of BCG Vaccine Effectiveness Studies. *Source:* Data from G.A. Colditz et al., Efficacy of BCG Vaccine in the Prevention of Tuberculosis: Meta-Analysis of the Published Literature, *Journal of the American Medical Association,* 271, pp. 698–702, © 1994, American Medical Association.

studies are too dissimilar. A National Research Council (NRC) evaluation of the evidence surrounding the efficacy of needle exchange programs to prevent HIV transmission provides an example.[14] The logic of this approach is clear—needles are an important vector of transmission among drug users because they are passed among users, so introducing clean needles into circulation should avert new infections. When asked by Congress to review the evidence on this issue in 1995, the NRC found dozens of evaluation studies that had been prepared. Each of these studies, however, addressed different aspects of the problem: how needles can be distributed when state laws prohibit their possession, the costs and logistics of distributing needles and condoms, knowledge of HIV risk factors, various changes in users' needle use and other HIV risk factors, referral to drug treatment, and so on. Other studies examined the concerns of community leaders and individuals living near the needle exchange sites. Only a handful of reports examined HIV infection rates, which are difficult to study because the annual number of new infections in any study group is generally rather small. Moreover, many of the existing studies were of poor quality, which is not surprising given that many of the existing programs were not legally sanctioned.

There were, however, two groups of studies that provided useful information. In New Haven, Connecticut, researchers had been evaluating a needle exchange program run out of mobile vans.[15] One unique aspect of this program was that every needle distributed was marked with an identifying number, and each needle returned was checked using biomedical measures for exposure to HIV. These two pieces of information showed that the program reduced the infectivity of needles in circulation by approximately one-third. Coupled with information from a survey of the needle exchange users, the researchers used a mathematical model to show that a needle exchange program could reduce the rate of new infections by approximately one-third.

Another series of studies took advantage of the fact that one of the first needle exchange programs in the United States was organized in Tacoma, Washington, which had a preexisting enhanced hepatitis B surveillance program.[16] Hepatitis B is transmitted through blood products and sexual activity, just as HIV, but has a higher infectivity rate and shorter latency period. As a result, a group of studies in Tacoma were able to establish that needle exchange programs were effective in preventing the transmission of a bloodborne virus.

The NRC panel reviewing this evidence used a logical model to synthesize the evaluation evidence. First, a series of process studies showing that needles could be distributed efficiently ruled in the plausibility of the idea. The New Haven studies showed that needle exchange programs can increase the availability of clean equipment and reduce HIV prevalence in needles in circulation. Logically, one expects that decreasing the fraction of needles in circulation that are contaminated will lower the risk of new HIV infections, and the Connecticut model quantified this effect. The Tacoma studies confirmed the logical analysis by showing that needle exchange programs can reduce the incidence of a bloodborne disease. The NRC panel concluded, therefore, that needle exchange programs can reduce the risk of HIV infection.

MEASUREMENT

Measurement is central to evaluation. Evaluations of program effectiveness can only assess the impact on the outcomes that have been measured, and measures of program inputs are critical for interpreting the results. The importance of measurement in performance improvement is clear from the management aphorism: what gets measured gets done. The development of measures for any evaluation involves the following four steps.

1. ***Clarify the goals and purposes of the evaluation.***

In general, the goals and purposes of an evaluation determine the types of measures that are needed. Outcome evaluations need measures of health outcomes, whereas feasibility evaluations must focus on costs and barriers to implementation. Evaluations of programs intended to be exported to other venues must include measures of the specific intervention so that it can be replicated. Evaluations based on quasi-experimental designs require careful measures of confounding factors for adjustment purposes. Efforts to ensure accountability often require financial measures.

As illustrated in Figure 13–3, various disciplinary lenses produce different approaches to health promotion and disease prevention. At the micro level, the *biomedical* lens focuses on biophysiological theories of disease causation and turns to biomedical interventions for solutions. The *psychosocial* lens focuses on the individual, investigating questions about individual and social behaviors such as self-efficacy and control. The *epidemiologic* lens examines disease patterns in populations and identifies differential risk factors, both biologic and environmental. The *society-and-health* lens aims to understand the way that cultural, social, economic, and political processes influence differential risks. The choice of lens underlying the intervention obviously determines the nature of the evaluation: what is measured, and so on.

An explicit "logic model" describing the logical sequence of events that connect an intervention to the desired change can be valuable in evaluating complex interventions or simple interventions in complex causal chains. Figure 13–4 illustrates a logic model for a community-based immunization program—part of a larger effort to reduce the impact of vaccine-preventable diseases. The upper component of the figure illustrates the different types of specific interventions that are possible: community-based educational programs designed to increase community demand for vaccinations, interven-

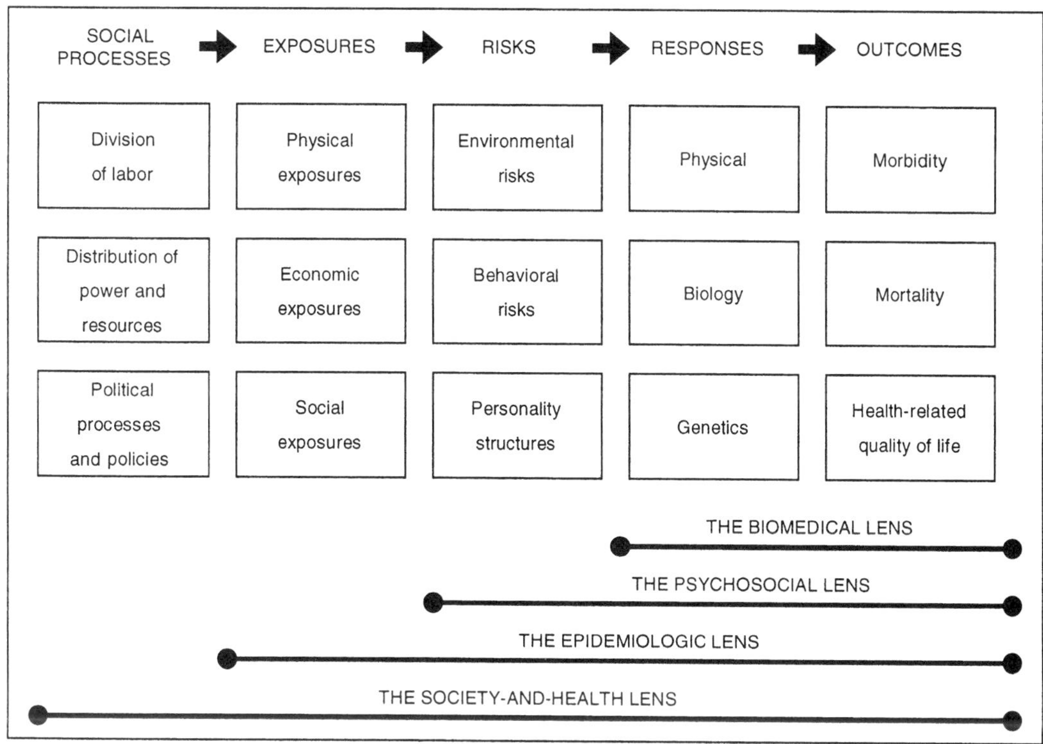

Figure 13–3 Alternative Disciplinary Lenses for Factors Influencing Health Outcomes. *Source:* Adapted, with permission, from the *Annual Review of Public Health,* Volume 19 © 1999 by Annual Reviews *www.AnnualReviews.org.*

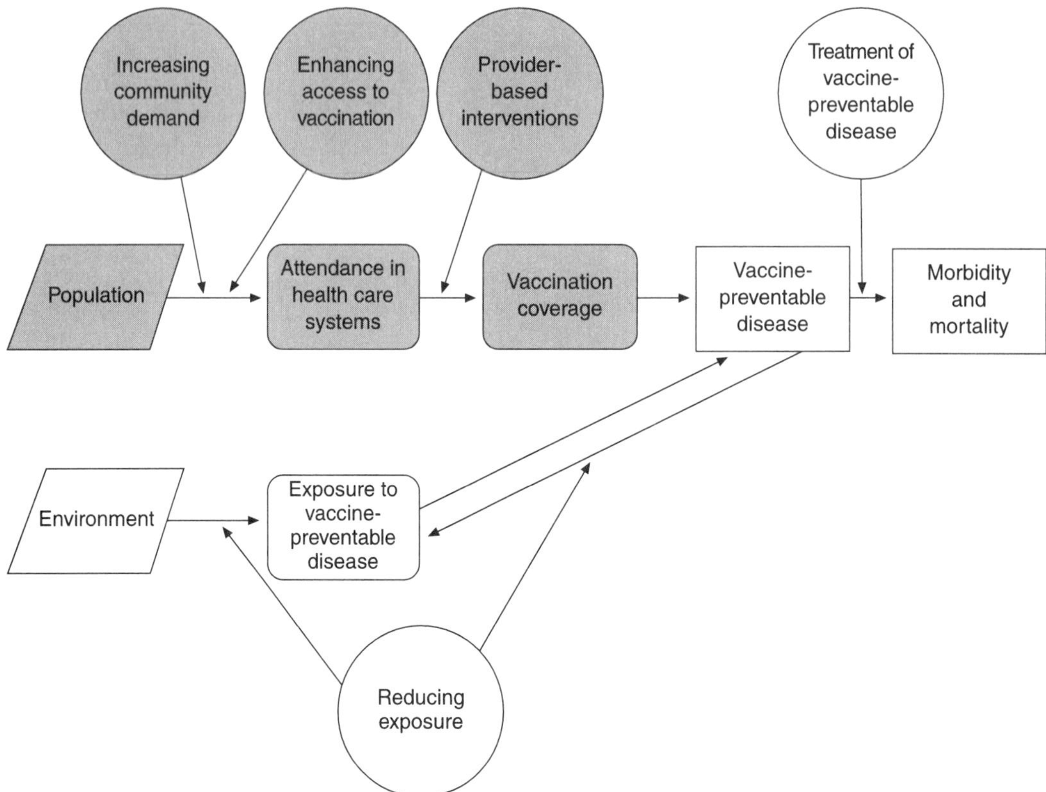

Figure 13–4 Evidence Model for Immunization Program Evaluations. *Source:* Adapted from Framework for Program Evaluation in Public Health, *Morbidity and Mortality Weekly Report,* 48 (No. RR-11), pp. 1–40, 1999, Centers for Disease Control and Prevention.

tions to enhance access to health care settings, and provider-based interventions to increase the use of vaccines among those who have access to care.

Evaluations of community-based interventions require measures of awareness and access in the community. Evaluations of provider-based interventions, on the other hand, require only measures of covered populations. A beneficial effect of vaccine coverage on vaccine-preventable disease and associated morbidity and mortality is assumed, based on previous clinical studies of the vaccines themselves. Intermediate measures of vaccine coverage, and not of morbidity and mortality, are thus sufficient for evaluations on efforts to improve immunization rates. Other interventions to reduce mortality and morbidity are possible (medical treatment of individuals who contract vaccine-preventable diseases, efforts to reduce contacts between infectious and noninfectious individuals). These are not, however, usually treated in evaluations of immunization programs.

2. ***Identify the concepts to be measured.*** Depending on the nature of the intervention and the purpose of the evaluation, measures should be chosen to reflect the logic of the process. In the immunization example in Exhibit 13–1, for instance, measures need to be developed for each of the major inputs and activities (availability of a registry), as well as the intermediate outcomes (births enrolled in a registry) and final outcomes (increased numbers of children immunized). In performance improvement processes (see below), it is important to identify responsibility for specific activities and choose measures that enable accountability for performance. It is also important to choose a set of measures that achieves a balance between short- and long-range goals and among levels and types of service.[17]

Complex programs require a variety of measures, relating to the logic of the intervention. As a condition of funding, the Health Resources and Services Administration (HRSA) maternal and child health programs, for example, require states to report their yearly performance on a number of performance measures distributed over both level and type of services, as illustrated in Exhibit 13–2.[18] States provide a variety of "types" of service: direct (immunizations), enabling (medical homes), population-based (lead screening), and infrastructure (Medicaid). Services can also be characterized by "level": capacity building (medical homes), process (lead screening), risk reduction (immunization), and outcome (infant mortality, low birth weight, and teen pregnancy). States must report on a minimum of 18 measures, distributed over level and type of service, including specific health outcomes.

3. ***Develop specific indicators for each concept.***

General concepts such as immunization coverage and low birth weight are not sufficient for program evaluation because they can be operationalized in many ways. Careful evaluation requires that each concept be measurable by one or more specific indicators, operationally defined in an unambiguous way.

Finding indicators that faithfully represent the critical concepts and can be calculated in a timely way from available data is often a challenge. Mortality, for instance, can be measured through general mortality rates or through disease-specific rates, which are available on a less timely basis. Health care costs can be measured by hospital and physician charges, but these may not accurately reflect the opportunity costs of these interventions consistent with economic theory. Quality of health care is sometimes measured through consumer satisfaction surveys, but such measures reflect only part of what policy analysts define as quality.[19] Table 13–1 illustrates the correspondence between some of the HRSA performance measure concepts and specific indicators for state maternal and child health programs.

4. ***Assess the performance of the proposed indicators with respect to validity, reliability, and sensitivity to change.***

Before an evaluation process goes forward, the indicators to be used must be assessed, especially in terms of validity and reliability. *Validity*

Exhibit 13–2 Examples of State Maternal and Child Health Performance Measures, Characterized by Type and Level of Service

	Level of Service			
Type of Service	*Capacity*	*Process*	*Risk Factor*	*Outcome*
Direct			Vaccine coverage	Infant mortality
Enabling	Medical home			Low birth weight
Population-based		Lead screening		
Infrastructure-building		Medicaid coverage		

Source: Maternal and Child Health Bureau, *Guidance and Forms for the Title V Application/Annual Report,* 1997, Health Resources and Services Administration, U.S. Department of Health and Human Services.

Table 13–1 Examples of Specific Indicators for State Maternal and Child Health Programs

Concept	*Specific Indicator*
Medical home	Percent of children enrolled in the state Special Health Care Needs program who have a "medical/health home." As defined by the American Academy of Pediatrics, this is children who have care that is accessible, continuous, comprehensive, family centered, coordinated, and compassionate (AAP, 1992).
Lead screening	Proportion of children aged 6 mo. to 5 years screened for excess blood lead
Medicaid coverage	Percent of potentially Medicaid-eligible children who have received a service paid by the Medicaid program
Vaccine coverage	Percent of children aged 19–35 months who have received the full schedule of age-appropriate immunizations against measles, mumps, rubella, polio, diphtheria, tetanus, H. influenza, and hepatitis B
Prenatal care	Percentage of infants born to pregnant women initiating prenatal care in the first trimester of pregnancy
Infant mortality	Number of infant deaths (< 1 year) divided by number of live births (per 1,000)
Low birth weight	Percent of very low birth weight infants (< 1500 grams at birth) among all live births
Teen pregnancy	Birth rate (per 1,000) for teenagers aged 15–17 years at the time of delivery

Source: Maternal and Child Health Bureau, *Guidance and Forms for the Title V Application/Annual Report,* 1997, Health Resources and Services Administration, U.S. Department of Health and Human Services.

is an indicator's capacity to measure the intended concept. *Reliability*, on the other hand, assesses whether the indicator consistently measures the concept. The relationship between the two is illustrated graphically in Figure 13–5.

Sensitivity to change assesses an indicator's ability to measure change that might be attributed to the intervention being evaluated. Some errors are related to chance fluctuations in epidemiologic rates. For most communities, for example, infant mortality rates fluctuate substantially from year to year simply because the numerator, the number of infant deaths, is small. Statistical measures can be used to assess the degree to which the indicator changes if and only if the concept being measured also changes. A common problem is when service records are used to assess changing disease burdens. Does a decrease in emergency department visits for asthma indicate the success of a prevention program, or measures to restrict access to individuals without insurance?

Compromises must generally be made among validity, reliability, data availability, and sensi-

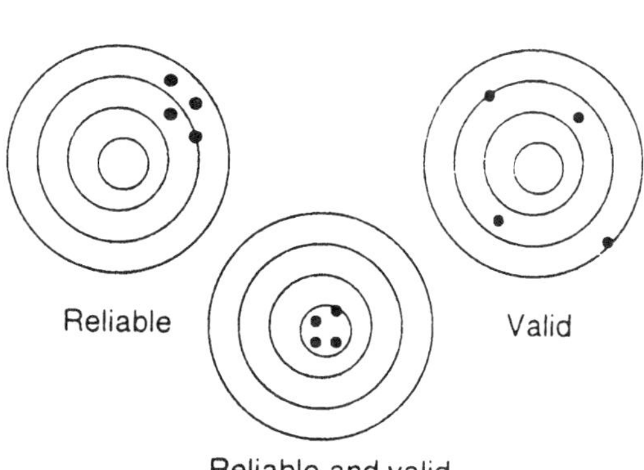

Figure 13–5 Illustration of the Concepts of Reliability and Validity

tivity to change. In the area of prenatal care, for example, evaluators often use the receipt of prenatal care in the first trimester, rather than more complex measures based on official recommendations of the U.S. Public Health Service, for the frequency and content of prenatal care, because the former measure is available on birth certificates and the latter is not.[20] This is a case of trading validity for increased data availability. In many communities, annual infant morality rates are not reliable due to the small number of infant deaths. Instead of annual rates, therefore, epidemiologists commonly calculate running averages by average infant mortality rate over three or five years. This is a case in which reliability is gained at the expense of timeliness and responsiveness to change. Another approach that is frequently used to deal with sparse data is to use proxy measures that reflect trends and differences. The percentage of infants born at low birth weight, for example, is used rather than infant mortality because low birth weight has been shown to be strongly associated with infant morality. This is a case of trading validity for reliability.

Data Sources

Data for evaluations in public health can be obtained from a wide variety of sources. (See Chapter 7 for an extensive description of various data sources.) The extended tobacco control example at the end of this chapter also illustrates the variety of data sources that can be accessed for evaluation efforts.

Capacity, process, and implementation measures can come from administrative records, existing reports and documents, and persons involved with the program. Administrative records provide good information on resources that are available and expended, the number of service providers assigned to a program, the number of clients served and the nature of services provided, and so on. Data of this sort can sometimes be derived from the management information systems used to run the program itself. In other cases, information can be obtained from clients, program staff, and others through surveys and focus groups. Documents such as grant proposals, newsletters, annual reports, and asset and needs assessments can also provide useful data for evaluations.

Outcome measures can also be derived from a variety of data sources, including vital statistics (birth and death records) and public health surveillance programs. Administrative and medical records from the health care system, because they are increasingly computerized and thus accessible, can also provide useful outcome measures. General- and special-purpose population surveys and client surveys can also provide useful information for program evaluation.

PRACTICAL ASPECTS OF PROGRAM EVALUATION

Improving the standards of evidence used in the evaluation of public health interventions is one of the most critical needs in this field. More rigorous studies are needed to better determine "what works," "for whom," "under what conditions," and "at what cost." According to a recent National Research/Institute of Medicine (IOM) report on family violence programs, which can be generalized to many other areas in public health, the road to improvement requires attention to: (1) assessing the limitations of current evaluations, (2) forging functional partnerships between researchers and service providers, (3) addressing the dynamics of collaboration in those partnerships, and (4) exploring new evaluation methods to assess comprehensive community initiatives.*

Interventions undergo an evolutionary process that refines theories, services, and approaches over time. In the early stages, interventions generate reform efforts and evaluations that rely primarily on descriptive studies and anecdotal data. As these interventions and evaluation efforts mature, they begin to approach the standards of evidence needed to make confident judgments concerning effectiveness and cost. For instance, current policy discussions are fo-

*This section draws heavily on the contributions of David Cordray to the NRC report *Violence in Families*.[21]

cused on determining the effectiveness or cost-effectiveness of selected programs or strategies, conclusions that require high standards of evidence. Existing evaluation studies, however, consist mostly of nonexperimental study designs, and thus provide no firm basis for examining the impact of programs or for considering the ways in which different types of clients respond to an intervention. Nonexperimental studies, however, can reveal important information in the developmental process of research. They can illuminate the characteristics and experience of program participants, the nature of the presenting problems, and the issues associated with efforts to implement individual programs or to change systems of service within the community. Although these kinds of studies cannot provide evidence of effectiveness, they do represent important building blocks in evaluation research.

A similar developmental process exists on the programmatic side of interventions. Many family violence treatment and prevention programs, for example, have their origins in the efforts of advocates who are concerned about children, women, and the family unit. Over several decades of organized activity, these efforts have fostered the development of interventions in social service, health, and law enforcement settings that program sponsors believe will reduce violent behavior or improve the welfare of victims. Some programs are based on common sense or legal authority; others are based on broad theories of human interaction or theory borrowed from other areas. All of these interventions were preceded by research studies that identified risk factors or critical decision points in the intervention process. As programs mature and become better articulated and implemented, evaluation questions and methods become more sophisticated and complex.

It is difficult for researchers to establish good standards of evidence in service settings because they cannot exert complete control over the selection of clients and the implementation of the interventions. But several strategies have emerged that can guide the development of evaluation research as it moves from its descriptive stage into the conduct of quasi-experimental and true experimental studies. An important part of this process is the development of a "fleet of studies."[21,22] The NRC evaluation of the effectiveness of needle exchange programs earlier provides one example. Although each individual study of a given project was insufficient to support a claim that the needle exchange program was effective, the collective strengths of the studies taken together provided a basis for a firm inference.

In order to overcome the technical challenges of conducting evaluations in public health service settings, several steps have been suggested.[21] Most importantly, research and evaluation need to be incorporated earlier into the program design and implementation process.[23] The use of innovative study designs, such as empowerment evaluation, described elsewhere in this chapter, can provide opportunities to assess the impact of programs, interventions, and strategies. Drawing on both qualitative and quantitative methods, these approaches can help service providers and researchers share expertise and experience with service operation and implementation.

Integration of the evaluation and practice perspectives requires creative collaboration between researchers and providers who are in direct contact with the individuals who receive services and the institutions that support them. Numerous points in the research and program development processes provide opportunities for such collaboration.[24] Practitioners, for example, have extensive knowledge of the needs of clients and the nature of existing services in the community. Service providers' knowledge of details concerning client flow, rates of retention in treatment, organizational capacity, and similar details are useful in developing new interventions and a logic model that provides the framework for the evaluation. Their participation can highlight differences between new services and usual-care situations, which are often a matter of degree. Practitioners can also help to ensure that the outcomes assessed are the ones of concern. Finally, service providers have knowledge of other services and factors in the community that affect outcomes of interest.

The dynamics of collaborative relationships between evaluators and program managers require explicit attention and team-building efforts to resolve different approaches and to stimulate consensus about promising models of service delivery, program implementation, and outcomes of interest. Creative collaboration requires attention to the following issues:[21]

- *Setting up equal partnerships*. Tensions between service providers and researchers may reflect differences in ideology and theory about the issues being addressed, or mutual misunderstandings about the purpose and conduct of evaluation research. Front-line service providers may resent the time and resources that research takes from the provision of services. True collaborative partnerships require a valuing and respect for the work of all sides. Both sides need to spend time observing each other's domains in order to better their constraints and risks.

  Recent collaborations in the evaluation of family violence interventions illustrate opportunities to address these concerns. Community agencies are beginning to realize that well-documented and soundly evaluated successes will help ensure their financial viability and even attract additional financial resources to support promising programs. Researchers are starting to recognize the accumulated expertise of agency personnel and how important they can be in planning as well as conducting their studies. Both parties are recognizing that, even if research fails to confirm the success of a program, the evaluation results can be used to improve the program.
- *The impact of ethnicity and culture on the research process*. Ethnicity and cultural competence influence all aspects of the research process and require careful consideration at various stages: formulation of hypotheses taking into account known cultural or ethnic differences, large enough sampling sizes to have enough power to determine differential impact for different ethnic groups, and analytic strategies that account for ethnic differences and other measures of culture. In evaluating family violence interventions, for example, there is a need for researchers who are knowledgeable about cultural practices such as parenting and care giving, child supervision, spousal relationships, and sexual behaviors in specific ethnic groups.
- *Exit issues*. The ideal relationship between a research team and the service agency is long term and sustained between large formal evaluations. Such informal collaborations can help researchers, for example, in establishing the publications needed for large-scale funding. Dissemination of findings in local publications is also helpful to the agency. Successful collaboration requires that all partners decide on the authorship and format of publications ahead of time. Thoughtful discussions are also needed before launching an evaluation about what will be released in terms of negative findings, and how the findings will be used to improve services.

  Another concern is the continuation of services when research resources are no longer available. Models of reimbursement and subsidy plans are needed to foster positive partnerships that can sustain services that seem to be useful to a community after the research evaluation has been completed.

Evaluation of Comprehensive Community-Based Interventions

In recent years, public health researchers have developed a series of comprehensive community-based interventions that reflect the growing appreciation of the social determinants of health and health-related behavior.[25,26] (See Chapter 25 for a more detailed discussion.) These interventions take place in schools, worksites, and even whole communities. They typically address smoking, diet, exercise, and other behavioral risk factors for cancer and cardiovascular disease.[4] Because of their complexity and scale, however, such interventions present special challenges to evaluators.

Moreover, public health interventions increasingly involve multiple services and the coordinated actions of multiple agencies in a community. The increasing prevalence of coexisting problems such as substance abuse and family violence or child abuse and domestic violence, for instance, has encouraged the use of comprehensive services to address multiple risk factors associated with a variety of social problems. In tobacco control, as illustrated below, the range of entities and activities involved is so great that in some senses, the community itself is the proper unit of analysis for evaluations.

As public health programs become a more integrated part of the community, the challenges for evaluation become increasingly complex.[21]

- Because participants receive numerous services, it is nearly impossible to determine which service, if any, contributed to improvement in their well-being.
- If the sequencing of program activities depends on the particular needs of participants, it is difficult to tease apart the effects of selectivity bias and program effects.
- As intervention activities increasingly involve organizations throughout the community, there is a growing chance that everyone in need will receive some form of service (reducing the chance of constituting an appropriate comparison group).
- As program activities saturate the community, it is necessary to view the community as the unit of analysis in the evaluation. Outcomes, however, are typically measured at the individual level. At a minimum, appropriate statistical models are needed to take the different levels into account.[5]
- The tremendous variation in individual communities and diversity in organizational approaches impede analyses of the implementation stages of interventions.
- An emphasis on community process factors (ones that facilitate or impede the adoption of comprehensive service systems), as opposed to program components, suggests that evaluation measures require a general taxonomy that can be adapted to particular local conditions.

Conventional notions of what constituted a rigorous evaluation design are not easily adapted to meet these challenges. Some authors have concluded that randomization is simply not feasible, and that conventional alternatives to randomization are technically insufficient.[27,28] Weiss proposed an alternative evaluation model based on clarifying the "theories of change" that explores how and why an intervention is supposed to work.[28] The evaluation should start with the explicit and implicit assumptions underlying the theory guiding the intervention efforts; this theory is generally based on a series of small steps that involve assumptions about linkages to other activities or surrounding conditions. By creating a network of assumptions, it is possible to gather data to test whether the progression of actions leads to the intended end point.

Other researchers note that the theory of change perspective provides some basic principles to guide collaborative evaluations.[29] First, the theory of change should draw on the available scientific information, and it should be judged plausible by all the stakeholders. Second, the theory of change should be doable—that is, the activities defined in the theory should be able to be implemented. Third, the theory should be testable, which means that the specification of outcomes should follow logically from the theory.

Community interventions are characterized by small relative effects. Strong interventions typically yield a two to five percent reduction in the prevalence of risk factors such as smoking or lack of exercise, or a similar percentage reduction in average serum cholesterol or blood pressure. As Rose observed, changes of this magnitude in entire populations are likely to have large effects on disease risk and the burden of morbidity and mortality.[30,31] Thus, from a public health perspective, the impact of an intervention is a product of both its efficacy in changing individual behavior and its reach, meaning the proportion of the population reached either through their direct participation or indirectly through diffusion of intervention messages throughout the community, worksite, or school.[32] Tosteson and colleagues, for instance, estimated that populationwide strategies to reduce serum cholesterol are cost-effective if cholesterol is reduced by as little as two percent.[33] Thus, although the effects of community interventions may appear small by standards of clinical research, these interventions can have a substantial public health impact.

Small effect sizes, however, create significant statistical difficulties in the evaluation of community interventions. Although the number of individuals involved in community trials is often large, the number of units of allocation that are randomized (schools, worksites, or whole communities) is typically very small. Furthermore, the power and precision of statistical tests depends more on the number of units of allocation than on the number of individuals.[5] Taken together with small effect sizes, these features of community interventions make it very difficult to achieve statistical significance in conventional terms. In other words, a true two percent reduction in a risk factor, which has great public health significance, might not achieve statistical significance in a study with thousands of individuals in a small number of communities.

A number of statistical approaches may help resolve this problem. First, more efficient statistical methods are needed to improve investigators' ability to detect small differences. This can come through increasing the number of units of allocation in studies or making better statistical use of the existing information through, say, the use of appropriate hierarchical statistical models.[34] Alternatively, where separate interventions have used parallel methods in similar populations, meta-analysis can be useful in increasing statistical power. Alternatively, future interventions might be planned with enough parallelism that meta-analysis is appropriate after the individual results are available.

Empowerment Evaluation

Empowerment evaluation represents a new use of evaluation concepts, techniques, and findings to foster improvement and self-determination. It has its roots in education and social services, but has many applications to public health. This form of evaluation draws on empowerment processes, in which attempts to gain control, obtain needed resources, and critically understand one's social environment are fundamental. It is designed to help people help themselves and improve their programs using a form of self-evaluation and reflection. Empowerment evaluation is necessarily a collaborative group activity, not an individual pursuit.[2]

As illustrated in Figure 13–6, empowerment evaluation involves six steps. These six steps are described below using the example of coalitions in three Kansas communities for the prevention of adolescent pregnancy and substance abuse.[35]

1. *Take stock—determine where the program stands, including strengths and weaknesses, and identify community concerns and resources.* A series of listening sessions—informal public meetings in which individuals identified problems, barriers to addressing the problem, resources for change, and potential solutions—were held to engage key leaders, people affected by the problem, and people who could contribute to addressing the problem. The groups included religious leaders, youth, parents, teachers, health officials, and representatives from informal neighborhood groups and community organizations.
2. *Focus on setting missions and establishing goals—determine where you want to go in the future with an explicit emphasis on program improvement.* In Kansas, the initial mission and goals were based on initiatives that had shown some success in reducing adolescent pregnancy and substance abuse in other Kansas communities. Following a shooting in one community, the coalition modified its objectives and action plan to reflect community concerns about youth violence associated with substance use.
3. *Develop strategies and action plans to accomplish goals and objectives.* Each community developed its own action plans, based on the model developed in other communities, consisting of proposed changes in programs, policies, and practices in a variety of sectors. Schools, for example, were to implement a "comprehensive K–12 age-appropriate sexuality education curriculum."

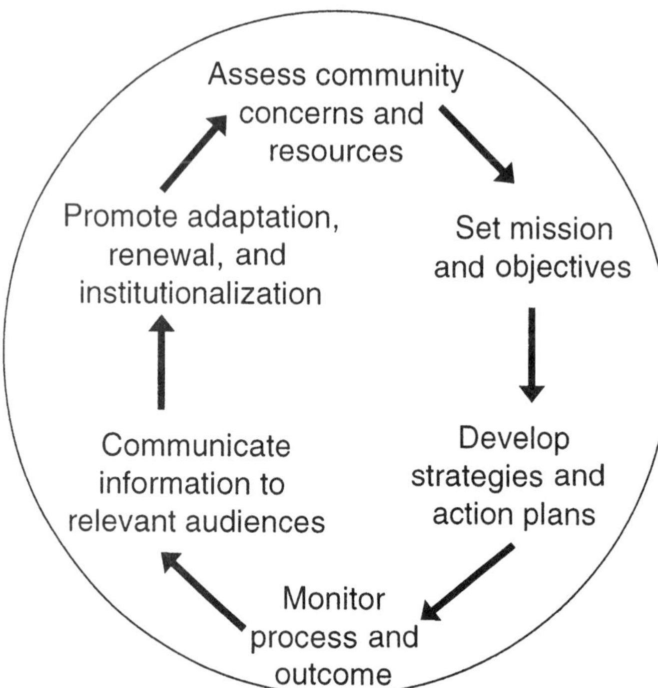

Figure 13–6 Process of Empowerment Evaluation. *Source:* Adapted from S.B. Fawcett et al., Empowering Community Health Initiatives Through Evaluation, in *Empowerment Evaluation: Knowledge and Tools for Self-Assessment and Accountability,* D.M. Fetterman et al., eds., p. 170, Copyright © 1996, Sage Publications, Inc. Reprinted by Permission of Sage Publications, Inc.

4. *Monitor process and outcome measures to document progress toward goals.* In Kansas, measurements were based on a monitoring system that was based on logs and administrative records to assess process and intermediate outcomes, constituent surveys of process and outcome, school-based behavioral surveys, community-level indicators such as the pregnancy rate, and interviews with key participants.
5. *Communicate information to relevant audiences.* Regularly sharing accomplishments and keeping constituents informed of progress are important to maintaining community support, obtaining additional resources, and ensuring accountability. In Kansas, data were shared with the coalition leadership, the community at large, and the Kansas Health Foundation, the primary sponsor.
6. *Promote adaptation, renewal, and institutionalization.* The monitoring data helped the Kansas coalition recognize accomplishments and redirect energies when necessary. In one community, for example, high levels of substance abuse service provision and low levels of community action indicated that the coalition was becoming a service agency rather than a catalyst for community change.

The Evaluation Process

A working group from the CDC recently published a set of standards and a framework for effective program evaluation in public health.[36] This framework derives both from the practical experience of the CDC and other public health practitioners and from the published standards and recommendations of practitioners in public health, social services, and education.

To be effective, evaluation efforts must meet the following four standards:

1. *utility:* Evaluation must serve the information needs of intended users.
2. *feasibility:* Evaluation efforts must be realistic, prudent, diplomatic, and frugal.
3. *propriety:* Evaluators must behave legally, ethically, and with regard for the welfare of those involved and those affected.
4. *accuracy:* Evaluation must reveal and convey technically accurate information.

The CDC's framework describes evaluation efforts as a cycle consisting of the following six steps (Figure 13–7). Although the steps are logically ordered, all are interrelated, and most actual evaluation efforts require iteration and feedback among the steps.

1. *Identify and engage stakeholders.* A number of different parties have an interest in the outcome of any evaluation; they include persons involved in and affected by the program, as well as the primary users of the evaluation, and especially those who will use it to make decisions about resources or policy. Some stakeholders are obvious: program participants, service providers, and so on. Other stakeholders, however, are less direct. Employers, for instance, may have an interest in a school-based drug prevention program if it increases the productivity of graduates hired by the company.

   Engaging these stakeholders means fostering input, participation, and power sharing in the planning and conduct of the evaluation and in the interpretation and dissemination of the findings. This en-

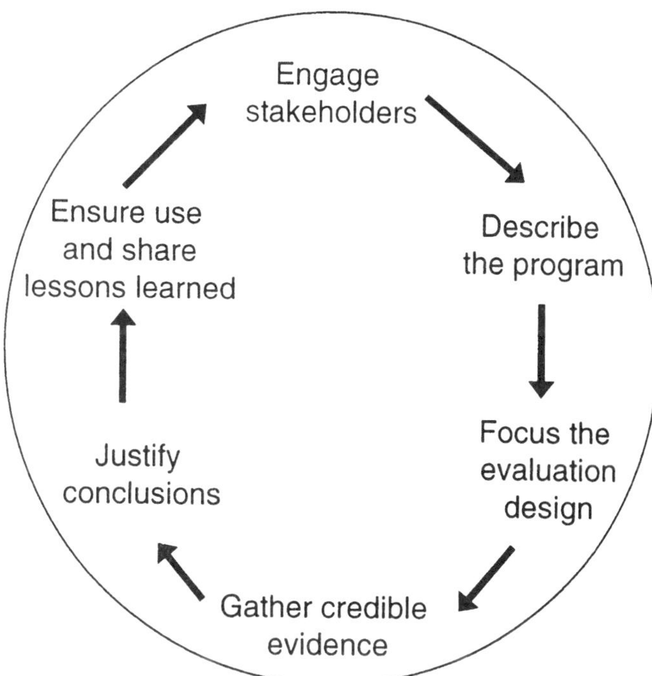

Figure 13–7 CDC Framework for Program Evaluation in Public Health. *Source:* Adapted from Framework for Program Evaluation in Public Health, *Morbidity and Mortality Weekly Report,* 48 (No. RR-11) pp. 1–40, 1999, Centers for Disease Control and Prevention.

gagement can improve credibility, clarify roles and responsibilities, ensure cultural relevance and understanding, help protect human experimental subjects, and avoid real or perceived conflicts of interest. Ultimately, it helps to increase the chance that the evaluation will be useful and have a positive impact.

2. *Describe the program.* Before a program can be evaluated, it must be described in terms of the needs it is to address and its purpose, activities, resources, and expected effects. Placing a program in a larger context and clarifying why program activities are believed to lead to the expected changes improves the evaluation's fairness and accuracy. It also permits a balanced assessment of strengths and weaknesses and helps stakeholders understand how program features fit together and relate to a larger context. A clear description of the program as actually implemented is especially important for new activities, which may be implemented in very different ways in different localities. Such descriptions are essential in assessing why interventions work in some settings and not in others.
3. *Focus the evaluation design.* If an evaluation is to be useful, it is important to clarify at the outset its purpose and uses, as well as the potential users of the results. Assessing the effectiveness of a new program may require different research designs than ensuring the accountability of contractors. Different users are interested in different research questions, depending on their interests, authority, and responsibility. Consider, for example, a communitywide campaign to educate people about the need to call 911 immediately after chest pains begin, and specifically not to worry about being embarrassed if the pain turns out not to be a heart attack. The local chapter of the American Heart Association, which may have been responsible for getting out the word through the media, would want to know how many people saw the ads and whether they understood and recalled the message. Emergency room staff would focus on how individuals were treated after they arrived, and look specifically at those individuals without heart attacks. Managed care organizations might look at the pretreatment approval process. Specific research methods for evaluation are discussed above.
4. *Gather credible evidence.* In order to ensure accuracy and meet the needs of users, evaluation efforts must be based on credible quantitative and qualitative indicators. Indicators are specific measures of program attributes or outcomes that pertain to an evaluation's focus or questions. An evaluation of an educational program to prevent teen violence would require, for example, information on the intensity of the intervention as well as the outcome. Specific indicators of program intensity might be the number of hours of student contact time in the ninth grade or the number of minutes of airtime on a specific group of radio stations that teens favor. Outcome indicators could be the percentage of students who recall the basic message of the program and the number of violent incidents in the targeted schools in the year following program implementation.

   Data that are timely must be identified or developed, and steps must be taken to ensure the credibility of the data to the intended users of the evaluation. If data are provided by an agency with a stake in the outcome of the evaluation, auditing or other steps to ensure accuracy may be necessary. Often, compromises must be made between validity, reliability, timeliness, and credibility.
5. *Justify conclusions.* The conclusions of an evaluation are justified when they are based on evidence that is credible to the stakeholders and that addresses their values and concerns. Standards are explicit statements of stakeholders' values that are operationalized in a way that allows evaluators to judge an intervention's success. A program to reduce the conse-

quences of sexually transmitted disease (STD), for example, might be evaluated in terms of its feasibility in public health clinics and managed care organizations, sensitivity to public values about sexuality, and reduction of disease burden in the population.

The conclusions and recommendations of an evaluation are the product of statistical analysis appropriate to the design of the evaluation and the synthesis of all of the available data, comparing indicators to appropriate standards. An STD evaluation might include an examination of the number of gonorrhea cases reported to the public health department before and after the intervention. This analysis, however, must be interpreted in context. Does a drop in reported cases reflect a decrease in disease, or in individuals getting treatment in private settings or not at all? Is a shift of cases from public clinics to private clinics a desired outcome? Analyses of this sort generally require a substantial amount of professional judgment by evaluation specialists.

6. *Ensure use and share lessons learned.* Evaluation results do not translate into informed decision making and appropriate action without deliberate efforts to ensure that the findings are appropriately disseminated and called to policy makers' attention. Evaluations must first be carefully designed with the concerns and interests of the stakeholders in mind, as discussed in step 3 above. Dissemination efforts must be planned to ensure that the evaluation results are brought to the attention of those persons or organizations that are in a position to use them in a form that is understandable and useful to that audience. Evaluations must follow up with stakeholders to ensure that the results are understood and not misused. Finally, opportunities for feedback can be useful to evaluators in creating an atmosphere of trust among stakeholders and in refocusing future evaluation efforts, if necessary.

Some managers in public health say, as a point of pride, that they always evaluate every program that they implement. Indeed, some federal agencies and private foundations require evaluation of all funded projects. How does this square with clinical medicine, where physicians do not "evaluate" every procedure that they perform? Having once shown that a procedure works, there is no need to evaluate it every time. The answer is that there are many forms of evaluation, and there is usually one appropriate for any situation in public health. If an intervention has been shown to work in another community, for instance, health officials might want to check that it is being properly implemented and works under the conditions in their communities. Evaluation techniques can also be useful to ensure that a program continues to be properly implemented, an approach known as "performance measurement."

PERFORMANCE MEASUREMENT AND IMPROVEMENT PROCESSES

In recent years, public health and health care policy makers have come to realize the importance of population-based data on health status and the determinants of health for effective policy determination, especially for improving the accountability of managed care organizations, public health agencies, and other entities that can contribute to the public's health. Part of this realization is due to the nature of public health and the emerging importance of preventive medicine: their impact can only be seen in statistical terms such as declining rates of lung cancer attributed to smoking reductions many years earlier. There are no grateful patients or families who know that they have been "saved" by the intervention of a particular physician or hospital. Managed care organizations and the purchasers of their services, moreover, have come to realize that performance measures based on data from the covered populations can be used to hold plans accountable for providing quality services. Similar approaches are beginning to be applied in public health settings as well.[37,38]

In response, a wide range of health data systems and approaches have been developed at the national level. *Healthy People, Healthy People 2000,* and *Healthy People 2010* have clarified the importance of specific, quantitative, population-based health measures for setting public health policy.[39–42] Other examples include the model standards developed by the American Public Health Association and others, the *Assessment Protocol for Excellence in Public Health* (APEXPH) developed by the National Association of County and City Health Officials and currently being revised, the measures used in A Planned Approach to Community Health (PATCH), and the measures proposed by the National Civic League's Healthy Cities/Communities project.[43–47] Taking this approach further, and consistent with the Government Performance and Results Act (GPRA), the U.S. Department of Health and Human Services has proposed a series of Performance Partnership Grants—to include specific performance measures for states receiving the funds—to replace a number of current block grants.[37] Although this specific approach has not been implemented, performance measurement has become increasingly common in the public health sector.[37] The HRSA's Maternal and Child Health Services Block Grants, for instance, now require annual performance measures at the state level, as discussed earlier.[18]

At the local level, many communities currently prepare community report cards for health, based in part on one or more of these efforts, but generally uncoordinated with their neighbors.[17,48] The availability of appropriate data is one of the common weaknesses of these approaches. The basic demographic and epidemiologic data available in communities, on which many of these report cards draw, often do not reflect the full spectrum of the dimensions of health or its determinants. Difficult technical problems with the existing measures and lack of data availability (especially for small geographic areas) have further limited the applications of population-based health assessment measures in public health practice.[49]

Performance Improvement in Managed Care

Managed care organizations and other organized health care delivery systems are increasingly using performance measures or report cards based on their defined populations to hold themselves accountable to members and purchasers. In recent years, the federal Health Care Financing Administration (HCFA), the Joint Commission on Accreditation of Healthcare Organizations, the National Committee for Quality Assurance (NCQA), and the Foundation for Accountability (FAcct) and other groups have developed a variety of performance measures for hospitals, providers, health plans, and managed care organizations.[50–53] Because it is responsible for delivering care to a defined group of enrollees, managed care makes possible, for the first time, accountability in terms of quality of care for populations, including access to care and health outcomes.[54] Going beyond current practices, Kindig has proposed that population-based health outcome measures should be the driving force in the market-based management of health plans, and that the health care for entire populations eventually should be managed with these measures.[55]

This trend presents an important opportunity for public health organizations as guarantors of the public's interest in the accessibility, content, and quality of health services. Rather than provide childhood immunizations directly through their own clinics, for example, public health organizations can work with branches of government responsible for the oversight of Medicaid and the regulation of health insurance to ensure that managed care immunization rates are audited and available to purchasers and the public.

The NCQA's *Health Plan Employer Data and Information Set (HEDIS)* is a prominent set of performance measures that deserves some attention here, in particular because of its increasing use in Medicaid and other publicly funded managed care.[51] (See Chapter 7 for a more detailed discussion.) *HEDIS* is a set of 20 standardized performance measures designed to ensure that purchasers and consumers have the information they need to compare the performance of managed health care plans reliably. The performance measures in *HEDIS* are related to many significant public health issues such as cancer, heart disease, smoking, asthma, and diabetes. The most recent version, *HEDIS 3.0,* also includes a standardized member satisfaction survey. The NCQA finds that managed care plans that consistently monitor and report on quality are showing significant improvements in quality, resulting in a substantial positive effect on the health of the American public.[51] Some of the measures most relevant to public health are shown in Table 13–2.

The partial list of *HEDIS* indicators in Table 13–2 illustrates two important points regarding performance measurement. First, there is a substantial overlap between the *HEDIS* measures and other public health performance measures. Childhood immunization and prenatal care measures, for example, are also included in the HRSA Maternal and Child Health Block Grant performance measures discussed above. The specific form of the indicators, however, can vary by application. The HRSA measure, for instance, calls for three hepatitis B and three Hib vaccinations, whereas the *HEDIS* measure requires only two of each. The HRSA measure applies to all children in the state aged 19–35 months; the *HEDIS* measure applies only to two-year-old children enrolled in the plan since birth. Lack of immunization associated with lack of access to health care, therefore, appears in the HRSA measure but not in the *HEDIS* measure.

Second, the breast cancer screening and diabetic eye exam measures illustrate two different approaches to incorporating clinical practice guidelines into performance measures. The U.S. Clinical Preventive Services Task Force recommends biannual mammography for women over age 50, so *HEDIS* focuses its indicator on "women between the ages of 52 and 69 who have had at least one mammogram during the past two

Table 13–2 Examples of Specific Performance in *HEDIS 3.0*

Issue	*Specific Indicator*
Advising smokers to quit	Percentage of smokers or recent quitters age 18 and older who received advice to quit smoking from a health professional.
Breast cancer screening	Percentage of women between the ages of 52–69 who have had at least one mammogram during the past two years.
Diabetic eye exams	Percentage of people with diabetes age 31 years and older who received an eye exam in the past year. (Note: Because some diabetics can safely be screened less frequently than annually, one would not necessarily expect a screening rate of 100%.)
Childhood immunizations	Percentage of two-year-old children who received appropriate immunizations by their second birthday, including four diphtheria-tetanus-pertussis, three polio, one measles-mumps-rubella, two hepatitis B, and at least two Hib vaccinations.
Prenatal care in first trimester	Percentage of women who began prenatal care during the first 13 weeks of pregnancy. Prenatal care consists of patient education, evaluation of the pregnant woman for physical or historic factors requiring special care, careful assessment of gestational age, and determination of the success with which the mother and fetus are tolerating the pregnancy.

Source: Reprinted with permission from the National Committee for Quality Assurance; State of Managed Care Quality 1999; *http://www.ncqa.org/pages/communications/news/somecqrel.html*; © 1999 by NCQA.

years."[51] The diabetic eye exam indicator, on the other hand, accommodates the possibility that not everyone in the target population does require the service by noting that "one would not necessarily expect a screening rate of 100%."[51]

Community Health Improvement Processes

The IOM has recently proposed a Community Health Improvement Process drawing on the existing use of evaluation tools in a community health setting.[17] Other authors describe similar processes using somewhat different terms, but the basic ideas and issues are typically the same: ownership by communities, a broad definition of health, a cross-disciplinary approach to intervention, and sharing of responsibility among stakeholders for both decision making and accountability. The IOM's model also can be thought of as an example of empowerment evaluation.*

The rationale for the community health improvement process (CHIP) model is that because a wide array of factors influence a community's health, many entities in the community share the responsibility of maintaining and improving its health. Responsibility shared among many entities, however, can easily become responsibility that is ignored or abandoned. At the level of actions that can be taken to protect and improve health, however, specific entities can and should be held accountable, with assignments made through a collaborative process. Because resources and concerns of communities differ, each will have to determine its own specific allocation of responsibility and accountability. Once accountability is assigned, communities can use performance monitoring to hold community entities accountable for actions for which they have accepted responsibility.

Growing out of this perspective, a CHIP that includes performance monitoring can be an effective tool for developing a shared vision and supporting a planned and integrated approach to improve community health. A CHIP offers a way for a community to address a collective responsibility and marshal resources of its individuals and families, the medical care and public health systems, and community organizations to improve the health of its members. A CHIP should include two principal interacting cycles based on analysis, action, and measurement (Figure 13–8). The overall process differs from standard models primarily because of its emphasis on measurement to link performance and accountability on a communitywide basis.

The health assessment activities that are part of a CHIP's problem identification and prioritization cycle should include production of a community health profile that can provide basic information to a community regarding its demographic and socioeconomic characteristics and its health status and health risks. This profile would provide background information that could help a community interpret other health data and identify issues that need more focused attention.

For example, the set of indicators for a community health profile might include

- *sociodemographic characteristics,* such as the high school graduation rate and median household income
- *health risk factors,* such as child immunization coverage, adult smoking rate, and obesity
- *health care resource consumption,* such as per capita health care spending
- *health status,* such as the infant mortality rate by race/ethnicity, numbers of deaths due to preventable causes, and confirmed child abuse and neglect cases
- *functional status,* such as the proportion of adults in good to excellent health
- *quality of life,* such as the proportion of adults who are satisfied with the health care system in the community

Within the CHIP framework, performance monitoring takes place in the analysis and implementation cycle. A community may have a portfolio of health improvement activities, each progressing through this cycle at its own pace. A

*This section draws heavily on the IOM report *Improving Health in the Community: A Role for Performance Monitoring.*[17]

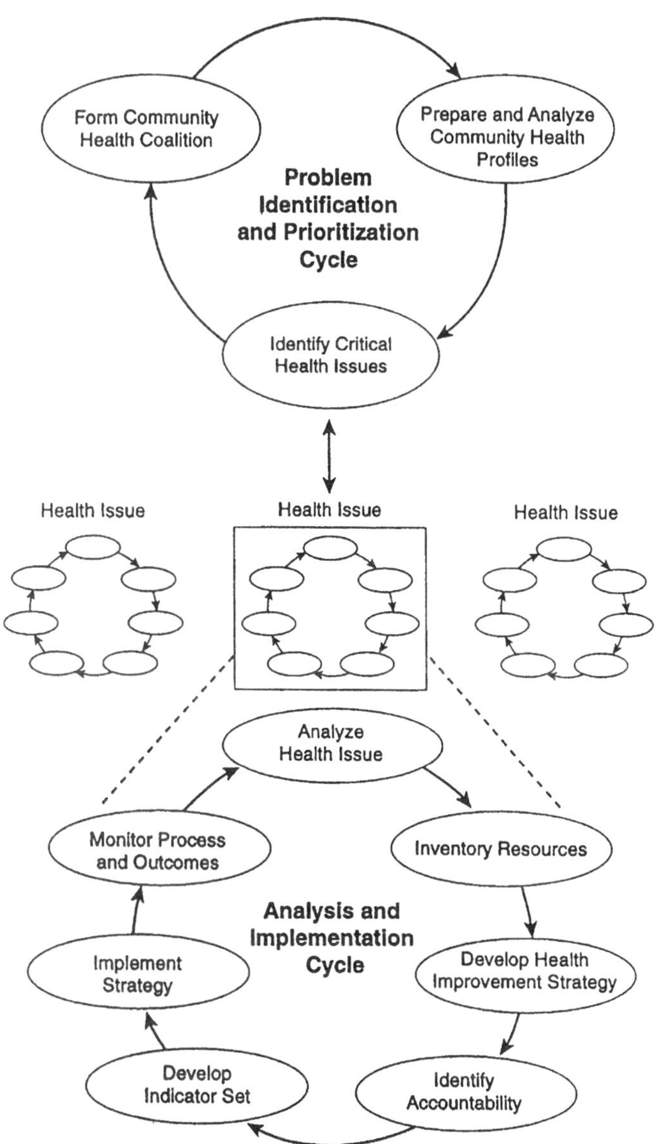

Figure 13–8 A Community Health Improvement Process. *Source:* Reprinted with permission from *Improving Health in the Community: A Role for Performance Monitoring,* © 1997 by the National Academy of Sciences. Courtesy of National Academy Press, Washington, D.C.

prototype performance indicator set for vaccine-preventable diseases is shown in Exhibit 13–3. Measures like these can be further articulated to clarify the accountability of individuals and families, the medical care and public health systems, and community organizations.

To make operational the concept of shared responsibility and individual accountability for community health, stakeholders need to know, jointly and as clearly as possible, how the actions of each potentially accountable entity can contribute to the community's health. Thus, a

Exhibit 13–3 Sample Prototype Indicator Set: Vaccine-Preventable Diseases

- Immunization rate for all children at 24 months of age.
- Immunization rate at 24 months of age for children currently enrolled in managed care organizations.
- Immunization rate at 24 months of age for children currently enrolled in Medicaid.
- Existence in the community of a computerized immunization registry that provides automated appointment reminders; if available, the percentage of children in the community included in the registry.
- Among children with commercial health insurance coverage, percentage with full coverage for childhood immunizations.
- Percentage of Medicare enrollees who received an influenza immunization during the previous calendar year; percentage who have ever received a pneumococcal pneumonia immunization.
- Pneumonia and influenza death rates for persons age 65 and older.
- Existence in the community of an active childhood immunization coalition involving health service providers, the local health department, parents, and interested parties.

Source: Adapted with permission from *Improving Health in the Community: A Role for Performance Monitoring,* © 1997 by the National Academy of Sciences. Courtesy of National Academy Press, Washington, D.C.

CHIP should include the development of a set of specific, quantitative performance measures that link accountable entities to the performance of specific activities expected to lead to the production of desired health outcomes in the community. Selecting these indicators will require careful consideration of how to gain insight into progress achieved in the health improvement process. A set of indicators should balance population-based measures of risk factors and health outcomes and health systems-based measures of services performed. Process measures (such as availability of insurance coverage for immunizations) might be included, but only to the extent that there is evidence that links them to health outcomes. To encourage full participation in the health improvement process, the selected performance measures should also be balanced across the interests and contributions of the various accountable entities in the community, including those whose primary mission is not health specific.

Example: Indicators for Tobacco Control Programs*

A concerted and coordinated youth-centered tobacco control effort must address all of the entities that have a stake in, and can influence, the use of tobacco and its effects, including federal, state, and local public health and other governmental agencies; health care providers and health plans; voluntary and professional organizations such as the American Cancer Society, the American Lung Association, and the American Heart Association; tobacco companies; and schools, workplaces, and other community-based organizations.[57,58] As the following example illustrates, one way to ensure that all of the possible opportunities for intervention are considered is to review the dimensions of the Evans and Stoddart field model.[25]

A concerted national effort will also require action at the national, state, and community levels. The proposed performance indicator sets (Table 13–3) thus also illustrate how to provide a mechanism at the national level, and a model for translation to state and local levels, to establish accountability for actions that can be taken to improve the health of the nation.[59]

This example also illustrates the kinds of data that must be used in a comprehensive evaluation effort. Two national sources can be used as a starting point for developing performance indicators for tobacco control: *Healthy People 2010,* which includes tobacco as one of its priority areas, and the recent Food and Drug Administration (FDA) regulations restricting the sale and

*This section draws heavily on a background paper prepared for the IOM/NRC National Cancer Policy Board.[56]

Table 13–3 National- and Community-Level Performance Measures for Tobacco Control

Issue/National Performance Measure	*Stakeholders/ Responsible Entity*	*Possible Corresponding Community Indicators*	*Possible Stakeholders/ Responsible Entities*
Smoking-related mortality:			
• Number of deaths nationally due to lung cancer, cardiovascular disease, emphysema, chronic bronchitis, respiratory infections; percentage of these deaths attributable to smoking	National health care providers and plans, federal government, business, national organizations, general public	• Number of deaths in the community due to lung cancer, cardiovascular disease, emphysema, chronic bronchitis, respiratory infections; percentage of these deaths attributable to smoking	Health care providers and plans, state and local health agencies, community organizations, business, special health risk groups, general public
Adult smoking:			
• Percentage of the adult population, ages 18 and older, who smoke regularly	Federal government, business, national voluntary organizations, general public	• Percentage of the adult population, ages 18 and older, who smoke regularly	State and local health agencies, business, community organizations, general public
Initiation of tobacco use:			
• Percentage of eighth, tenth, twelfth graders using cigarettes or smokeless tobacco in past 30 days • Percentage of eighth, tenth, twelfth graders using cigarettes or smokeless tobacco daily • Percentage of youth, ages 20–24, who smoke regularly • Percentage of males, ages 12–24, who use smokeless tobacco regularly	Federal government, national voluntary organizations, general public	• Percentage of eighth, tenth, twelfth graders using cigarettes or smokeless tobacco in past 30 days • Percentage of eighth, tenth, twelfth graders using cigarettes or smokeless tobacco daily • Percentage of youth, ages 20–24, who smoke regularly • Percentage of males, ages 12–24, who use smokeless tobacco regularly	State and local health agencies, schools community organizations, general public
Access of children and adolescents to tobacco:			
• Development of national regulations regarding youth access	FDA, Congress	• Effectiveness of local enforcement of laws prohibiting tobacco sales to youth (minimum age, minimum package size, vending machines, self-service displays, free samples)	State and local health agencies, local government, business, industry, public in general
• Implementation of regulations by manufacturers (minimum package size, self-service displays, mail order sales and coupons, free samples)	Manufacturers		

continues

Table 13–3 continued

Issue/National Performance Measure	Stakeholders/ Responsible Entity	Possible Corresponding Community Indicators	Possible Stakeholders/ Responsible Entities
Reduce appeal of tobacco to youth:			
• Development of national regulations regarding advertising to youth	FDA, Congress	• Implementation of regulations by manufacturers (billboards near schools and playgrounds) • Extent to which tobacco use prevention is incorporated into school curricula and activities	Local health agencies, local government, schools
• Implementation of regulations by manufacturers (text-only format, sponsorship of events, sales/distribution of nontobacco items)	Manufacturers		
Reduce exposure to environmental tobacco smoke:			
• Development of model ETS regulations • Prevalence of ETS regulations in federal government facilities	Federal government, national business organizations, national voluntary organizations	• State and local regulation of smoking in workplaces and enclosed public places • Enforcement of existing ETS regulations	State and local health agencies, local government, business, industry
Promote cessation of tobacco use:			
• Federal funding for development and evaluation of smoking cessation programs • Cessation attempts among the adult population, ages 18 and older, who smoke regularly	Federal government, national health care plans, national voluntary organizations, national business organizations	• Availability of smoking cessation programs • Cessation attempts among the adult population, ages 18 and older, who smoke regularly	Health care providers/plans, business, community organizations, general public
Smoking during pregnancy:			
• Federal funding for development and evaluation of smoking cessation programs for pregnant women • Cessation among pregnant women who smoke regularly	Federal government, national health care plans, national voluntary organizations, national business organizations	• Availability of smoking cessation programs for pregnant women • Cessation among pregnant women who smoke regularly	Health care providers/plans, business, community organizations, general public

continues

Table 13–3 continued

Issue/National Performance Measure	*Stakeholders/ Responsible Entity*	*Possible Corresponding Community Indicators*	*Possible Stakeholders/ Responsible Entities*
Health care system efforts to reduce tobacco use:			
• Percentage of smokers whose health care providers ask about smoking, provide cessation counseling, and assist cessation efforts • Proportion of nonsmoking youth counseled not to begin tobacco use • Percentage of health-care-plan covered lives with coverage for tobacco cessation programs	Federal government, national health care plans, national voluntary organizations, national business organizations	[For each health care plan:] • Percentage of smokers whose health care providers ask about smoking, provide cessation counseling, and assist cessation efforts • Proportion of nonsmoking youth counseled not to begin tobacco use • Percentage of health-care-plan covered lives with coverage for tobacco cessation programs	Health care providers/plans, business, community organizations, general public
Community-based programs to change social norms:			
• Federal funding for development and evaluation of community-based programs to change social norms and reduce tobacco use	Federal government, national business organizations, national voluntary organizations	• Existence of community-based anti-tobacco coalitions • Number of smoking cessation programs available and their use and success rate • Extent to which tobacco use prevention is incorporated into school curricula and activities • Students who associate physical or psychological harm with, and who perceive social disapproval of, regular use of tobacco	State and local health agencies, schools, community organizations, general public
Tobacco excise tax:			
• Federal excise tax per pack of cigarettes	Federal government, manufacturers, smokers, general public	• State excise tax per pack of cigarettes	State government, manufacturers, smokers, general public

Note: ETS, environmental tobacco smoke.
Source: Adapted with permission from *Taking Action to Reduce Tobacco Use,* © 1998 by the National Academy of Sciences. Courtesy of National Academy Press, Washington, D.C.

distribution of cigarettes and smokeless tobacco to protect children and adolescents.[60]

The first set of indicators on smoking-related mortality relates to disease outcomes. The specific measures used—the number of deaths due to lung cancer, cardiovascular disease, emphysema, chronic bronchitis, or respiratory infections; plus the percentage of these deaths attributable to smoking—are generally available for small geographic areas as well as nationally.[61]

The measures for the second and third issues relate to the individual behavior. Adult smoking is measured in terms of the percentage of the adult population, ages 18 and older, who smoke regularly. The same measure might be used locally as well as nationally. The state-based Behavioral Risk Factor Surveillance System, for which a standard question on adult smoking has been developed, might provide a basis for producing community-level data.[62] A second behavioral issue, initiation of tobacco use, is represented by four performance measures. Two of these measures—the percentage of youth, ages 20–24, who smoke regularly and the percentage of males, ages 12–24, who use smokeless tobacco regularly—are consistent with *Healthy People 2000*. Although technically they are measures of the prevalence of tobacco use, both indicators indirectly measure initiation of use because there is relatively little cessation in the age ranges in question. Two additional measures—the proportion of eighth, tenth, and twelfth graders using cigarettes or smokeless tobacco in the past 30 days and daily—are based on an annual survey of high school seniors.[63]

The next set of indicators deals with access of children and adolescents to tobacco, which is an aspect of the social environment. At the national level, the two measures proposed are: (1) the development of national regulations regarding youth access and (2) the implementation of regulations by manufacturers (regarding package size, self-service displays, free samples, etc.). The first relates to actions by the FDA, Congress, and other governmental agencies to develop national regulatory policies regarding access; the second monitors the performance of tobacco product manufacturers in complying with existing regulations. By their nature, these two indicators must be more qualitative than others proposed. At the community level, attention must focus on implementation of the regulations by public health and other governmental agencies, by business and industry, and by the general public. Indicators will need to be developed of the effectiveness of local enforcement of laws prohibiting tobacco sales to youth (e.g., regarding minimum age, minimum package size, vending machines, self-service displays, free samples). Depending on the community, compliance with these regulations might be measured through youth surveys, or perhaps by records of violations and enforcement activities.

Indicators relating to efforts to reduce the appeal of tobacco to youth address another issue reflecting the influence of the social environment. Similar to the previous measures, the national-level indicators focus on the development of national regulations regarding advertising to youth and the implementation of such regulations by manufacturers (e.g., regarding text-only format, sponsorship of events, sales/distribution of nontobacco items). At the local level, attention is focused on the implementation of regulations by manufacturers (especially regarding billboards near schools and playgrounds) and the extent to which tobacco use prevention is incorporated into school curricula and activities. Measures will need to be developed concerning the effectiveness of local implementation of the advertising regulations. Depending on the community, compliance with these regulations might be measured through youth surveys, or perhaps by records of violations and enforcement activities.

The next set of indicators on reducing exposure to environmental tobacco smoke relates to the influence of the physical environment on health. For the national level, one indicator addresses the development of model environmental tobacco smoke (ETS). Other steps that can be taken at the national level are represented by the indicator on the prevalence of ETS regulations in federal government facilities. For the state and local levels, measures are needed for the existence of state and local regulation of smoking in workplaces and enclosed public places, and the enforcement of existing ETS regulations at the local level.

The next two groups of indicators address smoking cessation, among adults in general and during pregnancy. In terms of the Evans and Stoddart model, they reflect an influence on health through both "individual response/behavior" and also interventions based in the health care sector and in the community to promote cessation.[25] For the national level, the indicators measure the efforts of the federal government and national organizations to develop and evaluate cessation programs as well as cessation attempts per se. The measures for development and evaluation efforts may need to be semiqualitative, but cessation attempts can be measured directly through population surveys. Cessation can also be measured directly at the community level. Additional performance measures must be developed for the availability of programs to help individuals stop smoking.

The next set of indicators relates to health care system efforts to reduce tobacco use. For three measures—the percentage of smokers whose health care providers ask about smoking, provide cessation counseling, and assist cessation efforts; the proportion of nonsmoking youth counseled not to begin tobacco use; and the percentage of health-care-plan covered lives with coverage for tobacco cessation programs—data can be obtained from national or community surveys or from health plan records. These indicators should be used at both the national and the community levels to assess overall practices of the health care sector, and used by individual health plans to guide their own efforts.

Other indicators might be used specifically at the national level to assess contributions that can be made by groups such as large health plans or national professional organizations or by academic health centers, which train health professionals who practice throughout the country. The suggested measures are: (1) the proportion of health plans or national professional organizations that have adopted policies or recommendations that during appropriate health care visits clinicians identify patients who use tobacco, provide cessation counseling, and assist in cessation efforts and (2) the proportion of academic health centers that include training in cessation counseling in undergraduate and continuing education curricula for health professionals (e.g., physicians, nurses, dentists, physician assistants).

The final two categories of indicators relate to changing social norms, which can be considered an aspect of the "social environment." With respect to community-based programs to change social norms, federal funding for development and evaluation of such programs must be monitored at the national level. At the local level, indicators can address the existence of community-based antitobacco coalitions, the number of smoking cessation programs available and their use and success rate, and the extent to which tobacco use prevention is incorporated into school curricula and activities. In addition, school surveys can be developed to measure the proportion of students who associate physical or psychological harm with, and who perceive social disapproval of, regular use of tobacco (a *Healthy People 2010* measure).[42] Data on the federal and state tobacco excise tax are available from industry sources.

• • •

A large and growing set of evaluation methods now exists to assist public health organizations in measuring and improving their programs and operations. These tools can be used to monitor the quality, outcomes, and efficiency of public health activities carried out by single and multiple institutions. These tools can also be used to examine the effects that interventions outside the domain of public health have on community health. Public health organizations must continually work to improve the standards of evidence used in evaluating public health interventions, so that results can inform managerial and policy decision making. Moreover, as an increasing share of public health interventions are carried out through multi-institutional partnerships, public health organizations must meet the growing imperative for collaboration in evaluation efforts. By doing so these organizations can move closer to the goals of evidence-based management and the gains in population health that it promises.

CHAPTER REVIEW

1. Evaluation addresses the following questions:
   - Which programs work, for whom, and under what conditions?
   - Which program variants work best?
   - Is the public getting the best possible value for its investment?
   - How can the impact of existing programs be increased?
2. All public health programs can be thought of in terms of *inputs, activities, outputs,* and *outcomes.*
3. Economic evaluations include costs and benefits in quantitative terms—for example, which program is most effective in terms of dollars per child immunized?
4. Formative evaluation refers to efforts to identify the best use of available resources, prior to a traditional program evaluation. Formative evaluation often employs qualitative methods such as focus groups or structured interviews.
5. *Statistical power* is the likelihood that an evaluation will detect the effect of an intervention, if there is one. Two factors affect statistical power: sample size and effect size, which is a quantitative measure of the program's impact.
6. Research synthesis—systematic reviews of existing studies, including meta-analysis—is increasingly used in public health to uncover robust effects.
7. The goals of an evaluation determine the types of measures that are needed. Outcome evaluations need measures of health outcomes whereas feasibility evaluations focus on costs and barriers to implementation.
8. A CDC framework for evaluation consists of a six-step cycle.
   - Identify and engage stakeholders.
   - Describe the program.
   - Focus the evaluation design.
   - Gather credible evidence.
   - Justify conclusions.
   - Ensure use and share lessons learned.

REFERENCES

1. P. DeCarlo, 1999. Project Access: Research That Feeds Back into the Community. *CAPS Exchange*. (San Francisco: Center for AIDS Prevention Studies, Undated).
2. D.M. Fetterman, "Empowerment Evaluation: An Introduction to Theory and Practice," in *Empowerment Evaluation: Knowledge and Tools for Self-Assessment & Accountability,* eds. D.M. Fetterman et al. (Thousand Oaks, CA: Sage, 1996), 3–46.
3. S.B. Green and D.P. Byar, "Using Observational Data from Registries To Compare Treatments: The Fallacy of Omnimetrics," *Statistics in Medicine* 3 (1984): 361–370.
4. G. Sorensen et al., "Implications of the Results of Community Intervention Trials," *Annual Review of Public Health 1998* 19 (1998): 379–416.
5. D.M. Murray, *Design and Analysis of Group-Randomized Trials* (New York: Oxford University Press, 1998).
6. D.C. Hoaglin et al., *Data for Decisions: Information Strategies for Policymakers* (Cambridge, MA: Abt Books, 1982).
7. D.A. Berry, "Benefits and Risks of Screening Mammography for Women in Their Forties: A Statistical Approach," *Journal of the National Cancer Institute* 90 (1998): 1,431–1,439.
8. T.A. Louis et al., "Findings for Public Health from Meta-Analysis," *Annual Review of Public Health 1985* 16 (1985): 1–20.
9. F. Mosteller and G.A. Colditz, "Understanding Research Synthesis (Meta-Analysis)," *Annual Review of Public Health 1996* 17 (1996): 1–23.
10. A. Shefer et al., "Improving Immunization Coverage Rates: An Evidence-Based Review of the Literature," *Epidemiological Reviews* 21 (1999): 96–142.

11. Task Force on Community Preventive Services. "Interventions To Improve Vaccination Coverage in Children, Adolescents, and Adults," *American Journal of Preventive Medicine 18,* no. 1S (2000): 92–96.
12. G.A. Colditz et al., "Efficacy of BCG Vaccine in the Prevention of Tuberculosis: Meta-Analysis of the Published Literature," *Journal of the American Medical Association* 271 (1994): 698–702.
13. G.A. Colditz et al., "The Efficacy of Bacillus Calmete-Guérin Vaccination of Newborns and Infants in the Prevention of Tuberculosis: Meta-Analysis of the Published Literature," *Pediatrics* 96 (1995): 29–35.
14. J. Normand et al., *Preventing HIV Transmission: The Role of Sterile Needles and Bleach* (Washington, DC: National Academy Press, 1995).
15. E.H. Kaplan and R. Heimer, "HIV Incidence Needle Exchange Participants: Estimated from Syringe Tracking and Testing Data," *Journal of Acquired Immune Deficiency Syndromes* 7 (1994): 182–189.
16. H.D.C. Hagan et al., "Risk for Human Immunodeficiency Virus and Hepatitis B Virus in Users of the Tacoma Syringe Exchange Program," in *Proceedings, Workshop on Needle Exchange and Bleach Distribution Programs* (Washington, DC: National Academy Press, 1994), 24–34.
17. J.S. Durch et al., *Improving Health in the Community: A Role for Performance Monitoring* (Washington, DC: National Academy Press, 1997).
18. Maternal and Child Health Bureau, *Guidance and Forms for the Title V Application/Annual Report* (Rockville, MD: Health Resources and Services Administration, 1997).
19. M.S. Donaldson, *Measuring the Quality of Health Care* (Washington, DC: National Academy Press, 1999).
20. Public Health Service, Expert Panel on the Content of Prenatal Care, *Caring for Our Future: The Content of Prenatal Care* (Washington, DC: U.S. Department of Health and Human Services, 1989.)
21. R. Chalk and P. A. King, *Violence in Families: Assessing Prevention and Treatment Programs* (Washington, DC: National Academy Press, 1998).
22. L.J. Cronbach and R.E. Snow, *Aptitudes and Instructional Methods: A Handbook for Research on Interactions* (New York: Irvington Publishers, 1981).
23. A.J. Reiss, Jr. and J.A. Roth, National Research Council, *Understanding and Preventing Violence* (Washington, DC: National Academy Press, 1993).
24. D.S. Cordray and G.M. Pion, "Psycho-Social Rehabilitation Assessment: A Broader Perspective," in *Improving Assessment in Rehabilitation and Health*, eds. R. Glueckauf et al. (Newbury Park, CA: Sage, 1993), 215–240.
25. R.G. Evans and G.L. Stoddart, "Producing Health, Consuming Health Care," in *Why Are Some People Healthy and Others Not? The Determinants of Health of Populations*, eds. R.G. Evans et al. (New York: Aldine De Gruyter, 1994).
26. D.L. Patrick and T.M. Wickizer, "Community and Health," in *Society and Health*, eds. B.C. Amick et al. (New York: Oxford University Press, 1995), 46–92.
27. R.G. Hollister and J. Hill, "Problems in the Evaluation of Community-Wide Initiatives," in *New Approaches to Evaluating Community Initiatives*, eds. J.P. Connell et al. (New York: The Aspen Institute, 1995), 127–172.
28. C.H. Weiss, "Nothing as Practical as Good Theory: Exploring Theory-Based Evaluation for Comprehensive Community Initiatives for Children and Families," in *New Approaches to Evaluating Community Initiatives*, eds. J.P. Connell et al. (New York: The Aspen Institute, 1995), 65–92.
29. J.P. Connell and A.C. Kubisch, *Applying Theories of Change Approach to the Evaluation of Comprehensive Community Initiatives: Progress, Prospects, and Problems* (New York: The Aspen Institute, 1996).
30. G. Rose, "Sick Individuals and Sick Populations," *International Journal of Epidemiology* 14 (1985): 32–38.
31. G. Rose, *The Strategy of Preventive Medicine* (New York: Oxford University Press, 1992).
32. D. Abrams, "Conceptual Models To Integrate Individual and Public Health Interventions: The Example of the Work-Place," in *Proceedings of the International Conference on Promoting Diet Change in Communities*, ed. M. Henderson (Seattle, WA: Fred Hutchinson Cancer Research Center, 1991), 173–194.
33. A.N.A. Tosteson et al., "Cost-Effectiveness of Population-Wide Educational Approaches To Reduce Serum Cholesterol Levels," *Circulation 95,* no. 1 (1998): 24–30.
34. D.M. Murray, *Design and Analysis of Group-Randomized Trials* (New York: Oxford University Press, 1998).
35. S.B. Fawcett et al., "Empowering Community Health Initiatives through Evaluation," in *Empowerment Evaluation: Knowledge and Tools for Self-Assessment & Accountability,* eds. D.M. Fetterman et al. (Thousand Oaks, CA: Sage, 1996), 161–187.
36. U.S. Centers for Disease Control and Prevention, "Framework for Program Evaluation in Public Health," *Morbidity and Mortality Weekly Report 48,* no. RR-11 (1999): 1–40.
37. E.B. Perrin and J.J. Koshel, *Assessment of Performance Measures for Public Health, Substance Abuse, and Mental Health* (Washington, DC: National Academy Press, 1997).
38. E.B. Perrin et al., *Health Performance Measurement in the Public Health Sector: Principles and Policies for Implementing an Information Network* (Washington, DC: National Academy Press, 1999).
39. U.S. Department of Health, Education, and Welfare, *Healthy People: The Surgeon General's Report on*

Health Promotion and Disease Prevention (Washington, DC: U.S. Government Printing Office, 1979).

40. U.S. Department of Health and Human Services, *Promoting Health/Preventing Disease: Objectives for the Nation* (Washington, DC: U.S. Government Printing Office, 1980).
41. U.S. Department of Health and Human Services, *Healthy People 2000: National Health Promotion and Disease Prevention Objectives* (Washington, DC: Office of the Assistant Secretary for Health, 1991).
42. U.S. Department of Health and Human Services, *Healthy People 2010: Understanding and Improving Health* (Washington, DC: U.S. Government Printing Office, 2000).
43. American Public Health Association et al., *Healthy Communities 2000: Model Standards.* (Washington, DC: American Public Health Association, 1991.
44. National Association of County and City Health Officials, *APEXPH: Assessment Protocol for Excellence in Public Health* (Washington, DC: 1991).
45. M.W. Kreuter, "PATCH: Its Origin, Basic Concepts, and Links to Contemporary Public Health Policy," *Journal of Health Education* 23 (1992): 135–139.
46. U.S. Centers for Disease Control and Prevention, *Planned Approach to Community Health: Guide for the Local Coordinator* (Atlanta, GA: 1995).
47. National Civic League, *The Healthy Communities Handbook* (Denver, CO: 1993).
48. J.E. Fielding et al., "Characteristics of Community Report Cards—United States, 1996," *Morbidity and Mortality Weekly Report* 46 (1997): 647–649.
49. M.A. Stoto, "Public Health Assessment in the 1990s," *Annual Review of Public Health 1992*, 13 (1992): 59–78.
50. Joint Commission on Accreditation of Healthcare Organizations, Oryx Fact Sheet (Oakbrook Terrace, IL: Joint Commission on Accreditation of Healthcare Organizations, 1998).
51. National Committee for Quality Assurance, *The State of Managed Care Quality 1999* (Washington, DC: 1999).
52. Foundation for Accountability (FAcct), *Reporting Quality Information to Consumers* (Portland, OR: 1997).
53. M. Darby, *Health Care Quality: From Data to Accountability* (Washington, DC: National Health Policy Forum, The George Washington University, 1998).
54. M.A. Stoto et al., *Healthy Communities: New Partnerships for the Future of Public Health* (Washington, DC: National Academy Press, 1996).
55. D.A. Kindig, *Purchasing Population Health: Paying for Results* (Ann Arbor, MI: The University of Michigan Press, 1997).
56. M.A. Stoto and J.S. Durch, Background paper prepared for the National Cancer Policy Board (1997).
57. Institute of Medicine and National Research Council, *Taking Action To Reduce Tobacco Use* (Washington, DC: National Academy Press, 1998).
58. B.S. Lynch and R.J. Bonnie, *Growing Up Tobacco Free: Preventing Nicotine Addiction in Children and Youths* (Washington, DC: National Academy Press, 1994).
59. M.A. Stoto, "Healthy People 2010 (letter)," *Public Health Reports* 113 (1998): 287–288.
60. "Children and Tobacco: Regulations Restricting the Sale and Distribution of Cigarettes and Smokeless Tobacco Products To Protect Children and Adolescents," *Federal Register*, 28 August 1996, 61, 44,395–44,618.
61. J.M. Schultz et al., "Quantifying the Disease Impact of Cigarette Smoking with SAMMEC II Software," *Public Health Reports* 106 (1996): 326–333.
62. U.S. Centers for Disease Control and Prevention, "State- and Sex-Specific Prevalence of Selected Characteristics —Behavioral Risk Factor Surveillance System, 1994 and 1995," *Morbidity and Mortality Weekly Report 46,* no. SS-3 (1997).
63. L.D. Johnston et al., *National Survey Results on Drug Use from the Monitoring the Future Study, 1975–1995. Volume I: Secondary School Students* (Rockville, MD: National Institute on Drug Abuse, 1997). NIH publication no. 97–4139.

CHAPTER 14

Public Health Research

Anne M. Gadomski

Public health organizations use research to produce new knowledge and interventions useful for improving population health. Health promotion research investigates the determinants of health and behavior change that are important to improving health status and quality of life. Other applications of public health research integrate clinical and population methods to identify innovations in public health practice and management. Public health organizations face many barriers in translating research findings into practice, including the complexity of real-life settings and the limited generalizability of many studies.

WHAT IS PUBLIC HEALTH RESEARCH?

The value of public health research from a practitioner's perspective lies in its ability to answer pragmatic questions, most often of the "what works?" variety. As described in Chapter 13, evaluation research can demonstrate the effectiveness of prevention, as in the case of teen pregnancy prevention. Politically, research can be very valuable in demonstrating the "market value" of public health (i.e., it enables one to show how dollars spent affect health outcomes). Research is often a key component in the evaluation of the community health improvement process in that it can increase community awareness of problems, enhance community mobilization efforts, and focus intervention efforts on areas of need. Public health research often extends beyond evaluation, by seeking new knowledge about the factors and mechanisms that shape population health. This chapter examines how public health organizations apply and use scientific research to improve management and practice within their institutions and within the larger field of public health.

In many ways, public health research is a vehicle for bridging the gaps between basic science and public health practice, between prevention and treatment, and between academic health institutions and public health organizations. If one of the goals of public health is to reduce population risks of disease, the success of public health interventions depends on the elucidation of causal pathways, including those that determine the effectiveness of public health interventions. The U.S. Centers for Disease Control and Prevention (CDC) defines prevention research as research that is designed "to yield results directly applicable to interventions to prevent occurrence of disease and disability, or the progression of detectable but asymptomatic disease."[1(p.50)] The Institute of Medicine broadened this definition to include health promotion research that addresses the underlying determinants of health and focuses on cultivating health and improving the quality of life.[1] Public health research includes but is not limited to evaluation research focused on public health interventions.

The complexity of public health necessitates the use of theories and conceptual frameworks to inform the design and conduct of useful research. One framework commonly used for public health research is the "health field model" (Figure 14–1), which elucidates the domains that influence community health as well as the interactions among these domains.[2,3] Focused on the macro level of community health, the model focuses on factors that affect the health of large segments of the population, rather than specific factors that result in small health changes at the level of the individual. Many interactions occur among the determinants of health, presenting challenges for empirical efforts to disentangle effects. Although complex, the model underscores the need for a population-based approach to community health research, one that includes the contextual variables (neighborhood, family, geographic location) as well as health system and individual-level determinants.[4]

Public health research is often directed toward preventing behavior-related morbidity and mortality, such as substance abuse, injury, sexually transmitted disease, and violence. Thus, theoretical constructs that focus on human behavior change are used to identify avenues of inquiry in empirical public health research. Social cognitive theory has been the underpinning for several successful behavioral-based prevention research programs.[5–7] An individual's characteristics, health behavior, lifestyle, and environment interact, producing "reciprocal determinism" that ultimately explains health behavior. The stages of change model in which "efficient self-change depends on doing the right things (processes) at the right time (stages)" has been successfully applied in studying addictive behaviors, particularly smoking.[8(p.1110)] Dryfoos recommends targeting the antecedents of high-risk behavior rather than presenting symptoms, a prevention strategy based on the social development model.[9,10]

Because individual behaviors are often influenced by aggregate constructs (media, commercial influences, environmental conditions), research based on behavior change models needs to incorporate contextual determinants, such as those included in the health field model. One example of a model that integrates these dimensions is the PRECEDE-PROCEED planning model for health promotion (see Chapter 12 for a full discussion of this model).[11] This model begins with several phases of social diagnosis, epidemiologic diagnosis, environmental diagnosis, and so forth, and ends in evaluation of each of these components with respect to an array of outcomes. Focusing on the process and effects of community interventions that follow commu-

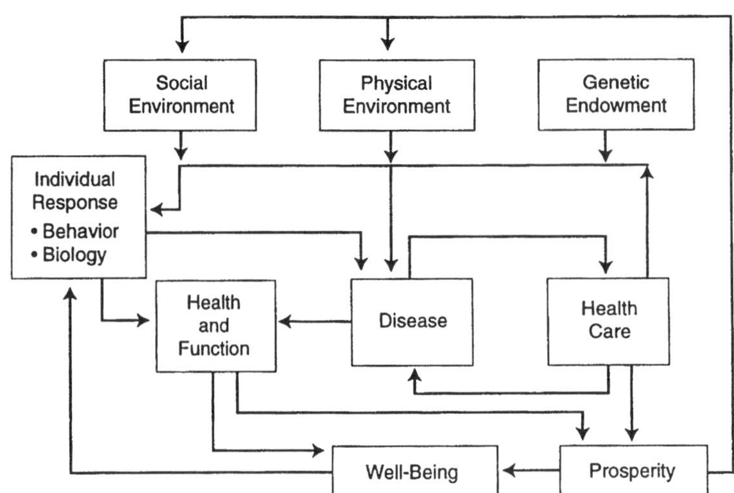

Figure 14–1 A Model of the Determinants of Health. *Source:* Reprinted from *Social Science and Medicine,* Vol. 31, No. 12, p. 1359, Copyright © Elsevier Science, Ltd., with permission from Elsevier Science, Ltd.

nity diagnosis is an approach currently promoted by the CDC for both research and practice activities.[12]

The many determinants of public health lead to broad areas of research (Exhibit 14–1). Traditionally, these have included health promotion, health education, disease prevention, behavior modification, and risk reduction. The breadth of public health research necessitates the integration of basic, clinical, and population approaches. This multidisciplinary approach usually includes concepts and methods from statistics, epidemiology, economics, communications, and education, as well as the pertinent biomedical fields. Given recent technical advances, expertise in more specialized fields such as behavioral genetics, health psychology, medical sociology, organizational science, medical anthropology, and computer sciences may be required. Research partnerships that recognize the interdependency of these fields are essential. The organizations and individuals that participate in such collaborative research require ability to communicate effectively and avoid or explain their disciplinary jargon. Community representation is also essential but often overlooked. Community-based research can facilitate the implementation of the most appropriate, effective, cost-effective, and culturally acceptable interventions.

Exhibit 14–1 Public Health Research Areas

- Policy analysis
- Disease prevention (risk factors)
- Health promotion (risk conditions)
- Social determinants
- Health services research: access to care, effectiveness and outcomes studies
- Operations research: how implementation is improved
- Environmental impact
- Community intervention
- Communication
- Dissemination
- Economic evaluation (cost-effectiveness, cost-benefit, and cost utility)
- Work force studies (supply, demand, distribution, competency)

At the community intervention level, the distinction between public health research and evaluation is often blurred. (See Chapter 13 for a more detailed discussion.) A rigorous program evaluation sometimes is equivalent to a research project, particularly if a new intervention is being implemented. Often, impact evaluation and research are terms that are used interchangeably when the focus of a study is an outcome. However, routine program evaluation that includes program inputs, processes, and expected outcomes sometimes falls short of the scientific rigor required for research evaluation. Some applications of public health research examine the impact of an intervention and therefore measure effectiveness. By contrast, some types of program evaluation studies focus on how well a program is implemented and are therefore more closely linked to quality assurance than to effectiveness research.

TRANSLATING RESEARCH INTO PRACTICE

"Real-time science...consists of loop after loop of trial, reflection, idea, and trial again."[13 (p. 877)]

In conducting and applying research, public health organizations implement an iterative cycle of problem identification, followed by research and then feedback to a community—arguably the most difficult step in the cycle. Translating research into practice is among the most daunting tasks faced by public health managers. The first challenge is to discriminate between valid information and misinformation. On this topic, Marcia Angell, former editor of *The New England Journal of Medicine*, cautions that "if it sounds too good to be true, it probably is."[14(p.1)] The next challenge is to shorten the time required for dissemination, application, and adoption of valid research findings in the field of practice. As new research results become available and are confirmed, the public health manager has to find ways to put these findings into practice. This may mean developing new messages for the public's education, advocating for legislation, changing health provider practices, or attempting to change public behavior directly.

Interestingly, temporal lags between research and practice can be paradoxical. On one hand, service delivery changes in advance of research. On the other hand, it is difficult to change clinical and public health practice. For example, market forces have rapidly changed health care service delivery. In response to the drive to reduce costs, the change makers have been managed care organizations rather than professional provider groups. These market forces have also resulted in the transfer of some public health functions to the private sector. The change in service delivery models and financing and managed care strategies is often so rapid that it eludes the researcher's ability to measure impact, develop messages for the public, or even fully understand what is happening.

On the other hand, clinical and public health practice is often difficult to influence or change. Unless legislated, incentivised, or otherwise compelled, attempts to change professional practice and incorporate new research findings are thwarted by competing demands at the practice level. Examples include the use of beta blockers for myocardial infarction, hypertension, or heart failure; the introduction of new vaccines or clinical practice guidelines; or screening for domestic violence. The lag between research findings and practical implementation is often many years. The question of how much evidence is needed to change professional practice is often debated in this context. How many clinical trials with what effect size are needed before practice guidelines can be constructed, agreed on, and disseminated?

This apparent paradox can be better understood and perhaps even addressed using the stages of change model to examine an organization's, provider's, or individual's readiness to change. The ease with which research is translated into practice depends on a readiness to change at potentially more than one level of practice: the individual patient or community member, the public health professional, and the public health organization. The organizational context influences individual and group management decisions. The stages of change model can be applied simultaneously to all these levels. The failure of an intervention can potentially be explained by a mismatch between stage and intervention. Thus, "ostensibly contradictory processes can become complementary when embedded in the stages of change."[8 (p.1112)]

Barriers to translating research into practice also include the complexity of real-life settings and the limited generalizability of some research findings. Clinical and community situations are much more complex than what is usually examined in research settings. There are simply too many variables to model or control in most studies. In addition, clinical and public health practitioners as well as other professionals face many competing demands that may inhibit the adoption of new knowledge and interventions. Using population-based research to inform clinical practice can be especially challenging because of the structural and professional differences between public health practice and medical practice.

Sometimes, specific integration processes speed the translation of research into practice. An example of this is the Guidelines for Adolescent Preventive Services (GAPS) questionnaires, produced by the American Medical Association for screening adolescents for risk behaviors. Prior to being seen for a regular visit, the adolescent and parent complete their own, rather lengthy questionnaires. Pertinent positives in terms of risk behaviors are lined up in the left column and negative answers are lined up in the right column. This allows the clinician to scan the form quickly, pick up the positives fairly rapidly, and target interventions where they are most needed. Drawbacks to such tools are the time it takes to fill them out and the limited health literacy one encounters among adolescents. Nevertheless, this tool enables one to move from a categorical to a comprehensive approach, from a disease to a health focus, from acute care to preventive care, and from medical dogma to population-based medicine. Hopefully, it also allows clinicians to move from what was learned in medical school to incorporation of new strategies and approaches throughout one's career.

Sometimes, translating research into practice and developing messages for the public requires empowerment strategies. For example, a rural myth is that rural areas are sheltered from substance abuse, violence, unsafe sex, and other risk behaviors. This notion was discovered in focus groups consisting of parents, school staff, and youth, as well as other studies that documented disparate views on risk behaviors between youth and parents.[15] In order to address this myth, the Otsego Public Health Partnership (OPHP) planned and helped schools in their area implement the *Youth Risk Behavior Survey (YRBS).* The prevalence of risk factors for adolescents in Otsego County was assessed using this self-administered survey that was conducted in 10 of 12 school districts in Otsego in 1997. More than 1,400 middle school students (response rate 87 percent) and more than 2,100 high school students (response rate 68 percent) completed this survey. Schools were assisted by the local public health partnership in conducting the survey, but had to buy into the effort.

The results of the Otsego study offered important but not surprising insight about the health issues facing students within the community. More Otsego County students were in a physical fight, ever tried cigarette smoking, ever drank alcohol, and ever used marijuana as compared to the average upstate New York 1996 estimates. The implications of the *YRBS* findings for schools and communities in Otsego County were clear: living in a rural area does not protect children from substance abuse, violence, or sexual activity. Putting these data in the hands of people who had never had to deal with such data before led to surprising reactions and empowerment. Thus, this *YRBS* research could be used as a community mobilization strategy. Although it was not statistically necessary to conduct the *YRBS* at a county level, it was necessary from the community development standpoint because the community needed to be convinced that these problems were real and they involved their children, their schools, and their neighbors.

A community's learning is a gradual process that can nevertheless be facilitated with sound and targeted public health research. This learning curve is a key determinant of the speed of the translation of research into practice. The temporal lag between research and practice is not only a function of where people are on their learning curves, but also of what barriers they face and what supports they have. This observation applies to clinicians, researchers, parents, public health practitioners, health and human service agencies, and consumers.

Another key issue in translating research into practice involves the trade-off between cost and effectiveness in public health practice, and community valuations of this trade-off. If research reveals strategies for achieving better health outcomes, but it is only with increased cost, is this research worth translating into practice? Will this translation take place? Unless the cost-effectiveness of changes in practice can be demonstrated clearly, new interventions can be difficult to implement. Thus, cost often limits research-driven innovation when resources are scarce.

KEY STEPS IN CONDUCTING RESEARCH

Exhibit 14–2 presents key steps in conducting research. However, it is important to realize that these steps are often iterative rather than sequen-

Exhibit 14–2 Doing the Research: Essential Component Checklist

- Identify the problem.
- Conduct a thorough literature review.
- Formulate the research question.
- Focus on modifiable risk factors.
- Develop the conceptual framework.
- Assemble the team.
- Refine the research question.
- Specify a testable hypothesis.
- Clarify the methods (design, target group, primary or secondary research).
- Select the measures.
- Calculate sample size.
- Train personnel.
- Collect/analyze data.
- Disseminate results.

tial, and they involve a multidisciplinary process that can be most rewarding if done properly. Successful research depends on correct identification of the public health problem and careful formulation of the research question and the hypothesis statement. Focusing on modifiable risk factors is essential if the research is designed to improve intervention efforts. The most time consuming aspect of the research design is defining the research question, applying theory and conceptual models to inform the research design, and finding the methods and measures commensurate to the task of answering the question.

The research question plays a dominant role in determining the design, methods, and sample size of the study. Therefore, each research project is somewhat unique in design and methodology. However, applying a theoretical model to local problems or community-specific research questions can be enlightening. Conceptual frameworks may lead to consideration of other factors or ways of specifying the original question that had been overlooked. For example, for youth smoking prevention research, are nonhealth care factors, such as effectiveness of local enforcement strategies, taken into consideration when attempting to measure the impact of a planned intervention? Such questions can be informed with the appropriate use of social and behavioral theory.

Primary and secondary research approaches can be used to answer public health research questions. Primary research methods offer more flexibility in tailoring the study design to the specific question of interest; however, these methods also involve a substantial effort in terms of data collection, training, staffing, funding, and time. By comparison, the indirect methods of secondary research rely on existing data and are therefore more feasible and timely approaches for answering some types of research questions. Secondary research approaches are somewhat opportunistic. For example, a time series analysis using death certificates and hospital discharge data was used to evaluate a community-based injury prevention program in New York City.[16] Linking existing databases to address a research question can be a particularly creative approach, but challenging in terms of the mechanics of linkage.[17] Secondary research using existing databases may encounter limitations that arise when using what was intended to be an administrative database for research purposes.[18] The specification of the outcome, reliability of the indicators used, and accuracy of data entry may be variable or suboptimal. Evidence reviews and meta-analyses are other examples of secondary research approaches that can be used to synthesize results of existing studies. Techniques for combining the results of studies have been developed that include qualitative assessment of each study as well as quantitative methods for adding up the effect size.[19]

In some cases research methods may offer only partial insight concerning a complex public health issue, such as the performance of a multifaceted public health intervention. For example, if several media channels are used in a campaign, isolating the impact of one of those channels can be difficult. Similarly, if a media campaign, professional training, and organizational policy changes are implemented in order to increase the awareness of and improve the management of domestic violence in a community, it is almost impossible to attribute changes in professional practices to any one of these measures. Most likely, the components of the intervention act synergistically and attempts to isolate the effects of one component may lead to misleading estimates of effect size. This problem arose when methods were sought for measuring a community's response to *YRBS* data, in an example provided earlier. Although certain changes in community awareness and perception were perceived by those disseminating *YRBS* data and facilitating community discussion of the results, measuring change at the community level was difficult. In this example, effective change would be multisectoral and originate in the family, with reinforcement by the school and enabling in the community, and expressed in a variety of ways.

Sample size and issues of sampling are of growing concern both to the producers and to the consumers of public health research. Margins of error for surveys are commonly cited in print media and other sources, and the public is becoming well versed in the nuances of sampling. Thus, sampling and sample size are often criticized and are subject to increasing public scrutiny. The issue of what is statistically significant versus what may be significant in terms of public health practice also arises in discussions concerning sample size.

The subjects to be studied in public health research efforts should be selected so as to be representative of the population of interest, and not selected based on convenience. This means that study subjects should meet specific selection criteria based on characteristics that define the population of interest (e.g., risk factors) and preferably based on randomized sampling from this population—as opposed to criteria based on whoever shows up or is available for study. Research projects that depend on convenience sampling alone can be compromised by selection bias that may or may not be measurable. For public health interventions, it is particularly important to look for effects in a target population and not chance missing these effects because the wrong population is used for the sampling frame, instead of those for whom the intervention was intended.

For outcomes that are determined by many factors, such as birth weight, it is important to gauge the impact of the intervention relative to the other determinants that are operative at the population level. For example, public health interventions designed to reduce the rate of low birth weight delivery face the challenge of demonstrating impact amidst a variety of proximal factors that appear to exert larger effects.[20] Thus, the attributable fraction of medical care as a determinant of birth weight is small, necessitating careful research designs, large sample sizes to demonstrate impact, and/or a focus on one proximate determinant of the outcome, in this case, preterm deliveries.

Methods for public health research include a variety of designs that comprise both experimental and nonexperimental (also termed quasi-experimental or observational) approaches. Nonexperimental research studies may employ cross-sectional or longitudinal designs, and they may rely on case-control or cohort methods of comparison. (See Chapter 13 for a more detailed discussion.) Hybrid nonexperimental designs, such as nested case-control and case cohort designs within a cohort study, compare cases to controls who also have risk factor information and offer advantages of both cohort and case-control studies. Experimental designs rely on randomization to produce intervention and control groups that are equivalent in terms of demographics, risk factors, and all other attributes except exposure to the intervention of interest. Randomization can occur at the level of the individual, clinic, local health unit, county, and so forth, depending on the research question. For nonexperimental research, multivariate statistical analysis is needed to control factors other than the intervention that may influence the outcome of interest (termed confounding factors). Because it is typically impossible to rule out the possibility that outcomes are influenced by other factors not measured in the nonexperimental research design, these types of studies are considered less scientifically rigorous and conclusive than the experimental design. However, multivariate methods may also be required for experimental studies if the randomization process fails to produce intervention and control groups that are equivalent in all attributes important to the outcome of interest.

Sometimes, research design is determined by the occurrence of "natural experiments" that are created by policy or program changes, natural or manmade disasters, or specific exposures delineated by geographic or other clustering phenomena. Given that the pace of change in communities is rapid, especially relative to the rate at which research progresses, it is important to consider secular trends in such situations. For example, including a comparison group that is not subject to a specific program allows the researcher to describe secular trends and therefore better estimate the effect size due to intervention. Other questions to consider include: What other external influences may affect the outcome under study? How does the delay in the occurrence of outcome of interest enter into the research design? How can exposure be measured more accurately? As with other types of nonexperimental studies, the natural experiment remains vulnerable to the influence of unobserved confounding factors and therefore provides less-conclusive evidence compared with the randomized experiment. Of course, it is often infeasible or at least unethical to conduct experimental research for many types of questions, such as those involving the effects of public policies, environmental shifts, or social and behavioral trends.

As alluded to before, multidisciplinary research teams are often needed to field research on complex public health issues. This variety in expertise presents group process challenges, such as communication barriers, increased time and resource demands, and complexity in terms of meeting the different agendas each representative brings to the research effort. Conveners of such groups are likely to feel as though they are losing control. However, setting goals, defining terms and measures, and reviewing prior research can be helpful group process activities that develop the team's effectiveness and operational efficiency.

The inclusion of community representatives in public health research efforts often enhances the design, implementation, and application of the study. Such inclusion allows process-level perspectives to be incorporated—at the level of the consumer and community as well as at the level of the provider and organization that will be implementing the proposed intervention. Including family representatives, patients, members of the target population, and/or advocates may require a trained group facilitator. Care must also be taken not to lose the operational and end-user perspectives in the drive to produce findings that are of scientific interest. Success of such research teams is often determined in part by the degree of each member's commitment to public health goals and objectives—a point to remember when assembling the team.

Collaboration should begin at the conceptual end of the research project rather than at the stage of research design and implementation. The research team should collectively visualize specifically what the product or endpoint of the research will be and how that can be applied. For example, if the contemplated research demonstrates that a given intervention for smoking prevention is effective, how can it be used, by whom, and at what cost? This mental exercise should also include consideration of whether the expected effect size is going to be large enough to convince policy makers and practitioners to adopt the intervention. Will the results be used to formulate managerial strategy, change policy, refine implementation, develop capacity, or community linkages? Also, the team needs to remember that statistical significance is not equivalent to practical significance from a public health perspective. Research that improves cost-effectiveness or increases cost efficiency is likely to be of more practical significance. Thus, the team must decide how the research will yield findings of an effect size that will be important from a public health perspective. A summary of the key implementation issues discussed above are listed in Exhibit 14–3.

MEASURING OUTCOMES

"The best advice to minimize both systematic and variable errors in measuring health is, in fact, to be aware of what a given perspective might either illuminate *or* fail to surface."[21(p.221)]

Key to a successful research project is choosing the right outcome measures. Do the indica-

Exhibit 14–3 Key Implementation Issues

- Who should be included on the research team?
- How can the project be funded?
- How can the project be staffed?
- Are consulting and/or contractual services needed?
- Are academic relationships needed?
- Should primary or secondary research approaches be used?
- Should quantitative or qualitative methods be used? (or both?)
- How are the results to be used?

tors measure what you want them to measure? The process outlined in the above paragraph should lead to a research question that is specific enough to allow the right measure to be chosen. The next step is to choose the right measure from the array of measures available. More often than not, a set of measures is included in order to address different facets of the research question. For example, media campaigns often include indicators that can reflect changes in awareness, exposure, or behavioral intention that may be attributable to the intervention.

There are tremendous advantages to be gained in using existing measures that have established validity and reliability. For example, in survey research, the use of existing instruments means that survey questions have been refined, instruments have been shortened, factor analysis has been completed, and benchmark data are available. On the other hand, the development of measures, such as survey instruments, takes time, and the right measure may not be available at the time the public health issue is most pressing at the local level. Thus, a research project may be faced with developing its own measures, with the attendant tasks of piloting, validity and reliability testing, and establishing constructs. In this case, partnering with content or survey experts in this area is essential to ensure that what the project intends to measure is measured.

Choosing between quantitative and qualitative measures in public health research can be controversial. Traditionally, quantitative measures have been favored in order to establish the market value of an intervention or demonstrate the effectiveness of an intervention. However, quantitative measures may not capture important intervention effects, particularly those related to more subtle behavioral change, transition from one stage of change to another, or changes in public perception. Also, quantitative measures may not be used appropriately. For example, a hemoglobin A1c measure may be used to measure quality of care for diabetes, but cannot be used as a proxy for the overall health status and functioning of a diabetic. Quantitation may yield the number of health visits but miss the quality of interaction during the visit. A qualitative assessment of the content of a visit and its impact on the outcome of interest may be more instructive and yield specific information that could lead to improvement in a PDSA cycle.

As an alternative research design, qualitative studies are helpful in building theories, generating hypotheses, identifying problems, and exploring different viewpoints. Qualitative data analysis techniques include ethnography, content analysis, and case studies. For example, case studies have been used to track and evaluate the rapid changes occurring in the Medicaid managed care programs at the state level.[22–24] For relatively new or underdeveloped areas of research, a mix of quantitative or qualitative approaches may be most instructive. In any case, these methods may complement each other in unexpected ways. For example, quantitative measures such as visit counts for domestic violence may demonstrate little statistically significant impact of training on medical care providers, whereas qualitative measures obtained from methods such as victim interviews, provider focus groups, or key informant interviews can elucidate why training efforts are having a limited effect.

AN OVERVIEW OF DATA ANALYSIS TECHNIQUES

Data analysis for any given outcome of interest usually includes two phases: univariate and multivariate analyses. *Univariate* analyses are used to identify individual predictors of the outcome of interest and to establish key relationships among the dependent and independent variables. For example, the relationship between categorical outcomes such as consumer satisfaction, and categorical independent variables such as insurance group, can be measured using the chi-square test or Fisher's exact test, as appropriate. For continuous outcomes, such as missed work days, the relationship to continuous independent variables, such as age, can be assessed by examination of X-Y scatter plots; if that relationship is linear, it can then be quantified using Pearson's correlation.

Multivariate analyses allow the researcher to control or adjust for known or new effect modifiers or confounders in predicting the outcome or describing an association. Multivariate models are built in which those variables found to be predictive in univariate testing are combined with known predictors in either linear or logistic regressions to identify which variables are independent predictors of the outcome or to estimate effect sizes. In simple multivariate models, linear regression is used for continuous dependent variables, for example, a blood pressure measurement, and logistic regression is used for dichotomous outcomes, for example, elevated blood pressure, no (0) or yes (1) using a predetermined cutoff. Logistic regression yields commonly used odds ratios that measure the association between the dependent and independent variable while controlling for the effects of other variables included in the model. Logistic regression also includes more complex modeling possibilities such as an ordered logic, for predicting an ordinal outcome that can be ranked higher than others, for example, normal (0), moderately elevated (1), or high blood pressure (2). Multichotomous variables, such as those reflecting discrete choices among multiple types of food or types of health care providers to visit, can be analyzed using a higher-order logistic model. Other types of multivariate methods exist for modeling outcome variables that assume other types of discrete and continuous distributions.

Geographic clustering of exposures or events introduce spatial or grouping factors that require special treatment. (See Chapter 10 for a more detailed discussion.) The quality of one's neighborhood environment is an example of a macrolevel risk factor that can influence an individual's self-reported health status.[25] Multilevel models can be developed in order to estimate the effect of such contextual variables measured at the aggregate level, such as geographic local or other cluster effects.[26] Similarly, randomization at the local health unit, county, or hospital level requires multilevel analysis, such as a mixed-effects linear model, to account for group effects.

Longitudinal or cohort studies, like the Nurses' Health Study, introduce time-related factors that also require specific analytic techniques.[27] Temporal factors include age, calendar date, time since exposure, or time of entry into the cohort, which introduces the problem of staggered entry times.[28] Relative risk models, which are based on the Cox proportional hazards model, deal with these time-dependent factors. Life table analyses and Kaplan-Meier curves are used to track changes over time in mortality; however, other outcomes may be used. Generalized estimating equations, logistic, log-linear, or Poisson regression techniques can also be used depending on the type, frequency, and distribution of the dependent variable. Longitudinal studies can also have problems related to repeated measurement, changes in measurement and/or exposure over time, missing data; and participant attrition that require specialized statistical techniques.

For newer areas of inquiry, certain statistical methods are used for exploratory composite and correlational analysis, such as factor analysis and principal component analysis. Factor analysis can be used to establish the psychometric properties of a survey instrument as well as to define the relationships between the dimensions measured in the survey. For example, factor analysis of a knowledge, attitudes, beliefs, and behavior survey of health care staff regarding domestic violence showed that two dimensions factored together: self-efficacy and familiarity with referral resources.[29,30] This finding led researchers to infer that health provider self-efficacy in responding to domestic violence victims was closely related to their ability to offer the victims access to resources the provider knew about and felt were effective. As a result, a programmatic emphasis was placed on developing linkages between health care providers and domestic violence referral sources.

Structural equation modeling with maximum likelihood estimates can be used to examine multiple causal relationships between risk factors and outcomes measured cross-sectionally or at different points in time in a longitudinal design. For example, a structural model of drug trafficking and illicit drug use among youth included in a two-year study documented a positive path between baseline drug trafficking to substance abuse at 24 months.[31] Although complex, such studies are helpful in elucidating important relationships among a variety of direct and indirect determinants and weighing their relative importance over time.

Statistical pitfalls are common in public health research but can be avoided. Large numbers of variables can lead to a large number of statistical comparisons that in turn can lead to spurious findings and inflated alpha or Type I errors (false positives). When using statistical tests, assumptions underlying the statistical methods should be reviewed and care should be taken that univariate analysis does not violate these assumptions. For example, if continuous variables, like missed work days, deviate markedly from normality, they may be logarithmically transformed. If this transformation does not achieve normality, other statistical tests may be necessary, such as the Wilcoxon rank-sums test for two group comparisons. For multivariate analysis, common statistical problems include violation of assumptions of normality in data, lack of testing for interactions between the independent variables, and fewer than 10 outcome events per independent variable in the model.[32] Inclusion of statistical expertise is essential in order to avoid these pitfalls, arrive at an adequate sample size, and properly represent research findings.

TARGETING PUBLIC HEALTH PRACTICE AREAS FOR RESEARCH

Given the competing demands public health organizations face, research tends to fall low on the desktop list of priorities. However, rather than be driven by current demands in more or less a reactionary mode, it helps to take a long-term view in determining the benefits of involvement in public health research. Reasons why public health organizations should participate in producing research rather than relying on others for published research are numerous. First, research adds ownership and accountability because it motivates staff to examine their issues, and provides answers that are relevant to their setting. Second, research increases effectiveness if the results are used as part of a performance improvement process (see Chapter 18 for further discussion). Third, research can facilitate collaborative relationships that gain a momentum of their own even after the research project is completed, resulting in several advantages that may accrue to a public health agency following a collaborative venture in research. These organizational incentives for involvement in public health research are illustrated in the following examples.

The use of *YRBS* data to address the myth that youth in rural areas are protected from substance abuse and other risk behaviors (an example used earlier in this chapter) represents strategic use of research data in community development. In 1997, parents, educators, and school staff were presented with county- and school-level data they had never had before. These data enabled them to focus on real issues facing youth (tobacco and alcohol use) as opposed to perceived ones (illegal drugs). It also provided a forum for education, school policy development, and community mobilization, although, as described previously, it has been difficult to assess the impact of this strategic use of data quantitatively.

The Public Health Priorities Initiative (PHPI) project was implemented in 1998 as a collaborative effort of the Departments of Health in Delaware, Otsego, and Schohaire counties and was funded by the New York State (NYS) Department of Health (DOH).[33] The purpose of the project was to identify the major public health and health care–related problems facing residents in the geographically similar and contiguous tri-county area. The PHPI implemented a number of surveys, focus groups, and print media queries that enabled data collection throughout the tri-county area. More than 3,000 residents in the tri-county area participated in the PHPI. Approaches to this assessment varied as needed to adapt to local conditions in each of the counties, but the basic approach was the same. This intercounty facilitation group process, charged with assessing the public health problems facing citizens of the tri-county region, generated the following conclusions:

- The most frequently cited category of problem was public health care programs and services (48 percent), followed by economic, social, and demographic factors (such as poverty, isolation, lack of services for youth, and aging of the region's population) (24 percent); access to health care system (14 percent); and disease and environmental factors (14 percent).

- Similar problems related to access to health care occur in the tri-county region. These include survival and viability of community hospitals, health care insurance costs, and limited access to medical and mental health care for low-income people.
- Due to aging of the population, economic problems, and increasing social isolation, significant burdens have been placed on the capacity of tri-county health care systems to meet the needs of residents.

The PHPI was a successful effort in tri-county collaboration and demonstrates the potential for organization and integrated planning. It also laid the groundwork for future collaboration in research, health promotion, and education in terms of intercounty health department communication, knowledge of partner county differences, as well as shared goals. This effort could also be viewed as a step toward achieving economies of scale and more efficient use of resources.

Another example of collaborative public health research is a population-based study of the adequacy of well-child care services.[34] This study was designed to examine the adequacy of well-child care and thereby assess the need for safety net services in a specific locale. The Otsego Public Health Partnership (a public–private partnership between Bassett Healthcare and the Otsego County Department of Health) collaborated with the NYS DOH Bureau of Immunization to address these issues. The study design was population based, using electronic birth certificates in order to identify a birth cohort born in Otsego County, New York. Electronic birth certificates were used to create a master list to which in-migrants were added as they were identified during the medical record review process. All providers in the county that render well-child care agreed to perform a chart review of all children aged 24–35 months in their practice. The collaboration with the local and state health departments enabled and facilitated access to the medical records. The medical record reviewers were Otsego County Health and NYS DOH immunization staff.

A total of 674 medical records were reviewed (57 percent belonged to a county birth cohort and 44 percent were in-migrants). Medical records of 64 percent of the birth cohort were located and reviewed. Among all 2-year-olds, 80 percent received DTP4, 89 percent Hib3, 75 percent Hib4, 77 percent HepB3, 85 percent MMR, 85 percent OPV3, and 17 percent varicella vaccine. The 4:3:1 rate was 75 percent at age two years. Sixty-eight percent had had 1 hematocrit, 74 percent had had one lead screen, and 43 percent had had two lead screens. By age two, 64 percent had had six well-child visits (the NYS DOH minimum standard) and 30 percent had had nine visits (the American Academy of Pediatrics' best practice standard). The birth cohort had significantly higher rates of documented immunization and preventive screening than in-migrants. This study demonstrated that immunization coverage in Otsego County was at or below the national average, and well-child care service provisions were below the American Academy of Pediatrics' standards in 1996.

Upon study completion, all participating clinics received copies of the immunization data entry and the analysis program (CASA), as well as a printed summary of their immunization rates. This study enabled individual primary care sites to assess their well-child care provision and provided a useful baseline for targeting the improvement of well-child care services in the county. For some clinics, this project facilitated reporting immunization rates to managed care organizations. For public health nurses, the project established a working relationship with the clinics and enabled ongoing practice-based immunization completion review as well as entrée to clinics to address other matters such as rabies, communicable disease follow-up, and health promotion. OPHP also included the results in a county report card that summarized health indicators and provided relevant health tips for the general public, thus completing the task of dissemination.

The budgets for the above projects were less than $50,000, including state funding and in-kind contributions. The specific research product in both cases was descriptive and provided baseline information that was useful for planning future efforts. The resulting collaborative ties, however, increase the reach of public health implementation efforts as well as the chance of receiving future funding for either research or implementation. Thus, the return on investments in public health research at the local level can be substantial if the right question is asked (and can be answered), the right people are involved, and results are used to further improve implementation.

• • •

Public health organizations have much to gain from involvement in public health research activities. Research creates new knowledge and identifies new approaches to public health management and practice—innovations that can be applied within the organization as well as disseminated to partners and peers in the field of public health. Much of the research that is directly relevant to public health organizations simply cannot be carried out in the traditional academic and scientific settings. Innovations in public health management and practice are derived most readily from practice-based and community-based research efforts. These efforts are designed and carried out in the settings where the research-derived innovations will ultimately be used, ensuring that any scientific findings are both statistically and practically significant. Public health organizations must take responsibility for leading and managing these types of efforts, in partnership with academia, community organizations, and other relevant institutions. These organizations and their managers have important roles to play as both the producers and beneficiaries of public health research.

CHAPTER REVIEW

1. A broad spectrum for public health research is motivated by the multiple determinants of health. Research areas include health promotion, health education, disease prevention, behavior modification, and other risk reduction, including environmental aspects. This breadth of potential studies requires
   - integration of basic research with clinical and population approaches
   - a multidisciplinary approach
   - partnerships including community representatives
2. At the community level, there may not be a sharp distinction between public health research and program evaluation. *Public health research* is often applied to examine the impact of an intervention and measuring effectiveness. *Program evaluation* often focuses on how well a program is implemented. When the focus of a study is an outcome, the two terms are often used interchangeably.
3. Public health research proceeds along an iterative cycle of problem identification, followed by research and then feedback to the community.
4. Successful research depends on correct identification of the public health problem and careful formulation of the research question and the hypothesis statement. Focusing on modifiable risk factors is essential to improve intervention efforts.
5. The research question dictates the design, methods, and sample size of the study.
6. Public health outcomes, such as birth weight, are determined by many factors. Gauging the impact of a public health intervention and distinguishing this effect from other determinants at the population level is a key challenge for research efforts.

REFERENCES

1. M.A. Stoto et al., eds., *Linking Research and Public Health Practice* (Washington, DC: National Academy Press, 1997).
2. M. Stoto, "Sharing Responsibility for the Public's Health: A New Perspective from the Institute of Medicine," *Journal of Public Health Management and Practice 3,* no. 5 (1997): 22–34.
3. R.G. Evans and G.L. Stoddart, "Producing Health, Consuming Health Care," in *Why Are Some People Healthy and Others Not? The Determinants of Health of Populations,* eds. R.G. Evans et al. (New York: Aldine De Gruyter, 1994).
4. C. Duncan et al., "Health-Related Behavior in Context: A Multilevel Modeling Approach," *Social Science and Medicine 42,* no. 6 (1996): 817–830.
5. A. Bandura, *Social Foundations of Thought and Action: A Social Cognitive Theory* (Englewood Cliffs, NJ: Prentice Hall, 1986).
6. B. Stanton, "Good News for Everyone?" *American Journal of Public Health* 87 (1997): 1,917–1,919.
7. T. Baranowski et al., "How Individuals, Environments and Health Behavior Interact: Social Cognitive Theory," in *Health Behavior and Health Education: Theory, Research and Practice,* eds. K. Glanz et al. (San Francisco, CA: Jossey-Bass, 1997), 153–178.
8. J.O. Prochaska et al., "In Search of How People Change: Applications to Addictive Behaviors," *American Psychologist 47,* no. 9 (1992): 1,102–1,114.
9. J.G. Dryfoos, "Preventing High-Risk Behavior," *American Journal of Public Health 81,* no. 2 (1991): 157–158.
10. J. Hawkins and J. Weis, "The Social Development Model: An Integrated Approach to Delinquency Prevention," *Journal of Primary Prevention* 6 (1985): 73–97.
11. L.W. Green and M.W. Kreuter, *Health Promotion Planning: An Educational and Environmental Approach,* 2d ed. (Mountain View, CA: Mayfield, 1991).
12. S.B. Cashman et al., "Carrying Out the Medicine/Public Health Initiative: The Roles of Preventive Medicine and Community-Responsive Care," *Academic Medicine 74,* no. 5 (1999): 473–483.
13. D.M. Berwick, "Harvesting Knowledge from Improvement," *Journal of the American Medical Association* 275 (1996): 877–878.
14. "If It Sounds Too Good To Be True…It Probably Needs a Second Look," *Food Insight* March/April 1999, 1 (newsletter available from the International Food Information Council Foundation, Washington, DC).
15. A.M. Gadomski et al., "Assessing Rural Community Viewpoints in Order To Implement a School-Based Health Center," *Journal of School Health 68,* no. 7 (1998): 304–306.
16. L. Kuhn et al., "Use of Poisson Regression and Time Series Analysis for Detecting Changes over Time in Rates of Child Injury Following a Prevention Program," *American Journal of Epidemiology 140,* no. 1 (1994): 943–955.
17. R.M. Bell et al., "The Urge To Merge: Linking Vital Statistics Records and Medicaid Claims," *Medical Care 32,* no. 10 (1994): 1,004–1,018.
18. C.J. McDonald and S.L. Hui, "The Analysis of Humongous Databases: Problems and Promises," *Statistics in Medicine* 10 (1991): 511–518.
19. S.N. Goodman, "Meta-Analysis in Health Services Research," in *Epidemiology and Health Services,* eds. H.K. Armenian and S. Shapiro (New York: Oxford University Press, 1998), 229–259.
20. N.S. Paneth, "The Problem of Low Birth Weight," *The Future of Children 5,* no. 1 (1995): 19–34.
21. L.A. Aday, *Designing and Conducting Health Surveys: A Comprehensive Guide,* 2d ed. (San Francisco, CA: Jossey-Bass, 1996).
22. S. Felt-Lisk et al., "Medicaid Managed Care in Rural Areas: A Ten-State Follow-Up Study," *Health Affairs 18,* no. 2 (1999): 238–245.
23. R. Slifkin et al., "Medicaid Managed Care Programs in Rural Areas: A Fifty-State Overview," *Health Affairs 17,* no. 6 (1998): 217–227.
24. T.A. Coughlini et al., "A Conflict of Strategies: Medicaid Managed Care and Medicaid Maximization," *Health Services Research 34,* no. 1 (1999): 281–293.
25. M. Malmstrom et al., "Neighborhood Environment and Self-Reported Health Status: A Multi-Level Analysis," *American Journal of Public Health* 89 (1999): 1,181–1,186.
26. C. Duncan et al., "Health-Related Behavior in Context: A Multilevel Modeling Approach," *Social Science and Medicine 42,* no. 6 (1996): 817–830.
27. G.A. Colditz, "The Nurse's Health Study: A Cohort of U.S. Women Followed Since 1976," *Journal of the American Medical Womens Association* 50 (1995): 40–44, 63.
28. T. Duncan, "New Techniques for the Analysis of Cohort Studies," *Epidemiologic Reviews 20,* no. 1 (1998): 122–134.
29. A.M. Gadomski et al., Impact of Health Care Provider Training in Domestic Violence Prevention (Paper presented at the American Public Health Association meeting, Chicago, November 1999), Abs 1034, 51.

30. A.M. Gadomski et al., Integrating Domestic Violence Management in a Rural Health Network (Paper presented at the Health Services Research meeting, Chicago, June 1999), Abs 592.

31. X. Li et al., "Drug Trafficking and Drug Use among African-American Adolescents: A Causal Analysis," *Journal of Adolescent Health 23,* no. 5 (1998): 280–288.

32. J. Concato et al., "The Risk of Determining Risk with Multivariate Models," *Annals of Internal Medicine 118,* no. 3 (1993): 201–210.

33. B. Warren, "Public Health Priorities Initiative" (report prepared for Otsego County Department of Health, Cooperstown, NY, March 19, 1998).

34. A.M. Gadomski et al., "Population-Based Study of the Adequacy of Well Child Care Services: A Rural County's Report Card," *Archives of Pediatric and Adolescent Medicine 152* (1998): 745–748.

Chapter 15

Protecting Human Subjects in Public Health Research

Patricia A. MacCubbin
Bruce Gordon
Ernest D. Prentice

Public health organizations play key roles in protecting the health and well-being of individuals and communities that participate in public health research. The protection of human subjects is an evolving concept. Federal regulations specify the responsibilities of Institutional Review Boards (IRBs). Key issues for protection from research risks are informed consent, subject selection, safeguards for vulnerable populations, and privacy and confidentiality assurances.

The evolving concept of the protection of human subjects from research risks has been well documented over more than a half-century. As the new millennium begins, it is useful to reexamine how and why the concept of human subjects protection gained attention and has become an everyday concern to researchers worldwide. Understanding the history of human subjects protection emphasizes how important it is to design public health research activities that minimize risks to research subjects and ensure that the potential subjects understand what the research entails before volunteering. Public health organizations are involved in the protection of human subjects both in reviewing the appropriateness of research by their staff and in evaluating research requests for confidential public health data under agency safeguard.

This chapter begins by reviewing some of the more infamous atrocities that were performed in the name of research, the public policies that resulted from recognition of the atrocities, and the institutional responsibilities and mechanisms that were created to ensure that research subjects are protected from risks. The federal definitions of research and human subjects, and their relationship to public health activities, are also explored. The required elements of informed consent are discussed, as are subject selection, vulnerable populations, and issues of privacy and confidentiality. This chapter will provide the public health administrator with a working knowledge of (1) the concept of human subjects protections, (2) the essential considerations in the review of research studies involving human subjects, and (3) the elements needed for preparing an application for submission to an IRB.

This chapter relies heavily on the National Institutes of Health (NIH) regulations Title 45, Code of Federal Regulations, Part 46, Regulations for the Protection of Human Research Subjects because public health organizations are less frequently involved in clinical trials of experimental drugs and medical devices not yet approved for use in the United States. Public health researchers involved in these types of trials are referred to the Food and Drug Administration (FDA) regulations at Title 21, Code of Federal Regulations, Part 50, Protection of Human Subjects and Title 21, Code of Federal Regulations, Part 56, Institutional Review Boards. The FDA regulations specify procedures for informed consent in studies involving new drugs or devices (21 CFR 50) and the role of IRBs (21 CFR 56). Many requirements are the same; however, there are differences. When in doubt, public health investigators should consult their IRBs and/or contact the FDA for advice and assistance.

RECOGNIZING THE NEED FOR HUMAN SUBJECTS PROTECTION

The need for human subjects protection as a basic public health function is readily evident from a review of the modern history of medical experimentation. This history clearly demonstrates that serious lapses in research ethics can occur in the quest for new public health and biomedical knowledge. Below we summarize some of the most notable historic developments and the lessons that public health organizations have learned from them. Exhibit 15–1 summarizes the significant events in human subjects research.

Nazi Medical Experiments

In the 1940s, Nazi doctors performed "experiments" using concentration camp prisoners as subjects. In this most infamous disregard for the human rights and welfare of research subjects, prisoners were subjected to freezing experiments at Dachau, high-altitude simulation experiments at Dachau, experimental surgery at Ravensbrook, mustard gas experiments at Sachsenhausen, and typhus experiments at Buchenwald. In the high-altitude simulation experiments, the physicians conducting the experiments used a German Air Force barometric chamber in which the unconsenting prisoners were subjected to low pressure and rapid changes in pressure. The objective was to study the physiological effects of pressure similar to the effects encountered when parachuting from high altitude. One of these experiments involved withholding oxygen from a prisoner while simulating high altitude. The results of the study were carefully recorded and revealed that the prisoner was observed from the time oxygen was withheld until death. The records detailed the physiological problems the prisoner experienced for approximately 30 minutes until his death, including perspiration, wiggling of the head, severe cramps, loss of consciousness, cyanosis, and foaming at the mouth. Following death, the prisoner was dissected.[1] This experiment, and the others, were performed on prisoners with no opportunity to consent, to decline to participate, or to withdraw. Coercion was the method routinely employed to recruit these study subjects.

Exhibit 15–1 Significant Events in Human Subjects Research

- Nuremberg Medical Trial—1946–47
- Dr. Andrew Ivy, American Medical Association rules—1946
- Nuremberg Code—1947
- Green Committee Report—1948
- Declaration of Helsinki—1964
- Surgeon General policy on prior peer review—1966
- Willowbrook—Late 1960s
- Tuskegee—1932–72
- National Research Act of 1974—1974
- Belmont Report—1978
- 45 CFR 46, subparts A, B, C, D—1974–83
- 21 CFR 50, 21 CFR 56—1981
- Common Rule—1991
- US General Accounting Office Report—1996
- US Department of Health and Human Services, Office of the Inspector General Report—1998

Nuremberg Medical Trial

In December 1946, the Nuremberg Medical Trial began. Twenty-three defendants went on trial for 32 known "experiments." Twenty of the defendants were physicians. In August of 1947, the tribunal found 16 of the 23 defendants guilty of war crimes and crimes against humanity.[1]

Dr. Andrew Ivy, a leading American medical researcher, was the medical consultant to the prosecution. Dr. Ivy prepared a summary of well-established "rules" involving human experimentation both for the prosecution and for the American Medical Association (AMA). The first rule involved obtaining consent from the human subject. The human subject must be a volunteer, the process of obtaining consent must be free from coercion, and the subject must be informed of any hazards before consenting. The second rule involved the design of the experiment. Results of prior animal experimentation and a knowledge of the natural history of the disease would justify performance of the experiment to obtain further knowledge for the good of society that could not be obtained otherwise. The third and final rule involved the conduct of the experiment. The researchers must be scientifically qualified. All unnecessary physical and mental suffering, as well as injury, must be avoided. No a priori reason may exist suggesting that death or disabling injury to the subject would occur.[2]

Nuremberg Code

In addition to the guilty verdict and sentencing of the war criminals, the tribunal formalized "certain basic principles [that] must be observed in order to satisfy moral, ethical and legal concepts [in] the practice of human experimentation."[1(pp.181–185)] These principles are contained in the Nuremberg Code. The first principle unequivocally states the role of informed, voluntary consent:[1(p.181)]

> The voluntary consent of the human subject is absolutely essential. This means that the person involved should have the legal capacity to give consent; should be so situated as to be able to exercise free power of choice, without the intervention of any element of force, fraud, deceit, duress, over-reaching or any other ulterior form of constraint or coercion; and should have sufficient knowledge and comprehension of the elements of the subject matter involved as to enable him to make an understanding and enlightened decision.

American physicians did not embrace the Nuremberg Code as might be expected. They regarded the Nuremberg Code as "a good code for barbarians but an unnecessary code for ordinary physicians."[3(p.151)] During the Nuremberg Medical Trial, American scientists were accused by the defendants of experimental improprieties in wartime malaria trials conducted on prisoners at Stateville Prison in Illinois. Despite the discussion of the Stateville Prison experiments, American physicians still did not recognize their own improprieties in medical research. Dr. Ivy chaired the Green Committee (named after the Governor of Illinois) to examine the ethics of malaria research on prisoners at Stateville. Conceding only possible coercion by reward, the Green Committee concluded that the experiments at Stateville were "an example of human experiments which were ideal because of their conformity" with the highest standards of human experimentation.[4(pp.457–458)]

Much discussion ensued during the next 16 years concerning portions of the Nuremberg Code. Most notably, in 1959, the National Society for Medical Research published a report suggesting that the first principle be softened. Henry Beecher, a Harvard-based researcher, agreed that "it is unethical and immoral to carry out potentially dangerous experiments without the subject's knowledge and consent," but he viewed the first Nuremberg principle as too extreme and not squaring with the realities of clinical research.[5] One of Beecher's colleagues, Joseph Gardella, the dean of the Harvard Medical School, agreed with Beecher and wrote that the Nuremberg Code was "not necessarily pertinent to or adequate for the conduct of medical research in the United States."[3(p.158)] Gardella also made a clear distinction between research on healthy volunteers and research conducted on sick patients that might have therapeutic value. He wrote, "It would be difficult and might prove to be impossible to devise one set of guiding principles that would apply satisfactorily to both of these two different categories."[3(p.158,159)]

Declaration of Helsinki

In 1964, the World Medical Association published the Declaration of Helsinki. The Declaration incorporated some of the first principles of the Nuremberg Code, but only included informed consent as the ninth point of the basic principles: "Each potential subject must be adequately informed of the aims, methods, anticipated benefits and potential hazards of the study and the discomfort it may entail. He should be informed that he is at liberty to abstain from participation in the study and that he is free to withdraw his consent to participation at any time."[6]

The Declaration also proposed two categories of clinical research—clinical research combined with professional care and nontherapeutic clinical research. Consent was absolute in nontherapeutic research. However, the Declaration allowed that, for clinical research with professional care, consent should be obtained "if at all possible, consistent with patient psychology."[6]

During the 1960s and early 1970s, many problems with medical research practices in the United States were discovered and publicized. Debates ensued, centered on oversight, the rights and welfare of subjects, informed consent, and risks versus benefits. In 1963, live cancer cells were injected into indigent elderly patients at Brooklyn Jewish Chronic Disease Hospital without their consent.[7,8] In the same year, NIH formed a committee to study problems of inadequate consent in research studies. The committee recognized the need for central oversight of research. NIH Director James Shannon recommended that NIH assume this responsibility and argued for prior peer review of research risks to subjects. By 1966, the surgeon general had accepted these recommendations and began requiring prior review for all U.S. Public Health Service grant-funded research involving human subjects.[3,7]

Willowbrook

In the late 1960s, the Willowbrook story broke. This involved a federally funded study of the natural history of hepatitis that was being conducted at the Willowbrook State School for the Retarded on Staten Island, New York. As part of this study, residents, nearly all profoundly retarded children, were injected with hepatitis-infected serum. Consent, obtained from parents, may have been misleading. The consent form suggested that the children were receiving a vaccine rather than the virus. Incentives for participation, such as more rapid admission to the school, and admission after the facility was closed to new residents, may be viewed as coercive.[3,7–9]

Tuskegee Syphilis Study

Following Willowbrook, in 1972, the *Washington Post*, and then the *New York Times*, exposed the Tuskegee syphilis study. This research study, which was sponsored and conducted by the U.S. Public Health Service, began in 1932. In this study, the natural history of untreated syphilis in 400 black men from the rural South was studied. In 1933, the study design was altered to extend the study indefinitely in order to follow these men until their death, at which point autopsies would be performed. The recruitment information may have been, as in Willowbrook, misleading and coercive. The men were not told the nature of their disease, nor that the research would offer no therapeutic benefit for them. They were offered free medical examinations and "special free treatments." The standard treatments of the 1930s, although ineffective and toxic, were withheld. However, in the 1940s, when penicillin was shown to be effective as a treatment for syphilis, treatment was again withheld. A 1969 Public Health Service blue-ribbon panel had reviewed the study and concluded that it was justifiable and should be continued because it offered "immense benefit to future patients."[3(p.179)]

In response to the revelations surrounding Tuskegee, the Department of Health, Education and Welfare (DHEW) appointed an ad hoc panel to review the Tuskegee syphilis study. The panel was also charged with reviewing the DHEW's policies and procedures for the protection of human subjects. The panel found the study "ethically unjustified." They recommended that the study be halted immediately and that the remaining subjects be given necessary medical care. The panel went on to recommend that Congress establish "a permanent body with the authority to regulate at least all federally supported research involving human subjects."[10]

Following the panel's recommendations, Congress, under the leadership of Senator Edward Kennedy, passed the National Research Act of 1974, establishing the National Commission for the Protection of Human Subjects of Biomedical and Behavioral Research. One of the National Commission's reports was *Ethical Principles and Guidelines for the Protection of Human Subjects of Research.*[11] This 1978 report, better known as the Belmont report, identified three basic ethical principles that should govern human subject research: respect for persons, beneficence, and justice. The DHEW published regulations in the *Federal Register,* which became codified as Title 45, Code of Federal Regulations, Part 46, Regulations for the Protection of Human Research Subjects (45 CFR 46). The regulations required grantee institutions to establish committees (called IRBs in later revisions) to review research with respect to the safety of the research proposed and adequacy of the informed consent as defined by the regulations. The DHEW established the Office for Protection from Research Risks (OPRR) in NIH as the oversight office, ensuring compliance with 45 CFR 46 for DHEW-funded research. Revisions in 1981 specified responsibilities of the IRBs and procedures that IRBs must follow. The regulations were further strengthened in the next nine years with the additions of subpart B (protections for pregnant women, fetuses, and human in vitro fertilization), subpart C (protections for prisoners), and subpart D (protections for children).

Additional regulations, similar to 45 CFR 46, were promulgated in 1981 by the FDA at 21 CFR 50 and 21 CFR 56. These regulations specify procedures for informed consent in studies involving new drugs or devices (21 CFR 50) and the role of IRBs (21 CFR 56). In 1991, an additional 16 federal agencies adopted the Final Common Federal Policy (also known as the "Common Rule") 45 CFR 46, subpart A.[3,7]

More recently, the IRB system has been undergoing close scrutiny.[12–14] In 1996, a report by the U.S. Government Accounting Office (GAO) described factors responsible for the weakening of institutional and federal efforts to protect human subjects from research risks, such as heavy workloads and limited funding for IRBs.[12] The report also addressed the concerns for potential conflicts of interest at the institutional or local level between the IRB and the institution and at the federal level between the OPRR and NIH. The 1998 report from the Office of the Inspector General (OIG) of the U.S. Department of Health and Human Services (DHHS, formerly DHEW) cited the following concerns:[14]

- IRBs review "too much, too quickly, with too little expertise."[13]
- IRBs conduct minimal continuing review.
- IRBs provide little training for investigators and board members.
- Potential conflicts of interest exist between universities and academic health centers and their IRBs.

The OIG recommended the following:[14]

- IRBs should undergo performance-based evaluations by the OPRR and the FDA.
- Institutions receiving funding from the Public Health Service should have programs for educating investigators and require written assurance from the investigators that they will uphold federal policies regarding human subjects protection.
- Institutions should provide sufficient resources to IRBs to enable them to carry out their responsibilities.
- NIH/OPRR and the FDA should revamp their assurance and inspection process.

THE IRB

The Common Rule, in §§ 46.107 through 108, specifies the minimum requirements for the structure, composition, and functions of an IRB. An institution must meet the minimum requirements of 45 CFR 46 in order to review and approve federally funded research, but may elect to exceed the minimum requirements of any section of 45 CFR 46, including the composition and size of the board.

IRB Composition

The IRB must have at least five members, all of whom must possess sufficient experience and expertise not only to review specific research activities, but also to understand the relationship between the proposed research and "institutional commitments and regulations, applicable law, and standards of professional conduct and practice" (45 CFR 46 § 46.107(a)).

Public health organizations range in size from the small local health units in rural locations with only a few employees to the large state and federal health agencies with thousands of employees. Each organization must determine its needs for human subjects review when establishing an IRB, and it must reevaluate these needs when reapplying for federal assurance. For a small organization, the minimum federal requirements may be sufficient for review and oversight of the quantity and diversity of research protocols generated annually. The much larger organization may decide that it needs a large board with membership representing major program research areas, or may elect to establish multiple boards, each of which would review specific types of research. For instance, one IRB may be established to review all behavioral research in the organization, and a second may review the biomedical research applications. The OPRR, in its oversight capacity, examines the burden on the IRB to determine if the board can function efficiently and provide adequate consideration for each protocol. At a recent seminar on OPRR compliance activities, Dr. Melody Lin, deputy director of the OPRR, suggested that an IRB with 2,000 protocols per year was overburdened.[15]

As part of the federal assurance process, the institution submits a roster of IRB members. For each member listed on the roster, earned degrees, representative capacity, indication of experiences relevant to anticipated contributions, and relationship to the institution are included. This information assists the OPRR in evaluating membership composition as it relates to the minimum requirements in 45 CFR 46 § 46.107.

The board must possess diversity in race, gender, cultural backgrounds, and knowledge of the subject area being reviewed. For research proposals involving vulnerable subjects, including children, prisoners, pregnant women, and persons with a physical or mental disability, the board should include one or more members with knowledge about, or experience working with, these subjects. For institutions conducting research involving prisoners, 45 CFR 46 § 46.304 requires that at least one member of the board be a prisoner or a prisoner representative.

The issue of diversity ensures that the IRB is not composed solely of members of one gender or of one profession. At least one member must have primary concerns in scientific areas, and at least one other member must have primary concerns in nonscientific areas. A meeting held to consider proposals not qualifying for "expedited" review must have at least one nonscientific member present. The members are expected to understand the elements of review, but, having diverse backgrounds, are not expected to have a working knowledge of every subject area for which projects are designed. The review of a protocol involving a subject area that is unfamiliar to all members is not unusual. In such a situation, the board has the option to enlist the advice of an individual with expertise in the subject area. The regulations allow for an individual with expertise to advise the board regarding a proposed project, but specifies that this individual may not vote.

The regulations in 45 CFR 46 § 46.107(d) require that the board be sensitive to community issues and that at least one member be appointed from outside of the institution, who is "not otherwise affiliated with the institution and...not part of the immediate family of a person who is affiliated with the institution." This is commonly understood to mean that a board must include at least one "community member." The community member is very important to the protection of human subjects from research risks. The community member functions independently of the institution, and, in this independence, is free to raise questions from the point of view of the subjects. Very often, a community member will have insight into potential problems, such as whether the community will accept or reject the protocol, whether the subjects are likely to understand the informed consent, or whether an incentive is coercive.

The community member may have a better understanding of recruitment methods that would be considered coercive to certain populations, regardless of the intentions of the researcher. Study subjects may not feel free to refuse enrollment in a study, or free to withdraw without any penalty, based on the "authority" of the person recruiting study subjects. A prisoner, for example, may find it difficult to decline enrollment in, or to drop out of, a study if the person recruiting subjects is a probation officer or prison guard. The elderly may not understand that they may choose not to enroll in studies that are recommended by their physicians, or they may not understand the difference between a study and standard treatment if their physicians are recruiting them.

Perhaps the researcher has designed a study involving tissue samples but has not worked closely with representatives of the community to be studied. Members of the community might be unwilling to participate in this study because of cultural or religious beliefs. Some cultural and religious groups believe that all of the human body is sacred. If blood, tissue, organs, or other body parts are used for research, the members of these communities should be included in determining the disposal process for specimens. If burial of the specimens would be the only acceptable method of disposal, and the researcher has not considered this, the community member would alert the researcher and the IRB to this issue.

Conflict of Interest

The regulations clearly state that an IRB member may not participate in the initial or continuing review of any project in which the member may have a conflict of interest. In practice, a member with a conflict may participate in providing information about the project, but may not participate in the voting for approval nor be present in the meeting while the discussion or vote is taking place. By not being present, the opportunity to affect the discussion or decision of the IRB is eliminated. The possibility exists, especially in an IRB of a small public health organization, for one board member to be the subordinate of another in the institution, such as having both the director and assistant director of a program on the board. If the supervisory member is the principal investigator for a research proposal under review, the subordinate might feel an unspoken pressure in the presence of the principal investigator to support the proposal. Without the investigator present during deliberation and voting, the subordinate has the opportunity to discuss the proposal and to vote freely.

Institutional Responsibility and the Federal Assurance

The Common Rule addresses IRB functions and operations, as well as the responsibilities of the institution. The institution negotiates an "assurance" with the OPRR at NIH as set forth in § 46.103. The assurance contains the principles, policies, and procedures that the institution will adhere to in the protection of human subjects from research risks. Institutional policies include the following (45 CFR 46):

- The institution will abide by 45 CFR 46 in all research regardless of funding source.
- All research will be reviewed by an approved IRB.
- No research will be permitted without prior IRB approval or informed consent from the subject or the subject's legal representative.
- The institution will conduct oversight to ensure that the policies regarding human subject protection from research risks are being followed in all research activities.
- The institution pledges to provide meeting space and sufficient staff to support the IRB.
- The institution will provide educational opportunities for investigators and IRB members.

The public health administrator should keep in mind that approval by an IRB does not necessarily mean approval by the institution. Officials of the institution have the right to disapprove the conduct of an approved project. A study might not be aligned with policies of the institution. In this case, the institution could prevent the study from being conducted at the institution, despite

IRB approval. However, once the IRB has declined to approve a study, the institution may not set aside the IRB decision and permit the study to begin.

State Laws

State governments as well as institutions have the right to promulgate rules and regulations and pass laws that are intended to provide more protection than is set forth in the Common Rule. The IRB members must be aware of applicable laws and regulations affecting human subjects protection in their jurisdiction. More restrictive state laws take precedence over the federal regulations. The following paragraphs present a few examples where IRB members must be aware of state laws.

Two conflicting California statutes, both more restrictive than the federal regulations regarding research on prisoners, caused a probe of a research study that was approved by the IRB of a California university. The study involved the test of a psychiatric drug on teenage inmates. One statute states, "no biomedical research shall be conducted on any prisoner in this state." The other statute allows the use of prisoners in drug studies if the drug is only available through a study and if it is in "the best interest of the patient."[16]

In New York State, Article 24A of the Public Health Law assigns the commissioner of the New York State Department of Health with the responsibility of reviewing and approving the policies and procedures, as well as the roster of the human research review committee, of any institution or agency conducting human research in the state. Article 24A also mandates that the conduct of human research involving minors, incompetent persons, persons with mental disabilities, and prisoners be approved by the commissioner of health. New York State courts recently interpreted Article 24A to apply to nonfederally funded research of greater than minimal risk.

Another New York State law that is more restrictive than the Common Rule is Section 79-*l* of the New York State Civil Rights Law (79-*l* CRL), the Genetics Testing Confidentiality Law. Under 79-*l* CLR, written informed consent to a genetic test must be signed and dated and contain at least eight elements specified in the law. These required elements are designed to ensure that the subject understands what the specific test is, the purpose of the test, the meaning and certainty of a positive result, and how long the biologic sample will be retained. The subject may designate to whom test results may be disclosed. The subject is encouraged to seek genetic counseling before consenting to take the test and to consider further testing, counseling, or obtaining medical advice if the test result is positive. The law further addresses the additional testing of anonymous samples, the role of the IRB, court-ordered testing and the release of information, and penalties for violating the provisions of the law.

APPLYING 45 CFR 46

Once the public health organization has an IRB in place, with documented policies and procedures, the actual review of protocols can take place. But not every activity is subject to review under 45 CFR 46. For every proposed study, two basic questions should be asked: Is it research? and Are human subjects involved?

Is It Research?

In 1993, the DHHS published a report that addressed the core functions of a public health organization.[17] Each of these functions (refer to Exhibit 2–3) is driven by data collected in some fashion. The data may be obtained through research, surveillance, program evaluation, or emergency response to a public health threat. Public health organizations that endeavor to collect health data or to study existing data for public health purposes must consider issues of human subjects protection. The answers to the questions "Is this research?" and "Are human subjects involved?" determine if human subjects research review is needed.

The first question asked by the public health manager, the researcher, and the IRB is whether the project is research or nonresearch. *Research* is defined in the Common Rule (45 CFR 46 § 46.102(d)) as follows:

> *Research* means a systematic investigation, including research development, testing and evaluation, designed to develop or contribute to generalizable knowledge. Activities which meet this definition constitute research for the purposes of this policy, whether or not they are conducted or supported under a program which is considered research for other purposes. For example, some demonstration and service programs may include research activities.

The interpretation of this definition has generated much debate. However, a definitive answer proves to be elusive. Federal agencies, public health institutions, and researchers alike strive to understand the Common Rule's definition.

The Centers for Disease Control and Prevention (CDC), requires investigators conducting CDC-sponsored public health research to follow the Common Rule. The CDC has published guidelines to assist investigators in understanding what constitutes public health research and public health nonresearch. These guidelines are available on the Internet.[18] The U.S. Agency for International Development (USAID) has also produced an interpretive guide to the Common Rule that addresses the research question.[19]

Research versus Nonresearch

To continue the discussion of research versus nonresearch, some definitions related to nonresearch activities may be useful.

- *Surveillance* is the ongoing systematic collection, analysis, and interpretation of outcome-specific data, closely integrated with timely dissemination of these data to those persons responsible for preventing or controlling disease or injury.[18,20]
- *Surveillance of infectious diseases* is the regular collection, summarization, and analysis of data on newly diagnosed cases of any infectious disease for the purpose of identifying high-risk groups in the population, understanding the mode(s) of transmission of the disease, and reducing or eliminating its transmission.[21]
- *Emergency response* is a public health activity that is undertaken in an urgent or emergency situation, usually because of an imminent threat to the population, but sometimes because the public and/or government authorities perceive an imminent threat that demands immediate action. The primary purpose of the activity is to determine the nature and magnitude of a public health problem in the community and to implement appropriate measures to address the problem.[18,22]
- *Program evaluation* is the systematic application of scientific and statistical procedures for measuring program conceptualization, design, implementation, and utility; making comparisons based on these measurements; and using the resulting information to optimize program outcomes.[18,23,24]

The two important pieces of the Common Rule definition of research are *designed* and *contribute to generalizable knowledge.*

Research Design. The USAID interpretive guide explains that in order to be considered research, a study must have a systematic design in advance for the definite purpose of contributing to generalizable knowledge.[19] The key is *designed in advance.* A public health surveillance activity that is carried out during an outbreak, which happens to contribute to generalizable knowledge as a result of the surveillance, would not be considered research because the investigation was not designed to contribute to generalizable knowledge, but rather to determine the cause of that particular outbreak in order to prevent further spread of the disease.

The USAID guide provides examples of activities that might be considered research and those that might not. Activities that might be considered research include the following:[19]

- experiments
- observational studies
- surveys

- tests
- recordings

Activities that might not be considered research include the following:[19]

- routine outbreak investigations
- disease monitoring
- program evaluation
- quality assurance
- medical care
- quality improvement
- fiscal or program audits

Contributes to Generalizable Knowledge. Generalizable knowledge is knowledge that can be applied to others beyond the study participants. In a public health setting, contributing to generalizable knowledge cannot be the only determinant of whether the study is research or not. In an emergency response to a public health threat, investigators use standard public health methods to uncover the cause of an outbreak. In the public health activities following the toxic shock syndrome outbreak, for example, surveillance quickly uncovered one brand of superabsorbing tampons as the major contributing factor in the outbreak. This knowledge was generalizable to all women using that brand of tampon, and the tampon was taken off the market. However, the surveillance activities were not intended to be research; the public health investigators wanted to find the cause of the epidemic in order to halt the spread of toxic shock.

NIH guidelines provide additional useful advice regarding research versus nonresearch: "The primary intent of non-research or practice in public health is to prevent disease or injury and improve health.... In some cases knowledge may be generalizable but the primary intention of the endeavor is to benefit a population by controlling a health problem in the population from whom the information is gathered."[18]

A common misinterpretation of *contributes to generalizable knowledge* is whether or not a study can be published. This should not be one of the criteria to judge whether the study is research. Many nonresearch activities result in publications (e.g., program summaries), while many research efforts fail to generate publishable findings.

Consider the Following Scenario. An outbreak of *mycoplasma pneumoniae* occurs in a closed community. In this community, most residents take meals and worship together. The children attend a school for community residents. All residents use the same health care facility, located within the community, with one primary care provider who is well respected by all members of the community. Approximately one-half of the community is diagnosed with the disease. The state health department is alerted. Anecdotal information suggests that one medication used to treat the illness may also be preventive. The public health physician assigned to the outbreak by the state health department would like to administer this medication prophylactically to those residents who have yet to manifest the disease. The community health care provider agrees. There is another similar closed community in another state experiencing an outbreak of the same disease. This medicine will not be given prophylactically in that community. Comparing the results in the two communities would be interesting and may have a major public health impact.

Is this research? On one hand, it is an outbreak threatening the health of a community. The outbreak must be controlled quickly. On the other hand, although a study design has been formalized, administering the medication and comparing the experience of this community to the community without the medication may lead to better control of mycoplasma in future outbreaks. Is this research? The IRB, in this case, decided this was research and required review.

Are Human Subjects Involved?

Once it is determined that the answer to the question "Is it research?" is yes, the next question is "Are human subjects involved?" Again, the Common Rule (45 CFR 46 § 46.102(f)) provides definitions to assist in the determination:

> *Human subject* means a living individual about whom an investigator

> (whether professional or student) conducting research obtains (1) data through intervention or interaction with the individual, or (2) identifiable private information.
>
> *Intervention* includes both physical procedures by which data are gathered (for example, venipuncture) and manipulations of the subject or subject's environment that are performed for research purposes. *Interaction* includes communication or interpersonal contact between investigator and subject. *Private information* includes information about behavior that occurs in a context in which an individual can reasonably expect that no observation or recording is taking place, and information which has been provided for specific purposes by an individual and which the individual can reasonably expect will not be made public (for example, a medical record). Private information must be individually identifiable (i.e., the identity of the subject is or may readily be ascertained by the investigator or associated with the information) in order for obtaining the information to constitute research involving human subjects.

Using this definition, the researcher should be able to decide if human subjects are involved. An investigator who is unsure whether the study is research or involves human subjects should consult the IRB for advice. The IRB members are conversant with the regulations and have the experience to recognize whether review is necessary. One of the responsibilities of the IRB is to educate research staff regarding human subjects protection. Requesting assistance from the IRB would begin a dialogue between the IRB and the researcher that would facilitate the educational opportunity.

Is the Study "Exempt"?

The concept that research involving human subjects may be exempt from the regulations is difficult for the new investigator to understand. After going through the process of determining if it is research and if human subjects are involved, there is a whole class of research that is clearly exempt from the regulations. Exhibit 15–2 presents the six categories of research that are defined as exempt by 45 CFR 46 § 46.101. Paragraph (c) states "Department or Agency heads retain final judgement [sic] as to whether a particular activity is covered by this policy." "Department or Agency heads" refers to federal department or agency heads. However, many institutions require that investigators apply to their IRB for the determination of exempt status. Investigators who are unsure of their institution's policy in this regard should consult the IRB rather than assume that their research is exempt.

ELEMENTS OF REVIEW

The federal regulations list seven required elements of review, all of which must be satisfied in order to approve research (Exhibit 15–3)(45 CFR 46 §46.111). The first requirement is that *risks to subjects are minimized*. When reviewing a protocol, the reviewer must evaluate whether the study procedures to be used are consistent with sound research design and are also procedures that do not unnecessarily expose the study subject to risk. The risks are also minimized when the procedures being used are those that are already being performed on the subject for diagnostic treatment purposes.

The second requirement for human subjects review is that the *risks to subjects be reasonable in relation to anticipated benefits*. In assessing risk, the IRB evaluates whether the anticipated risks of the research are matched by, or outweighed by, the potential benefit to the individual subject or to society as a whole. Research that carries risks and no individual benefit can be allowed if there is enough societal benefit and if the subject gives legal, informed consent. A higher standard for the risk/benefit relationship is applied to research involving children. Societal benefit is not enough justification. For children, the risk must only be a minor increase over minimal risk and be commensurate. For research

Exhibit 15–2 Six Categories of Exempt Research

1. Research conducted in established or commonly accepted educational settings, involving normal educational practices
2. Research using educational tests, survey procedures, interview procedures, or observations of public behavior, unless human subjects can be identified, directly or indirectly, and any disclosure could place the subject at risk for criminal or civil liability or damage the subject's financial standing, employability, or reputation
3. Research involving educational tests, survey procedures, interview procedures, or observations of public behavior, not exempt by the category above, if the human subjects are elected or appointed public officials or candidates, or if federal statute(s) require(s), without exception, that confidentiality be maintained
4. Research involving the collection or study of existing data, documents, records, pathological specimens, or diagnostic specimens, if these sources are publicly available or if the information is recorded in such a manner by the investigator that subjects cannot be identified directly or through identifiers linked to the subjects
5. Research or demonstration projects designed to study, evaluate, or otherwise examine public benefit or service programs, procedures for obtaining benefits or services under those programs, possible changes in or alternatives to those programs or procedures, or possible changes in methods or levels of payment for benefits or services under those programs
6. Taste and food quality evaluation and consumer acceptance studies if wholesome foods without additives are consumed or if a food is consumed that contains a food ingredient, agricultural chemical, or environmental contaminant at or below the level found to be safe by the Food and Drug Administration, Environmental Protection Agency, or U.S. Department of Agriculture

Source: 45 CFR 46 § 46.101

on children involving greater than minimal risk and no prospect of direct benefit to the individual subjects, but likely to yield generalizable knowledge about the subject's disorder or condition at 45 CFR 46 § 46.406(c), the regulations state "the intervention or procedure presents experiences to subjects that are reasonably commensurate with those inherent in their actual or expected medical, dental, psychological, social, or educational situations." In evaluating the risks to subjects in relation to anticipated benefits, the importance of the knowledge that may be expected to result also has to be evaluated to determine whether the risk is justified.

The third required review element is that the *selection of subjects is equitable.* In order to ensure that the benefits and burdens of research are fairly distributed, the researcher must design the selection procedure to be equitable. The potential subjects should be told how and why they were selected for the study. This element of review is important because a researcher might find it more convenient to select from certain populations, such as selecting from a Medicaid enrollee population, a prison population, or Women, Infants, and Children (WIC) clients. Unless the research is designed to study that population, every effort should be made to select a more equitable population. A researcher might propose to select participants from a population with a lower educational or lower literacy level in order to mask the true study intentions in a consent form. Many populations are considered "vulnerable," such as children, prisoners, pregnant women, persons with mental disabilities, or economically or educationally disadvantaged persons. Although researchers are encouraged to include protected classes in research, especially children and pregnant women, additional scrutiny by the IRB must be taken to ensure that the selection of these populations is appropriate and justifiable.

The next two requirements for research review involve the concept of informed consent.

Exhibit 15–3 Elements of Review

- Risks to subjects are minimized.
- Risks to subjects are reasonable in relation to anticipated benefits, if any, to subjects and the importance of the knowledge that may reasonably be expected to result.
- Selection of subjects is equitable.
- Informed consent will be sought from each prospective subject or legally authorized representative.
- Informed consent will be appropriately documented.
- The research plan makes adequate provisions for monitoring the data collected to ensure the safety of subjects. The research plan makes adequate provisions to protect the privacy of subjects and to maintain the confidentiality of data.
- Additional safeguards have been included in the study to protect the rights and welfare of subjects likely to be vulnerable to coercion.

Source: 45 CFR 46 § 46.111

The informed consent process provides the opportunity to ensure that the subject, or representative, has been told and understands what participation in the research study entails. Following a comprehensive informed consent process, the potential subject is able to choose whether to volunteer to participate in the study. This process is described in detail later in this chapter. The two review requirements related to informed consent are that (1) *informed consent must be sought from each subject or his or her legally authorized representative*, as required by § 46.116, and (2) *informed consent must be appropriately documented* as required by § 46.117. In most cases, informed consent should be documented with a written consent form that has been previously approved by the IRB. This form must be signed by the subject or the subject's legal representative. A copy of the signed form must be given to the subject, and a copy must be retained by the research team for documentation.

Before a research plan can be approved, the plan must contain *adequate provisions for monitoring data collected to ensure the safety of the subjects*. In other words, the plan must show how the data will be monitored throughout the progress of the study so that any problems affecting the safety of the subjects will be identified. Making a note of each problem and filing it does not meet the intent of monitoring the data. Without a process to identify, quantify, or analyze patterns of problems, the investigator may not be able to ensure the safety of the study subjects. As soon as an investigator recognizes a problem, the IRB must be notified.

The research plan must also demonstrate that there are *adequate provisions to protect the privacy of subjects and to maintain the confidentiality of data*. Protection of privacy involves such issues as ensuring that the subject's disease status is not revealed to anyone, and ensuring that the subject's public benefits status is not revealed (such as health insurance coverage, Medicaid, welfare, and WIC). Recruiting only human immunodeficiency virus (HIV)–positive clients to participate in a survey of risky sexual behaviors while the client is sitting in a crowded waiting room of a family planning clinic could violate the client's right to privacy because the recruitment procedure could reveal the client's HIV status. The privacy of next of kin should also be considered. Revealing a newborn subject's positive HIV status automatically reveals the positive status of the mother. In genetics research, the privacy of the next of kin of subjects must be respected to prevent inadvertent identification of their genetic status.

Confidential data are data containing identifiable information. Medical records, birth records, abortion records, and other registry-type data contain identifiers and must remain confidential. Confidentiality of identifiable paper and computer information may be protected through methods such as restricted access to files, recoding or removing identifiers from computerized data, automatic deletion of phone numbers at the successful completion of a telephone survey call, destruction of files, and prohibition on faxing of identifiable data.

In addition to the seven required elements of review, the proposal must also be scrutinized to *ensure that no subjects will be vulnerable to coercion or undue influence to participate in the study.* Special precautions need to be taken to protect vulnerable populations. The study proposal should provide safeguards to protect the rights and welfare of the subjects in the study. Coercion may be very subtle. The researcher, in an effort to ensure adequate participation, may offer incentives to potential subjects. However, the incentive may affect the voluntary nature of study participation. Not all incentives are coercive. A $5 coupon for participating in an anonymous survey of healthy behaviors would not be considered coercive for most populations. However, an $800 cash payment to participate in a drug trial would be a coercive incentive for a homeless person. The incentive does not have to be monetary. It might involve a service or an opportunity. The researcher must take care in designing the incentive package to avoid any coercive inducements.

Informed Consent

Informed consent is one of the most important principles in human subjects protection. As discussed at the beginning of the chapter, in 1946, Dr. Andrew Ivy, the medical consultant to the prosecution in the Nuremberg Medical Trial, formulated rules involving the protection of human research subjects. His first rule involved obtaining consent from the research subject.[2] As policies designed to protect human research subjects evolved, informed consent was an essential element. The Common Rule specifies both the general requirements for informed consent (45 CFR 46 § 46.116) and the requirements for the documentation of informed consent (45 CFR 46 § 46.117). The regulations at § 46.116 are quite clear:

> Except as provided elsewhere in this policy, no investigator may involve a human being as a subject in research covered by this policy unless the investigator has obtained the legally effective informed consent of the subject or the subject's legally authorized representative. An investigator shall seek such consent only under circumstances that provide the prospective subject or the representative sufficient opportunity to consider whether or not to participate and that minimize the possibility of coercion or undue influence.

This introduction continues, specifying that the language must be understandable to the subject or representative. This is generally interpreted to mean presented in no greater than an eighth grade reading level, which is about average for U.S. adults. Medicaid enrollees have an average reading level of fifth grade.[25] For those potential subjects who do not speak or understand English, the consent form should be prepared in a language the subject speaks or reads. The informed consent may not include exculpatory language waiving any of the subject's rights or releasing the investigator, sponsor, institution, or its agents from liability for negligence.

This section of the regulations (45 CFR 46 § 46.116) lists eight basic elements that must be included in the informed consent and an additional six elements to be included when appropriate. The OPRR provides a useful informed consent checklist, as well as guidance on obtaining informed consent from subjects who do not speak English, on its Web site at www.nih.gov/grants/OPRR/humansubjects.

The required basic elements of informed consent are listed in Exhibit 15–4. These basic elements are intended to ensure that subjects who enter research studies are fully aware of what is to take place, how they will be affected by participation, and that they may decline to participate or may withdraw at any time without penalties or loss of benefits of any sort.

Presenting a potential subject with a properly prepared informed consent form, however, does not ensure that the subject is informed. The form should be used as an integral piece of the discussion of the research study with the potential subject. The potential subject should feel free to ask questions and receive further clarification about any aspect that he or she is uncomfortable with or does not understand. Likewise, the investiga-

Exhibit 15–4 Basic Elements of Informed Consent

- A statement that the study involves research, an explanation of the purposes of the research and the expected duration of the subject's participation, a description of the procedures to be followed, and identification of any procedures which are experimental;
- A description of any foreseeable risks or discomforts to the subject;
- A description of any benefits to the subject or to others which may reasonably be expected from the research;
- A disclosure of appropriate alternative procedures or courses of treatment;
- A description of the extent to which confidentiality of records identifying the subject will be maintained;
- For research involving more than minimal risk, an explanation as to whether any compensation or medical treatments are available if injury occurs and, if so, where further information may be obtained;
- An explanation of whom to contact for answers to pertinent questions about the research and research subjects' rights, and whom to contact in the event of a research-related injury to the subject;
- A statement that participation is voluntary, and that the subject may refuse to participate or may discontinue participation at any time without penalty or loss of benefits to which the subject is otherwise entitled.

Source: 45 CFR 46 § 46.116

tor should assess comprehension by questioning the individual concerning his or her understanding of all the elements of informed consent. Just as the informed consent form should be prepared in a language and at a reading level that is appropriate to the subject, the discussion of the research with the study subject should also be understandable to the subject.

Coercion

The informed consent procedure must also occur in a way that is not coercive. As discussed earlier in the chapter, the potential subject may feel coerced to participate because of the position of authority of the person conducting the informed consent procedure, such as a personal physician, school nurse, probation officer, prison guard, workplace supervisor, or professor. Despite assurances of the right to refuse to participate or the right to withdraw, in this scenario, the subject may be concerned about the consequences of not enrolling in the study.

Consider the following example: an offer to be entered into a "lottery" for $750 is the incentive to recruit low-income mothers at a WIC site. The well-intentioned researcher does not see this incentive as coercive. The researcher assumes that a potential subject would understand that she may or may not "win" the $750. However, the mother might misunderstand the lottery concept and believe that she will be paid $750 to participate, just as many people misunderstand their chances of winning the lottery or a magazine sweepstakes. A perceived incentive of $750 for a mother struggling to provide for her family may be something she cannot refuse. If she enrolls for this reason, the incentive is coercive. A fairer, less coercive incentive might be for the investigator to divide the $750 into smaller but equal incentives offered to all potential participants.

If an excessive incentive is only available upon completion of the study, then the right to withdraw is also compromised. One complicated example of a potentially coercive incentive to participate and to remain in the study involves an indigent teen being recruited into a study while the teen is a client of an HIV clinic in New York City. In New York State, a teen seeking services in an HIV clinic does not need parental permission. Because requiring permission from a parent for the teen to participate in a study of sexual practices would violate the subject's right to privacy, the teen may be enrolled in the study without parental permission. Offering a $100 gift certificate to a shop frequented by local teens as an incentive for participation in the study becomes such an attractive incentive for an indigent teen that it would be difficult for the teen to choose not to participate. The coercive nature of the incentive increases if the teen is then told that every question must be answered in order to be paid. Recognizing that this incentive is, in effect, coercive, the investigator who wishes to offer an incentive then must decide what a proper incentive would be. Where do you draw the line? The incentive should not be so desirable that the potential subject, who might not participate without an incentive, is compelled by the incentive itself to enroll in the study.

Waiver or Alteration

The regulations allow some research projects to alter or waive some or all of the basic elements of informed consent. Alteration or waiver of elements is allowed: (1) in research related to public benefit or service programs where the research could not practically be carried out without the waiver or alteration, and (2) in research involving no more than minimal risk, where the rights and welfare of subjects would not be adversely affected by the waiver or alteration, the research could not practically be carried out without the waiver or alteration, and subjects would be provided with additional pertinent information after participation whenever appropriate.

Permission

When recruiting children, there are additional considerations for obtaining informed consent. In research involving children, the investigator seeks *permission* from the parent or legal guardian to include the child or ward in the research (45 CFR 46 § 46.408). All of the elements of informed consent would be presented to the parent or legal guardian to ensure that the parent or guardian clearly understands what the child will be committed to as a participant in the research.

Assent

In addition to obtaining permission, the investigator must also solicit the assent of the child, when the child is capable of assenting. *Assent* is defined in 45 CFR 46 § 46.402 as "a child's affirmative agreement to participate in research." Further, "[m]ere failure to object should not, absent affirmative agreement, be construed as assent." The child's capability to assent can be determined by age, maturity, and psychological state. Obtaining assent may be waived for children with limited capability or if an "intervention or procedure involved in the research holds out a prospect of direct benefit that is important to the health or well-being of the child and is available only in the context of the research" (45 CFR 46 § 46.408).

Dissent is the refusal to assent. If the child dissents, is this binding? The answer has been debated. The American Academy of Pediatrics Committee on Bioethics has stated that in the research context, the persistent refusal to assent by a child may be ethically binding. Whether the dissent is binding may be affected by the potential direct benefit to the child if he or she is enrolled in the research.[26]

SPECIAL PROTECTIONS FOR VULNERABLE POPULATIONS

It is well recognized that vulnerable populations require special protections against the risks posed by research involving human subjects. Looking back to the history of abuses in research, it is clear that the subjects selected in those studies were subjects who had little or no choice concerning participation in the research—prisoners of Nazi concentration camps, inmates at Stateville Prison, retarded children at Willowbrook, the indigent elderly at Brooklyn Chronic Disease Hospital, and poor black men in the Tuskegee study. Special considerations must be given to children, prisoners, pregnant women, persons with mental disabilities, or economically or educationally disadvantaged persons because these groups may be vulnerable to coercion or undue influence (45 CFR 46 § 46.111). The regulations (45 CFR 46) provide additional protections for fetuses, pregnant women, and human in vitro fertilization in subpart B, prisoners in subpart C, and children in subpart D. Each subpart describes the additional duties of the IRB, the research allowed involving each group, and the research not eligible for exemption.

Pregnant Women

NIH encourages the inclusion of women in research.[27] Because the fetus has a unique relationship with the mother and is an unconsenting research subject, subpart B provides additional protections to ensure that the research meets the health needs of the woman and minimizes risks to the fetus. The informed consent process must obtain consent from the mother and father, or just the mother in certain situations, and must provide information on the possible impact of the research on the fetus. In research involving termination of a pregnancy, investigators may not have any role in decisions regarding the termination of the pregnancy or in determining the viability of the terminated fetus.

Prisoners

Incarceration puts the prisoner in a unique situation as a potential study subject. The prisoner is vulnerable to coercion and undue influence as a result of the prison culture. Prison guards, probation officers, and other prisoners have the opportunity to exert influence on decisions the prisoner makes. Because of this situation, even though a prisoner may be properly informed about the research, he or she may not be free to choose whether to enter a study, to withdraw from a study, or to question his or her rights as a study subject. Care must be taken to eliminate possible coercion, to protect the prisoner's right to privacy, and to protect confidentiality. Subpart C of 45 CFR 46 addresses the additional protections that apply to prisoners as potential research subjects. In order to review research protocols involving prisoners, the IRB must have at least one member who is either a prisoner or prisoner representative. Subpart C also restricts the types of research that can use prisoners as subjects.

Children

Children and minors are afforded special protections under subpart D of 45 CFR 46 because they have not reached the legal age for consent and, in most cases, have not achieved the maturity to understand the risks and benefits of participating in research. Because a child cannot consent, provisions are made for a parent or guardian to give permission for the child to become a research subject and the child's assent is requested. Assent and permission were discussed earlier in this chapter.

When reviewing research protocols involving children, IRBs must evaluate the level of risk to the subjects and the potential benefits. The four categories of research the IRB may approve are (45 CFR 46)

1. research not involving greater than minimal risk
2. research involving greater than minimal risk but presenting the prospect of direct benefit to the individual subjects
3. research involving greater than minimal risk and no prospect of direct benefit to individual subjects, but likely to yield generalizable knowledge concerning the subject's disorder or condition
4. research not otherwise approvable that presents an opportunity to understand, prevent, or alleviate a serious problem affecting the health or welfare of children

On March 6, 1998, NIH promulgated a new policy to ensure the inclusion of children in NIH-sponsored research, *NIH Policy and Guidelines on the Inclusion of Children as Participants in Research Involving Human Subjects*.[28] This policy resulted from concern that medical treatments used for children are often treatments that are developed through testing only on adults. This policy, however, is not absolute. Exceptions to the policy include studies involving diseases not seen in children, studies that would more appropriately be conducted as pediatric studies, and studies where a comparable study in children is already underway. It is important to note that all protections provided for under subpart D should continue to be followed.

Acquired Immune Deficiency Syndrome (AIDS) Studies

In December 1984, the OPRR issued *Guidance for Institutional Review Boards for AIDS Studies* as part of the OPRR Reports series.[29] No special federal regulations exist for persons with AIDS. However, this guidance document covers the portions of 45 CFR 46 to which special attention should be paid when dealing with AIDS studies. Of particular concern is the protection of confidentiality. Research participants could suffer serious consequences as a result of improper disclosure of their disease status. With mandatory AIDS/HIV reporting in most states, public health agencies regularly conduct some form of AIDS studies, such as surveys, seroprevalence studies, and studies comparing diagnostic techniques. When study design allows, blinded or unlinked studies provide useful information while ensuring the protection of confidentiality. In the conduct of AIDS-related research, the OPRR advises that possible benefits accrued from the study must be maximized and the potential harm to the subjects must be minimized.

Many states have laws or regulations providing special protections for persons with AIDS or HIV. Public health agencies may also have internal policies designed to provide additional protections for these subjects. The IRB and investigators should be aware of any applicable state laws or regulations or agency policies when designing and reviewing AIDS protocols.

Individuals with Questionable Capacity To Consent

In many states, the public health agency may be a separate agency from the mental health agency, but in some states, the two functions are combined in one agency. As a result, the public health manager in a combined agency may have the opportunity to include individuals in a study who may lack the capacity to consent.

In subparts B, C, and D of 45 CFR 46, specific regulations apply to conducting research on pregnant women, prisoners, and children. However, the regulations do not provide additional protections for potential research subjects who may lack the decision-making capacity to consent to the research. NIH provides guidance in *Protecting Human Research Subjects: Institutional Review Board Guidebook*[30] and an Internet document, *Interim Research Involving Individuals with Questionable Capacity to Consent: Points To Consider*.[31] In the guidebook, *cognitively impaired* is defined as follows:

> Having either a psychiatric disorder (e.g., psychosis, neurosis, personality or behavior disorders), and organic impairment (e.g., dementia) or a developmental disorder (e.g., mental retardation) that affects cognitive or emotional functions to the extent that capacity for judgement [sic] and reasoning is significantly diminished. Others, including persons under the influence of or dependent on drugs or alcohol, those suffering from degenerative diseases affecting the brain, terminally ill patients, and persons with severely disabling physical handicaps, may also be compromised in their ability to make decisions in their best interests.[30(p.26,sec.6)]

When reviewing a protocol involving persons with questionable capacity to consent, the IRB and the investigator should be sure that additional safeguards are in place to protect the health and well-being of these subjects. In NIH's *Points To Consider,* the IRB and investigator are cautioned that potential and actual research subjects could easily be confused by dual roles of the researcher, as both investigator and clinician, and could easily misunderstand the difference between treatment and research.[31] Therefore, the consent process must be conducted to ensure that the differences are clearly indicated. An assessment of competence may assist the investigator in determining the best consent process to follow. The guidebook recommends that the investigator should presume that adults are competent to consent "unless there is evidence of serious mental disability that would impair reasoning or judgement [sic]."[30(p.29,sec.6)]

The subject who does not have the capacity to consent should, as in research with children, be allowed the opportunity to assent. The subject may dissent or ask to withdraw. The subject's wishes should be respected in most instances. The National Commission for the Protection of Human Subjects recommends that the subject's wishes be honored based on the risk level of the research study and the likelihood of benefit to the subject as a result of participation.[30]

Selection of subjects should be conducted to ensure that the research has a direct relationship to the conditions or circumstances of the potential subjects. When selecting subjects from an institutionalized population, the issues of voluntariness and competence must be considered. Some institutionalized persons may not understand that participation is voluntary, or they may feel compelled to participate when someone of authority or someone they might want to please asks them to participate.[30]

The subject of legal guardianship must be carefully examined. Not all legal guardians have the authority to consent on behalf of the subjects to be enrolled in a research study. The guardianship may be limited to consent to medical care. The guidelines also caution that an institutional official who is a subject's court-appointed guardian is not the appropriate person to give consent for the subject to enroll in research because of the potential conflict of interest.[30]

In January 1999, the National Bioethics Advisory Commission submitted the report *Research Involving Persons with Mental Disorders That May Affect Decisionmaking Capacity* to President Clinton. This report discusses, in detail, topics involved in research with incapacitated persons, such as informed consent, surrogate decision making, assent or objection, assessment of risks and benefits, and recommendations and guidance.[32]

Students and Employees

Research designed to enroll students or employees as subjects should be carefully examined to ensure that voluntariness is maintained. Both groups might be subject to coercion, whether expressed or only perceived. Students and employees may not believe that they have the right to refuse to enroll or to withdraw at any time. Students might feel that their grades would be affected by not participating; employees might worry about job status or career. Just as with prisoners and other institutionalized subjects, the IRB must scrutinize the consent process to ensure voluntariness.

• • •

One of any research instutition's key responsibilities under its assurance with OPRR is the training of research investigators and IRB members in strategies to protect individuals and populations that participate in public health research. This chapter is intended to assist public health managers, investigators, and IRB members in understanding and applying regulations and laws designed to protect human subjects from research risks.

Many other resources for protecting human subjects in public health research exist. The OPRR has an excellent Web site (http://grants.nih.gov/grants/oprr/oprr.htm) that includes the regulations, the guidebook, OPRR Reports/Dear Colleague letters with updates and clarifications, a directory of staff to contact for assistance, information on OPRR-sponsored national conferences, and links to other useful sites. The FDA Web site contains their information sheet series of clarifying documents, tips, and fact sheets, along with regulations and a staff directory (http://www.fda.gov/oc/oha/IRB/toc.html). The Medical College of Wisconsin maintains an IRB-related Web site (www.mcwirb.org) with a free e-mail–based discussion list for IRB subscribers. IRB members and administrators share experiences and solicit guidance from their peers through this e-mail service. Two human subjects protection–related associations, Public Responsibility in Medicine and Research (PRIM&R) and Applied Research Ethics National Association (ARENA), maintain Web sites (www.aamc.org/research/primr and www.aamc.org/research/primr/arena) with information on publications and related conferences and provide a forum for addressing biomedical and bioethical issues. There are many professional journals that deal with ethics: *IRB* is a journal dedicated to IRB issues, published by The Hastings Center. Finally, with a wealth of printed and electronic information available to assist investigators, and IRB members and administrators, the staff at the OPRR and the FDA are always available to answer questions.

CHAPTER REVIEW

1. Following the National Research Act of 1974, a 1978 report by the National Commission for the Protection of Human Subjects (Belmont report) identified three basic principles that govern human subjects research.
   - respect for persons
   - beneficence
   - justice
2. The DHEW-published regulations in the *Federal Register* (Title 45, Code of Federal Regulations, Part 46) require grantee institutions to establish IRBs to review research with respect to risks to subjects, equitable subject selection, adequacy of informed consent, provisions for data monitoring, protection of privacy and maintenance of confidentiality, and coercion and undue unfluence.
3. The "Common Rule" specifies the minimum requirements for the structure, composition, and functions of IRBs. The research institution's assurance normally affirms that the institution will abide by 45 CFR 46 in all research regardless of funding source, and all research will be reviewed.
4. Once the public health organization has an IRB in place (or arrangement for availability of IRB review), two questions are asked to determine if a proposed activity does indeed require review.
   - Is it research?
   - Are human subjects involved?
5. In distinguishing research from nonresearch activities, public health organizations may classify the following activities as nonresearch:
   - surveillance for disease control efforts
   - emergency response
   - program evaluation

   In many cases the information generated from these types of activities is subsequently used for research. At that time, the information falls within the purview of human subjects review requirements.
6. Research activities are defined for the purposes of human subjects review to include efforts that are *designed in advance* to *contribute to generalized knowledge.*
7. Vulnerable populations needing special protections include pregnant women, prisoners, children, persons with AIDS, individuals with questionable capacity to consent, students, and employers.

REFERENCES

1. *The Medical Case, Trials of War Criminals before the Nuremberg Military Tribunals under Control Council Law 10* (Washington, DC: U.S. Government Printing Office, 1949).
2. "Supplementary Report to the Judicial Council," *Journal of the American Medical Association* 132 (1946): 1,090.
3. *Advisory Committee on Human Radiation Experiments: Final Report* (Washington DC: U.S. Government Printing Office, 1995).
4. "Ethics Governing the Service of Prisoners as Subjects in Medical Experiments: Report of a Committee Appointed by Governor Dwight H. Green of Illinois," *Journal of the American Medical Association* 136 (1948): 457–458.

5. H. Beecher, "Experimentation in Man," *Journal of the American Medical Association* 169 (1959): 461–478.
6. World Medical Association, "Declaration of Helsinki: Recommendations Guiding Medical Doctors in Biomedical Research Involving Human Subjects," adopted by the Eighteenth World Medical Assembly, Helsinki, Finland, 1964.
7. R.R. Faden and T.L. Beauchamp, *A History and Theory of Informed Consent* (New York: Oxford University Press, 1986).
8. J. Katz, *Experimentation with Human Beings: The Authority of the Investigator, Subject, Professions, and State in the Human Experimentation Process* (New York: Russell Sage Foundation, 1972).
9. D.J. Rothman, "Were Tuskegee and Willowbrook 'Studies in Nature?'" *Hastings Center Report* 12 (1982): 5–7.
10. U.S. Department of Health, Education and Welfare, *Final Report of the Tuskegee Syphilis Study Ad Hoc Panel* (Washington, DC: U.S. Government Printing Office, 1973).
11. National Commission for the Protection of Human Subjects of Biomedical and Behavioral Research, "The Belmont Report: Ethical Principles and Guidelines for the Protection of Human Subjects of Research" [DHEW Pub. No. OS 78–0012] (Washington, DC: 1978).
12. U.S. General Accounting Office, *Scientific Research: Continued Vigilance Critical to Protecting Human Subjects* [GAO/HEHS-96–72] (Washington, DC: U.S. Government Printing Office, 1996).
13. C. Marwick, "Institutional Review Boards under Stress: Will They Explode or Change?" *Journal of the American Medical Association* 276 (1996): 1,623–1,626.
14. U.S. Department of Health and Human Services, Office of the Inspector General, *Institutional Review Boards: A Time for Reform* [OEI-01–97–00193] (Washington, DC: U.S. Government Printing Office, 1998).
15. Dr. Melody Lin, seminar communication, Dartmouth College, 7 October 1999.
16. T. Weber, "1997 Drug Test on Teenage Inmates Probed," *Los Angeles Times*, 16 August 1999.
17. U.S. Department of Health and Human Services, *Health Care Reform and Public Health—A Paper on Population-Based Core Functions: The Core Function Project* (Washington, DC: Public Health Service, 1993).
18. U.S. Centers for Disease Control and Prevention, "Guidelines for Defining Public Health Research and Public Health Non-Research," 17 June 1999. URL: http://www.cdc.gov/od/ads/opspoll1.htm.
19. U.S. Agency for International Development, "How To Interpret the Federal Policy for the Protection of Human Subjects or 'Common Rule,'" (Part A) 2 February 1999. http://www.info.usaid.gov/pop_health/commonrule.htm.
20. S.B. Thacker and R.L. Berkelman, "Public Health Surveillance in the United States," *Epidemiolgy Review* 10 (1988): 164–190.
21. J.S. Mausner and S. Kramer, *Mausner & Bahn Epidemiology, An Introductory Text,* 2d ed. (Philadelphia: W.B. Saunders Co., 1985).
22. A.D. Langmuir, "The Epidemic Intelligence Service of the Centers for Disease Control," *Public Health Reports* 95 (1980): 470–477.
23. P.H. Rossi and H.E. Freeman, *Evaluation: A Systematic Approach* (Newbury Park, CA: Sage Publications, 1993).
24. A. Fink, *Evaluation Fundamentals* (Newbury Park, CA: Sage Publications, 1993).
25. B.D. Weiss and C. Coyne, "Communicating with Patients Who Cannot Read," *New England Journal of Medicine 337,* no. 4 (1997): 272–274.
26. American Academy of Pediatrics Committee on Bioethics, "Informed Consent, Parental Permission, and Assent in Pediatric Practice," *Pediatrics 95,* no. 2 (1995): 314–317.
27. G.B. Ellis, "Inclusion of Women and Minorities in Research," *OPRR Reports 94,* no. 1 (1994).
28. National Institutes of Health, *NIH Policy and Guidelines on the Inclusion of Children as Participants in Research Involving Human Subjects,* 6 March 1998. http://grants.nih.gov//grants/guide/notice-files/not98-024.html.
29. Office for Protection from Research Risks, *OPRR Reports: Guidance for Institutional Review Boards for AIDS Studies,* 26 December 1984. http://www.nih.gov/grants/oprr/humansubjects/guidance/hsdc84-dec.htm.
30. Office for Protection from Research Risks, *Protecting Human Research Subjects: Institutional Review Board Guidebook* (Washington, DC: National Institutes of Health, 1993).
31. National Institutes of Health, *Interim Research Involving Individuals with Questionable Capacity To Consent: Points To Consider.* http://www.nih.gov/grants/policy/questionablecapacity.htm.
32. National Bioethics Advisory Commission, *Research Involving Persons with Mental Disorders That May Affect Decisionmaking Capacity* (Rockville, MD: National Bioethics Advisory Commission, 1998).

PART III

Administrative Processes and Strategies for Public Health Organizations

Population-based management requires managerial decisions and actions by public health professionals across multiple interventions, institutions, and risk groups rather than within them. The chapters in Part III move beyond operational issues to explore strategies for managing population health across functional areas and organizational boundaries. These cross-cutting strategies involve issues in human resources management, financial management, performance measurement and improvement, communications and media relations, marketing, constituency building, academic partnerships, legislative relations, and leadership. The chapters in this section examine issues in designing, implementing, and sustaining administrative strategies that target populationwide goals and objectives. The strategies examined here enable public health professionals to move from managing internal operations to managing population-based performance.

CHAPTER 16

Human Resources Management

Lee Thielen

The purpose of human resources management is to enhance the effectiveness of the work force in meeting organizational and community goals. Personnel management consists of a variety of functions including recruitment, compensation, position classification, and performance appraisal. Work in public health organizations is best accomplished through teams. Attention to diversity, mentoring, and training of the work force are integral components of a successful human resources strategy.

The purpose of human resources management is to realize the full potential of the public health work force in achieving the goal of population-wide health improvement. Successful human resources management motivates workers and results in enhanced effectiveness. This chapter addresses the basic principles that all or most human resources systems need for success. The employees of any organization determine its failure or success, its strengths or weaknesses, its accomplishments, and its disappointments. Public health administrators often place emphasis on the management of financial resources, information resources, and human resources, but often the most important determinant of institutional success is how well human resources are managed.

Personnel management includes all of the functions and activities that allow an organization to manage its work force. These functions include recruitment, selection, promotion, succession planning, position classification, compensation, benefits, recordkeeping, counseling, disciplinary and corrective actions, training, identification of competence requirements, coaching, staffing planning, performance planning, and performance appraisal. In addition, it is through personnel management that organizational procedures, policies, and values related to the work force are determined and implemented. Although core personnel management activities are usually organized in a designated human resources office, all managers and all supervisors engage in personnel management every day. These midlevel managers rely on a centralized human resources office to provide information, guidance, and support with difficult personnel issues.

Most organizations hire and staff a human resources or personnel office with professional staff members. Qualified staff understand both the theory and the practice of personnel management, but they must also understand current employment law and the practices and policies of any parent organization, such as the county or state government. These individuals also require strong interpersonal and technical skills to develop and implement human resources strategy. Due to the many laws governing employment practices, recordkeeping requirements and advancing information technologies often drive the kinds of new skills needed to staff a successful human resources office.

Staff in human resources offices require a basic understanding of employment law, personnel selection, counseling, mediation, position classification, compensation, and information management. The office should be positioned in a central part of the organization, such as directly reporting to the director or to a director of administration. For an organization to accomplish its mission and objectives, the practices and policies of human resources must support the organization's direction. In addition, the human resources office must work closely with the accounting, budgeting, and payroll functions of the organization so that all units can accomplish their objectives.

WORK PERFORMANCE

Important to work performance is a set of variables that include characteristics of the individual, the job, and the environment (Exhibit 16–1).[1,2] Katz and Kahn described three behavioral requirements basic to the functioning of people in the workplace.[3]

1. People must be attracted not only to join the organization, but also to remain in it.
2. People must perform the tasks for which they are hired and must do so in a dependable manner.
3. People must go beyond this dependable role performance and engage in some form of creative, spontaneous, and innovative behavior at work.

Human resources are especially important to the public health organization because staff are undoubtedly the most important asset in achieving improvements in population health. A chief priority of both senior and middle managers within the organization is to excel at the motivational challenge to increase employee participation and production at work. Managerial approaches to motivation are examined in this chapter as specific human resources functions, including employee development, mentoring, job training, quality management, and recruitment. Additionally, human resource systems and processes frequently encountered by public health managers are examined, including merit systems, job classification systems, labor relations processes, and contract development processes.

Patterns of managerial motivation are shown in Table 16–1. According to the Porter and Lawler model, employee effort is determined by two factors: (1) the value placed on certain outcomes by the individual and (2) the extent to which the person believes that his or her effort will lead to at-

Exhibit 16–1 Variables Affecting the Motivational Process in Organizational Settings

I. Individual Characteristics	II. Job Characteristics (Examples)	III. Work Environment Characteristics
1. Interests 2. Attitudes • toward self • toward job • toward aspects of the work situation 3. Needs • security • social • achievement	1. Types of intrinsic rewards 2. Degree of autonomy 3. Amount of direct performance feedback 4. Degree of variety in tasks	1. Immediate work environment • peers • supervisor(s) 2. Organizational actions • reward practice • systemwide rewards • individual rewards • organizational climate

Note: These lists are not intended to be exhaustive but are meant to indicate some of the more important variables influencing the employee motivation.

Source: Adapted with permission from L.W. Porter and R.E. Miles, Motivation and Management, in *Contemporary Management: Issues and Viewpoints,* J.W. McGuire, ed., © 1974.

Table 16–1 General Patterns of Managerial Approaches to Motivation

Traditional Model	*Human Relations Model*	*Human Resources Model*
Assumptions		
1. Work is inherently distasteful to most people. 2. What they do is less important that what they earn for doing it. 3. Few want or can handle work that requires creativity, self-direction, or self-control.	1. People want to feel useful and important. 2. People desire to belong and to be recognized as individuals. 3. These needs are more important than money in motivating people to work.	1. Work is not inherently distasteful. People want to contribute to meaningful goals that they have helped establish. 2. Most people can exercise far more creative, responsible self-direction and self-control than their present jobs demand.
Policies		
1. The manager's basic task is to closely supervise and control subordinates. 2. He or she must break tasks down into simple, repetitive, easily learned operations. 3. He or she must establish detailed work routines and procedures, and enforce these firmly but fairly.	1. The manager's basic task is to make each worker feel useful and important. 2. He or she should keep surbordinates informed and listen to their objections to his or her plans. 3. The manager should allow subordinates to exercise some self-directions and self-control on routine matters.	1. The manager's basic task is to make use of "untapped" human resources. 2. He or she must create an environment in which all members may contribute to the limits of their ability. 3. He or she must encourage full participation on important matters, continually broadening subordinate self-direction and control.
Expectations		
1. People can tolerate work if the pay is decent and the boss if fair. 2. If tasks are simple enough and people are closely controlled, they will produce up to standard.	1. Sharing information with subordinates and involving them in routine decisions will satisfy their basic needs to belong and to feel important. 2. Satisfying these needs will improve morale and reduce resistance to formal authority—subordinates will "willingly cooperate."	1. Expanding subordinate influence, self-direction, and self-control will lead to direct improvements in operating efficiency. 2. Work satisfaction may improve as a "by-product" of subordinates making full use of their resources.

Source: Adapted with permission from R.E. Miles, L.W. Porter, and J.A. Craft, Leadership Attitudes Among Public Health Professionals, *American Journal of Public Health,* p. 1990–2005, © 1966, American Public Health Association.

tainment of these rewards.[4,5] Other theories of successful managerial motivation also emphasize the role of individual expectancy with respect to the assigned job. If people are assigned to tasks for which they lack capability, their expectancy for accomplishment and resulting performance will be low. Human resources managers sensitive to the importance of these self-efficacy beliefs in job performance typically rely on four methods to strengthen employee confidence.[5]

1. Performance successes strengthen a person's perception of his or her capability. Building experience through staged successes can help to overcome limitations in training, supervision, and mentoring.

2. Modeling ideal performance using other employees can convey to observers effective strategies for responding effectively to different work situations.
3. Social persuasion, including realistic encouragement, can increase individuals' beliefs that they possess the necessary capabilities to do the job.
4. Reducing job stress levels using staged successes, performance models, and social persuasion can improve performance over time.

The foundation of the human resources model is positive reinforcement of employee performance, rather than use of punishment for undesirable behaviors, and concentration on building strengths. Positive reinforcement is a widely recommended strategy that is supported in both the scientific and professional literatures on human performance. Positive reinforcement enhances an individual's commitment to the organization and can be achieved by fulfilling the individual's core professional needs for job security, social support, and achievement.

Guidelines for positive reinforcement include the following:[6]

- Don't reward every worker in the same way; differentiate rewards based on performance.
- Do something. Nonaction by managers also influences employee behavior, but there may be negative consequences to nonaction on performance.
- Tell the individual worker what he or she can do to receive positive reinforcement.
- Tell the worker what he or she is doing wrong.
- Do not correct the worker in front of others.
- Make the consequences equal to the behavior; reward good workers and counsel employees with unsatisfactory performance.

ORGANIZATIONAL COMMITMENT

After the newly recruited employee becomes a member of the organization, preparation is needed so that the former applicant learns and becomes committed to the organization's goals, objectives, and operations.[7] Organizational commitment involves three factors: (1) belief in the goals and values of the organization, (2) willingness to exert considerable effort on behalf of the organization, and (3) desire to continue work with the organization. This concept is not limited to organizational loyalty, but rather it reflects a desire by the individual to further the success of the organization. Better work performance is correlated with the employee's commitment to the organization.[8] There is also a positive relationship between organizational tenure and job commitment.[9] High levels of organizational commitment are associated with low levels of employee turnover.[10]

What enhances employee commitment to organizations, including public health organizations? The attachment the employee brings to the organization on the first day of work correlates with the employee's propensity to develop a stable attachment and long stay with the organization.[7–9] The implications for astute recruitment and employee orientation are evident.

Public health organizations need to have mechanisms in place to develop organizational commitment among new employees. The mission of public health is conducive to the development of an organizational culture with improved health as the goal. The skills and professional identity of multiple members of the work force facilitate this culture. The role of the human resources staff is to develop core personnel functions to support this culture, including training managers and supervisors in the principles of goal setting, positive reinforcement, employee participation, and communication.

Goal Setting

Goal setting must be specific and designed to occur within an appropriate time frame. Participation by the supervisor and staff in determining goals leads to acceptance and increased clarity of the goals. Group goal setting promotes cooperation and team cohesion; nonetheless, goals must also promote individual understanding through "contracts" that outline specific tasks to be accomplished. Contracting processes have been used successfully by local and state public health organizations for many years. As part of this process, overall organization goals are translated into specific objectives. The accomplishment of specific objectives is contracted with individuals and teams over a defined time period, often a year. Quarterly milestones can also be set. Both the supervisor and staff understand the task at hand, how performance is measured, and what deliverables are expected. Employees can be encouraged to go beyond baseline performance in setting contract objectives. For example, a lead poisoning program supervisor could contract to achieve a specific screening rate of children under five years of age in a community. The contract might further seek that a specific proportion of children with high blood lead levels receives environmental follow-up and hazard abatement. Additional provisions could include the improvement of lead testing performance in specific settings such as managed care organizations, as well as the implementation of geographic information systems mapping lead exposures within the community served.

A supportive manager does not use goals to threaten subordinates, but rather to clarify what is expected and to motivate performance improvement. The employee experiences satisfaction from attaining goals.[11] Rewards for the individual include pay increases and promotion. However, recognition and approval from leaders is also key to staff motivation.[3] Another type of individual reward is peer group social approval. This factor is particularly important in mission-oriented public health organizations staffed by multidisciplinary teams of professionals including epidemiologists, environmental specialists and engineers, laboratory workers, and nurses.

Teams

Work in public health agencies is often accomplished best by groups and teams, where the stimulus to perform is increased by peer interaction. This strategy is commonly used in response to particular public health challenges. Using an array of individuals from different departmental units can help develop a team with broad categorical perspectives and harness the energy of various disciplines.

There are many successful examples of team-based approaches to human resources management. In 1991, a major increase in syphilis in one state led the state health department to form a multidisciplinary team to devise a response to the problem.[12] This team-based approach was better than relying solely on the sexually transmitted disease bureau staff because the problem transcended categorical functions within the organization. Therefore, personnel from maternal and child health programs, family planning services, human immunodeficiency virus (HIV) and acquired immune deficiency syndrome (AIDS) programs, laboratory services, health education services, public relations offices, outreach services, and health care facility regulation divisions were represented on the task force. The different perspectives, orientations, and services resulted in an improved approach to the problem. To be successful, multidisciplinary teams must be given adequate resources, time, and authority to proceed on tasks. Information is also critical to productive team-based strategies. Information for human resources management is a two-way process. The manager must receive input from workers and teams concerning needs, conditions, and recommendations. The workers and teams, in turn, need clear directions to reduce uncertainty and provide feedback about performance.

Effective human resources management strategies rely on principles of positive reinforcement, reward, organizational commitment, team-building, and information exchange.

DIVERSITY IN THE WORK FORCE

There are many legal reasons why public health organizations should strive for diversity in the workplace. None of these reasons is as compelling, however, as the potential talent and skill that are brought to the workplace when the staff reflects the reality of the population served. Customers to public health organizations include people of myriad languages and cultures. In addition to issues of ethnicity, religion, color, sexual orientation, and culture, a well-balanced organization includes a broad range of age levels and people with disabilities. The recruitment, testing, and selection of staff need to be designed to reduce any potential adverse effects on protected classes. Adverse effects are defined as using a "selection process for a particular job or group of jobs that result in the selection of members of any racial, ethnic, or sex group at a lower rate than members of other groups."[13(p.197)] Agencies and organizations that work proactively to encourage diversity incorporate fair selection practices, targeted recruitment, and employee training in diversity. They also use an employee–manager committee to encourage diversity in the work force and appoint a staff member to function as an equal opportunity counselor. Some of the laws governing equal opportunity and affirmative action include Title VII of the Civil Rights Acts of 1964 and 1990, Executive Order 11246 (amended by Executive Order 11375), the Equal Pay Act of 1963, the Age Discrimination in Employment Act of 1967, the Americans with Disabilities Act, and state and local laws.[14]

PROFESSIONAL DEVELOPMENT

There are two key motivations for investing in the professional development of employees. First, such development leads to greater job satisfaction by the employees, improved morale, reduced turnover, and enhanced performance. Second, the organization benefits from a staff with a breadth of skills, knowledge, and attitudes. Creativity and ownership in the success of the organization come from enhancement of the quality of the work force. There are many ways to further employee development. These include training and education, mentoring programs, and employee involvement in organizational improvement and decisions. Public health organizations are often at a competitive disadvantage in the pay and working conditions that they are able to offer employees relative to other employers. However, the intrinsic satisfaction that can come from making a difference in the community is a highly motivating characteristic of public health work. Employees who feel valued and see tangible investments in their growth will often develop a commitment to the organization that is as powerful a motivator or more powerful than compensation.

Training and Education

Every organization needs a training budget that is recognized as being just as important as other expenses, such as utilities and equipment maintenance. A common error in organizations is to assume that the training budget is discretionary and thus subject to reduction during difficult budgetary times. Each employee needs a personal development plan that includes both specific skills and personal growth components. This plan should be negotiated during each annual work planning session and updated to reflect changing roles in the organization and new technologies. For example, clinical responsibilities within an organization may be declining as these responsibilities are assumed by private sector managed care plans, but the need for community health assessment may be growing. This shift in organizational and community needs should be reflected in the skills that management makes available to staff through training opportunities.

Training initiatives must also reflect the evolving competencies required of public health professionals, such as designing and interpreting health status indicators or surveillance data for specific risk factors and disease outcomes and crafting and monitoring service contracts to achieve specific results consistent with the rules and laws of the local jurisdiction. These examples of professional competencies may be quite different from the tasks that were expected of staff in the recent past, when more clinical services were directly provided by public health organizations. As the role of public health organizations changes, staff must be transitioned to new responsibilities. New technologies create a constant need for new skills as information tools and scientific options evolve. A developmental plan for each employee needs to recognize these changes.

Mentoring of Employees

The word mentor comes from Homer's Greek mythology and refers to the god, Mentor, who was the guardian and tutor of Odysseus' son when he left for his extended journey. To be a mentor is to provide to others the knowledge, wisdom, and skills learned from experience. An example of useful mentoring in a public health organization is the senior environmental inspector who is asked to help a new inspector for the first six months of the job. This experience may be priceless in preventing mistakes and embarrassment to the organization, and in developing a valuable new employee.

An organization may use formal or informal methods for mentoring new or younger staff. A mentoring program can strongly influence both the success of new employees and their job satisfaction. Mentoring often occurs naturally within organizations. Mentoring relationships may be informal and based on a junior employee seeking help or on-the-job training, or characterized by a senior employee helping new or younger employees. Mentoring, whether formal or informal, should be encouraged in an organization. The employees who receive the advice and guidance of a more experienced staff member learn the organizational culture, rules, procedures, and job skills quicker than those who do not. The experienced staff members may enjoy greater job satisfaction as they help employees. Assigning staff to assist newer employees is helpful to the agency.

Quality Management

There are many ways to involve employees in shaping and improving the organization. One of these is by using the techniques of total quality management, or TQM. This technique owes much of its success to the work of Dr. W. Edwards Deming, who used quality improvement in postwar Japan. TQM received much later acceptance in the United States as corporations realized that quality improvements were needed to compete in an international marketplace. TQM is based on the use of employees to create constant improvement in work systems. The assumption is that quality improvement can only come from constantly challenging and improving systems. It does not come from inspections or from fixing problems after they occur. Although a thorough use of TQM techniques requires extensive training and skill development to understand how to empower work teams and to identify where systems need changing, any organization can benefit from the basic assumption that most improvements can be achieved with existing staff and by creating an atmosphere of self-improvement.

Other areas in which employee teams can add to the productivity of organizations include policy development, program design and implementation, and workplace reengineering. Top–down imposition of change will usually meet more resistance than strategies that empower staff to problem solve for the benefit of both employees and the organization. Employee councils, customer service teams, diversity committees, safety committees, and workplace enhancements are all avenues for achieving enhanced employee involvement in the organization.

RECRUITMENT OF A PUBLIC HEALTH WORK FORCE

The ease in recruiting public health workers is heavily dependent on issues such as salary, the supply of workers with the needed skills, the strength of the private sector, the responsiveness of the personnel system to changes in the marketplace, the reputation of the organization, the morale of the current work force, and the skill of those charged with recruiting. The most difficult person to recruit is usually the organization's senior administrator. A local or state health official is ideally a doctoral-level professional, with either an MD or a PhD in another health profession. Experience in public health practice and public sector administration is often helpful to administrators in these positions. Significant public health experience may offset the need for extensive academic training. The ability to offer tenure in office, such as a contract for a specified period of appointment, promotes continuity and increases the supply of qualified applicants willing to serve in these high-level positions.[15]

According to Dr. Kristine Gebbie of Columbia University, two-thirds of the public health work force falls into five professional groups. These groups include physicians, nurses, environmental professionals, administrators, and health educators. These professions are in high demand in the private sector as well as the public sector, making recruitment and retention important to the success of the public health organization.

Many of the limitations imposed by merit systems and comparable civil service systems are not always under the control of the public health organization, but some are. For example, the supply of workers with the skills needed may be limited, so the challenge lies in how to increase the supply. One way is to develop relationships with academic institutions and their faculty to help channel referrals to the organization. Another technique is to "grow your own" and create opportunities for existing staff to increase their skill level within the organization. A third example is to pay for employees to enhance their professional and technical skills through external education and training, perhaps even paying the tuition for graduate programs.

Managers should never assume that personnel systems are unchangeable. They are only unchangeable if the managers never seek flexibility or improvements. An important role for senior administrators and other high-level managers is to develop relationships with decision makers that allow input into the process of developing rules, procedures, and laws that govern the personnel systems of the organization. For example, following difficult recruitment efforts by one state health agency for a high-level regulatory manager, the agency suggested that out-of-state moving expenses be included in the state's fiscal rules. At the next hearing for changes in fiscal rules, that change was made for the state. This effort was appreciated by all of the state agencies. Managers of other agencies simply had not thought to ask.

Another creative solution includes the incorporation of private sector techniques for recruitment. In the past, these techniques might have been viewed as foreign to the public sector, but in fact they allow greater success in recruiting difficult-to-find talent. They include sign-on bonuses, pay matching to allow a counteroffer when an employee or potential employee is being recruited by others, referral awards to existing staff for helping recruit hard-to-fill positions, and temporary pay differentials to compensate for such responsibilities as acting duties or special projects. These types of incentives in the public sector are fairly recent phenomena and are driven by talent shortages that can occur in such areas as nursing and computer specialists.

Recruitment may be targeted or broad reaching. Traditional recruitment techniques have included newspaper ads, professional organizations' job lines or newsletters, and the posting of announcements through bulletin boards. A new and particularly powerful approach involves Internet-based recruiting, especially on the Web site of the organization or related institutions. Most governmental agencies now include Internet announcements as a way to notify potential applicants of opportunities. Asking employees to assist with recruitment is especially useful because staff will often have a developed network of contacts in their field and enjoy being part of the promotion of the agency. Job fairs may be helpful for certain types of recruitment, and using internships to identify talented individuals who are still in training is an excellent technique that allows both the intern and the organization to see if there is a good fit.

Minimal information to include in any job announcement includes a brief and accurate job description, minimal qualifications, salary range, how to apply for the position and receive additional information, and a closing date for applications. It is also helpful to open the announcement with a positive description of the agency that creates the image of an exciting place to work.

THE CONCEPT OF A MERIT SYSTEM

Many public health organizations exist in the public sector at the local, state, and federal level. They also exist in the nonprofit sector and can even be found within some investor-owned corporations. Indeed, a growing array of public health functions is delivered in the private sector through health care organizations, hospitals, and other partners within the public health community. Most public health agencies in the public sector operate under similar personnel systems for governmental employees. A merit system, or civil service system, helps minimize the patronage that can exist in a political organization. The Pendelton Act of 1893 established the United States Civil Service Commission.[12] Included in the act were requirements such as protection from political pressures, the establishment of competitive examinations, and mandatory probationary periods. These practices have carried forward into most state and local governmental units.[13] Many public agencies have allowed additional flexibility to occur at higher-level positions so that a change of administration may mean a number of changes in leadership. This is sometimes achieved through a designation of certain positions as senior executive service or a similar name, or through the use of annual contracts for high-level positions.

There are three principal differences between employment within a merit system and employment in the traditional private sector: (1) the rigorous nature of the selection, (2) the separation of top candidates from the appointing authority or supervisor, and (3) the protections that employees have once they are permanent or tenured into the merit system. These protections often make it more cumbersome and complex for supervisors or managers to dismiss or demote the employees. However, the protections can also help prevent undue political interference or involvement in the selection and promotion of the work force. The key to any merit system is understanding how to make it function efficiently and effectively within the constraints of the law.

Frequently, the head of a governmental public health agency is a political appointee. This is typical for state health officials who are often appointed by their governor (Table 16–2). At the local level, the head of the county, city, or regional health district may be appointed by a county manager, a city manager, a mayor,

Table 16–2 State and Territorial Health Officials' Position Requirements

Official State/ Territorial Requirement	*Number in 1997*	*Number in 1995*	*Number in 1992*	*States/Territories Reporting in 1997*
MD only	7	5	15	CA, IL, IN, MS, NE, NJ*, TN
MD and MPH Experience	6	5	5	FL, GA, KS, MO, MT, VT
MD and Board Certification or State Licensure	6	7	4	AL, AR, KY, LA, OK, VA
MD and MPH or Experience in Public Health	3	5	2	IA**, RI, UT
MD, MPH, and Experience in PH or Board Certification	4	2	2	DE, NH, NC, TX
MPH or Public Health Experience	9	9	2	AK, AZ**, IA**, CT, MD, ND, OR, SC, WA
Administrative/Mgmt. Experience	10	8	2	AZ, CO, HI, ID, MA, NV, NM, OH, SD, WY
Doctorate Degree	0	0	1	
Other	5	7	n/a	Guam, MI, MN, PA, WV
Total Number of Agencies Responding	50	48	33	

*Only required if the deputy commissioner is not an MD
**Falls in two categories
Source: Copyright © 1988 by the Association of State and Territorial Health Officials (ASTHO).

county commissioners, or a local board of health. Although it is very desirable for a local health official to be trained and experienced in public health, frequently, physicians with board certification in other areas are appointed as local health officials, sometimes serving on a part-time basis.

As a result of serving at the pleasure of their governors, the average tenure of state health officers ranges from 18 to 30 months, depending on whether the years examined include a large number of gubernatorial elections. A similar scenario can occur at the local level. As noted in *A Guide for the Recruitment, Selection and Retention of a State Health Officer*, "The lack of continuity in public health leadership is a serious problem, particularly at the state agency level. The average tenure is less than two years. This high turnover is caused by 'political-technical conflict, inadequate pay, the effect of reorganization, frustrations with the structure of decision-making, and low professional prestige' (The Future of Public Health by the Institute of Medicine)."[15(p.1)] This instability of leadership has historically been a deterrent to talented public health professionals in accepting high-level public health positions. The directors or health officials are expected to be leaders both within and outside of the organization, be a spokesperson for the agency to stakeholders and citizens, and provide a vision for employees to embrace and seek to implement.

JOB CLASSIFICATIONS AND JOB ANALYSIS

The federal government adopted a system of job classifications after the passage of the Civil Service Commission legislation in 1912.[12] This basic concept has remained a part of the personnel management at all levels of government in an effort to minimize or eliminate political favoritism. Positions are to be based on actual duties performed, and compensation is to be based on comparable work both within and outside of government. Thus, for example, a microbiologist in a local health department will have a job description that is unique to that type of scientific work with a pay scale that reflects similar work. Under this system, the position is classified, not the individual. Duties are the key to setting classifications, not how well the work is accomplished. Some agencies use a system of evaluation of the position based on factors. These may include such items as job requirements, difficulty of work, responsibility, independent decision making, number of employees supervised, budget managed, relationships with other decision makers, complexity of work, working environment, and accountability. Although qualifications and education can be set for the type of position, the system usually does not provide for additional compensation for additional education and training beyond that which is required at a minimal level for the position. The classification system puts the classifier in the human resources office in a dual position—that of enforcer and that of serving management. This frequently creates a tension where management wishes to respond to particular individual employees or applicants and the classification system puts limitations on such factors as compensation, required qualifications, and incentives for retention. Some agencies have created greater flexibility through mechanisms such as performance pay to provide management with additional options and tools.

SELECTION OF APPLICANTS

The most important decisions that any manager makes are those of selecting and promoting employees. Unfortunately, the personnel selection process is too often hurried, incomplete, and inappropriate, resulting in huge costs in productivity and morale, as well as potential legal actions. The selection process in any organization is usually governed by specific rules and laws. The intent in the public agency is to maintain a system that is based on merit or the meeting of minimal qualifications. Most agencies will use a combination of reviewing résumés, testing for knowledge or skills, role playing, and checking references prior to interviewing the final candidates. The human resources office will usually wish to partner with the program manager or senior administrator to determine the best techniques to match the candidates with the job requirements.

Interviewing candidates for employment is key to wise selection. The interview process is usually limited to the final few (usually three) candidates who have survived the screening process that has occurred. It is usually advisable to invite peers to attend the interview, perhaps a team of stakeholders and others with whom the applicant must work and interact in order to provide input to the appointing authority. The appointing authority is defined as the individual who has the authority to make the actual offer of employment. This may be a department head, a program manager, or perhaps the senior administrator or health officer.

A good interview is conducted in a comfortable setting and includes introductions to all the parties involved, along with an explanation of why they have been asked to participate. Questions that are open-ended are usually most helpful. There are many questions that cannot be asked, and the human resources office may have guidance regarding the questions to avoid.

The Mountain States Employers Council, Inc. has identified 10 common errors made when interviewing candidates.[16]

1. *Failing to establish rapport with the applicant:* There are two excellent reasons to put the applicant at ease. First, he or she will respond better to the interview and provide a clearer representation of talents and experience. Second, while the interviewee is marketing him- or herself to the organization, the interviewer is also marketing the agency as a good place to work. Having the applicant think positively about the interviewer and the organization is important for successful recruiting. Some ways to ease into the interview are to offer the applicant a cup of coffee, or to show the candidate the office, laboratory, or site where the candidate will be working.
2. *Asking direct instead of open-ended questions:* Applicants will offer more information if they are asked questions that cannot be answered with yes, no, or a similar brief statement. For example, "Have you ever investigated a disease outbreak?" is less useful than, "Tell me what experience you have had with disease investigations."
3. *Asking questions that are too general:* Questions that are too general provide too little useful or specific information to assist in the selection process. Requiring an answer that lends itself to specific time frames, experience, skill, events, and so forth will yield more useful information. For example, "Tell me about your nursing career" may reveal less than, "Please discuss your last position as a visiting nurse for a local health department."
4. *Asking multiple questions:* If lengthy and complex questions are asked, the applicant is likely to answer only a portion of the question or answer the question as he or she interpreted its meaning.
5. *Failing to ask reflective questions:* If an answer is not clear or seems incomplete, the interviewer should ask for additional information. For example, if asked why he or she left a previous position, a brief answer of "There were layoffs due to reduced funding" might not provide sufficient information to evaluate the reasons why the individual left. By adding another question such as "Tell me more about the agency's decision to terminate your position," additional information may be obtained regarding the termination.
6. *Asking leading questions:* Too much information included in the question can lead the applicant in the direction that will yield the most acceptable answer. However, that answer may not be indicative of how the applicant really feels about the topic. For example, the question, "Our agency is very interested in keeping abreast of the latest technology. How do you feel about learning new software when we upgrade our computers?" can bias the applicant toward a positive response.

7. *Not allowing enough time for the applicant to respond to questions:* The interviewer should avoid rushing the applicant. Providing sufficient time to give a complete answer is important.
8. *Asking questions that identify or single out a candidate's protected group status:* Only questions that are related to the job should be asked. Questions that tend to identify or discuss a person's race, religion, sex, age, disability, or national origin should not be mentioned.
9. *Spending too much time talking:* The purpose of the interview is to hear from the applicant, not the interviewer. A good rule of thumb is that the applicant should be talking approximately 80 percent of the time.
10. *Failing to demonstrate active listening:* The interviewer should provide both verbal and nonverbal messages that show whether he or she is listening, attentive, and interested in the answers.

Reference Questions

A key part of the selection process includes the verification of previous employment and the discussion that occurs with previous employers or other references. Applicants might typically provide three or more references. These should be in addition to references from previous supervisors. Applicants should be asked for written authorization to contact previous employers and references. Many agencies or companies have a policy to release only the dates of employment and the titles of the positions held. Other organizations will be more cooperative. Questions asked of references should include how the individuals know the applicants and how they might have worked together, as well as questions that will indicate the work ethics and skills of the applicant. One way to elicit useful information is to describe the qualities and skills sought and then ask if the applicant has those qualities and skills. Objective questions are useful, such as "Did the applicant use Excel spreadsheets in his work in your office?" Work attendance history may be useful to indicate work practices. It is sometimes useful to ask the individuals whether they would hire the applicant themselves, and, if so, why. Just as in an interview, any questions that appear to indicate an attempt to determine religion, race, age, or national origin should be avoided.

UNIONS AND PUBLIC HEALTH ORGANIZATIONS

Unions are a major force in some public health organizations, but may have a limited role in others. The role they play is often influenced by the history of unionization and corresponding laws that are different in various states and communities. One public health organization may be under collective bargaining with several unions; another may have no true unionization practices, but employee organizations may lobby for increased benefits, salaries, and so forth. Union organizing is growing in the health care industry due to several factors: the growing instability in the industry, the movement of labor from manufacturing to service industries, and the desire for higher wages among many job classifications involved in the health care industry. Unionization is also growing in certain aspects of governmental jurisdictions, particularly at the local level. Generally, unionizing is most successful when communications within the organization are considered weak or untrustworthy. In those cases, employees will seek both an ear and a voice outside of the organization. The sympathetic ear will listen to grievances and concerns; the voice will speak for the employees in corrective and disciplinary issues and advocate for improved conditions, pay, and benefits.

Employees join unions for job security, improved wages, and/or better benefits, or in response to poor working conditions, unequal treatment, limited opportunities for advancement, lack of recognition, and petty work rules and procedures. Dealing with labor unions requires an understanding of labor law and the details of any labor contracts, as well as knowledge of acceptable procedures and practices. The organization's lawyers and human resources specialists are well suited to detailed bargaining and grievance processes. It is incumbent on management to provide an outlet for employee issues and concerns within the organization so employees will use the internal processes to settle issues first. If unions are part of the organization, regular meetings with management and union representatives can be very productive in solving issues before they reach serious levels.

There are guidelines that should be followed regarding what can and cannot be done by management when union organizing occurs. Management can[14]

- Tell employees about current wages and benefits and how these compare with other organizations.
- Tell employees the disadvantages of union dues, assessments, and practices.
- Advise employees that management does not favor unionization.
- Explain the unionization process.
- Prevent union materials from being distributed during work hours in the work area.
- Continue to enforce rules in a consistent manner.

Management cannot[14]

- Reward employees with pay increases or promotions for voting against the union.
- Threaten employees with termination for supporting the union.
- Spy on union meetings.
- Ask employees how they will vote on unionization.
- Urge employees to persuade others to vote against the union.

More detailed guidance can be provided by the organization's attorneys and human resources specialists.

PERFORMANCE MANAGEMENT AND PERFORMANCE APPRAISALS

Managing employees is the greatest responsibility of any administrator. Although most managers will eagerly agree that personnel management is a key responsibility, many do not relish the tasks and roles required for effective performance management. Formal performance appraisals are an important part of supervisory responsibilities in most organizations. Appraisals are for the benefit of the organization, and ideally, for the benefit of the employee. They are used to inform organizational decisions that determine salary, promotions, transfers, layoffs, demotions, and terminations. They also provide the mechanism and opportunity for employees to receive useful coaching and suggested changes in behavior, attitudes, knowledge, and skills. However, if left to their own devices, many managers and supervisors would never administer a performance appraisal. Therefore, the organization usually creates prescribed procedures with common forms and other tools. The most successful systems are designed with the recognition that

- Performance improves most when specific goals are established.
- Coaching is needed on a regular basis, not once a year.
- Mutual goal setting by the employee and the supervisor improves performance.
- Criticism and praise have less effect than participation in goal setting by the employee.

Successful performance appraisal systems take time to implement, and yet most supervisors spend only four to eight hours a year per employee in performance management, including preparation, paperwork, and discussion.[17] It is, therefore, not surprising that most employees do not see a link between their performance and their pay.

There are many options available to an organization regarding the instrument used for appraisals. These can include a numeric rating scale or a non-numeric rating. For example, the instrument may be developed with a maximum number of points set at 100. Other instruments may focus on categories of performance such as *exceeds objectives, fully meets objectives, partially meets objectives,* and *unsatisfactory.* One agency uses *unsatisfactory, fully competent,* and *peak performer,* which also match numeric ranges. Some instruments focus on behavior;

others focus on traits and skills. Factors evaluated, such as communications, leadership, or problem solving, may be weighted so that some are recognized as more crucial than others. The instrument is less important than how it is administered and how plans are developed against which the employee is evaluated.

An organization is more likely to have successful performance management if: (1) both supervisors and employees are trained regarding the appraisal process and how to develop meaningful objectives and work plans, (2) supervisors are trained to be coaches and mentors, and (3) performance management is seen as a meaningful mechanism for development. Performance management starts with the job, not the form, and both parties have a responsibility regarding its success.

The phases of performance management include[16(p.21)]

- performance planning, where objectives, standards, competencies, and a development plan are mutually determined
- performance execution, which involves the actual work being accomplished
- performance assessment, which includes both parties independently assessing how the plan was achieved
- collection of data from other parties, such as subordinates, peers, or customers
- performance review, where the results are discussed
- the renewal of the agreement or contract for the following performance period

There are mutual responsibilities for a successful review. The employee needs commitment to the objectives and goals, solicitation of feedback from others, communication that is open and regular with the supervisor, the collection of performance information or data, and preparation for the review. The supervisor is responsible for creating an environment that encourages open communication and motivation, observing and documenting performance, updating and revising objectives and standards, explaining the relationship between the overall goals of the organization and the employee's objectives, creating developmental paths, and reinforcing effective behavior. The employee's work plan should reinforce and integrate with a unit or program work plan. Objectives at both the program and the employee level should be specific, measurable, achievable, results oriented, and timely.

Some of the most common errors in performance management include the following:[17]

- *Contrast effect:* The employee is compared with another employee or employees.
- *First impression error:* An initial observation rules the supervisor's thinking even though it is no longer applicable.
- *Halo or horns effect:* One aspect of the employee's performance is generalized to the entire performance.
- *Like me effect:* The supervisors may rate employees who are similar to him or her higher than others.
- *Skews to the center, negative, and positive:* The supervisor has a tendency to rate employees in the middle, or at the high or low end of the scale.
- *Attribution bias:* The supervisor has a tendency to attribute failing to factors that are under the control of the employee and successes to outside causes.
- *Recent effect:* The supervisor remembers the most recent event instead of the full performance period.
- *Stereotyping:* The supervisor ignores the individual and generalizes across groups or work units.

Some organizations directly link pay to performance; others do not. In governmental agencies, salary increases are often based more on seniority than on performance. In unionized organizations, union rules and contracts may dictate salary levels to a greater extent than the supervisor. The success of performance management does not require a link to pay, although that link may make both employees and supervisors more aware of the importance of appraisals and planning activities. The need to include as much objectivity as possible in appraisals increases with the link to pay. If there is no obvious linkage, supervisors may have a tendency toward "grade inflation" or leniency in ratings. Supervisors generally find it more comfortable to discuss positive ratings and results than to focus on areas where objectives are not being met. This tendency leads to a sense of unfairness in the work force and discounts the opportunities that performance planning and appraisal provide.

CONTRACTING FOR SERVICES

State and local law, regulations, and union agreements often place limits on the ability of an organization to contract for services. If local practices allow, it is often advisable to contract for services that are not at the core of the organization's mission. A general rule is that the organization or agency should do those tasks for which the agency is particularly suited. Accountability may also influence which services can be contracted. For example, it is not a core service for a local health department to provide janitorial services, and an outside service may provide a cost-beneficial approach to providing that service. It is, however, a core function of the agency to administer environmental regulations, such as the permitting of individual septic systems. Therefore, the public may want the department to be accountable for those regulatory services directly. Unique technical skills may be best obtained through contractual services due to high cost and infrequent use. These might include the maintenance of scientific equipment or programming for an information system. The keys to contracting for services successfully are to respect current personnel and union restrictions; bid all services to several potential providers, if possible; and allocate time and resources to monitor the contract and results of the work. The most common errors in contracting for services are in writing contracts that are not sufficient for results and accountability and underestimating the need to monitor results and take action if results are not produced.

PERSONNEL POLICIES

Policies that implement basic rules of the organization and provide management intent are important to successful personnel management. At a minimum, an organization should have specific agency or organizational policies on such topics as affirmative action, violence in the workplace, the use of drugs and alcohol by employees, outside employment, use of the various types of leave, work hours, disability accommodations, employee grievances, and sexual harassment. Many of these policies are determined by the need to clarify how the agency or organization will respond to legal questions and challenges. With specific policies in place, an organization is better equipped to deal with employee behavior issues and lawsuits. It is important that each employee has a copy of the current policies. These should be provided at a new employee orientation and followed with periodic issuance of policies to all staff members. Policies should be signed by the top-level manager to illustrate that they are organizationwide policies and decisions. Policies should cite relevant law and other directives such as state or local rules.

CHAPTER REVIEW

1. The foundation of the human resources model is positive reinforcement of the employee accompanied by supervision, performance appraisal, mentoring, and training.
2. Although personnel management responsibilities are the overall responsibility of the human resources office, all managers and all supervisors deal with personnel management every day. The human resources office provides guidance and direction with the various personnel functions and deals with the most difficult personnel issues.
3. Diversity is encouraged so as to yield skills and experience in the work force that are appropriate for the populations served.

4. TQM is a technique that involves employees in shaping and improving organizations.
5. The most important decisions for a manager are those of *recruiting, selecting,* and *promoting* staff. Advertising, interviewing, and questioning references are key activities to be carried out by the manager in collaboration with the human resources office.
6. Dealing with labor unions requires an understanding of labor law and the details of any labor contracts, as well as knowledge of acceptable practices and procedures. Managers should meet regularly with union representatives and take steps to resolve issues and concerns within the organization by internal processes.
7. Contracting for services can be associated with sizeable benefits to the public health organization but needs to be undertaken after careful consideration of personnel and union restrictions. Contracts for services are to be awarded subsequent to a bid process involving potential providers and with terms explicitly specified to ensure results, accountability, and ease of monitoring.
8. Personnel policies should spell out the basic rules of the organization, including those pertaining to affirmative action, violence in the workplace, the use of drugs and alcohol, outside employment, employee grievances, work hours, various types of leave, and sexual harassment.

REFERENCES

1. D.J. Cherrington, "Need Theories of Motivation" in *Motivation and Work Behavior,* 5th ed., eds. R.M. Steers and L.W. Porter (New York: McGraw-Hill, 1991), 31–34.
2. L.W. Porter and R.E. Miles, "Motivation and Management" in *Contemporary Management: Issues and Viewpoints,* ed. J.W. McGuire (Englewood Cliffs, NJ: Prentice Hall, 1974).
3. D. Katz and R.L. Kahn, *The Social Psychology of Organizations* (New York: John Wiley & Sons, 1966).
4. R.E. Miles et al., "Leadership Attitudes among Public Health Professionals," *American Journal of Public Health* (1966): 1,990–2,005.
5. C.C. Pinder, "Valence-Instrumentality-Expectancy Theory" in *Motivation and Work Behavior,* 5th ed., eds. R.M. Steers and L.W. Porter (New York: McGraw-Hill, 1991), 144–164.
6. W.C. Hammer, "Reinforcement Theory and Contingency Management in Organizational Settings" in *Motivation and Work Behavior,* 5th ed., eds. R.M. Steers and L.W. Porter (New York: McGraw-Hill, 1991), 61–87.
7. M.A. Neale and G.B. Northcraft, "Factors Influencing Organizational Commitment" in *Motivation and Work Behavior,* 5th ed., eds. R.M. Steers and L.W. Porter (New York: McGraw-Hill, 1991), 290–297.
8. R.M. Steers, "Antecedents and Outcomes of Organizational Commitments," *Administrative Science Quarterly* 22 (1977): 46–56.
9. J.L. Koch and R.M. Steers, "Job Attachment, Satisfaction and Turnover among Public Employees," *Journal of Vocational Behavior* 12 (1978): 199–228.
10. H. Angle and J. Perry, "An Empirical Assessment of Organizational Effectiveness," *Administrative Science Quarterly* 26 (1981): 1–14.
11. G.P. Latham and E.A. Locke, "Goal Setting—A Motivational Technique That Works" in *Motivation and Work Behavior,* 5th ed., eds. R.M. Steers and L.W. Porter (New York: McGraw-Hill, 1991), 357–370.
12. L.F. Novick, "Syphilis: A Broad Initiative to Control New York State's Epidemic [editorial]," *New York State Journal of Medicine* 92 (December 1991): 524–525.
13. J.M. Shafritz et al., *Personnel Management in Government, Politics and Process* (New York: Marcel Dekker, Inc., 1986), 28–30.
14. C.R. McConnell, *The Effective Health Care Supervisor,* 4th ed. (Gaithersburg, MD: Aspen Publishers, Inc., 1997), 461–471.
15. L. Thielen et al., *A Guide for the Recruitment, Selection and Retention of a State Health Officer* (Washington, DC: Association of State and Territorial Health Officials, 1993).
16. *Top Ten Errors Made by Interviewers* (Denver, CO: Mountain States Employers Council, Inc., 1999).
17. D. Grote, *The Complete Guide to Performance Appraisal* (New York: Amacon, 1996).

Chapter 17

Financing the Public's Health

Perri S. Leviss

Approximately 1 percent of the nation's total health expenditures is devoted to public health activities. Of the funds spent by public health organizations, a considerable amount is spent for personal health services. New players in providing public health services include community-based providers, hospitals, and managed care organizations. Local health departments (LHDs) are now forced to share limited funding sources, identify nongovernmental funding streams, and develop new alliances. In the past, public health organizations have not expended significant effort in evaluating the costs of providing their services.

Public health organizations across the country are responsible for ensuring the health of the public. The discussion of these responsibilities often comes in the form of legislative mandates, regulations, executive orders, and public mission statements. But, how does anyone know if public health organizations are adequately funded to carry out this large and looming task? Additionally, with the billions of dollars spent on health care services each year nationally, what is the right amount of monies allocated to public health?

The financing of public health services is complicated by the unique organization of public health delivery within each state and locality. Some states have active LHDs that receive significant funding for the provision of comprehensive preventive and primary care services; others have no organized local governmental units and the majority of governmental public health funding resides with the state health departments (SHDs). More recently, nongovernmental players in the health system have taken growing responsibility in providing some public health services as a cost-effective way to prevent disease, morbidity, and mortality. This chapter will first explore the history and the current trends for financing public health services and then discuss the critical tools necessary to deliver public health services effectively in the twenty-first century.

WHY LOOK AT PUBLIC HEALTH FINANCING?

Understanding the financing of public health services is critical for private and nonprofit health providers as well as public health organizations. However, the body of literature on this subject is slim compared to the available sources on health care financing. This is consistent with how the majority of Americans view public health services. Many do not understand the dif-

Acknowledgment: The author would like to extend her appreciation to Richard Naeder, Assistant Commissioner of Finance, New York City Department of Health, for his review and comments on the chapter, and to Kim Harrison, Senior Consultant, American Express Tax and Business Services Inc., for her data collection efforts.

ference between public health and health care services; some don't know they even have a governmental body that oversees public health activities; and others equate public health with research. In an era of managed care, the growing number of uninsured individuals, and the recent passage of policies that regulate the level of care offered to the general public, it is increasingly important to evaluate who is delivering public health services and how the services are financed in order to maximize the "bang for the buck" that Americans get for their health care dollar. In addition, reviewing how public health services are financed in different parts of the country provides public health organizations operating at national, state, and local levels with useful information that may influence future funding and organizational decisions. Finally, if governmental public health organizations want to continue to participate actively and help steer health policy in collaboration with other parts of the health system, they must pay more attention to the costs of the services that they deliver as well as the funding streams that support these services.

PUBLIC HEALTH VERSUS PERSONAL HEALTH EXPENDITURES

Compared to most other industrialized countries, the U.S. government expends the least amount of public funds on health services as a percentage of total expenditures. At the same time, the United States spends a much larger proportion of its gross domestic product on health care services than most other industrialized countries. Additionally, unlike other industrialized nations, the United States has historically placed a greater emphasis on hospital services than on primary and preventive care services; other industrialized countries have historically allocated a greater percentage of health dollars to ambulatory care services.[1] The U.S. government has invested significant resources into building the acute care/hospital-based infrastructure in the post-World War II period. In 1929, the United States spent 17 percent of its total health expenditures on hospital care; in 1990, this number was at 43 percent.[1]

The history of hospital-based spending in the United States began in the turn of the twentieth century as the combination of many factors including increased urbanization, industrialization, and immigration; new medical discoveries (e.g., anesthesia, vaccines); and the production of new medical equipment (e.g., radiographs) gave rise to large health care institutions to treat Americans. With more people involved in health care, and more permanent physical structures to support the delivery of services, hospital-based health care workers began organizing themselves and created significant lobbying forces over the years that have directed additional funding to support these acute care institutions as well as the workers themselves.[1]

As this medical enterprise grew throughout the early half of the twentieth century, public health was left out of the health care formula. At this point, health care and public health split, with health care being relegated substantially to the private sector and public health being directed as largely a governmental responsibility. And equally as important, the health insurance system (both publicly and privately funded) provided incentives for hospital-based care and for diagnostic and therapeutic procedures, rather than for clinical preventive services (e.g., immunizations, screening tests).[2] It is only recently with the advent of managed care that some of these clinical preventive services are considered covered services. Finally, the research-oriented funding streams encouraged biomedical research instead of population-based and behavioral studies. In her book, *Medicine and Public Health: The Power of Collaboration,* Roz Lasker surmises, "reflecting public demand for biomedical advances (in the post-World War II period), funding was considerably less generous for population-based public health programs than for medical care; for health departments than for hospitals; for epidemiological and social science investigation than for clinical studies and basic science research; and for the education and training of public health professionals than for those in medicine."[2(p.19)] The combination of these factors has led to a public health infrastructure that is underfunded and undervalued.

HISTORY OF PUBLIC HEALTH FINANCIAL DATA COLLECTION

In 1993, approximately $8.4 billion, or 1 percent of the nation's total health spending, was spent on public health. This includes federal, state, and local revenues as well as Medicaid payments, patient fees, and regulatory fees.[3] Routinely measuring how much is spent on public health services is a difficult task. Over the years, there have been a variety of local and national studies on the subject (Exhibit 17–1). However, there is no existing system to capture these data comprehensively or longitudinally. Below are a select numbers of activities that have taken place over the past century in order to measure the amount of dollars spent on public health.

- The Public Health Service (PHS) collected data on cities and programs in the early 1900s.[4]
- In 1923, the American Public Health Association's (APHA) Committee on Administrative Practice (CAP) collected data from 83 city health departments on expenditures, organization, and public health practice. In 1943, the CAP published the *Health Practices Indices,* charts that included the range of services provided at LHDs as well as budgetary information.[5]
- In the late 1940s, states that received federal funding as part of the Hill-Burton Act were required to report the staffing levels for public health departments. The PHS often examined these data in combination

Exhibit 17–1 Timeline for Public Health Financing Data Collection Activities

1923	The American Public Health Association (APHA) Committee on Administrative Practice (CAP) collects expenditure data from 83 city and local health departments.
1943	The APHA CAP publishes *Health Practice Indices* that include budgetary information.
1960	The Health Care Financing Administration begins estimating public health expenditures based on census data and other local/state data sources.
1970	The National Public Health Program Reporting System is developed to collect longitudinal public health expenditure data.
1990	The National Association of City and County Health Officials (NACCHO) publishes estimates of national public health expenditures as part of the first *National Profile of Local Health Departments.*
1991	The Centers for Disease Control and Prevention (CDC) begins a study to estimate expenditures on health promotion and disease prevention activities.
1992	The Public Health Foundation issues an inventory of the block grant expenditures for state health departments.
1993	The CDC and NACCHO conduct a second survey of local health spending.
1994	The Public Health Foundation begins a series of studies to track expenditure data for state and local health departments.
1995	A second study by the Public Health Foundation in collaboration with the Public Health Service focuses on state health expenditures.
1996	Urban Institute's Assessing the New Federalism Project evaluates the public health system and its financing in 13 states.
1997	The Public Health Foundation in collaboration with the NACCHO and the National Association of Local Boards of Health evaluates local health spending.

with other expenditure information provided by state health agencies.[4]

- Beginning in 1960, the Health Care Financing Administration (HCFA) has used a combination of Bureau of the Census data and other local/state data sources to develop an estimate of public health expenditures in its reporting of national health expenditures.[4]
- In the 1970s, the National Public Health Program Reporting System (the Association of State and Territorial Health Officials Reporting System) was developed and funded by the PHS to provide longitudinal public health expenditure data by categorical public health programs.[4]
- In 1990, the National Association of County and City Health Officials (NACCHO) published the *National Profile of Local Health Departments*, which provided limited financial as well as programmatic data from 1989 on local public health. This study was undertaken in part to support the *Assessment Protocol for Excellence in Public Health (APEXPH)* project. This study was later revised to include more financial data and other modifications and reissued once again in 1995 under the title *1992–1993 National Profile of Local Health Departments* (see bullet below).[5]
- In 1991, the Centers for Disease Control and Prevention (CDC) began a study to estimate health promotion and disease prevention activities nationally. The results demonstrated that in 1988, there was approximately $32.8 billion devoted to these activities, which represented 3.5 percent of the total national health expenditures. However, the CDC recognized that the study lacked clear definition of public health expenditures.[4]
- In 1991, the Public Health Foundation (PHF) issued *Public Health Agencies 1991: An Inventory of Programs and Block Grant Expenditures,* which compiled financial and programmatic data on SHD expenditures and funding sources.[6] The data compiled from the study indicated that more than $118 billion was spent in 1989 for public health by both state health agencies and LHDs ($77.5 billion in direct state dollars, $17.5 billion in pass-through grants to LHDs, and $23.0 billion in additional LHD expenditures).[6] The study reported that in FY 1989, state funds accounted for 53.7 percent of state health agency expenditures, federal grants/contracts 36.5 percent, local funds 1.9 percent, fees and reimbursements 5.1 percent, and other sources 2.8 percent. SHDs spent approximately 75 percent of their funds on personal health services, with smaller amounts for environmental health, health resources, and other public health functions. Nineteen percent of the state health organizations' expenditures were directed at LHDs. Additionally, the study reported that 28.1 percent of the LHDs' expenditures came from state funds, 33.6 percent from local funds, 15.5 percent from federal grants and contracts, 12.9 percent from third-party reimbursements, 2.3 percent other, and 7.6 percent unknown. More than 50 percent of LHD expenditures were for personal health services. Finally, the study evaluated the health organizations' spending for two of the largest federal block grant programs and found that the majority of the $434 million in Maternal and Child Health Services (MCH) Block Grant dollars and $84 million in Prevention Block Grant dollars were spent on personal health services (95.4 percent for MCH and 63.7 percent in Prevention).[6]
- In 1992–93, the CDC, along with the NACCHO, collected data through a national mail survey on the spending characteristics of LHDs. The *1992–1993 National Profile of Local Health Departments* study found that the average annual per capita spending for LHDs was $32.[5(p.31)] Additionally, the data showed that there was a wide range of spending among LHDs, and that the size of the population was the greatest predictor of the amount spent on local health services. According to the NACCHO survey, in 1992–93, 13 percent

of LHDs reported that they spent less than $100,000, 53 percent reported expenditures greater than $500,000, and 34 percent reported expenditures greater than $1,000,000. Other factors that explained variability in expenditures included the number of staff, the number and types of programs provided, and the available funding sources. Additionally, the study captured data similar to that of the PHF's earlier study, but in this case, the data indicated that LHDs rely more heavily on state funds and less on federal sources (Table 17–1). The study also found that as population size increases, the percentage of an LHD's funding from state/local sources increases and the percentage from Medicaid and Medicare decreases.[5]

- Beginning in 1994, a series of studies was funded by the PHS (performed in coordination with the PHF and other bodies) to establish and track a comparable set of expenditure data for public health services. The first of these studies involved a sample of health departments in Connecticut, Iowa, Missouri, Oregon, and Rhode Island and later Illinois, Texas, and New York. The study resulted in a set of guidelines describing and distinguishing core public health activities and detailing the expenditures of government agencies (public health agencies, mental health agencies, environmental health agencies, and substance abuse agencies) on public health services. Results from the study indicated that the eight states reported spending $2.8 billion or $44 per capita (ranging from $31 to $57) on core public health services (not including personal health services). This figure was significantly higher than that from the earlier NACCHO study, which reported an average of $32 per capita. Additionally, the study concluded that core public health services accounted for only 27 percent of the total expenditures by these government agencies.[4]
- In 1995, a second study was undertaken by the PHS in collaboration with the Public Health Foundation and a group of other federal agencies and national associations to improve on the original study methodology. This study included six of the original states that had participated in Phase I (Illinois, Iowa, New York, Oregon, Rhode Island, and Texas) with the addition of Arizona, Louisiana, and Washington. Additionally, the study included data from local governmental agencies as well as their state counterparts. Results from this study indicated that $8.8 billion was spent in 1995 on essential/core public health services, but of this, $6.1 billion (or 69 percent) was spent for the provision of personal health/primary care. On a per capita basis, the study concluded that $137 (ranging from $51 to $219) was spent on average for health services (now including population-based health at $42 per capita and personal health services at $95 per capita).The study identified that a number of public health services were being delivered by organizations other than the public health departments. The study also demonstrated that state sources accounted for 50 percent of expenditures for population-based health

Table 17–1 Sources of Local Health Department Expenditures

Funding Source	*1991 Public Health Foundation Study*	*1992–93 CDC and NACCHO Study*
State funds	28.1%	40%
Local funds	33.6%	34%
Federal funds	15.5%	6%
Third-party reimbursements	12.9%	10%
Fines and fees	*	7%
Other	2.3%	3%
Unknown	7.6%	Not listed
Total	100%	100%

*Fines and fees may be included in local funds or the unknown category, but were not specifically broken out during the study.

services, local sources (tax levy appropriations and fines/fees) accounted for 16 percent, federal funds for 32 percent, and Medicaid and other funds accounted for 2 percent in the nine participating states.

- In 1996, as part of the Urban Institute's *Assessing the New Federalism Project*, the public health system was evaluated in 13 selected states. This study demonstrated the wide range of state public health funding that is controlled and administered on the local level. Of all the study states, Wisconsin had the greatest percentage (79.1 percent in 1994) of state and local public health dollars that were locally administered; Massachusetts had just 7.4 percent of the dollars administered locally. Additionally, the study found that the sources of funds for LHDs varied tremendously. In Massachusetts and New Jersey, more than 85 percent of the LHDs' funding came from local revenue sources, with the remainder being spread between state, federal, Medicaid, Medicare, and other sources. Contrasting data were gathered from Alabama and Florida, where the largest percentage of revenues came either from the state (in Florida's case) or from Medicaid and Medicare (in the case of Alabama). The study observed that the ways in which LHDs get and spend their dollars was related to their individual organizational structures or that in some cases the financing structures had supported the development of specific organizational structures. Through evaluating the intersection between how LHDs get their revenue and how they expend dollars, the Urban Institute scholars developed four categories of states:[3]
    1. states where LHDs receive the majority of revenues locally, but the majority of spending statewide happens at the state level
    2. states where LHDs receive a large percentage of revenues locally and spending is also locally controlled
    3. states where the largest percentage of revenues come from nonlocal sources and spending is controlled by the state
    4. states with low levels of revenue from local sources, but a relatively high degree of local control over public health expenditures
- The third and most recent study by the PHS was jointly conducted by the NACCHO, the National Association of Local Boards of Health (NALBOH), and the Public Health Foundation in 1997–98 and involved three case studies of Onondaga County, New York; Northeast Tri-County, Washington; and Columbus, Ohio, in order to test the ability of LHDs to use a standard data tool for collecting public health expenditure information and to compare the expenditure patterns of the three localities. The study results showed that, on average, approximately 21.4 percent of the LHDs' expenditures were for personal health services, 67 percent were for population-based services, and 11.6 percent were for administration and other services. However, the range among the three participating counties was very wide.[7]

Although the studies highlighted above note the number of important limitations in the work, the data gathered through the studies provide a marker and a lens within which to evaluate the allocation of public health dollars among the different range of health services. In summary, the national trend appears to be that

- Public health services continue to represent a small percentage of the total amount spent on health care.
- Of the funding spent on public health services, a considerable amount is expended for personal health services.
- There is a significant variation in the amount spent as well as the financing sources for local public health services.
- There is a wide range of organizations that deliver public health services (both population-based and personal health services).

All the data collection activities thus far speak to the need for a routinized and consistent way of capturing public health expenditure data and an evaluation of how differences in public health expenditures may impact health outcomes.[3]

ORGANIZATION OF PUBLIC HEALTH FINANCING

The way public health is financed follows the structure of public health delivery. The federal agencies that distribute public health funding and provide oversight of the funding are fragmented and at times uncoordinated. State and local public health departments receive federal public health dollars from a combination of agencies under the U.S. Department of Health and Human Services (DHHS) (including the Food and Drug Administration, the Indian Health Service, the Agency for Healthcare Research and Quality, the Office of the Assistant Secretary for Health, the PHS, the CDC, the Health Resources and Services Administration, the Substance Abuse and Mental Health Services Administration, HCFA, and the National Institutes of Health), the Department of Housing and Urban Development, the Department of Agriculture, the Environmental Protection Agency, and the Department of Education.

In addition, the organization of public health at the state level differs across the country. Usually, there is one central government body that oversees public health services in each state; however, in some cases, the agency may have more or less expansive programmatic responsibilities. In recent years, the power of public health at the state level has been diluted as many state public health agencies have either merged with human services/social service agencies or mental health agencies. Other public health functions have been fractionalized as the responsibilities were split up among many different state organizations. However, the actual delivery of many public health services is local and, in most cases, the county, city, and municipal government entities are the bodies that directly deliver public health services. There are more than 3,000 organized LHDs nationally, with a wide range of structures, staffing levels, and programmatic responsibilities. More than 50 percent of these governmental bodies have populations less than 25,000 and therefore support limited activities.

Even with all these different organizations participating in public health, the last part of the twentieth century brought important new players to public health. In addition to governmental organizations, community-based providers, and, most recently, hospitals and managed care organizations have begun to participate actively in providing and overseeing public health services. With the addition of these new players, LHDs have been forced to share limited funding sources, identify nongovernmental funding streams, and develop new strategic alliances in order to ensure the public's health.[3]

There are a variety of factors that have affected how public health funding is organized locally and nationally. Public health has never "made it" to the public agenda. Although some categorical public health issues have received local and national attention (e.g., cholera, tuberculosis [TB], human immunodeficiency virus [HIV]/acquired immune deficiency syndrome [AIDS], *E. coli*) due to large outbreaks of disease or public health emergencies, public health is not a high-priority public policy issue for Americans. There are a variety of factors that may have contributed to the lack of public attention surrounding public health, including the large number of diverse programs and services included under the auspices of public health and the absence of advocacy/lobbying groups who work on public health (they are mostly organized around a specific population or disease). As opposed to other social issues including welfare, foster care, and education, there has been little comprehensive or national planning to address the public health system, and therefore little financing associated with building the public health infrastructure. Federal and state funding has continued to follow specific programs and services of the day or of the year, and state and local public health agencies have continued to operate in reactive as opposed to proactive modalities.

Federal Funding Streams and Expenditures

The movement toward organized public health services began at the end of the nineteenth century and continued at a fast pace throughout the 1950s and 1960s. In this period, state and federal funding streams were developed to support local health services. During the early part of the century, federal funding was only made available on a special case-specific basis in order to conduct research and demonstrations in sanitation fields. In these programs, the federal government funded the salaries for these activities directly and did not flow the monies through the state or local governments. In 1918, the first federal "grant" program was created through the PHS for venereal disease control services, but the funding stream quickly dissipated a few years later. However, it was the 1935 passage of Titles V and VI of the Social Security Act that provided institutional funding for public health activities. The Social Security Act created "general health grants" that supported state and local public health services; special grants for maternity, child health, and disabled children were approved soon afterward in 1936. A flood of specialized and categorical programs were created through the late 1930s and through the 1940s around issues of venereal disease, emergency maternity and infant care, TB, cancer, heart disease control, mental health, and industrial waste studies. Grants for capital construction of health facilities were also created during this boom (post–World War II) period.[8]

After the initiation of federal public health financing, there was significant variability in the amount and comparable percentage that states received for public health services. In a 1955 article published in the *American Journal of Public Health,* Jay Haldeman wrote, "There is considerable variation among the states in the proportion which federal grant funds constitute state and local expenditures for public health purposes. Although variation in state wealth has narrowed since health grants were first instituted, the state having the highest per capita income is still more than twice as well off financially as the state with the lowest per capita income."[8(p.967)] In 1953, federal contributions ranged from 9 percent of the state's total public health expenditures in California and New York compared to 54 percent in Arkansas and 55 percent in Wyoming. In the median state, federal grants consisted of 28 percent of the total expenditures, with the low-income states still contributing a larger percentage of their own resources to public health services than the wealthier states.[8]

Federal grants totaling more than $63 million reached a relative high during the early 1950s. With the Korean War, grant dollars were diminished for public health services, and the trend toward federal financing of hospital-based acute care services began and continued for many decades. At the same time that federal funding was declining, state and local appropriations for public health services began increasing. From 1946 to 1955, the ratio of state and local health appropriations to federal grants rose from 2:1 to 6:1. However, even through this growth period, public health advocates maintained that public health services were underfunded and that the federal government had an obligation to support the assurance of the public's health.[8(pp.968–970)]

From the 1950s through today, the financing of local public health services has become more and more of a regionally based decision, resulting in part from historical relationships between individual states and localities. The federal government continued to finance categorical public health programs based on the emergence of new diseases (e.g., HIV/AIDS), the priorities of Congress, and the needs of individual localities. Although many advocates were and continue to be supportive of state and local government determining the local health needs and programs for its own communities, the lack of a standard structure for local public health and the absence of a mandated set of national public health programs have over the years led to a fragmented public health infrastructure that differs from community to community and state to state.

In the 1980s and 1990s, new federal dollars for public health services were limited, and existing funding streams were not secure. Under President Ronald Reagan, many public health programs were either reduced, eliminated, or combined in the form of block grants. It was during this period that the MCH block grants and other block grants were developed, phasing out dozens of categorically based programs. It was not the block granting itself that reduced public health funding; rather, combining the public health programs allowed lawmakers to make future reductions to the block grants without constituents being able to attach a specific public health program to the dollar losses. It is difficult to develop a constituency for a "block grant" as opposed to an advocacy group for a low birth weight prevention program. In 1989, the largest federal grants supporting state and local public health activities were the MCH Block Grant, Family Planning—Title X, Preventive Health and Health Services Block Grant, HIV/AIDS (Ryan White), and the Immunization Action Grant.[6]

Most recently under President Bill Clinton, the federal government has again proposed various scenarios to "block grant" some of the available funding and provide greater flexibility to LHDs. But these efforts have stopped and started many times; at this stage, the changes have not provided LHDs with what they need in order to finance core public health programs.[9] Specifically, in 1996, President Clinton submitted a proposed budget that included a consolidation of 108 public health programs into 16 block grants that the states would have the authority to distribute to localities. Within the 108 programs, the CDC's 32 programs were slated for consolidation into three "performance partnership" grants.[10]

Over the years, two of the largest federal health programs (Medicaid and Medicare) have provided little support to state and local health departments. Congress did, however, expand Medicaid coverage to pregnant women and children in the late 1980s, which did provide some additional revenue for traditional public health providers.[10] However, most recently, the small amount of revenue that came from these programs has begun to disappear. With the predominance of Medicaid managed care, Medicaid revenue has been declining for many LHDs as patients obtain services with providers who are in network and local public health agencies discontinue some of the Medicaid-reimbursable clinical services they have historically provided.

States, however, continue to rely heavily on federal funding to support their public health departments and services. In many states and cities, federal grants make up a large percentage of their operating budgets. Due to their budgetary prominence, federal grants drive programmatic policies and priorities at the state and local levels. In some states, federal dollars have "compensated" for diminishing state support in certain public health areas. The Special Supplemental Food Program for Women, Infants, and Children (WIC) Program and other related nutrition programs make up the largest percentage of SHD budgets. Other large federal grants today include the MCH Block Grant, the Family Planning (Title X) Grant, and the Prevention Block Grant.[3]

Medicare

Medicare has not provided significant funds to public health organizations nationally, in part because many of the personal health services that health organizations provide are not geared to the Medicare-eligible population. Additionally, Medicare recipients have many other options for receiving personal health services and do not choose to go to the LHDs or SHDs for care. Historically, many public health organizations have operated home health agencies; in some cases, these organizations collect Medicare revenue. Recently, many of the public health organizations that did own and operate home health agencies have either privatized or contracted out these services, and the small amount of Medicare dollars flowing to public health organizations has declined. In some cases, public health organizations may have developed other public health programs that Medicare will finance, but these are few and far between. For the most part, those population-based public health services that are directed at the elderly population (such as an elderly falls prevention program) are not reimbursable by Medicare.

Medicaid

Medicaid was enacted in 1965 as part of the War on Poverty programs to provide health care coverage for the poor. Over the past 30 to 40 years, Medicaid has provided a small but important revenue stream for many LHDs. Encouraged by the passage of the Omnibus Budget Reconciliation Acts of 1986 and 1987, many states expanded traditional Medicaid coverage for pregnant women and infants with incomes that were at or above poverty. With this expansion, maternal health and family planning–related public health activities obtained a new funding source. Since its inception, Medicaid has provided increased access to personal and public health services for these designated populations. Many public health departments that are providers of personal health services (including primary care, MCH services, and home health services) have historically depended on Medicaid revenues to help support other population-based public health programs or to help reduce local tax levy contributions for public health. The introduction of and emphasis on Medicaid as a funding stream for public health services have in some ways contributed to public health's ongoing identity battle about whether or not it is a personal health care provider or a population-based care provider. Medicaid dollars have supported many safety-net personal health services that public health departments have and continue to provide. The advent of medical managed care has had a significant impact on the public health agency and is discussed further in this chapter and in Chapter 30.

State Funding Streams and Expenditures

SHDs provide both categorical grant funding and base funding for the provision of public health programs. The amount of funding provided by states to localities, the form of the funding, and the requirements of the financing differ among states. In 1996–97, the New York State Association of County Health Officials, the New York City Department of Health, the New York State Department of Health, and the New York Academy of Medicine, with the assistance of the Association of State and Territorial Health Officials, conducted 25 open-ended telephone surveys with representatives from SHDs nationwide. Eligibility criteria for survey participation were aimed at identifying those SHDs that had embarked on a formal process to evaluate the roles of state and local health units in providing and ensuring public health services in the eight years prior to survey administration. In the majority of states contacted ($n = 18$), public health services were provided exclusively or primarily at the county or multicounty level. Four states had a large number of municipal public health units; in three states, the SHD was responsible for the provision of all public health services.[11]

Among the participating states, significant variation existed in the level of state funding and in the method used to distribute state funds to the local health units. Funding, for the purpose of this study, referred only to discretionary or base funding of local health units and did not include pass-through contracts or state and federal categorical grants. From the surveys, funding patterns were categorized into seven core methodologies that were employed across jurisdictions. The history of how one financing mechanism was chosen over another was in many cases influenced by the history of the state and local relationship, the makeup of the legislative and executive branches, and the baseline funds that were available for local distribution. Brief descriptions of these different financing methods are included in the following paragraphs:[11]

- *Combination funding: the use of more than one funding mechanism to fund LHDs.* Usually, this involves some per capita funding for basic public health services and specific grants for discrete local activities or staff.
- *Contract funding: the use of a negotiated contract to fund the public health services provided at the local level.* Usually, LHDs submit a funding application annually to the SHD to receive funds available through the local health maintenance fund.
- *Formula funding: the distribution of funds to local health units based on a formula that incorporates variables that correlate with the health status and the financial resources of the population.* The formulas may include different variables, such as per capita income, assessed land value, and disease rates, in an attempt to account for dif-

ferences in localities' resources and population-level health indicators.

- *Local funding: the almost exclusive use of locally collected funds and grants to support the public health services provided by the local health department.* LHDs in these states are usually funded primarily through local taxes, inspection fees, and categorical and outside grants.
- *Per capita funding: the distribution of state funding to local health units based solely on the population base served by the local health unit.* In some states, per capita funding is not available to part-time health departments, but full-time municipal health departments are eligible for a sliding level of per capita funding depending on the size of the health department. The goal of the funding differential where most health departments are currently organized at the municipal level is to encourage the consolidation of municipal health departments while simultaneously increasing the capacity of LHDs.
- *Reimbursement funding: LHDs are reimbursed for a specific set of services based on the expenditures associated with providing the services.* The types of services that are allowable for reimbursement are usually preestablished by the state, and a complete programmatic and financial documentation of expenditures is required in order to process the reimbursement. The SHD usually requires the LHDs to predefine the set of services and strictly ensures that the localities are performing the said services described in the plan.
- *State funding: the LHDs are extensions of the SHDs and the state is responsible for funding and providing all the public health services at the local level.* This usually occurs in smaller or more rural states, where there are less formally organized governmental units.

Local Funding Streams and Expenditures

In addition to federal and state funding, most LHDs receive varied amounts of local support to carry out basic public health services. Local funding usually comes in the form of tax levy contributions from residents and businesses that reside in the community and therefore are the "users" of services. The amount of funds chiefly depends on the local tax base (in essence, the makeup of the locality that is served), its taxing policies, and the level of importance local governments place on public health programs and services.[3] These funds are appropriated by the local legislative and executive branches through a routine and formal process that usually occurs annually, at a minimum. LHDs usually have an opportunity to request additional local tax levy dollars for new programs, mandated services, or other emergencies. Tax levy funds may also be reduced due to budget issues in any given jurisdiction.

Permits and Licensing Fees/Fines

Many of the larger LHDs rely heavily on the fees and fines that they may collect directly from their regulatory activities. Fees and fines result from inspections, permits, and licensing, largely from environmental health activities. Specific programs and activities that typically generate fees and fines include day care, lead poisoning prevention, inspections (food, water, camps, and beaches), and vital records.

Patient Services Revenue

Over the past decade, many public health organizations have begun to implement sliding fee scales in order to support the continued operation of their programs. Sliding fee scales usually assess a copayment based on a client's reported income as well as family size. In cases where the patient cannot pay, the fee scale is brought to zero in order to ensure that everyone receives the health services that he or she needs. For public health organizations that have not routinely collected fees, the shift in both thinking and process required by the implementation of fee scales has meant significant time and effort in training staff and installing new billing systems. However, if public health organizations want to remain cost-competitive, they must be able to collect patient revenue effectively while maintaining their strong mission-driven organizations.

Indigent Care/Charity Care Pools

Some public health organizations obtain reimbursement for uncompensated clinical and primary care services through indigent care pools. The eligibility criteria, structure, and amounts available for and from these pools differ state to state, but some LHDs have been able to access these pools to support their personal health or safety-net services.[12]

Private Foundations/Corporations

Public health organizations have only recently joined the crowd of organizations seeking new sources of funding (other than governmental sources). Foundations, philanthropies, and corporations provide alternative financing options for local public health services. However, the drawbacks to these funding sources are that they are usually time sensitive, they are allocated for a specific project with a defined time period, and they do not provide ongoing support for operations of a public health program. Additionally, some localities may not look favorably at financing core public health services through nongovernmental means, further limiting the types of programs that would be appropriate for this funding stream. However, private foundations or corporations provide an ideal testing ground for new programs in order to generate a proven track record so that the program can eventually receive local, state, or even federal funding.

KEY FINANCIAL OPERATIONS IN LHDs

LHDs are facing difficult decisions about their programs and services. As health care has become more and more business-like, LHDs are being forced to enhance key financial capacities in order to operate more efficiently and effectively.

Strategic Financial Planning and Budgeting

Public health organizations must develop an integrated program planning and financial process to ensure that fiscal issues are incorporated into the organization's planning activities. The staff in the fiscal office should be involved in programmatic development from the initial stages and not as an afterthought. In order to support this integrated process, LHDs should place their financial staff/office in prominent positions. Budgeting should be a proactive, routine, and comprehensive process that begins at the program level and works its way up centrally. The process for developing and monitoring LHD budgets should be clear and concise, with a few designated review points along the way. Capital budgets should be considered in coordination with the operating budgets. The budgeting process should be completed annually in conjunction with an organization's strategic planning activities so as to enable the LHD to define its internal and external priorities and shift dollars to support these activities. Finally, the budget process should account for and monitor all activities of an LHD, including those funded by grant dollars.

Budget Development

The budget should be developed initially by each of the major program areas within the LHD with the technical assistance of the finance staff. In small LHDs, the budget may be developed more centrally. The program budgets should each be submitted in a uniform format (preferably in an electronic format). Within the program budgets, there should be two distinct types of requested dollars: those for existing programs and those for new programs. Dollars requested for existing programs should detail the percentage increase or decrease based on last year's funding allocation and explain the change (e.g., there was a sharp increase in the costs of asthma drugs or fewer patients came to the TB clinic). Dollars requested for new programs should be accompanied by a detailed description of the following items: reason for the request (e.g., new federal mandate or an emergent public health need), requested funding source (tax levy or grant dollars), description of the request, five-year budget projections (including both revenues and expenses associated with the request), and an impact statement if the funding request is denied. Along with the requests for new funds, programs should be required to submit a list of activities that could be reduced or eliminated if necessary. This information should be submitted to a central committee in the LHD for consolidation and review. The public health director or health commissioner should be intimately involved in the review and approval of the LHD's budget (as well as the LHD's personnel and finance directors). The executive staff of the LHD should communicate the organization's final recommendations to key program staff before the budget is submitted to any outside party. In some jurisdictions, the budget should be submitted to the local board of health for approval as well.

Budget Negotiations

Typically, the budget that has been developed by the LHD is then submitted to the budget or finance office of the executive branch. Usually, the only part of the budget that is negotiated with the executive and legislative branches is the tax levy portion of the LHD's budget because the local government does not have decision-making authority over state and federal grants/contracts. The negotiation between the LHD and the executive branch is usually a back and forth process that may involve the development of supplemental materials to support a budget request, telephone conversations between the parties, and sometimes even face-to-face meetings. During this period, politicking becomes fierce and LHDs may call on advocates, the research community, or other supporters to lobby their cause. Once the budget or finance office approves the LHD's budget, it is submitted to the jurisdiction's chief executive (e.g., mayor, county executive) for consideration. Usually, the LHD will have an opportunity to present its budget to the chief executive, but this depends on the jurisdiction. Once the chief executive has approved the budget, it is submitted to the legislative branch of government for consideration. Usually, part of the legislative review involves meetings with the LHD to discuss the budget submission. The legislative and executive branches may have different budget priorities and this is the time when they must reach consensus. It is during these negotiations that the LHD may find items added, deleted, or modified in its budget based on the priorities of the legislative branch.

Budget Adoption

When the two branches of government reach consensus, a final budget is passed and the LHD is notified of its final spending authority. The adopted budget is usually published and made available for public review. The LHD can then begin implementing new programs or eliminating activities in accordance with what was included in the budget.

Budget Modification

Usually during the budget year, there are several scheduled opportunities for external modifications in the budget (meaning that the LHD can obtain new dollars or can lose existing dollars based on the decisions of the legislative and executive branches of government). The frequency of these changes depends on the individual locality. Additionally, the amount of internal flexibility that an LHD has to modify its own budget (shifting dollars among and between LHD programs) during the budget period is also dependent on the jurisdiction. Larger health departments may have a higher ceiling on the amount of dollars they can shift without obtaining approval from the executive branch.

Types of Budgets

There are many different types of budgeting techniques. The type of budget that an LHD uses will most likely depend on the budgeting system in operation for the entire local governmental structure. Some different types of budgets include performance-based budgets, zero-based budgets, line-item budgets, and program budgets. A jurisdiction may also employ a combination of types. Additionally, most LHDs will usually have both an operating budget and a capital budget that follows the process that is described above. The *operating* budget funds those items that are required in order to maintain the daily operations of the LHD, including the staff and materials/supplies. The operating budget includes both the revenues and the expenses associated with the health department's activities. The *capital* budget finances equipment purchases and facility construction. In order for equipment to be capitally eligible, it usually has to last for a certain number of years and be greater than a certain dollar amount. The exact requirements are set by the individual locality.

The Budget Cycle

The cycle for developing the LHD's budget follows the cycle that has been established for the local government. In most counties and cities, the budget cycle is annual, although in some small jurisdictions, it may be longer. The budget cycle follows the jurisdiction's fiscal year so that a new budget is adopted prior to the beginning of the new fiscal year. The dates of fiscal years also differ by jurisdiction, with most following either the calendar year (January 1 to December 31) or another set of dates determined by the local government.

Expenditure and Revenue Monitoring

In addition to developing the budget, the LHD must routinely monitor its spending and revenues (both tax levy and grant dollars) to ensure that its public health programs stay within their allocated spending limits and that the LHD is collecting anticipated revenues. Developing a central system for systematically monitoring expenses and revenues is critical for any LHD. In many cases, the LHD will use a system that has been centrally designed for all government agencies within its jurisdiction, but in other cases, the complexity in the LHD's funding streams may require that a system be designed specifically for the LHD. Additionally, as with any arm of government, the LHD must monitor its budget in order to be accountable to the taxpayers. Any monitoring system that is developed must have both central control by the LHD's finance office as well as decentralized access to the system by program staff. Actual spending and revenue collections should be reconciled against the budget on a monthly basis to ensure early detection of problems. As part of the monitoring process, the LHD may have some of its grant programs audited by outside organizations or the LHD may choose to audit some of its subcontractors. In either case, the LHD should see the audit as an opportunity to get its financial data in order and help plan for future public health programs.

Revenue Generation

When developing new programs or evaluating old programs, LHDs should evaluate how they can generate revenues associated with the public health service. Many health departments are constrained from generating any profits, but in many cases, the health departments are not currently able to recover their costs. Additionally, health departments should look for new customers to purchase existing or new public health services. This may include for-profit corporations, hospitals, community-based organizations, managed care organizations, individuals, and many others.

Sliding Fee Scales

Historically, many public health organizations have not charged for their services based in most part on a belief that cost sharing may have a detrimental effect on the patients continuing to come to public health departments to receive care. However, in today's environment of new safety-net providers, the implementation of Medicaid managed care, and declining public health resources, organizations should establish fees for a variety of clinical and nonclinical services. LHDs may choose to set fee schedules for a unique range of services based on the services provided, the services chargeable under law, the local political environment, and a variety of other factors.

Billing/Collections and Other Financial Systems

Many public health organizations have antiquated systems that support the collection and monitoring of financial data. In order to compete in the new health environment, public health departments must have more advanced information systems and staff to support these systems in order to capture advanced financial as well as billing-related data. The development and maintenance of these systems are complicated by the fact that LHDs often have a number of funding sources that each have different cycles of allocating dollars and different reporting requirements. Additionally, public health organizations must change the attitude of their work force to integrate billing and fiscal monitoring activities into routine workflow processes.

THE YEAR 2000: PUBLIC HEALTH FINANCING CHALLENGES

Public health organizations are being forced to reinvent themselves due to a variety of confounding environmental and political factors coming together at one time: additional safety-net providers, fewer dedicated public health dollars, Medicaid managed care, and public demand for less government. Public health organizations across the country are evaluating which services they should continue to provide, which they should expand, which they should minimize, and which they should eliminate. As public health organizations grapple with decisions about the right mix of services to be provided, these organizations continue to be faced with difficult financial conditions. The challenge for public health as it decides what it wants to look like in the twenty-first century is to develop a financing methodology that consistently and securely supports core activities. Although the financing structure for public health services is fragmented at best, historically, there have been dollars to support specific categorical public health services, which have cross-subsidized some of the core population-based services. However, many of these funding streams are disappearing, or the organizations are no longer providing the services that received funding. It is the core population-based public health services such as disease surveillance, outbreak investigations, emergency response programs, and environmental health services that need to be financed nationally and locally. In addition to identifying a financing mechanism for the public health infrastructure, there are several other discrete financial challenges for public health.

Medicaid Managed Care Implementation

As states continue to implement Medicaid managed care, public health departments are faced with continuing declines in Medicaid revenues due to decreasing numbers of Medicaid-eligible patient visits. Although public health advocates should be encouraged that new health providers are now available to provide these services to the underserved population, some LHDs had relied on Medicaid dollars to support core public health activities. These health departments must now identify new funding streams to supplant the loss of Medicaid revenue. Medicaid managed care also provides health departments with some new funding opportunities. As managed care organizations are required to provide preventive services, LHDs can play a role in providing some (or in limited cases, all) of those services under contract with the managed care organization or can be a monitor of the services delivered by other providers.

Privatization of Public Health Services

In reaction to the current climate, many health departments are privatizing public health services. The privatization of public health services has taken many different forms across the country. Some health departments have contracted out entire personal health programs (e.g., child health, dental health, primary care) to other public or private sector providers or even networks of providers (e.g., local hospitals, community-based organizations); others have contracted out the clinical parts of personal health programs and maintained a monitoring oversight/quality assurance role for the programs; and others have eliminated the programs altogether. As health departments reduce their spending on specific privatized services, it is critical that they invest resources (both financial and personnel) in identifying revenue to support those remaining public health services. Additionally, privatization presents an opportunity for LHDs to develop new partnerships for the provision of public health services. Although the LHD may not have the funding to provide the public health service itself, it may play an important role in coordinating the activity or developing the public health policies supporting the activity.

Cost-Competitiveness

As arms of government, public health organizations generally have not spent significant energy evaluating the costs of providing public health services. Many governmental public health organizations develop program-based budgets (not budgets based on the unit costs of services) and evaluate the costs only for those services that they charge for. As part of the process of reinventing themselves, health departments must have data on the costs of their services. Although there is no oversight or regulatory body that requires this information (although there may be in the not-so-distant future), understanding the costs of all public health services has significant value for organizations as an internal management tool, as a way to negotiate more funding, and as a public relations opportunity. By knowing what an individual unit of service costs an organization to deliver and quantifying these services, public health organizations can

- Compare themselves to similar organizations.
- Compare the cost of one type of public health service to another within the organization.
- Comprehensively evaluate the components (both personal services and other than personal services) of cost to identify areas of efficiency and inefficiency.
- Analyze their internal organization and infrastructure.
- Understand the range and demand for services delivered.
- Lobby local, state, or national organizations for the reimbursement of discrete public health services.
- Demonstrate the value of public health services to the public.

Increasing Numbers of Uninsured

As public health organizations continue to privatize public health services, the number of uninsured individuals continues to rise across the country. This poses an inherent challenge to public health organizations as they have historically served as safety-net providers to the uninsured and underinsured population. As the assurers of the public's health, public health organizations must take an active role in developing the public policies and the financing mechanisms to support health care coverage for this growing population.

Information Technology Innovations

Public health organizations are the collectors and analyzers of data. Over the past decade or two, organizations have begun to use new technology to support these activities, but in many cases, the systems that were built were ad hoc and not central to the daily operations of public health organizations. In order for public health organizations to participate actively as leaders in promoting and protecting the public's health, they must invest significant dollars in building local, state, and national systems to support information exchange. Many other health organizations are implementing computer-based patient records; installing sophisticated systems for billing, management, and data tracking; using handheld tablets for field work; and developing Internet strategies for accessing and monitoring health data. Public health organizations must be active designers and purchasers of technology and be committed to spending the necessary resources to update their operations to twenty-first century standards. The up-front costs for technology may pose a challenge for organizations to manage because much of the technology will only show returns after several years, but it is a worthwhile investment.

Changes in Grant Funding

The recent trend of declining grant dollars for core public health services will most likely continue. As a result, LHDs may have to develop creative solutions for financing those services that may have previously been supported through grant funds. Additionally, LHDs may have to think very carefully about using grant dollars to support core public health activities. The continued shift away from categorical funding will force LHDs to develop more intense partnerships with other members of the community and more integrated public health programs.

The Business of Public Health

Public health organizations have not thought of themselves as businesses and therefore have not acted as them. This has meant that public health organizations have not focused energy or resources on understanding their customers, marketing services to their customers, actively collecting revenues for their services/programs, or maintaining a productive and happy work force—some of the key tenets of any business. But health is one of the largest business sectors in the United States and in the world, and has gained significant prestige and market share over the past century. If public health organizations want to survive as an important force in the health arena, they need to be prepared to change attitudes as well as shift resources in order to support some core business-related activities.

Public health organizations have the unique challenge of trying to inform the general public about what they do routinely to protect the public's health. Many of the public health services that are provided by government go undetected unless there is an emergency. Most Americans would not know that a public health organization's surveillance activities are used to identify when there is an outbreak of encephalitis-carrying mosquitoes or when hamburger meat in the supermarkets or at the butcher's is infected with a strand of *E. coli.* Public health organizations must take this opportunity to identify the erosion of the public health infrastructure as an issue that needs public support and one that requires national standards for the organization and delivery of public health services. Only when these issues reach the policy agenda will the development of a secure and comprehensive financing mechanism for public health be realized.

• • •

Understanding the financing structure of public health services is an important and difficult task that is complicated by the lack of literature on the subject. Although there are volumes of texts published on health care financing, there are no books and few scholarly journal articles that have been dedicated to the financial structure of public health services. The disorganization and the haphazardness of the public health financing structure nationally present significant risks to the future of public health. Without institutionalized and consistent financing systems for public health services, these activities can be eliminated without significant public attention. Additionally, the lack of organized systems for public health financing prevents the collection of comprehensive and national data sets on public health activities. With financial data in hand, public health advocates may be able to develop stronger arguments in support of enhanced public health activities. As public health continues to compete with health care services for funding and public attention, it is essential that public health arm itself with as much information as it can about its programs and services. By financially accounting for its activities, public health practitioners can demonstrate the true bargain that public health really is.

CHAPTER REVIEW

1. The financing of public health services is complicated by the unique organization of public health delivery within each state and locality.
2. There is no existing system that can comprehensively measure the amount of spending on public health services or evaluate how differences in public health expenditures may impact health outcomes.

3. The financing of local public health services varies and is related to historical relationships between states and their localities.
4. Under President Reagan, many public health programs were combined into block grants followed by reductions in overall funding; they were no longer explicitly tied to an individual and recognizable public health problem.
5. Public health organizations must develop an integrated program planning and financial process. The budget process should be completed annually in conjunction with the organization's strategic planning activities to enable the public health organization to define priorities and shift its resources accordingly.
6. The public health organization must monitor its spending and revenues to ensure that programs are within allocated spending limits and that the organization is collecting anticipated revenues.
7. As states continue to implement Medicaid managed care, public health organizations are faced with continuing declines in revenues due to decreasing numbers of Medicaid-eligible visits.
8. Public health financing challenges include identifying a financing mechanism for infrastructure and the core population-based health services.
9. Public health organizations must gather data on the costs of providing services to identify areas of efficiency and inefficiency and demonstrate the value of public health to the public.

REFERENCES

1. G.F. Anderson and S. Maxwell, "The Organization and Financing of Healthcare Services," in *The AUPHA Manual of Health Services Management,* eds. R.J. Taylor and S.B. Taylor (Gaithersburg, MD: Aspen Publishers, Inc., 1994), 87–101.
2. R.D. Lasker and the Committee of Medicine and Public Health, *Medicine and Public Health: The Power of Collaboration* (New York: The New York Academy of Medicine, 1997).
3. S. Wall, "Transformations in Public Health Systems," *Health Affairs 17,* no. 3 (1998): 64–80.
4. K. Eibert et al., "Public Health Expenditures: Developing Estimates for Improved Policy Making," *Journal of Public Health Management and Practice 3,* no. 3 (1997): 1–9.
5. *1992–1993 National Profile of Local Health Departments* (Washington, DC: Centers for Disease Control and Prevention with the National Association of County and City Health Officials, 1995), 7–19, 21–23, 31–37.
6. *Public Health Agencies 1991: An Inventory of Programs and Block Grant Expenditures* (Washington, DC: Public Health Foundation, 1991), 3–5, 115.
7. M. Barry et al., Where Do the Dollars Go? Measuring Local Public Expenditures (Paper presented to the Office of Disease Prevention and Health Promotion, Office of Public Health and Science, U.S. Department of Health and Human Services, Washington, DC, March 1998).
8. J. Haldeman, "Financing Local Health Services," *American Journal of Public Health 45,* no. 8 (1955): 967–971.
9. C. Kent, "Budget-Cutting Ax Slashes Public Health (1996 Congressional Budget Resolutions)," *American Medical News 38,* no. 21 (1995): 3–4.
10. L. Jones, "State by State Approach to Public Health," *American Medical News 38,* no. 8 (1995): 1–2.
11. New York State Association of County Health Officials et al., *Public Health Assessment Project Final Report* (Albany, NY: 1997).
12. E. Brown et al., "State Approaches to Financing Health Care for the Poor," *Annual Review of Public Health* 11 (1990): 377–400.

CHAPTER 18

Performance Measurement and Improvement

Bernard J. Turnock
Arden S. Handler

Public health organizations use performance measurement activities to track the work produced and results achieved through their internal and interorganizational efforts. Increasingly, organizations rely on performance measurement activities both to achieve internal quality improvement goals and to demonstrate accountability to external stakeholders. A growing array of management tools and processes is available to assist organizations in carrying out performance measurement activities on a routine basis. Organizations should adapt measurement approaches to fit their specific institutional capacities and priorities, and to address the needs and concerns of the communities they serve.

Public health leaders and managers face issues related to performance at many different levels of the public health system, including the performance of individuals, programs, agencies, interorganizational collaborations, and the systemwide enterprise itself. Although these levels represent different aspects of public health performance, each can be assessed using common approaches that focus on the work produced and the results achieved. Performance measurement is an important management tool with an impressive record in improving performance throughout both the public and private sectors. These accomplishments derive from fundamental principles of the improvement science field: to improve something we must be able to control it; to control it we must be able to understand it; and to understand it we must be able to measure it.[1] This link between performance measurement and performance improvement provides a context for understanding the lessons and implications of performance measurement efforts in public health during the twentieth century. This chapter examines these lessons, as well as various applications using performance standards to improve the performance of public health organizations and systems, including the accreditation of public health agencies.

PERFORMANCE MEASUREMENT AND PERFORMANCE MEASURES

Performance measurement, performance monitoring, performance management, and performance improvement are topics that are extensively addressed in the literature.[2-4] Although performance measurement is a simple concept, it lacks a simple or single definition. Basically, performance measurement is the selection and use of quantitative measures of critical aspects of activities, including their effect on the public and other customers. Put more simply, it is the regular collection and reporting of data to track work that is produced and results that are achieved.

An expert panel convened by the National Resource Council concluded that performance measurement involves three major activities: (1) developing an explicit set of goals and objectives and articulating a strategy for their achievement, (2) establishing and implementing strategies for performance measurement, and (3) using performance information to improve management and resource allocation.[5] The panel also identified principles to guide performance measurement efforts for publicly funded health programs.[5]

- Performance measurement activities must proceed from clearly defined goals and be viewed as tools for monitoring and promoting progress toward these goals.
- Because health needs and priorities vary, performance measurement should promote the development and use of measures that can be adapted for differing priorities and strategies. Measures should be valid, reliable, and responsive to change, and have agreed-on definitions.
- Performance measurement activities must recognize and meet information needs for different functions (e.g., program operation, management, policy making, funding). Ideally, measures for specific functional purposes should be linked, conceptually or in practice, to provide a consistent assessment of performance across these different functions.
- Performance measurement must consider the feasibility and cost of data collection and analysis for proposed measures.
- Performance measurement activities, including the measures used and their supporting data, should be evaluated periodically to ensure their continuing appropriateness and usefulness.
- Performance measurement should be viewed as a developmental and evolving activity. Measures should be refined or replaced as new information on the linkages between outcomes and processes becomes available, as better sources of data are developed, and as priorities change.

An effective performance measurement process incorporates stakeholder input; promotes top leadership support; creates a clear mission statement; develops long-term goals and objectives; formulates short-term goals and interim measures; devises simple, manageable approaches; and provides support and technical assistance to those involved in the process. In this light, performance measurement serves several important purposes, providing information concerning the capacity to perform, results of current efforts, and effectiveness of current performance. Potential benefits from measuring performance include

- better goals and objectives
- identification of strengths and weaknesses
- opportunities for collaborative approaches
- clearer lines of accountability
- improved quality
- better tracking of progress over time
- more effective communication
- better resource deployment

Performance measurement focuses on what is occurring, but it does not extensively address why or how. Evaluative research (sometimes called program evaluation) provides more in-depth assessment of the conceptualization, design, implementation, and utility of social interventions.[6] (See Chapter 13 for a more detailed discussion.) Performance measurement can be viewed as one component of a comprehensive evaluation, but its primary purpose is to inform managers so that changes can be instituted within the life cycle of a set of activities. In sum, performance measurement is a management and oversight tool to facilitate positive change and improvement in performance.

The terminology used in performance measurement is often inconsistent and confusing; the definitions used in this chapter are adapted from several sources.[5,7] In general, a *performance measure* is the specific quantitative representation of a capacity, process, or outcome that is deemed relevant to the assessment of performance. Similar to the concept of prevention, performance measurement requires an object. It is critical to specify what (or whose) performance will be measured. In public health, performance measurement most frequently occurs within the context of a particular program (e.g., childhood immunizations or retail food safety). However, the performance of an agency (e.g., a state or local health department), partnership, community public health system, or even an individual is also an appropriate target for performance measurement. Because the prime focus of this chapter is on measuring and improving performance in organizations and even more complex public health systems, the term *performance measurement* will mean the selection and use of quantitative measures of public health system capacities, processes, and outcomes to inform public health leaders and managers and the public about critical aspects of the public health system.

Performance measures can take several different forms. A performance measure that takes the form of a generally accepted, objective standard of measurement—such as a rule or guideline against which the level of performance can be compared—is often termed a *performance standard*. In essence, a performance standard is an expectation of what will be done or accomplished. Performance measures that are used to determine whether or to what extent a performance standard is achieved are often called *performance indicators*. For example, a performance standard might call for a comprehensive community health assessment to be completed every three years. Performance indicators for this standard could take one of several forms. The administrator of the local public health agency could be asked whether this standard was met, or perhaps a review team might look for a completed assessment at the time of a site visit. The agency administrator's response (yes or no) and the actual document are both performance indicators in this example.

The definition of performance measurement acknowledges critical dimensions of performance, including capacities, processes, and outcomes. It is important to consider the meaning of these terms as they relate to performance measurement for public health organizations and systems.

- *Capacities* refer to the resources and relationships necessary to carry out the important processes of public health; this capacity to perform is made possible by the maintenance of the basic infrastructure of the public health system, as well as by specific program resources.
- *Processes* refer to what is done to, for, with, or by defined individuals or groups to identify and address community or population-wide health problems. The performance of key processes (e.g., monitoring health status, investigating health hazards, and building constituencies) leads to the development of other processes that can also be viewed as outputs. In public health practice, these outputs take the form of interventions (e.g., policies, programs, and services) intended to achieve outcomes that are important to the system. The formulation known as the essential public health services, which embodies these key processes and outputs, serves as the framework for public health practice: the identification and addressing of important health problems and the implementation of interventions intended to impact outcomes.
- *Outcomes* reflect the immediate and long-term changes (or lack of change) experienced by individuals and populations as a result of the processes. Measures of outcome reflect the magnitude and direction of the effect of processes on health status, risk reduction, social functioning, or consumer satisfaction outcomes.

The *Public Health in America* framework addresses both the general outcomes and the key processes of public health practice; the link between this document and performance measurement is presented in Exhibit 18–1.[8]

Performance measures provide information concerning the capacity to perform, process performance (including outputs), and ultimate results. Although useful by themselves, performance measures provide richer information when multiple dimensions are measured and related to each other. For example, relating capacities to outcomes (such as the cost-effectiveness or cost per case of disease prevented) is a common approach to assessing effectiveness. Similarly, measures relating capacities to processes

Exhibit 18–1 Links between *Public Health in America* Framework and Performance Measurement

Public Health in America Elements*	Usefulness for Performance Measurement Activities**
Healthy people in healthy communities Promote physical and mental health and prevent disease, injury, and disability	Vision statement Mission statement *Useful for formulating vision and mission statements*
Public health: • prevents epidemics and the spread of disease • protects against environmental hazards • prevents injuries • promotes and encourages healthy behaviors • responds to disasters and assists communities in recovery • ensures the quality and accessibility of health services	Broad categories of outcomes affected by public health activities; sometimes viewed as what public health does *Useful for developing performance measures for public health outcomes*
Essential public health services 1. Monitor health status to identify community health problems. 2. Diagnose and investigate health problems and health hazards in the community. 3. Inform, educate, and empower people about health issues. 4. Mobilize community partnerships to identify and solve health problems. 5. Develop policies and plans that support individual and community health efforts. 6. Enforce laws and regulations that protect health and ensure safety. 7. Link people with needed personal health services and ensure the provision of health care when it is otherwise unavailable. 8. Ensure a competent public health and personal health care work force. 9. Evaluate effectiveness, accessibility, and quality of personal and population-based health services. 10. Research for new insights and innovative solutions to health problems.	Processes of public health practice that affect public health outcomes; sometimes viewed as how public health does what it does *Useful for developing performance measures for public health processes; these can be linked with capacity measures and with outcome measures for more comprehensive assessment of public health performance*

Source: Data from *Public Health Functions Steering Committee, *Public Health in America,* at *www.health.gov/phfunctions,* 1994, Public Health Service; and **authors.

(as in the cost per unit of service delivered) provide useful insights into efficiency. Ideally, measuring and relating measures for all of these dimensions provide the most useful information for improving performance.

Performance measurement and performance improvement initiatives have proliferated in the public sector in the final decades of the twentieth century fueled, in part, by the potential for improving the quality of public programs and services. Federal agencies have been subject to the Government Performance and Results Act since the mid-1990s; state and local governments have adopted a variety of accountability systems.[3,5]

Performance measurement has gained widespread acceptance in the health sector, both public and private, as well. Accreditation programs based on principles of performance measurement are in place for a wide variety of health care organizations and settings, including community networks providing health services.

Paralleling these developments, specific interest in performance measurement within the public health system has matured steadily during the twentieth century, especially after the Institute of Medicine's (IOM's) 1988 report, *The Future of Public Health.*[9] This interest is advanced by aspirations of improving quality, enhancing accountability, and strengthening the science base of public health practice.[10–12] The evolution of this interest is a revealing story in its own right.

Measuring Public Health Performance through 1990

Over the past century, efforts to measure public health performance have ranged from simple accounting to more sophisticated strategies in which performance is judged against already established expectations or standards.[13] Much of the early activity focused on local public health practice, although the very earliest attempt targeted state health departments. In that 1914 effort, Chapin completed a survey of state health agencies for the American Medical Association (AMA) in order to describe the services of those agencies and their role in fostering the development of local health departments (LHDs). Chapin's report concluded that state public health agencies were "mostly ill-balanced. Much of what is done counts little for health and much is left undone which would save many lives."[14(p.96)] He proposed the use of relative values for various preventive services and rated the state agencies on each service and in the aggregate. This quantitative approach was later incorporated into local public health practice appraisal initiatives orchestrated by the American Public Health Association (APHA).

In 1921, the first report of APHA's Committee on Municipal Health Department Practice called for the collection of information on local public health practice to provide the basis for the development of standards of organization and achievement for LHDs serving the nation's largest municipalities.[15,16] The committee concluded that "few standards are available to the health officers who would pattern their departments after those which predominate in American practice or achieve most satisfactory results."[15(p.7)] A survey instrument was developed and applied to 83 cities through site visits involving various committee members, including public health giants Winslow (committee chairman), Chapin, and Frost.

The committee soon saw the need to examine local public health practice more broadly, and in 1925 was reconstituted as APHA's Committee on Administrative Practice. The new committee developed an appraisal form to be used as a self-assessment tool by local health officers.[17] Both strengths and weaknesses of this initiative are apparent in its aspirations:

> The idea was to measure the immediate results attained—such as statistics properly obtained and analyzed, vaccinations performed, infants in attendance at instructive clinics, physical defects of school children discovered and corrected, tuberculosis cases hospitalized, laboratory tests performed—with the confidence that such immediate results would inevitably lead on to the ultimate end of all public health work, the conservation of human life and efficiency.[17(p.1)]

Successive iterations of the appraisal form appeared throughout the 1920s and 1930s; these were well received by LHDs, although there were occasional concerns that quantity was being emphasized over quality.[18] Using these forms, local health officers were able to compare their ratings with other agencies and submit their assessment to the Health Conservation Contest and its successor, the National Honor Roll. The basis for comparison was a numerical rating score based on aggregated points awarded across key administrative and service areas. Comparative ratings were to be used to improve health programs, advocate for resources, summarize health agency activities in annual reports, and engage other health interests in the community.[17] Agency ratings often attracted considerable media interest, resulting in both good and bad publicity for local agencies. Despite the initial intent to emphasize "immediate results," the major focus of the ratings remained on measuring public health capacity and the intervention or output aspects of public health processes.

In 1947, a new, and still voluntary, instrument, the evaluation schedule, which included capacity, process, and outcome measures and was scored centrally by the APHA Committee on Administrative Practice, replaced the appraisal form (Exhibit 18–2).[18,19] No longer was the focus on good or bad scores; results were presented for health agencies of varying size and type so that individual LHDs could directly compare their performance in meeting community needs with that of their peers. The use of these tools lost momentum in the 1950s when APHA's interest in public health performance and its measurement diminished.[20]

Prior to 1990, there were several other efforts to assess public health performance across the entire national public health system. One focused primarily on capacity factors, such as the presence or absence of an LHD in a jurisdiction and the full- or part-time availability of health

Exhibit 18–2 Measures of Public Health Performance Used in the 1947 Evaluation Schedule

1. Hospital beds: percentage in approved hospitals
2. Practicing physicians: population per physician
3. Practicing dentists: population per dentist
4. Water: percentage of population in communities over 2,500 served with approved water
5. Sewerage: percentage of population in communities over 2,500 served with approved sewerage systems
6. Water: percentage of rural school children served with approved water supplies
7. Excreta disposal: Percentage of rural school children served with approved means of excreta disposal
8. Food: percentage of food handlers reached by group instruction program
9. Food: percentage of restaurants and lunch counters with satisfactory facilities
10. Milk: percentage of bottled milk pasteurized
11. Diphtheria: percentage of children under two years given immunizing agent
12. Smallpox: percentage of children under two years given immunizing agent
13. Whooping cough: percentage of children under two years given immunizing agent
14. Tuberculosis: newly reported cases per death, five-year period
15. Tuberculosis: deaths per 100,000 population, five-year period
16. Tuberculosis: percentage of cases reported by death certificate
17. Syphilis: percentage of cases reported in primary, secondary, and early latent stage
18. Syphilis: percentage of reported contacts examined
19. Maternal: puerperal deaths per 1,000 total births, five-year rate
20. Maternal: percentage of antepartum cases under medical supervision seen before sixth month
21. Maternal: percentage of women delivered at home under postpartum nursing supervision
22. Maternal: percentage of births in hospital
23. Infant: deaths under one year of age per 1,000 live births, five-year rate
24. Infant: deaths from diarrhea and enteritis under one year per 1,000 live births, two-year rate
25. Infant: percentage of infants under nursing supervision before one month
26. School: percentage of elementary children with dental work neglected
27. Accidents: deaths from motor accidents per 100,000 population, five-year rate
28. Health department budget: cents per capita spent by health department

Source: Reprinted with permission from Committee on Administrative Practice, *Evaluation Schedule for Use in the Study and Appraisal of Community Health Programs,* pp. 53–54, © 1947, American Public Health Association.

officers.[21] The Emerson report in 1945 advanced several national standards, including one calling for complete coverage of the population by full-time LHDs (meaning those with full-time health officers).[22] Several other targets established in the Emerson report also provide interesting insights into the capacity of the national public health system at the time. For example, the committee concluded that the nation had 64 percent of the public health personnel and 63 percent of the financial resources needed to ensure full coverage of the population with six basic public health services (vital statistics, communicable disease control, environmental sanitation, public health laboratory services, maternal and child health services, and public health education).[22]

Another of these efforts provided extensive information on state health agencies. The Association of State and Territorial Health Officials (ASTHO) established a national public health reporting system, which functioned throughout much of the 1970s and 1980s. Although useful in terms of expenditures and programs for the official state health agencies, these reports had very little information on the public health activities of LHDs. Information on state-level environmental protection, substance abuse, and mental health services was also incomplete if these services were the responsibility of agencies other than the official state health agency.

In retrospect, a major limitation of the public health performance measurement activities before 1990 was the lack of emphasis on the more fundamental processes of public health practice, such as building constituencies and assessing and prioritizing community health needs, and the inability to link measures of capacities, processes, and outcomes in order to understand their relationships. The lack of a conceptual framework that explicates these relationships was the root cause for this limitation. As a result, the basic assumption expressed in the appraisal form that "immediate results would inevitably lead on to the ultimate end of all public health work, the conservation of human life and efficiency" remained largely untested.[17(p.1)]

The 1988 IOM report, which focused on the core functions of public health, was followed by a series of initiatives to facilitate operationalization of this framework including, for the first time ever, a national health objective for coverage of the population by an effective local public health presence. By the year 2000, objective 8.14 called for 90 percent of the population to be served by an LHD that was effectively carrying out public health's core functions in that community.[23] Despite little consensus as to what was meant by "effectively" addressing the core functions of public health, it was clear that the performance of key public health processes in public health organizations and systems was the focus of this new objective. Subsequent efforts to rally around this national performance measure, however, suggest that the public health community had not learned the lessons of its performance measurement history.

Measuring Public Health Performance after 1990

Much of what is known concerning current public health performance in the United States has been developed within the context of various initiatives established after the appearance of the IOM report. Unfortunately, many of these experiences remain unpublished, and few can be transported and replicated elsewhere. However, more than a dozen reports on various aspects of public health performance were published during the 1990s. Although these studies used somewhat different panels of performance measures, their contribution to public health performance measurement largely resides in their focus on performance measures for key processes related to the public health core functions and essential public health services (Exhibit 18–1).

Public health practice performance data focused on process performance (including outputs) were reported by the National Association of County and City Health Officials (NACCHO) in its 1990 and 1993 surveys of LHDs.[24,25] For 48 questions associated with the three core functions from the 1990 NACCHO survey, mean LHD performance was 50 percent. For 96 questions linked with the core functions in the 1993 NACCHO survey, mean performance was similar at 46 percent. Studies using practice measures based on the core functions reported performance scores of 57 percent performance for 14 LHDs in 1992, 56 percent for 370 LHDs in 1993, and 50 percent for 208 LHDs in 1993.[26-30] When similar performance measures were used on a statewide basis in Iowa in 1995, the overall performance score was 61 percent.[31]

Based on a variety of field tests and performance studies completed in the early 1990s, a consensus set of 20 practice performance measures (Exhibit 18–3) was established by leading researchers in the field. Other investigators have also used these performance measures in published reports, and more than a dozen states have examined public health performance within their state–local public health system using these measures. These studies consistently demonstrate suboptimal performance of key public health practices and considerable variability in the performance of specific measures.

Using the 20 consensus measures with a random sample of 298 LHDs stratified by population size and type of jurisdiction, an effort was made to assess the extent to which the U.S. population in 1995 was being effectively served by the public health core functions identified in the IOM report (assessment, policy development, and assurance).[32] Performance for these 20 measures ranged from 23 to 94 percent. The most frequently performed measures were investigating adverse health events, maintaining necessary laboratory services, implementing mandated programs, maintaining a network of relationships, and providing information regularly to the public. The least frequently performed measures were assessing the use of preventive and screening services in the community, conducting behavioral risk factor surveys, regularly evaluating the effect of services on the community, allocating resources consistent with community action plans, and deploying resources to meet identified needs (Table 18–1). The overall weighted mean performance score for all 20 measures was 56 percent. Subscores for assessment, policy development, and assurance measures were similar to the overall mean. City- and county-based LHD jurisdictions with populations greater than 50,000 performed these measures more frequently (65 percent) than other LHJs in this study (Table 18–2).

Another study in 1998 using the same 20 measures found similar levels of performance (65 percent) in 356 jurisdictions with populations of 100,000 or more.[33] Although the performance of the more populous jurisdictions was somewhat higher than the combination of large and small jurisdictions included in the 1995 national study, both the relative rankings and the population size–specific scores were quite similar in these two studies.

Although the various studies conducted throughout the 1990s used somewhat different methods and measures, they consistently demonstrate practice (process and outputs) performance in the 50–70 percent range and paint a picture of less than optimal functioning of the public health system nationally and in many states. Notably, this range is consistent with conclusions of the Emerson report a half-century earlier as to effective public health coverage of the nation based on an assessment of capacity factors. Although the precise status is not known, it is clear that the United States fell well short of its year 2000 target of having 90 percent of the population residing in jurisdictions in which public health's core functions are being effectively addressed. Two studies of practice performance conducted nationally in the 1990s concluded that only approximately one-third of the U.S. population in the 1990s was effectively served.[30,32]

These efforts to measure core function performance have served several important purposes. By providing information on both key processes and outputs of public health practice, many state–local systems have initiated public health practice improvement strategies. These efforts also provide the opportunity for measures of public health practice performance to be linked with measures of capacity and outcomes, furthering understanding of the relationships between and among these key dimensions of the public health system.

The relationship between capacity and process performance (including outputs) has been examined in two studies. One study linked prac-

Exhibit 18–3 Core-Function-Related Measures of Local Public Health Practice Performance Developed Collaboratively by University of North Carolina and University of Illinois-Chicago Investigators: 1995

Assessment

1. For the jurisdiction served by your local public health agency, is there a community health needs assessment process that systematically describes the prevailing health status and needs of the community?
2. In the past three years in your jurisdiction, has the local public health agency surveyed the population for behavioral risk factors?
3. For the jurisdiction served by your local public health agency, are timely investigations of adverse health events, including communicable disease outbreaks and environmental health hazards, conducted on an ongoing basis?
4. Are the necessary laboratory services available to the local public health agency to support investigations of adverse health events and meet routine diagnostic and surveillance needs?
5. For the jurisdiction served by your local public health agency, has an analysis been completed of the determinants and contributing factors of priority health needs, adequacy of existing health resources, and the population groups most impacted?
6. In the past three years in your jurisdiction, has the local public health agency conducted an analysis of age-specific participation in preventive and screening services?

Policy Department

7. For the jurisdiction served by your local public health agency, is there a network of support and communication relationships, which includes health-related organizations, the media, and the general public?
8. In the past year in your jurisdiction, has there been a formal attempt by the local public health agency at informing elected officials about the potential public health impact of actions under their consideration?
9. For the jurisdiction served by your local public health agency, has there been a prioritization of the community health needs that have been identified from a community needs assessment?
10. In the past three years in your jurisdiction, has the local public health agency implemented community health initiatives consistent with established priorities?
11. For the jurisdiction served by your local public agency, has a community health action plan been developed with community participation to address community health needs?
12. During the past three years in your jurisdiction, has the local public health agency developed plans to allocate resources in a manner consistent with the community health action plan?

Assurance

13. For the jurisdiction served by your local public health agency, have resources been deployed, as necessary, to address the priority health needs identified in the community health needs assessment?
14. In the past three years in your jurisdiction, has the local public health agency conducted an organizational self-assessment?
15. For the jurisdiction served by your local public health agency, are age-specific priority health needs effectively addressed through the provision of/or linkage to appropriate services?
16. In the past three years in your jurisdiction, has there been an instance in which the local public health agency has failed to implement a mandated program or service?
17. For the jurisdiction served by your local public health agency, have there been regular evaluations of the effect that public health services have on community health status?
18. In the past three years in your jurisdiction, has the local public health agency used professionally recognized process and outcome measures to monitor programs and to redirect resources as appropriate?
19. For the jurisdiction served by your local public health agency, is the public regularly provided with information about current health status, health care needs, positive health behaviors, and health care policy issues?
20. In the past year in your jurisdiction, has the local public health agency provided reports to the media on a regular basis?

Source: Reprinted from B.J. Turnock, A.S. Handler, and C.A. Miller, Core Function-Related Local Public Health Practice Effectiveness, *Journal of Public Health Management and Practice,* Vol. 4, No. 5, pp. 26–32, © 1998, Aspen Publishers, Inc.

Table 18–1 Percentage of Local Health Jurisdictions (LHJs) Performing 20 Core-Function-Related Measures of Local Public Health Practice: 1995 and 1998

Core-Function-Related Performance Measures	*LJHs National Sample,* 1995 n = 298*	*LHJs > 100,000 population,** 1998 n = 356*
1. Community needs assessment process	53.0	71.5
2. Behavioral risk factor surveys	29.2	45.8
3. Timely investigations of adverse health events	93.6	98.6
4. Necessary laboratory services available	89.3	96.3
5. Analysis of determinants, resources, and populations most impacted	45.0	61.3
6. Analysis of preventive and screening services	22.8	28.4
7. Network of relationships	82.6	78.8
8. Inform elected officials	73.2	80.9
9. Prioritization of community health needs	52.7	66.1
10. Implemented community health initiatives	68.8	81.9
11. Community health action plan	39.6	41.5
12. Plans for resource allocation	36.6	26.2
13. Resources deployed to meet needs	37.3	48.6
14. Organizational self-assessment	50.3	56.3
15. Provision/linkage of services for priority needs	64.1	75.6
16. Implemented all mandated programs	82.9	91.4
17. Evaluations of effect of services in the community	30.5	34.7
18. Programs monitored and resources redirected	42.3	47.3
19. Public provided information regularly	78.8	75.4
20. Provide reports to media regularly	68.5	75.2
Average: Assessment measures (#1–6)	54.9	66.7
Average: Policy development measures (#7–12)	58.2	60.2
Average: Assurance measures (#13–20)	55.4	64.4
Average: All activities	56.1	63.8

Source: Data from *B.J. Turnock, A.S. Handler, and C.A. Miller, Core Function-Related Local Public Health Practice Effectiveness, *Journal of Public Health Management and Practice,* Vol. 4, No. 5, pp. 26–32, © 1998, Aspen Publishers, Inc.; and **G.P. Mays et al., *Performing Essential Public Health Services in the Nation's Most Populous Communities: Who Contributes?* (in press).

tice performance measures from a 1993 national survey with NACCHO profile information for 264 LHDs.[34] Capacity factors linked to higher levels of practice performance included full-time agency head, larger annual expenditures, greater number of total and part-time staff, budgets derived from multiple funding sources, private health insurance as a significant budget component, and female agency heads.

A 1998 study of LHDs in the most populous jurisdictions identified several capacity factors associated with higher levels of practice performance.[33] These were population size, presence of a local board of health, existence of mixed or shared arrangements with a state health agency, and participation in public health activities by managed care plans and universities. This study also documented the substantial contribution (one-third of the total effort) to practice performance made by parties other than the governmental health agency in these jurisdictions. The most important contributors to process performance were state agencies, hospitals, local governmental agencies, nonprofit organizations, physicians and medical groups, universities, federally funded community health centers, managed care plans, and federal agencies.

The link between key processes and programs and services (outputs) offered by LHDs has also been examined. One study linked higher levels

Table 18–2 Mean Performance Scores for Local Health Jurisdictions by Population Size and Jurisdiction Type: 1995 ($n = 298$)

Local Health Jurisdiction Strata (by Population Size and Jurisdiction Type)	*Mean Performance Score (%)*
City 50,000 ($n = 12$)	47.9
City > 50,000 ($n = 10$)	77.0
County 50,000 ($n = 80$)	56.4
County > 50,000 ($n = 43$)	66.9
City–County 50,000 ($n = 34$)	57.1
City–County > 50,000 ($n = 24$)	59.2
Multicounty 50,000 ($n = 6$)	60.8
Multicounty > 50,000 ($n = 7$)	60.7
All other LHDs (all population sizes) ($n = 26$)	36.9
Jurisdiction unknown ($n = 56$)	54.8
Weighted sample total	56.1

Source: Reprinted from B.J. Turnock, A.S. Handler, and C.A. Miller, Core Function-Related Local Public Health Performance, *Journal of Public Health Management and Practice*, Vol. 4, No. 5, pp. 26–32, © 1998, Aspen Publishers, Inc.

of performance of key processes with a greater percentage of services directly provided, as well as with the following specific services: personal preventive and treatment, maternal and child health, chronic disease personal prevention, health education, injury control, dental health, case management services, and human immunodeficiency virus (HIV)/acquired immune deficiency syndrome (AIDS) testing.[34] In another study, only the provision of behavioral health services was linked with higher levels of performance of key public health processes.[33]

Lessons from Twentieth-Century Efforts

During the 85-year period from 1914 to 1999, an increasing body of information has been assembled on various aspects of public health system performance, its capacity (LHDs, expenditures, health officers, boards of health, state–local relationship, size and type of jurisdiction, agency staff, professional disciplines of staff, organizational structure, etc.), its processes (including key processes and outputs), and its outcomes. However, meaningful comparisons between the findings of the Committee on Administrative Practice's evaluations in the mid-1940s and those from the 1990s are not possible due to differences in approaches, methods, and measures. The earlier studies largely examined capacity, outputs (services), and outcomes, whereas later efforts focused on the essential public health services and emphasized key processes and outputs. These different approaches are evident in Exhibits 18–2 and 18–3, which provide key measures from the evaluation schedule and the 20 public health practice consensus measures described earlier.

Several lessons are apparent. The first is that measurement for the sake of measurement has never been the purpose of these activities. The intent has consistently been to gather information that would be useful for the improvement of local public health practice. However, the early instruments—including the appraisal form and evaluation schedule—placed considerable emphasis on the performance of specific services (outputs) rather than on more basic public health processes, such as community assessment or constituency building. None of these efforts has comprehensively examined the links between capacity, processes, and outcomes and their relationship to an effective governmental presence. Over more than eight decades of efforts, it has been easier to measure specific aspects of the public health system than to develop consensus as to what these measurements tell us about public health performance.

Although the efforts throughout the twentieth century have included outcome measures, most have failed to link capacity and process measures to these health outcomes. Prior to 1990, there was no real effort to do so. After 1990, only one study has attempted to relate LHD practice performance levels to some general community health status indicators.[35] No clear links were found, in part because the study did not focus on health outcomes that were targeted by community needs assessments. It is now possible to perform such an examination in environments where practice performance has been tracked over time, and where community needs assessments have led to interventions for high-priority community health problems. Various levels of practice performance can now be related to changes in key outcome measures in order to identify the effectiveness of the various practices. As suggested by the framework depicted in Figure 18–1, performance measurement in the public health system can now begin to measure capacities, processes, and outcomes in ways that allow for changes in one to be linked with changes in others.

APPLICATIONS USING PUBLIC HEALTH STANDARDS

Public health performance standards, when used prior to 1990, primarily related to capacities and the output aspects of public health practice rather than the key processes necessary to carry out the public health core functions characterized in the IOM report. Standards, or performance expectations, for public health practice developed after 1990 have focused on both key processes and outputs and have proven useful in a variety of applications, including agency self-assessment for capacity building, measures of performance in state–local public health systems, and state and national surveillance vis-à-vis objective 8.14. Still, these standards remain in an early stage of development, with poorly developed links to outcome standards established in national health objectives for the years 1990, 2000, and 2010.

The 1990s witnessed many public health organizations conducting organizational self-assessments, identifying strengths and weaknesses, and channeling this information into organizational capacity-building plans. The panel of performance expectations for local public health practice in the *Assessment Protocol for Excellence in Public Health (APEXPH)* has served as a blueprint for many public health agencies seeking to focus and strengthen their roles in their communities.[36] *APEXPH* adoption and implementation experience has been substantial, although not universal. Where *APEXPH* has been implemented widely, public health practice performance has been found to be substantially higher than where it is less frequently used. Evidence from the most extensive implementation of an *APEXPH* derivative on a statewide basis showed actual performance nearly doubling in Illinois over a two-year time frame.[37] However, few self-assessment tools

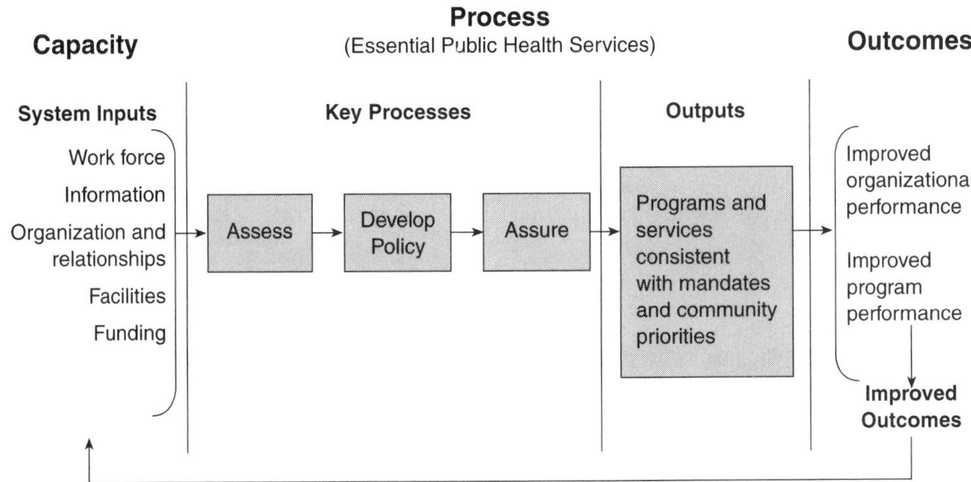

Figure 18–1 Framework for Measuring Public Health System Performance

other than *APEXPH* have been widely used within the public health community, and even *APEXPH* has lacked a strategic planning component and a focus on community public health systems. Only modest progress has been made toward the establishment of a framework for continuous improvement strategies, which facilitates the identification of best practices, identifies common causes of system performance, and promotes greater uniformity and consistency of public health activities.

Nonetheless, the evolving interest in, and growing acceptance of, performance measurement and quality improvement strategies among public health professionals and organizations appears evident in several recent developments. A prime example is the evolution of *APEXPH* into MAPP (Mobilizing for Action through Planning and Partnerships), with its increased emphasis on local public health systems rather than on community public health agencies.[38] MAPP will serve to promote broader community health improvement efforts that link public and private community partners to specific performance expectations in addressing priority health needs in the community.

Other examples of increased interest in performance measurement in public health are reflected in expanded community-driven collaborations, such as the local partnerships initiated under the National Turning Point Program and the enhanced community health improvement process outlined by the IOM in its 1997 report on performance monitoring to improve community health.[10] Both promote the use of performance measures and performance monitoring to link accountable partners to community improvement efforts. Although progress has been slow, the trend has been toward increasing the use of performance measurement as a tool for improving public health practice.[13]

There have been only a few attempts to use performance measures to examine the national public health system on a nationwide basis.[30,32,33] After a decade, there is little attention paid to whether the nation has achieved its year 2000 objective calling for 90 percent of the population to be effectively served. As a result, the potential for a nationwide performance measurement system to serve as a stimulus for reengineering and systemwide improvement remains yet unrealized. Without national leadership, states have struggled with how best to measure and improve public health practice in the 50 widely varying state–local systems that make up the national public health system.

Nearly 90 percent of the states reported some level of involvement in local public health performance assessment in 1997, although only one-half had an active and ongoing process.[39] Frameworks based on the core functions or essential public health services were used as the basis for these assessments in 22 states. However, few states use these assessments to allocate state funds across program areas and local jurisdictions, inform budget appropriation decisions made by the state legislature, or evaluate public health programs.[39] However, some states are using various combinations of capacity and process (including outputs) standards as a way to improve performance. The following examples from the states of Washington and Illinois illustrate some of these approaches.[40–43]

The state legislature in Washington adopted a framework for a statewide public health improvement plan in 1994 and directed the public health community to identify clearly the capacities needed to carry out core functions, the total cost associated with these capacities, the extent to which the capacities were in place, the difference between current and necessary capacity, and the funding needed to close the gap.[40,41] Capacity categories needed to address public health core functions were identified and capacity standards were developed. Subsequent concerns emerged that these capacity standards were overly subjective and not equally applicable for local health jurisdictions with different characteristics. This prompted the development of process and output standards for state and local public health agencies organized around community health assessment and four broad output-related categories (preventing communicable diseases, protecting against environmental risks, promoting healthy behaviors, and ensuring quality health services). These performance standards are described in Exhibit 18–4; they are to be used as the basis for contracts between the state and its LHDs.[40,41]

Exhibit 18–4 Proposed Standard for Public Health in Washington State, 2000

Protecting people from communicable disease

1. A surveillance and reporting system is maintained to identify emerging health threats.
2. Response plans delineate roles and responsibilities in the event of communicable disease outbreaks and natural disasters that threaten the health of people.
3. Communicable disease investigation and control procedures are in place and actions are documented.
4. Urgent public health messages are communicated quickly and clearly.
5. Communicable disease and disaster responses are routinely evaluated for opportunities for improving public health system response.

Understanding health issues

1. Public health assessment skills and tools are in place in all public health jurisdictions and their level continuously maintained and enhanced.
2. Information about environmental threats and community health status is collected, analyzed, and disseminated at intervals appropriate for the community.
3. Public health program results are evaluated to document effectiveness.
4. Health policy choices are guided by health assessment information, with involvement of representative community members.
5. Health data are handled so that confidentiality is protected and health information systems are secure.

Assuring a safe, healthy environment for people

1. Environmental health education is planned component of environmental health programs.
2. Services are available throughout the state to respond to environmental events or natural disasters that threaten the public's health.
3. Both environmental health risks and environmental health illness are tracked, recorded, and reported.
4. Compliance with environmental health regulations is sought through enforcement actions.

Prevention is best: Promoting healthy living

1. Public policies are adopted that support prevention priorities and that reflect consideration of scientifically based public health literature.
2. Active involvement of community members is sought in addressing prevention priorities.
3. Access to high-quality prevention services for individuals, families, and communities is encouraged and enhanced by disseminating information about available services and by engaging in and supporting collaborative partnerships.
4. Health promotion activities are provided.

Helping people get the services they need

1. Information is available at both the state and local level that describes the local health care system, including resources critical for public health protection and information about health care providers, facilities, and support services.
2. Information is collected, monitored, and disseminated regarding trends that, over time, affect access to critical health services.
3. Plans to reduce specific gaps in access to critical services are developed, implemented, and addressed through collaborative efforts.
4. Measures that address capacity, process, and outcomes for critical health care services are developed, monitored, and maintained.

Example

Protecting People from Disease and Injury

Standard 3

Communicable disease investigation and control procedures are in place and actions are documented.

Local public health indicators

1. Disease investigations begin within one working day, according to the disease investigation protocol.
2. Disease-specific investigation and control protocols are readily available to and implemented by staff. The protocols may include direct treatment, or referral to care, depending on the disease.
3. When control necessitates medical treatment, individuals are linked to private and public sources for treatment.
4. A procedure is documented for securing emergency biologics.

continues

Exhibit 18–4 continued

State public health indicators

1. Consultation and staff time are available for local support of disease investigation management during outbreaks or public health emergencies.
2. Procedures for obtaining state or federal assistance are written and disseminated.
3. Guidelines for communicable disease investigation and control are developed and shared with local jurisdictions, including model forms and records.

Source: Reprinted with permission from Public Health Systems Planning and Development, *Proposed Standards for Public Health in Washington State,* © 2000, Washington State Department of Health.

LHDs in Illinois have been subject to performance standards that were established by the state since the 1970s. After a series of strategic planning activities beginning about 1985, these performance standards were revised effective in 1993, changing the basis of certification by the state to standards based on processes (including outputs) related to public health core functions. The revised certification requirements call for LHDs to implement an adaptation of *APEXPH* known as IPLAN (Illinois Plan for Local Assessment of Needs), including both the organizational self-assessment and community health improvement planning components of *APEXPH.*[42,43] This produced a substantial change in patterns of performance of core-function-related practices, nearly doubling performance scores over a two-year period from 1992 to 1994.[37] Performance measures for Illinois LHDs are similar to those described in Exhibit 18–3. There is explicit authority in state law for the state health agency to establish performance standards for LHDs. The standards are promulgated through the state rule-making process with compliance reviews conducted every five years by the state health agency. Longitudinal assessments of performance of these practices in 1992, 1994, and 1999 have been linked with selected capacity factors as well as outcomes related to community health priorities identified in the first round of IPLAN implementation. This will enable an examination of the relationship between the various components of the public health system.

Experiences such as those found in these states, as well as in Missouri, Oregon, Florida, Michigan, South Carolina, and others, have laid the foundation for the development of a national public health performance standards program. The overall lack of uniformity and consistency among these various state efforts reflects the different needs, values, and circumstances of the relatively autonomous state–local public health networks across the United States. In part due to this diversity in type and focus of performance standards, the U.S. Centers for Disease Control and Prevention's Public Health Practice Program Office has promoted the development of national public health performance standards for use in several complementary applications. These applications include: (1) self-assessment and continuous improvement of local public health systems as part of the MAPP process, (2) surveillance of the public health system nationally and longitudinally, (3) accreditation of public health organizations, and (4) performance standards for use in state–local systems.[44]

The National Public Health Standards Program represents a partnership among national and state public health organizations to improve the public health delivery system through the development of local and state-based performance standards focused on capacity and processes, the systematic collection and analysis of performance-based data, and a national leadership effort to improve systemwide performance.[44] The NACCHO has coordinated the development of standards for local public health systems, the ASTHO has led the development of standards for state health agencies, and the National Association of Local Boards of Health (NALBOH) has guided the development of governance standards for local boards of health. Exhibit 18–5 provides examples of performance measures for local public health practice that may result from this process. Complementary to these standards is an extensive panel of national health objectives for the public health infrastructure, which is included in *Healthy People 2010* (Exhibit 18–6).[45] Primary goals for both of these efforts are to improve quality, enhance accountability, and strengthen the science base of public health practice.

A variety of salutary effects have been cited as potential benefits of a nationwide public health performance standards initiative. These include improved accountability; better resource deployment; enhanced capacity building for

Exhibit 18–5 Example of Public Health Performance Standards from Local Public Health Systems Draft Instrument: 1999

Essential service 2

Diagnose and investigate health problems and health hazards in the community

Indicators:

1. Identification and surveillance of health threats
2. Emergency preparedness and response plan
3. Investigate and respond to public health emergencies
4. Laboratory support for investigation of adverse health events and diagnosis of disease and injury

Standard for Indicator 3

The local public health system has:

- a team of public health workers and other professionals who analyze relevant data when an adverse public health event or potential threat occurs
- current, science-based protocols to guide the immediate investigation of communicable disease outbreaks, environmental health hazards, potential biologic agent threats, and large-scale disasters
- a community response team that updates and follows written protocols for emergency response, including implementing a program of contact and source tracking

Measures for Indicator and Standard 3

Does the local public health system maintain science-based protocols to guide an immediate investigation of public health threats?

If so, do these protocols address:

Communicable disease outbreaks?

If so, have these protocols been evaluated and updated within the past year?

Environmental health hazards?

If so, have these protocols been evaluated and updated within the past year?

Biologic agent threats?

If so, have these protocols been evaluated and updated within the past year?

Large-scale disasters?

If so, have these protocols been evaluated and updated within the past year?

Does the local public health system maintain written protocols for implementing an emergency program of contact and source tracking?

Have these protocols been evaluated and updated within the past year?

Have they been employed or tested within the past year?

Using a five-point scale (1 = low and 5 = high), rate the current status for your local public health system protocols to guide an appropriate response to adverse health events.

Source: Reprinted from Public Health Practice Program Office, *Draft Local Public Health Assessment Tool,* October 1999, Centers for Disease Control and Prevention.

Exhibit 18–6 *Healthy People 2010* Public Health Infrastructure Objectives

Data and Information Systems

- Increase the proportion of public health agencies that provide Internet and e-mail access for at least 75 percent of their employees and that teach employees how to use the Internet and other electronic information systems to apply data and information to public health practice.
- Increase the proportion of public health agencies that have made information available to the public in the last year on the leading health indicators, health status indicators, and priority data needs.
- Increase the proportion of all major national, state, and local health data systems that use geocoding to promote the development of geographic information system (GIS) at all levels.
- Increase the proportion of population-based Healthy People 2010 objectives for which national data are available for all population groups identified for the objective.
- Increase the proportion of leading health indicators, health status indicators, and priority data needs for which data—especially for select populations—are available at the tribal, state, and local levels.
- Increase the proportion of Healthy People 2010 objectives that are tracked regularly at the national level.
- Increase the proportion of Healthy People 2010 objectives for which national data are released within 1 year of data collection.

Skilled Workforce

- Increase the proportion of public health agencies that incorporate specific competencies in the essential public health services into personnel systems.
- Increase the proportion of schools for public health workers that integrate into their curricula specific content to develop competency in the essential public health services.
- Increase the proportion of public health agencies that provide continuing education to develop competency in essential public health services for their employees.

Effective Public Health Organizations

- Increase the proportion of public health agencies that meet national performance standards for essential public health services.
- Increase the proportion of tribes, states, and the District of Columbia that have a health improvement plan and increase the proportion of local jurisdictions that have a health improvement plan linked with their state plan.
- Increase the proportion of state and local public health agencies that provide or ensure comprehensive laboratory services to support essential public health services.
- Increase the proportion of public health agencies that provide or ensure comprehensive epidemiology services to support essential public health services.
- Increase the proportion of federal, state, and local jurisdictions that review and evaluate the extent to which their statutes, ordinances, and bylaws ensure the delivery of essential public health services.

Resources

- Increase the proportion of federal, state, and local public health agencies that gather accurate data on public health expenditures, categorized by essential public health service.

Prevention Research

- Increase the proportion of public health agencies that conduct or collaborate on population-based prevention research.

Source: Reprinted from *Healthy People 2010: Understanding and Improving Health,* 2000, U.S. Department of Health and Human Services.

community, state, and national public health systems; widespread use of best practices; and greater focus on mission and goals.[46] Depending on the lens used, each of these can be viewed as quality improvement, although their implementation presents formidable challenges.

CRITICAL ISSUES FOR SUCCESS

Several major issues challenge efforts to improve performance within the public health system through a national public health performance standards initiative. Resolution of these issues will require consensus on the purpose or purposes of the effort, the definition and components of quality, and the ability to effect widespread change.

For public health performance standards to succeed, their purpose must be clear. Although performance standards afford many potential benefits for improving the quality of public health practice, choices must be made with the selection of some benefits over others. At the most basic level are decisions about whether performance standards will be used primarily to improve quality, provide accountability, or strengthen the science base of public health practice. The particular aspects of the public health system to be improved must also be clear in order to avoid widely varying expectations of what is being improved, as well as subsequent dissatisfaction over the relevance of changes made.

There is increasing consensus that the key processes and outputs of public health practice are embodied in the essential public health services framework. But there is far less agreement as to what constitutes reasonable performance expectations for those key processes and outputs, and even less consensus as to the best approaches for their improvement. Some states such as Illinois and Missouri have developed performance standards based on the core functions and essential public health services. Others such as Oregon and Florida have developed standards that are organized only around programs and services. Some states have developed standards that cover both core functions and programs, such as the Michigan initiative accrediting LHDs. Washington State's efforts represent yet another approach by addressing both essential public health services and broad categories of public health outcomes. The optimal approach for organizing public health systems around public health standards is not clear. It is clear, however, that the focus and structure of those systems will establish the context in which decisions will be made as to the type of standards (minimum, best practices, optimal achievable), who will measure them (the practitioners, experts, or lesser expert outsiders), the form of disclosure (internally, among partners, fully public), who will act on the results (internal parties, outside enforcers), and even who or what is to be measured (individual organization, network, population-based community).

For performance measurement to foster quality improvement, there are several aspects of quality that must be considered. Performance measures must meet a variety of important tests, including validity, reliability, sensitivity, functionality, credibility, availability, and low potential for misuse. The first three of these are traditional criteria for performance indicators. *Validity* assesses the extent to which an indicator measures what it seeks to measure. *Reliability* assesses the extent to which an indicator will provide the same information if it is applied again. *Sensitivity* assesses whether an indicator is responsive or sensitive to changes in that which is being measured. *Functionality* implies the development of measures that are consistent with the overall purpose and goals of the public health system and that facilitate planning and evaluation efforts. Measures of performance must also be readily *available*, comprehendible, and *credible* to various audiences, and provide *minimal opportunity for misuse.* From a practical perspective, the potential for performance information to be misused, and actually used against the organization courageous enough to undertake performance measurement, is one of the greatest deterrents to performance measurement in the public health community today. Although these are considered basic criteria for performance measures, there have been relatively few attempts to test the public health performance measures that have been used to date for these attributes.

An important issue related to quality is whether the component qualities of a practice add up to quality or, in other words, which specific subqualities are important. For example, it is widely acknowledged that prenatal care improves perinatal outcomes, but little is known as to which aspects or qualities of that larger practice really make a difference. It is very possible that measuring broad practices such as those delineated in the core functions and essential public health services will yield the same dilemma. To date, there has been only limited consensus as to the best approaches for measuring public health practices. Several instruments use a series of yes/no responses as indicators of performance. Scaled responses assessing the degree to which a measure is performed have also been used. Another approach provides a detailed list of components of a practice and assesses quality based on the presence or absence of various components. Still another approach uses different respondents, such as non-LHD respondents in the community and LHD staff other than the agency director, as a strategy to obtain different perspectives on public health performance. Measurement efforts that use several or all of these strategies may provide a multidimensional snapshot of performance and quality that is more meaningful than those using only one. Exhibit 18–7 provides examples of various performance measures for one of the essential public health services: diagnosing and investigating public health problems and hazards in the community.

In order to understand better which qualities are important, there must be consensus within the public health community on a theoretical and conceptual model that explicates the relationships of the essential public health services to each other, to the capacity factors of the public health infrastructure, and to important community outcomes. Agreement on the key research issues and questions to be used to test this research framework is also necessary.

Another major consideration in terms of improving quality is whether performance measurement will be limited or widespread. If limited implementation leads to only scattered local data or piecemeal state and national information, there will be only minimal opportunities to improve quality. It is important to consider mechanisms and incentives for performance standards to be widely used. This may require expanded system-building efforts at the state and local level involving greater use of mandates, such as in statutes and rules. Other incentives, such as grants in aid and direct financial support, or the establishment of professional standards of practice and accreditation initiatives, may also be necessary. Without these kinds of system incentives, goodwill alone may not be enough to improve overall quality in the public health enterprise.

The establishment of a national accreditation or certification initiative for LHDs through either the national public health organizations or the Joint Commission on Accreditation of Healthcare Organizations (Joint Commission) has only recently been given serious consideration. Absent a federal initiative to support and fund core functions and essential public health services in state–local public health systems through block grants to states, a voluntary national accreditation program for LHDs may emerge as the most realistic approach to promoting widespread adoption of practice standards related to the core functions.

ACCREDITATION OF PUBLIC HEALTH ORGANIZATIONS

Interest in strategies to accredit public health organizations has arisen from several sources. Public health organizations, with the notable exception of academic programs leading to graduate degrees in public health, remain one of the few health-related entities that are not subject to national standards and review from an external accrediting body. Credentialing of both individuals and organizations has become such an accepted means of fostering quality improvement and accountability throughout the health sector that its absence from the public health system is noteworthy.

Accreditation of educational and health care organizations generally involves several steps. Initially, major stakeholders develop an independent entity that establishes the standards and review process to be applied. For example, the Joint Commission developed through the efforts of organized medicine and the hospital industry. Institutions of higher learning saw accreditation as a means to facilitate transferring credits earned at one institution to be used toward a degree at another. The Council on Education in Public Health (CEPH) now operates as a collaboration between the APHA and the Association of Schools of Public Health. Accreditation of public health organizations would almost certainly require the participation of the ASTHO and the NACCHO, as well as perhaps the NALBOH, the APHA, and possibly other na-

Exhibit 18–7 Performance Measure Examples for Essential Public Health Service 2: Diagnose and Investigate Health Problems and Health Hazards in the Community

1. Capacity measure
The health agency has trained staff and current science-based protocols to guide the immediate investigation of communicable disease outbreaks, environmental health hazards, potential biologic agent threats, and large-scale disasters. (Yes/No)

2. Practice measure (key processes and outputs)
For the jurisdiction(s) served by the health agency, timely investigations of adverse health events, including communicable disease outbreaks and environmental health hazards, are conducted on an ongoing basis. (Yes/No)

3. Outcome measure
No preventable deaths occur as a result of communicable disease outbreaks, environmental health hazards, biologic agents, or large-scale disasters. (Yes/No)

4. Components (key processes and outputs)
Which of the following characterize your health agency's efforts to diagnose and investigate health problems and health hazards?

A. Epidemiologic surveillance systems (such as sentinel physicians, hospital reporting, disease registers) are in place and linked with state and national surveillance systems.
B. Laboratory services necessary to support investigations of adverse health events and routine diagnostic and surveillance needs are available on a timely basis.
C. There is a written emergency response plan that describes the role of participating entities in the event of specific public health emergencies.
D. The community response team actively updates and follows written protocols for emergency response, including implementing a program of contact and source tracking.
E. Sanitation and environmental expertise are available for investigations and emergencies.
F. Epidemiologic expertise is available for investigations and emergencies.
G. Evidence-based protocols guide investigations.
H. Health-related hazards, behaviors, and risk factors are analyzed in terms of their impact on disease and morbidity.
I. Epidemiologic and behavioral science techniques are used to collect and analyze disease, injury, and environmental trends and patterns.
J. A formal monitoring process exists to track persistent threats and to alert communities to possible environmental assaults or biologic agent outbreaks.
K. Current, evidence-based protocols are in place to guide the immediate investigation of communicable disease outbreaks, environmental health hazards, potential biologic agent threats, and large-scale disasters.

5. Extent needs met
How effective are the activities in your health district to diagnose and investigate health problems and health hazards in the community? (Meets all/most/half/some/no needs)

6. Contributors
Which of the following stakeholders contribute to the performance of this essential public health service? (state health agencies, hospitals, local government agencies, nonprofit organizations, physicians and medical groups, universities, federally funded community health centers, managed care plans, federal agencies)

7. Percent contribution measure
What percentage of the total effort for performance of this essential public health service is attributed to each of the contributing parties?

8. Multiple respondents
Additional respondents inside health agency and community respondents outside health agency provide responses to questions 1–7 above.

tional public health organizations as major stakeholders in the process.

Most accreditation activities commence with a self-study or self-assessment by the entity seeking to be accredited. The self-assessment document is submitted to the accrediting body and examined by staff and experts who then site visit the applicant in order to verify compliance with the standards. Decisions as to full or conditional accreditation are based on the extent to which standards are addressed. Finally, the results are made public. The highest levels of compliance generally result in longer time frames until the next cycle begins. If plans of correction are required, these are generally reviewed on an interim basis or examined at the time of the next review. In this elaborate process, the key elements are the standards and the reviewers. Considerable costs accrue to the applicant organization, which pays a fee to the accrediting body and absorbs the considerable costs of preparation, on-site review, and follow-up.

Although accreditation is considered to be voluntary, in many applications, it is anything but that. Both hospitals and schools of public health, for example, perceive accreditation as essential to doing business. Accreditation has its greatest demand where there are multiple parties that value and/or require it. Third-party payers and governmental regulatory agencies require accreditation of hospitals. A variety of federal grants and contracts can only be awarded to accredited schools of public health. Creating a variety of end users for accredited status is a formidable challenge for the public health system.

At the national level, there are two organizations with experience in accrediting activities related to public health: the Community Health Accreditation Program (CHAP) of the National League for Nursing and the Joint Commission. A third model is the state-based accreditation program that was developed in Michigan.

The National League for Nursing's CHAP initially established standards for public health nursing and later for home health services.[47,48] After 1996, the focus extended to public health organizations in order to establish standards for a wide variety of public health programs in a more flexible format, emphasize the importance of the interests and rights of individual consumers of public health services, strengthen the long-term viability of public health organizations, and give recognition to the importance of public health programs in relation to the entire health care system. Standards of excellence are organized around structure and function, quality of services and products provided, resources, and long-term viability. LHDs in South Carolina are accredited through the CHAP with several levels of function and services reviewed by external survey teams following a self-study performed by the agency. The process is mandatory (LHDs in South Carolina are offices of the state agency) and is implemented as a method to ensure standardization across the state as well as to monitor the quality of services offered statewide. The state health agency is also accredited under these standards.

The Joint Commission does not currently have standards for LHDs, but does have a Network Accreditation Program for managed care organizations and integrated delivery systems. Applicants must clearly define the population served and include an accountable entity that complies with standards for health promotion and disease prevention services for the defined population. Standards address the establishment of the network's role in the delivery of primary, secondary, and tertiary preventive services. They also address collaboration with community leaders and organizations in the design of services, preventive services that are both efficacious and appropriate to the needs of the community, and educational needs relating to health promotion and disease prevention.[49,50]

In Michigan, LHDs voluntarily participate in an accreditation program consisting of a self-assessment and an on-site review.[51] An extensive set of accreditation standards is available in published form addressing requirements for core capacity, cost shared, and categorical services. The on-site review serves to validate and verify self-reported compliance. Although voluntary, there are links with state funding. An external accreditation commission housed in the Michigan Public Health Institute and based on authority conferred in state statutes coordinates the entire process. Additional information on the Michigan accreditation program is provided in Exhibit 18–8.

Accreditation initiatives often favor optimal rather than minimal standards and prefer to focus on clearly accountable entities (e.g., a local public health department rather than a community public health system).[52] Their experiences also suggest that the value of accreditation is derived from how extensively the credential is accepted and used by

Exhibit 18–8 Michigan Local Health Department Accreditation Self-Assessment Instrument: 1997

A. Health assessment (1 standard, 4 indicators)
B. Policy development (2 standards, 5 indicators)
C. Quality improvement (1 standard, 4 indicators)
D. Health promotion (1 standard, 1 indicator)
E. Health protection (4 standards, 8 indicators)
F. Administration (9 standards, 30 indicators)
G. Competent work force (2 standards, 4 indicators)
H. Food service sanitation (10 standards, 12 indicators)
I. Communicable disease control (3 standards, 10 indicators)
J. Hearing (6 standards, 11 indicators)
K. Immunization (6 standards, 20 indicators)
L. On-site sewage treatment management (7 standards, 13 indicators)
M. Sexually transmitted disease (4 standards, 4 indicators)
N. Vision (6 standards, 13 indicators)
O. HIV/AIDS prevention and intervention (1 standard, 4 indicators)
P. Maternal and infant support services (1 standard, 5 indicators)
Q. Family planning (28 standards, 55 indicators)

Example: Health protection (E above)

Standard

The local health department ensures a system for monitoring, inspection, intervention, and enforcement activities that eliminates or reduces exposure and risk from environmental threats and communicable diseases.

Indicators

The local health department employs epidemiologic tools such as sampling, cluster analysis, biomapping, interview techniques, or computer software to perform epidemiologic analysis, either on-site or through an agreement with the state or other qualified entity, in order to monitor the environmental and communicable disease risks to the public. (Fully Met, Not Met)

The local health department employs legal mechanisms to ensure compliance with health protection standards. (Fully Met, Not Met)

Source: Reprinted from *Michigan Local Health Department Accreditation Self-Assessment Report,* © 1997, Michigan Department of Community Health, Michigan Public Health Institute.

external stakeholders. For accreditation to be successful, there must be both short- and long-term benefits. Public health goals for a healthier population reflect appropriate long-term benefits. However, short-term and measurable benefits of accreditation to public health organizations must also be articulated, if for no other reason than to provide a reasonable counterbalance to the cost in time, dollars, and political energy needed for the effort.[53] Some potential benefits might include simplified interstate or intrastate transfer of data, legislative exemptions from restrictions on access to confidential data, ability to compete directly for federal funds, contracting advantages with Medicaid and other state agencies, or even a market advantage in competition for directly contracting with the private sector for some services. Also, peer pressure on localities that do not adequately support their public health responsibilities could serve as an inducement. There is a growing consensus that self-assessment is now well established in the public health system and that the time has come to make the process formal and public.[54]

Voluntary accreditation of public health organizations could lead to greater interest in the possibility of credentialing various segments of the public health work force. In one form or another, there are already credentials for some public health workers, including sanitarians, health educators, public health nurses, and public health physicians. Interest in credentialing public health administrators has also grown, with New Jersey licensing local public health administrators and Illinois developing an independent competency-based certification program for public health administrators working in a variety of public and private agencies. These developments are consistent with one public health leader's observation: "There is a compelling need to view professional preparation programs, the public health workforce, and operating public health units as parallel but interested partners that share a common mission: protecting and promoting health."[54(p.23)]

• • •

Although reports of the demise of the public health infrastructure may have overstated the case, the outlook for its spontaneous improvement remains bleak. To some extent, public health has undermined its own credibility by holding itself out to be the guardian and protector of the public's health while lacking the capacity to deliver on its promise, or to measure its ability to do so.

Performance measurement leading to performance improvement initiatives has been undertaken in many different settings during the twentieth century, including the public sector, where they have been applied to improving governmental processes, programs, and services. Its application to improving the performance of public health core functions, although only being undertaken in a few locales, has been largely positive, however, suggesting that a national public health performance standards program based on the essential public health services framework could also be successful. "What gets measured gets done" is the performance measurement analogy for what is known in research as the Hawthorne effect.[55] Its lesson for the public health community is that the measurement process itself influences the credibility and consistent performance of that which is measured.

With interest increasing inside the public health community and broader participation in public health improvement efforts evolving in many states and localities, the opportunity for a national public health performance standards program emphasizing performance measurement and quality improvement strategies has never been greater. Critical factors that must be addressed in order for this effort to be successful include agreement as to the ultimate purpose of performance improvement efforts, delineation of the specific measures to be used, and mechanisms to promote their widespread use. It is unlikely that any one set of measures and one single process can accomplish all three goals (quality improvement, enhanced accountability, and strengthened science base) of a national public health performance standards initiative. Rather, it is likely that different formulations of standards and measures based on the essential public health services framework will be necessary.

Short of a national system for public health performance measurement, there is a continuing need for concerted efforts to reform state–local public health systems, organizing them around the core functions and essential public health services rather than categorical programs and services. At the core of these systems should be tools such as MAPP, community health improvement processes linked to *Healthy People 2010* objectives and leading health indicators.[56,57] It is only within this context that accreditation initiatives for organizations and individuals, grant funding linked to the performance of essential public health services, report cards, and evaluative research activities will be meaningful and valued.

In sum, public health performance standards will improve quality if the performance standards focus on all aspects of the public health system—its capacity, its processes, and the links between these and important community health outcomes—and if the public health community accepts and uses them. Early attention to and consensus around these issues will determine the quality of public health practice in the twenty-first century.

CHAPTER REVIEW

1. Measurement for the sake of measurement has never been the purpose of public health performance measurement activities conducted in the United States. The intent has consistently been to gather information that is useful to administrators, policy makers, and practitioners in improving public health practice.
2. Most of the public health performance measurement strategies developed since 1990 are based on the framework identified in the 1988 IOM report, *The Future of Public Health.* These strategies consist mainly of process- and activity-based measures of performance linked to one of the IOM's core public health functions of assessment, policy development, and assurance.
3. Prior to 1990, public health performance standards related primarily to capacities and the output aspects of public health practice rather than the key processes necessary to carry out the public health core functions characterized in the IOM report. Standards, or performance expectations, for public health practice developed after 1990 have focused on both key processes and outputs and have proven useful in a variety of applications, including agency self-assessment for capacity building. Still, these standards remain in an early stage of development, with poorly developed links to outcome standards as established in national health objectives for the years 1990, 2000, and 2010.
4. Several factors appear critical to the success of performance measurement efforts that are carried out within individual organizations and across multiple public health systems.
   - The purpose of measurement must be clear. At the most basic level, administrators must decide whether performance measures will be used primarily to improve quality, demonstrate accountability, or strengthen the evidence base for public health practice.
   - Consensus must be reached among the major stakeholders involved as to what the key processes and outputs to be measured are, what constitutes reasonable performance expectations in these domains, and what the best approaches for improving performance in these domains are.
   - Performance measures must meet several important criteria, including measurement validity, reliability, sensitivity, functionality, credibility, availability, cost-effectiveness, and low potential for misuse. Some of these criteria can be verified through objective empirical tests; others are necessarily subject to the judgments of the stakeholders involved.
5. Accreditation programs may assist public health organizations in improving internal quality and demonstrating external accountability through the application of effective performance measurement activities.

REFERENCES

1. H.J. Harrington, *The Improvement Process: How America's Leading Companies Improve Quality* (New York: McGraw-Hill, 1978).
2. J.S. Wholey and H.P. Hatry, "The Case for Performance Monitoring," *Public Administration Review* 52 (1992): 604–610.
3. J.S. Wholey and K.E. Newcomer, "Clarifying Goals, Reporting Results," *New Directors for Evaluation* 75 (1997): 91–98.
4. C.E. Trott and J. Baj, *Building State Systems Based on Performance: The Workforce Development Experience, A Guide for States* (Washington, DC: National Governors Association, 1996).
5. E.B. Perrin et al., eds., *Health Performance Measurement in the Public Sector: Principles and Policies for Implementing an Information Network* (Washington, DC: National Research Council, National Academy Press, 1999).

6. P. Rossi and H. Freeman, *Evaluation: A Systematic Approach* (Thousand Oaks, CA: Sage Publications, 1994).
7. Joint Commission on Accreditation of Healthcare Organizations, *Primer on Indicator Development and Application: Measuring Quality in Health Care* (Oakbrook Terrace, IL: 1990).
8. Public Health Functions Steering Committee, *Public Health in America* (Washington, DC: Public Health Service, 1994). <http://www.health.gov/phfunctions>
9. Institute of Medicine, Committee on the Future of Public Health, *The Future of Public Health* (Washington, DC: National Academy Press, 1988).
10. Institute of Medicine, Committee on Using Performance Monitoring To Improve Community Health, *Improving Health in the Community: A Role for Performance Monitoring* (Washington, DC: National Academy Press, 1997).
11. National Research Council, Panel on Performance Measures and Data for Public Health Performance Partnership Grants, *Assessment of Performance Measures for Public Health, Substance Abuse, and Mental Health* (Washington, DC: National Academy Press, 1997).
12. Northwest Prevention Effectiveness Center and the Health Policy Analysis Program, School of Public Health and Community Medicine, University of Washington, *Enabling Performance Measurement Activities in the States and Communities* [USDHHS Grant no. U48/CCU009654] (Seattle, WA: University of Washington, 1998).
13. B.J. Turnock and A.S. Handler, "From Measuring to Improving Public Health Practice," *Annual Review of Public Health* 18 (1997): 261–282.
14. H.F. Vaughan, "Local Health Services in the United States: The Story of CAP," *American Journal of Public Health* 62 (1972): 95–108.
15. American Public Health Association, Committee on Municipal Health Department Practice, "First Report, Part 1," *American Journal of Public Health 12,* no. 2 (1922): 7–15.
16. American Public Health Association, Committee on Municipal Health Department Practice, "First Report, Part 2," *American Journal of Public Health 12,* no. 2 (1922): 138–347.
17. American Public Health Association, Committee on Administrative Practice, "Appraisal Form for City Health Work," *American Journal of Public Health 16,* no. 1 (suppl.) (1926): 1–65.
18. W.W. Walker, "The New Appraisal Form for Local Health Work," *American Journal of Public Health 29,* no. 5 (1939): 490–500.
19. W.L. Halverson, "A Twenty-Five Year Review of the Work of the Committee on Administrative Practice," *American Journal of Public Health 35,* no. 12 (1945): 1,253–1,259.
20. American Public Health Association, Committee on Administrative Practice, *Evaluation Schedule for Use in the Study and Appraisal of Community Health Programs* (New York: American Public Health Association, 1947).
21. F.W. Krantz, "The Present Status of Full-Time Local Health Organizations," *Public Health Reports* 57 (1942): 194–196.
22. H. Emerson and M. Luginbuhl, *Local Health Units for the Nation* (New York: Commonwealth Fund, 1945).
23. U.S. Public Health Service, *Healthy People 2000: National Health Promotion and Disease Prevention Objectives* [DHHS Pub. No. (PHS) 91–50212] (Washington, DC: U.S. Government Printing Office, 1990).
24. National Association of County and City Health Officials, *1990 National Profile of Local Health Departments* (Washington, DC: 1992).
25. National Association of County and City Health Officials, *1992–1993 National Profile of Local Health Departments* (Washington, DC: 1995).
26. C.A. Miller et al., "A Screening Survey To Assess Local Public Health Performance," *Public Health Reports 109,* no. 5 (1994): 659–664.
27. C.A. Miller et al., "A Proposed Method for Assessing the Performance of Local Public Health Functions and Practices," *American Journal of Public Health 84,* no. 11 (1994): 1,743–1,749.
28. T.B. Richards et al., "Assessing Public Health Practice: Application of Ten Core Function Measures of Community Health in Six States," *American Journal of Preventive Medicine 11,* no. 6 (suppl.) (1995): 36–40.
29. T.B. Richards et al., "Evaluating Local Public Health Performance at a Community Level on a Statewide Basis," *Journal of Public Health Management and Practice 1,* no. 4 (1995): 70–83.
30. B.J. Turnock et al., "Local Health Department Effectiveness in Addressing the Core Functions of Public Health," *Public Health Reports* 109 (1994): 653–658.
31. J.E. Rohrer et al., "Assessing Public Health Performance in Iowa's Counties," *Journal of Public Health Management and Practice 3,* no. 3 (1997): 10–15.
32. B.J. Turnock et al., "Core Function-Related Local Public Health Performance," *Journal of Public Health Management and Practice 4,* no. 5 (1998): 26–32.
33. G.P. Mays et al., *Performing Essential Public Health Services in the Nation's Most Populous Communities: Who Contributes?* (submitted for publication).
34. A.S. Handler and B.J. Turnock, "Local Health Department Effectiveness in Addressing the Core Functions of Public Health: Essential Ingredients," *Journal of Public Health Policy* 17 (1996): 460–483.
35. S.E. Schenk et al., "Public Health Performance Related to Selected Health Status and Risk Measures," *American Journal of Preventive Medicine 11,* no. 6 (suppl.) (1995): 55–57.

36. National Association of County Health Officials, *An Assessment Protocol for Excellence in Public Health* (Washington, DC: 1990).
37. B.J. Turnock et al., "Capacity-Building Influences on Illinois Local Health Departments," *Journal of Public Health Management and Practice 1,* no. 3 (1995): 50–58.
38. National Association of County and City Health Officials, *Mobilizing for Action through Planning and Partnerships* (Washington, DC: NACCHO, 2000, in press).
39. G.P. Mays et al., "Assessing the Performance of Local Public Health Systems: A Survey of State Health Agency Efforts," *Journal of Public Health Management and Practice 4,* no. 4 (1998): 63–78.
40. Washington State Department of Health, *Public Health Improvement Plan: A Blueprint for Action* (Olympia, WA: 1996).
41. Washington State Department of Health, *Proposed Standards for Public Health in Washington State* (Olympia, WA: 2000).
42. Illinois Roadmap Implementation Task Force, *Improving the Public Health System: The Road to Better Health for All of Illinois* (Springfield, IL: Illinois Department of Public Health, 1990).
43. Illinois Local Health Liaison Committee, *Project Health: The Reengineering of Public Health in Illinois* (Springfield, IL: Illinois Department of Public Health, 1994).
44. Centers for Disease Control and Prevention, Public Health Practice Program Office, National Public Health Performance Standards Program, <http://www.phppo.cdc.gov/dphs/nphsp> (31 March 2000).
45. U.S. Department of Health and Human Services, *Healthy People 2010: Understanding and Improving Health* (Washington, DC: USDHHS-PHS, 2000).
46. B.J. Turnock, "Can Public Health Performance Standards Improve the Quality of Public Health Practice? *Journal of Public Health Management and Practice 6,* no. 5 (2000).
47. Community Health Accreditation Program, *Standards of Excellence for Public Health Organizations* (New York: CHAP, National League for Nursing, 1997).
48. T. Ayer, "Accreditation through Standards of Excellence for Public Health Organizations," *Journal of Public Health Management and Practice 4,* no. 4 (1998): 24–27.
49. Joint Commission on Accreditation of Healthcare Organizations, *1996 Comprehensive Accreditation Manual for Health Care Networks* (Oakbrook Terrace, IL: 1996).
50. Joint Commission on Accreditation of Healthcare Organizations, *Assessing and Improving Community Health Care Delivery* (Oakbrook Terrace, IL: 1994).
51. Michigan Public Health Institute, *Michigan Local Health Department Accreditation Self-Assessment Report* (Lansing, MI; Michigan Department of Community Health, 1997).
52. P.M. Schyve, "Joint Commission Perspectives on Accreditation of Public Health Practice," *Journal of Public Health Management and Practice 4,* no. 4 (1998): 28–33.
53. E.L. Greenberg, "How Accreditation Could Strengthen Local Public Health: An Examination of Models from Managed Care and Insurance Regulators," *Journal of Public Health Management and Practice 4,* no. 4 (1998): 33–37.
54. P.P. Evans and C.W. Keck, "Accreditation Well-Established in Higher Education; Offers Useful Lessons for Other Arenas," *Journal of Public Health Management and Practice 4,* no. 4 (1998): 19–23.
55. F.J. Roethlisberger and W.J. Dickson, *Management and the Worker* (Cambridge, MA: Harvard University Press, 1947).
56. E.L. Baker et al., "Health Reform and the Health of the Public: Forging Community Health Partnerships," *Journal of the American Medical Association 272,* no. 16 (1994): 1,276–1,282.
57. J.A. Harrell and E.L. Baker, "The Essential Services of Public Health," *Leadership in Public Health 3,* no. 3 (1994): 27–31.

CHAPTER 19

Communication and Media Relations

Douglas Hirano
Brad Christensen

Developing and managing successful public health activities require the ability to communicate effectively with the variety of stakeholders involved in these efforts. Increasingly, public health organizations rely on explicit communication strategies to manage relationships with the media, policy makers, and the public. Key channels of communication include press releases, news conferences, radio, cable and satellite television, pamphlets, posters, videotaped messages, and town meetings. Media relationships can be especially helpful in mounting populationwide health promotion and disease prevention interventions. External communication strategies should be coordinated with internal communication processes to ensure organizational performance.

COMMUNICATION IN PUBLIC HEALTH

Robert Frost once wryly noted that "good fences make good neighbors." Nothing could be further from the truth in the effective practice of public health. Effective communication is in fact vital to the ability to improve the quality and quantity of life locally, nationally, and globally. And although the science of public health has continued to advance, the concomitant ability to communicate results and accomplishments has lagged behind.

This is one reason why public health practice—for all its success in improving life expectancy over the past 100 years—continues to toil in relative obscurity compared with organized medical practice. As a result, population-based approaches to health improvement continue to suffer from poor funding and limited advocacy. It has been estimated that health promotion and disease prevention expenditures constitute 3 percent of health care expenditures.[1]

An added difficulty is the fact that public health activities such as the prevention of epidemics, assurance of safe water and food, and maintenance of health statistics are largely transparent to the general public and, consequently, undervalued. Thus, although former Surgeon General C. Everett Koop's well-known comment, "Health care is vital to all of us some of the time, but public health is vital to all of us all of the time," resonates with public health professionals, it often falls on deaf ears when aimed at the public, the media, and policy makers.

Fortunately, the realization that "good communication equals good public health" is growing. Three decades ago, public health communication was generally limited to sterile brochures, pamphlets, and early morning public service announcements (PSAs). Modern public health organizations use social marketing and entertainment education techniques to encourage lifestyle changes, media advocacy to transform health policy making, and risk communication to better characterize health risks.[2] Public health administrators are also becoming increasingly aware that organizational efficiency and employee morale are dependent on effective organizational communication.

Nonetheless, the effective use of communication to improve public health practice is still the exception rather than the rule. Public health administrators continue to learn on the job about communication strategies and do admirably well under many circumstances. However, given the importance of communication in public health, these strategies should not be left to chance. Academic institutions and continuing education programs need to offer pragmatic training in effective communication strategies to improve public health practice.

In the long run, the ability to develop and carry out a strategic communication plan at program, organization, and population levels will go a long way toward strengthening public health practice and also providing public health professionals with the visibility and credibility that are needed to lead health system change.

This chapter describes strategies for public health administrators to improve organizational performance through enhanced communication. This includes a major focus on relations with the media, as well as strategies for effective communication with policy makers, the public, and stakeholders within the organization. Basic principles of social marketing, media advocacy, and risk communication are examined briefly for their roles in communication strategies. These concepts are covered in more detail in other chapters.

Communication Purposes

Communication undergirds almost all of public health practice. Listed below are some examples of intended outcomes of effective public health communication. This listing is not meant to be comprehensive, but instead to suggest the scope of the role of communication in public health practice.

- *Increased service utilization:* To ensure that available services target at-risk populations, outreach is necessary. Examples of services requiring publicity include immunizations, primary care, family planning, and tobacco cessation. Targeted communication regarding service availability can ensure that populations access these services appropriately.
- *Healthier lifestyles:* Public health organizations play critical roles in informing the public about the important role of personal lifestyle and behaviors in determining health status. Modifiable behaviors such as tobacco use, lack of physical activity, and poor nutrition contribute to 700,000 premature deaths a year in the United States.[3] Effective communication strategies can convey the risks of such activities to population groups most affected by them.
- *Improved organizational performance:* Public health organizations, like other bureaucratic institutions, require effective internal and external communication strategies to ensure that the organization functions at optimum efficiency and effectiveness and that employee morale remains high.
- *Supportive health policies:* Effective public health policy development requires regular communication with the media, elected officials, lobbyists, and community groups, among others.
- *Effective emergency management:* The threat of public health emergencies (e.g., natural disasters, bioterrorist activities, and communicable disease epidemics) requires a strong and rapid emergency communication system among public health organizations, emergency care providers, public safety agencies, medical care providers, and many others.

How pervasive is the need for effective communication in public health? An analysis of more than 300 objectives for the *Healthy People 2000* goals identified 219 objectives in which health communication played a primary or secondary role in their accomplishment.[4] Exhibit 19–1 shows the 10 essential public health services and the potential role of communication in each of these services.

Exhibit 19–1 The Role of Communication in Performing the Essential Public Health Services

1. Monitor health status and solve community health problems.
   Communication role: Deliver relevant health status information to communities, particularly changes in rates that suggest the need for intervention; provide an opportunity for communities to voice concerns about perceived health problems.
2. Diagnose and investigate health problems and health hazards in the community.
   Communication role: Notify individuals and communities of potential health hazards (e.g., issue traveler's advisories in areas with known vectorborne disease transmission).
3. Inform, educate, and empower people about health issues.
   Communication role: Use multiple levels of communication, including social marketing and community education, to bring about healthy lifestyles.
4. Mobilize community partnerships and action to identify and solve health problems.
   Communication role: Assist in the development of coalitions and partnerships that will lead to collaborative action.
5. Develop policies and plans that support individual and community health efforts.
   Communication role: Inform the public about new laws that affect health, such as laws protecting the confidentiality of human immunodeficiency virus/acquired immune deficiency syndrome information; share draft planning documents with stakeholders as a means to receive input and to generate investment in outcomes.
6. Enforce laws and regulations that protect and ensure safety.
   Communication role: Share information with the regulated community to facilitate the adherence to proper licensing and safety standards; ensure easy access (e.g., Web site availability) to the required forms and rules relating to licensing and regulation.
7. Link people to needed personal health services and ensure the provision of health care when otherwise unavailable.
   Communication role: Inform medically underserved populations about opportunities for health care and the need for preventive services.
8. Ensure a competent public health and personal health care work force.
   Communication role: Inform public health practitioners and health care providers about training opportunities, such as satellite videoconferences.
9. Evaluate effectiveness, accessibility, and quality of personal and population-based health services.
   Communication role: Inform policy makers about the efficacy of population-based health services.
10. Research for new insights and innovative solutions to health problems.
    Communication role: Publish results of applied research in peer-reviewed journals so that other agencies can translate findings into more effective public health practice.

Source: Essential Public Health Services Work Group of the Public Health Functions Steering Committee.

Channels of Communication

The practice of public health offers a variety of ways to communicate information, called *channels* of communication (the term *media* is also used). A channel defines the route or method by which communication occurs. A channel of communication can be in writing (e.g., a scientific manuscript, a memorandum, newsletter, or news release) or by verbal means (e.g., news conference, radio interview, or conference call). During recent decades, additional avenues for communicating have evolved, including cable and satellite television, computer networking, electronic mail, automatic message systems, and videotaped messages. Other channels include health fairs, pamphlets, posters, and PSAs. Each mode may have certain advantages in certain situations. Table 19–1 includes a list of typical communication purposes with channels and intended audience.

Table 19–1 Typical Communication Purposes with Channels and Intended Audience

Purpose	*Communication Channel*	*Intended Audience*
Disease outbreak announcement	News media	General public
Research study results	Scientific journal	Public health practitioners
Policy recommendation	Newspaper (op-ed piece)	Policy makers
Behavioral change/ social marketing	Television spots/commercials	General public
New program initiative	Press conference	General public
Outreach	Lay health workers	Ethnic communities
Strategic planning	Community meeting	Community members
General health information	Health fair	Community members

The choice of an appropriate channel depends on content as well as audience. Certain audiences prefer certain communication channels. For instance, the preference of video-age young people for short, visually oriented messages—what futurist John Naisbett called "blips"—has prompted some public health agencies to create short, visual PSAs targeting teens. In contrast, technical audiences prefer written documents, often with oral explanation available.

Channels can be used to receive information as well as to transmit information. Town halls, advisory groups, focus groups, and customer satisfaction surveys are means to gather information. Receiving useful information from a number of sources is often as critical as sending information.

Principles of Effective Communication

The field of communication is broad in scope, and a large body of literature is available on the topic. The purpose of this section is to describe the key characteristics of good communication and to stimulate further research and practice in this area. Listed below are several key principles of communication that are particularly relevant to public health practice.

- *Keep messages and language simple.* There are few reasons to try to communicate information in a manner that is complex. In general, complexity will only obscure the central message and important supporting points. Simple and short messages are more memorable and easily understood. Plain language is best. One state epidemiologist, in describing an outbreak of a fecal-orally transmitted disease, used the term *poop* in numerous television and radio interviews. This may not have sounded scholarly, but it communicated effectively. In developing written materials, it must be remembered that almost half of the population reads at very basic levels—approximately eighth grade or below.[5]
- *Ensure cultural competency.* Society is becoming increasingly diverse. Estimates suggest that by the year 2050, the majority of Americans will be racial/ethnic minorities. Conceptually, cultural competence is expressed by communicating acceptance, deep understanding, and responsiveness to the needs and concerns of members of special populations.[6] This requires "the willingness and ability to utilize community-based values, traditions, and practices in developing and evaluating interventions, communication, and other activities."[7(p.4)]
- *Strike while the iron is hot.* Sometimes, timing is everything in effective communication. For example, during the 1996 out-

break of bovine spongiform encephalopathy, otherwise known as "mad cow" disease, Hawaiian health officials staved off cuts to the state laboratory by emphasizing the need for strong laboratory capacity to detect emerging pathogens such as that causing "mad cow" disease.[8]

- *Use multiple communication channels.* Studies indicate that messages provided in multiple ways (e.g., radio, television, newspapers) are more likely to be remembered than those provided through a single medium. Studies indicate that people retain 20 percent of what they read; however, if they read and hear, they retain 65 percent of the message.[9]
- *Listen.* Communication efforts that include an opportunity for interactive dialogue can be effective. This is true for town halls, forums, and other types of meetings where input is the main goal. The purpose of the interaction is to receive useful information from policy makers, constituents, and others to shape policies and programs and to establish a relationship based on openness and shared understanding.

Target Audiences

One of the most critical factors in effective communication is knowing to whom you are trying to communicate. Although this seems a simple principle, it is violated on almost a daily basis in the field of public health. All too frequently, one-size-fits-all messages are crafted for broad delivery to the public. Thinking of the general public as an audience may make sense conceptually, but it makes little sense for many communication strategies.

As in business marketing, customizing communication strategies to smaller subgroups (i.e., audience segments) of a larger population often pays dividends in terms of information dissemination. Audiences tend to vary by factors (e.g., race/ethnicity, socioeconomic status, age, and educational level) that will affect communication effectiveness. Examples of potential public health target audiences include health care providers, women of childbearing age, older adults, individuals with disabilities, monolingual individuals, policy makers, other public health practitioners, and the media.

Audience segmentation involves breaking a larger group into smaller, more homogeneous audiences and targeting those audiences with appropriate messages, using appropriate channels. Segmentation avoids sending the same message through the same channel to a large heterogenous group, resulting in inefficiency and suboptimal communication. For instance, in developing its tobacco prevention campaign, the Arizona Department of Health Services used focus groups to gather information from adolescents regarding potentially effective media messages targeted at teens. The result was a media campaign that led to a 96 percent statewide prompted recall among adolescents of the campaign slogan: "Tobacco: tumor-causing, teeth staining, smelly, puking, habit."[10]

Segmentation can also help avoid information gaps caused by selective attention. For instance, audiences who are better informed about and more favorably inclined toward good nutrition are more likely to be reached by community education programs than those who are less informed, less favorable, and less likely to seek out, receive, or retain nutrition information. Community education campaigns can inadvertently widen the information gap unless uninformed populations are targeted and specific media and messages are tailored for the hard-to-reach.

BUILDING CONSTITUENCY AND VISIBILITY

Public health practitioners have made great strides in improving communication effectiveness, but there are still areas in need of further improvement. This section will discuss strategies for communicating with three separate constituencies: communities, policy makers, and stakeholders within the organization itself. Although numerous other constituencies must be engaged, these three are important to effective public health practice in any setting.

Communicating with Communities

One of the most difficult challenges in the practice of public health is for agencies to maintain good communication with the communities they serve. This task is difficult for a number of reasons. Communities can be somewhat diffuse, made up of numerous health advocacy groups, nonprofit associations, health care providers, professional associations, and neighborhood groups. Communities can also be suspicious of governmental agencies; at times, community advocates can be more emotional than rational. Therefore, effectively communicating in this environment takes patience and persistence.

A good model for communicating with communities was originally developed for *risk communication,* that is, communicating environmental and health risks to communities. Exhibit 19–2 provides the "seven cardinal rules of risk communication."[11] Adherence to these rules in all communication contexts (i.e., in addition to risk communication) can greatly assist public health practitioners in their efforts to establish strong relationships with communities.

A word should be added regarding community meetings. The use of town halls, regular public forums, open meetings, public advisory groups, and other types of group processes presents opportunities to gather input from community stakeholders. In implementing these processes, there are a few keys to success.[12] These may seem self-evident, but are frequently overlooked by public health practitioners.

- Ensure that the process has objectives and a specific target audience.

Exhibit 19–2 Seven Cardinal Rules of Risk Communication

1. *Accept and involve the public as a legitimate partner.* Demonstrate your respect for the public and underscore the sincerity of your effort by involving the community early, before important decisions are made. Involve all parties that have an interest or a stake in the issue under consideration.
2. *Plan carefully and evaluate your efforts.* Begin with clear, explicit risk communication objectives—such as providing information to the public, motivating individuals to act, stimulating response to emergencies, or contributing to the resolution of conflict. Classify and segment the various groups in your audience. Aim your communications at specific subgroups in your audience.
3. *Listen to the public's specific concerns.* Do not make assumptions about what people know, think, or want done about risks. Take the time to find out what people are thinking: use techniques such as interview, focus groups, and surveys.
4. *Be honest, frank, and open.* State your credentials, but do not ask or expect to be trusted by the public. If you do not know an answer or are uncertain, say so. Get back to people with answers. Admit mistakes.
5. *Coordinate and collaborate with credible sources.* Take time to coordinate all interorganizational and intraorganizational communications. Devote effort to the slow, hard work of building bridges with other organizations.
6. *Meet the needs of the media.* Be open with and accessible to reporters. Respect their deadlines. Do not hesitate to follow up on stories with praise or criticism, as warranted. Try to establish long-term relationships of trust with specific editors and reporters.
7. *Speak clearly and with compassion.* Use simple, nontechnical language. Be sensitive to local norms, such as speech and dress. Use vivid, concrete images that communicate on a personal level. Use examples and anecdotes that make technical risk data come alive. Avoid distant, abstract, unfeeling language about deaths, injuries, and illnesses.

Source: Reprinted from V.T. Covello and F. Allen, *Seven Cardinal Rules of Risk Communication,* April 1988, U.S. Environmental Protection Agency.

- Select a time, date, and meeting location consistent with the meeting objectives and audience. Public hearings often exclude people who work during normal business hours.
- Notify target audiences of the meeting or hearing through appropriate, multiple media. Notification should include this basic information: who the meeting affects and why; purpose of the meeting; what is likely to result from the meeting; date, time, and place of the meeting; and directions to the site.
- Make sure the meeting site is ready; select an alternate location in case the audience is too large or small, or in the case of sound, lighting, or other problems.
- Use a carefully planned agenda; this ensures that the meeting does not exceed available time or attention span and also that certain information is provided before deliberations begin.
- Clarify meeting ground rules. This includes issues such as time limits for speakers, acceptability of written transcripts in testimony, and use of Robert's Rules of Order.
- Follow through after a meeting to ensure that results and feedback are forthcoming. Important steps include scrutinizing the minutes or transcripts to identify promises, requests, or issues that require follow-up.

It is also important for public health practitioners to be visible within the community. This includes being routinely present at relevant community health meetings, as well as attempting to build bridges with nonhealth organizations, such as seeking speaking opportunities with organizations such as the Rotary Club, Sierra Club, and the League of Women Voters. Physician managers and directors should consider joining the local medical society.

A variety of communication strategies was used in the investigation of a potential cluster of chronic disease along the United States/Mexico border.[13] In this particular situation, which was highly charged and politicized, the Arizona Department of Health Services coordinated the conduct of an epidemiologic study of potential cancer and lupus clusters in the community of Nogales, Arizona. There was community suspicion that these illnesses were the result of environmental pollution. Within this process, the Arizona Department of Health Services met with key community members and identified community needs. In the short term, an identified need was medical care for community members with lupus and cancer. The department director personally participated in these meetings.

The department also supported community-based education through a contract with a local nonprofit agency. In collaboration with the state environmental quality agency, the department held environmental health open houses and health fairs. Lastly, upon completion of the health study, the department ensured that the community was the first to receive and review the study. The department maintained its credibility throughout this process while drawing attention to the health problem along the Arizona/Mexico border. Strategic communication was the key to resolving this potentially explosive situation.[13]

Communicating with Policy Makers

A review of the nation's public health system more than a decade ago concluded that "public health agency leaders should develop relationships with and educate legislators and other public officials on community health needs, on public health issues and on the rationale for strategies advocated and pursued by the health department."[14(p.14)] This observation came from the Institute of Medicine's (IOM's) groundbreaking 1988 report *The Future of Public Health* and serves to emphasize the importance of effective communication with policy makers.

Many experienced public health practitioners describe their relationships with policy makers (e.g., state legislators, county supervisors, and city officials) as love/hate. Practitioners love policy makers when they approve programmatic budget increases or important public health legislation, and are severely disappointed when they do not. In either case, it cannot be denied that positive and productive communication with policy makers can reap great benefits for public health agencies.

However, communication with policy makers is made difficult by a number of factors: policy makers are generally busy people with numerous issues to confront; policy makers also hear from the "other side" (e.g., the tobacco industry); and policy makers must take into account public opinion and partisan concerns. Combined, these factors make communication with policy makers tricky at best, potentially dangerous at worst. This, however, is not a reason to avoid communication with policy makers. On the contrary, regular communication is in order. Some suggestions for maintaining open channels with key policy makers include the following:

- Put legislators and other relevant policy makers on the mailing list for the program or agency newsletter.
- Place periodic phone calls to bring elected officials or staff up to date and to keep the agency's agenda part of their agenda.
- Provide reports, both written and oral, of how citizens complaints referred to the agency have been handled.
- To the extent possible, put a personal face on issues; personal stories should be culled from successful population-based program activities.

Another strategy is to invite policy makers to attend ceremonies (e.g., new program launches, groundbreaking ceremonies, etc.). This provides an opportunity for educating the official and an added bonus for the official to be associated with a successful public program.

In general, it is important to be responsive to requests from policy makers. Competent and timely responses from state agencies are greatly appreciated and can enhance agency credibility.

Communicating within the Organization

Many analysts have examined communication in the workplace. This literature consistently emphasizes that good internal communication is key to good employee morale and to peak operating efficiency in any organization. It is certainly true within a small or large public health organization or program. However, little attention has traditionally been given to this area of public health practice.

From a management perspective, it is important to maintain contact with staff. In addition to standard staff meetings, there are a number of strategies to promote staff interaction. Informal activities such as brown-bag lunches can be effective. One state public health agency instituted a Monday morning informal coffee that allowed all members of the staff to chat, network, and raise issues in a nonthreatening, nonbureaucratic atmosphere. One state health department uses the "employee communique" as a less formal mechanism to provide employee-based human interest updates (e.g., news on employee-related births, retirements, awards). This weekly update is a single sheet that is strategically placed on the walls of the restroom stalls, thus ensuring that all employees have a chance to review the latest edition.

Computer technology has assisted greatly in sharing information among and within organizations. The electronic posting of management team meeting minutes can ensure that all employees with a computer can stay abreast of the latest management discussions. At least one public health organization has used satellite technology to allow the state health department director to speak to department staff across the state. The Centers for Disease Control and Prevention uses compressed digital technology to communicate visually and interactively between its sites in Atlanta, Georgia; Cincinnati, Ohio; and Morgantown, West Virginia.[15]

A department newsletter can also serve as a means to communicate internally, and also to inform constituencies such as the medical community, service providers, local health organizations, and policy makers about important department activities.

MEDIA RELATIONS

"The trouble is that the stupid people—who constitute the grand overwhelming majority of this and all other nations—do believe and are molded and convinced by what they get out of a newspaper," Mark Twain wrote nearly one hundred years ago. He also said there are "only two forces that can carry light to all corners of the globe—the sun in the heavens and the Associated Press down here."

Both Twain quotes, with a little updating, ring true today. Now 30-second television snippets do much of the molding and convincing. And to the Associated Press, you can add CNN, NBC, CBS, ABC, Reuters, and the Internet, for starters.

So since Twain's days, the influence of the media has broadened enormously. But the news has become more simplified as the world has grown ever more complex. As a result, the job of the public health communicator has become more critical and much, much more difficult.

The first step to success is to embrace the fact that interaction with the media is desired and often necessary for the effective communication of a health message. News correspondent Daniel Schorr once said, "If you don't exist in the media, for all practical purposes, you don't exist."[16] Too many public health professionals seem content to steer clear of the news media, limiting themselves to strategies that might include PSAs and stacks of brochures at health fairs. But some say PSA stands for "people sound asleep" because they usually air in the wee hours. And how many of those brochures are actually read? PSAs, brochures, and other back-roads message carriers can be useful, but they need to be augmented whenever possible with travels along the superhighway of the six o'clock news.

In Arizona, the state health department's efforts to engage the press at every opportunity on the issue of lead poisoning clearly demonstrate that the news media offer the cheapest and most effective means of reaching the public *and* influencing public policy.

Separate news releases were issued to alert the public about discoveries of dangerous levels of lead in bulk water storage tanks, crayons from China, folk remedies called *azarcon* and *greta*, Mexican candy wrappers, two brands of pool cue chalk, and imported plastic mini-blinds. All of the releases prompted radio, television, and print coverage throughout the state. The crayon and mini-blinds news releases sparked media inquiries from coast to coast, effectively warning a nation and spurring the federal Consumer Product Safety Commission (CPSC) into action. A dozen brands of Chinese crayons were recalled and vinyl mini-blinds manufacturers were required by the CPSC to discontinue the use of lead as a stabilizer. It was estimated that at least 25 million sets of the leaded mini-blinds were being imported annually from China, Taiwan, Mexico, and Indonesia.[17]

The total printing, postage, and fax-line cost of producing and distributing all six of the lead-warning news releases was approximately $500. Consider how many PSAs and brochures would have been needed—and at what cost—to have even a fraction of the impact.

Once the decision has been made to think of the news media as an opportunity rather than an unwanted intrusion, both the possibilities and challenges are enormous. One of the toughest tasks is to reach the media's overloaded radar screen with your health message. The two major tools used to engage the media proactively are news releases and news conferences.

News Releases

Newspapers and television and radio stations often are flooded with hundreds of news releases each day. Only a few manage to stay out of the trash. Those that do contain a headline and lead paragraph that grab the attention of a harried assignment editor or reporter—a task sometimes akin to capturing lightning in a jar. Successful news releases are written in third-person news style. They are not overly enthusiastic or bloated with self-praise. Exclamation marks are barred completely, but action verbs are spread about freely. The text is easily understood and does not require the reader to wade through a swamp of technical complexities, medical terms, and bureaucratic jargon. But most importantly, releases that earn news coverage are based on actual news.

Well, what is and is not "news?" The announcement of virtually any grant is news, as long as the news release explains why the grant is important to the public. The launching of any public health outreach or advertising campaign or promotion is also news. Or an enforcement action against a licensed facility such as a child care center, nursing home, or hospital. The introduction or passage of a public health legislative proposal or budget item can prove worthy fodder. So can (and should) any public health warning—from rabies in foxes to excessive fecal coliform in a popular lake. The release of any statistical report is news, too, as long as the report's major points are summarized and presented in a compelling manner.

For example, here is how a news release announcing the completion of a statistical report on playground equipment safety began:

> Thousands of trips to emergency rooms and doctors' offices and more than 6,000 days of absenteeism are caused each year by playground-related injuries at Arizona elementary schools, according to a new study by the Arizona Department of Health Services.
>
> The study indicated that reportable injuries are occurring at rates of 275 per week and 10,500 per academic year, and that more than 1 out of every 50 elementary school students is injured each year. The study's report called the findings "alarming," especially since schools reported only those injuries severe enough to require hospitalization, restricted activity, absenteeism, or visits to a physician or clinic. The report described the situation as an "injury epidemic."[18]

The release sparked enormous news coverage, including segments on all four major Phoenix television stations and a report on the front page of the state's major daily newspaper that included a bar graph and a photo of a child on a swing set. Most of the reports used the hot-button terms "alarming" and "injury epidemic," both of which had been extracted from deep within the statistical report for the news release. Suddenly the issue of playground safety existed, and the ensuing interest of state, city, and school administrators and policy makers sparked quite a run for copies of the report.

What, then, does not pass muster as news? It is often impossible to stir much interest with a news release announcing a conference on any health topic. Conferences are educational, not newsy, in nature, and reporters generally do not have time to sit through them.

Breast Cancer Awareness Month, by itself, is not news. Neither is National Nutrition Month, Infant Immunization Week, Child Health Day, or any of the other special days, weeks, and months that stir whereas-laden blather from elected officials. The problem is that there are more than 9,000 special days, weeks, and months each year, according to *Chase's Annual Events*.[19] They include everything from Humpback Whale Awareness Month to National Baked Beans Month.

The media are overwhelmed to the point that no special occasion is special. A news release touting a celebratory cause will head straight for the assignment editor's wastebasket unless the release contains, and is dominated by, an actual news hook. Here are the headlines and lead sentences of two news releases that do inject news into a celebratory event.

> SAFETY STRESSED IN FOOD CODE REWRITE
>
> To help set the stage for September's Food Safety Education Month, the Arizona Department of Health Services today announced it is rewriting the state's Food Code, a reference that guides restaurants, grocery stores and institutions such as nursing homes on how to prevent food-borne illness.[20]

The release went on to say that the new Food Code "will address the most critical risk factors that cause food-borne illness—unsafe food temperatures, cross-contamination, and poor handwashing practices." Information specific to Food Safety Education Month began in the sixth paragraph.[20]

> LATINO 5-A-DAY NUTRITION CAMPAIGN LAUNCHED
>
> A campaign to promote fruit and vegetable consumption among Hispanics was launched today—the first day of National 5-A-Day Week—by the Arizona Department of Health Services.[21]

The release also noted the health benefits of fruit and vegetable consumption and the fact that Hispanics are lagging behind the general population in terms of achieving the 5-a-day goal.[21]

A few final strategies for effective news releases include:

- Avoid firing off releases too frequently because there will be a diminution of overall interest. Overabundance of any item reduces the value of each unit. This is possibly the only notion on Earth in which economists and reporters are of like minds. The ideal frequency of news releases will depend on the size of the respective public health agency, the number of programs it operates, the quantity of reports produced, and so on. Generally, however, try not to issue two releases in the same day, look for a spacing of at least two or three days between releases, and vary the subject matter of the releases. The Arizona Department of Health Services, for example, averages approximately six or seven releases per month and rarely frequents the same well (i.e., immunizations or tobacco prevention) twice during any given month.
- Fax or e-mail the news release. A faxed or e-mailed news release stands a better chance of coverage than a mailed news release. News is, well, "new," and a faxed release conveys more of a sense of immediacy.
- List a contact person on the news release and make sure that person is immediately available on the day the release is issued. That means the contact person needs to clear his or her slate of meetings. Don't expect a seasoned reporter to simply go with a quote from a news release rather than to solicit fresh comments from the contact person.

News Conferences

News conferences, if planned and conducted properly, can prove extremely useful for elevating the importance of an issue, introducing a new campaign, or spotlighting an important accomplishment or enterprise. Unlike separate interviews with reporters, news conferences are economical in terms of the interviewee's time requirements, and they allow the conveyance of the same message to a whole group of broadcast and print reporters. Also, because there is a herd mentality among the media, feeding all of them the same message at the same time reduces the risk of a reporter falling out of step and overplaying a minor point or a negative element. Additionally, a news conference can achieve much broader coverage than a news release because it can offer television reporters an interesting, colorful, and relevant visual setting. In short, a news conference can provide the perfect forum to present your side of the story to a captive audience.

News conferences proved tremendously valuable during the startup of a massive, tobacco-tax-funded tobacco-prevention campaign in Arizona that initially targeted youth. Although Arizona is among the most conservative states in the Union, the campaign's planned ad campaign would have ruffled feathers in some of the trendiest spots in New York City. It employed intense visual images, humor, and stomach-turning grossness to reach the MTV generation. In one ad, a boy's date absentmindedly takes a swallow from his spit-tobacco cup at a movie theater. In another, a teenage girl transforms into a rotting apparition as she puffs away. In a radio ad, a boy tells a graphic tale about how pus from a dead bird reminds him of spit tobacco. The word "puking" is featured prominently in the campaign's slogan. It would have been political suicide to simply unleash a campaign of this nature on an unsuspecting public without justifying its cost and tactics.[22]

The solution was to educate the media (and by extension adults and policy makers) concurrently about the severity of the youth tobacco problem and the strategy behind the ad campaign. Eleven news conferences were held during the first 16 months of the campaign. Every new wrinkle in the campaign, from the latest commercial to the startup of a merchandise center selling T-shirts and other antitobacco gear, offered another opportunity to repeat two points.

1. Tobacco use is the nation's number 1 killer and it begins almost all the time as a childhood addiction.
2. The ads and other elements of the campaign are geared toward capturing the attention of teens and are not intended to appeal to adults.

The news conferences produced massive positive news coverage—more than 200 newspaper articles and 226 minutes of television news in the first 10 months alone. The coverage fostered an understanding of the campaign by the general public, and it spawned fawning editorials in many newspapers, including the major Phoenix and Tucson dailies.

The editorial support and public goodwill that had been established helped enable the campaign to weather a storm that erupted 15 months into the effort when "Maggot," the most controversial and intense of all the ads, aired. It featured a teenage girl going through her morning ritual of brushing her teeth and putting on her makeup. All the while she is smoking, and her beautiful face transforms into a grotesque sight of rotting flesh. Worms appear on her toothbrush, in the sink, and in her mouth. The spot closes with a stylized shot of somebody spewing green vomit.

Within two days, 100 telephone calls were received about the ad, and almost all were critical. The spot, however, was defended editorially and by a columnist for the *Tribune*, a major Phoenix-area newspaper. Already on the wane, the negative phone calls then dropped to a trickle when a written statement was added to the beginning of the commercial warning parents that the contents may be offensive to young children.

Now that the value of a news conference as a communication tool has been established, how does one go about setting up a successful conference? The main challenges are selecting a visual and appropriate site, luring the media to the site, packaging your message into something they can use, and avoiding embarrassment. Here are some tricks of the trade.

- *Think visual.* Four blank walls in an office building won't lure any television cameras. Nor will any spokesperson behind a podium, unless that podium is situated in an area the helps tell the story. Examples of thinking visually include the selection of a neonatal unit of a hospital for the announcement of a campaign to promote folic acid, the staging of a healthy cooking demonstration in a grocery store for the launching of a campaign to promote fruit and vegetable consumption, and the operation of a children's fashion show to introduce a line of antitobacco T-shirts, bandannas, and other gear.
- *Bait the hook.* A communication director's/public information officer's worst nightmare is to call a news conference and then have nobody show up from the media. In fishing for reporters, consider your line and hook to be a faxed "media advisory" and your bait to be the headline and first paragraph of that advisory. Make it grab you and reveal a visual element if you can. Also, don't throw the line in the water too soon. To most editors and reporters, advance planning means scheduling something after lunch rather than before. Therefore, fax the media advisory no more than two days before the event to reduce the chances it will be lost or forgotten. And make sure a copy is sent to the local AP bureau, which enters such information in a "daybook" calendar of activities that is sent to broadcast and print media outlets.

The following is a sample of the bait that was used to attract reporters to the announcement of a campaign to promote folic acid among women of childbearing age.

BIRTH DEFECTS TARGETED BY
NEW STATE CAMPAIGN

A major campaign will be launched to encourage women in Arizona to greatly reduce their risk of having a baby with a disabling or deadly defect of the spine or brain. The campaign will urge all women of childbearing age to consume folic acid. Sufficient amounts of folic acid can reduce the risk of a neural tube birth defect by up

> to 70 percent. However nearly half of all women of childbearing age in Arizona—about half a million women—are unaware of the critical role played by folic acid.[23]

The advisory went on to list the date, time, and location of the event.

The bait lured six television cameras, four radio stations, and three print reporters to the event.

- *Package the information in sound bites.* Television and radio reporters rely exclusively on sound bites, which encapsulate a key thought in maybe two sentences often running less than 10 seconds. Some reporters even cut the bite to a "sound bark" of two or three words. Print reporters like quotes that are colorful, clever, and to the point. Nobody likes long explanations. Therefore, package your message so that it can be received by your audience. That doesn't mean everything needs to sound like a sound bite. It does, however, mean that the main message you want to get across needs to be stated at least once in a clear, clever, and concise manner. Throw enthusiasm into the mix, too. If your spokesperson shows no passion for the message he or she is pitching, why should anyone else?
- *Avoid embarrassment.* Preparation is the key to avoiding embarrassment. Make sure the main speaker's knowledge of the news conference topic extends well beyond his or her written text. It is also wise to have a bona fide expert on the subject on hand as a safety valve. Otherwise, even a simple question-and-answer session might destroy the speaker's credibility by revealing an emperor with no clothes.
- *Provide backup materials.* Make a news release and other backup materials available at the news conference. These might include fact sheets, written texts of prepared speeches, reports, graphs, videos, and other documents. Such materials help reporters flesh out the details and background of a topic that might only be glossed over at the news conference. They also seem to add a sense of legitimacy to the news conference.

PLAYING DEFENSE

Although proactive relations with the media should keep reporters from dwelling on the negatives, there will be times when an action, inaction, or error by a public health organization does come under fire. After all, easily more than half of today's news stories are negative in tone and contain elements of conflict, criticism, and controversy. For example, a story headlined "Immunization Rate Plummets to All-Time Low" is almost a sure bet for the front page, whereas one headlined "Immunization Rate Posts Record High" might get buried near the obituaries.

When a reporter calls for an interview on a negative story, any good defensive strategy requires an advance understanding of what the story is about, the development of one or two major messages you intend to stress throughout the interview, and thorough preparation for the toughest questions that may be asked.

Before agreeing to an interview, the public health administrator should interview the interviewer. Ask what the story is about, how you fit in, what other parties have been interviewed, what documents are involved, when the story will run, and so on. Find out as much as you can.

In developing your main message(s) before the interview, always favor positive language that defines or explains over defensive statements. The message should be in the form of a compelling and quotable sound bite. Ideally, it should begin with the conclusion and then move to an example or supporting information, followed by a sentence explaining what it all means to the audience. Don't wait for a specific question to deliver your main message. On virtually any question from a reporter, it is possible to simply touch on the answer and then use a bridging phrase such as "it's also important to know" to go to your message. Prepare beforehand for the toughest questions and for the "bridges" you may use. Finally, when you've answered a question, stop talking. Do not feel compelled to fill silence with sound.

Also remember that how a person looks and sounds can often be more important than what he or she says, especially when a camera is involved. Maintain steady eye contact with the reporter, speak confidently, smile whenever you can, and stay away from gaudy jewelry, loud colors, and checkered or striped patterns in your wardrobe. If you can, avoid wearing eyeglasses, and never wear dark glasses. Vests also should be avoided.

MEDIA INTERACTION GUIDELINES

Regardless of the forum—from a news conference to a phone interview—and whether the nature of the reporter's questions have you playing offense or defense, the following guidelines will help you get your point across effectively and earn the reporter's respect:

- *Accuracy:* It is paramount. If you do not know the answer to a question, say so and offer to get back to the reporter with the answer as quickly as possible. Also, do not use words or phrases that make you appear uncertain. These include "apparently," "it seems," and "to the best of my knowledge."
- *Preparation:* Never risk being ill-prepared in an interview with the news media. If a reporter calls and you are not prepared or are caught off guard, buy yourself some time—even if it is just five minutes—by saying you need to pull a file or obtain relevant information and will call him or her right back.
- *Promptness:* Remember that reporters operate under strict deadlines. Return their phone calls promptly. One of the performance measures for the public information office at the Arizona Department of Health Services is the percentage of reporters' calls that are returned within five minutes.
- *Completeness:* Answer questions fully and offer to provide copies of relevant documents. Tell the whole story. Take the time to provide background and be sure to explain the factors that led to a certain situation, condition, or controversy.
- *Honesty:* Do not shade the truth because in the long run, the truth always prevails. Remember that half-truths and errors of omission can place the credibility of your agency and yourself at risk. Also, never downplay or overplay the severity of a disease threat or outbreak. The former may provoke angry reactions of government whitewashing, insensitivity, and inaction; the latter may prompt complaints of scare tactics and grandstanding.
- *Clarity:* Speak plain English. Do not use technical terms, acronyms, or abbreviations that are not familiar to the general public.
- *Admit a mistake:* Do not be afraid to admit to a mistake or to say that a program or service could have been operated better or more efficiently, if that is the case, but be sure to emphasize efforts to correct a problem.
- *Never say "No comment":* Rather than leave the reporter guessing, explain why you cannot disclose information. If barred by privacy laws, for example, explain that fact and fax the reporter a copy of the statutory restriction.
- *Avoid unforgivables:* The public will not forgive arrogance, indifference, or incompetence. The price for failure to avoid the unforgivables can be steep.

BUILDING A MODEL COMMUNICATION/PUBLIC INFORMATION OFFICE

The ideal structure and responsibilities of a model communication/public information office of course depend on whom you ask. However, the National Public Health Information Coalition (NPHIC), which is an affiliate of the Association of State and Territorial Health Officials and is funded through a grant from the U.S. Centers for Disease Control and Prevention, has developed a model communication office for a state health department.

According to the NPHIC model, the communication/public information office should be established as a branch of the office of the agency's chief executive administrator "so that any and all consultation offered and/or instructions given carry the necessary weight."[24] The NPHIC further recommends that the director of the communication/public information office be directly answerable and have direct and complete access to the agency's chief executive administrator. According to the NPHIC, "dangerous breakdowns in communication are a given with every layer of administrative responsibility created between the agency's top policy maker and the staff person(s) responsible for communicating those policies internally or externally."[24]

The NPHIC recommends that the director of communication/public information be considered a member of the first team of advisors to the chief executive administrator. "Involved daily in contacts with agency staff, external publics and inquiring reporters, the insight offered and queries posed by the director of public information/communication can be invaluable in spotting the strongest approach, as well as the weakest links, in a public policy issue," stated NPHIC's Model Office document.[24] "The importance of direct and frequent access to and briefing of the chief executive administrator cannot be overemphasized. As much as any element of a successful management team, the top spokesperson must be able to anticipate the needs of the top policymaker to get the message out, and in many cases, must carry, as an advisor, that very need to the policymaker."[24]

Responsibilities of the model communication/public information office, again according to the NPHIC, should include[24]

- news releases
- news conferences
- agency photographic services
- media interview requests relating to agency policy
- speech consultation and/or writing
- employee newsletter
- design development and content consultation for all brochures, booklets, posters, and other graphics art materials that are not of a staff training nature
- production and content consultation for all audio/video materials that are designed for the general public or specific segments of the population
- public education/awareness campaigns, including planning of campaign scope, materials, timing, and target audiences

To perform the above responsibilities, the communication/public information office should be composed of, at a minimum, a director, all of the agency's public information writers, a photographer, videographers and graphic design personnel, and at least one administrative support person for every five total staff in the unit, according to the NPHIC.[24] In terms of overall numbers, one public information office staff member for every 200 employees of an agency may be sufficient to handle all of the above responsibilities adequately.

• • •

Throughout the past century, public health organizations have played key roles in extending the quality and quantity of life in the United States. Nonetheless, efforts to communicate the importance and value of these advances have not been as successful. Public health programs still suffer from limited public understanding and advocacy. Administrators need to communicate effectively with a wide variety of constituencies, including community groups, health care providers, policy makers, and the media. In particular, effective relationships with the media can be helpful in promoting healthy behaviors and marketing program efforts and policy decisions. Further progress in developing effective programs and policies depends on health communication strategies such as media advocacy, social marketing, entertainment education, and risk communication. Public health administrators must stay abreast of technological communication advances and use the Internet and interactive communication systems (e.g., satellite and compressed digital videoconferencing) to maximize communication effectiveness and efficiency.

CHAPTER REVIEW

1. The effective use of communication in public health practice is still the exception rather than the rule.
2. There are a number of ways to communicate information, called *channels* of communication denoting the route or method used. Each mode may have certain advantages in certain situations.
3. Principles of communication include
   - Keep the method simple.
   - Ensure cultural competency.
   - Strike at the best opportunity.
   - Use multiple channels keyed to the target audience.
4. Good communication with communities should be maintained by seeking opportunities to gather input at meetings in town halls, regular public forums, and open meetings.
5. Strategies for communicating with staff to improve employee morale and increase operating efficiency should be devised.
6. News releases and press conferences should be developed in a manner that will engage the media proactively with a newsworthy subject presented in a clear and compelling manner. Relationships with media contact representatives are important.
7. Effective media-interaction guidelines stress honesty, clarity, preparation, and completeness. Never appear arrogant, indifferent, or incompetent.
8. The communication/public information office should be structured so that it relates directly and frequently to the organization's chief executive and is continuously available to the media.

REFERENCES

1. R. Brown, A. Elixhauser, J. Corea, B. Luce, and S. Sheingold (Battelle), *National Expenditures for Health Promotion and Disease Prevention Activities in the United States* (Atlanta, GA: Centers for Disease Control and Prevention, 1991).
2. E. Maibach and D.R. Holtgrave, "Advances in Public Health Communication," *Annual Review of Public Health* 16 (1995): 219–238.
3. M. McGinnis and D. Foege, "Actual Causes of Death in the United States," *Journal of the American Medical Association* 270 (1993): 2,207–2,212.
4. Office of Disease Prevention and Health Promotion, *Healthy People 2010 Objectives: Draft for Public Comment* (Washington, DC: U.S. Department of Health and Human Services, 1998).
5. I.A. Kirsch et al., *Adult Literacy in America* (Princeton, NJ: Educational Testing Service, 1993).
6. F.G. Castro, "Cultural Competence Training in Clinical Psychology: Assessment, Clinical Intervention, and Research," in *Comprehensive Clinical Psychology,* eds. A.S. Bellack and M. Hersen (Oxford: Pergammon, 1998), 127–140.
7. Arizona Department of Health Services, *Cultural Competency in the Administration and Delivery of Behavioral Health Services* (Phoenix, AZ: Arizona Department of Health Services, 1995), 4.
8. B. Levy, "Communicating Public Health Challenges for the 21st Century." Presentation at the University of Texas, School of Public Health, Houston, TX, February 1997.
9. B. Maude, *Practical Communication for Managers* (White Plains, NY: Longman, 1974).
10. M. Eisenberg, H. Lee, M. Burgoon, B. Beach, E. Alvaro, and R. Givens, "Evaluation of the TEPP Media Campaign: Report No. 1 (October 1998): Historical Impact of the TEPP Media Campaign" (Tucson, AZ: University of Arizona Cancer Center, 1998).
11. V.T. Covello and F. Allen, *Seven Cardinal Rules of Risk Communication* (Washington, DC: U.S. Environmental Protection Agency, 1988).
12. J.L. Garnett, *Communicating for Results in Government* (San Francisco: Jossey-Bass Publishers, 1992).
13. J. Dillenberg and D. Hirano, "Confronting a Border Health Crisis: A Comprehensive Approach," *Journal of*

Public Health Management and Practice 3 (1997): 12–19.

14. Institute of Medicine, *The Future of Public Health* (Washington, DC: National Academy Press, 1988), 14.
15. Personal Communication. Brian Siegmund, Centers for Disease Control and Prevention, April 14, 2000.
16. Communications Consortium Media Center, *Strategic Communications for Nonprofits: Strategic Media—Designing a Public Interest Campaign* (Washington, DC: Benton Foundation and the Center for Strategic Communications, 1991), 7.
17. U.S. Consumer Product Safety Commission, Office of Information and Public Affairs, News release #96–50, June 25, 1996, Washington, DC.
18. B. Christensen, *ADHS Study Finds School Injury Epidemic*, news release (Phoenix, AZ: Arizona Department of Health Services, November 1998).
19. H.M. Chase and W.D. Chase, *Chase's Annual Events* (Lincolnwood, IL: NTC Publishing Group, 1999).
20. P. Simeri, *Safety Stressed in Food Code Rewrite*, news release (Phoenix, AZ: Arizona Department of Health Services, August 1999).
21. B. Christensen, *Latino Nutrition Campaign Launched*, news release (Phoenix, AZ: Arizona Department of Health Services, September 1999).
22. A. Dominy, *Pus*, radio commercial (Phoenix, AZ: Riester-Robb Advertising and Public Relations, 1996).
23. B. Christensen, *Media Advisory* (Phoenix, AZ: Arizona Department of Health Services, January 1999).
24. NPHIC Executive Board, *Model Communications/Public Information Office* (Atlanta, GA: National Public Health Information Coalition, 1994).

CHAPTER 20

Public Health Marketing

Lynne Doner
Michael Siegel

The discipline of marketing offers public health organizations a variety of concepts and strategies for motivating behavior change in specific populations of interest. Public health organizations use these techniques not only to influence individual health behavior, but also to mobilize public support for core public health policies and institutions. Marketing strategies can therefore enable organizations to improve the effectiveness of specific public health interventions and to strengthen the institutional capacity of the public health system as a whole.

This chapter provides an introduction to marketing concepts and the ways they can be applied in a public health environment to help bring about changes in personal health behaviors and in policies affecting public health institutions and practice. Marketing is sometimes criticized as working "downstream" (e.g., asking members of the public to make changes in their behavior) when effective change takes place "upstream" (e.g., changing policy). In fact, a combination of downstream and upstream efforts often works best, and the marketing framework is an appropriate way to plan, develop, implement, and assess the entire spectrum of activities that may be necessary to bring about social change successfully.

WHAT IS MARKETING?

Marketing is a disciplined, audience-focused, research-based *process* to plan, develop, implement, and assess activities that are designed to influence the behavior change of target audiences. It emphasizes developing a comprehensive strategic approach based on a thorough understanding of the problem to be addressed, the audience to be reached, the action to be taken, and the environment in which the action will take place. In a public health context, marketing efforts are undertaken to improve societal health, either through influencing changes in the health behaviors of individuals, in policies that impact health behaviors, or in perceptions of and support for public health as an institution.

Traditionally, marketing techniques have been used in public health primarily to influence changes in individual health behaviors, such as seeking prenatal care, getting screened for a particular health condition, or improving eating and physical activity habits. This type of marketing is often termed *social marketing*, which has been defined as "the application of commercial marketing technologies to the analysis, planning, execution, and evaluation of programs designed to influence the voluntary behavior of target audiences in order to improve their personal welfare and that of their society."[1(p.7)]

This type of marketing has played a part in some of the world's most successful efforts to influence personal health behaviors, beginning in 1972 with the National Heart, Lung, and Blood Institute's formation of the National High

Blood Pressure Education Program to increase awareness, prevention, treatment, and control of hypertension.[2] One measure of success: hypertension treatment rates increased from 31 percent during 1976–80 to 54 percent during 1991–94. Other successful uses of marketing techniques include the Pawtucket Heart Health Program, which led to more than 10,000 people getting their blood cholesterol measured in a two-year period; the Philippines National Urban Immunization Program, which helped increase the proportion of children who had all vaccinations by age one from 32 percent to 56 percent; and the U.S. 5 A Day for Better Health Program, which has seen an increase from 8 percent to 40 percent in the percentage of people who know how many servings of fruits and vegetables to eat each day.[3–6]

Today, the field of public health is moving toward a broader use of marketing techniques to help bring about policy change or increase support for public health as an institution. For example, the marketing framework has provided a strong foundation for many of the advocacy activities that have been undertaken to support tobacco control, as well as for efforts to preserve or increase public health funding.[7] The U.S. Centers for Disease Control and Prevention (CDC) recently called for the application of marketing strategies to promote public support and secure increased funding for public health programs.[8,9]

Marketing can be distinguished from other approaches to influencing individual and policy change by its emphasis on the following concepts:

- exchange relationships
- behavior change
- competition
- consumer orientation and audience segmentation
- formative and process evaluation
- product, price, place, and promotion

Exchange Relationships

Marketers believe that *exchange* is central to the actions people take: a person gives something in order to get something in return. Before entering into an exchange, a person weighs the benefits to be received against the costs (in money, time, or psyche). Only if the benefits are greater than the costs will the person make the exchange. It is important to understand that the only relevant costs and benefits are those that are important to the person contemplating the exchange. These may or may not be health-related costs and benefits. Generally, immediate tangible benefits such as looking or feeling better are more compelling to people than longer-term, intangible benefits such as potentially reducing the risk of cancer or heart disease.

The idea of weighing costs and benefits is not unique to marketing; many models and theories that are used to understand or predict health behavior change incorporate a similar concept. For example, the transtheoretical model of stages of change includes a decisional balance construct that is described as the pros and cons of changing a behavior.[10] Social cognitive theory includes outcome expectancies, which "influence behavior according to the hedonic principle; that is, if all other things are equal, a person will choose to perform an activity that maximizes a positive outcome or minimizes a negative outcome."[11(p.163)]

Behavior Change

> The bottom line of all marketing strategy and tactics is to influence behavior. Sometimes this necessitates changing ideas and thoughts first, but in the end, it is behavior change we are after. This is an absolutely crucial point. Some nonprofit marketers may think that they are in the "business" of changing ideas, but it can legitimately be asked why they should bother if such changes do not lead to action.[12(p.110)]

The emphasis on behavior change is one way marketing efforts can be distinguished from some other health education and health promotion efforts. Depending on the situation in which a marketing approach is being applied, that behavior may be colleagues' attendance at a meeting, at-risk individuals coming in for screening for sexually transmitted diseases, or policy makers' support of a new public health initiative; but the end goal is always getting the audience to take an action, not merely increasing knowledge or changing attitudes. Marketers will increase knowledge to the extent that such activities are precursors to behavior change (i.e., parents are unlikely to get children immunized unless they know they need to do so), but the focus is on identifying exactly what is necessary for the behavior change to take place.

One challenge as public health administrators is to select a specific behavior to change; often, a number of behaviors can lead to desired outcomes. Integral to this decision is selecting a behavior that is perceived as "doable" by target audience members. Sometimes this means focusing on one step toward the desired behavior. For example, the national 5 A Day campaign asked the target audience to *add two* servings of fruits and vegetables each day, even though the program goal was *eating five* servings each day. This decision was made because target audience members were already eating two to three servings a day, and adding an additional two was more reasonable to them.[13] Appropriate models and theories of behavior change can help practitioners make such decisions.

Competition

> Every choice of action on the consumer's part involves giving up some other action. Thus, campaigns must keep in mind not only what the marketer is trying to get across but also what the customer sees as the major alternatives.[1(p.17)]

For a public health initiative, competition can be defined as anything that limits resources, diverts attention from the subject of the initiative, or calls for contrary behaviors. There are three main sources of competition: other organizations conducting programs on the same subject, other behavior changes, and commercial sources.[7] Identifying competition allows planners to identify a niche in which to position a program or activity vis-à-vis the competition. Sometimes, another organization—even a "friend"—may be promoting a product, message, or practice that is in conflict with your organization's goals. At other times, a commercial opponent may encourage the very behavior that public health practitioners are trying to stop, such as smoking or ownership of certain types of firearms. More often, commercial advertising, television programs, or magazines emphasize behaviors or choices that have negative health consequences if they are not moderated or balanced by other behaviors, such as having nonmonogamous sex without using condoms or eating only "junk" foods.

Consumer Orientation

> Social marketing provides a problem-solving process from which behavior change strategies are formulated and translated into discrete and integrated tactics aimed at specific behavior change. The point of social marketing is that these tactical approaches are selected and implemented based on what has been discovered in the consumer research phase as being most relevant and potentially effective with the target, not what self-designated experts believe to be important for the target population to know or practice.[14 (p.147)]

An organization's consumer orientation manifests itself in how the organization approaches the exchange and how it approaches the consumer. Andreasen discussed a number of characteristics that are typical of an organization-centered (rather than consumer-centered) mindset.[1]

- The organization's mission is seen as inherently good.
- Customers are seen as the problem (e.g., assuming they are not doing something they should be doing, rather than determining if in fact they are not doing something and, if so, how that could be fixed).

- Marketing is seen as communications (rather than a broader range of potential solutions).
- Marketing research has a limited role.
- Customers are treated as a mass.
- Competition is ignored.
- Staffers are drawn from those with product (the behavior itself) or communications skills.

In contrast, consumer-oriented organizations analyze the transaction from the consumer's point of view rather than the organization's. They define the "problem" in terms of what the target audience needs and wants, not what the organization would like to provide. They use marketing research to group the audience into segments based on their needs and wants, and to take a broader look at potential obstacles to the behavior change, rather than assuming that consumers are in some way at fault (due to ignorance or stubbornness) and telling them what to do to remedy the problem. In many instances, "fixing" a problem behavior involves much more than communicating with consumers about it. In addition to education, policy and/or technological changes may be necessary.

For example, when it became apparent that many child safety seats were improperly installed in the United States, the National Highway Traffic Safety Administration (NHTSA) and many local community and law enforcement agencies worked together to educate parents and caregivers about proper installation procedures and sponsored events where installation could be checked and corrected, if necessary.[15] A product usability study, however, illustrated that the reason so many safety seats were installed wrong had more to do with technology than with parents.[15] Therefore, NHTSA used its educational efforts as an interim approach while it used its policy-making ability to mandate a technological change. In 1999, NHTSA issued a final rule (federal regulation) mandating a standardized anchorage system (separate from the seat belts) in passenger vehicles and corresponding standardized attachments on child safety seats.[16]

The consumer orientation also means that marketers make extensive use of formative research to analyze all aspects of the exchange transaction from the consumer's viewpoint. "Their mission in life is to know who their customers are, what they want and need, and where and how to reach them."[7(p.204)] They do this by following a careful process of audience analysis, and then using this analysis to segment the audience along key dimensions, such as readiness or ability to change behavior. They then select audience segments and determine what is necessary to facilitate behavior change for each segment. This may require changing any of the marketing variables—the product itself, the price, the experience of getting it, or communication concerning it. This process is described in more detail later in this chapter.

The Four Ps: Product, Price, Place, and Promotion

On even a casual foray into the marketing literature, the reader is likely to come across references to "the marketing mix" or "the four Ps." *Product, price, place,* and *promotion* constitute the marketing mix—the group of variables that a marketer can alter to sell a product. Although not all of them transfer equally well to a public health setting, where the attempt is to bring about behavior change that is not always tied to a tangible product or service, understanding these variables is central to understanding the marketing approach. Exhibit 20–1 presents definitions for each variable and key questions that public health practitioners should answer as part of planning marketing strategy and activities.

Two Other "Ps" To Consider: Partners and Policy

Because almost every public health issue has a number of organizations addressing aspects of it, it is most expedient to understand and consider the activities of these actual or de facto "partners" when planning an organization's marketing activities. Partners can be other organizations involved with a social change effort or

Exhibit 20–1 The Marketing Mix (as Applied in Social Change Settings)

Product

The behavior, good, service, or program exchanged for a price; ultimately, the behavior change sought

- What are the benefits of the behavior change to members of the target audience—what needs or wants do they have that the product (behavior change, program, or policy) can fulfill?
- What is the competition for the product?
- What legal, technological, and/or economic policy changes can facilitate individual behavior change?
- What accomplishments can reasonably be expected independent of policy changes?

Price

The cost to the target audience member, in money, time, effort, lifestyle, or psyche, of engaging in the behavior

- What will the behavior change "cost" each target audience?
- Do target audience members perceive the cost to be a fair exchange for the benefit they associate with the behavior change?
- How can costs be minimized?

Place

The outlet(s) through which products are available—or situations in which behavior changes can be made

- What are target audience members' perceptions of place?
- What barriers (costs) does the place create, and how can they be overcome?

Promotion

Some combination of advertising, media relations, promotional events, personal selling, and entertainment to communicate with target audience members about the product

- What is the current demand among target audience members for the behavior change?
- What messages can best influence demand?
- What promotional materials and activities are appropriate for the message?
- How can those materials and activities best be delivered to target audience members?

Source: Adapted from M. Siegel and L. Doner, *Marketing Public Health: Strategies to Promote Social Change,* p. 217, © 1998, Aspen Publishers, Inc.

serving as conduits to target audiences. Questions to ask about partners include the following:

- What other organizations are conducting activities addressing the social change?
- What organizations are credible to the target audience?
- What are the opportunities to work together with either type of organization?

Policy is important because with some public health issues, a policy change is necessary before behavior change can occur; with other issues, policy changes can support individual behavior change efforts. Two examples of the first situation are the child safety seat issue discussed earlier and exposure to secondhand smoke. Members of the public cannot reasonably avoid secondhand smoke in public places, such as restaurants, shopping malls, and airports, without policy changes restricting smoking to confined areas. An example of policy changes that can support individual behavior changes is limiting consumption of dietary fat. The U.S. Food and Drug Administration's (FDA's) rule mandating "Nutrition Facts" labels on most foods provides consumers with the information they need to select foods that are lower in fat. On a smaller scale, restaurants that have a policy of identifying lower-fat menu items provide a similar service.

Questions to ask about policy include the following:

- What policy changes *are necessary* for individuals to improve their health behaviors?
- What policy changes *could support* individuals in their efforts to improve their health behaviors?

- What policy changes can this organization bring about?

WHY INTEGRATE MARKETING INTO PUBLIC HEALTH PRACTICE?

Over the past century, the nature and role of public health practice have changed significantly, especially in developed countries. Many basic public health functions became widespread during the nineteenth century as industrialization and immigration led large numbers of people to move from low-density rural areas to high-density cities where inadequate public water supplies and waste disposal systems led to repeated outbreaks of cholera, dysentery, tuberculosis (TB), and other infectious diseases.[17] In contrast, although today's public health practitioners continue to address infectious disease, they also confront a chronic disease epidemic rivaling the infectious epidemics of the past, a medical climate that emphasizes treatment over population-based prevention, and a lost vision of public health among public health practitioners and society. The appropriate use of marketing can help public health practitioners be more effective in today's environment.

Preventing and Controlling Chronic versus Infectious Disease

With the widespread deployment of improved sanitation (particularly clean water and adequate waste disposal in cities), the development of vaccines, and the discovery of antibiotics, the twentieth century has seen enormous drops in morbidity and mortality resulting from infectious diseases. Today, chronic diseases pose the major threats to public health in developed countries, although some new and reemerging infectious diseases continue to extract a heavy toll on the quality and quantity of life (e.g., human immunodeficiency virus (HIV)/acquired immune deficiency syndrome (AIDS), drug-resistant TB). (Refer to Figure 1–3 in Chapter 1.) In recent years, some conditions that were previously thought to be chronic have been determined to have infectious causes (e.g., ulcers caused by *H. pylori* and cervical cancers caused by the human papilloma virus), and, as the CDC has noted, "ongoing research on the possible role of infectious agents in causing or intensifying certain chronic diseases (including diabetes mellitus type 1, some cancers [Montesano, Hainaut, & Wild, 1997; Di Bisceglie, 1997; Muñoz & Bosch, 1996], and heart conditions [Danesh, Collins, & Peto, 1997; Mattila, Valtonen, Nieminen, & Asikainen, 1998])...is imperative."[17(p.627)]

However, unless and until today's leading chronic diseases are found to have infectious causes, preventing and controlling them often require fundamentally different strategies than those that would be used with infectious diseases. Table 20–1 presents some common differences between infectious and chronic diseases and the steps needed for control (the differences shown will not apply to every infectious or chronic disease).

As the table shows, preventing and controlling infectious disease are often more straightforward than doing the same for chronic disease. For infectious diseases with an available vaccine, public health programs can focus on convincing target audiences to get themselves or their children immunized one time, or, at most, periodically. From the consumer's perspective, the action is clear and relatively low cost in terms of money, time (at most, a few trips to the doctor; in some developing countries, immunization campaigns go door-to-door), psychological (fear), and physical costs (some immunizations cause discomfort). In addition, there is a clear, definite benefit that outweighs the cost: avoidance of, at the least, a disease that will have higher time and physical costs, and, at the most, death.

In contrast, the consumer behaviors required to prevent or treat chronic disease generally have higher financial, time, psychological, and physical costs, and the corresponding benefits are less definite and often less immediate. Public health programs must convince consumers to initiate *and maintain* a single behavior change, or, more often, a series of behavior changes (e.g., various changes in diet and physical activity, compliance with monitoring and treatment) in the hopes that these changes might lessen the possi-

Table 20–1 Common Differences between Preventing and Controlling Infectious versus Chronic Disease

	Infectious Disease	*Chronic Disease*
Cause	Straightforward (once infectious agent is discovered)	Complex; often unknown
Taking preventive action	Will prevent transmission	May reduce risk of developing condition
Availability of one-time preventive behavior versus permanent behavior modification	Depends on disease — one-time or single-series vaccines available for some; periodic immunization required for others (e.g., influenza) — permanent lifestyle modification required for those with no vaccine	If prevention is possible, generally requires permanent lifestyle modification
Treatment complexity	Ranges from simple one-time treatment (e.g., course of antibiotics) to ongoing and complex treatment (e.g., HIV/AIDS)	Usually complex and ongoing treatment or monitoring for recurrence is required
Force of law	In some instances (e.g., childhood immunizations)	No
Public outcry/concern	Spikes when new outbreaks occur	No
Possibility of eradication from population	Sometimes yes, if vaccine is available	No

bility of developing the condition or lessen its severity.

Other factors that complicate chronic disease control are the lack of public reaction to chronic diseases and the limited tools available to public health practitioners. When there is an unexpected outbreak of infectious disease, especially a relatively uncommon disease, the outbreak generally gets significant media coverage. People become concerned, often take actions to avoid infection, and expect public health officials to take the necessary steps to limit transmission. For example, the West Nile virus outbreak in New York City and surrounding counties resulted in a large number of human cases, including multiple deaths, and, appropriately, substantial media coverage.[18] To contain the outbreak, the departments of health in New York City and surrounding locales availed themselves of the tools at their disposal, such as Malathion spraying.[19]

In contrast, during the same period of time, many more cases of cancer and other chronic disease were undoubtedly diagnosed in New York. Yet, because these were expected and not quickly preventable, there was no public outcry, and public health officials were not expected to do anything beyond their usual activities. Even in times when there is no immediate crisis, public health officials are likely to have more tools available to them, such as regulations requiring immunizations before children can enter school, to help fight infectious disease as compared to chronic disease.

Need for Population-Based Prevention

In general, health resources in the United States are disproportionately allocated to medical treatment rather than prevention. Although many of the pioneering advances in medical diagnosis and treatment result from these expenditures, this inequitable allocation jeopardizes the nation's health for a number of reasons.

- Despite the widely held perception that recent advances in medical treatment have resulted in a dramatic decline in mortality, there is substantial evidence that the observed decline in mortality in the developed world during the eighteenth to twentieth centuries was attributable largely to public health and not medical interventions.[7,20–23] Supporting this conclusion, other authors have attributed declines in mortality to improvements that are in the purview of public health, not medical treatment: the purification of water, efficient sewage disposal, and improved food, hygiene, and nutrition in the eighteenth century; and rising standards of living, improved hygiene, and improved nutrition in the nineteenth century—with only five percent of the second half of the century's decline in mortality attributed to immunization.[24,25] In the twentieth century, the U.S. Public Health Service estimated that of the 30 years that have been added to life expectancy since 1900, only 5 years are the result of improvements in clinical medicine, with the remaining 25 years being attributable to population-based public health programs.[26]
- Prevention is often cheaper than treatment. For example, an analysis of the U.S. Department of Agriculture's Special Supplemental Food Program for Women, Infants, and Children (WIC) revealed that for mothers and newborns during the first 60 days after birth, the government saves more money on Medicaid than it spends for prenatal care through WIC.[27]
- Treatment advances tend to benefit the socioeconomically advantaged disproportionately, and, as a result, to increase the gap in health status between rich and poor Americans.
- As the CDC recently noted, "the emergence of drug resistance in many organisms is reversing some of the therapeutic miracles of the last 50 years and underscores the importance of disease prevention."[17(p.3)]

Emphasizing prevention, not just treatment, requires a commitment to changing a wide range of governmental and commercial policies that shape the physical, social, and political environment in which people live, because their behavior is a product of the social conditions and social norms in their community.[28] For example, all of the following policy changes have a role to play in improving public health, although some would have more of an effect than others: reducing poverty, increasing the percentage of children (and adults) covered by health insurance, facilitating physical activity during the work day, and decreasing the mass media portrayals of unsafe behaviors and unrealistic body types.

LOST VISION OF PUBLIC HEALTH

The Institute of Medicine (IOM) has defined the mission of public health as to fulfill "society's interest in assuring conditions in which people can be healthy."[29(p.7)] Yet a 1999 survey conducted among registered voters revealed that "approximately half (57%) of the respondents could not define public health as either protecting the population from disease or policies and programs that promote healthy living conditions for everyone."[30(p.258)] In recent years, a number of factors have contributed to a lost vision—among public health practitioners, policy makers, and the public—of public health's role in society. These factors include

- illusions about the role of health care reform and managed care vis-à-vis public health
- political and economic factors that directly threaten public health funding
- practitioners backing away from advocating for public health causes

Illusions about Health Care Reform and Managed Care vis-à-vis Public Health

Discussions concerning health care reform and managed care have dominated the American health policy agenda for the past decade. Although some public health practitioners believe that health care reform and the continued rise of managed care present opportunities for public health, in reality, the objectives of each are in opposition. Public health has a broad focus: to deliver adequate population-based disease and injury prevention and control programs to the American people, with the goal of ensuring a basic level of well-being for all, regardless of age, race, income, social status, or health status. Because programs must be administered repeatedly, consistently, and over many years (often decades) before the necessary changes in social conditions, norms, behavior, and policy take place, the public health view is inherently long term. In contrast, health care reform and managed care both have a comparatively narrow emphasis on controlling the costs of medical care, either by changing how hospitals and health care providers are reimbursed or by limiting patient care. Because employers often switch plans (sometimes yearly) in an effort to reduce costs, and for-profit managed care organizations must answer to stockholders, this view is fundamentally short term.

Consequently, although it was initially thought that managed care organizations would be receptive to funding prevention programs because prevention is cheaper than treatment over the long term, the reality is that managed care organizations perceive no short-term benefit to funding expensive prevention programs because of high patient turnover and because denying treatment, not expanding prevention programs, is the most effective way to increase short-term profits.[31]

Political and Economic Factors that Directly Threaten Public Health Funding

In recent years, antiregulatory sentiment among members of the public and policy makers in the United States has increased. For example, the percentage of Americans who believe that the federal government can be trusted to "do what is right" most or all of the time declined from 76 percent in 1964 to a low of 14 percent in 1994.[32] Consequent efforts to decrease the regulatory power of the federal government and return control back to the states have had major ramifications for public health funding. For example, during 1995–96, congressional bills were introduced that would have eliminated or severely weakened the authority of nearly every major federal health agency to protect the public's health.[7] And, as always, special interest groups, such as the National Rifle Association and the tobacco industry, are mobilized to fight or repeal legislation that compromises their interests. Public health practitioners have difficulty wielding comparable influence because they do not have the same tools available: they cannot make campaign contributions and, if they are federal or state employees or recipients of federal grants, they are prohibited from lobbying.

As Mullan noted, "It will be the response to this challenge—the stewardship of the public trust despite the siren calls of devolution and privatization—that will render the ultimate commentary on the leadership of federal public health at the end of the 20th century." [33(p.24)]

Practitioners Backing Away from Advocating for Public Health Causes

The IOM has described public health's history as "one of identifying health problems, developing knowledge and expertise to solve problems, and rallying political and social support around the solutions."[29(p.70)] Yet today's public health practitioners are increasingly hesitant to "rally" political and social support. Some hesitancy is due to concerns that this rallying may constitute lobbying, which is restricted by federal law; other hesitancy stems from special interest group pressure, exemplified by the tobacco industry's accusations of illegal activity and use of the Freedom of Information Act (FOIA) to force state practitioners to copy hundreds of documents.[34,35]*

CHALLENGES OF PUBLIC HEALTH MARKETING

In using the marketing process and marketing techniques, public health practitioners confront a number of challenges that commercial marketers can often avoid. Rothschild outlined some problems that are encountered more frequently by all nonbusiness entities: "the intangibility of nonbusiness products, the nonmonetary price of purchase, the extreme lack of frequency of purchase, the lack of behavioral reinforcers, the need to market to an entire but heterogeneous society/market, and the extreme levels of involvement varying from very low to very high."[36(p.12)] In addition, public health practitioners frequently encounter the following challenges:

- unfavorable state of demand
- lack of marketing orientation
- limited professional training
- better-financed competition
- limited ability to assess impact

*Policy advocacy activities, such as researching, developing, planning, implementing, enforcing, and evaluating public health policy, are not lobbying unless they involve the promotion of a specific vote on a specific legislation.[7] As defined in the Internal Revenue Service Code, lobbying refers to an attempt to influence the outcome of legislation through communication with a legislator, government official, or the public (26 U.S.C.S. 4911). Generally, a communication is considered lobbying only if it: (1) refers to specific legislation and (2) promotes a specific vote on that legislation.[37]

Unfavorable State of Demand

As Table 20–2 illustrates, there are eight possible states of demand for a product. Unfortunately, public health products are usually in one of the last three demand states (negative, no demand, or unwholesome), although some may experience irregular demand (e.g., influenza vaccines) or faltering demand (e.g., "mature" products, such as HIV/AIDS prevention behaviors, that are no longer as salient due to improved treatment or simply the fact that they are no longer new).

Unwholesome demand occurs when an alternative product or behavior is more appealing than the public health product or behavior. On an individual level, tobacco products, alcohol, and drugs are three examples of unwholesome demand. At the policy level, the desire for freedom from gun controls is an instance of unwholesome demand. Other public health programs or products confront a situation of *no demand*—an instance where people are not necessarily against the product, but simply are not interested. Some policies to further chronic disease prevention and control might fall into this category; for example, many employers may not be particularly interested in (or even aware of) policy changes that would help employees get more physical activity during the work day.

Rangan and colleagues outlined the following reasons why social changes are so often in states of *negative demand*:[38]

- The target community opposes the change being advocated (e.g., efforts to reduce family size often conflict with a population's current way of life).
- Adoption costs often exceed tangible benefits.
- Early adopters stand to lose (in the family planning example, if only a few couples choose to have smaller families, they will be at a disadvantage among their peers).
- Benefits accrue only when a large percentage of the target community accepts the proposed change.

Table 20–2 States of Marketing Demand

Demand State	*Marketing Approach*
Full demand (demand is at the desired level)	Maintenance
Overfull demand (demand is too high)	Demarket (temporarily or permanently discourage customers without impugning the product)
Latent demand (people have a strong need for a product that does not yet exist)	Developmental marketing (create and market a product to satisfy existing demand)
Irregular demand (seasonal or widely fluctuating)	Synchromarket (synchronize fluctuations in demand and supply)
Faltering demand (lower than former level)	Remarket/revitalize (alter the product, the target audience, or the marketing effort)
Negative demand (public dislikes the product, does not want it, is not willing to pay a price for it)	Conversional marketing (design a marketing effort to cause demand to rise, perhaps by fulfilling other needs)
No demand (no interest in the product)	Stimulational marketing (alter the product or marketing effort to fulfill other existing needs; alter the environment so the product becomes valued; promote in more places in hopes that the problem is actually a lack of exposure)
Unwholesome demand (for an alternative product)	Countermarket (designate the product as intrinsically unwholesome)

Source: Data from P. Kotler, *Marketing Management: Analysis, Planning, and Control,* 3rd ed., © 1976, Prentice-Hall.

For all three unfavorable demand scenarios, the marketer's job is to identify appropriate target audiences and ferret out benefits that they can or do associate with the desired behavior or policy change so that a way can be found to position it as superior to the competing behavior or policy. To do this, solid consumer research—especially in terms of core values and benefits that people can associate with a product or behavior change—becomes even more important for public health practitioners than for commercial marketers.

Lack of Marketing Orientation

The indicators of an organization mindset, rather than a consumer/marketing mindset, were presented early in this chapter. This nonmarketing orientation creates a number of difficulties when public health practitioners attempt to market a product or behavior. First, "unlike commercial marketers, who develop products based on what customers are most likely to purchase, public health institutions often allocate resources based on legislative priorities as reflected in mandates or current funding streams (i.e., if tax money or grants are available for tobacco control, then the institution focuses on tobacco control), rather than on an analysis of what behavior changes might best impact a population's health—let alone what changes are most likely to be made by the population served."[7(p.205)] Furthermore, those charged with the marketing function within a public health organization are rarely in a position to influence or change the organization's priorities or institute other changes to support the behavior or policy change being sought.

Second, public health practitioners often hesitate to target, or focus on, specific groups of people because of a mandate to serve "the general public." However,

> trying to appeal to everyone is problematic for a number of reasons. One, it wastes resources because not everyone needs a particular intervention. Often, particular subgroups of the population are reached by other entities, have a very low incidence of the problem the intervention addresses, or have already embraced the behavior being promoted. Two,...even if "everyone" needs a particular intervention, some subgroups are likely to be closer to actually changing their behavior, while others are not nearly ready. And different groups will associate different costs and benefits with the behavior in question. Finally, social change resources are often extremely limited. By trying to stretch them to include "everyone," no audience group will be reached with any intensity.[7(p.206)]

Limited Professional Training in Marketing

Very few public health employees charged with marketing functions have a marketing background, although some have training as health educators or are drawn from communication and public information departments. As might be expected, this lack of experience can lead to poorly conceived marketing efforts, or an excessive dependence on communication when at times adjusting another variable in the marketing mix would do more to bring about change. For example, if a clinic is underutilized because the hours are inconvenient for clients, all the promotional activities in the world are unlikely to increase usage as much as adjusting the clinic hours to meet client needs.

Similarly, most public health practitioners have limited, if any, training or expertise in advocacy skills, including coalition building, community organizing, media advocacy, and political activity. As the IOM has noted, "effective public health action for many problems requires organizing the interest groups, not just assessing a problem and determining a line of action based on top-down authority."[39(p.122)]

Better-Financed Competition

The competition may be an unwholesome product, behavior, or policy, but it almost always has more money behind it than the public health effort. And this financing often extends beyond the money spent by the product sponsors. For example, tobacco products and alcohol, in particular, make regular appearances in the story lines of television and movie programming; likewise, drug use is often featured in popular music. Although much of this is not necessarily paid for by the obvious competition, it nonetheless creates a more pervasive "unhealthy" environment and reinforces the idea that use of such products is normative. In fact, the mass media often portray such product use, particularly cigarette smoking, as far more common than it actually is.

Because public health marketing budgets are often modest at best, when promotional efforts are used, it is difficult to attain sufficient reach (percentage of the target audience reached with promotional messages) and frequency (number of times a member of the target audience is reached) to support behavior change. Most public health organizations do not have the funds to pay for advertising placement; consequently, they must rely on media-donated time for ads and editorial (nonadvertising) coverage. Media-donated, or public service, time is problematic because the donated time slots often do not correspond to when the target audience is viewing or listening, and because the few slots that are donated do not provide sufficient frequency. Editorial coverage (e.g., news or feature stories) can be very effective but is often difficult to obtain because the issue being promoted is "evergreen," meaning that a story on it could run at any time—there is no urgency. In addition, public health practitioners lose control of the message when it appears in news or feature stories rather than in advertising. Commercial marketers, on the other hand, have the resources to put together an appropriate mix of advertising, public relations, and other media components.

Limited Ability To Assess Impact

Although commercial marketers can tie many of their activities directly to changes in product sales, public health practitioners often have a much more difficult time linking marketing activities to behavior or policy changes, let alone to ultimate changes in morbidity and mortality. The reasons for this are discussed in more detail under "Issues in Evaluating Outcomes" later in this chapter.

THE MARKETING PROCESS

The marketing process generally follows a defined set of steps. These steps are often depicted as a circle, or wheel, to symbolize the iterative nature of the process: everything learned at one stage feeds into the next, and often something learned in a subsequent stage will feed back into an earlier stage. In the example in Figure 20–1, the four major stages of planning, development, implementation, and assessment are depicted, with research and evaluation in the center to illustrate that they play a role in, and provide a strong foundation for, each stage.

Exhibit 20–2 lists the essential activities that take place during each stage. As can be seen, the planning process is extensive because it provides the framework for all subsequent activities. Although portraying marketing as a linear process is the easiest way to present and understand it, it should be pointed out that the process is not so sequential in practice. For example, planning and development decisions are often driven to some degree by limited funds available for development or implementation. Or monitoring data may suggest a need to revise the plan or create or revise a tactic, necessitating a return to a previous stage. The following sections discuss fundamental aspects of each stage.

Planning

A more apt title might be *iterative planning*, because as new knowledge is gained from each

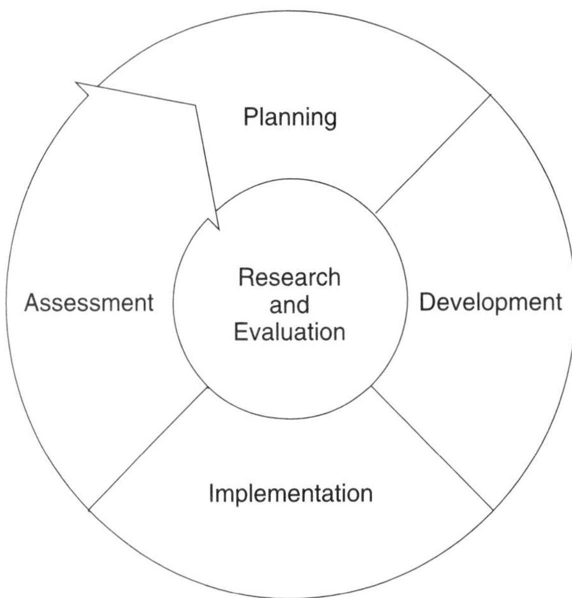

Figure 20–1 Stages of Marketing Initiatives. *Source:* Reprinted from M. Siegel and L. Doner, *Marketing Public Health: Strategies To Promote Social Change,* p. 200, © 1998, Aspen Publishers, Inc.

Exhibit 20–2 Planning, Developing, Implementing, and Assessing a Marketing Effort

Stage 1: Planning

- Analyze the situation.
  - Identify and prioritize problems based on public health burden.
  - Assess the social change environment, including the competition.
  - Identify interventions most likely to be effective.
- Set goals and objectives: specify behaviors, conditions, or policies to be changed.
- Segment and select target audiences: determine the target populations for each desired social change.
- Understand target audiences.
  - Identify and prioritize basic needs, desires, and values.
  - Identify the current behavior and attributes of the behavior that satisfy those needs, desires, and values.
  - Explore ways of framing the desired behavior to reinforce core values.
- Develop a strategic plan addressing product, price, place, promotion, and partners.
  - Redefine the product as offering a desired benefit.
  - Package and position the product as offering the benefit.
- Develop a communication strategy.
  - Frame the communication to reinforce (not to conflict with) the audience's core values.
  - Focus on the promise (the benefit) and support for it.
- Conduct message concept testing.

Stage 2: Development

- Develop product and/or promotion plans.
- Develop prototype products and/or communication materials.
- Pretest with target audience members.
- Refine the products and materials.
- Build in process evaluation measures.

Stage 3: Implementation

- Produce the products and materials.
- Coordinate with partners.
- Implement the intervention.
- Conduct a process evaluation.
- Refine the products, materials, and delivery channels as needed.

Stage 4: Assessment

- Conduct an outcome evaluation.
- Refine the program.

Source: Reprinted from M. Siegel and L. Doner, *Marketing Public Health: Strategies To Promote Social Change,* p. 226, © 1998, Aspen Publishers, Inc.

planning activity, previous ideas or assumptions often require revision. The major goal of all planning activities is to clearly identify

- the problem that marketing activities will address (e.g., *what* changes need to be made and *who* needs to make them)
- all possible components of a solution (e.g., *how* changes can be made, and what will facilitate change)
- of those components, what components the marketing effort will include

One way to do this is to create a model, or map, of how the problem realistically needs to be addressed. This model will help everyone involved clearly see what individual, social, or policy changes will be necessary in order to lessen or control the problem. It also helps determine what roles are appropriate for a particular organization and what roles will have to be played by others. The model can be used throughout an initiative to make sure the effort stays focused on the objectives. It is also helpful when crafting evaluation efforts because it provides a blueprint of who is doing what and what the result of each activity should be. Figure 20–2 provides the beginning of such a model for increasing the percentage of child safety seats that are properly installed in passenger cars. It will be used as a case study throughout the remainder of this chapter.

Such a model should begin as a synthesis or depiction of what is learned when the situation is

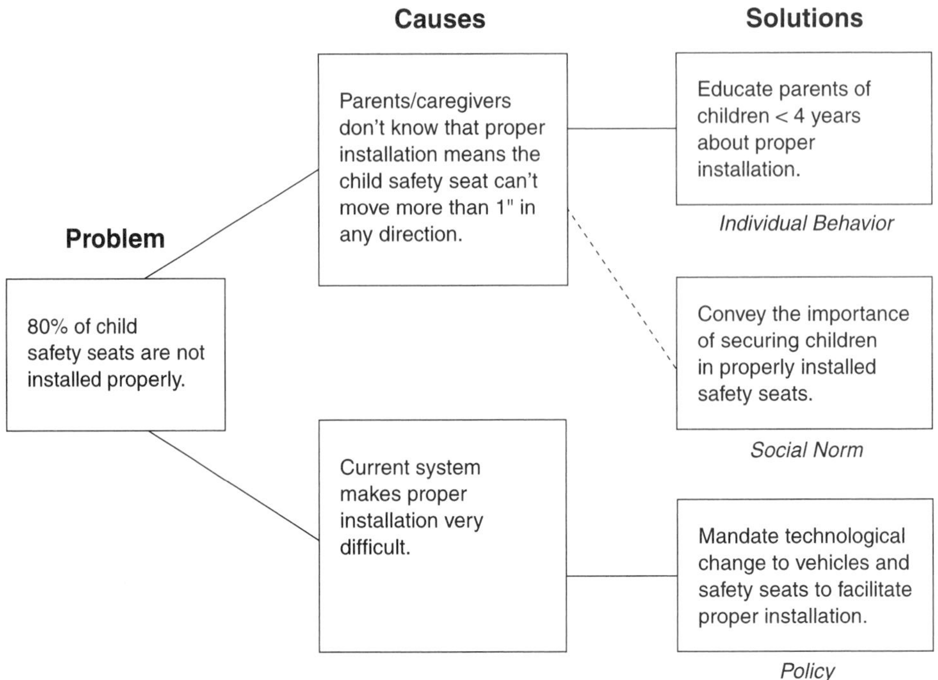

Figure 20–2 Modeling the Child Safety Seat Initiative

analyzed (see Exhibits 20–2 and 20–3). As the planning process continues, it can be fleshed out and revised: goals and objectives can be added, target audiences can be more carefully defined, and strategies for each component of the solution can be crafted.*

Problem Definition: Making Sure the Real Problem Is Addressed

Many marketing efforts, in public health and in other disciplines, fail because planners do not thoroughly explore and define the problem and its potential solutions. Adequate problem definition requires a thorough understanding of the current behavior, the desired behavior, and the environment—current policies, social norms, and competing behaviors—in which the change will take place.

In the child safety seat example, inadequate problem definition would have occurred if planners had not recognized that two marketing mix variables needed to be addressed: product and promotion. If planners had "blamed" parents and other caregivers for the improper installations without recognizing that the existing product technology made proper installation exceedingly difficult, they might have relied on promotional efforts as a solution. At best, this approach would not be very effective; at worst, it might exacerbate the problem by increasing the number of caregivers who became frustrated or who lost confidence in the safety of existing child restraint systems. In the short term, planners did rely on promotional activities, because fixing the product was a multiyear process. (Although one of the initial studies was conducted in 1996, all aspects of the final regulation will not go into

*More detail on conducting the steps involved in the planning process can be found in other sources.[7,40,41]

Exhibit 20–3 Key Aspects of the Child Restraint System Situation Analysis

Problem

- Child restraints are 71 percent effective in reducing the likelihood of death in motor vehicle crashes. However, actual average effectiveness of restraints in use is 59 percent, due to
  - Incorrect use, and/or
  - Vehicle seat and/or seat belt incompatibility issues
- Consumer frustration with installation and compatibility may lead to eroding confidence in the safety of child restraint systems and decreased usage of the systems.

Causes

- Incorrect use. A 1996 four-state study found that 80 percent of participants made at least one significant error in installation. Seventy-two percent did not use a locking clip when necessary, or used it incorrectly; 17% used the vehicle seat belt incorrectly.
- Vehicle seat and seat belt incompatibility. Advances in seat and seat belt design features to protect older children and adults have led to increased difficulty with child restraint installation. In consumer clinics (somewhat similar to focus groups) conducted in the United States and Canada, virtually all participants expressed high levels of dissatisfaction with conventional means of attaching child restraints in vehicles.

Source: Data from *Federal Motor Vehicle Safety Standards; Child Restraint Systems; Child Restraint Anchorage Systems,* 64 Fed. Reg. 10785, 1999, National Highway Transportation Safety Administration.

effect until 2002.) Conversely, if they had relied only on changing the product, they probably would not have made as much progress because: (1) even with the new products, parents and other caregivers still need to know what "properly installed" is, and (2) communicating with parents and caregivers about installing safety seats is likely to influence the social norm regarding their use (e.g., if the target audience constantly hears about the importance of installing the seats correctly, it reminds them to use the seats).

The other half of adequately defining a problem is adequately defining the solutions to the problem—and then determining which of those solutions the organization can actually implement. Ultimately, these solutions become the goals and objectives for the marketing activity. In the child safety seat example, NHTSA could implement the policy solution (albeit by working with consumer advocacy groups and vehicle and child safety seat manufacturers) and aspects of the individual behavior change and social norm solutions, but the latter require partnerships with many local organizations to be effective. In contrast, an advocacy group would have been wise to concentrate on marketing the policy change to NHTSA and manufacturers while marketing individual behavior change to parents and caregivers. A local public health agency, on the other hand, might concentrate on promoting individual behavior change through materials, publicity, and local checkpoints.

When selecting approaches to addressing a public health problem, it is important to recognize that there are many problems that communication alone cannot solve. If, during the planning process, it is discovered that major policy changes are needed to address the problem adequately, there are three options.

1. Work for the policy changes, or find a partner who can make the policy changes.
2. Proceed with the communication activity, but carefully limit objectives to what communication can reasonably be expected to accomplish in the absence of other changes.
3. Allocate resources to a different topic where the organization's efforts can make more of a difference.

When taking the second course, be aware that there are some situations where promotion will only make matters worse. One example is increasing demand when supply is inadequate, as might have been the case with child restraints: educating consumers about proper installation would drive up demand for it, but the existing child restraint systems could not deliver, ultimately leading to consumer frustration, and potentially, abandonment of the product or efforts to install it properly. Or, let's say a local health department wants to promote a new vaccine for children during National Child Health Month, but shipments of it have been delayed. If the promotion effort goes forward, people will be exposed to the promotion and try to get the vaccine, only to be turned away and told to return when there is more vaccine. They will find the experience frustrating and some will not come back again, so the promotion will have backfired.

Understanding How a Behavior or Issue Is Framed

Understanding how the behavior or issue is *framed* in the minds of the target audience(s) is an important aspect of developing useful approaches to solving the problem. Framing involves packaging and positioning an issue to convey a certain meaning.[39,42–48] Schon and Rein defined frames as "the broadly shared beliefs, values, and perspectives familiar to the members of a societal culture and likely to endure in that culture over long periods of time, on which individuals and institutions draw in order to give meaning, sense, and normative direction to their thinking and action in policy matters."[46(p.xiii)] Often, frames can be used to define the problem in a different way and suggest solutions to it.[45,48,49]

To illustrate how to identify and analyze how an issue is framed, Exhibit 20–4 provides an example from the tobacco policy debate. The process of using frames to package and position a behavior or issue so that the target audience is motivated to take action is discussed in more detail in the "Framing Messages" section of this chapter.

Exhibit 20–4 The Tobacco Policy Debate

BACKGROUND

Menashe and Siegel prepared a framing memo on tobacco policy issues, attempting to identify and analyze the frames used to support and oppose tobacco policy interventions during the past decade. They identified these frames by analyzing all front-page articles relating to tobacco that appeared in the *Washington Post,* the *New York Times,* the *Los Angeles Times,* and the *Wall Street Journal* from 1985 to 1996. A summary table from their framing memo outlines the five dominant tobacco industry frames (Table 20–3) and the five dominant tobacco control frames (Table 20–4) they identified.

In their analysis of how protobacco control and antitobacco control groups framed the issue, Siegel and Menashe found that the tobacco industry has been much more successful in developing frames that appeal to the most compelling core values of the American public: freedom, independence, civil liberties, individual rights, control, autonomy, equality, fairness, economic opportunity, capitalism, and democracy (Table 20–3). In contrast, most of the public health community's frames have been based on the core value of health (Table 20–4).

TOBACCO INDUSTRY APPROACHES

The tobacco industry has been steadfast in framing tobacco policy in terms of core human values. Their dominant framing strategies—big government/civil liberties, moralizing/hostility, accommodation, choice, and health vs. wealth—elicit more of a passionate gut response than those put forth by tobacco control frames. The core frames of the tobacco industry conjure up images of a free America, anti-Big Brother sentiment, freedom of the American citizen, the freedom of choice, strengthening the economic prosperity of America and its citizens, supporting the economic livelihood of the tobacco farmer and the farmer's family, and also concern about America's youth. With the power of these images, it is no wonder that the tobacco industry has been able to remain so supported and successful.

TOBACCO CONTROL APPROACHES

Over the past decade, tobacco control advocates have increasingly used frames that appeal much more to the most compelling core values. For example, the deceit and manipulation frame (Table 20–4) appeals to the core values of equality, fairness, and justice. Its core position is that the to-

continues

Exhibit 20–4 continued

bacco industry intentionally manipulates people to smoke by controlling nicotine levels, using deceptive advertising, denying tobacco's harmful health effects, and targeting specific population subgroups. The core position of the nonsmokers' rights frame is that exposure to secondhand smoke violates people's right to a safe working environment and clean air in public places, and this frame appeals to the values of individual freedom, individual rights, and equality.

In addition, tobacco control frames that have been used most recently tend to attribute responsibility for the problem to society—that is, to the tobacco companies for producing, marketing, and selling an addictive product and to the government for failing to control the sale and marketing of this drug to youth. For example, the smokers at risk frame and illicit drug for minors frame attribute responsibility for the tobacco problem to individual smokers, individual youth, and individual merchants. In contrast, frames such as deceit and manipulation, nonsmokers' rights, and drug delivery device attribute responsibility to the tobacco companies and to the government.

CONCLUSIONS

The increased use of frames that are based on the most deeply ingrained core values and that shift the attribution of responsibility from the individual to society may, in part, explain the increased success of the tobacco control movement in obtaining unprecedented policy gains at the federal, state, and local levels. As Wallack, Dorfman, Jernigan, and Themba suggested, "one of the great successes of the antitobacco movement has been to win the framing battle with the tobacco companies and erode the credibility and legitimacy of the tobacco interests. As a result of the movement's efforts, the general public increasingly views the tobacco industry as 'merchants of death.'"[2(p.71)]

Now that the dominant tobacco industry and tobacco control frames have been identified and analyzed, tobacco control practitioners can use formative research to test the effectiveness of alternative frames in garnering support for specific tobacco policies. They can also test the effectiveness of new tobacco control frames and attempts to reframe tobacco industry arguments so that they support, rather than oppose, tobacco control policies.

Source: Reprinted from M. Siegel and L. Doner, *Marketing Public Health: Strategies To Promote Social Change,* pp. 241–244, © 1998, Aspen Publishers, Inc.

Role of Theory and Models of Behavior

Once the problem has been clearly defined, theories and models of behavior can be helpful in discerning how best to approach solving it. These theories and models can guide the segmentation and selection of audiences as well as the content of the intervention. Some theories and models that practitioners often find useful include diffusion of innovations, social cognitive theory, and the transtheoretical model of stages of change.[10,11,50,51] Diffusion of innovations can help planners understand how an innovation (new behavior or policy) is likely to move through a population or an organization (or series of organizations). Social cognitive theory and the stages of change model are of particular help in determining how individual behavior will change and the role that an intervention can play to facilitate that change (i.e., increasing self-efficacy or confidence in ability to change behavior, affecting the cost–benefit equation by decreasing costs or increasing benefits). Glanz, Lewis, and Rimer's *Health Behavior and Health Education* provides a good overview of many theories and models that can be used to help guide efforts to bring about health behavior change.[52]

Some practitioners shy away from theory, perhaps in part because the often complex terminology makes them think they will not understand it or that it cannot be applied in the "real world." However, judicious use of theory can keep planners from reinventing the wheel, provide additional support for the recommended approach, and fill in some missing pieces on what to do in a given situation. Applying theory does not have to involve an unfamiliar vocabu-

Table 20–3 Dominant Tobacco Industry Frames: 1985–96

Frame	*Big Government/ Civil Liberties*	*Moralizing/Hostility*	*Accommodation*	*Choice*	*Health vs. Wealth*
Core position	Big government is interfering with personal lifestyle decisions, taking away smokers' rights.	Antismoking zealots are moralizing to us, discriminating against us, telling us what to do.	We can and should accommodate both smokers and nonsmokers.	Smoking is a matter of choice like any other choice in life.	Business will suffer if tobacco is regulated.
Metaphor	Big Brother Prohibition	Puritanism Holocaust	Accommodation of customers Negotiation Etiquette	Drinking alcohol Sex	Government regulation of small businesses
Images	Prohibition era *1984*	Puritan era Holocaust Prohibition era	Negotiation Hospitality Environments	Prison cell	The Depression Small "mom and pop" stores
Catch phrases	Prohibition, big government, Big Brother, government off our backs, goes too far, red meat, candy, fat	Second-class citizens, cultural war, hostility, accommodation, tolerance, bombarded, antismoking zealots, fascists, health Nazis, attacking smokers, under siege	Accommodation, fair, balanced, reasonable, compromise, customers, clientele, hospitality	Choice, mature adults, judgments, clientele, already know the risks	Economic impact, jobs, out of business, tourists, making a living, difficult times, recession, suffering, hardship
Attribution of responsibility for problem	Big government Bureaucracy	Antismoking zealots	Hard-nose, uncompromising antismoking advocates	Individual smokers who make bad choices	Antismoking advocates who don't care about business
Implied solution	Keep government out of tobacco regulation.	Demand tolerance for smokers.	Demand accommodation of smokers and nonsmokers.	Let people decide whether to smoke, where to eat and work.	Let the market operate without intervention.
Core values	Freedom Civil liberties Autonomy Control	Freedom Civil liberties Autonomy Control Democracy	Fairness Equality	Freedom Autonomy Control	Free enterprise Capitalism Economic opportunity

Source: Reprinted from M. Siegel and L. Doner, *Marketing Public Health: Strategies To Promote Social Change,* p. 243, © 1998, Aspen Publishers, Inc.

Table 20–4 Dominant Tobacco Control Frames: 1985–96

Frame	*Smokers at Risk*	*Illicit Drug for Minors*	*Drug Delivery Device*	*Deceit and Manipulation*	*Nonsmokers' Rights*
Core position	Smokers are putting themselves at great risk by smoking.	Cigarettes are not legal until age 18; thus we must punish merchants who sell them and youth who smoke.	Companies manipulate nicotine levels; therefore FDA must regulate the product for consumer safety.	The tobacco industry now manipulates people to smoke through deceptive advertising and lies.	Nonsmokers have a right to be protected from secondhand smoke in workplaces and public places.
Metaphor	Unhealthy habits, like drinking alcohol, eating high-fat foods	Illegal drugs: marijuana, alcohol	Regulation of medical devices and drugs, deceptive packaging, food labeling	Untruthful advertising	Environmental toxins; workplace hazards
Images	Making love with death; disgusting, dirty habit	Undercover investigations, law enforcement, speeding tickets, fines	Corporate fraud and deceit; painstaking investigation; vultures out to addict people	Secret plans; lying under oath; hiding	Smoke, hazardous workplaces, chemicals, pollution
Catch phrases	Unhealthy habit, discourage smoking	Crack down, sting operations, possession, use, supply, caught, punishment	Manipulation, fraud, deceit, jurisdiction, addictive, consumer watchdog	Lies, deceit, manipulation, targeting, denial, conceal, hide, secret	Nonsmokers' rights, health hazard, protection, danger, secondhand, involuntary, passive, smoke-free
Attribution of responsibility for problem	Individual smokers	Merchants Teenagers	Greedy, sneaky corporations that lie, mislead, and deceive	Tobacco industry	Workplace owners; government
Implied solution	Smokers should quit.	Merchants should not be allowed to sell cigarettes to youth; kids should not smoke.	Public must be protected by federal government.	Advertising and other aspects of tobacco business must be regulated.	Voluntary or legislative policies should restrict smoking in public places.
Core values	Health	Health	Health	Equality Fairness Justice	Freedom Civil liberties Equality Justice

Source: Reprinted from M. Siegel and L. Doner, *Marketing Public Health: Strategies To Promote Social Change,* p. 244, © 1998, Aspen Publishers, Inc.

lary: drawing on various theoretical constructs regarding determinants of behavior, Bill Smith of the Academy for Educational Development argues that the goal should be to make individual behavior changes fun, easy, and popular:[53]

- *fun:* Provide perceived benefits the audience cares about.
- *easy:* Remove barriers to action; make behavior as simple and accessible as possible.
- *popular:* Influence social norms; help the audience feel that this is something others are doing, particularly others who are important to them.

Using the ideas in the child safety seat example might yield the following:

- *fun:* Convey to parents that this is something they can do simply, to help their children and feel like a good parent/caregiver.
- *easy:* Fix the product so child restraint systems can be easily and quickly installed correctly; provide motorists with a simple test they can use to see if installation is correct.
- *popular:* Use mass media, community events, and other venues to show that other caregivers and protectors of children (e.g., law enforcement officers) think this is important.

Crafting the Plan

As potential solutions (target audiences, the actions they should take, and the means of getting them to take these actions) become clear, a strategic plan can be assembled. Such a plan should be tailored to the situation, but typically looks something like the outline shown in Exhibit 20–5. The plan closely follows the activities presented in Exhibit 20–2. If multiple approaches are being used (e.g., a policy change and individual behavior changes, as in our example), then separate goals, objectives, target audiences, strategy, and components sections might be developed for each approach. The plan should be used to develop and assess tactics and implementation plans. Also, it (or the executive summary of it) can be shared with partners and other interested parties as a quick way of explaining what the organization is doing.

Exhibit 20–5 Outline of a Strategic Plan

Executive summary
Background and mission
Challenges and opportunities
Goals
Objectives (measurable outcomes)
Target audiences
Core strategy
Components for implementing and monitoring strategy:
  Product development
  Managing perceived price
  Improving access (place)
  Promotion (including communication strategy)
  Partnerships
  Evaluation

Source: Adapted from M. Siegel and L. Doner, *Marketing Public Health: Strategies To Promote Social Change,* p. 235, © 1998, Aspen Publishers, Inc.

Formative Research

"Formative research is foremost. It provides more value for the effort than any other kind of research."[54(p.63)]

Marketers place so much emphasis on formative research because it underpins how the problem is defined and how strategies to address it are crafted (selection of target audiences, actions they should take, and the approaches that will be used to help them). If a strategy is wrong or incomplete, every tactic can be executed flawlessly, but program objectives are unlikely to be accomplished. As a result, marketers tend to allocate a large proportion of their research and evaluation dollars to studies that are conducted to understand the problem and the audience, and to develop and assess reactions to proposed strategies, including products, service delivery approaches, messages, and materials used to implement the intervention.

Common Marketing Research Methods. Marketers tend to rely on a mixture of qualitative and quantitative research. *Qualitative research* allows the exploration of potential strategies and perceived benefits of and barriers to taking a particular action. It is also a good forum for assessing target audience reactions to new or existing products and potential ways of framing messages. Qualitative research typically supports the planning and development stages. Common qualitative methodologies include focus groups and one-on-one, in-depth interviews. Because of the way in which participants are selected and the relatively unstructured questioning (qualitative methods are more akin to a conversation than a structured questionnaire), findings from qualitative methods are not quantifiable or projectable to the population from which participants were drawn.*

In contrast, *quantitative research* provides measures of *how many* members of a population have particular knowledge, engage in a particular behavior, or would be willing to take a specific action. During the planning process, it is particularly useful for audience segmentation and selection; it can also be used to test positioning and messages in some instances. Quantitative methods are most often some type of survey, although observational studies (e.g., observing people and counting how many engage in a particular behavior) or methods such as medical chart review are also in this category. If quantitative studies are conducted with a census or a probability sample (and, for surveys, appropriately constructed questionnaires), the results can be representative of and projectable to the population.[7]

Because of the cost and time involved in obtaining solid quantitative data, market researchers often look first to secondary data sources (information that has already been collected for some other purpose). Useful federal and/or state data sources can include the *Behavioral Risk Factor Surveillance System (BRFSS),* the *Youth Risk Behavior Survey (YRBS),* the *National Health Interview Survey (NHIS),* and *the National Health and Nutrition Examination Surveys (NHANES).** Useful commercial sources include the annual studies conducted by Mediamark Research Inc. (MRI) and Simmons Market Research Bureau. Some market research companies, such as Claritas Corporation, provide geodemographic segmentation systems that allow neighborhoods to be categorized and mapped according to demographic and lifestyle characteristics.

Selecting and Understanding Target Audiences. Earlier in this chapter, the importance of segmenting and selecting target audiences was presented (see "Challenges of Public Health Marketing"). Marketers begin selecting target audiences by segmenting the population into groups and then studying each group to determine which one(s) would be the most appropriate target audiences. If possible, it is usually best to segment the population based on its current behavior, or a combination of its current behavior and willingness to make a particular change in it.

One useful exercise is to compare "doers" (those who already engage in the behavior) with "nondoers" (those who do not), to see what other differences exist between the two groups. Often, such an analysis provides insights into the determinants of each group's behavior. These determinants can then be addressed by the marketing initiative. For example, perhaps the child safety seat initiative's program planners discovered that caregivers who install the safety seats properly know that they should not move more than one inch in any direction, and a large percentage of those who install them improperly do not have this knowledge.

The sources discussed in the previous section (or in other studies) may have the necessary variables for a behavioral segmentation of "the general public"; if not, a custom study would have to be conducted in order to segment on behavior. Additional factors to consider when selecting target audience segments are shown in Exhibit 20–6.

---

*Details on qualitative methodologies and how to use them are provided in other sources.[7,55,56]

*More information on these studies can be found on CDC's Web site (http://www.cdc.gov), under "surveillance" and "National Center for Health Services."

Exhibit 20–6 Factors Influencing the Selection of Target Audiences

- Audience size
- Extent to which the group needs or would benefit from the behavior change
- How well available resources can reach the group
- Extent to which the group is likely to respond to the program
- For secondary audiences, the extent to which they influence primary audiences

Source: Reprinted from M. Siegel and L. Doner, *Marketing Public Health: Strategies To Promote Social Change,* p. 271, © 1998, Aspen Publishers, Inc.

In general, it is important to consider the likelihood of progress toward the initiative's objectives when selecting audience segments. For example, the audience should be large enough that if a reasonable percentage of the members take action, noticeable progress will be made. Sometimes, practitioners want to choose the group that is most "in need" of a particular action (e.g., their current behavior is farthest from it). But often, this group may be least likely to respond; choosing a group closer to taking the action may require fewer resources, result in more progress toward objectives, and positively influence the social norm regarding the behavior.

In the child safety seat example, if only occasional caregivers such as grandparents or baby sitters who have a child safety seat in their vehicle infrequently were targeted, not much progress would be made toward increasing the percentage of child safety seats that are properly installed. Yet this audience might seem to be a logical choice if they are least likely to be familiar with proper installation and therefore most "in need" of the knowledge. This selection can be particularly critical when the audience is policy makers: persuading those who are undecided, especially if many are, is likely to be far more productive than trying to reach those who are definitely opposed to a change.

Once target audience segments have been selected, they need to be profiled thoroughly to determine the best intervention strategies to help or convince them to take action. In the child safety seat example, the planners took two courses of action: a policy change to improve the product (and therefore make the behavior easier), and education to give people the knowledge they need to engage in the behavior. Next, they needed to figure out how to reach the target audience and persuade them to take the action of installing a safety seat correctly. In order to do this, they needed to understand the benefits and barriers the audience associates with the behavior, where and when to reach the audience, and the types of messages they would find compelling. Qualitative research is often used to help craft this understanding.

On the policy side, a consumer preference clinic (somewhat similar to a focus group) was conducted by U.S. and foreign vehicle manufacturers to assess consumer reactions to various technological changes that would enable the seat to attach to an anchorage designed specifically for it (a variety of rigid bar anchorage systems vs. a flexible latchplate system). They found that all the systems were strongly preferred over current designs that use vehicle seat belts to attach the restraint to the vehicle. When making its final decision, NHTSA considered the results of this research, the preferences of vehicle and safety seat manufacturers and other interested parties, cost implications of the various designs, and compatibility with the systems approved or likely to be approved in other countries.

Framing Messages: Crafting Communication Strategies

> The communications strategy describes how the behavior or issue will be framed and positioned in the consumer's mind. It spells out the target audience(s), the action they should take and how they will benefit, and how to reach them with messages. It is based on a thorough understanding of the audience and their wants, needs and values coupled with knowledge of the types of appeals likely to work in a given situation.[7(p.312)]

Good communication is focused, specific, and personal. When done properly, it will be compelling to the target audience—whether that audience is some segment of the general public, health professionals, or policy makers. Many professionals recommend drawing a picture (or finding a photograph) to represent the target audience, and then designing communication as though having a conversation with that person. Some version of the questions shown in Exhibit 20–7 helps many commercial and health communicators develop focused, specific, and personal communication.

Activities conducted throughout the planning process (see Exhibits 20–3 and 20–4) generally provide a starting point for determining how an issue or action should be framed and developing the communication strategy. In particular, these activities generally shed light on how competing behaviors are framed (or on how competitors frame an issue), what the target audience is like, and what openings can be used to reach them. However, some amount of custom formative research (even if it is small and informal due to budget constraints) is generally necessary to determine if audience members think the suggested actions are reasonable, planners' initial thinking about benefits and barriers is accurate and believable, and image is appropriate.

Exhibit 20–7 Questions To Guide Communication Strategy Development

- Who should be in the target audience, and what are they like?
- What is the action they should take—and what are they doing now?
- What are the obstacles that stand between the audience and the desired behavior?
- What is the benefit to the audience of engaging in the behavior?
- What is the support for that benefit—what will make it credible to the audience?
- What are the best openings for reaching the audience—and are the channels available appropriate for conveying the message?
- What image should communications convey?

Source: Reprinted from M. Siegel and L. Doner, *Marketing Public Health: Strategies To Promote Social Change,* p. 315, © 1998, Aspen Publishers, Inc.

A detailed discussion of how to develop communication strategy is not possible here. Good sources for additional information include an article entitled "Strategic Questions for Consumer-Based Health Communications," by Sutton and colleagues, and Maibach and Parrott's *Designing Health Messages*.[57,58] However, each question can be elaborated on a bit.

- *Who should be in the target audience, and what are they like?* Demographic characteristics are only the beginning. As Sutton and colleagues wrote, "What's important to this person? What are his or her feelings, attitudes, and beliefs about the behavior change and its benefits and barriers? What can motivate this person to do something different?"[57(p.728)]
- *What is the action they should take, and what are they doing now?* Roman and Maas observed that "overambition is the pitfall of most strategies."[59(p.5)] To select an action, you need to understand the competition (what are they doing now?) and identify, from among the possible actions a person could take, what the audience perceives to be reasonable.
- *What are the obstacles that stand between the audience and the desired behavior?* Common barriers include perceived conflicts between the desired action and beliefs, current practice, social norms, or how the issue is typically framed.
- *What is the benefit to the audience of engaging in the behavior?* The goal here is to find the most motivating benefit. In most circumstances, personal benefits that will be attained immediately or in the very near future are more compelling than longer-term benefits that may or may not directly reward the target of the communication.
- *What is the support for that benefit—what will make it credible to the audience?* Support is the reason the benefit outweighs the

obstacles, and it can take many forms: hard data, demonstrations of how to perform the action (to convey "easy" or increase self-efficacy by showing audience members they can do it), or demonstrations of the valued benefits associated with the action (e.g., a mother feeling like she is "being a good mom" after correctly installing a child safety seat). Executional detail, such as music, colors, design, typeface, and paper stock, or the degree to which people depicted are like target audience members in speech, dress, and action, can all support or detract from the promised benefit.[57]

- *What are the best openings for reaching the audience—and are the channels available appropriate for conveying the message?* Openings include the times, places, and states of mind when a person is most receptive to a message.[57]
- *What image should communication convey?* "The symbols, metaphors, and visuals linked to the behavior or positioning of an issue convey image, as do the types of actors, language, and/or music used."[7(p.323)] Image tells target audience members whether or not the communication is for them or someone they would like to be.

When developing a communication strategy, common errors include the following:[7]

- including multiple actions or framing an issue in multiple ways rather than focusing on one
- focusing on long-term public health benefits rather than short-term consumer benefits
- appealing to noncritical values (e.g., good health) rather than core values (freedom, autonomy, control, independence)
- supporting the message with facts alone when an emotional appeal would be more compelling
- using mass media to convey complex messages
- developing strategies for different audiences that conflict or send mixed messages

Development, Testing, and Implementation

> In the final analysis, textbooks can offer little on implementation that will improve upon a good plan, an adequate budget, good organizational and policy support, good training and supervision of staff, and good monitoring in the process evaluation stage.... The key to success in implementation beyond these six ingredients is experience, sensitivity to people's needs, flexibility in the face of changing circumstances, and eye fixed on long-term goals, and a sense of humor.[40(p.205)]

Selecting Appropriate Tactics

Tactics are the short-term, detailed steps that are used to implement a strategy.[7] For example, changing a clinic's hours, holding a community event, or producing a particular ad are all tactics. Selecting tactics for a marketing effort involves considering the model of how change is expected to occur, the marketing strategy, available resources, and the initiative's time line. Because different social change efforts employ a wide range of tactics, it is impossible to review all possible considerations here. However, the following list of questions can be used to help assess the appropriateness of each tactic.

- Is it on strategy? It may be a great idea, but if it doesn't fit with the strategy, save it for another program.
- To what degree does it complement and reinforce other tactics?
- Can it be created and implemented in a time frame that works with the overall time line and with other tactics that may need for it to be in place before they are put into place (e.g., training staff prior to implementing other program elements)?
- Will the tactic's contribution to achieving objectives be worth its cost?
- For each promotional tactic, what will it contribute to reach and frequency? The goal should be to reach as many target audience members as possible *as often* as pos-

sible. For example, radio ads can be a better solution than television ads because the costs of producing and placing them are far lower, so the same budget (or a much lower budget) can pay for far greater frequency on radio than on television.

- Does it make sense for the organization to develop or sponsor this tactic, or would it be a better fit for one of the partner organizations?

With complex, multifaceted programs, it is important to have "reality check" meetings periodically to make sure that the various components will work together and reinforce each other conceptually, that nothing has drifted off strategy, that everything can be rolled out in a time line that makes sense, and that each tactic will cost a reasonable amount relative to what it is expected to accomplish.

Mass Media Tactics

Space limitations preclude an in-depth discussion of mass media approaches. However, it is important to mention the following approaches because practitioners often use the mass media to communicate directly with target audiences in an effort to bring about individual behavior changes or to influence social norms or policy changes.

Advertising is most commonly used to communicate about individual-level behavior changes, although it can also be used to influence social norms or communicate about societal-level policy changes. It is most appropriately used to create awareness, provide reminders, or disseminate simple messages that require little context or explanation. Traditionally, public health communicators have produced the advertisements and then relied on the media to run them for free (i.e., as a public service). This approach has always been problematic because, even if sufficient reach was obtained, frequency tended to be less than optimal. However, over the past 20 years, three developments have simultaneously eroded the effectiveness of public service advertising.

1. More and more social causes use the mass media to disseminate messages, leading to increasing competition for available public service placement.
2. Deregulation ended government oversight of television and radio stations' broadcast of public service advertising (magazines and newspapers were never required to run public service ads).
3. The increasing number of media vehicles (e.g., more cable stations and magazines, the advent of the Internet) has led to smaller, ever more fragmented audiences. In response to these changes in the public service advertising environment, more and more of today's public health initiatives are purchasing advertising placement.*

Practitioners also attempt to gain *news or feature coverage* of public health issues. This approach often includes working with the media to get coverage of messages targeting individual health behaviors (e.g., a story on how to incorporate physical activity into one's day, or how to avoid transmitting an infectious disease). However, news and feature coverage (and some advertising) can also be used to shape how an issue is framed on the public agenda, an approach referred to as *media advocacy*. Media advocacy involves taking steps to frame an issue to gain media attention and suggest societal policy change as the appropriate solution to the problem.[48] Effectively gaining access to the media involves using appropriate tactics to frame an issue so that it is perceived as newsworthy by news reporters, editors, and producers. Elements of a public health story that may increase its newsworthiness include irony, controversy, celebrity, human interest, or a local angle.[54] The challenge is to work with the reporters, editors, and producers to frame the issue as a societal problem with societal causes, rather than an isolated incident or a problem brought on by individuals themselves (see Exhibit 20–5 for an example). Such an approach supports societal-level public policy changes to address

*For a good introduction to developing effective advertising, see 1992's *How To Advertise* by Kenneth Roman and Jane Maas.[59]

the problem rather than simply individual-level behavior changes.

A third way to involve the mass media in public health issues is through *entertainment education*, or the process of embedding social change messages in entertainment media (i.e., movies, television programs other than news, some radio programs, comic books, popular music). This approach is important because: (1) it provides an additional channel for reaching target audiences and (2) as Signorielli observed, "many if not most of the images in the media are in serious conflict with realistic guidelines for health, nutrition, and medicine. Research on the contributions of these portrayals to people's conceptions about health and medicine, although scarce, nevertheless indicates that those who spend more time with the media may have beliefs about health-related issues that are in conflict with the things they should do to remain healthy and/or improve the current status of their health."[60(p.153)] Organizations considering this approach, however, should carefully consider how controversial the subject and their organization is, and how (if at all) the approach can be implemented without causing unease. For example, when the U.S. Office of National Drug Control Policy returned advertising time to television broadcasters in exchange for programming that included on-strategy anti-drug messages, it was described as an "arrangement under which the federal government was covertly working with the networks to boost the quotient of anti-drug material in their entertainment programming," and members of the news media decried the approach as an infringement on free speech.[61(p.A29)]

Common Pretesting Methods

Before producing or implementing a new (or updated) product, product or service delivery change, or messages and materials, pretesting should be conducted with target audience members to ensure optimal results.

Messages and Materials. Pretesting messages and materials (e.g., advertisements, message points, pamphlets, brochures, instructions, forms, etc.) will not ensure success, but it can identify potential misinterpretations and, for materials, problems with executional details (e.g., readability of typeface or type size, reactions to colors, music, voices, timing, etc.), as well as assess the extent to which materials are clear, true to the strategy, and understood by the intended audience.

Common pretesting methods include *central-site (or intercept) interviews, in-depth interviews,* and *theater-style testing;* some detail on each is presented in Table 20–5. In some instances, quantitative, statistically projectable surveys can be used to explore or test message strategies; taking such an approach with materials tests is generally cost-prohibitive but may be useful at times.[7,62]

Focus groups, although often used for pretesting, generally are not appropriate because people do not typically view and react to materials in groups. They see or hear the material alone and draw conclusions about it alone. In addition, focus groups are more subjective and open to interpretation than methods involving consistent administration of a standard questionnaire.

Peer or professional review can be used to ensure that materials are scientifically accurate and that stakeholders are comfortable with them, or to obtain buy-in from others involved with the activity. Draft materials and a self-administered questionnaire can be distributed to reviewers, or reviewers can be convened and work as a group.

Topics typically covered in a pretest are shown in Exhibit 20–8.

Products. If a new product has been created, such as in the child restraint example, it is desirable to develop a prototype and conduct usability tests prior to production. Usability testing is also a good idea for Internet Web sites. This process can reveal problems, some of which may need to be corrected through design changes; others can be addressed in accompanying instructions. It is wise to test accompanying instructions for any product (new or old) included in an initiative, using the materials testing methodologies outlined above, to ensure that directions for use are clear and understandable and that they address common questions and misperceptions.

Changes in Product or Service Delivery. When a new process for obtaining products or services

Table 20–5 Comparison of Common Pretesting Methodologies

Method	*Description*	*When To Use*
Central-site (intercept) interviews	60–100 one-on-one interviews conducted in shopping malls, at community events, or at other places people gather. Quasi-quantitative: most questions closed ended; interview typically lasts 10–20 minutes; 100 or more respondents. Convenience sample; not projectable.	Used to test print, radio, and television advertising; posters; and pamphlets. Not good for longer materials because the interview length would be excessive. Used to learn *how* a target audience is reacting without great detail on *why.*
In-depth interviews	One-on-one interviews at a central site or at audience members' locations. Can be in person or by telephone.	Used to test long materials or large numbers of materials, or when intercepting people or getting them to a central site is not feasible.
Theater-style testing	60–100 or so audience members brought to a theater or other central site to view material, then complete a self-administered questionnaire or use more sophisticated response systems. Convenience sample; not projectable.	Used to test final (or nearly final) television ads or programming. Ads can be tested using a syndicated service; custom theater-style tests can be set up yourself.

Source: Data from authors; and M. Siegel and L. Doner, *Marketing Public Health: Strategies To Promote Social Change,* © 1998, Aspen Publishers, Inc.

has been designed or an old process has been streamlined, pretesting any forms (using the materials testing methodologies outlined above) and pilot testing the process itself can allow areas of confusion or bottlenecks to be identified and resolved prior to wider implementation.

Exhibit 20–8 Topics Commonly Included in Materials Pretests

- What is the main idea of the (ad, booklet, etc.)?
- What is the (ad, booklet, etc.) asking you to do?
- Did you have any questions? (What?)
- What, if anything, did you particularly like?
- What, if anything, did you particularly dislike?
- Was anything offensive? (What? Who would it offend?)
- Was anything hard to believe?
- Who is this (ad, booklet, publication, etc.) for?

Source: Reprinted from M. Siegel and L. Doner, *Marketing Public Health: Strategies To Promote Social Change,* p. 417, © 1998, Aspen Publishers, Inc.

Working with Partners

Supporters, intermediaries, coalitions, and partnerships are critical to the success of many social change efforts. They can be governmental agencies, community-based nongovernmental organizations, health voluntaries, professional associations, foundations, the media, large corporations, or local businesses. They can provide additional resources, entrée into target audience populations, and means of extending the scope, reach, and frequency of social change efforts. Successfully involving other organizations in an initiative requires patience, flexibility, and a commitment to making it work. Exhibit 20–9 lists some issues to consider when working on developing partnerships for a marketing initiative.

Assessment

Evaluation is a critical aspect of marketing. However, the marketing approach uses evalua-

Exhibit 20–9 Suggestions for Developing Successful Partnerships

- Think of potential partners as target audiences: What is the benefit to them of helping you?
- Consider the partner's impact on the initiative's credibility.
- Find out what your organization can legally and ethically do before exploring possibilities with partners
  - What partners are appropriate?
  - What can you ask partners to do?
  - What can you do for partners in return?
  - What activities can partners undertake that your organization cannot?
- Develop clear ideas of the roles you want partners to play—and an understanding of what roles they should not have (from your organization's perspective).
- Be flexible—losing prospective partners can limit a program's effectiveness.
- Put agreements in writing.
- Understand the challenges of working with partners.

Source: Reprinted from M. Siegel and L. Doner, *Marketing Public Health: Strategies To Promote Social Change,* p. 369, © 1998, Aspen Publishers, Inc.

tion to *improve* efforts, not just *assess* them. Beyond "How are we doing?" marketers expect evaluation data to help them answer "How can we do better?"

Earlier in this chapter, *formative* research and evaluation were discussed, as was their importance in crafting successful intervention components. This section highlights two additional types of evaluation:

- *process* evaluation, which "typically tracks and documents implementation by quantifying what has been done; when, where and how it was done; and who was reached."[7(p.449)] This type of evaluation allows ongoing monitoring and refinement of implementation.
- *outcome* evaluation, which examines the degree to which an intervention achieved its objectives, or had the effects it was planned to have

Importance of Monitoring and Refinement

The marketing approach is to use process evaluation data to monitor and refine an intervention constantly once it is in place. Doing so allows tactics to be adjusted in response to changes in audience needs, competitive activities, or environmental factors, thereby maximizing progress toward objectives. However, constantly refining implementation can require using alternative outcome evaluation designs because many standard evaluation designs expect a static intervention. This issue is discussed in more detail in the next section.

Some form of process information should be available for each tactic included in a marketing effort. Ideally, these data will go beyond providing statistics on how often a message was sent out, and also provide information on who was motivated enough to take action as a result. The best way to ensure that adequate monitoring information will be available is to build it into or set it up for each tactic from the beginning. For example, if materials are being distributed, inventory tracking systems can be set up to capture not only how many copies were distributed, but where and when they went. The results provide information on gaps in coverage (e.g., where the materials are not going). If materials are requested by target audience members (rather than intermediary organizations), looking at the information in conjunction with information on the time and place of other promotional activities provides a sense of which promotional activities are more effective.*

Issues in Evaluating Outcomes

Evaluating the results of marketing efforts is challenging for a number of reasons.

*Other examples of integrating process data collection into tactics are provided in Siegel and Doner, 1998.[7]

- Marketing efforts do not occur in isolation. Because other organizations and secular trends usually address the same social change, it is difficult, and often impossible, to attribute effects to a particular intervention.
- Standard evaluation techniques are not designed to assess interventions that are constantly being refined (e.g., tactics that are not working are altered or dropped, and new tactics may be introduced).
- Measuring statistically significant change may require unreasonable outcome expectations.

How, then, to approach the need to evaluate and assess how well an intervention did or is doing? In Exhibit 20–10, a series of questions to consider when planning an intervention and its corresponding outcome evaluation is offered.[7]

What outcomes are reasonable to expect? The crucial word here is *reasonable*. Often, public health marketing efforts are expected to attain unrealistically large effects. As Beresford and colleagues noted in discussing populationwide efforts to change eating habits, "The public health model, or population strategy, consists of shifting the entire distribution of a risk factor, including the mean, down. The diminution in risk for a given individual is typically small and may not even be clinically important. Nevertheless, because the entire distribution is affected, the impact on morbidity and mortality can be substantial."[63(p.615)]

If an intervention needs to have large effects in order to be considered a success, ask why. Sometimes this happens because expectations concerning appropriate effects sizes have been carried over from expectations for clinical studies. At other times, the power (or lack thereof) of the evaluation drives expectations of effects. Measuring statistically significant change with a small margin of error on a populationwide basis is prohibitively expensive. One way to reduce the cost is to reduce the evaluation's sample size. However, when sample size is reduced, the margin of error increases, which means that larger effects are required before observed changes can be considered statistically significant. If large effects are expected, can the intervention be structured so that it is of sufficient intensity and duration to achieve this level of success?

Commercial marketers generally have far greater resources yet expect modest effects. As Fishbein remarked, "Thus, while a condom manufacturer would be more than happy if an advertising campaign increased the company's share of the market by 3% or 4%, a public health intervention that increased condom use by the 3% or 4% probably would be considered a failure."[64(p.1075)]

One of the major factors influencing outcome expectations should be the type of intervention. Is it reasonable to expect slow, gradual changes or rapid, large changes? For most public health interventions, an expectation of slow, gradual changes is much more likely.[65] However, as Hornik noted, it is possible to see large, rapid changes in behaviors that are very easy to change and that result in sharply reduced risks of devastating events (i.e., preventing Reye's syndrome by using an aspirin substitute rather than aspirin, and reducing sudden infant death syndrome by putting babies to sleep on their backs rather than on their stomachs).[66]

How is the intervention expected to work? Is it expected to impact individuals' behavior directly? Influence social norms around that behavior? Result in a policy change to facilitate a behavior? Many evaluations are designed to

Exhibit 20–10 Questions To Guide Outcome Evaluation Plans

- What outcomes are reasonable to expect?
- How is the intervention expected to work?
- What type of evaluation design is most appropriate for the intervention setting?
- How will outcomes be measured?
- What was actually implemented?

Source: Data from M. Siegel and L. Doner, *Marketing Public Health: Strategies To Promote Social Change,* © 1998, Aspen Publishers, Inc.

measure a behavior change among target audience members when in fact the intervention was not designed to induce such change directly.

What type of evaluation design is most appropriate for the intervention setting? The gold standard is a randomized controlled trial. That is, target audience members are randomly assigned to treatment and control groups, outcome variables are measured to establish a baseline, the intervention is implemented (usually remaining constant through the implementation period), and outcome variables are measured again. In this way, any differences between the two groups can be attributed to the intervention. Quasi-experimental designs are similar, but assignment to each group is not random. Examples of quasi-experimental designs include community interventions where treatment and control communities are matched on key variables or populations within a community are divided into groups (this approach might be used with a school-based intervention).

A big problem with any experimental approach is what Durlak termed "the fantasy of untreated control groups."[67(p.76)] With most public health initiatives, it is very unlikely that members of the control group are receiving no intervention. They may not be receiving a particular organization's intervention, but they are almost certainly receiving something. As Feinlieb observed, "Science does not operate in a vacuum; the forces that operate to justify large, expensive community intervention studies also are operating among the general public to get them to accept the evidence and act on it even before the scientific establishment does."[68(p.1697)]

Alternatives to experimental and quasi-experimental designs are designs for full-coverage programs, or programs that are delivered to all members of a target population.[69] Such designs include comparisons between cross-sectional studies (e.g., independent surveys taken at different points in time), panel studies or repeated measures designs (measuring outcomes multiple times among the same group of people), and time-series analyses (taking many measures of outcome variables prior to intervention, using those measures to project what would have happened without the intervention, and comparing the results to repeated measures taken after the intervention).

How will outcomes be measured? The measures should be consistent with what the initiative attempted to accomplish. For example, if the child safety seat intervention was designed to get caregivers to attend a local event where the installation of the safety seat could be checked, the outcome measure should be what percentage of them did that, not what percentage of them have properly installed safety seats.

Measures also need to be sufficiently sensitive to capture progress toward outcomes. Commenting on a community intervention designed to increase safer sex that used as an outcome measure the proportion of young men who engaged in *any* act of unprotected anal sex, Fishbein wrote, "Was it fair to view a person who reduced unprotected sex acts from 100 to 0 as no more of a success than one who reduced such acts from 1 to none?"[64(p.1076)]

What was actually implemented? A surprising number of outcome evaluations conclude that an approach or program failed when in fact it was not adequately implemented or was not measured as implemented.[70] This disconnect between implementation and evaluation can occur when the evaluation and implementation teams are totally separate and do not communicate well, or when insufficient process evaluation data were collected, so it becomes impossible to determine the degree to which various tactics were implemented.

BUILDING MARKETING CAPACITY

Elsewhere in this chapter it was noted that few public health practitioners charged with marketing functions have a marketing background. How does a public health professional effectively integrate marketing into public health practice and acquire the necessary training and skills?

To begin, Smith advocates mastering a core of fundamental ideas that can be used to benefit any program of social change:[53]

- Keep the audience and the behavior in the picture constantly (e.g., decide who your audience should be and what you want them to do, then never lose focus of that audience and that behavior).
- Try to make the behavior fun, easy, and popular; using these three words focuses everyone on giving people what they want, in addition to what public health practitioners think they need.
- Base decisions on hard fact, or at least recognize when hard fact is not available, and monitor implementation closely.

Smith calls these core fundamentals *minimalist marketing*, and argues that they can be used to integrate marketing into many of the activities that public health professionals might undertake to support a social change effort, giving the following as examples:[53]

- Organize meetings: Invite members of the audience to meetings; identify and discuss both structural and internal barriers to the behavior to ensure that the real problem is identified.
- Build partnerships: Ask people what they *want* instead of what they *need.*
- Give presentations: Think about the audience, what they expect, and what you want them to do after the meeting.
- Review proposed programs: Focus on the audience and the behavior or action, the benefits that will be offered, and the evidence that the approach is right.
- Speak up: Every interaction is a marketing opportunity if you believe that the person(s) are an audience that you have to understand and offer something to in order to get what you want from them.

Beyond these basic practices, marketing capacity can be built in a number of ways.

- Take advantage of opportunities to partner with organizations with more marketing expertise.
- Look for marketing experience when making new hires, including interns, technology transfer fellows, and interagency personnel exchanges.
- Apply for federal or state grants that include training or technical assistance in marketing.
- Look for other relevant training opportunities.
- Require demonstrated marketing experience for appropriate contractors and grantees.
- Invite qualified experts to review grant or contract proposals, or to sit in on strategic planning sessions (get recommendations for such experts from others who are more familiar with marketing whose judgment you trust).
- See if a local college or university class would consider working on an initiative as class project.

For those who are interested in learning more about the marketing process and its applications in public health, a list of suggested reading has been included at the end of this chapter. In addition, the University of South Florida's School of Public Health sponsors an annual conference, "Social Marketing in Public Health" (held every June), and a variety of training sessions in conjunction with the conference and at other times during the year. Those with more marketing experience may be interested in the "Innovations in Social Marketing" conference; its locale changes from year to year, but information is generally published in *Social Marketing Quarterly*.

USING MARKETING APPROACHES ON LIMITED BUDGETS

Planning, designing, implementing, and assessing large-scale, sophisticated marketing initiatives require a lot of training and experience in a variety of disciplines—and a lot of money. But, as Smith observed, not all public health problems require elaborate, highly expert marketing efforts or vast resources.[53]

Although the importance of adequate formative research has been stressed, many local and state programs, in particular, do not have the funding to conduct extensive primary research. In such a situation, it is best to look for research that has already been conducted on the topic. Often, other states, the federal government, or other organizations are addressing the same topic and may have conducted studies that will inform your initiative, even if they are not a perfect fit. Involving members of the potential audience(s) in planning and design can be helpful, as long as it is remembered that individual opinions cannot be considered representative of an entire population. Audience members can also serve as a "reality check" for tactical ideas and can review materials for cultural and language appropriateness, relevance, and impact. Finally, depending on the target audience, small-scale pretesting can consist of a few intercept interviews conducted where people already gather—for example, a health care facility waiting room, senior center, community center, or church.

Local community resources can sometimes provide help with developing tactics. For example, many graduate students are interested in freelance projects. College or university professors of marketing, marketing research, advertising, and public relations often look for "real-world" class projects, although keep in mind that they proceed more slowly than paid contractors and their involvement generally will be confined to a quarter or semester. Some students might be interested in an ongoing internship for the experience it would provide. Another option is local professionals who may be willing to donate some time pro bono, perhaps in exchange for recognition of their contributions.

CHAPTER REVIEW

1. Marketing can be distinguished from other strategies for influencing health status and policy change by its emphasis on the following:
   - exchange relationships
   - behavior and policy change
   - competition
   - consumer orientation and audience segmentation
   - formative and process evaluation
   - program components beyond communication (e.g., product, price, and place)
2. Product, price, place, and promotion constitute the marketing mix—the group of variables that a marketer can alter to achieve the desired public health outcome of behavior change.
   - The *product* is the specific behavior change, good, service, or program of interest.
   - The *price* is the cost that must be borne by the target audience in terms of monetary expenditure, time, discomfort, inconvenience, and so forth.
   - The *place* includes the outlets through which the product is available or situations in which behavior changes can be made.
   - The *promotion* involves some combination of advertising, media relations, promotional events, advocacy, and entertainment used to communicate with target audience members about the product.
3. Public health organizations confront a number of challenges in marketing interventions and policies to the intended target audience, including
   - intangible products
   - nonmonetary costs
   - extreme levels of audience involvement, from very low to very high
   - unfavorable states of demand within the target audience

- lack of marketing orientation within the organization
- limited professional training in marketing within the organization
- better-financed competition
- limited ability to assess the impact of marketing

4. The marketing process consists of four major activities: planning, development, implementation, and assessment. Each of these major activities is facilitated and supported by research and evaluation.
5. Marketers rely on information from a combination of qualitative and quantitative research activities to design appropriate marketing strategies. *Qualitative* research activities often involve focus groups and key informant interviews conducted with members of the target audience. *Quantitative* research activities typically involve surveys of the target population and the use of secondary data that reveal attitudes and behaviors of the target population.
6. Understanding how a behavior or health issue is *framed* in the minds of the target audience is an important aspect of developing a successful marketing strategy. Framing involves packaging and positioning an issue to convey a specific meaning.
7. Key steps in developing and implementing a marketing process include the following:
   a. Determine what changes need to be made, who needs to make them, and how they can be made effectively.
   b. Set realistic marketing goals and objectives.
   c. Segment, select, and profile target audience(s).
   d. Develop a strategic plan addressing product, price, place, and promotion (including how to frame messages).
   e. Develop and pretest prototype products, tactics, and/or materials.
   f. Implement intervention, using process evaluation to monitor and refine as needed.
   g. Assess outcomes and refine efforts as needed.

REFERENCES

1. A.R. Andreasen, *Marketing Social Change: Changing Behavior To Promote Health, Social Development, and the Environment* (San Francisco: Jossey-Bass Publishers, 1995).
2. National High Blood Pressure Education Program, *The Sixth Report of the Joint National Committee on Prevention, Detection, Evaluation, and Treatment of High Blood Pressure* [NIH Pub. No. 98–4080] (Bethesda, MD: National Institutes of Health; National Heart, Lung, and Blood Institute; National High Blood Pressure Education Program, 1997).
3. R.C. Lefebvre and J.A. Flora, "Social Marketing and Public Health Intervention," *Health Education Quarterly* 15 (1988): 299–315.
4. R. Hornik et al., *The HealthCom Project in the Philippines: The National Urban Immunization Program 1989–1990* (Washington, DC: Academy for Educational Development, 1991).
5. R.C. Lefebvre et al., "Use of Database Marketing and Consumer-Based Health Communication in Message Design: An Example from the Office of Cancer Communications' '5 A Day for Better Health' Program," in *Designing Health Messages: Approaches from Communication Theory and Public Health Practice,* eds. E. Maibach and R.L. Parrott (Thousand Oaks, CA: Sage Publications, 1995), 217–246.
6. National Cancer Institute, *Unpublished Tables* (Bethesda, MD: 1999).
7. M. Siegel and L. Doner, *Marketing Public Health: Strategies To Promote Social Change* (Gaithersburg, MD: Aspen Publishers, Inc., 1998).
8. U.S. Centers for Disease Control and Prevention, "Public Opinion about Public Health—California and the United States, 1996," *Morbidity and Mortality Weekly Report* 47 (1998): 69–73.
9. F. Kroger et al., "Marketing Public Health: The CDC Experience," in *Social Marketing: Theoretical and Practical Perspectives,* eds. M.E. Goldberg et al. (Mahwah, NJ: Lawrence Erlbaum Associates, 1997), 267–290.
10. J.O. Prochaska et al., "The Transtheoretical Model and Stages of Change," in *Health Behavior and Health Edu-*

cation: Theory, Research and Practice, 2d ed., eds. K. Glanz et al. (San Francisco: Jossey-Bass Publishers, 1997), 60–84.

11. T. Baranowski et al., "How Individuals, Environments, and Health Behavior Interact: Social Cognitive Theory," in *Health Behavior and Health Education: Theory, Research and Practice,* 2d ed., eds. K. Glanz et al. (San Francisco: Jossey-Bass Publishers, 1997), 153–178.
12. P. Kotler and A.R. Andreasen, *Strategic Marketing for Non-Profit Organizations,* 2d ed. (Upper Saddle River, NJ: Prentice-Hall, 1996).
13. National Cancer Institute, *"5 A Day for Better Health": NCI Media Campaign Strategy* (Bethesda, MD: 1993).
14. R.C. Lefebvre et al., "Social Marketing and Nutrition Education: Inappropriate or Misunderstood," *Journal of Nutrition Education 27,* no. 3 (1995): 146–150.
15. National Highway Traffic Safety Administration, *Patterns of Misuse of Child Safety Seats: Final Report* [Rep. No. DOT HS 808–440] (Washington, DC: 1996).
16. National Highway Traffic Safety Administration, *Federal Motor Vehicle Safety Standards; Child Restraint Systems; Child Restraint Anchorage Systems;* 64 Fed. Reg. 10785 (1999).
17. U.S. Centers for Disease Control and Prevention, "Achievements in Public Health, 1900–1999: Control of Infectious Diseases," *Morbidity and Mortality Weekly Report* 48 (1999): 621–629.
18. U.S. Centers for Disease Control and Prevention, "Update: West Nile Virus Encephalitis—New York, 1999," *Morbidity and Mortality Weekly Report* 48 (1999): 944–946, 955.
19. U.S. Centers for Disease Control and Prevention, "Outbreak of West Nile-Like Viral Encephalitis," *Morbidity and Mortality Weekly Report* 48 (1999): 845–849.
20. R.G. Evans et al., eds., *Why Are Some People Healthy and Others Not? The Determinants of Health of Populations* (New York: Aldine DeGruyter, 1994).
21. P.R. Lee and C.L. Estes, eds., *The Nation's Health,* 5th ed. (Sudbury, MA: Jones and Bartlett, 1997).
22. S. Levine et al., "Does Medical Care Do Any Good? in *Handbook of Health, Health Care, and the Health Professions,* ed. D. Mechanic (New York: Free Press, 1983), 394–404.
23. B.J. Turnock, *Public Health: What It Is and How It Works* (Gaithersburg, MD: Aspen Publishers, Inc., 1997).
24. T. McKeown, "Determinants of Health," *Human Nature*, April (1978): 60–67.
25. T. McKeown et al., "An Interpretation of the Decline of Mortality in England and Wales during the Twentieth Century," *Population Studies* 29 (1975): 391–422.
26. U.S. Public Health Service, *For a Healthy Nation: Returns on Investment in Public Health* (Washington, DC: 1995).
27. "WIC Decreases Medicaid Costs, USDA Study Shows," *Nutrition Week 20*, no. 41 (1990): 6–7.
28. S.N. Tesh, "Hidden Arguments: Political Ideology and Disease Prevention Policy," in *Dominant Issues in Medical Sociology,* 3d ed., ed. H.D. Schwartz (New York: McGraw-Hill, 1994), 519–529.
29. Institute of Medicine, Committee for the Study of the Future of Public Health, *The Future of Public Health* (Washington, DC: National Academy Press, 1988).
30. U.S. Centers for Disease Control and Prevention, "Public Opinion about Public Health—United States, 1999," *Morbidity and Mortality Weekly Report* 49 (2000): 258–260.
31. J. Mallozzi, "Consumer Advocacy in Medicare HMOs," *States of Health 6*, no. 8 (1996): 1–9.
32. J. Weisberg, *In Defense of Government: The Fall and Rise of Public Trust* (New York: Scribner, 1996).
33. F. Mullan, "Federal Public Health, Semi-Reinvented," *American Journal of Public Health* 87 (1997): 21–24.
34. M. Levin, "Legal Weapon: Tobacco Companies, Facing Increasingly Strong Opposition, Have Turned to Open-Records Laws To Fight Back, Inundating State Offices with Requests for Documents," *The Los Angeles Times*, 21 April 1996, D1, D4.
35. J. Mintz, "3-Year-Old U.S. Program Cuts Smoking, Draws Fire," *The Washington Post*, 19 April 1997, A1.
36. M.L. Rothschild, "Marketing Communications in Non-business Situations or Why It's So Hard To Sell Brotherhood Like Soap," *Journal of Marketing* 43 (1979): 11–20.
37. National Cancer Institute, *Restrictions on Lobbying and Public Policy Advocacy by Government Contractors: The ASSIST Contract* (Bethesda, MD: 1993).
38. V.K. Rangan et al., "Do Better at Doing Good," *Harvard Business Review 74,* May–June (1996): 42–54.
39. S. Chapman and D. Lupton, *The Fight for Public Health: Principles and Practice of Media Advocacy* (London: BMJ Publishing Group, 1994).
40. L.W. Green and M.W. Kreuter, *Health Promotion Planning: An Educational and Environmental Approach,* 2d ed. (Mountain View, CA: Mayfield, 1991).
41. National Cancer Institute, *Making Health Communication Programs Work: A Planner's Guide* [NIH Pub. No. 89–1493] (Bethesda, MD: 1989).
42. R. Entman, "Framing: Toward Clarification of a Fractured Paradigm," *Journal of Communication* 43 (1993): 51–58.
43. S. Iyengar, *Is Anyone Responsible? How Television Frames Political Issues* (Chicago: University of Chicago Press, 1991).
44. P. Kaniss, *Making Local News* (Chicago: University of Chicago Press, 1991).
45. C. Ryan, *Prime Time Activism: Media Strategies for Grassroots Organizing* (Boston: South End Press, 1991).

46. D.A. Schon and M. Rein, *Frame Reflection: Toward the Resolution of Intractable Policy Controversies* (New York: Basic Books, 1994).

47. L. Wallack and L. Dorfman, "Media Advocacy: A Strategy for Advancing Policy and Promoting Health," *Health Education Quarterly* 23 (1996): 293–317.

48. L. Wallack et al., *Media Advocacy and Public Health: Power for Prevention* (Newbury Park, CA: Sage Publications, 1993).

49. P. Watzlawick et al., *Change; Principles of Problem Formation and Problem Resolution* (New York: Norton, 1974).

50. E.M. Rogers, *Diffusion of Innovations*, 4th ed. (New York: Simon & Schuster, 1996).

51. A. Bandura, *Social Foundations of Thought and Action* (Englewood Cliffs, NJ: Prentice-Hall, 1986).

52. K. Glanz, F.M. Lewis, and B.K. Rimer, eds., *Health Behavior and Health Education: Theory, Research and Practice*, 2d ed. (San Francisco: Jossey-Bass, 1997).

53. B. Smith, "Notes from the Field: Marketing with No Budget," *Social Marketing Quarterly* 5, no. 2 (1999): 6–11.

54. G.I. Balch and S.M. Sutton, "Keep Me Posted: A Plea for Practical Evaluation," in *Social Marketing: Theoretical and Practical Perspectives,* eds. M.E. Goldberg et al. (Mahwah, NJ: Lawrence Erlbaum Associates, 1997), 61–74.

55. R.A. Krueger, *Focus Groups: A Practical Guide for Applied Research,* 2d ed. (Thousand Oaks, CA: Sage Publications, 1994).

56. D.L. Morgan and R.A. Krueger, *The Focus Group Kit.* (Vols. 1–6). (Thousand Oaks, CA: Sage Publications, 1998).

57. S.M. Sutton et al., "Strategic Questions for Consumer-Based Health Communications," *Public Health Reports* 110 (1995): 725–733.

58. E. Maibach and R.L. Parrott, eds., *Designing Health Messages: Approaches from Communication Theory and Public Health Practice* (Thousand Oaks, CA: Sage Publications, 1997).

59. K. Roman and J. Maas, *How To Advertise,* 2d ed. (New York: St. Martin's Press, 1992).

60. N. Signorielli, *Mass Media Images and Impact on Health: A Sourcebook* (Westport, CT: Greenwood Press, 1993).

61. M. Williams, "...But Really, What Was Sold?" *The Washington Post*, 21 January 2000, A29.

62. R. Hornik and K.D. Woolf, "Using Cross-Sectional Surveys To Plan Message Strategies," *Social Marketing Quarterly* 5, no. 2 (1999): 34–41.

63. S.A.A. Beresford et al., "A Dietary Intervention in Primary Care Practice: The Eating Patterns Study," *American Journal of Public Health* 87 (1997): 610–616.

64. M. Fishbein, "Editorial: Great Expectations, or Do We Ask Too Much from Community-Level Interventions?" *American Journal of Public Health* 86 (1996): 1,075–1,076.

65. A.R. Kristal, "Choosing Appropriate Dietary Data Collection Methods To Assess Behavior Changes," in *Charting the Course for Evaluation: How Do We Measure the Success of Nutrition Education and Promotion in Food Assistance Programs? Summary of Proceedings,* ed. L. Doner (Alexandria, VA: USDA Food and Nutrition Service, 1997), 39–41.

66. R. Hornik, "Public Health Education and Communication as Policy Instruments for Bringing About Changes in Behavior," in *Social Marketing: Theoretical and Practical Perspectives,* eds. M.E. Goldberg et al. (Mahwah, NJ: Lawrence Erlbaum Associates, 1997): 45–58.

67. J.A. Durlak, *School-Based Prevention Programs for Children and Adolescents* (Thousand Oaks, CA: Sage Publications, 1995).

68. M. Feinlieb, "Editorial: New Directions for Community Intervention Studies," *American Journal of Public Health* 86 (1996): 1,696–1,698.

69. P.H. Rossi and H.E. Freeman, *Evaluation: A Systematic Approach,* 5th ed. (Newbury Park, CA: Sage Publications, 1993).

70. C.E. Basch et al., "Avoiding Type III Errors in Health Education Program Evaluations: A Case Study," *Health Education Quarterly* 12 (1985): 315–331.

CHAPTER 21

Building Constituencies for Public Health

Michael T. Hatcher
Ray M. Nicola

Public health organizations are challenged to develop effective relationships with the complex constellation of constituents who are involved in or affected by community health issues. An effective constituency-development process allows public health organizations to develop relationships that facilitate community health improvement. Using such a process, public health organizations identify major public health constituents, delineate participation factors, develop and manage effective interactions with constituency groups, and apply strategies for evaluating and improving constituency engagement in public health issues. Each of these tasks requires explicit analytic and management strategies for linking constituency-building activities to community health improvement.

Public health organizations operate within complex institutional environments that include many different types of constituents. The consumers of public health services in any given community are many and diverse, as are the individuals and organizations involved in producing these services. Improving health within communities and populations requires coordinated decision making and problem solving by all of these constituents. Such problem solving occurs most readily and successfully when constituents are actively engaged in addressing health issues that matter to them.[1(p.5)]

Problem solving in public health rarely occurs through spontaneous consensus. In a democratic society, change is produced through the tensions of multiple interests and the opinions of differing societal segments. These segments represent constituencies for public health organizations seeking action on community health issues. All too frequently, public health professionals rely on a false dichotomy in developing relationships with constituents—they approach each constituent as either an adversary or an ally. Adversarial situations stimulate defensive responses that stalemate progress. These situations often arise because communication is limited to debate and entrenched positions instead of dialogue, negotiation, and solution development. On the other side of the coin, public health professionals focus on attracting and sustaining the attention of allies and other uninvolved constituents on health issues requiring community-based decisions. Allies are typically sought among individuals and organizations that pursue similar missions and that engage in similar types of activities involving public health issues. However, this dichotomous approach to constituency development can severely limit the actions and outcomes that public health organizations achieve. To transcend this false dichotomy, public health organizations require an analytic and

Source: The material in this chapter appeared previously in M. Hatcher and R. Nicola, Building Constituencies for Public Health, *Journal of Public Health Management and Practice,* Vol. 6, No. 2, © 2000, Aspen Publishers, Inc.

management framework for linking constituency building with community health improvement goals.

This chapter outlines a framework for constituency development in public health that focuses on achieving sustained improvements in community health. Within such a framework, public health organizations identify public health constituencies explicitly and broadly, delineate constituent participation factors, develop and manage effective interactions with constituency groups, and apply models for evaluating and improving the engagement of constituencies in public health issues (Figure 21–1). Each of these tasks requires explicit analytic and management strategies for linking constituency-building activities to community health improvement.

The constituency development framework begins with the understanding that people need a reason to invest their energy in processes that address community health. If people and the community they are a part of are not motivated and ready to participate, action will not occur. The second aspect of the framework is focused on managing the constituency-building processes and factors for constituent involvement. This segment of the framework addresses the responsibility of public health leaders to manage and enable effective constituent engagement and participation. The third aspect of the framework focuses on approaches or models that facilitate constituent and community involvement and lead to interventions. The fourth aspect of the framework includes public health intervention sciences that are available to produce community-based results. The remaining portion of the framework demonstrates how constituent-based actions are linked to producing behavioral, systems, and environmental impacts, which in turn produce desired health outcomes and quality-of-life improvements. Discussions of the first three aspects of the framework that influence and move constituents and their communities to action are the focus of this chapter. Identifying public health interventions and the resulting health effects such interventions produce is presented in the framework to establish an operational link between constituency building and community health improvement.

WHO IS PUBLIC HEALTH'S CONSTITUENCY?

A "constituency" (in addition to the meaning of "a body of voters") is: (1) a group of supporters or patrons and (2) a group served by an organization or institution; a clientele.[2] By definition, therefore, people who benefit from public health actions and people who support improved health of the public are the constituency. Because public health serves the entire population, everyone

Know	Do			Produce		
Constituent Participation Factors	Organizational Practice	Constituent Improvement Approaches	Public Health Interventions	Health Impacts	Health Outcomes	Quality-of-Life Improvements
• Motivations • Readiness	• Know the community • Develop positions and strategies • Build network linkages • Mobilize for action	• PRECEDE PROCEED model • *APEXCPH* • *PATCH* • *Healthy People* in Healthy Communities 2010 • *Healthy Cities*	• Clinical • Behavioral • Systems • Environmental	• Clinical • Behavioral • Systems • Environmental	• Decreased morbidity • Decreased mortality	• Physical • Mental • Social • Spiritual • Environmental

Figure 21–1 Linking Constituency Building to Community Health Improvement

in the country is part of the public health constituency. There are, however, certain groups in the constituent population who are in a special position to influence public health outcomes; these include public health workers, policy makers, business leaders, and others.

Building on the concepts of supporters and clients, an operational definition of constituency building can be established. For purposes of this chapter, *constituency building* is the art and science of establishing relationships among a public health agency and the public it serves, the governing body it represents, and other health-related organizations in the community. Relationships are established to generate debate, dialogue, decisions, and actions among constituent groups in addressing community health needs and issues. Key points of this definition acknowledge that sciences such as political science, interpersonal communications, media advocacy, and others can be applied to building linkages and relationships with constituents. Applying the appropriate science at the right time, however, requires artful application. Complicating the simplicity of this definition is the fact that people and organizations are often members of multiple constituencies, and their movement between groups is fluid and frequently based on alignment of issues within the groups.[1,3] Due to the fluid nature of constituent alignment on community health issues, public health leaders must develop a strategic understanding of individual and organizational values, missions, and assets held by constituents affected by or having influence over decisions and actions required to address community health concerns. Such influence may be constituted through a position of power that shapes opinions and directs organizations, controls resources and information, or possesses key technology. Such an understanding is critical in managing constituency relationships.

INCENTIVES FOR CONSTITUENCY PARTICIPATION

An understanding of why people participate in community activities provides the first guidance for constituency building. Factors include the sociopolitical environment, community needs, community attitudes and beliefs, and existing leadership and organization in the community.[4] The literature from various fields of study and authors such as Brown, Schwartz, Mattessich, and Monsey offer insight on the motivations that move people to act.[4-6] For example, people participate when they feel a sense of community, see their involvement and the issues as relevant and worthy of their time, believe that the benefits of participation outweigh the cost, and view the process and organizational climate of participation as open and supportive of their right to have a voice in the process.[1] The issue itself also influences participation. People are motivated to work for change when conditions of the issue are no longer acceptable to them. The readiness of constituents to take action can be determined by understanding the perception of, and support for, the issue within the community. For example

- Are there perceptions that a problem or threat that affects health exists?
- Is the issue perceived to be important, achievable, and deserving of community action?
- Is there a science base to resolve the issue?
- Is community collaboration likely due to political and public interest and community history for leadership and collaboration?
- Are resources available for action?
- Is the political and social climate supportive of the constituency's goals?
- Is there a community infrastructure to sustain interest and community action?

Answers to these and related questions are necessary to help public health leaders determine constituent readiness and the level of action that may be possible.[7] Public health leaders who understand the motives for constituent participation and the attributes of readiness can stimulate action with appropriate information and public processes that fulfill individual and group needs for participation.

ORGANIZATIONAL MANAGEMENT FOR EFFECTIVE CONSTITUENCY INTERACTION

A public health leader who seeks constituent participation on a public health issue can design organizational structure and management processes within his or her agency that facilitate and direct interactions with constituents, for purposes of:

- Knowing the community and its constituents.
- Establishing positions and strategies that guide the agency's interaction with constituents.
- Building and sustaining formal and informal networks necessary for maintaining relationships, communicating messages, and leveraging resources.
- Mobilizing constituencies for community-based decision making and social action.

Performance of these processes is likely to be shared across the agency, with specific roles delegated to organizational units such as an assessment and planning unit, a senior management group, and an education and outreach group. The organizational structures or units tasked with creating or delegating the management and performance of these processes are dependent on existing forms and functions within the agency.

By managing these processes, public health leaders can consistently address factors that produce effective constituent involvement, including[1,5]

- the clarity of initiative goals
- the defined roles for constituent involvement
- constituent ownership of both initiative process and outcome
- the design of capacity-building elements incorporated into processes and structures used to facilitate individual and group actions of constituents
- the overall feeling of satisfaction, rather than frustration, a process achieves in fulfilling a constituent's reasons for participating in community activities

Knowing the Community and Its Constituents

Knowing the community and its constituents is more than an epidemiologic assessment. It involves coordinating and directing activities that are necessary to identify constituent groups, analyzing group characteristics and factors that generate constituent involvement, and assessing current and potential assets (including fiscal, physical, informational, and human resources) constituents and their organizations can direct toward resolving community health issues. The tasks involved in constituent identification and analysis of group characteristics include demographic groupings; individual and organizational beliefs, values, missions, and goals; and organizational and leadership structures of constituent groups as well as their history of working with others. Through this assessment, it is possible to determine the roles and type of support (political, financial, manpower, etc.) constituents can reasonably provide to a public health initiative, as well as possible conflicts of interest that may arise among groups.[8]

To be most effective, public health leaders must determine which constituents are affected by specific issues, assess their probable response to these issues, and use the most effective methods to involve each constituent group in appropriate activities. Constituent skills should match those needed for resolving the public health issue on which the agency is facilitating dialogue and action. If the skills do not match, a determination must be made concerning training and education necessary to increase constituent involvement. In identifying and recruiting a constituent base for public health, the agency must have policies, structures, resources, and leadership to assess community mobilization efforts and assist in developing human and other constituency resources for public health action. Mechanisms that enable the identification and analysis of the agency's constituent base provide essential information concerning potential collaborators on public health issues. From a leadership perspective, knowing the community is essential because social programs tend to fail due to a lack of appropriate management and an oversimplified view of constituent motivations.[9]

Establishing Positions and Strategies To Guide Interaction with Constituents

Another important process area is focused on organizational decision making that results in the establishment of a position and strategy for bringing a health issue before constituents. The purpose of this decision making and planning is to initiate constituent dialogue and action. Public health leaders must make their decisions based on understanding multiple domains of influence on health such as social, epidemiologic, behavioral, environmental, ecologic, and political factors.[10] Through such analysis in decision making, public health leaders are better equipped to consider the position options available and weigh each option's effect on the different constituencies. Specific attention should be given to the perceived needs of customers served, attitudes of policy-making bodies, application of public health science, public health delivery system capabilities, and appropriate community health data. A position is established against this pool of competing interests. Through this practice element, the agency prepares itself to participate in the democratic process of decision making with constituents. The result is stimulation of community debate, dialogue and involvement around the health issue, and a determination of the community's expectations. This internal organizational position development is not intended to exclude constituent input. Instead, it provides a starting point for dialogue with constituents and enables the public health leader to communicate clearly.

Once an agency position has been reached, strategy options can be evaluated and selected based on the best chance for achieving dialogue and action. Four organizational strategy types can be considered: authoritative, competitive, cooperative, and disruptive.[11]

1. The *authoritative* strategy applies rules and regulations to require a desired action. It is used when an organization has control over its environment. Successful authoritative strategies demand an ability to monitor and enforce its directives. This strategy was used effectively by the National Highway Traffic Safety Administration in the early 1980s when it was announced that airbags would be required in automobiles unless a specified percentage of the U.S. population was subject to mandatory seatbelt laws requiring occupant restraint use. This prompted policy debate and the passage of vehicle occupant protection across the nation.
2. *Competitive* strategies attempt to make an organization's position more desirable and attractive to constituents. The successfully competitive organization attracts adequate support to accomplish its purpose and avoids pressures from others that promote actions that are incongruent with the desired public health goals. Public health officials often apply this strategy when funding is sought and there is competing interest for the same dollars. Success is won by demonstrating why the proposed program spending is needed, the quality and impact of the program over others, and external support for the program.
3. *Cooperative* strategies establish agreements that offer mutual benefits to constituents and their organizations. An organization may use one of three cooperative strategy forms: (1) *contracting,* which is a negotiated agreement between two parties for exchanging resources or services; (2) *coalition,* which is a pooling of resources by several organizations for a joint venture; or (3) *co-optation,* which is the absorption (or conversion) of representatives from key (opposition or competitive) constituent groups into the leadership or policy-making structure of an organization to moderate or avoid opposition or competition.
4. *Disruption* strategies are "the purposeful conduct of activities which threaten the resource-generating capacities" of an adversary.[11(p.79)] The most visible public health example of this strategy is antitobacco initiatives that seek to limit the sales and market base of tobacco companies in an effort to prevent the use of tobacco by children.

Throughout the position development and strategy development process, it is essential to focus on the needs and interests of the agency's constituency. The question of when to enlist direct constituent involvement is of critical concern. Is constituent input advisable during the problem analysis phase or as strategy and objectives are being weighed? Although early constituent involvement is usually indicated, agency time and resource constraints may dictate that constituents are most appropriately brought in during the implementation phase. Some considerations in determining the time most appropriate for involving constituents are

- *operating time frame:* How much time is there to achieve the goal?
- *level of constituent knowledge:* How much education will constituents need?
- *constituent commitment:* How much of a time commitment are constituents willing to make?

Whatever the judgment on a point of entry for constituent participation, public health leaders must establish direction for the interaction and involvement of agency staff with constituents acting on important health issues in the community.

Building and Sustaining Networks

Network development is the third process area public health leaders must consider in the operations of an agency. Developing networks is focused on establishing and maintaining relationships, communication channels, and exchange systems that promote linkages, alliances, and opportunities to leverage resources among constituent groups. Effective performance results in open channels of communication to constituents, enables active and ongoing interactions, and accelerates resource and community mobilization efforts on service and policy issues. If public health leaders view networking as an ongoing and essential activity in the agency's operations, constituency mobilization can be productive and require minimal effort. If agency leaders only communicate with constituents as a crisis management technique, however, they may find that communication channels that were once useful no longer exist.

The challenge for public health is to establish ties with a network of diverse constituency supporters that will respond to public health issues. Key to a successful network is identifying and assessing the network structure in place and understanding the effect of structure on the availability of resources for public health. Public health has access to both formal and informal constituent groups. The formal groups or organizations have recognized stability and influence in the community; informal groups may represent less structured and influential constituents who are often very resourceful. Each group brings with it important considerations that public health leaders need to be aware of if true networking potential is to be realized.[12] Thus, the ability of public health leaders to develop and direct networking activities relies heavily on identifying and assessing the existing networking structure.

Assessment of formal to formal ties should reveal interactions of information flow, resource allocation, service delivery, or policy endeavors with influential individuals and organizations serving on boards, committees, coalitions, and governing bodies. If the leader finds that formal ties are weak, he or she may choose to concentrate on strengthening formal ties with key partners to improve relationships and increase the agency's influence and its resource potential.

A highly involved constituency base may allow an agency to have several ties with informal and voluntary groups. A lack of ties with informal community groups may impede agency outreach performance. Public health leaders may then choose to pursue more informal community ties to enlarge the constituency base and improve service outreach. In this situation, management needs to provide adequate resources to ensure the development, participation, and retention of informal and volunteer organizations.

Mobilizing Constituencies

Mobilizing constituencies for community-based decision making and social action is the fourth process area. Mobilization is bringing into readiness or organizing people and resources for active service.[2] An agency can prepare or organize the community to act. Making the community ready in this case means organizing constituencies to act through social pressure and community involvement to meet the health needs that exist. Through mobilization, community interest on health issues is stimulated, constituents are prepared to act, and, if necessary, constituents are assisted to respond in resolving the public health issue.

The ability to mobilize the constituents around a particular issue reflects not only the agency's structural capability to mount such an effort, but the community's ability and readiness to respond. Based on an understanding of the community and its constituents, a public health leader must answer key questions in selecting a mobilization approach.

- Who are the constituents and stakeholders within the community?
- Does the community believe itself capable of affecting its environment?
- Will the community hear and absorb the information that is supplied by the public health agency?
- Does the community have the capability to mount a response?

The answers to these questions provide the framework that the agency can use to analyze its social mobilization options. The mobilization option chosen to bring dialogue and action on a public health issue must support the agency position and be consistent with the strategy selected so as to guide constituent interaction and the constituents' capacity to act. Specific models for mobilization will be discussed later in this chapter.

ASSESSING THE EFFECTIVENESS OF PUBLIC HEALTH CONSTITUENCIES

Assessing the effectiveness of a public health constituency means evaluating the group's ability to have a positive impact on the community's health. Because effectiveness in this case means reaching public health objectives, any such assessment should also examine the clarity of the objectives. Clarity of political appeal and intervention science, including mobilization approaches, is central to the assessment.

Political appeal is measured against any competing actions that are proposed to achieve the same objective. If the competing actions are equally as effective at accomplishing the objective, and one does not cost more than the other, a compromise rather than opposition is appropriate. If the competing action is not built on good public health science, then opposition may be necessary though unfortunate because all involved in a fight become injured. Given the choice between compromise and opposition, it is necessary to apply a competitive strategy to raise the appeal of the advocated action.

Clarity of science is achieved with selection and use of effective interventions and mobilization approaches. Appropriate use of science enables identification of measures to establish objective targets and evaluate collaborative actions and intervention outcomes. The health objectives and outcomes require an adequate assessment of the community's health status. Although this chapter is not focused on assessment tools, many approaches described in the following sections are useful in assessing health status. Some of the resources available to aid in establishing objective targets and monitoring progress are *Healthy People 2010,* the National Commission for Quality Assurance's *Health Plan Employer Data and Information Set (HEDIS),* and the National Center for Health Statistics' (NCHS') leading health indicators.[13–15]

Literature is also available that describes methods for assessing the competency and effectiveness of constituency groups based on group interaction and its components of process, structure, and organizational content.[5] These methods describe how effective a constituency is in working together as a group.

INTERVENTIONS FOR IMPROVING PUBLIC HEALTH CONSTITUENCIES

Once there is an understanding of the participation "drivers" of constituents and a knowledge of the organizational factors that contribute to effective constituency interactions, it is time to move to action. Public health constituencies become stronger by taking effective action to improve the public's health; that is, the success of group goals in itself provides reinforcement of participation in constituency efforts.

There are different applied public health interventions for specific disease issues and many resources available to provide guidance on interventions. *The Clinical Preventive Services Guidelines* provide the evidence base for the effectiveness of individual public health interventions in a clinical setting.[16] The *Guide to Community Preventive Services*, an analogous U.S. Public Health Service project now under development, provides the evidence base for the effectiveness of public health interventions in a community setting.[17]

Several broad cross-cutting interventions are available that facilitate constituent involvement in planning for health actions; examples of these are described in the next section.

TOOLS FOR DEVELOPING EFFECTIVE PUBLIC HEALTH CONSTITUENCIES

Public health practitioners at local, state, federal, and global levels have developed different tools to assist in achieving long-term health improvements in populations by working with constituency groups in improving communities, including *Healthy People 2010*; *Healthy People 2010 Toolkit: A Field Guide to Health Planning*; *Assessment Protocol for Excellence in Public Health (APEXPH)*; the U.S. Centers for Disease Control and Prevention's (CDC's) Planned Approach to Community Health (PATCH); and the World Health Organization's (WHO's) "Healthy Cities" initiative.[13,18–21] These approaches all facilitate constituent involvement.

Healthy People 2010 Tools

Healthy People 2010 lays out the prevention agenda for the nation and provides direction for local programs as they identify and set priorities and develop health objective targets.[13] The *Healthy People 2010* framework builds on initiatives that have been pursued over the past two decades. *Healthy People: The Surgeon General's Report on Health Promotion and Disease Prevention*[22] provided targets to reduce premature mortality in four life age groups during the 1980s and was supported by objectives with 1990 endpoints. *Healthy People 2000: National Health Promotion and Disease Prevention Objectives*[23] guided efforts toward health targets for the year 2000. Like its predecessors, *Healthy People 2010* was developed through a broad consultation process characterized by intersectoral collaboration and community participation. It is the action agenda for the first decade of the twenty-first century. *Healthy People 2010* is the U.S. contribution to the WHO's "Health for All" strategy.

The *Healthy People 2010 Toolkit* is a resource developed to support state and local leaders in establishing participatory plans to address priority health objectives over this decade. The Toolkit is organized around seven action areas that address building a leadership and structural foundation, addressing resource issues, engaging community partners, establishing health priorities and objectives, addressing measurement issues, managing and sustaining the participatory process, and communicating health goals and objectives to those who can influence accomplishment of the objectives. This Toolkit was developed by the Public Health Foundation in cooperation with the U.S. Department of Health and Human Services' Office of Disease Prevention and Health Promotion and Office of Public Health and Science.[18]

APEXPH and *MAPP*

Since 1991, local public health officials have used the *APEXPH* to assess internal organizational capacity and to begin a community process of consensus building around health issues.[19] In 1999, a national work group under the leadership of the National Association of County and City Health Officials (NACCHO) and the CDC started developing *Mobilizing for Action through Planning and Partnership (MAPP)*.[24] This new tool is an evolution of *APEXPH* and provides community and local health department leaders with a robust tool to guide their creation of a local health system that ensures the delivery of services essential to protecting the health of the public. The *MAPP* tool provides several new features. One feature provides indicators to measure community capacity for providing public health services rather than examining only the capacity of the local health department. These indicators closely mirror the local health system measures used by the CDC National Public Health Performance Standards Program. A second feature has a strategic planning component. A position paper and case studies on strategic planning support this feature. The feature addressing the community health assessment process has been revised to add a stronger focus on environmental health, behavioral risk factor data, and health-related quality of life.

PATCH

The CDC's PATCH tool helps communities plan, assess, conduct, and evaluate health programs for preventing and controlling chronic diseases.[20] Representatives from the community, state and local health departments, and the National Center for Chronic Disease Prevention and Health Promotion of the CDC have formed a partnership to identify and address the community's priority chronic disease needs. Using the PATCH process, such a partnership organizes the community, collects and uses local area data, sets priority goals, carries out interventions, and evaluates program effectiveness and its impact on community health.

Healthy Cities

The original Healthy Cities model began as a demonstration project of the WHO and has been adapted and applied in more than 30 states in the United States.[21] California, Indiana, South Carolina, and Massachusetts are states where this model of health and quality-of-life improvement is applied most frequently. The Healthy Cities model uses a broad definition of health. It promotes broad public–private partnerships through processes of social and environmental change designed to improve the health and quality of life of populations through interventions addressing ecological determinants of health such as education, recreation, employment, health services, transportation, and housing.[25]

The above tools and models are frequently incorporated into academic syllabi for public health students and into ongoing practice education such as leadership and management development programs for practicing public health professionals. For example, the Public Health Leadership Institute and many of the state and regional public health leadership development programs require participants to perform an individual project during the life of the program, which uses constituency engagement as a principal feature.

INITIATING THE CONSTITUENCY-BUILDING PROCESS

The body of knowledge concerning public health constituency building continues to grow. A recent publication developed by the CDC reviews the existing literature and examines the practical experiences of public health practitioners and researchers. The following principles are identified by the Committee for Community Engagement in the CDC's *Principles of Community Engagement*:[1]

Before starting a community engagement effort:

- Be clear about the purposes or goals of the effort and the populations and/or communities you want to engage.
- Become knowledgeable about the community (Figure 21–1) in terms of its economic conditions, political structures, norms and values, demographic trends, history, and experience with engagement efforts. Learn about the community's perceptions of those initiating the engagement activities.

For engagement to occur, it is necessary to:

- Go into the community, establish relationships, build trust, work with the formal and informal leadership, and get commitment from community organizations to create processes for mobilizing the community.
- Remember and accept that community self-determination is the responsibility and right of all people who make up a community.

No external entity should assume that it can bestow to a community the power to act in its own self-interest.

For engagement to succeed:

- Partnering with the community is necessary to create change and improve health.
- All aspects of community engagement must recognize and respect community diversity. Awareness of the various cultures of a community and other factors of diversity must be paramount in designing and implementing community engagement approaches.
- Community engagement can only be sustained by identifying and mobilizing community assets, and by developing capacities and resources for community health decisions and action.
- An engaging organization or individual change agent must be prepared to release control of actions or interventions to the community, and be sufficiently flexible to meet the changing needs of the community.
- Community collaboration requires long-term commitment by the engaging organization and its partners.

These guidelines underscore the importance of knowing constituency groups within a community and establishing constituent engagement plans within a health organization. Building constituencies is neither an automatic nor an intuitive process for public health organizations and their managers to undertake. Nonetheless, effective constituencies can be formed and sustained through explicit managerial strategies combined with sound evaluation tools. Because constituent interaction is critical for effective organizational performance and community health improvement, constituency building cannot be overlooked as a strategic action for public health organizations.

CHAPTER REVIEW

1. Constituencies for public health organizations include the *individuals* and *institutions* that benefit from public health actions and that support improved health within the population.
2. Constituency building is the process of establishing relationships between a public health organization and the public it serves, including consumers, governing bodies, and other health-related organizations in the community. Relationships are established to facilitate decision making and action for addressing community health needs or issues.
3. An effective constituency-building process involves the following steps:
    - Identify major constituents within the community and their interests.
    - Establish positions and strategies that guide the organization's interaction with constituents.
    - Build and sustain formal and informal relationships necessary for communication, resource sharing, and joint decision making among constituents.
    - Motivate constituencies to engage in community-based decision making and collective action.
4. Key issues that must be considered in developing strategic relationships with constituents include
    - *operating time frame:* How much time is there to achieve the goal?
    - *level of constituent knowledge:* How much education will constituents need?
    - *constituent commitment:* How much resources are constituents willing and able to commit to the effort?
5. Explicit strategies for evaluating and improving constituency engagement must be used continuously by public health organizations. Assessment and planning tools, such *as Healthy People 2010, Healthy People 2010 Toolkit, APEXPH, MAPP,* PATCH, or Healthy Cities, may be helpful to structure some interactions with constituents.

REFERENCES

1. U.S. Centers for Disease Control and Prevention, *Principles of Community Engagement* (Atlanta, GA: 1997).
2. *The American Heritage Dictionary of the English Language,* 3d ed. [Electronic version] (Boston: Houghton Mifflin Co., 1992).
3. Institute of Medicine, National Academy of Sciences, *Assessing the Social and Behavioral Science Base for HIV/AIDS Prevention and Intervention: Workshop Summary and Background Papers* (Washington, DC: National Academy Press, 1995).
4. E.R. Brown, "Community Action for Health Promotion: A Strategy To Empower Individuals and Communities," *International Journal of Health Services 21,* no. 3 (1991): 448–451.
5. R.M. Schwartz, *The Skilled Facilitator: Practical Wisdom for Developing Effective Groups* (San Francisco: Jossey-Bass Publishers, 1994).
6. P.W. Mattessich and B.R. Monsey, *Collaboration: What Makes It Work; A Review of Research Literature on Factors Influencing Successful Collaboration* (St. Paul, MN: Amherst H. Wilder Foundation, 1992).
7. S.B. Kar, ed., *Health Promotion Indicators and Actions, Indicators for Individual and Societal Actions for Public Health* (New York: Springer Publishing Co., 1989).
8. Public Health Foundation, *Constituency Building: Partnerships for Public Health* (Washington, DC: 1987).
9. M. Wilson, "The New Frontier: Volunteer Management Training," *Training and Development Journal,* July (1984): 50–52.
10. L.W. Green and M.W. Kreuter, *Health Promotion Planning: An Educational and Ecological Approach,* 3d ed. (Mountain View, CA: Mayfield, 1999).
11. Y. Hasenfeld, *Human Service Organizations* (Englewood Cliffs, NJ: Prentice-Hall, 1983).
12. B. Wellman, "Applying Network Analysis to the Study of Support," in *Social Networks and Social Support,* ed. B.H. Gottlieb (London: Sage Publications, 1983), 173–181.
13. U.S. Department of Health and Human Services, Public Health Service, *Healthy People 2010* (Conference Edition in Two Volumes) (Washington, DC: Office of Public Health and Science, 2000).
14. National Committee for Quality Assurance, *HEDIS Report Cards*, <http://www.ncqa.org/pages/policy/hedis/intro.htm> (20 April 2000).
15. National Center for Health Statistics, *Health, United States, 1998 with Socioeconomic Status and Health Chartbook* (Hyattsville, MD: 1998).
16. U.S. Department of Health and Human Services, *Release of the Guide to Clinical Preventive Services*, 2d ed., <http://158.72.20.10/pubs/guidecps/release.htm> (20 April 2000).
17. U.S. Department of Health and Human Services, Task Force on Community Preventive Services, *Guide to Community Preventive Services,* <http://web.health.gov/communityguide/default.htm> (20 April 2000).
18. Public Health Foundation, *Healthy People 2010 Toolkit: A Field Guide to Health Planning,* <http://www.phf.org/hp2010asst.htm> (23 April 2000). Additional information is available at <http://www.health.gov/healthypeople/state/toolkit/> (23 April 2000). (This tool was developed by the Public Health Foundation in cooperation with the U.S. Department of Health and Human Services' Office of Disease Prevention and Health Promotion and Office of Public Health and Science, August 1999).
19. National Association of County and City Health Officials, *Assessment Protocol for Excellence in Public Health* (Washington, DC: 1991).
20. P. Hanson, "Citizen Involvement in Community Health Promotion: A Role Application of CDC's PATCH Model," *International Quarterly of Community Health Education 9,* no. 3 (1988–89): 177–186.
21. World Health Organization, *Promoting Health in the Urban Context, Five-Year Planning Framework, A Guide to Assessing Healthy Cities* (Copenhagen, Denmark: World Health Organization Regional Office for Europe, 1988).
22. U.S. Department of Health and Human Services, Public Health Service, *Healthy People: The Surgeon General's Report on Health Promotion and Disease Prevention* (Washington, DC: 1979).
23. U.S. Department of Health and Human Services, Public Health Service, *Healthy People 2000: National Health Promotion and Disease Prevention Objectives* (Washington, DC: 1990).
24. National Association of County and City Health Officials, *Mobilizing for Action through Planning and Partnership* (Washington, DC: 2000).
25. M.F. Katz and M.W. Kreuter, "Community Assessment and Empowerment," in *Principles of Public Health Practice,* eds. E.D. Scutchfield and C.W. Keck (Albany, NY: Delmar Publishers, 1997).

Chapter 22

Academic Partnerships in Public Health Practice

Stephen H. Linder
Beth E. Quill
Lu Ann Aday

The public health agency can only achieve its objectives by successfully mobilizing other stakeholders in the community. Characteristics of partnerships are described in various models of collaboration, with special attention given to academic–practice partnerships in public health. Academic linkages with public health organizations are a vital component of the community partnerships and consortiums that are increasingly used for health improvement.

Partnerships in public health are rapidly increasing in importance. Financial and programmatic restraints of government have stimulated public health organizations to form alliances and consortiums with other entities in their communities.[1] The evolving role of local health departments (LHDs) from delivering services to performing population-based essential functions has necessitated new modes of involvement with health care providers, community-based organizations, and the public. Public health organizations must interact with the full range of factors that influence community health, requiring collaboration and community partnerships that also include nonhealth agencies.[2]

The increasing recognition of the value of partnership is fueled by the realization that the public health organization can achieve its objectives only by successfully mobilizing other stakeholders in the community. Virtually all new sources of competitive funding now available to public health organizations specify a requirement for a consortium of community entities participating in a partnership to implement the initiative.

This chapter examines the characteristics of partnerships and various models of collaboration. Emphasis is directed to the academic partnership in public health practice. (Public health partnerships are discussed in Chapter 3.) A set of 20 cases describing partnerships is presented to illustrate various modes of forging partnerships among academics, public health professionals, community health services professionals, and community residents. Academic linkages with public health practice are a vital component of partnerships committed to community health improvement.

THE NATURE OF PARTNERSHIPS

Consistent with recent federal designs for "reengineering" government, administrators in public sector organizations are forming new partnerships with both nonprofit and for-profit entities as a means of leveraging their resources and broadening support for their programs. Pub-

---

The authors gratefully acknowledge permission to adapt and/or reprint selected text from the following: L.A. Aday and B.E. Quill, "A Framework for Assessing Practice-Oriented Scholarship" (pp. 38–46), and B.E. Quill and L.A. Aday, "Toward a New Paradigm for Public Health Practice and Academic Partnerships" (pp. 1–3), *Journal of Public Health Management and Practice 6,* no. 1 (2000), 1–3.

lic health partnerships are best viewed as a part of this movement. Much of the writing on partnering, however, conveys the impression that partnerships of this kind are new to government. Along with the image of newness and innovation, we are led to believe that partnering, as a management practice, deserves wide emulation both inside government and out. And although subject to local adaptations, the more of this practice that is seen, the better off programs will be. Not wanting to dampen this enthusiasm, it is important to consider where this new strategy came from, why it has caught on, and how easily it can be distorted.

The etymology of the term "partnership" offers a few solid clues as to its current meanings. It has Middle English origins in the practice of partitioning property; earlier Latin roots find a close relative in Roman Law where multiple heirs can be stipulated as "partners" in an estate. The common notion of partnering, as joining in some shared endeavor, springs from these roots. And yet, the partnering that is associated with management practice adds more formal connotations of rule-governed, strategic relationships. This augmented meaning is more likely drawn from technical definitions employed by the professions to order the complexities of organizational relationships; in this instance, partners are separated formally by explicit role expectations from other actors, such as competitors, customers, clients, and so on. Professional terms with narrow technical meaning will occasionally grow into positive idioms and make their way into the vernacular, in part because of the status afforded the professions in today's technological society.

The technical sense of a partnership, however, appears to originate in business law (via the Uniform Commercial Code), where it applies exclusively to a type of contractual arrangement for the sharing of profits and losses from doing business together.[3] The essential feature is the jointness of the arrangement—every partner bears some of the risk, pays some of the cost, and can claim a portion of the gain. Hence, there is an implicit notion of fair division among the parties to some common enterprise, agreed to ahead of time, and enforced, when necessary, through the courts. This idea of setting out a fair division of responsibilities and burdens beforehand carries over into the efforts of nonprofits, forming collaboratives as a means of pooling both resources and risk. With no profits to divide (and symbolic gains, such as status, difficult to partition), much of the activity of partnering among nonprofits, as will be shown, relates to defining and sustaining that fair division.

The term partnership probably first enjoyed semantic extension in international trade. Here, nation–states assume the status of partners, cooperating for mutual advantage or loans linked to diplomacy. Partnerships, then, entered the vernacular with connotations of peace, neighborliness, and prosperity. These connotations appear next in another set of federal efforts to cultivate trading partners of a sort, this time in economically depressed urban areas. The partnering of local developers with city government, by most accounts, was not accompanied by shared prosperity. The ill effects of these partnership efforts seemed to discourage government's use of the term, that is, until the recession-based austerity of the late 1970s. The new thinking was that government's responsibilities could be maintained in the face of resource cuts, so long as "partners" could be found to help share the burdens.[4]

The conservative political realignment in the early 1980s created a more favorable climate for seeking partners, this time with the idea of them eventually assuming government's responsibilities as their own. In this case, partners were organizations that stood to inherit governmental functions through a process known as privatization.[5,6] The formation of partnerships, in this instance, served as a stage in the process. Eventually, government would withdraw, and the private organization would either maintain the service or not. For those committed to an activist government, partnerships offered a way of compensating for dwindling resources. For those desiring a smaller governmental role, partnerships served as a transitional device along the way to privatization. In either event, the rubric seemed to invoke good business practices and market-like discipline under the auspices of greater efficiency and more responsive customer service. For government, partnering not only signaled a capacity to operate like a thriving business, but an effort to stretch public resources through collaboration of some sort in lieu of seeking more tax dollars.

From the earlier discussion of the legal definition, what distinguishes partnerships from other sorts of contractual arrangements is the notion of fair division; there are at least two parties who devise a means to share both a resource commitment and a measure of control. By implication, what makes them partners, rather than principals and agents or buyers and sellers, is the expectation of symmetry in their relationship. The symmetry extends from having an equal say in the fairness of the division, to parity in the contribution that each party makes. If one party dictates the terms of the division to the other, this moves away from partnering toward a principal–agent relationship. Relatedly, if one party provides all of the cash and contracts and the other does all of the work, this moves toward the familiar buyer–seller relationship. In each case, the terms will differ, as will the incentives and intent. Principal–agent relationships are built on the assumption that opportunism on the part of the agent is to be expected and guarded against; buyer–seller relationships typically assume self-interested gain seeking by both parties. In contrast, partnering assumes shared fate—that each party's interest coincides with, and is best served by, the collective interest of the partnership.

In this context, the symmetry implied by the core definition of partnering, as resting on fair division, has two aspects. The first relates to formulation. Do all of the parties contribute to fashioning the terms of the relationship in ways that reflect their capabilities and eventual contribution? Or conversely, are the most important terms specified by a single, directive party, prior to the formation of the partnership itself? Symmetry in formulation demands shared control over terms, as opposed to having it concentrated in one of the parties, whose goals effectively dictate them for all. The second relates to function. Does each of the parties assume a share of the costs and responsibilities (and among for-profits, the gains)? Or is the assumption lopsided, with one party providing all of the funds, and another, all of the know-how?

A key advantage of partnering arrangements is that parties share control and a similar stake in the outcome. In this way, not only are participating organizations more likely to cooperate, but they are also more likely to have complementary motives that reduce the chances of shirking or self-seeking behavior, and consequently, the need for coercive terms. In short, partnering in the face of symmetry builds on and, at the same time, relies on, mutual trust.

Aside from having a clearer picture of what is going on in arrangements that claim to be partnerships, this determination of symmetry might also serve as a threshold test for those individuals or organizations considering whether "partnering" suits their needs. As will be shown, not all relations calling themselves partnerships are mutually beneficial, despite the gloss of the rhetoric. Accordingly, not all partnerships are worth forming or joining. More partnering is not necessarily better, nor in the public's interest, for example, when it serves as a euphemism for government sharply reducing funds while diverting responsibilities to less accountable, private parties. And finally, much of what passes as partnerships are not partnerships at all; rather, they are efforts to win public endorsement for relationships among parties of diverse motives, formulated and executed in highly directive ways. Calling these arrangements partnerships conveys a false sense of unity, inviting public trust while disguising the coercion, perhaps on the part of a large, bureaucratic funder, necessary to hold it together.

MODELS OF PARTNERSHIP IN PUBLIC HEALTH

In public health, the federal government, foundations, and for-profit health care providers are more likely to be offering funds and looking for partners willing to listen to how they want it spent. Those who have the money, and are seeking partners, typically assume a higher level of control than those who need the money and are willing to do what they are asked in order to get it. In turn, their partners are most likely those in need of resources to meet their responsibilities: the professional schools, LHDs, nonprofit service providers, and voluntary civic associations. Accordingly, they are willing to listen.

The typical federal "partnership" in public health involves a competitively bid contract for services whose content is either fully specified or subject to periodic review. Depending on the experience in the area, the prototype can either be the procurement process or research and development funding. In either case, the discretion of the "partner" is highly structured, and the resources flow in one direction. If the prototype is research and development, continued funding may be contingent on identifying other funding sources, perhaps with complementary commitments, to help defray future costs should the activity prove worthwhile to the federal sponsors. As will be shown later, federal partnerships with schools of public health have followed this pattern. This is a principal–agent relationship without the symmetry conditions that define partnering. And yet, partnering is invoked, perhaps to convey a sense of unity of purpose and trust that would garner public support.

In contrast, the foundations seldom become partners themselves, preferring to broker partnerships that can sustain a given activity after a temporary infusion of start-up funding. This protects the foundation from long-term commitments that would eventually stifle new initiatives and builds in concerns for the sustainability of the activity once the foundation chooses to withdraw. Although the brokering of partnerships among nonprofit providers and civic associations has been a traditional pursuit, in public health areas, the foundations' most recent strategy has been to urge the professional schools to join in the partnering. The most interesting feature of this strategy is that it combines the old-style funding of technical assistance and training with a new-style paternalistic appeal to a different kind of professional identity. Not only are the schools counseled to partner for their own good, but now they are convinced that partnering is the only way for them to accomplish their basic mission of serving the field of practice. Once devoted to academic research, professional education, and technical assistance, the schools are now encouraged by the Carnegie Endowment, Kellogg Foundation, and Pew Charitable Trust to be more practice oriented, to be aware of the problems faced by their fellow professionals who do public health work, and to lend assistance. These reports are examined more closely in a subsequent section.[7(pp.7,35)]

This appeal was reinforced by a federal effort in parallel reports to get more technical assistance to LHDs without necessarily increasing federal funding. The federal appeals, through the Institute of Medicine (IOM) and an interagency forum, sounded the same theme as the foundations: linkages to practice, partnerships for service, scholarship for the practice community, and so on.[8,9] In effect, partnering with underfunded practitioners was elevated to a civic virtue. From the perspective of the underfunded program manager at the LHD, this kind of partnering is very attractive.

The technical assistance provided by schools of public health tends to be subsidized in two ways. First, academics are more likely to provide in-kind contributions out of loyalty to the missions of their profession and its service ethos; as will be shown, incentives for these contributions have been built into the reward structures of many schools. And second, most universities have restrictions of some sort on outside funding, limiting salary levels, per diem rates, or cost recovery. In contrast, for-profit consultancies will not only price out these subsidies, but typically charge a higher rate for indirect costs. The program manager, then, is likely to get a bargain in dealing with academics and perhaps some voluntary contributions as well. The downside is that most academics are protective of their autonomy and may believe in the symmetry that partnering officially promises. A later section will address the problems attending this partnering.

Academic partnering was neither a spontaneous outbreak nor a natural evolution, but was grafted onto the schools' missions by a combination of external pressure and internal reform. As a brief look at the historical missions of the schools of public health reveals the internal tensions between training for professional tasks and generating new knowledge occupied the formative decades—not concerns over finding partners to do either.[10] Moreover, over the span of the last century, partnering rhetoric and activity appear concentrated in the post-Reagan decades and largely in the United States and post-Thatcher Britain, at least until quite recently. For the most part, the pressures to partner originated with the principal funder of public health services, the federal government, and gathered momentum through the large foundations.[4] The partnership device served as a means not only of directing academic work toward areas of increasingly unmet public need, but also of managing the fiscal austerity afflicting nonprofit providers and local governments alike. Partnering in other sectors, such as transportation and housing, served as a reprise of sorts from the drive for full-scale privatization of public services. Schools seemed willing to provide technical know-how and professional assistance at a rate that was far below that charged by the profit-making consultancies, and often did so with a service ethic tied to professional ideals. Bringing schools in as partners could be seen as less costly for government than privatizing either the provision of services or the transfer of know-how to the field of practice.

The next section examines the efforts by foundations and the federal government to transform schools of public health into willing partners with local providers and program officers. Part of this effort involved moral suasion. Report after report claimed that partnering with community providers was a central responsibility of the schools. Not only was it consistent with their historical missions, but it was crucial to their scholarship and to the way they trained their students. These arguments went beyond a reinterpretation of roles, however, to advocate the restructuring of reward systems within academic organizations so that proper incentives could be provided for this partnering work. Next, some of the features that make up the partnership landscape, at least in public health, are presented. Finally, the chapter returns to the assessment of partnering relative to core public health functions and to the question of when a "partnership" is not a partnership, as it has been defined for purposes of this chapter.

THE HISTORICAL ROLE OF SCHOOLS OF PUBLIC HEALTH

Historically, the basic tension between research and practice in schools of public health paralleled the similar but older tension in medicine. Should the principal role of the schools be to educate researchers and scientists or to train practitioners? Relatedly, should programs emphasize education for specialized research or general training in practical skills? As Elizabeth Fee noted, the early schools of public health contended with the demand from the field for professional training and pressure from within academe to develop research to advance the science.[11] It was not long before scientific research predominanted in public health education and the needs of the public health work force remained unmet, despite the growth of the number of schools of public health through the 1930s and 1940s.

The missions of schools of public health would again be reordered as a comprehensive plan to provide public health services at the local level was developed by the American Association of Public Health.[12] This demand for new public health professionals was further exacerbated by the military demands for training in the Second World War. By 1950, an American Public Health Association (APHA) survey revealed that the existing schools of public health were crowded to capacity.[13] And yet, although the emphasis on scientific research continued to grow, training dollars to support students fell by approximately one-half. From after WWII until approximately 1960, 40 percent of the budget across the schools went for teaching, 40 percent for research, 10 percent for community service, and 10 percent for administration.[10,14]

Demographic changes, changing patterns of disease, the expansion of hospitals, and biomedical research had a profound influence on public health after the Second World War. The predominance of medicine and the need for changing curricula to address community health problems focused attention on funds for training. Federal training funds permitted schools to expand and tailor their curriculum to an increasingly diverse student population and evolving areas of inquiry. Despite the general growth of schools of public health, now supported by federal funds, and expanded research in the biologic sciences, a large number of studies questioned their performance.[10] Ultimately, the schools would face the same pressures for fiscal austerity and accountability that drove the retrenchment of federal efforts in human services generally.

Nonetheless, the changing climate for federal and state support of public services was not the only impetus toward partnering as a means to leverage dwindling resources. There was also a concerted effort by foundations and federal agencies to reframe the roles of the professional schools in ways that supported the partnering idea. In effect, partnering took on symbolic value as a desirable means of carrying out one's obligation to the public. Accordingly, it was promoted as an innovative reform for better realizing the schools' service ideals, rather than as a transitional device toward further privatization of public health.

THE PARTNERING REPORTS

The IOM's report, *The Future of Public Health,* released in 1988, captured the concerns raised about the mission and charge of public health schools and their relationships to communities.[8] Among the report's recommendations was a primary emphasis on stronger linkages among universities, communities, government, and practicing professionals. The premise that improved communication and sharing of resources would result in improved health of the community, better-trained public health professionals, and more relevant research undergirded the framework of the document. The call for the academy to revisit its missions of teaching, service, and research was echoed in several foundation and government reports of the early 1990s.[7,15,16] William C. Richardson, president of Johns Hopkins University, commented on the imperative to improve partnerships.

> The university in partnership with the community can play a significant, though probably less immediate, role in addressing these fundamental problems. In fact, we would argue that those universities located in the midst of urban disintegration must do so if they are to be successful themselves. Undeniably, community health is tied to the health of the community; it is just as undeniable that the contemporary urban university, ready or not, must become an active participant in the efforts to resuscitate local economies that are very often in dire need of critical care.[17(p.12)]

Two federal agencies (the U.S. Centers for Disease Control and the Prevention [CDC] and the Health Resources and Services Administration [HRSA]) collaborated to form the Public Health Faculty/Agency Forum to study specifically how public educational institutions and public health practice agencies collaborate. The objectives of the forum were to: (1) strengthen relationships between public health academicians and public health; (2) improve the teaching, training, and practice of public health; (3) establish links between schools of public health and practice agencies; and (4) collaborate with others in achieving the year 2000 objectives for the nation.[9,18] The report of this group and the implementing body convened in 1992—the Council on Linkages Between Academia and Public Health Practice—emphasized the need for linkages and disseminated recommendations that served to guide change within academia and practice. In concert with the Association of Schools of Public Health, substantial efforts toward implementing the IOM and forum recommendations have been made. Expanded technical assistance and research activities partnering schools with government, private sector, and community-based organizations are now chronicled as successes.[14]

Nonetheless, with claims of success have come criticisms of shortcomings. And yet, these criticisms take the "Why partnership?" question as settled and merely ask how partnering can be made bigger and better.[7,16] The frictions experienced in the first generation of partnering arrangements are attributed not to flaws in the device, but to deficits on the part of the participants, who may operate according to different cultural norms, missions, and historical incentives. Arguments have centered on the continued valorization of the role of service in university work; fundamental redefinitions of research, teaching, and service in ways that better support partnering; and a reconsideration of the obstacles that the academy often brings to partnerships.

Despite assets including technical expertise, nonpartisanship, dissemination capability, and social status, practitioners appear to mistrust faculty attempts to develop partnerships. Tensions often make partnerships difficult:

> If there is mistrust on one side, there is on the other an equally long history of disregard for the importance of telling our neighbors what it is that we do and how our actions can benefit all members of our society. Part of this has to do with the sophisticated, highly technical nature of our work and the challenge of explaining it to anyone outside our specialty. Part of it has to do with the incredible demands of modern research and the little time it seems to leave for any activities outside the lab. And part of it comes from that cultural chasm mentioned earlier, the inability of the two groups to find common ground on which to base a discussion.[17(pp.15–16)]

As Lancaster pointed out, there are gaps between the research mission of universities and the interests of practitioners that make partnering difficult.[19] He specified these gaps as: (1) a communication gap, whereby lack of shared language and different emphases prevent joint definition of research questions and identification of mutual priorities; (2) an access gap, whereby practitioners in some parts of the country have little or no access to university faculty skilled in public health; (3) a credibility gap, whereby practitioners discount the observations of academicians as unrealistic and academicians discount the observations of practitioners as simplistic; and (4) an expectation gap, whereby the practitioner's view of what it takes to operate effectively in the real world fails to meet the standards of scientific rigor demanded by the researcher.[19] These gaps continue to demand attention and circumscribe efforts to conduct practice-oriented research within a partnership model.

The solution, for some, was provided by the Carnegie Endowment's effort to restructure the reward system in higher education as a way of directing intellectual energy toward the solution of societal problems. Here, the internal obstacles to practice-oriented partnering were addressed.

RESTRUCTURING ACADEME FOR PARTNERSHIPS

In 1990, the Carnegie Foundation for the Advancement of Teaching released a report by its president, Ernest L. Boyer, entitled *Scholarship Reconsidered: Priorities of the Professoriate.*[20] The report highlighted trends toward excessive specialization in higher education and argued that greater insularity was the result. An advocate of the classical, humanistic conception of the liberal arts, Boyer wanted to restore the university to its prewar position of social and cultural leadership. Ironically, he would, at the same time, bolster the rationale for professional schools to reassert their leadership over their respective professions by remedying their own excesses of specialization and insularity. The report set out distinctive criteria for assessing scholarship that could be applied within the professional schools, and redefined domains of scholarly activity in ways that were intended to counteract insularity. He concluded that the key culprit was the reward structure within universities that inhibited scholarly engagement with the community.

As the level of support from taxes and endowments dwindled, the source of financial support for schools shifted to a reliance on external research funding. The reward structure for faculty then came to emphasize research productivity over more traditional concerns, such as teaching and practice-oriented contributions, in hiring, promotion, and tenure decisions. The Carnegie Endowment's report offered a new rationale for schools to partner with community professionals by advocating new missions of community leadership and outlining a reward system to support them.

Engagement in practice-oriented scholarship, along the lines that Boyer suggested, was quickly adapted to the core functions of public health. Those on the practice side would be able to benefit from an infusion of expertise at little or no cost, whereas those on the academic side could be reassured of their importance and worth. The redefinition of practice put the academic at the center.

> Public health practice involves the linkage of academic information to the realities of community health by forging partnerships among academics, public health professionals through their agencies, community human services professionals through their agencies, and empowered community residents in order to improve the public's health.... The activities involved in practice may include such things as community assessment; assurance activities as represented by the development of interventions, training and education programs, and dissemination of health information; and help in the policy development arena.[21(p.82)]

The significance and impact of the faculty member's role in improving the field of practice is also more sharply highlighted in evaluating scholarly contributions. In practice-oriented scholarship, service to the community is seen to depend on the strength of collaborative ties between academics and practice. Partnering, then, comes to the foreground as the device of choice in making and sustaining interactions with the practice community.

After a decade of federal and foundation promotion, the partnering concept won the endorsement of the Association of Schools of Public Health's Practice Council. Its report, *Demonstrating Excellence in Academic Public Health Practice,* recommended that schools encourage and promote partnerships under the auspices of practice-oriented scholarship through new funding, faculty incentives, revised promotion criteria, and more outlets for scholarly findings.[22] By this time, the transformation of the schools from the inside out was largely complete. Faculty were now guided not only by professional norms exhorting academics to partner, but also by a reformed system of internal incentives that rewarded the practice work that partnering entailed. As mentioned earlier, however, not all partnerships are alike. And some that claim to be are not "partnerships" at all.

DEPLOYING PARTNERSHIPS FOR PUBLIC HEALTH

As noted earlier, the test for partnering hinges on evidence of symmetry in two senses: first, *symmetry in formulation*, indicated by shared control over resources, commitments, and purposes; second, *symmetry in function*, or shared fate with respect to possible risks and rewards. Rather than convey a false precision in claiming to identify partnering as varying degrees of either, the intent is to separate examples, where neither condition is met, from those where either or both are plausibly satisfied. In short, this chapter divides the nonpartnerships that invoke the rhetoric from the plausible ones. To be sure, there is a wide variety of arrangements in public health that have assumed the title of partnerships. The motives for doing this, on the part of both public health organizations and professional schools, should be clearer from the earlier discussion. By way of illustration, however, only a small set of cases will be necessary. Twenty cases will be presented. Ten lack evidence of symmetry, with one "partner" typically operating unilaterally. Another 10 involve multilateral partnerings, offering some evidence of symmetry in formulation, function, or both. Because the level of detail varies widely in these case accounts, any finer designations of partnership traits would be uneven and potentially biased. This task is left to other investigators.

Part I: The Nonpartnerships

The first 10 cases of nonpartnerships (or only nominal ones) are arranged in Exhibit 22–1. In each instance, there is a unilateral effort by one would-be partner to find another participant willing to serve its purposes. In each instance, the unilateral seekers provide all of the resources and rely on the other partner to perform the desired functions. Depending on the "strings" that can come attached to these arrangements, they resemble either principal–agent relations (more strings) or buyer–seller ones (fewer strings) rather than partnerships as they are defined in this chapter. In this sample of cases, government at all levels and private (family) philanthropic organizations are the unilateral seekers. The majority of the partners sought are nonprofit providers of one kind or another, rather than voluntary community organizations or for-profit businesses. A brief description of the cases follows the ordering of the table. The unilateral seekers appear in the rows, and the set of possible participants in their projects is arrayed across the columns. As the descriptions make clear, there is a concentration of arrangements between government and various service providers that more closely resembles principal–agent relationships than partnerships.

Federal Government

- *Association of Schools of Public Health-Council on Linkages:* The CDC and the HRSA have supported and continue to support academic projects at schools of public health through cooperative arrangements with the Association of Schools of Public Health. This can be documented at the federal level through the participation of the CDC and the HRSA in the Council on Linkages Between Academic and Public Health Practice in 1992.[22,23] Other federal agencies such as the Agency for Toxic Substances Disease Registry have also participated through this process to link with academic institutions.
- *Prevention Research Centers (PRCs):* The development of PRCs marks another significant federal effort to unite the academic missions with public health and community interests. In 1984, Congress enacted Public Law 98–551, legislation that authorized the creation of the Health Promotion and Disease Prevention Center Program designed to establish a national network of academic centers for prevention research.[24,25] These 23 centers, which are implemented through the CDC, included multidisciplinary faculty emphasis on community-based training in health promotion. The multidisciplinary public health expertise and the community involvement are distinguishing characteristics of the program. PRCs have stimulated research in cancer prevention, injury control, tobacco control, mortality and morbidity measures reduction in chronic and acute illness, and others directly related to the health of the community. Highly variable in their research activities, PRCs raise fundamental questions concerning the partnership relationships.[24,26] Baker articulated two of these for consideration: "Can practice/community/academic teams be created to solve urgent, practical problems in the real world of public health? Can this be done in such a way that new knowledge is generated?"[27(p.13)]

State Government

- *Maryland State Health Departments-MCO:* The necessity to interface with multiple provider settings and governmental agencies to achieve effective services is emphasized in the Medicaid managed care case of Maryland. Medicaid recipients are managed under two primary mechanisms: Medicaid health maintenance organizations and the Medicaid Access to Care Program. Three private corporations in Mary-

Exhibit 22–1 Nonpartnership Cases

Unilateral Seekers	Partners	For-Profit Providers		Nonprofit Providers			Voluntary Community Organizations		
		Managed Care Organizations	Private Business	Professional Schools	Medical	Service Organizations	Civic	Specialty	Ad Hoc
Government	Federal			Association of Schools of Public Health-Council on Linkages Prevention Research Centers					
Government	State	Maryland State Health Department-MCO		Missouri					
Government	Local	Baltimore		Akron Academic Health Department		Healthy LA			
Government	Local	Denver		Columbia Public Health Scholars					
Philanthropy	Public								
Philanthropy	Private					Medicine and Public Health			
Providers	Managed Care Organizations								

land have contracts to serve Medicaid clients. The advantages of the contracts are continuity of care and preventive services. However, the system acknowledges gaps in the number of screenings and enrollments of new patients with providers.

- *Missouri:* The partnership of the Missouri Department of Health, the Saint Louis University School of Public Health, Washington University, and the University of Missouri conducted data collection and analysis on work disability using the key indicator of arthritis. This effort identified rural geographic areas of the state with high prevalence of arthritis and provided a framework for providing the core activities to deal with disability, including assessment, policy development, and assurance.[28] This project underscores the important role of research and service of universities in defining community need, developing health measures, assessing the health delivery system, defining the role of its health professionals, and designing ways to improve it that will be beneficial.[14,29]

Local Government

- *Baltimore:* The Baltimore City Health Department is participating in a demonstration project called Total Health Plan. Under this plan, the health maintenance organization reimburses the health department for family planning and emergency services and reimburses the school-based health centers for services to enrollees. The demonstration model has been successful in using established community-based entities in the public/private partnerships. These examples from the Total Health Plan demonstration illustrate both the potential and the shortcomings of managed care partnerships.[30]
- *Denver:* Denver reveals a health care market that is large, consolidated, and economically healthy. An independent health care authority integrates public health functions in a quasi-governmental health system with managed care organizations, health maintenance organizations, hospitals, and health centers serving residents with and without insurance.[31] Private health care organizations noted significant community health efforts, including care of medically indigent and Medicaid beneficiaries. Although there has been substantial progress, a competitive market and role transitions reflect limited interaction with the Denver Department of Health.[32]
- *Akron Academic Health Department:* The development of linkages between universities and LHDs is evidenced by the relationship between the Akron Health Department and the Northeastern Ohio Universities College of Medicine. The agreement of 20 years includes the health department as a teaching department of the College of Medicine, training medical students in community health. In addition, faculty appointments and shared staff positions enhance the teaching and research capabilities of both institutions and suggest a stronger alliance with communities in solving public health problems.[33]
- *Columbia Public Health Scholars:* The New York City Health Department has had an extensive history of collaboration with the Joseph L. Mailman School of Public Health of Columbia University. Recent initiation of a Public Health Scholars Program provides a unique opportunity for exceptional staff from the New York City Health Department to obtain formal education at the Columbia University School of Public Health.[34] This project follows a five-year Model Health Department School of Public Health Collaboration supported by funds from the HRSA that resulted in 10 specific projects designed to meet the *Healthy People 2000* objectives. Such initiatives can be noted in other schools of public health.
- *Healthy LA:* The Healthy Los Angeles 2000 initiative partnered the Southern Area Clergy Council, a group of 75 churches, and the Los Angeles County Health Department and other groups to develop projects addressing controlling violence, the use of tobacco, and lead poisoning.

These priorities selected by the churches culminated in a major conference of faith and health leaders to establish partnership networks across the country. The size of churches, and their influence in the community, suggest that the faith community can be instrumental in promoting the health and social agenda. In Los Angeles, one million residents formally belong to churches and religious institutions.[35]

Private Philanthropy

- *Medicine and Public Health:* Given the challenges of the current health care environment, several queries emerged that stimulated the Medicine and Public Health Initiative by the American Public Health Association and the American Medical Association in 1994. The gap, commonly noted between medicine's focus on individuals and public health's on populations, was examined in the 1997 report, *Medicine and Public Health: The Power of Collaboration,* supported by the Robert Wood Johnson Foundation through the New York Academy of Medicine.[36] The report claims that: (1) both sectors are concerned about the direction of the health care system, (2) both are under economic and performance pressure, and (3) neither can accomplish its mission alone.[36] This initiative collected more than 500 cases of collaboration, most at the community level. These cases were advanced as models of partnerships to improve the delivery of health care services. The initiative itself, however, was not a partnership.

Part II: Plausible Partnerships

The next set of 10 cases appears to satisfy one or the other conditions of symmetry. Here, the same actors are involved, but this time, the partnering tends to be multilateral rather than a product of some unilateral design for participation. The partnership seekers tend to play less directive roles, typically acting as intermediaries among potential partners or helping to promote the partnering activities of others. Further, new participants are included—private business, nonprofit medical care organizations, and voluntary community organizations. Because there are multiple partners involved, and a dominant partner is less likely to emerge, the brief case summaries have been ordered across the columns of the second table rather than across the rows. The 10 cases of plausible partnerships are summarized in Exhibit 22–2. Although each case appears in multiple columns, only its first appearance will be discussed in the narrative.

Managed Care Organizations

- *Clark County:* The critical importance of community needs assessments in defining community health priorities stimulated the partnership of the Clark County (Washington) Health Department, the CDC, the county hospital, the managed care organization, city and county government, and community residents called Community Choices 2010. This group conducted a year-long assessment project and identified six health domains in which to intervene. This process, involving more than 400 people, evolved into a "Healthy Communities" project and subsequent programmatic changes by area health organizations.[36]
- *Albuquerque:* The University of New Mexico formed a partnership with the Albuquerque City Human Services Department and the local department of public health, university hospital, college of nursing, and community leaders to develop a network of primary care providers in an impoverished area of the city. From this effort, a new building was designated and contracts for service providers from the university and county providers were established. The focus on academic medical centers highlights several tensions surrounding the public/private partnerships in health care. The first is the changing complexion of privatization within the hospital system. As more hospitals achieve for-profit status, the market influences begin to dictate the partnership arrangements. With

Exhibit 22–2 Plausible Partnership Cases

Multilateral Seekers	Partners	For-Profit Providers		Nonprofit Providers			Voluntary Community Organizations		
		Managed Care Organizations	Private Business	Professional Schools	Medical	Service Organizations	Civic	Specialty	Ad Hoc
Government	**Federal**	Clark County	ENCORE	ENCORE WE ACT		ENCORE	Healthy Communities		
Government	**State**				Healthy Communities	Turning Point	Turning Point		
Government	**Local**	Clark County Albuquerque	Turning Point Healthy Communities	Monroe County WE ACT Albuquerque	Clark County	Monroe County	WE ACT Clark County	Monroe County* (*Ad hoc for this purpose)	Turning Point
Philanthropy	**Public**								
Philanthropy	**Private**		University of Hawaii Turning Point	Healthy Communities Mass Coalition University of Hawaii Health of the Public	Healthy Communities University of Hawaii	Mass Coalition	Turning Point Mass Coalition Health of the Public		
Providers	**Managed Care Organizations**								

managed care altering the structures and incentives of health services delivery systems, the public health/private sector distinctions become less clear. The linkage of medicine and public health as academic disciplines points out the public/private tension as well as collaborative efforts.[36]

Private Business

- *ENCORE:* The ENCORE Program is a breast and cervical screening program delivered through a nonprofit organization (YWCA), a for-profit entity (AVON), the CDC, and the University of Texas School of Public Health. Part of a national program, ENCORE findings support the program's effectiveness in screening low-income and minority women and the benefits of an academic/private/nonprofit/public partnership.[37]
- *Turning Point:* Although there is limited evidence that collaboration improves health, and there is a distinct need for evaluation and testing of models, collaborations/partnerships offer significant benefits. Supported jointly by the W.K. Kellogg Foundation and the Robert Wood Johnson Foundation, Turning Point is a national project in 14 states and 41 communities. These projects develop a state coalition of leaders across sectors to address complex systems that support and deliver health services. At the community level, local leaders and a broad array of sector interests, businesses, government, and faith and community organizations are working together to strengthen the community infrastructure. A fundamental interest of this national project is to develop, test, and evaluate partnership models that emphasize health improvement using state, local, and community recommendations. Key to the success are the state–local linkages.[38]
- *University of Hawaii:* The University of Hawaii developed a model of multidisciplinary care systems for teaching, service, and research to strengthen three existing clinics. The clinics each had a separate focus: family practice, primary care, and nurse practitioner approach. A nonprofit corporation was established to formalize the association with the health centers and create a 14-member board with community members. This project demonstrates commitment to the philosophy of community-based education requiring students to participate in community education and realizing the role of community members in community-based research.[39]

Professional Schools

- *WE ACT:* After a decade of tentative collaboration between Columbia University's School of Public Health and the civic organization, West Harlem Environmental Action (WE ACT), the parties formed a partnership to improve environmental quality and environmental justice for residents in Harlem, New York. The benefits of researchers sharing in community problem solving were a fundamental contribution of academia. The community brought knowledge of the community culture and resources and an instruction in community success. The project was enhanced by funding from governmental agencies (the Environmental Protection Agency and the CDC). The lessons of this experience are expressed in the maturation of the relationship from one of skepticism to one of productive interchange and accomplishment. Further, the focus on understanding the elements of the relationship and the impact on project outcomes supports careful attention to the building, tending, and patience required in developing partnerships that are mutually respectful.[40]
- *Monroe County:* The collaboration of the Monroe County Health Department, the Monroe County Medical Society, the University of Rochester, the American Cancer Society, and Cancer Action developed a partnership (Women's Health Partnership) to coordinate 41 providers with the goal of promoting breast and cervical cancer screenings in Monroe County, New York,

especially in uninsured and minority groups. Since the partnership's communitywide campaign began, the mammography rates for women 50–70 years of age in Monroe County have increased from 43 percent to 62 percent, with the greatest improvement in those neighborhoods that had low rates at baseline.[36]

- *Healthy Communities:* Projects designated as "Healthy Communities" can be traced to the 1986 meeting of the World Health Organization (WHO), where the development of the WHO Europe Healthy Cities Project marked a serious effort to change the quality of life in European cities. The concept itself can be noted as far back as 1844 in England, where there was a Healthy Towns Association.[41] Thus, the understanding of the role of local government in establishing the conditions of a healthy city coupled with a contemporary notion of health promotion has resulted in a variety of approaches in European cities; most of the 29 projects are in cities of more than 100,000 population. In the United States, the first statewide healthy cities project was established in Indiana by the University of Indiana School of Nursing in partnership with the W.K. Kellogg Foundation. Subsequent projects have received the support of state government, such as California and the California Healthy Cities Project. A governmental partnership by the U.S. Office of Health Promotion and Disease Prevention with a nonprofit organization, the National Civic League, created the Healthy Cities initiative. This expansion of city models resulted in more than 200 self-proclaimed Healthy Cities and Communities in the United States by mid-1995.[42] Subsequent initiatives included the Voluntary Hospitals Association of America and the Healthcare Forum. These partnerships had local variability and local partnership distinctions, but induced cross-sector participation.
- *Mass Coalition:* The W.K. Kellogg Foundation also funded a Community Partnership/Health Professions Education Project in 1989 that desired to create partnerships with academic centers and community health centers. The premise was to create new organizational structures to be the basis for new primary health care–oriented funding patterns and the advancement of community focus in health professionals' education.[39] The following example illustrates the tenor of these projects. Four community-based coalitions located in central and western Massachusetts (Athol/Orange, Holyoke, Northern Berkshires, and Worcester), the Massachusetts Association of Health Boards, the Area Health Education Centers, Community Partners, the University of Massachusetts School of Public Health, and the University of Massachusetts Medical Center joined together to serve Latin Americans and other underserved populations. Partners focused on projects to develop multicultural community-based approaches, improve the capacity of communities to solve their own problems, promote the capacity of local boards of health to assess and ensure the health of their communities, initiate policies that would have an impact on public health, and institute sustainable linkages among schools of public health and medicine, boards of health, and community based-organizations.[43]
- *Health of the Public:* The Health of the Public Project supported by the Pew Charitable Trust and the Rockefeller Foundation represents another initiative to broker partnerships among academic health centers, private foundations, and the community. This project, which was initiated in 1993, included 17 universities charged with designing health care systems for the health of the community.[44]

PROSPECTS

Among advocates of partnering, there is a tendency to assume that partnerships arise spontaneously as opportunities present themselves and that partners cooperate as collaborators with shared purposes in a common enterprise. For the most part, this is a myth. Partnering involves complex organizations, not autonomous individuals; motives are mixed; and experiences and commitments are reinterpreted as membership changes. Further, because of the risks that organizations face from opportunism and manipulation, there is a residue of strategic wariness in their dealings with unfamiliar entities. Partnerships, then, are built slowly and with repeated showings of good faith by those involved; otherwise, symmetry breaks down, and one partner either assumes control or is left with most of the work. Symmetry is seldom automatic; purposes will differ among entities, as will resource capabilities, creating pressures toward asymmetry. Among the professional schools, asymmetry tends to accompany expertise rather than financial resources. With government, the asymmetry may be financial or legal. When symmetry does exist, it is probably more likely among similar kinds of entities, say, professional schools or grassroots organizations, which have had successful dealings with each other in the past.

More importantly, symmetry is never free. Resources, as well as expectations, must be invested in the partnering itself. The more diverse the entities involved, the more attention is needed to maintain the basic framework of cooperation. Accordingly, the most diverse of the partnerings described here, say, the Mass Coalition or Turning Point, required the services of a broker to bring the partners together, to promote common purposes, and to offer some assurances against opportunism. Of course, this means that the broker can also act as a gatekeeper, deciding who is included and excluded by default. In the extreme, then, this comes to resemble the unilateral partnership seekers, who look for partners to participate on preset terms for certain financial support.

The discussion presented here regarding partnerships in public health practice suggests several lessons for the public health practitioner. The first lesson elucidated by the historical review of partnerships and analysis of partnership relationships is how crucial it is to conduct an inquiry regarding the nature of the partnership and the utility of the partnership model in addressing the public health concerns of the new century. As previously noted, a fuller understanding of partnerships by public health practitioners (types, motives, symmetry, etc.) within the community predisposes a refined criterion for choosing and sustaining true partnerships that are advantageous to all participants and promise long-term benefits. Public health practitioners are instrumental in convening and stimulating partnership development. Practitioners will be challenged to apply enhanced skills to partnering and coalition building that are consistent with the new paradigms of the "new public health" to engage community and develop civic involvement as means to create healthy citizens and communities.

Second, the tools of the public health administrator are ideally suited to evaluate the community's capabilities and capacities and hence design successful partnerships. Community health assessments, asset mapping, and community development skills are well suited for determining the merits and obstacles of potential partnerships in public health practice. Public health administrators need to apply the conventional assessment tools used in the community to the assessment and development of partnerships. This new perspective on partnering promises more enlightened and productive models of partnerships in these communities. Public health administrators can be leaders in promoting careful assessments as precursors to partnership development.

The final lesson speaks to the development of best practices in public health. Partnerships between academe and practice have been promoted as a model of best practice in public health. To truly achieve partnerships, the relationships must be based on symmetry of power rather than on asymmetry. In the examples suggested, successful models can be developed when the tenets of academe, practice, and the community are considered.

In summary, the prospect is favorable for organizations committed to public health that desire to partner if the full dynamics of the partnership are acknowledged and partnership rhetoric is replaced by well-defined partnership roles.

CHAPTER REVIEW

1. The essential feature of partnership is the *jointness* of the arrangement; every partner bears some of the risk, pays some of the cost, and can claim a portion of the gain.
2. There are at least two parties to a partnership who devise a means to share resource commitment and a measure of control. What makes them partners is the expectation of *symmetry* in their relationship.
3. Academic partnering was grafted onto schools' missions by external pressure and internal reform. The federal government and foundations—principal funders—exerted pressures to partner.
4. Partnership directed academic work toward areas of increasingly unmet public need and also was viewed as a means to manage the fiscal austerity afflicting nonprofit providers and local governments.
5. Six key national reports issued by government or foundations in the early 1990s encouraged partnering.
6. There are gaps between the research missions of universities and the interests of practitioners that make partnering difficult and result in tension. Mistrust of faculty by practitioners is a recurring theme.
7. Partnerships between academe have been promoted as a "best practice" in public health. Success has been achieved when these relationships are based on a symmetry of power rather than asymmetry.

REFERENCES

1. E.L. Baker et al., "Health Reform and the Health of the Public," *Journal of the American Medical Association* 272 (1994): 1,276–1,282.
2. Institute of Medicine, *Healthy Communities: New Partnerships for the Future of Public Health* (Washington, DC: National Academy Press, 1996).
3. *Uniform Partnership Act* (1997). <http://www.law.upenn.edu/bll/ulc/fnact99/1990s/upa97fa.htm> (25 May 2000).
4. M. Bendick and P.M. Levinson, "Private Sector Initiatives or Public–Private Partnerships?" in *The Reagan Presidency and the Governing of America*, eds. L. Salomon and M. Lund (Washington, DC: The Urban Institute, 1981), 455–479.
5. E.S. Savas, *Privatization: The Key to Better Government* (Chatham, NJ: Chatham House Publishers, 1987).
6. P.K. Halverson et al., "Privatizing Health Services: Alternative Models and Emerging Issues for Public Health and Quality Management," *Quality Management in Health Care 5*, no. 2 (1997): 1–18.
7. Pew Health Professions Commission, *Critical Challenges: Revitalizing the Health Professions for the Twenty-First Century* (San Francisco: 1995).
8. Institute of Medicine, *The Future of Public Health* (Washington, DC: National Academy Press, 1988).
9. A.A. Sorenson and R.G. Bialek, *The Public Health Faculty/Agency Forum: Linking Graduate Education and Practice: Final Report* (Gainesville, FL: University Press of Florida, 1991).
10. E. Fee and B. Rosenkrantz, "Professional Education for Public Health in the United States," in *History of Education in Public Health*, eds. E. Fee and R.M. Acheson (New York: Oxford University Press, 1991), 230–271.
11. E. Fee, "Designing Schools of Public Health for the United States," in *History of Education in Public Health*, eds. E. Fee and R.M. Acheson (New York: Oxford University Press, 1991), 155–196.
12. H.C. Emerson, *Local Health Units for a Nation* (New York: The Commonwealth Fund, 1945).
13. L.S. Rosenfield et al., *Report on Schools of Public Health in the U.S. Based on a Survey of Schools of Public Health in 1950* [Pub. #270] (Washington, DC: Public Health Services, U.S. Department of Health, Education, and Welfare, 1953).
14. Association of Schools of Public Health, *Strong Schools, Strong Partners: A Report on Practice Activities of Schools of Public Health* (Washington, DC: 1998).
15. A. Kaufman and R.E. Waterman, *Health of the Public: Strategies for Reorienting Academic Health Centers toward Community Health Needs* (San Francisco: Health of the Public Program, 1993).

16. E.H. O'Neil, *Health Professions Education for the Future: Schools in Service to the Nation* (San Francisco: Pew Health Professions Commission, 1993).
17. W.C. Richardson and M.P. Field, "The Role of the University in Urban Health," in *The University in the Urban Community: Responsibilities for Public Health,* eds. T.R. Hogness et al. (Washington, DC: Association of Academic Health Centers, 1993), 7–28.
18. U.S. Department of Health and Human Services, Public Health Services, *Healthy People 2000: National Health Promotion and Disease Prevention Objectives* [DHHS Pub. No. (PHS) 91–50212] (Washington, DC: 1991).
19. B. Lancaster, "Closing the Gap between Research and Practice," *Health Education Quarterly* 19 (1992): 408–411.
20. E.L. Boyer, *Scholarship Reconsidered: Priorities of the Professorate* (Princeton, NJ: Princeton University Press, 1990).
21. L. Rowitz, "An Academic Linchpin," *Journal of Public Health Management and Practice 1*, no. 3 (1995): 82–84.
22. Association of Schools of Public Health Practice Council, *Demonstrating Excellence in Academic Public Health Practice* (Washington, DC: 1999).
23. R. Bialek, "A Decade of Progress in Academic/Practice Linkages," *Journal of Public Health Management and Practice 6*, no. 1 (2000): 25–31.
24. Institute of Medicine, *Linking Research and Public Health Practice* (Washington, DC: National Academy Press, 1997).
25. P.L. Riley and J.P. Kaplan, "Prevention Research Centers: The Academic and Community Partnership," *American Journal of Preventive Medicine* 16 (suppl. 3) (1999): 5–6.
26. N.M. Clark, "Community/Practice/Academic Partnerships in Public Health," *American Journal of Preventive Medicine* 16 (suppl. 3) (1999): 18–19.
27. E.L. Baker and C.W. Tyler, "Research Linkages between Academics and Public Health Practice: Can They Become a Practical Reality?" *American Journal of Preventive Medicine* 11 (suppl. 3) (1995): 13.
28. E. Anderson et al., "The Missouri Disability Epidemiology and Health Project," *American Journal of Preventive Medicine* 16 (suppl. 3) (1999): 63–71.
29. G.S. Omenn, "The Context for a Future School of Public Health," in *The University in the Urban Community: Responsibilities for Public Health,* eds. T.R. Hogness et al. (Washington, DC: Association of Academic Health Centers, 1993), 93–116.
30. Bureau of Primary Care, *Medicaid Managed Care: A Handbook for Public Health Agencies* (Washington, DC: National Association of County and City Health Officials, 1995).
31. G.P. Mays, "Case Study: Integrating Public and Private Health Care Systems in Denver, Colorado," in *Managed Care and Public Health,* eds. P.K. Halverson, A.D. Kaluzny, and C.P. McLaughlin (Gaithersburg, MD: Aspen Publishers, Inc., 1997), 201–221.
32. P.K. Halverson, A.D. Kaluzny, and C.P. McLaughlin (eds.), *Managed Care and Public Health* (Gaithersburg, MD: Aspen Publishers, Inc., 1997).
33. C.W. Keck, "Lessons Learned from an Academic Public Health Department," *Journal of Public Health Management and Practice 6*, no. 1 (2000): 47–52.
34. D. Greene et al., "Creating Training Opportunities for Public Health Practitioners," *American Journal of Preventive Medicine* 16 (suppl. 3) (1999): 80–85.
35. C. Evans, "The Role of City, County and State Health Departments in the University–Community Interaction," in *The University in the Urban Community: Responsibilities for Public Health,* eds. T.R. Hogness et al. (Washington, DC: Association of Academic Health Centers, 1993), 123–142.
36. R.D. Lasker, *Medicine and Public Health: The Power of Collaboration* (New York: The New York Academy of Medicine, 1997).
37. M.E. Fernandez et al., "Evaluation of ENCORE Plus: A Community-Based Breast and Cervical Screening Program," *American Journal of Preventive Medicine* 16 (suppl. 3) (1999): 35–49.
38. B. Berkowitz, "Collaboration for Health Improvements: Models for State, Community and Academic Partnerships," *Journal of Public Health Management and Practice 6,* no. 1 (2000): 67–72.
39. R.W. Richards et al., *Community Partnerships: A Kellogg Initiative in Health Professions Education* (Battle Creek, MI: W.K. Kellogg Foundation, 1991).
40. M.E. Northridge et al., "The Adolescent Years: A Partnership in Harlem Comes of Age," *Journal of Public Health Management and Practice 6,* no. 1 (2000): 53–60.
41. T. Hancock, "The Evolution, Impact and Significance of Healthy Cities/Healthy Communities Movement," *Journal of Public Health Policy 14*, no. 1 (1993): 5–18.
42. B.C. Flynn, "Healthy Cities: Toward Worldwide Health Promotion," *Annual Review of Public Health* 17 (1996): 299–309.
43. W.K. Kellogg, *Community-Based Public Health Initiative* (Battle Creek, MI: W.K. Kellogg Foundation, 1993).
44. L. Dessau and M. Fischbuch, *Academic Health Centers and the Community: A Practical Guide for Creating Shared Visions* (Hamilton, Ontario, Canada: Dixon Desktop Publishing, 1992).

CHAPTER 23

Legislative Relations in Public Health

Stephanie A. Kennan

The federal government plays a significant role in public health through the enactment of legislation that creates, authorizes, and funds programs. States, in addition to their own legislative roles, are often responsible for implementing federal health programs and regulations. The federal budget and appropriations processes determine what public health programs become national priorities and what resources become available to states in carrying out these functions.

OVERVIEW

The public health legislative process reflects the federalist system of government from which it derives. States have traditionally been responsible for performing regulatory health functions such as provider licensure, insurance regulation, and promulgation of public health standards for ensuring environmental safety. The federal government establishes national health priorities by creating and authorizing public health programs and by allocating federal funds to these programs. Increasingly, states become the regulators and implementers of health programs, standards, and regulations established through federal legislation. Local public health organizations tailor these larger programs and initiatives to specific communities and populations.

Understanding the federal budget process and the roles of the president, Congress, and the states can help public health professionals and advocates shape these priorities. A hypothetical example illustrates the importance of such knowledge. Congress could create a program to assist states in creating or enhancing trauma programs, authorizing such a program to operate for five years. However, in year four Congress provides no funding for the program through the annual appropriations process, effectively ending the program and making reauthorization a more difficult task. To respond effectively to such legislative developments, public health organizations require an intimate knowledge of the legislative process and the opportunities for shaping legislative outcomes. For some programs, such as the Older Americans Act, Congress fails to reauthorize the act for several years, and yet continues to fund the programs under that act. This development means that the programs can continue to operate but cannot be updated or changed to reflect different needs or priorities. Thus, the federal budget and appropriations processes often determine what public health programs become national priorities and what federal funds become available to the states to carry out health functions. Understanding the steps of the federal budget process and how the appropriations process stems from the budget process can help public health organizations to know at what points they can be most effective in providing information and expertise. This knowledge also helps organizations to know when to look for potential changes in programs.

THE FEDERAL BUDGET PROCESS

When applied to the federal government, the term *budget process* actually refers to a number of processes that have evolved separately and that occur with varying degrees of coordination. In its most elemental form, the federal budget is a comprehensive accounting of the government's spending, revenues, and borrowing. Ultimately, however, the budget and the appropriations processes also represent the country's priorities by what is funded, how it is funded, and by how much.

Article 1 of the U.S. Constitution grants the "power of the purse" to Congress, but does not establish a specific procedure for the consideration of budgetary legislation. The Budget and Accounting Act of 1921 established the statutory basis for an executive budget process by requiring the president to submit to Congress annually a proposed budget for the federal government.[1] It also created the Bureau of the Budget (later reorganized as the Office of Management and Budget [OMB]) in 1970 to assist the president and the General Accounting Office (GAO) to assist Congress as the principal auditing agency of the federal government.

The Congressional Budget and Impoundment Control Act of 1974 established a statutory basis for a congressional budget process and provided for the annual adoption of resolution on the budget as a mechanism for facilitating congressional budgetary decision making.[2] It also established the House and Senate Budget Committees and created the Congressional Budget Office (CBO) to provide budgetary information to Congress independent of the executive branch.

The key terms in federal spending are budget authority, obligations, outlays, and spendout rate. Congress enacts *budget authority* in law. Budget authority allows federal agencies to incur *obligations,* such as entering into contracts, employing personnel, and submitting purchase orders. *Outlays* represent the actual payment for these obligations, usually in the form of electronic transfers or checks from the Treasury Department. The rate at which budget authority becomes outlays in a fiscal year is called the *spendout rate* or the outlay rate. The spendout rate varies among agencies' accounts depending on the timing of activity in each account.[3]

Typically, new budget authority is provided in the form of appropriations. Permanent appropriations provide new budget authority each year without any annual legislative action. Usually, this type of new budget authority is provided in legislation authorizing or creating the program, such as in the case of most entitlement programs (e.g., social security benefits). Annual appropriations, on the other hand, generally provide new budget authority for the particular fiscal year for which they were enacted. In rare cases, appropriations are made available for more than one year.

Within the budget, there are two categories of spending: mandatory spending and discretionary spending.[3] *Mandatory* spending includes interest, entitlement programs, and programs funded by permanent appropriations. In either case, the spending amounts of mandatory programs are based on benefit levels or other factors that have been established by laws that created the program rather than through the appropriations process. Medicare and Social Security are examples of mandatory spending and are entitlement programs. These programs bypass the appropriations process completely. *Discretionary* programs' spending levels are established by Congress through 13 general appropriations bills and other appropriations bills like emergency appropriations bills that occur during the annual appropriations process.[4]

For fiscal year (FY) 1997, federal outlays totaled $1,601.2 billion. Mandatory spending, not including net interest, accounted for 51 percent of total federal outlays. Discretionary spending for all programs across the functions of the government accounted for 34 percent of the federal budget for the same time period. Most public health programs fall into the category of discretionary spending. Net interest outlays accounted for the remaining 15 percent of spending.[5] Therefore, funding for such vital programs as research, immunizations, and drug abuse and prevention compete for dollars within the federal budget with other programs such as Head Start, Special Supplemental Food Program for Women, Infants, and Children (WIC) feeding program, and other priorities of government in a relatively small part of the federal budget.

Table 23–1 lists the 21 largest mandatory and discretionary spending activities, each of which has outlays greater than $10 billion. This table does not include "offsetting collections," which may reduce the total spent. The 11 largest mandatory programs account for 51.7 percent of total federal outlays; the 10 largest discretionary spending activities account for 21.6 percent.

The amount of federal funds available for discretionary programs is minimal. This explains why Congress continues to worry about the growth of Medicare and Social Security as the baby boomers age. Growth in entitlements, if not slowed or reformed, will squeeze the amount of funds available for worthwhile priorities.

Steps to Creating the Federal Budget

The Congressional Budget and Impoundment Control Act of 1974* as amended establishes the congressional budget process, which coordinates the legislative activities on the budget resolution appropriations bill, reconciliation legislation, revenue measures (taxes), and other budgetary legislation. Section 300 of this act provides a timetable so that Congress may complete its work on the budget by the start of the

*The Congressional Budget and Impoundment Control Act of 1974 has been amended several times. The full authority is listed as 2 U.S.C. 601-688 (1988 & Supp. IV 1992); PL 93-344 (88 Stat.297); amended by the Balanced Budget and Emergency Deficit Control Act of 1985, PL 99-177 (99 Stat.1037, 1038; further amended by the Balanced Budget and Emergency Deficit Control Reaffirmation Act of 1987, PL 100-119 (101 Stat.754); further amended by the Budget Enforcement Act of 1990, PL 101-508 (104) Stat.1388-573 to 1388-630); further amended by the Omnibus Budget Reconciliation Act of 1993, PL 103-66 (107 Stat.312); and further amended by the Budget Enforcement Act of 1997, PL 105-33 (111 Stat.251).

Table 23–1 Discretionary/Mandatory Spending Outlays (in billions of dollars)

Fiscal Year	*Discretionary Spending*	*Entitlement/ Mandatory Spending*	*Net Interest*	*Offsetting Receipts*	*Total*
1981	307.8	339.6	68.8	–37.9	678.2
1982	325.8	370.9	85.0	–36	745.8
1983	353.1	410.7	89.8	–45.3	808.4
1984	379.2	405.8	111.1	–44.2	851.9
1985	415.7	448.4	129.5	–44.7	946.5
1986	438.4	462.0	136.0	–45.9	990.9
1987	444.0	474.4	138.7	–52.9	1,004.1
1988	464.2	505.3	151.8	–56.8	1,064.5
1989	488.6	549.6	169.3	–63.8	1,143.7
1990	500.3	627.3	184.2	–58.7	1,253.2
1991	533.0	702.6	194.5	–105.7	1,324.4
1992	534.0	716.6	199.4	–68.4	1,381.7
1993	540.4	736.8	198.8	–66.6	1,409.4
1994	543.3	784.0	203.0	–68.5	1,461.7
1995	545.1	818.2	232.2	–79.7	1,515.7
1996	533.8	857.5	241.1	–71.9	1,560.5
1997	548.3	896.3	244.0	–87.3	1,601.2
1998	553.6	938.6	243.4	–84.1	1,651.4

Source: Reprinted from Congressional Budget Office, *The Economic and Budget Outlook: Fiscal Years 2000–2009,* Table F-8, p. 132, January 1999, U.S. Government Printing Office.

fiscal year on October 1. If the budget and appropriations bills are not completed by October 1, the federal government could shut down.

What is usually the case is that some of the 13 appropriations bills are completed and others are not. Those programs that are not funded by October 1 may shut down. However, Congress may also provide funding through a continuing resolution (CR). A CR permits Congress to continue funding at current levels through a specified time period. This means that programs receive no increase but can continue operating. This device is often used if Congress feels that it needs a few more days or weeks to finish its work but does not want programs to be discontinued, or if Congress runs into political stumbling blocks and cannot complete work but does not want to shut down the government. Should either Congress or the president believe that the appropriations bills will be vetoed by the president, politics can come into play in determining whether Congress considers passing a CR or allows the federal government in part or in whole to shut down.*

Preparing the President's Budget Submission

As required by the Budget and Accounting Act of 1921, the president prepares and submits a comprehensive budget to Congress by the first Monday in February.[1] Due to the size and complexity of the federal budget, however, the president must rely on the departments and agencies to bear the primary responsibility of formulating their budget requests.

Federal agencies typically rely on their own internal process to prepare their initial budget requests, with the agencies usually beginning work on the budget approximately 10 months before the president submits his budget to Congress (approximately 17–18 months before the start of the fiscal year). This means that at any given point, each agency and department in the federal government is working on three budgets: implementing the current budget, defending the proposed budget, and preparing a future budget.

To prepare a budget submission, agencies estimate the resources necessary to continue the existing programs at current levels for the next fiscal year. This includes spending estimates for personnel, equipment, and other program expenses. Then, agencies include estimates for new initiatives funded with any available incremental resources. In addition, the OMB will inform an agency of any presidential initiatives to be incorporated into its initial budget. All the lower-level budget requests are then consolidated into an agencywide budget to be submitted to the OMB.

The Government Performance and Results Act (GRPA) of 1993 established a statutory framework to link the formulation of the budget with government performance.[6] Under the GRPA, agencies are also required to prepare strategic plans, annual performance plans, and annual program performance reports. The strategic plans must cover at least six years and must be revised and updated at least once every three years. Beginning with the FY 1999 budget, agencies were required to prepare and submit annual performance plans to the OMB with their budget requests. Last, agencies will be required to prepare annual performance reports beginning with the FY 2001 budget cycle. The first performance reports will cover FY 1999 and must be submitted to the president and Congress by March 31, 2000.

The agencywide budget requests and performance plans are viewed by the OMB staff responsible for the particular program area. During this review process, agency officials clarify policy and technical questions with OMB staff. The OMB director makes decisions on the budget requests and performance plans, and agencies are notified of these decisions through what is known as the OMB "passback." Agencies are then given an opportunity to appeal if they disagree with aspects of the passback.

Once final decisions are made by the OMB and the president, federal agencies and depart-

*For an overview of the principles of the federal appropriations process, see U.S. General Accounting Office, *Principles of Federal Appropriations Law: Vol II*, 2d ed. [GAO report GAO/OGC-92-13] (Washington, DC: December 1992, Ch 8. "Continuing Resolutions.")

ments must revise their budget requests and performance plans to conform with these decisions. The materials prepared for the president's budget submission to Congress include program descriptions, the requested spending levels, and the proposed appropriations language for each "account." This information is contained in the appendix volume of the president's budget submission each year.

Although the president's budget does not have the force of law, it is a way in which the president can tell Congress and the public what the executive branch believes to be important. It is also a comprehensive examination of federal revenues and spending. For example, the budget submitted for FY 1999 by the president included major increases for Ryan White Acquired Immune Deficiency Syndrome (AIDS) programs, the Substance Abuse and Mental Health Services Administration (SAMHSA), Child Care and Development Block Grants, and the National Institutes of Health (NIH).[5]

Congressional Action Begins with the Budget Committees

Within six weeks of the president's budget submission, congressional committees are requested to submit their "views and estimates" of spending and revenues within their respective jurisdictions to the House and Senate Budget Committees. These views and estimates, along with information from other sources, are then used by each budget committee in drafting and reporting a resolution of the budget to its respective body. Other information is gathered through hearings by each budget committee. That information includes budget and economic projections, programmatic information, and budget priorities. This information comes from the CBO, the OMB, the Federal Reserve, executive branch agencies, and outside interest groups. It is interesting to note that, often, the projections from the CBO differ from those from the OMB. This is because the different budget agencies use varying assumptions concerning the economy and the cost of programs. This difference is often a source of friction between the legislative and executive branches.

The Chairman's Mark

After hearings, each budget committee chairman creates an individual budget proposal known as the "chairman's mark" and presents that proposal to the respective committee. This proposed budget is usually developed in consultation with other members of the political party and leadership. In recent years, this has not been a bipartisan effort and has in many instances ignored the president's proposed budget completely. In addition, it is possible for the House Budget Committee chairman and the Senate Budget Committee chairman to have very different views of the budget. This means that the House and Senate chairman marks may have very different approaches and assumptions.

Next, each committee meets and amends the chairman's proposal of the respective committee. This is known as mark-up, because the proposal is literally marked up and changed. Because the budget resolution created in committee deals with aggregate numbers, it is important to understand what assumptions go into the creation of the budget. The assumptions are not spelled out in the legislation. For example, a proposed budget resolution could state that the growth of Medicare would be reduced by 10 percent over five years. The budget committee makes assumptions about where the reductions will be made within Medicare, such as the reductions should come from reimbursement to hospitals and home health agencies. The committees with jurisdiction over Medicare—the Senate Finance Committee, the House Ways and Means Committee, and the House Commerce Committee—would be responsible for figuring out specifically how to achieve those reductions and may at times ignore the budget committee assumptions. This process is known as budget reconciliation.

Passing the Budget Resolution

When the House and Senate pass their respective budget resolutions, they are then "conferenced" just as any other legislation would be. This means that representatives of the Senate and House Budget Committees meet to resolve differences in the resolutions passed by the House and Senate. The final resolution that is the product of this conference is then passed by both the House and Senate and is not signed into law. In essence, the budget resolution serves as a blueprint in establishing budget priorities and defines the parameters for all subsequent budgetary actions for that year. The spending, revenue, and public debt laws necessary to implement decisions agreed to in the budget resolution are subsequently enacted separately as part of the "budget reconciliation" process or as part of the appropriations process.

Budget Reconciliation

Traditionally, budget resolutions contain what are known as budget reconciliation instructions. These are instructions to the committees of a jurisdiction concerning the spending of programs in their jurisdiction. This should not be confused with the appropriations process. Budget reconciliation contains programmatic changes that will achieve the desired effect—usually programmatic changes that will reduce the amount needed to be spent or ways in which to raise revenues (taxes or user fees).

For example, in 1999, because a budget surplus was projected, the only budget reconciliation instructions were to the Senate Finance Committee and House Ways and Means Committee to reduce taxes.[7] The tax cut bill was vetoed by the president because the president did not believe the surplus was large enough to support the size of tax cut that was passed by Congress. The budget resolution established aggregate spending levels for each broad category of functions for the federal government in relation to the desire to provide a broad tax cut. It was left to the committees with jurisdiction over taxes to determine how to achieve that cut.

It is not uncommon for reconciliation instructions to affect every committee in Congress and for the reconciliation bill to become an omnibus bill that creates sweeping programmatic changes because it often is the only legislative vehicle that will be sure to pass Congress. Sometimes, such legislation is called a "Christmas tree" because it becomes so loaded with different provisions that are on the bill solely because members of Congress and interest groups know that if attached to reconciliation they are usually assured that it will be enacted into law.

Entitlements and Appropriated Entitlements in the Federal Budget Process

Entitlements are programs that require the payment of benefits to persons, states, or local government, or to other entities if specific criteria established in the authorizing law are met. Entitlement spending currently makes up more than half of total federal spending and is growing faster than other types of spending.[3] Spending on entitlements is not controlled directly through the annual appropriations process. Instead, entitlement spending is based on the benefit and eligibility criteria of individual benefits and bypasses the appropriations process. Because most entitlement spending is required by permanent laws, the level of spending on these programs is often referred to as mandatory or direct spending. Congress and the president have created procedures to control entitlement spending though the congressional budget process. Social Security, Medicare, and federal employee retirement are examples of such programs.

The Congressional Budget and Impoundment Control Act (CBA) prohibits consideration of any new entitlement legislation prior to the adoption of a budget resolution.[2] Once the budget resolution has been approved, entitlement spending is subject to the same controls as discretionary spending—that any expansion must be paid for within that function of the government. The CBA also prohibits consideration of any new entitlement legislation or amendment that would cause the aggregate spending levels of the government to be exceeded.

In addition to these general spending controls, Congress usually uses the reconciliation process to create significant changes in the existing permanent laws of entitlement programs. These changes are often needed in order to reduce growth rates in spending on these programs to ensure their long-range solvency. This process requires the "authorizing" committees responsible for the entitlement programs to recommend legislative language to achieve the spending levels allocated to them under the reconciliation instructions in the budget resolution. Reconciliation allows Congress to package these changes into one measure, which is then considered under expedited procedures that limit debate and place restrictions on amendments.

Spending and the Pay-as-You-Go Process

In 1990, Congress established a control mechanism for new entitlement spending called "pay-as-you-go" (PAYGO) rules.[8] These rules apply to new direct spending and revenue legislation for the purpose of holding Congress and the president accountable for any increase in the federal deficit due to legislative action. In other words, any increase in spending resulting from new legislation must be paid for (offset) by spending reductions, revenue increases, or a combination of both.

If the net effect of new legislation enacted during a congressional session causes an increase in the deficit, the president is required to issue an order for across-the-board cuts in programs. This is known as a sequester. Some programs such as Social Security and veterans benefits are exempt from the sequester. However, the majority of public health programs are subject to the potential of a sequester regardless of whether it was a federal health program or some other program that caused the deficit to increase.

In the Senate, PAYGO rules are also enforced by a "point of order."[8] The free-standing point of order prohibits the Senate from considering any direct spending or revenue legislation that would violate the PAYGO requirements by increasing the deficit. The Senate may waive this point of order by a three-fifths vote (60 senators) or by unanimous consent. Much of the votes you may see in Senate budget debate are motions to waive the point of order. If the motion to waive the point of order fails, then the amendment cannot be considered. The House has no similar point of order.

THE APPROPRIATIONS PROCESS AND HEALTH PROGRAMS

Not counting emergency appropriations bills and continuing resolutions, the bulk of the discretionary spending of all functions of the government is subject to the annual appropriations process. This process includes consideration of 13 different bills to fund the government. This process is overseen by the House and Senate Appropriations Committees. Each committee is divided into subcommittees. Each committee has a subcommittee that has jurisdiction over public health funding. In the House and Senate, that subcommittee is known by the same name: the Subcommittee on Labor, Health and Human Services, and Education. On Capitol Hill, the bill that funds most of the health functions of the budget (but not entitlement) is referred to as the "Labor-H bill." It funds programs in the Department of Labor, the Department of Health and Human Services (DHHS), and the Department of Education. Funding for veterans' health programs is overseen by the Subcommittee on Veterans Affairs and Housing and Urban Development for each committee. Because the Labor-H bill frequently is among the most controversial of the appropriations bills, it is usually the last or nearly the last appropriations bill to be considered by the full House and Senate. It is often views on social policy that become controversial in this bill. For example, whether or not to fund fetal tissue research has been controversial, and debate on this kind of issue slows consideration even at the committee level.

Known as "appropriators," the Appropriations Committees in fact control only about one-third of the total federal spending provided for a fiscal year. These committees hear from interest groups, government agencies, and other members of Congress regarding specific funding levels for each program or "account" as they are called in appropriations parlance. It is these committees that are the focus of many interest groups who want funding for disease-specific issues or are looking for funding for specific projects in specific locations. Not only is what is funded at question, but what the funding levels are in the final package is key to determining the nation's priorities.

By the end of March or early April, members of Congress submit to these committees lists of programs or special projects they wish to see funded through the appropriations process. Members' "wish lists" are based on requests from constituents including individuals, state governments, businesses, and institutions such as universities and libraries. Members are asked to attach priorities—high, medium, or low—to these requests. The Appropriations Committees decide each year how they want to handle member requests and timetables for these requests. If a request is important from a state perspective, a frequent lobbying strategy is to not only ensure that individual members have placed a request on their list, but to ensure that the entire congressional delegation, including House and Senate members, includes the request in their wish lists. In addition, members are often asked to write letters with other members of Congress to reflect broad support for funding for national programs or priorities.

For example, funding for specific research within NIH is often subject to this kind of lobbying tactics. Diabetes, Alzheimer's disease, heart and stroke, cancer, and other disease-specific groups will ask grassroots members to contact members to support increases in funding research for their particular research while the national organization works on getting a letter with as many different members of both political parties signed on to show the appropriators the support for such increases. In the case of NIH funding, the budget resolution would have specified an aggregate spending level and not listed specific increases for particular institutes or research. The appropriators would hear through testimony and information requests from NIH, the DHHS (which oversees NIH), and interest groups concerning how to divide the money available under the budget resolution for the specific programs under NIH's jurisdiction. For FY 1999, the budget resolution provided the promise of doubling the amount of funds available for NIH in the aggregate within five years and included a significant increase for FY 1999. (However, neither the president's budget nor the budget resolution for FY 2000 included a large increase for NIH to keep the promise of doubling research within five years. The president's budget proposed only a two percent increase.)[9] Interest groups had lobbied for a 15 percent increase. The small increase specified in the budget resolution led groups to ask appropriators to ignore the budget resolution aggregate amount, which would require cutting other health programs, and to lobby heavily for increases within their specific disease research interests. Appropriation Committee members literally have to decide line by line how to distribute these funds and in doing so set very specific priorities.

Should Congress begin to run out of time to consider each of the 13 bills separately on the floor of the Senate or House, it is not uncommon for the leadership to put together several bills and create an "omnibus appropriations" bill. This occurred before the November 1998 elections. Although some of the individual appropriations bills had been considered, and the committees had not completed work on the rest of the bills, less than half of the 13 bills had been considered by the full House or Senate. Congress needed to recess in order to let members up for reelection to have time to campaign. So the leadership permitted the rest of the appropriations to be considered as one single bill.[10]

After each body has passed its version of an individual appropriations bill, it goes to conference so that members of the House and Senate can resolve differences. The final product is known as the "conference report." It is this report that is sent back to each body for final passage.

Earmarks

Appropriations legislation does at times specifically "earmark" spending. Earmarking is a way in which the appropriators can ensure that funds are spent for a specific project or in a specific location. For interested parties who want to ensure that funding is spent on a specific project, such earmarks are vital. For example, if a university wants federal money to assist in developing a new building to do biotechnology research and development, it might want to seek an earmark to ensure that the money is spent on their building as opposed to anyone who might qualify for construction funds for health research labs.

Report Language

A conference report contains more than the legislative language of a bill. It also contains an explanation of what Congress' intent was in specific provisions. Although report language does not hold the force of law, it is useful in establishing a legislative history. In addition, report language serves as a useful tool in providing specific directions to the agencies that will have to implement the budget or new program. Report language is written in narrative form, and in many instances, can be as important as the legislative language should there be questions concerning the intent of the legislative language. Conference reports cannot be amended on the floor of the House or Senate and must be voted up or down by a simple majority. Generally, before the House considers a conference report on an appropriations measure, it adopts a special rule waiving all points of order against the conference report and its consideration. The rule usually does not provide for amendments either.[11,12]

Health Appropriation Anomaly

Most federal domestic health programs are administered through or in consultation with agencies that are under the DHHS. This includes the Food and Drug Administration (FDA). However, the FDA is the only agency within the DHHS that does not receive its appropriation from the Labor-DHHS-Education appropriations bill. The FDA once was part of the U.S. Agriculture Department. When it was moved to the DHHS, the appropriators never moved jurisdiction of the funding of that agency to the Labor-DHHS-Education Subcommittees. Instead, the FDA and all of the programs that agency oversees still receive appropriations as part of the Agriculture appropriations bill.[13]

Legislating on Appropriations Bills

Technically, appropriations bills are charged specifically with determining spending levels for programs rather than with delineating programmatic changes. In fact, the Senate and House have rules that prohibit legislating—or making changes in policy—on an appropriations bill. By attaching a "rider," a provision that does not affect the spending level but changes policy, a member can bypass the committee legislative and hearing process. What is considered legislating on an appropriations bill, however, can be the subject of debate. In the Senate, a point of order can be brought against a provision by a member who believes that a provision is legislation on an appropriations bill.[13] The point of order is subject to a ruling by the parliamentarian and a vote by the Senate on whether or not the provision violates the rules. The House of Representatives has its own rules that also in theory prohibit legislating on an appropriations bill.[14]

However, what is considered legislating on an appropriations bill may be simply a measure of expediency. For example, within the Agriculture appropriations bill for the FDA for FY 2000, the House version attached a provision prohibiting the use or research of the controversial drug RU486. This provision did not impact the FDA's program spending levels, but was a prohibition on certain agency activities concerning the agency's role in overseeing the safety and effectiveness of drugs. Such a prohibition could be considered legislating on an appropriations bill because the proposal was aimed at eliminating the availability of RU486 for which the primary use is as an abortifacient. However, it could be argued that the actual language was only a directive concerning how the FDA organizes its spending priorities. Because similar language was not included in the Senate version, it would be left to conference to determine if that provision made it into the final conference report, which would not be subject to amendment and would have to be voted up or down. This is also an example of how a social issue can impact spending allocations and priorities.

The Relationship between Authorization and Appropriations Measures

Congress has established an authorization–appropriations process that provides for two separate types of legislative measures to be considered. Authorization legislation is legislation that establishes, continues, or modifies agencies or programs. For example, an authorization act may change the structure or establish or modify programs within the jurisdiction of the DHHS. Authorization legislation can also specify the specific maximum amount that can be spent on a program and for how long. For example, authorizing legislation could create a program to be funded at $18 million over three years. At the end of three years, Congress would have to decide to reauthorize the program or end the program. If Congress decided to renew the program, it would have to determine new spending or budget authority specifying how much may be spent for future years during the length of the reauthorization. The appropriations process would decide how much money would actually be spent per year, knowing that $18 million is the ceiling for the life of the program.

CREATING HEALTH PROGRAMS—AUTHORIZING COMMITTEE JURISDICTIONS

Health care issues can be considered in any number of committees depending on how the legislation or issue is crafted. The usual breakdown for health legislation falls among four committees within the House and Senate.

In the Senate, Medicare and Medicaid are within the jurisdiction of the *Senate Finance Committee.* The Senate Finance Committee also has jurisdiction over social security issues. In the House of Representatives, Medicare Part A and B, both benefits and spending issues, are under the jurisdiction of the *House Ways and Means Committee.* Like the Finance Committee, this committee also has jurisdiction over social security. However, Medicare Part B benefit issues only also fall under the jurisdiction of the *House Commerce Committee,* which also has jurisdiction over Medicaid. This split jurisdiction of Medicare Part B has meant that House budget reconciliation proposals have contained policy changes that are very different within the same bill and are left unresolved until the conference with the Senate.

Public health programs are under the jurisdiction of the *House Commerce Committee* and the *Senate Health, Education, Labor and Pensions Committee* (formerly known as the Senate Labor and Human Resources Committee). These committees deal with issues like FDA reform, NIH research, medical data privacy, the Public Health Service Act, health professional training, and so forth.[11,13]

There are times, however, in which the political leadership can assign health issues that may cut across several committees' jurisdiction to one committee. For example, in 1998, when Congress was considering a global tobacco settlement, the tobacco issue could have cut across several committees. However, this would have slowed down the consideration of such comprehensive legislation. In the Senate, the leadership decided to allow the Senate Commerce Committee to have jurisdiction over the entire issue even though this committee had no usual jurisdiction over health programs.

The 1994 attempt at health care reform was hampered in part because so many House committees were given jurisdiction over different sections, including the House Education and Labor Committee and the House Judiciary Committee, in addition to the traditional health committees. The more committees a bill is referred to, the less likely it is that the bill will be considered outside the committee process. In the Senate, Senate rules prohibit referral to more than one committee.

HOW A BILL BECOMES A LAW—REALLY

The Constitution requires that bills that raise taxes start within the House of Representatives. Otherwise, any bill can begin in either body by first being introduced by a member and then being referred to a committee that holds hearings. After hearings, a committee holds a mark-up in which committee members can offer amendments. The bill is then "reported" to the full body for consideration, where it can be subject to further amendment. Then the same thing happens in the opposite legislative body. When the two versions are completed, they are then conferenced and a conference report is sent for final passage in the House and Senate. After final passage, the bill is sent to the president for his signature or veto. If the president vetoes a proposal, the bill is sent back to the House and Senate to be voted on again. Three-fourths of the House and three-fifths of the Senate are needed to override a veto. See Exhibit 23–1 for an explanation of the rule-making process.

As referred to in instances in this chapter, the House and Senate have different rules for the consideration of different kinds of legislation. What is important to note is that a little-discussed committee in the House controls what amendments are offered to legislation on the floor of the House and in fact scripts the consideration of bills before the full body. This committee, known as the House Rules Committee, is one of the most powerful committees in the House.

Exhibit 23–1 The Rule-Making Process

- Congress has passed a law and it has been signed into law by the president.
- A federal agency proposes rules/regulations to implement the law.
- The proposal is cleared through the agency and the department.
- The proposal is sent to the Office of Management and Budget (OMB) for clearance concerning budget impact.
- Once cleared through the OMB, the proposal is published in the *Federal Register* for a public commentary period.
- Public comments are received and considered.
- Revisions to the proposed regulations are made.
- The revised regulations are cleared through the agency and department.
- The OMB provides final clearance.
- The revised regulations are published as final regulations in the *Federal Register*.

All legislation in the House must go before the House Rules Committee before it can be considered on the floor of the House. If a bill has been referred to and considered by different committees within the House, those different versions can be pieced together into one proposal by the House Rules Committee. The committee also decides the length of time for consideration of a bill and what amendments will be permitted to be considered. This makes ensuring that specific issues and interests are addressed at the committee with jurisdiction level that much more important because if an issue is not addressed and a floor amendment is needed, there is always the possibility that the House Rules Committee can block a floor amendment. Before each bill is voted on in the House of Representatives, the House votes to adopt the rule. It is in the debate on the rule that members can make the case for defeating the rule if the House Rules Committee has proposed a rule that blocks the consideration of an amendment that the majority of the House thinks should be considered.[15]

In the Senate, the Senate Rules Committee does not have the same kind of authority or power.[13] Instead, the Senate operates under a set of rules designed to protect the rights of the minority and reflects that the Senate is a smaller body than the House. Most often, the Senate leadership works together to develop a time agreement for the consideration of a specific bill. A time limit can specify how many amendments can be offered. That agreement is usually adopted by unanimous consent.

Unanimous consent is also used for the passage of bills without taking up debate time on the floor. Therefore, if a bill contains a provision that is particularly onerous, interests groups will often seek out a member to object should a unanimous consent agreement on that bill be offered. It takes only one member to object in such instances and delay consideration of a bill.

The Senate also has a mechanism where an individual senator can block the consideration by the full body of a bill or nomination. This process is known as a hold. This process was once secret, so that it was difficult to discover who had placed a hold on a bill. Under a new agreement that began in 1999, if a senator wants to place a hold, he or she must notify the leadership, the sponsor of the bill, the chairman of the committee with jurisdiction, and the committee's ranking minority member.[16] This means that the proposal can be considered at the committee level, but cannot be brought to the floor as a free-standing specific bill until the hold is released. A member with a bill that has a hold on it could try to bring it to the floor as an amendment to legislation the full body is considering, if the amendment is germane to the issues in the bill or is part of an agreement that permitted the legislation to come to the Senate floor. Holds can be placed indefinitely.

The Senate also has rules that allow members to filibuster.[13] This is an example of how the Senate rules protect the rights of the minority. Filibustering is more than simply holding the floor and talking as some Hollywood movies portray it. It can be a series of parliamentary procedures that slows the process down, preventing the Senate from consideration of other legislation. Using such procedures to slow the process requires members to be on the floor, throwing off the Senate schedule and delaying other members' ability to get work done.

LEGISLATION AND REGULATION

Federal agencies are authorized to issue regulations by their enabling statutes, statutes establishing new programs, and statutes amending and extending the duties and responsibilities of those agencies. Most regulations are issued under the notice-and-comment procedure established by the Administrative Procedure Act (APA).[17] Less commonly, some agencies are required to add such elements of adjudicatory proceedings as cross-examination and rebuttal witnesses to the notice-and-comment requirements when promulgating regulations. These agencies include the Federal Trade Commission, the Consumer Product Safety Commission, and the Occupational Safety and Health Administration.

It is important to note that to challenge the federal authority on a regulation, thorough research must be done beyond the legislation creating the program, but including all the enabling legislation of the powers and duties of the department.

Informal Notice-and-Comment Rule Making

The informal notice-and-comment rule-making process requires that an agency publish a notice of proposed rule making in the *Federal Register;* afford all interested parties an opportunity to participate in the proceeding through the submission of written comments, or, at the discretion of the agency, by oral presentations; and when consideration of the relevant matter presented is completed, incorporate in the final rules "a concise general statement of their basis and purpose."[18] A final rule must be published in the *Federal Register* not less than 30 days before its effective date. Interested persons have the right to petition for the issuance, amendment, or repeal of a rule.[18] The APA does not specify a minimum period for public comment. However, Executive Order 12866, which was issued on September 30, 1993, requires a period of no less than 60 days.[19] An agency may extend or reopen the period for public comment at any time. Agencies are also free to grant additional procedural rights to interested persons. Much of the bare bones rule-making requirements in the APA have been fleshed out in detail by federal court rulings that have sought to make the rule-making process more accessible to the interested public and to ensure fair and meaningful input.

Approximately 75 percent of all regulations are issued by agencies over which the president exercises considerable oversight and supervision and are subject to Executive Order 12866.[20] These agencies are also the ones issuing the more costly social regulations. They include the Environmental Protection Agency (EPA), the Occupational Safety and Health Administration and the Mine Safety and Health Administration (both in the Department of Labor), the FDA (DHHS), the Department of Energy, the Department of the Interior, the Department of Agriculture, and the Department of Transportation.

Unfunded Mandates

The Unfunded Mandates Reform Act (UMRA) seeks to address some of the issues raised by state and local officials about the costs of carrying out federal programs and regulations.[21] Since the mid-1980s, Congress debated legislation to slow or prohibit the enactment of unfunded federal mandates. Under the UMRA, federal mandates include the provision of law or regulations that impose enforceable duties, including taxes. They also include provisions that reduce or eliminate federal financial assistance available for carrying out existing local or tribal government and "private sector mandates." The act establishes requirements for committees and the CBO to study and report on the magnitude and impact of mandates in proposed legislation. Under the UMRA, congressional committees have the initial responsibility to identify federal mandates in measures under consideration. Committees may have the CBO study whether proposed legislation could have a significant budgetary impact on nonfederal governments or a financial or employment impact on the private sector.[22] When an authorizing committee orders that a bill containing a federal mandate be reported, it must provide the measure to the CBO. The CBO must then report on an estimate of mandate costs to the committee.[21] For each reported measure with costs greater than $50 million (for intergovernmental mandates or $100 million for private sector mandates), the CBO must provide an estimate of the direct costs of federal mandates in it or in any necessary implementing regulations and the amount of existing federal funding the legislation authorizes to pay these costs.[21] The committee is to include the CBO estimate in its report or publish it in the *Congressional Record.*

The *Federal Register*

The *Federal Register* is much like an executive gazette, published each work day, consisting of public documents issued by the president and federal agencies that announce and describe actions, either taken or proposed, that affect or will affect the public. Each document, depending on the subject matter, is printed in one of four sections of the *Federal Register*. The four sections include a rules and regulations section, a proposed rules section, a notices section, and a presidential documents section. In addition, the *Federal Register* contains a corrections section and a jumps and blanks section.

The number of pages and of documents in the *Federal Register* that are devoted to regulatory actions constitutes only a small number of the total pages and documents printed in that publication. It is difficult if not impossible to determine precisely the number of federal regulations issued each year. Regulatory action taken by an agency may involve issuing a new regulation, revising, or abolishing an existing regulation, or a combination of the three. Moreover, each regulatory action may create several new regulations or affect a number of existing regulations.

The *rules and regulations* section of the *Federal Register* contains regulatory documents announcing and describing final regulatory actions taken by the federal agencies. Some of the documents have general regulatory applicability and legal effect, and are listed in the *Code of Federal Regulations (CFR)*. The *CFR* is the annual codification of the general and permanent rules published in the *Federal Register* by federal departments and agencies. Its purpose is to present the official and complete text of agency regulations and thereby provide a comprehensive and convenient reference for those regulations. The documents in the rules and regulations section are the documents having the greatest regulatory impact on the public. The section also contains two other types of rule documents. One type of document, termed ministerial and informational/administrative, does not affect regulations. These documents include notices of meetings, notices that proposed regulatory action is being terminated, corrections of previous rule documents, and changes in comment periods and similar matters. These documents deal with such matters as airworthiness directives, quarantine actions and related measures to prevent the spread of animal and plant pests and diseases, and similar ongoing regulatory activities.

The *proposed rules* section contains notices to the public of regulatory actions proposed by the federal agencies. The purpose is to give the interested public an opportunity to participate in the rule-making process.

Except for one section, the remaining four sections of the *Federal Register* generally have little to do with federal regulations. The *notices* section is the largest of the sections and contains material other than rules or proposed rules that is applicable to the public. Included in this section are notices of hearings and investigations, committee meetings, agency decisions and rulings, delegations of authority, filing of petitions and applications, and agency statements of organization and functions.

The *presidential documents* section contains such documents as proclamations, executive orders, and similar instruments of national interest. Occasionally, an executive order may impact the regulatory process. For example, Executive Order 12291, issued in February 1981, established the policy of requiring agencies to conduct a cost–benefit analysis on regulations imposing yearly costs of $100 million or more, and centralized the review of regulations in the OMB.[23] Executive Order 12866, issued in October 1994, revoked the earlier order, but continued the requirement for cost–benefit analysis of major regulations and review by the OMB.[19]

The *corrections* section consists of corrections to previously published information, and the *jumps and blanks* section consists of pages left blank to enable the agency to maintain the integrity of an accurate page count of the other sections.

Some commentators have expressed concern that each year, the number of regulatory actions imposing new requirements of revising existing requirements far surpasses the number of new laws established. That the number of regulatory actions surpasses the number of laws should not be surprising. Generally, a new law establishes broad goals and sets general standards, such as protecting the public's health and safety by improving the regulation of nursing homes. Congress has neither the time nor the expertise necessary to develop the specific conditions and circumstances required to administer statutes. In addition, it is generally easier to enact controversial laws when they establish general goals and leave to each federal agency responsible for implementing a law the more specific cases to develop and issue regulations to achieve the goals and standards. Frequently, many regulatory actions are required to carry out one law. Consequently, each year, the number of final regulatory actions taken is far greater than the number of new laws passed.

Accountability of Federal Agencies

It is important to note that contrary to what many members of the public may believe, federal agencies are not independent entities free of external constraints and oversight. Most of the agencies are under the supervision and direction of the president. All are subject to congressional oversight and dependent on Congress for their statutory authority and usually appropriations. Almost all of their regulatory actions are subject to judicial review. Federal agencies act only under authority that is delegated to them by specific laws or by presidential directives. In addition, the APA establishes the framework under which the agencies engage in rule making, and subjects that rule making to judicial review.

Since 1981, regulatory action of federal agencies has been closely monitored by the OMB. The OMB, which is part of the executive office of the president, reviews and clears the most important regulatory actions in order to ensure that, in general, among the various alternatives, the regulatory action is most likely to achieve its goals with the least cost and burden to the public.

In addition, congressional review of regulations is required. The Congressional Review Act of 1997 requires agencies to send their final regulations to Congress for review 60 days before they take effect.[24] A regulation may be rejected within the review period if Congress passes a joint resolution of disapproval and the president signs it, or, if he vetoes the resolution,

Congress overrides the veto. Critics of congressional review argue that it encroaches on agency independence, delays unnecessarily the issuance of regulations, and requires expertise that Congress does not have. Proponents respond, however, that congressional review enables Congress to make the final decision on the need for specific regulations and makes agencies more sensitive to congressional intent. Since the law's enactment, seven joint resolutions of disapproval have been introduced, but none has been passed.

More often what occurs is that members of Congress are contacted by interest groups or state governments to point out that a particular proposed regulation is unfavorable. Members of Congress frequently write agencies asking for changes in regulations as members of the public during the public comment period.

Judicial Review of Rule Making

The APA subjects agency actions to judicial review except where a statute precludes such review or "where agency action is committed to agency discretion by law."[17] Any person adversely affected by an agency action "within the meaning of the relevant statute" may challenge that action.

THE DHHS

The DHHS is the principal agency within the federal government with the responsibility for protecting the health of all Americans and providing essential human services. The DHHS includes more than 300 programs covering a variety of activities, including

- Medicare and social science research
- the prevention of outbreaks of infectious disease, including immunization services
- food and drug safety assurance
- Medicare (health insurance for elderly and the disabled)
- Medicaid (health insurance for low-income individuals)
- financial assistance for low-income families
- child support enforcement
- maternal and infant health improvement
- Head Start (preschool education and services)
- child abuse and domestic violence prevention
- substance abuse treatment and prevention
- services for older Americans including home-delivered meals
- comprehensive health services delivery for American Indians and Alaska Natives
- national health data collection

DHHS programs are administered by 11 DHHS operating divisions (see Chapter 3 for more information). The DHHS is the largest grant-making agency in the federal government. The DHHS must work with state and local government because many of the DHHS-funded services are provided at the local level by state or county agencies, or through private sector grantees. The overall budget for the DHHS in FY 1999 was $387 billion.

DHHS Operating Divisions

U.S. Public Health Service operating divisions include NIH, the FDA, Centers for Disease Control and Prevention (CDC), the Agency for Toxic Substances and Disease (ATSDR), Indian Health Service (IHS), the Health Resources and Services Administration (HRSA), the SAMHSA, and the Agency for Health Care Policy and Research (AHCPR).

- *NIH* is the world's premier medical research organization, supporting more than 35,000 research projects nationwide in diseases like cancer, Alzheimer's, diabetes, arthritis, heart ailments, and AIDS. NIH includes 17 separate health institutes. It was established in 1887 as the Hygienic Laboratory. Its main campus is outside of Washington, D.C., in Bethesda, Maryland. Its FY 1999 budget was $15.7 billion.
- The *FDA* ensures the safety of foods and cosmetics as well as the safety and efficacy of pharmaceuticals, biologic products, and medical devices—products that represent

25 cents of every dollar in U.S. consumer spending. Originally established in 1906, it is headquartered in Rockville, Maryland, and its FY 1999 budget was $1.1 billion.

- The *CDC* maintains national health statistics and works with states and other partners to provide a system of health surveillance to monitor and prevent the outbreak of diseases. The CDC also provides for immunization services and guards against international disease transmission, with CDC personnel stationed in more than 25 foreign countries. In addition, the CDC supports research into disease and injury prevention. Originally established in 1946, it is headquartered in Atlanta, Georgia, and its FY 1999 budget was $2.7 billion.
- The *ATSDR* works with states and other federal agencies to prevent exposure to hazardous substances from waste sites. The agency conducts public health assessments, health studies, surveillance activities, and health education training in communities around waste sites on the U.S. EPA's National Priorities List. The ATSDR has also developed toxicologic profiles of hazardous chemicals found at these sites. Founded in 1980, it is headquartered in Atlanta, Georgia, and its FY 1999 budget was $74 million.
- The *IHS* has 37 hospitals, 60 health centers, 3 school health centers, and 46 health stations. It also assists 34 urban Indian health centers. Services are provided to nearly 1.5 million American Indians and Alaska Natives of the 557 federally recognized tribes through a work force of approximately 14,500 employees and an additional tribal and urban Indian health work force of approximately 10,000. Annually, there are approximately 90,000 hospital admissions and 7 million outpatient visits, 4 million community health representative client contacts, and 2.4 million dental services. Established in 1924 as part of the Department of the Interior, the IHS was transferred to the DHHS in 1955. It is headquartered in Rockville, Maryland, and its FY 1999 budget was $2.6 million.
- The *HRSA* helps provide health resources for medically underserved populations. A nationwide network of 643 community and migrant health centers, plus 144 primary care programs for the homeless and residents of public housing, serve 8.1 million Americans each year. The HRSA works to build the health care work force and maintains the National Health Service Corps. The HRSA also provides services to people with AIDS through the Ryan White CARE Act programs and oversees the organ transplantation system. It also oversees the National Practitioners Data Bank, which contains reports on physicians and other providers who settle malpractice suits or lose clinical privileges or their license to practice. The HRSA was established in 1982 and is headquartered in Rockville, Maryland. Its FY 1999 budget was $4.3 billion.
- The *SAMHSA* oversees programs concerning the quality and availability of substance abuse prevention, addiction treatment, and mental health services. It provides funding through block grants to states for direct substance abuse and mental health services, including treatment for more than 340,000 Americans with various substance abuse problems. This agency also helps improve substance treatment through its Knowledge Development and Application Grant Program. It was established in 1992 and is headquartered in Rockville, Maryland. Its FY 1999 budget was $2.5 billion.
- The Agency for Healthcare Research and Quality (AHRQ formerly *AHCPR*) supports research on health care systems, quality and cost, and the effectiveness of medical treatments. It was established in 1989 and is headquartered in Rockville, Maryland. Its FY 1999 budget was $171 million.

Human Services Operating Divisions

Three divisions within the DHHS administer human services. These agencies are the Health Care Financing Administration (HCFA), Administration for Children and Families (ACF), and Administration on Aging (AOA).

- *HCFA* administers two entitlement programs, Medicare and Medicaid, which provide health care to approximately one in every four Americans. Medicare provides health insurance for more than 39 million elderly and disabled individuals. Medicaid, a joint federal–state program, provides health coverage for more than 34 million low-income persons, including nearly 18 million children, and nursing home coverage for low-income elderly. HCFA also administers the new State Child Health Insurance Program (S-CHIP) through approved state plans that cover more than 2.2 million children. HCFA was established in 1977 and is headquartered in Baltimore, Maryland. Its budget for FY 1999 was $342.8 billion.[25]
- The *ACF* is responsible for more than 60 programs that provide services and assistance to needy children and families. The agency administers the new state–federal welfare program, Temporary Assistance to Needy Families, providing assistance to an estimated 12.2 million persons, including 8.4 million children. The ACF also administers the National Child Support Enforcement System, collecting $11.8 billion in 1996 in payments from noncustodial parents. This agency also administers the Head Start Program, serving approximately 800,000 preschool children. Programs under this agency assist low-income families with child care funds and support state programs to provide for foster care and adoption assistance. Its programs also fund child abuse and domestic violence prevention programs. Established in 1991, the agency brought together several existing programs and is headquartered in Washington, D.C. Its FY 1999 budget was $38.3 billion.[25]
- The *AOA* supports a nationwide aging network, providing services to the elderly to enable them to remain independent. The AOA supports nearly 240 million meals for the elderly each year, including home-based delivered "meals on wheels." The AOA programs provide transportation and at-home service. In addition, the AOA helps fund ombudsman services for the elderly and provides policy leadership on aging services. Its FY 99 budget was $883 million.[25]

BLOCK GRANTS AND FUNDING PROGRAMS

There is no legal definition for the term "block grant," but block grants are characterized by a federal–state or local relationship in which there is considerable discretion in grant administration within a broadly defined program area. Typically, block grants have less "red tape" in their applications and administrative requirements. They apply to broad purposes such as "public health" rather than to narrow (categorical) purposes such as lead poisoning or rodent control. They consolidate a number of existing narrowly based programs into one grant instrument. They frequently are associated with budget reductions, although that is not necessarily the outcome.

Block grants blend the characteristics of categorical grants and general revenue sharing. This blending of attributes and expectations associated with each type of grant leads to a constant tension, and is a major factor explaining why block grants are sometimes characterized as "unstable." There are almost always compromises—the products of trade-offs made in the process of enactment.

The debate over block grants has historically focused on design, implementation, and evaluation to the heart of the federal system, including what role the federal government should play in domestic government and where responsibility should be shared among the various levels of government and the private sector, including decision-making authority.

Some believe that block grants are a more efficient and effective mechanism for achieving federal purposes. For example, in its report, *Strengthening the Partnership in Intergovernmental Service Delivery,* the National Performance Review recommended support for the National Governors' Association and the National Conferences of State Legislators' proposal for Federal-State Flexibility grants.[26] Flexibility and the ability to package a number of related programs into a workable arrangement are often mentioned as objectives by those individuals who advocate block grants. In addition, block grants promote long-term planning by providing formula-based funding and eliminating funding uncertainties that are endemic to competitive categorical programs.

Some proponents of block grants also view categorical grants as an instrument of an overreaching national government and block grants as a devolving of power to subnational governments. The objective, then, would be to not make the federal government work more effectively, but to get the federal government out of the picture. The Reagan administration took this position and the block grants President Reagan proposed were a major tool in the administration's blueprint for American government.

Opponents of block grants fear that financial support for blocked programs will diminish, as it is thought to be more difficult to get support for broad purposes. In addition, many fear that the interests of certain groups such as the urban poor will be neglected in the absence of social targeting requirements. Still others believe that the government that collects the taxes should be the government that determines how the money is spent.

Both opponents and proponents of block grants may view them as a way to reduce expenditures. Originally, funds were increased, not decreased, in order to gain support; however, it was thought that future program growth could be curbed.

Today, many view block grants as a synonym for budget cuts, in large part because of the experiences during the Reagan administration, when funds for newly created block grants were reduced by 13 percent from the previous year's (FY 1981) total appropriation for 57 categorical grants. This 13 percent reduction was lower than the 25 percent saving the Reagan administration had sought to achieve through its block grant proposal.[27]

Since then, Congress has not given much consideration to the block grant option, although several proposals were made during the Bush administration. In his 1991 State of the Union message, President George Bush proposed a turnover to the states of $15 billion worth of federal aid programs in one large block. The criteria used to select the programs were programs judged by the states to be of continuing value, but whose federal funding priority was declining, and programs that were candidates for flexible management by the states.

State and local organizations developed their own proposal for turnovers, using the following criteria:

- The programs selected should have some broad degree of commonality.
- The programs should be either categorical grants to state governments or project/competitive grant programs in which states currently reviewed most of the funds awarded.
- Priority should be given to grants that have unduly limiting mandates and overly detailed administrative regulations.
- The programs should generally be national in scope and not benefit primarily certain regions or states.

The debate, then, centered on what criteria to use to determine what should be included in a block grant (Table 23–2).[28]

The Substance Abuse Prevention and Treatment (SAPT) Block Grant is an example of this shared federal–state responsibility using funding as the lever. SAPT is administered by the SAMHSA and is the primary tool the federal government uses to support state substance abuse prevention and treatment programs. In FY 1999, appropriations for the block grant were $1.585 billion. Funds go directly to states, which have broad discretion to decide how to use them, within federal guidelines. Funds are allocated to states under a formula reflecting several factors: state personal income data, state financial resources, state population estimates, and the cost of providing services in each particular state. By law, the SAMHSA must update the cost of services index every three years.[29] The Omnibus Consolidated and Emergency Supplemental Appropriations Act of 1999 established minimum state allotments.[30]

States participating in the substance abuse block grants are required to spend 35 percent of their grant on alcohol prevention- and treatment-

Table 23–2 Block Grants

Program	*Recipient*	*Match Requirements*	*Administrative Federal Agency*	*FY 1995 Funding (in millions)*
Job Training Partnership Act	States	None	DOL	$1,653.50
Community Development Block Grants	Metropolitan cities and urban counties and states	None	HUD	$4,484.00
HOME Investment Partnership Grants	Metropolitan cities and urban counties and states	25%	HUD	$1,400.00
Surface Transportation Program	States	20%	DOT	$352.00
Federal Transit Capital and Operating Assistance	Local governments	Capital 20% Operating 50%	DOT	$1,500.00 $710.00
Federal, State, and Local Partnership for Education Improvement	States	None	ED	$347.20
Community Services Block Grants	States	None	DHHS	$473.00
Social Services Block Grant	States	None	DHHS	$2,800.00
Community Mental Health Services Block Grants	States	None	DHHS	$275.40
Prevention and Treatment of Substance Abuse	States	None	DHHS	$1,200.00
Preventive Health and Health Services Block Grants	States	None	DHHS	$158.00
Maternal and Child Health Services Block Grants	States	None	DHHS	$684.00
Low-Income Home Energy Assistance Block Grants	States	None	DHHS	$1,319.00
Child Care Development Assistance Block Grants	States	None	DHHS	$935.00
Local Crime Prevention Block Grants	States	None	DOJ	Program first authorized in FY 1996

Source: Reprinted from U.S. Advisory Commission on Intergovernmental Relations, *Block Grants: A Comparative Analysis*, Report A-60, 1997, U.S. Government Printing Office.

related activities; 35 percent for drug prevention- and treatment-related activities, and 20 percent to provide primary prevention and education services to at-risk populations.[31] The agency monitors states' implementation of the prevention set-aside portion of the block grant.

States are required to spend at least as much as they spent in FY 1994 to furnish and improve treatment services to pregnant women and women with dependent children. States are also required to offer prenatal and child care services, and allow children to live with their mothers while in treatment if necessary. States must ensure that treatment facilities receiving block grant funds give preference to pregnant women seeking treatment.

Due to the rising incidence of tuberculosis (TB) in the United States, substance abuse programs supported under this grant are required to provide TB services to individuals in their programs. Because of the high numbers of substance abusers who are human immunodeficiency virus (HIV) positive, states with more than 10 cases of AIDS per 100,000 persons must set aside at least two percent of their grant for outpatient HIV services.

States may not use grant funds to provide inpatient services except when it is medically necessary for substance abuse treatment and when these services cannot be provided in the community. In addition, SAPT block grant funds may not be used to provide financial assistance to any entity other than a public or nonprofit private entity. Not more than five percent of the funds may be used for administration.

To receive their full block grant allocation, states must have a law providing that it is unlawful for any manufacturer, retailer, or distributor to sell tobacco products to individuals under 18. States must also have a mechanism for measuring compliance with its requirement and for reducing noncompliance to specified levels. States are required to maintain a level of spending on substance abuse prevention and treatment programs that is at least as high as the average spending for two years preceding any particular year. If a state does not meet this requirement, it will lose a portion of its grant funds.

In addition, these funds are then subject to what is known as the Synar amendment. This amendment, passed in 1992 as part of the ADAMHA Reorganization Act,[29] requires states to enforce their tobacco minimum-age-of-sale laws or risk losing substance abuse block grant funds. The Synar amendment is administered by SAMHSA and has been an important catalyst for the passage of state tobacco-control legislation. Under Synar, state officials are supervising random, unannounced visits to retail outlets by minors as a means of monitoring retailer compliance. Retailers caught selling tobacco to minors may be fined or have their tobacco licenses suspended. So although this block grant is not directly aimed at tobacco smoking prevention, additional federal legislation has established a health priority by using the loss of federal funds as the hammer to get the state to establish reduction in youth smoking as a state priority.

Through this grant, the federal government can direct in general the categories of individuals who should receive service priority and additional services beyond the strict meaning of alcohol- or drug-related services, and the state is free to design a program around the broad requirements of the grant. In addition, this grant is used as leverage to ensure another public health goal—reductions in teen smoking.

MEDICAID

Medicaid is the largest joint federal/state entitlement program and is not subject to the annual appropriations process. The program provides payment for health care for certain groups of low-income individuals. Medicaid can be thought of as three distinct programs: one program funds long-term care for the chronically ill, disabled, and aged; another program provides comprehensive health insurance for low-income children and families; and the Disproportionate Share (DSH) Program assists hospitals with the cost of uncompensated care. In FY 1997, HCFA estimated that Medicaid enrolled 41.4 million persons at a total cost of almost $166 billion. The federal share of the cost was $95.6 billion.

Each state establishes its own eligibility within broad federal guidelines. States must cover certain population groups such as recipients of Supplemental Security Income (SSI), that is, the aged, blind, and disabled, and have the option of covering others. Historically, Medicaid eligibility for poor families (generally women with dependent children) was linked to the receipt of cash welfare payments. In recent years, Medicaid ties to welfare benefits have been loosened. The trend culminated in the creation of the Temporary Assistance for Needy Families (TANF) Program in 1996. The new welfare law included provisions severing the automatic link with Medicaid but allowed states to maintain the link as an option.[32]

Medicaid does not cover everyone who is poor, reaching only 46 percent of persons in poverty in 1996. Eligibility is also subject to "categorical restrictions"; benefits are available only to members of families with children and pregnant women and to persons who are aged, blind, or disabled. Beginning in 1984, Congress expanded eligibility for pregnant women and children. Partly as a result, the number of beneficiaries grew by 60 percent over the next 10 years. Over the past 2 years, however, enrollment has declined, probably due at least in part to a healthy economy and welfare program reforms. Some speculate that families exiting the TANF program are losing Medicaid due to the confusion about eligibility and administrative error. Some preliminary exit surveys suggest that many of those individuals are becoming uninsured.

Special eligibility rules apply to persons who receive care in nursing facilities and other institutions. Many of these persons have incomes that are well above the poverty level but qualify for Medicaid because of the high cost of their care. Medicaid had thus emerged as the largest source of third-party funding for long-term care. It is also a major source of federal support for programs to serve individuals with mental retardation or developmental disabilities. Older adults and individuals who are blind or who have disabilities represent 26 percent of Medicaid enrollment, but account for 60 percent of the program spending. In contrast, poor families make up 72 percent of enrollment but only 26 percent of spending.[33]

The State Child Health Insurance Program (S-CHIP) created in 1997 is another new program that is likely to impact the Medicaid landscape. S-CHIP provides federal matching funds for states to expand health benefits coverage for modest-income children though Medicaid, a separate state program, or a combination of both. The federal matching percentage for S-CHIP children—whether covered through Medicaid or a separate program—is between 65 and 85 percent. S-CHIP is focusing more attention on the rate of participation among eligible children in Medicaid and S-CHIP. It has been suggested that many currently uninsured children are actually eligible for Medicaid but do not participate. If S-CHIP as well as Medicaid is unable to enroll a significant percentage of eligible children, criticism of the two programs is likely to increase.

Each state defines its own package of Medicaid-covered medical services. Federal law mandates some, such as hospital nursing facility and physician care; others such as prescription drugs and dental care are at state option. States also set their own reimbursement rules. Many states pay considerably less under Medicaid than providers' costs or customary charges. As a result, many medical care providers refuse to accept Medicaid patients or limit the number of such patients they will treat. Still, Medicaid beneficiaries appear to have significantly better access to care than comparable uninsured individuals.

Before 1990, most Medicaid services were provided on a fee-for-service basis by any health care practitioner who was willing to accept Medicaid payment. By 1999, more than half of Medicaid recipients were enrolled in some kind of prepaid managed care organization. This shift to managed care provided the impetus for a set of laws passed as part of the Balanced Budget Act of 1997 (which was the budget reconciliation legislation for that year).[34] Among other things, these laws make mandatory enrollment into managed care organizations easier for states and establish quality and other standards for Medicaid managed care organizations. Recent press suggests that a growing number of health maintenance organizations that have accepted large numbers of Medicaid beneficiaries are now pulling out of the Medicaid program due to the low negotiated per capita payments from which many states have claimed Medicaid savings.

States are often concerned when Congress enacts legislation that establishes unfunded mandates. Unfunded mandates are responsibilities or duties imposed by the federal government on state and local governments without providing funding for the costs incurred. The issue touches on the proper role of federalism—the responsibility of the federal government to establish priorities and national standards and the responsibility of local governments to determine their own priorities and standards. Advocates of mandates that may incur costs at the state and local levels contend that such mandates are often designed to address problems that are found nationwide. They argue that regulations set uniform standards for all localities, and that requiring localities to pay at least some of the costs will motivate them to cease such violations. State and local government officials, on the other hand, have expressed alarm at the increasing cost of complying with the mandates.

Throughout the 1980s, Congress frequently created unfunded mandates in Medicaid. For example, Congress passed provisions creating a new category of individuals for which states would be responsible for a portion of the cost of their care. This group, known as dual eligibles, is poor and elderly and therefore eligible for both Medicare and Medicaid. The states are required to pay the beneficiaries Medicare premiums and cost sharing. It is thought among national policy makers that the reason the rate of enrollment for these individuals in Medicaid is so low is not only due to the stigma of Medicaid, but also because the states do not want to have to expend dollars for these individuals' care.

To demonstrate the importance of report language, when the provision was originally passed, the legislative language did not specify at what rate cost sharing would be based on. States decided to reimburse providers on the lower Medicaid rate rather than the Medicare reimbursement rate. Drafters of the provision had assumed the higher Medicare rate, but neither the legislative language nor the report language made clear what rate was to be used.

LONG-TERM CARE

Financing issues in long-term care for the elderly have commanded the attention of Congress and state governments for more than two decades. Although Congress had debated different approaches for changing the way in which these services are financed, the cost of expansion of long-term care coverage under public programs has been the central focus of the debate.

Federal and state governments already spend large sums of money on long-term care for the elderly. In 1995, federal and state spending for nursing home care—largely through the Medicaid program—amounted to $34 billion, and an additional $21 billion was spent on home care.[35] Because so much of the long-term care dollars are now coming from Medicaid, states have been in the forefront of studying and experimenting with innovative ways in which to provide cost-effective long-term care.

THE ROLE OF STATES

The current role of states in public health is a mixed set of signals in which the state may choose its priorities and has more flexibility but in an ever more demanding environment reflecting a rapid evolvement of a new thinking of the relationship between states and the federal government within the past 30 years.

The relationship of the states and the federal government has been characterized by many shifts over the history of the United States. In 1964, the federal government sought "creative federalism" in which the Johnson administration's Great Society programs sought to end the national government's role in meeting the administration's goals to achieve socially desirable goals in reducing poverty and the elimination of hunger. Medicare was created during this time. Under the theory of creative federalism, federal involvement was justified as a necessary evil in order to legitimate intrusion into state and local affairs. Under the new theory, federal involvement was justified as long as Congress could establish a national purpose for such actions. The Great Society programs used states' and local governments' intermediaries or agents to implement national policies, and the volume of federal regulations increased as the federal government became increasingly involved in areas that had previously been the purview of state and local governments or the private sector.

This period was followed by the kind of contemporary federalism that is experienced now.

This period is characterized by shifts in the intergovernmental grant system, growth of unfunded federal mandates, and concerns about federal regulations. In the 1970s, presidents tried to respond to the concerns raised about the intergovernmental grant system, particularly duplication, fragmentation, overlap, and confusion.[36] The administrations of Richard Nixon and Gerald Ford attempted to redirect the relationship of the federal government to the states. The administrations' principal tools were revenue sharing and consolidating federal aid programs into six special revenue-sharing programs. The intent was to shift funds, authority, and responsibility to states and local governments in an effort to manage the intergovernmental grant system more effectively. Though not completely successful, the Nixon era did recast the debate on the roles of various levels of governments.

In 1976, the Supreme Court in *National League of Cities v. Usury* addressed one of the fundamental issues in federalism: to what extent Congress may impose on the sovereignty of the states.[37] The Supreme Court ruled that the Fair Labor Standards Act's 1974 amendments, which extended hour and wage coverage to state and local public employees, violated state sovereignty as protected under the 10th Amendment's enumerated powers class. This clause limits the federal government's power to those specified in the Constitution. This case was important in that it provided thinking that federal powers could be checked.

With the Reagan administration, new initiatives stimulated the debate on the appropriate roles of federal, state, and local government. President Reagan, rather than attempt to manage federal government more rationally, as was the case in the Nixon administration, sought to restructure the system of governance fundamentally. In his 1981 inaugural address, President Reagan raised an issue as old as the Republic: What is the nature of the union? The president stated that the federal government did not create the states; the states created the federal government.[38]

In 1981, Congress passed the Omnibus Budget Reconciliation Act, which consolidated a number of social programs into nine block grants, allowing for greater state and local autonomy and flexibility in the fashioning of strategies to address federal objectives and local needs. The administration was not successful in the second phase, which would have reallocated federal–state responsibility and resources for welfare, food stamps, and Medicare, and would have turned back revenue sources to the states.

In 1985, the Supreme Court revisited the issue of state sovereignty and state and local government protection from the imposition of federal actions. In the *Garcia v. San Antonio Metropolitan Transit Authority* case, the Court reversed its previous holding from the *National League of Cities v. Usury* case.[39] *Garcia* has had two significant impacts on federalism, according to some scholars. First, under *Garcia,* the Supreme Court held that the 10th Amendment does not protect state and local governments from compliance with the Fair Labor Standards Act. Two, the Court seems to be backing away from its role as final arbiter or interpreter of the Constitution in disputes between political branches of the federal government and the states. The Court appears to be allowing such disputes to be resolved by the political—that is the legislative—branch of government.

With the Clinton administration's initiative of reinventing government and the House Republicans' Contract with America, there were efforts to rearrange the relationship of the federal government and the states. The present debate has resulted in the passage of unfunded federal mandate legislation that required the federal government to assess the cost/benefit impact of federal legislation on states, local governments, and the private sector; has fueled discussions concerning the possible elimination of several federal departments; has prompted consideration of how to reform the regulatory process; and has caused the consideration of legislation that would eliminate, downsize, consolidate, or block grant a number of federal programs in an effort to foster greater flexibility and control by state governments.[6] This debate has been driven by fiscal and philosophical factors including the desire to reduce the federal deficit, to achieve management efficiencies at the federal level, and to reconsider the proper role of the federal, state, and local governments.

So where does that leave the states when it comes to establishing public health policy and implementing new and innovative strategies for meeting the health needs of populations within the states' and localities' borders? In the current climate, states have options that they might not have had in the 1960s and 1970s. At the same time, states may face the continued challenge of reductions in funds from both federal and state governments and meeting other requirements placed on them from the federal level.

For example, more states are seeking waivers from Medicaid and Medicare to find different ways of providing care for dual eligibles, and many states have sought Medicaid waivers to either expand or operate Medicaid programs differently. Some states are looking at waivers from programs that would permit them to address the needs of the disabled and to assist them in getting back to work without losing health care coverage.

Because long-term care is becoming a larger Medicaid burden for the states, some states are looking at the use of state dollars for different types of services. For example, assisted living has been pioneered in the state of Oregon, which now leads the country in the amount of state dollars used to provide home- and community-based care services.

In addition to trying to address state and local needs, states are also charged with more responsibility in their role as agents for the federal government. For example, states are under criticism because of the way in which they have acted to ensure the quality of nursing homes under federal quality standards. States, in turn, charge that the resources given them by the federal government to do the job of quality surveys are not enough to ensure quality.

States have led the federal government by showing that one strategy to fight teen smoking is to use the power of tax to increase the cost of tobacco products. In fact, in the recent tobacco settlement, states fought with Congress over the use of the money. States believed that because they had led the battle with tobacco companies and expended their resources doing so, all funds should go to them without any federal requirements concerning how the money would be spent. However, some individuals in Congress and the administration believed that a portion of the funds were federal funds, and that Congress should waive the federal government's right to the funds but then stipulate how that money should be spent by states. These efforts failed, and the federal right to the money was waived without specific requirements on how the funds could be spent.

States have traditionally held the authority to regulate insurance and to provide state licensure to qualified providers. Yet even in these areas, actions on the federal government can have impact. For example, in state licensure, many states have moved to provide more authority for non-MD health providers to act more independently. However, Medicare's conditions of participation do not recognize these differences. For example, a classic fight continues between certified registered nurse anesthetists (CRNAs) and anesthesiologists over Medicare reimbursement. Although many states permit CRNAs to have independent practices, Medicare does not recognize this. Therefore, Medicare policies can impact not only the reimbursement, but also the growth of specialties and non-MD health providers who often provide access to care in rural areas. Another example is that nurse practitioners under some state laws can order hospice services. However, the Medicare program does not recognize this authority for the Medicare hospice benefit.

The passage of the S-CHIP also showed a willingness on the part of Congress to provide states with flexibility even while trying to require that more children be covered. States were free to design plans within guidelines. Most began to design plans that were either an expansion of state Medicaid programs or stand-alone components. A growing number of states explored statutory options provided under S-CHIP to include family coverage. Many states examined how to develop innovative outreach strategies to provide families with applications and program information.

Other examples of recently passed health legislation are the opposite. The Mental Health Parity Act of 1996, for example, mandated private insurance coverage requirements concerning mental health services.[40] The Health Insurance Accountability and Portability Act of 1996 also placed requirements on health insurance coverage that the states must oversee.[41] In this legislation, however, it specified that if the state does not provide adequate oversight, HCFA would be authorized to become the entity that ensures that requirements of the act are followed.

In recent years, states have experienced strong revenue growth. However, that growth has been below that of the federal government. During the five-year period from 1993 to 1998, federal revenues increased 7.7 percent, whereas states experienced only 5.2 percent revenue growth per year. The federal government is dependent on income tax, which is sensitive to underlying economic activity. In contrast, states depend heavily on sales tax, which is an eroding tax base because states do not tax most services—the major growth sector in the economy. Further, more states are losing increasing amounts of revenues from both mail order and Internet sales, which generally are not taxed.

This strong economic growth has permitted states to have resources that they might not have in bad economic times. Health programs are often at risk in federal government's need to address budget deficits and when states have fewer resources. Those dependent on federal and state grants to run programs, and state and local government dependent on federal funding to ensure the continuance of specific programs, have to be aware of what economic conditions will mean for the funding sources.

THE ROLE OF ADVOCATES

Who are advocates? News articles refer to various interest groups either helping or defeating specific legislative issues. Armies of well-heeled paid lobbyists are often pictured in the halls outside important committee meetings. However, advocacy goes on every day in the form of letters and conversations with federal and state officials and their staff by ordinary citizens.

Officials can only know from the people they serve what the concerns of their communities are going to be, and this information helps officials determine priorities. Providing information to officials cannot be underestimated in helping both the official and the staff who advise them in understanding the needs of localities. Whether the information is describing a problem, or simply letting them know of a program's success, the value of information directly from those using or administering programs cannot be underestimated.

It is important to understand the funding process at the federal level—and what latitude states can have through block grants and waivers to redirect health priorities into what is needed in state and local communities. If a federal health program can make a significant impact on a state or local community, it is important to know when to contact a federal official for help. For members of Congress, it is the funding issues that drive the process. Knowing that funding is needed for a project in June for the next fiscal year instead of in early March makes the official's job harder if it is determined that this should be a priority.

STATE LEGISLATION

Legislative authority is operative in both federal and state government. For the states, government authority is based on "police power" to provide for the health, safety, and welfare of the population.[42] In terms of public health, police powers include all laws and regulations that improve morbidity and reduce mortality of the community. (For more information see, Chapter 5.) These powers cover the wide range of areas that enable public health agencies to pursue their most fundamental missions of protection from communicable disease transmission, requiring immunization for school entry, ensuring confidentiality essential to preventive programs, and implementing environmental protections including those for air, water, and waste disposal. As illustrated in Chapter 5, this legislation also serves to protect health sometimes in conflict with private interests. For example, it is state legislation that provides for the detention of individuals with active pulmonary TB who refuse to take medications, thus endangering the community from transmission of this disease and the development of resistant organisms.

Legislation to protect from injury is also enacted at the state level, including requirements for bicycle helmets. Again, state legislation is critical to an agenda to improve population health and also can be controversial, balancing public and private interests in areas such as HIV reporting and partner notification and immunization requirements that can exclude unimmunized children from school. Public health administrators require skills in both fostering and advocating for legislators who advance this agenda and conversely resisting legislative attempts at the state level, which can compromise their objectives. This principle was emphasized in the 1988 IOM Report *Future of Public Health*.[43] Duties of the state were enumerated including the assurance of an adequate base for health activities.

Legislative priorities culminating in the enactment of state statute are the result of a concerted effort by a number of involved parties. Public health agencies formulate legislative priorities and work with executive staff of the chief executive office (governor), legislators and legislative staff, advocates, and other interested individuals. Legislative support or nonsupport of public health does not occur by accident or spontaneously. Ascertaining the impact of the proposed bill on the spectrum of those persons affected and the associated costs is a necessary part of this preparation. In considering or crafting new legislation, an ongoing partnership between the public health specialist and the lawyer or legislative draftsman must be formed early. Also, a decision may need to be made if a new statute rather than new regulation is needed to accomplish the objective.[42] These efforts should best begin long before the opening of the legislative session.

In advocating for legislation, public health proponents will need to relate to legislators and often, more importantly, to more accessible legislative staff. It is often more effective to make a point with legislators by encouraging other individuals and interests in the community to make their views known to legislators rather than rely on state health staff. State staff are providing information and "educating" legislators. Generally, state law or regulations prohibit all public officials from engaging in political activities or lobbying. As Grad pointed out, "it has never been held under any state 'Hatch Act' that a public health officer or employee may not bring the need for legislation to the attention of the appropriate legislative officers."[42]

If the legislative proposal is of importance, the program may be included in the governor's annual message. When the draft legislation has been prepared by the state health department or governor's office, an interested legislator can introduce it into the legislative process. By a similar route, outside groups can get health legislation introduced into the system. It is the public health director's (or staff's) responsibility to take a position and be available for testimony on the proposal.[42]

Using New York State as an example, a bicameral legislature (like most states) has 150 members of the Assembly and 61 members of the Senate. All are elected in even-numbered years; members of both houses serving two-year terms.[44] Major players are the governor (and executive staff), the majority party in each house, and its leadership. The Speaker of the Assembly and Senate Majority Leader wield enormous power and also appoint all chairpersons of committees. There are 36 Assembly and 34 Senate Standing Committees. Health bills will be considered in Health Committee, but may be considered in other committees as well because of split jurisdiction of the subject or need for fiscal review. Also, a Rules Committee plays a special role in each house and are chaired by the Speakers of each house. A bill must pass both houses before it can be sent to the governor, who must sign or veto the bill within 10 days. Also, budget bills are enacted by the legislature after the governor presents a proposal two months before the end of the fiscal year. In New York State, specific items added to the budget by the legislature are subject to the governor's approval. The budget process is key to state public health agencies because of the resources appropriated, and also because the accompanying language is statute and can commit the agency to new or varied courses of action.

• • •

Because the federal government can set so many priorities by what it chooses to fund, and at what level it chooses to fund programs, the federal government plays an instrumental role in determining what a state must do concerning health policy. The states, on the other hand, enjoy enormous flexibility in meeting health policy goals, while at the same time acting as the federal government's agent in overseeing many more programs. Public health organizations increasingly find it necessary to become actively involved in health policy development in order to shape federal, state, and local public health priorities. Knowledge of legislative processes and legislative relationships is requisite for developing a policy environment that supports population health improvement.

CHAPTER REVIEW

1. The federal budget is a comprehensive accounting of the government's spending, revenues, and debts.
2. Within the budget, there are two categories of spending: *mandatory* and *discretionary*. Most public health programs fall into the discretionary category.
3. The budget resolution serves as a blueprint in establishing budget priorities for that year. The spending, revenue, and public debt laws necessary to implement decisions agreed to in the budget resolution are subsequently enacted separately as part of the "budget reconciliation" process or as part of the appropriations process.
4. The appropriations process is overseen by the House and Senate Appropriations Committees; each has a subcommittee with jurisdiction over public health spending.
5. Except for tax bills, which must begin in the House of Representatives, any bill can originate in either body after it is first introduced by a member. After referral to a committee and hearings, the bill is "reported" to the full body for consideration. After the same thing happens in the other legislative body, the two emerging versions are brought to a conference and a final conference report is voted on by the House and Senate.
6. Federal agencies are authorized to issue regulations by their enabling statutes, statutes establishing new programs, and statutes amending and extending the duties and responsibilities of those agencies.
7. The federal government plays an instrumental role in determining what a state must do concerning health policy by setting priorities for funding. The states serve as the agent of the federal government in overseeing federally legislated programs. In addition, states enact their own legislation, which shapes a broad scope of public health activities.

REFERENCES

1. *The Budget and Accounting Act of 1921,* 42 Stat. 20.
2. *The Congressional Budget and Impoundment Control Act of 1974,* Public Law 93-344 (88 Stat. 297).
3. Congressional Budget Office, *The Economic and Budget Outlook: Fiscal Years 2000–2009* (Washington, DC: U.S. Government Printing Office, 1999).
4. R. Ketih and A. Schick, *Manual on the Federal Budget Process* [CRS Report 98-720 GOV] (Washington, DC: U.S. Library of Congress, Congressional Research Service, 1998).
5. U.S. Office of Management and Budget, *Budget of the United States Government: Fiscal Year 1999* (Washington, DC: Government Printing Office, 1998).

6. *Government Performance and Results Act,* Public Law 103-62, codified at 31 U.S.C. 1011nt.
7. House Concurrent Resolution 68, as reported by House Report 106-91. Conference Report adopted by the House of Representatives on April 14, 1999 and by the Senate on April 15, 1999.
8. *The Balanced Budget Act and Emergency Deficit Control Act of 1985,* Public Law 99-177, codified at 2 U.S.C. 901 *et. seq.*
9. Office of Management and Budget, *Analytical Perspectives, Budget of the United States* (Washington, DC: U.S. Government Printing Office, 1999).
10. *Congressional Record,* vol. 144, 105th Cong., 2d sess., p. S12659 (October 16, 1998) and p. S12810 (October 21, 1998).
11. House Rule XXII, clause 9, *U.S. House of Representatives Rules and Manual,* H.R. 105-358 (1998).
12. Senate Rule XXVII, *Senate Manual,* Senate Document 104-1 (January 1997).
13. Senate Rule XVI, *Senate Manual,* Senate Document 104-1 (January 1995).
14. House Rule XXI, *House Practice: A Guide to the Rules, Precedents and Procedures of the House of Representatives.* 104th Cong., 1st sess. (1996).
15. *House Practice: A Guide to the Rules, Precedents and Procedures of the House of Representatives.* 104th Cong., 2d. sess. (1996).
16. Statement of Senator Ron Wyden, *Congressional Record,* vol. 145, 1st sess., p. S14498 (November 10, 1999).
17. *Administrative Procedure Act,* 60 Stat. 237, codified at 5 U.S.C. 701-710.
18. 5 U.S.C. 553.
19. Executive Order 12866, *Federal Register,* vol. 58, no. 190, p. 51735 (September 30, 1993).
20. *Federal Regulatory Reform: An Overview* [CRS Issue Brieft IB 95035] (Washington, DC: U.S. Library of Congress, Congressional Research Service, March 16, 2000), 3.
21. *Unfunded Mandates Reform Act,* Public Law 104-2 (109 Stat. 48).
22. 2 U.S.C. 602(c)(2); Section 202 of *Congressional Budget Act of 1974,* Public Law 93-344, as amended.
23. Executive Order 12291, *Federal Register,* vol. 46, p. 13193 (February 17, 1981).
24. *Congressional Review Act of 1997,* 5 U.S.C. 801-808.
25. "Department of Health and Human Services: HHS Agencies." http://www.hhs.gov/progorg (18 February 2000). Accessed 15 June 2000.
26. A. Gore, *From Red Tape to Results: Creating a Government that Works Better and Costs Less.* Report of the National Performance Review (Washington, DC: U.S. Government Printing Office, 1993).
27. American Enterprise Institute for Public Policy Research, *Rethinking Federalism: Block Grants and Federal, State, and Local Responsibilities* (Washington, DC: 1981).
28. U.S. Congress Joint Economic Committee, *Block Grants and the Intergovernmental System,* 97th Cong., 1st sess. (July 15 and 22, 1981).
29. *Alcohol, Drug Abuse, and Mental Health Administration (ADAMHA) Reorganization Act of 1992,* Public Law 102–321, replaced DAMHA with the Substance Abuse and Mental Health Services Administration (SAMHSA).
30. *The Omnibus Consolidated and Emergency Supplemental Appropriations Act of 1994,* Public Law 105-277.
31. C.O. Echeverria, "The Substance Abuse and Mental Health Services Administration," [CRS Report 97-844 GOV] (Washington, DC: U.S. Library of Congress. Congressional Research Service, March 19, 2000), 2–3.
32. *The Personal Responsibility and Work Opportunity Reconciliation Act of 1996 (PWORA),* Public Law 104-193.
33. Congressional Research Service Review of Budget Information, 1999.
34. *Balanced Budget Act of 1997,* Public Law 105-33. For more information concerning Medicaid and managed care, see Health Care Financing Administration, *National Summary of Medicaid Managed Care Programs and Enrollment* (February 17, 1998).
35. U.S. General Accounting Office, *Long-Term Care: Diverse, Growing Population Includes Millions of Americans of All Ages* [GOA./HEHS-95-26] (Washington, DC: 1996).
36. E. Boyd, *American Federalism: 1976 to 1997 Significant Events* [CRS Report 95-518 GOV] (Washington, DC: U.S. Library of Congress, Congressional Research Service, January 6, 1997).
37. *National League of Cities v. Usury,* 96 SCT 2465, 426 US 833, 49 LED 2d 245 (1976).
38. General Services Administration, National Archives and Records Service, Office of the Federal Register, *Public Papers of the President—Ronald Reagan 1981: Inaugural Address, January 20, 1981* (Washington, DC: U.S. Government Printing Office, 1982).
39. *Garcia v. San Antonio Metropolitan Transit Authority,* 105 SCT 1005, 83 LED 2d 1016 91985.
40. *Mental Health Parity Act of 1996,* Public Law 104-204, Title VII.
41. *Health Insurance Accountability and Portability Act of 1996,* Public Law 104-191.
42. F. Grad, *The Public Health Law Manual,* 2d ed. (Washington, DC: American Public Health Association, 1990), 1–137.
43. Institute of Medicine, *The Future of Public Health* (Washington, DC: National Academy Press, 1988), 1–225.
44. E. Stock, *The Citizen Lobbyist* (Albany, NY: The League of Women Voters of New York State, 1997), 1–32.

CHAPTER 24

Leadership in Public Health

Vaughn Mamlin Upshaw
William A. Sollecito
Arnold D. Kaluzny

Changes in population health and the health care system increasingly require public health organizations to take actions that are beyond their traditional scope of activity. Successfully accomplishing these actions requires public health administrators to go beyond competent managerial decision making by providing leadership both within and outside their organizational settings. This chapter examines key leadership concepts and strategies that administrators can use to transform public health challenges into opportunities for improving organizational and community performance.

Despite a growing arsenal of administrative skills and technical resources, public health professionals routinely face health issues that far surpass their organizations' spheres of control. These challenges derive from changes in the organization and financing of health services, as well as changes in the populations that require those services. Professionals must address an expanding array of health problems and risks in the population using limited human, capital, and intellectual resources that are often inadequate and unstable over time. The complex developments influencing public health practice in the current environment include the following:

- *Population shifts:* More people are immigrating to the United States, bringing with them cultural beliefs, languages, and health practices that are different from the traditional ones. The population is also aging, bringing increases in chronic disease and disability. And, more people are uninsured, particularly low-wage earners and their families.
- *Changes in the financing of health services:* Managed care is rapidly replacing fee-for-service as the standard for payment of health services. Risk is shifting from insurers to providers and health service organizations.
- *Restructuring of health care organizations:* Integrated delivery systems, alliances, and mergers have reshaped the health care marketplace. Fewer hospitals operate independently, and most physicians have joined provider groups to improve their bargaining power.
- *Information revolution:* Information is knowledge and is essential to population health planning and policy development. Epidemiology uses information to understand and build evidence for public health problems and programs. An advantage will go to those individuals who are technologically sophisticated and to those organizations that build information management capacities.[1]
- *Greater consumer choice:* With increased access to information, consumers are more

The authors would like to acknowledge Dr. Elizabeth Tornquist, Adriane Terrell, and Marleen Sturgill for their assistance in the preparation of this manuscript.

active in decisions concerning their health, and they often reject traditional medicines for alternative approaches.

- *Community empowerment:* Successful change in community health requires the participation of those individuals who have a stake in the outcome. Moving away from clinical care and toward population health must, therefore, involve families and communities in determining what solutions will work.
- *Redefinition of government's role:* There is increasing pressure to privatize the provision of public health services and improve public health through a combination of public and private delivery systems.[2] Being accountable for the health of communities, however, means that government must have the capacity to collect, analyze, and report health status data across health and services systems. A public health challenge is to maintain oversight and accountability for services that are provided by private organizations.
- *Scientific breakthroughs and emerging threats:* Mapping genetic predisposition to chronic diseases such as cancer, arthritis, and diabetes will move public health interventions away from a focus on populations to a focus on at-risk individuals. At the same time, diseases are emerging and re-emerging in new and drug-resistant forms. These diseases are occurring globally, and with high mobility between countries, they are becoming local public health threats.
- *The complex political and social context for public health:* Multiple constituents with varying amounts of power compete within a political environment for resources, position, and authority over public health issues. As political support becomes more important in addressing public health problems, individuals, families, and communities become more dependent on professionals and governments to resolve public health issues.
- *Invisibility of public health:* Public health is often said to be "most effective when nothing visible happens to the health of a community."[3(p.12)] Communicating what public health is and sustaining the public's interest long enough to "build the understanding and support that is essential to good public health practice" is critical for the future of public health.[4(p.20)] Public health must develop the necessary infrastructure and capacity to communicate health status measures in an understandable and useful manner to policy makers, community leaders, and the public through multiple sources, including the media.

These developments present significant challenges for public health organizations and the professionals who manage them (Exhibit 24–1). For example, public health professionals are asked to justify their programs, but the benefits of public health programs are often uncertain because there is a lack of clear evidence that these programs have a positive impact on the population's health. State and local officials are called on to provide more services with greater efficiency and effectiveness, yet few public health professionals receive training in how to identify, design, and implement continuous quality improvement efforts. Public health agencies provide care to diverse populations and must juggle multiple complex demands for attention and resources. As the world becomes more dependent on access to information and

Exhibit 24–1 Public Health Challenges

- Uncertain benefits of public health programs
- Demand for more services with greater efficiency and effectiveness
- Diverse population with complex demands
- Limited information system capacity
- Perceived poor quality and value of public health
- Competitive health care market
- Accountable for public health outcomes with limited resources

technology, many local and state public health agencies are still limited in their access to information systems and software applications. The public assumes that public health departments provide low-quality services to poor people, yet the primary mission of public health agencies typically is to provide services that improve the health of populations. Growing competitiveness in health care markets places greater pressure on public health agencies to provide reimbursable services, often diverting public health from its primary mission of population-based health care. Finally, calls for reduction in the size of government are frequently coupled with increased interest in accountability, which places public health agencies in the difficult position of having to demonstrate that they are improving public health outcomes with fewer resources.

These challenges have pervaded public health for many years and have fostered a growing recognition of the need for effective leadership—not simply effective management—within the public health community. The well-publicized report, *The Future of Public Health*, by the Institute of Medicine (IOM), concluded that the field of public health was in disarray and called for enhanced leadership and leadership training.[5] Unfortunately, leadership is a term that means different things to different people, and therefore requires a clear definition of its purpose, functions, and actions necessary to provide leadership training. The objective of this chapter is to examine the role of leadership within a changing public health environment and demonstrate how various challenges may be transformed into leadership opportunities. The chapter concludes with a case study (Appendix 24–A) demonstrating the role of leadership in crafting effective institutional responses to an evolving public health system.

LEADERSHIP AS INFLUENCE

The challenges currently faced by public health organizations and professionals have several characteristics in common. First, they demonstrate that the infrastructure of public health is never able to address all of the health needs and demands of the community. The very nature of organizations is such that their design and written policies are incomplete and require modification or judgment to accommodate the real work of the organization. Second, as an organizational entity, public health operates within a complex and changing external environment. Over time, processes often become inefficient or infeasible; when this occurs, individuals need to function beyond their specified roles in the organization. Simply put, organizations are composed of people, and dynamic organizational relationships require individuals to accommodate and function beyond their prescribed roles.

For these reasons, leadership is more than the attributes of a position in an organization or the personal characteristics of an individual. Leadership is behavior that goes beyond required performance. Specifically, leadership "is the influential increment over and above mechanical compliance with the routine directives of the organization."[6(p.302)] Thus, leadership is a generic process within an organization, and all professionals have an obligation to provide leadership and thereby enhance the functions of the organization. In public health, going beyond routine directives means going beyond mandated services and traditional organizational boundaries to meet the challenges of improving the health of the community.

Sustaining a Vision

Leadership occurs at multiple levels and in a variety of contexts. At the *individual* level, leadership is demonstrated by someone who is conscious of his or her values, goals, relationship, and influence to the larger organization. Individuals who inspire others are able to communicate their vision of how the world should be and to organize processes and systems to make this vision a reality; these individuals are clearly demonstrating leadership.

At the *organizational* level, the leadership challenge is to ensure that individuals understand the mission and functions of the organization and motivate and direct people within the organization to accomplish key goals and objectives. Here, public health professionals need to understand the potential for improvements or change within the organization and inspire others to realize this potential.

Public health professionals must also be able to demonstrate leadership within the larger community. Unlike individual leadership, which focuses on a person's self-awareness and motivation, or organizational leadership, which requires public health professionals to direct people's activities and design more effective and efficient systems, *community* leadership requires that public health professionals exhibit skills in listening, communication, conflict resolution, negotiation, and political strategy given the various constituencies involved within the community. Public health professionals must develop competencies in each of these areas in order to turn challenges successfully into opportunities.

Building Trust

Public health leadership depends on the individual's ability to build a culture of trust and commitment within the organization and through community partnerships. Public health professionals who blame managed care, politicians, or community members for public health failures are missing an opportunity to provide leadership in dealing with the challenges facing the community. Establishing successful public health programs begins with establishing trust and cultivating strong community relationships. Effective public health professionals make relationships a top priority. They resist competitive nonproductive behaviors, create openness, destroy organizational boundaries, and adopt principles that support public health policy objectives.[7] Engaging the local health and human services system and expanding participation into the community help to develop shared responsibility for achieving public health improvements.

Creating Partnerships

Public health professionals exercise leadership to ensure that everyone within the organization is empowered to achieve the organization's goals. Public health professionals exercise leadership within their organizations by generating useful information, identifying more effective and efficient work processes, developing systems for reporting and improving performance, and emphasizing activities that improve public health. A key leadership strategy is to ensure that every employee participates in building partnerships and alliances with others to achieve community public health goals. (See Chapter 22 for a detailed discussion on partnerships in public health.) Leaders ensure that internal operations enhance successful external partnerships by doing the following:[8–10]

- Select the right partners (internal and external) and get the right partners to do the right job.
- Plan for sequential, small advances toward achieving larger goals.
- Align incentives within and between organizations to achieve goals.
- Establish procedures that support and continually improve practices.
- Look for and encourage boundary spanning between organizations.
- Set realistic time frames for accomplishing goals.
- Establish performance expectations for individuals, teams, and organizations.

There is a growing recognition within the health care community that health-related organizations must work collectively to improve the health of populations. As part of President Clinton's health care reform initiative in 1994, the American Hospital Association, Voluntary Hospital Association, Inc., and Catholic Health Association of the United States outlined a framework for Community Care Networks (CCNs).[11] Their commitment to CCNs has continued even though the national health care reform effort failed. The goal of CCNs is to help health care providers envision a country that ensures affordable access to health services by "reforming health care delivery locally so patients, communities and their resources, needs and problems drive the reconfiguration of local health care."[11(p.xxviii)]

To improve health at the population level, leadership skills are needed in both the public and the private health sectors. The ability to form effective coalitions, to see the whole and its parts simultaneously, and to be tenacious are essential leadership skills for the twenty-first century.[12] Public health professionals must be able to build relationships with multiple partners, manage complex relationships, and successfully work with diverse groups.[7,10]

Building Infrastructure

Within their organizations, public health professionals need to foster an environment that rewards discovery, learning, and improvement in networking and shared activities. Leadership requires that organizations are able to attract, recruit, train, and retain a skilled public health work force. Public health organizations need personnel systems that accommodate the changing nature of work and the growing interdependence between organizations and the public. Public health professionals need to ensure that public health systems have the necessary human and capital infrastructures to improve communications, build partnerships, and bridge functions across relevant organizations and community groups, including the media, to improve health outcomes.

Leadership within the community requires an infrastructure capable of responding to enduring and emerging public health problems, so leaders must communicate this need and routinely provide evidence of how the system is working. Professionals in public health must build an infrastructure and evidence base for effective public health programs and services, and develop a means to share public and private accountability for achieving these. For example, public and private health professionals can share information about best practices using the U.S. Preventive Services Task Force *Guide to Clinical Preventive Services*.[13] They can also use this tool to monitor community progress toward preventive health goals.

Concerns about the adequacy of the public health infrastructure have been growing for some time. The disarray in public health infrastructure that was documented by the IOM did not occur instantaneously, nor has it disappeared. There are no clear estimates of what would be required to establish an optimal public health system, but any estimate would certainly be costlier than efforts to prevent specific public health problems. Increasingly, the effects of social and environmental problems are being felt in the health services, but understanding their causal factors and prevention opportunities requires more than the available information. Many community health problems are the focus of public health interventions, yet there is a lack of credible evidence that these activities actually produce the intended results. Consequently, accountability for public health activities is difficult to demonstrate because no part of the public health system has sufficient resources, knowledge, or capacity to resolve complex health and social problems independently.

LEADERSHIP AS AN INTEGRATING THEME

Effective leadership ensures that all of the individuals who affect the health of the population share in common public health goals. A vision that inspires others must do more than simply urge people to accomplish individual and organizational goals. A vision for public health must foster the desire to create systems that improve public health: this is the responsibility of all individuals in the public health community. Although public health professionals and elected officials sometimes claim victory over public health problems, they need only consider the resurgence of tuberculosis to be reminded of how dangerous it is to declare victory before the war is over.

Because public health is a shared goal rather than a defined discipline, achieving public health objectives requires community partnerships.[14] But public health operates within a very complex political economy that often complicates interorganizational relationships. (See, for example, Chapter 22's discussion of community–academic partnerships.) As described by

Bailus Walker, "Health policy formulation and health program planning and development involve a continuous series of interactions between health officials, governmental and private sector participants, and others in the health policy and program development process."[15(p.4)] Adopting controversial public health measures, such as tobacco ordinances, for example, requires participation not only from the governing authority empowered to adopt such ordinances, but also from the business community and the public. The potential for controversy is just one of the major challenges facing modern public health organizations. Organizations may fail to address such challenges for a variety of reasons, including[7]

- challenges that go unaddressed for extended periods of time, creating effects that are difficult to arrest and reverse
- costs that far exceed what has been budgeted for ameliorating challenges
- unknown interdependencies and complications that become apparent as challenges develop over time
- challenges that make cause and effect impossible to track, such that responsible agents and viable solutions are difficult to identify

FROM CHALLENGES TO OPPORTUNITIES

Faced with an incomplete and evolving infrastructure, a dynamic environment, and the nature of human relationships, public health requires acts of leadership from all people working in the public health profession. That is, successful public health organizations depend on decision makers who can assess challenges and derive opportunities from them. Reframing public health problems as opportunities gives public health professionals a means to motivate and mobilize employees, communities, and partners to change the future of public health. Some of the most pressing challenges and associated opportunities facing public health organizations include the following (Exhibit 24–2):

- *Build evidence of prevention's effectiveness:* The difficulty of documenting the benefits of prevention suggests that we need to redouble our efforts to build an evidence base for public health initiatives. In-

Exhibit 24–2 Public Health Challenges and Opportunities

Public Health Challenges	Public Health Opportunities
• Uncertain benefits of public health programs	• Build evidence and knowledge of population-based interventions.
• Demand for more services with greater efficiency and effectiveness	• Create systems that foster innovation and continuous quality improvement.
• Diverse population with complex demands	• Create unique programs and services that improve health for individuals, families, and communities.
• Limited information system capacity	• Develop infrastructure for collecting, managing, analyzing, and reporting epidemiologic, clinical, administrative, and financial data.
• Perceived poor quality and value of public health	• Create and sustain a positive public health image.
• Competitive health care market	• Convene and collaborate with multiple partners.
• Accountable for public health outcomes with limited resources	• Share performance standards, responsibility, and risk for public health.

terventions cannot simply be advocated; they must be subject to well-designed evaluation. Empirical evaluation can constantly build evidence of the effectiveness and efficiency of public health initiatives.

- *Innovation and improvement:* One of the basic tenets of continuous improvement is the need to create optimal systems. An optimal system produces a synergy, which translates into greater efficiency and effectiveness. The development and improvement of performance standards require leadership at all levels in public health organizations. When coupled with a virtual organization approach, standards, new techniques, and accountability for improvement of public health performance can be shared among partners. Risks can be minimized and responsibilities for achieving public health objectives can be distributed among partners using performance standards.
- *Programs for communities, families, and individuals:* Appropriate access to and use of services demand innovation by public health agencies. This can be facilitated by connecting public health practitioners and academic research and by implementing and extending demonstration programs that have achieved success in a community environment. Public health professionals must be able to identify successful programs and take the necessary steps to promote similar innovations. For example, the Children's Primary Care Research Group at the University of North Carolina recently completed a communitywide system intervention linking clinical and public health methodology to improve the delivery of preventive services to mothers and children in a community. This program is an integrated approach that links researchers, policy makers, and practicing health professionals so that what has been learned in research can be implemented more rapidly in the community. It was initially implemented in two counties in North Carolina and is now being extended to the entire state.[16] Achieving the full potential of such programs will also require ongoing evaluation to ensure that access and appropriate services continue to be provided as programs move from academic modeling to real world applications.

  Also critical is a multidisciplinary approach to meeting diverse needs. For example, states in the eastern United States are using social workers and other professionals to help them understand and better meet the health needs of Hispanic populations, who have immigrated into these areas in very large numbers. Public health agencies are also recruiting and training workers who are bilingual and knowledgeable of cultures that are experiencing rapid growth.[17] The complexity of needs in diverse populations requires innovative methods for carrying out community assessments. Once again, a bridge between practice-based research and real-world applications is critical. This requires public health professionals who have the knowledge and vision to take advantage of technological advances in new approaches. Continuous improvement in the application of these methods will help to ensure that tools are sensitive enough to measure needs accurately. The use of innovative evaluation strategies will aid in making adjustments when necessary.
- *Develop infrastructure for public health:* Improving information system capabilities is possible through the application of innovative, user-friendly, Web-based technology. Use of the Internet facilitates both data collection and the dissemination of results. Health departments and health workers are now becoming more familiar with Web-based technology. Linking health departments and other health organizations in "virtual organizations" will permit greater sharing of information and greater availability of resources across broader systems.[18] Technology also allows individuals to gain access to resources that were previously "out of reach," such as public health

databases and medical libraries. Health applications can be implemented using technology that has been developed for other purposes. For example, geographic information systems (GIS) offer a beneficial way to identify and locate public health problems more rapidly and with greater accuracy. Public health efforts after the Hurricane Floyd disaster in North Carolina in September 1999 were improved by the use of GIS to pinpoint potential sources of infectious disease and monitor the emergence of health and environmental problems.[19]

- *Creating and sustaining a positive public health image:* To develop a positive image for public health requires public health professionals to be engaged with communities at multiple levels. At the population level, public health marketing can promote positive behaviors and discourage individuals from taking unnecessary health risks. At the community level, public health professionals can integrate community assessments with other public health activities and ensure that assessed needs receive appropriate responses. Effective public health professionals can communicate public health goals and priorities to wide audiences and work effectively with the media and press to ensure that public health information is readily available. A good example of using public health information to create greater public awareness is the "Whole Hog Web site" developed by the Environmental Resource Program at the University of North Carolina School of Public Health.[20] This Web site is a tool for elementary and secondary teachers who teach environmental education. It provides case studies, games, facts, and simulations illustrating the complex interplay of health, economic, and social factors in creating healthy communities. For communities in North Carolina where hog production is both a source of economic strength and a public health management issue, the Web site brings an important public health issue to the forefront in a way that has great impact without creating controversy.
- *Collaborate with others:* A key opportunity for public health is to create multiple partnerships, bringing together people with different types of specialization. In recent years, health departments have begun to outsource more services. With proper leadership, this approach can bring the advantages of virtual organizations[18] that share complementary resources and skills with mutual trust. As in other industries where partnerships have been successfully applied, the key requirement is entrepreneurial individuals who are willing to take risks in order to achieve maximum benefits. A critical mechanism for this is using technology to link partners in a seamless manner. For example, virtual drug development models have been very successful by linking biotechnology and pharmaceutical companies with contract research organizations.[21]
- *Resource constraints:* The fact that demands for public health are unrelenting while resources remain constant or diminish suggests that systems of continuous improvement need to be created. In some cases, public health systems simply need to be redesigned or reengineered in order to meet expectations. As described by Ellen Gaucher (1994), the director of quality improvement at the University of Michigan Hospitals, "Within health care, some of our processes are so bad that we could spend the rest of our professional careers trying to continuously improve them. We need to throw them out and begin with a clean sheet of paper and make sure we understand what the elements of each of these processes are. We need to redesign them to be effective in the long run."[22]

BUILDING LEARNING RELATIONSHIPS

The challenges and opportunities facing public health form an essential reality that is shared among all of the health professions. Describing how these challenges and opportunities affect medicine, Ed O'Neil, co-director of the Center for the Health Professions and executive director of the Pew Health Professions Commission, observed that,

> In this period of transformation, when what was certain and established will become vague and unpredictable, the essential leadership task will be to bring coherence, structure and meaning to a world of changing norms and expectations. What leadership skills and competencies will be needed to understand, survive and thrive in such an environment? Will they be tied to those that have existed before, or will this be a period of discontinuity with the recent past?[23(p.271)]

Examples of the competencies that public health leaders need in order to address these emerging challenges appear in Exhibit 24–3. They include the ability to evaluate programs, a focus on quality improvement and organizational learning, and skills in program design and communication, to name a few. To the extent that public health professionals have training and ability in the areas that equip them to provide leadership—regardless of their position in the organization—they will be able to make a difference in the community.

A new generation of leadership is needed to span the traditional domains of public health, medical care, and human services and to forge the alliances that will make sustained improvement possible. This new leadership requires individuals who can exert influence beyond organizational expectations. A good share of the burden of producing these individuals falls on

Exhibit 24–3 Public Health Challenges, Opportunities, and Leadership Competencies

Public Health Challenges	Public Health Opportunities	Public Health Competencies
• Uncertain benefits of public health programs	• Build evidence and knowledge of population-based interventions.	• Program evaluation
• Demand for more services with greater efficiency and effectiveness	• Create systems that foster innovation and continuous quality improvement.	• Continuous quality improvement, organizational learning, and innovation
• Diverse population with complex demands	• Create unique programs and services that improve health for individuals, families, and communities.	• Program planning and design linked to community and organizational goals
• Limited information system capacity	• Develop infrastructure for collecting, managing, analyzing, and reporting epidemiologic, clinical, administrative, and financial data.	• Understanding of the appropriate applications for information technology, including GIS, biostatistics, data management, epidemiology, and financial management
• Perceived poor quality and value of public health	• Create and sustain a positive public health image.	• Management communications skills to allow for translating and communicating community and organizational plans to diverse audiences
• Competitive health care market	• Convene and collaborate with multiple partners.	• Building coalitions, negotiating conflicts, and honoring diversity
• Accountable for public health outcomes with limited resources	• Share performance standards, responsibility, and risk for public health.	• Gaining commitment from multiple groups; contract negotiation

the academic community, which has the flexibility and perspective to move beyond the conventional boundaries of public health to meet health needs better in a changing health care system. The development of leadership requires that faculty and students participate in communities to gain a better understanding of the challenges of serving radically different populations, working in public health settings, and governing health care institutions.

The recently created North Carolina Institute for Public Health (NC-IPH) provided leadership in the manner it responded to Hurricane Floyd. Hurricane Floyd was a major public health crisis. Twenty inches of rain within a 24-hour period resulted in more than $6 billion worth of damages in 27 counties in eastern North Carolina. The hurricane was responsible for 51 deaths, more than 57,000 damaged homes (10,000 being condemned), and the loss of millions of hogs, turkeys, and chickens. Thirty communities were submerged for weeks, disabling water and waste treatment facilities.[24]

The University of North Carolina School of Public Health (SPH) played a key role in the response to the crisis through its recently established NC-IPH. This institute was developed in order to make the resources of the SPH available to the public health practice community of the entire state, thereby meeting the needs of the citizens of North Carolina. The NC-IPH was designed to provide various forms of assistance to local health authorities in the form of consulting, as well as specific services requested by local health agencies. These services are provided in collaboration with, and drawing on, the resources of the SPH.[25]

Although the goals of the NC-IPH were to anticipate and prevent public health crises, the procedures for accomplishing these goals were embryonic at best. Within days of the institute's creation, Hurricane Floyd challenged the faculty and staff to assist the citizens of eastern North Carolina. And indeed they did! Faculty, staff, and students responded to the challenge and the NC-IPH played a major role in coordinating relief efforts, and also in providing a full range of public health services from community assessment to water testing.

This example illustrates one of the most critical characteristics of leadership—the ability to mobilize quickly to address challenges when they occur and make a difference in the outcome, beyond simply complying with a formalized set of roles, rules, and procedures. The NC-IPH, although it had clear goals and a clear mission, did not have time to develop specific working relationships with relevant faculty and state agencies. Nonetheless, individuals clearly went beyond their prescribed roles to address the challenges confronting the citizens in the affected communities. Collaboration among the numerous organizations involved created a synergy in which agencies and academic institutions functioned effectively in a manner that went far beyond their traditional roles. Public health practitioners at the state level and in the academic community clearly exhibited many of the leadership characteristics described in this chapter and created a model for ongoing collaboration.

To convert challenges into opportunities, attention needs to be given to building the knowledge and skills that equip individuals to exceed required performance. Leadership training in public health must help individuals better leverage and manage community resources, understand diversity and its role in both the provider and consumer communities, and function in the emerging world of public–private partnerships. Through understanding and skill, individuals will be able to exert leadership when faced with incomplete and evolving infrastructures, changing and complex environments, and a diverse interplay of cultures and relationships within the public health community. Key components of public health leadership training include the following:

- A new multidisciplinary curriculum in community health improvement must involve faculty beyond schools of public health together with key stakeholders in the health industry, the public health community, and the larger business community. Leading scholars and practitioners from academia, public and private health care organizations, industry, government, and community-based organizations need to focus on "civic entrepreneurship," which emphasizes diversity training, the assessment of growing inequality and its impact on public health, and the creation of new revenue streams for agencies and organizations above and beyond traditional grant applications and government support.[26,27]

- A diverse and talented student body capable of encompassing the breadth and depth of public health should be actively recruited. In addition to selecting individuals with leadership potential from mid- and upper-level positions in public health agencies, private health care organizations, and community-based health and human services organizations, special efforts need to be made to recruit students from places that are not normally associated with public health. Students with unique expertise may help public health meet the challenges of the future. For example, digitization and computer networking are changing the world. Recruiting students from Microsoft and Silicon Valley to study public health may provide opportunities for new approaches and applications. Getting others to use the concepts and methods of public health within the context of their organizations may affect how public health programs are designed and implemented in the future.[28]
- Career development programs are needed to ensure that current and future faculty members design curricula that are relevant to contemporary public health challenges and opportunities within communities. Faculty from schools of public health and other professional schools need to be encouraged to pursue in-depth study of community health issues and organizations. Such study can provide opportunities for individuals to develop the leadership skills that are needed in the community. Special attention needs to be given to building and nurturing public–private partnerships, which leverage resources to benefit the health and well-being of the larger community.
- To strengthen the links between academic institutions and the community, health professionals from the community need to be involved with academic institutions at multiple levels. Community partners need to interact with students and faculty and carry out practice-based research and educational activities. These interactions can serve as a continual source of new material for curriculum content, case-based learning, practitioner-oriented publications, and pilot data for larger studies in community health improvement.
- The creation of leadership laboratories can bring a core group of faculty and students together with a national network of community health organizations that are committed to leadership development and organizational improvement. In such laboratories, faculty and students can address real-world community health issues through partnerships with participating organizations. The leadership laboratory can serve as a forum for exchanging ideas and experiences, testing model programs and processes, providing consultation and technical assistance, and obtaining real-time observations on changing community demographics and health trends, policies, and marketplace changes.
- Expanded opportunities to participate in continuing education on leadership are needed for public health professionals. The CDC sponsors a Public Health Leadership Institute for state and local health officials, and schools of public health from across the country have created a public health training network that includes regional leadership institutes based in schools of public health. The Management Academy for Public Health at the University of North Carolina at Chapel Hill is a year-long program for teams of public health and community professionals interested in improving their skills to implement

public health programs. Opportunities such as these offer public health professionals a means to improve their management and leadership skills, expand their professional networks, and develop expertise that they can use to mentor and support other public health workers.

Converting challenges to opportunities requires competent leadership at all levels of the organization and within all of the various disciplines of the public health community. Leadership requires the commitment and dedication of both academic and practice communities; through these partnerships, leaders can bring "coherence, structure and meaning to a world of changing norms and expectations."[23(p.271)]

• • •

Leadership in public health occurs within a rapidly changing environment and is required at every institutional and community setting. Leadership exists when individuals and organizations exceed the performance levels that are required or expected in public health. In doing so, public health leaders motivate the larger community of professionals, organizations, and citizens to work toward enhancing and improving population health.

Leadership occurs in many forms, but includes the following tasks at a minimum:

- Ensure that adequate resources and techniques are present to accomplish key objectives.
- Link public health programs and interventions to relevant public health problems.
- Promote public health programs that are evidence based.
- Facilitate continual innovation, improvement, and learning within organizations and communities.
- Engage diverse partners with multiple skills in public health planning, implementation, and evaluation.
- Communicate public health goals within the organization, the community, and political arenas.

It is unlikely that public health will ever operate in environments that are predictable and stable. Building the skills and competencies to move from challenges to opportunities is an ongoing leadership task. Emerging programs for public health leadership in academic institutions, coupled with emerging Web-based technologies, make education and training available to individuals across the country and the world. No longer is any public health worker isolated from information and resources that can be used to improve the public's health. Now is the time for public health leaders to define the value of public health and engage others in making public health a public priority!

CHAPTER REVIEW

1. *Leadership* is defined generally as the incremental activities carried out over and above mechanical compliance with the routine directives of an organization. In public health, exceeding routine directives requires going beyond mandated services and traditional organizational boundaries to meet the challenges of improving the health of the community.
2. Leadership is exercised to accomplish a number of activities that are considered to be instrumental in improving the delivery of public health services.
   - Build trust among major stakeholders in public health and health care delivery.
   - Develop a shared vision of public health goals and priorities among stakeholders.
   - Forge interorganizational partnerships to accomplish shared objectives.
   - Strengthen the public health infrastructure and resources that are available within a community.

3. Effective leadership strategies allow public health decision makers to transform challenges into opportunities for improving performance among public health organizations and professionals. Such transformations are possible in a number of important domains of public health activity, including
    - demonstrating the effectiveness of public health interventions
    - addressing resource constraints
    - expanding access to public health services
    - assessing health needs in the population
    - ensuring that public health activities involve and benefit diverse populations within the community
    - improving the availability and utility of public health information
    - engaging community members in public health decision making
    - redesigning administrative processes and systems in public health to improve performance
4. Leadership skills must be continually developed and refined over time through "learning relationships" among public health organizations and professionals. These relationships should encourage public health professionals to think and act beyond organizational expectations when complex problems are encountered. In many cases, these relationships entail partnerships between public health organizations and academic public health institutions, which allow a continual exchange of ideas and experiences based on theory, empirical research, and practical knowledge.

REFERENCES

1. J. Goldsmith, "Leading across the Network," in *The 21st Century Health Care Leader*, ed. R.W. Gilkey (San Francisco: Jossey-Bass Publishers, 1999), 301–307.
2. P.K. Halverson et al., "Privatizing Health Services: Alternative Models and Emerging Issues for Public Health and Quality Management," *Quality Management in Health Care 5,* no. 2 (1997): 1–18.
3. R.H. Sewell, "New Challenges Facing Public Health Leadership: Chronic Disease Intervention and Health System Monitoring," *Leadership in Public Health 4,* no. 2 (1999): 12 [On-line]. URL: http://www.uic.edu/sph/chs/php/Ldrv4n2.htm.
4. T.L. Schlenker, "Sustaining the Public's Interest in Public Health," *Leadership in Public Health 4,* no. 2 (1999): 20 [On-line]. URL: http://www.uic.edu/sph/chs/php/Ldrv4n2.htm.
5. Institute of Medicine, *The Future of Public Health* (Washington, DC: National Academy of Sciences Press, 1988).
6. D. Katz and R. Kahn, *The Social Psychology of Organizations*, 2d ed. (New York: John Wiley & Sons, 1978), 302.
7. M. Wheatley, *Leader to Leader* Winter, no. 11 (1999): 28–34.
8. A.D. Kaluzny and H.S. Zuckerman, "Alliances in a Changing Industry," in *The 21st Century Health Care Leader*, ed. R.W. Gilkey (San Francisco: Jossey-Bass Publishers, 1999), 149–157.
9. J. Kotter, "Winning at Change," *Leader to Leader* Fall, no. 10 (1998): 27–33.
10. J. Elders, "The Community Role in Public Health Leadership," *Leadership in Public Health 4,* no. 2 (1999): 7–11 [On-line]. URL: http://www.uic.edu/sph/chs/php/Ldrv4n2.htm.
11. R. Bogue and C. Hall, eds., *Health Network Innovations: How 20 Communities Are Improving Their Systems through Collaboration* (Chicago: American Hospital Publishing, Inc., 1997).
12. W. Foege and M. Rosenberg, "Public and Community Health," in *The 21st Century Health Care Leader*, ed. R.W. Gilkey (San Francisco: Jossey-Bass Publishers, 1999), 85–90.
13. T.P. Houston et al., The U.S. Preventive Services Task Force Guide to Clinical Preventive Services, 2d ed. AMAM Council on Scientific Affairs. *American Journal of Preventive Medicine 14,* no. 4 (1998): 374–6.
14. A. Sommer, "W(h)ither Public Health?" *Public Health Reports 110,* no. 6 (1995): 657–661.
15. B. Walker, Jr., "Political Dimensions of Public Health Leadership," *Leadership in Public Health 4*, no. 2 (1999): 1–6 [On-line]. URL: http://www.uic.edu/sph/chs/php/Ldrv4n2.htm.
16. P.A. Margolis et al., "Linking Population and Practice-Based Strategies To Improve the Health and Development of Mothers and Children: Implementation of a

Community-Level Intervention" (Unpublished manuscript, 1999).

17. J. Johnson, K. Johnson-Webb, and W. Farrell, "A Profile of Hispanic Newcomers to North Carolina," *Popular Government* Fall (1999): 2–12.
18. J. Byrne, "The Virtual Corporation." *Business Week* 3304 (1993): 98–102.
19. North Carolina Department of Health and Human Services, "Public Health Response Post Hurricane Floyd," 30 September 1999, <http://www.dhhs.state.nc.us/docs/floydplan.htm>.
20. The Carolina Health and Environment Community Center, "Whole Hog" (1999), <http://checc.sph.unc.edu/rooms/education/Whole Hog>.
21. W.A. Sollecito and M.M. Dotson, "Getting the Most from a Contract Research Organization," *Proceedings of the Annual Project Management Institute Symposium* (Vancouver, BC: Project Management Institute, 1994).
22. E. Gaucher, World Class Healthcare (Paper presented at the National Conference on Benchmarking, San Diego, CA, 14 July 1994).
23. E. O'Neil, "Core Competencies for Physicians," in *The 21st Century Health Care Leader*, ed. R.W. Gilkey (San Francisco: Jossey-Bass Publishers, 1999), 271. (Citing J. Taylor and W. Wacker, *The Hundred Year Delta* [New York: HarperCollins, 1997].)
24. L. Copeland, "North Carolina Is Still Reeling from Floods," *USA Today*, 17 December 1999, 03A.
25. W.L. Roper and R. Stevens, "The North Carolina Institute for Public Health: Science into Service," *Public Health Reports 115,* no. 1 (2000).
26. W.C. Farrell, Jr., and J.H. Johnson, Jr., "Demographic and Social Change in Urban America: Towards an Urban Health Initiative," in *The University in the Urban Community: Responsibilities for Public Health*, eds. J.R. Hogness et al. (Sun Valley Forum on National Health, Washington, DC: Association of Academic Health Centers, 1995), 33–60.
27. J.H. Johnson, Jr., and W.C. Farrell, Jr. "Growing Income Inequality in American Society: A Political Economy Perspective," in *The Inequality Paradox: Growth of Income Disparity*, eds. J.A. Auerbach and R.S. Belous (Washington, DC: National Policy Association, 1998), 133–180.
28. M. Brown, "Strategic Thinking: Considerations for Public Health—A Personal Perspective" (Paper presented at the Symposium on Public Health Leadership, School of Public Health, University of North Carolina at Chapel Hill, March 1999).

Appendix 24–A

Leading Organizational Change in Public Health: The Case of the Cabarrus County Public Health Authority

The following case study illustrates some of the key leadership principles in public health by showing public health professionals functioning beyond their traditional roles to address public health challenges. This case study describes the process for creating the Cabarrus County Public Health Authority. It illustrates leadership at individual, organizational, and community levels in addressing long-term challenges resulting from changes in public health systems and support mechanisms.

CABARRUS COUNTY, NC

In 1996, Cabarrus County, in North Carolina's western piedmont, faced the familiar public health problems associated with a growing population, including a growing Latin American population with associated cultural and language barriers. Educational needs, a lack of public transportation, and fragmented human services made it difficult for citizens to access health care services within the county.

The delivery system in Cabarrus County includes one hospital, which opened in 1937 as a county hospital but reorganized as a nonprofit corporation in 1991. The hospital is a full-service hospital system that is accredited by the Joint Commission on Accreditation of Healthcare Organizations. It is licensed for 457 beds and 30 bassinets, with a daily census of approximately 270 beds. Located in the county seat, it provides comprehensive health services to residents in a five-county region. There are also a medical society and a physicians' organization in the county.

The Cabarrus County Health Department (CCHD) was established in 1911. A local board of health, appointed by the county commissioners, hired the current health director in 1981. In 1997, the agency operated with a budget of $6,540,508 and employed 85 people in 13 program areas. A home health agency was a part of the health department until early 1992, when it was reorganized as a unit independent of the county government with its own advisory board. Emergency medical systems also operate under the oversight of a separate county advisory board.

CHANGING TIMES FOR PUBLIC HEALTH CHALLENGES

Reductions in federal and state spending have shifted public health costs onto local governments, prompting elected officials to explore options for reducing the size of government, privatizing public services, and limiting the governmental burden for providing public health services (especially care for the indigent). As long as health departments remain a unit of county government, public health services tend to shift from the county into the private sector in a piecemeal fashion, eroding the continuity of population-based services and compromising the county's public health agency.

Source: Adapted from V. Upshaw, *The Changing Face of Public Health: A Case Study,* © 2000, Aspen Publishers, Inc.

In Cabarrus County, a number of factors—including an existing legal structure, the political will to act, and a leader with a vision of change—prompted exploration of an alternative option for the provision of public health services: the creation of an authority for public health in Cabarrus. The change process was initiated by the local health director, who was interested in strengthening the efficiency and effectiveness of the local health department (LHD). During the process, several other community stakeholders contributed vision and leadership to ensure success, including government officials, health care professionals, the local board of health, and the governing board of the newly created authority.

North Carolina statutes allow counties to establish organizations that operate as independent governmental units or authorities at the local level. There are many types of authorities—hospital, airport, sewer, and water—and they are all relatively independent of local elected officials. Authorities typically have some revenue source on which they can rely, and they tend to operate with a fairly flexible set of rules. They are not as tightly controlled as county health departments, and they often have rules that are designed specifically for them by the state's General Assembly.

In 1996, the CCHD director found it increasingly difficult to keep public health services operating at an optimal level as a unit of county government. At the same time, for-profit entities were beginning to compete with health departments for paying patients. The director knew that that would eventually lead to the county's inability to finance health department costs, which could result in significantly reduced public health services and increased risk to public health. A potential solution was privatization.

National estimates of private involvement in the provision of public health services range from 24 to 31 percent.[1] In Cabarrus, the county commissioners had already considered privatizing the county home health agency, EMS, and Medicaid managed care. Thus, the commissioners agreed to a joint meeting with the board of health and unanimously voted to adopt a proposed public health authority "in concept." The commission established an ad hoc task force to outline specifics, prepare a detailed financial analysis, and recommend candidates for appointment to the authority board (i.e., to lead the change process).

The ad hoc task force included 20 individuals with differing interests. A professor in health administration from the University of North Carolina at Charlotte was chair. Other key players included the new hospital chief executive officer and the new county manager. In addition, the chief of medicine at the hospital played a significant role in the group's deliberations.

In six months, the task force approved a plan for a public health authority to provide preventive and primary care services with a seven-member board representing providers, the county, and the community.

The ultimate responsibility for health issues was transferred from the county commissioners to the authority board, allowing the commissioners to avoid balancing health care against other county services. The authority was a mechanism for the commissioners to retain oversight, yet still give the authority sufficient freedom to do the job in a creative fashion that it could not do as a department of county government. The public health authority also offered the health department flexibility to coordinate with the hospital and other providers while ensuring that county commissioners retained accountability.

CHALLENGES AND OPPORTUNITIES FOR THE PUBLIC HEALTH AUTHORITY

In order for leadership to be successful, it must seize opportunities and develop sustainable solutions. To be sustainable, the new public health authority had to define itself as a new entity (issues of autonomy), ensure services and accessibility (issues of flexibility), and become fiscally solvent and viable (financial control). The new authority also needed to ensure that public health remained a visible and influential entity within the local health care system. To accomplish these goals, a number of key organizational issues had to be resolved.

To survive in the competitive health care market, it was agreed that the authority should be able to extend beyond the county's geopolitical boundaries and benefit from economies of scale. Expanding its reach was also seen as a way for the public health authority to improve its public image and expose a larger segment of the community to its services.

An explicit goal of the public health authority was to carry out essential population-based health services such as outreach, screening, and prevention.[2] Task force members recognized that government's public health activities and infrastructures would continue to be necessary to protect the public from outbreaks and epidemics, prevent problems before they start, and ensure a clean environment. Government had to have a presence, and "do what others won't," one member of the task force noted. People agreed that the authority had to ensure that health services were available to disadvantaged members of the community, and at the same time, increase businesslike practices in order to pay for those services. The authority was expected to expand opportunities for new services and new delivery systems significantly, increasing the public role in providing primary care and preventive health services.

It was decided that the authority would be funded through an annual per capita allocation from the county commissioners, and additional revenues would be secured through federal grants, private foundations, direct contributions, and contracts with managed care organizations. In addition, Medicaid managed care was expected to increase the organization's financial options. Forming a public health authority also enabled employees to establish new personnel and management systems designed to meet their needs.

TRANSITION TO THE CABARRUS PUBLIC HEALTH AUTHORITY

The resolution to establish the Cabarrus Public Health Authority (CPHA) was officially signed by the county commissioners on October 21, 1996. The resolution cited the rapidly changing health care system and the need for a flexible public health system as the reasons for creating a semi-independent organization. The new entity was established under the Hospital Authorities Act, but was titled as a "public health authority," with responsibility for all the traditional public health functions the county assigned to the board of health.

THE AUTHORITY'S BOARD OF COMMISSIONERS

Unlike private organizations, federal, state, and local governments have the responsibility for public health assessment, policy development, and assurance functions, and these fundamental roles cannot be privatized or abdicated.[3] Although public and private organizations may deliver individual and population-based health services, government must be responsible for ensuring their adequacy and availability.

Typically, the local board of health and its appointing board of county commissioners share responsibilities in leadership and decision making for local public health issues in North Carolina. A board of health hires the local public health director and establishes public health rules and policies. The county commissioners finance public health at the local level. In Cabarrus, the CPHA board was created as a quasi-governmental body responsible for ensuring the availability of essential public health and personal health services. The CPHA model gives private health providers, community representatives, and local government joint accountability for accomplishing public health activities. By getting key stakeholders involved in establishing goals, allocating resources, and ensuring public health and population-based services, the CPHA fosters shared responsibility and participation in accomplishing public health goals. The CPHA model is not a threat to existing providers or a burden on the county commissioners. The authority is a means to overcome the traditional tensions between the public and private health care sectors. The strength of the authority's governance structure "is that it brings citizens, government, and providers together," said the chair of the county commissioners.[4(p.44)] The authority therefore functions as an important vehicle for public health leadership development and leadership practice within the county.

TRANSITION ISSUES

A critical element in leading change is managing the transition process. In Cabarrus County, the major challenges in making the transition from an LHD to a public health authority were establishing trust, creating personnel and financing systems, and building organizational capacity.

Trust issues were present at many levels. People had to learn to trust one another and at the same time learn to trust in a new organizational structure. Moving out of county government also meant that the CPHA had to create new personnel and financing systems. Under the new authority, employees were exempt from the State Personnel Act, and the county personnel system and administrators had more flexibility to create job classifications, establish temporary positions, and institute new compensation schedules. The CPHA was also financially independent of the county. The county made a commitment to provide resources annually at a fixed percentage on a per capita basis, but it was clear that these resources alone would be insufficient to support the CPHA—meaning that the organization would need to increase revenues through expanding reimbursable services, gaining new contracts, and securing grants.

To carry out its responsibilities and fulfill its mission, the authority needed additional organizational capacity. Employees expressed needs for additional expertise, training, technology, and information systems. Combining the health department and home health agencies meant that the organizational leaders needed to establish clear roles, responsibilities, managerial expectations, lines of authority, and accountability.

The transition issues in the reorganization were met through visionary leadership coupled with good management skills. As in other examples of organizational change, the key leadership task was to maintain a focus on the overall vision while moving carefully and deliberately with concern for the needs of all stakeholders.

CONCLUSION

The Cabarrus case illustrates how changes in federal and state health care delivery and financing systems influence the way in which local public health agencies deliver services, structure their organizations, and acquire adequate financing. This case provides one example of how, with the proper leadership, local officials and providers can redesign their public health system to address the needs of uninsured and underinsured individuals while limiting the financial burden on local government.

Through the establishment of an independent, quasi-governmental entity, public health officials sought to gain greater advantage for public health activities in the health care marketplace. Ultimately, the decision to create an authority for public health occurred only because leaders from the private and public sectors were willing to take a risk in creating an alternative public health model.

There are many questions to answer before the success of the CPHA can be determined, but an evaluation of the first year's activities reveals that many goals have been met or exceeded, suggesting that public health can survive and thrive in the emerging health care marketplace. The leadership challenges for this new entity will be ongoing; only with a clear focus on the long-term vision can such challenges be met.

REFERENCES

1. P.K. Halverson et al., "Performing Public Health Functions: The Perceived Contribution of Health and Other Community Agencies," *Journal of Health and Human Services Administration 18,* no. 3 (1996): 288–303.
2. J.A. Harrell and E.L. Baker, "The Essential Services of Public Health," *Leadership in Public Health 3,* no. 3 (1994): 27–30.
3. Institute of Medicine, *The Future of Public Health* (Washington, DC: National Academy of Sciences Press, 1988).
4. V.M. Upshaw, "The Changing Face of Local Public Health: A Case Example," *Journal of Public Health Management and Practice 6,* no. 2 (2000): 39–45.

PART IV

Applications in Public Health Administration

The principles of population-based management can be applied effectively in a variety of specific institutional and community settings. The chapters in Part IV examine applications of contemporary managerial decision making in a variety of specific practice settings. Although it is impossible to cover all of the relevant practice settings in public health, the settings examined here reflect the diversity of issues and activities that make up modern public health practice. These applications include community-based prevention initiatives, environmental health programs, public health laboratory settings, disaster preparedness and response initiatives, human immunodeficiency virus prevention and control programs, and public health responses to managed care and the uninsured. Together, these chapters demonstrate how core managerial concepts and strategies can be used to address a variety of contemporary public health problems and issues.

CHAPTER 25

Community-Based Prevention

Elizabeth A. Baker
Ross C. Brownson

Community-based programs and policies differ from other health interventions in that their development, implementation, and evaluation are informed by both community perspectives and professional expertise. To develop and sustain community-based programs, public health organizations must mobilize and engage community members in collaborative processes to design, implement, and evaluate interventions. In doing so, public health organizations use existing resources, skills, and relationships with the community, while also cultivating new capacities and partnerships among organizations and individuals. Community-based strategies offer opportunities for public health organizations to improve both the effectiveness and the efficiency of traditional health interventions.

Public health has traditionally taken a population-based approach to health promotion and disease prevention, with its main functions being recently defined as assessment, policy development, and assurance.[1] Because of the complex web of individual, social, and environmental factors that influence health, these public health functions have been performed by individuals in a variety of public agencies and private organizations.[2] However, in order for public health practitioners to fulfill these functions, the Institute of Medicine has suggested that practitioners learn to be more responsive to the public's needs, to be more inclusive of community expertise, and to work in interdisciplinary teams with individuals from multiple agencies.[1,3] Public health practitioners and administrators have moved toward community-based prevention programs and policies as a way to accomplish these tasks.

Community-based programs and policies are distinguished from other types of programs because their development, implementation, and evaluation are informed by both community and scientific expertise. This chapter describes two broad areas necessary to gather and use this expertise (community and agency coalition development and evidence-based planning), and points to specific tools or resources that can assist practitioners in their efforts to create community-based prevention programs.

DEFINING KEY TERMS: COMMUNITY AND COALITION

Before discussing community-based prevention efforts, it is important to define and distinguish the important concepts of *community* and *coalition*. For some, a *community* may be defined as a geographic area or neighborhood. For others, in order to be considered a community, members of the community must have a sense of shared identity with other members of the community, a sense of belonging and emotional connection to the community, and a set of shared values and norms.[4] Lastly, some people consider communities to be defined by formal and informal collective associations or organizations.[5] Therefore, many practitioners consider themselves to be working with "the community" when they are working with community-based organizations (CBOs) or associations. For purposes of community-based prevention efforts, it is critical to involve both members of the community itself as well as representatives of organizations that work with, or benefit, members of the community.

A *coalition* is defined as a group of community members and/or organizations that join together for a common purpose.[6] Coalitions may differ considerably in the roles and responsibilities of each coalition member, and in the types of activities they wish to engage in (level of integration). Some coalitions are focused on categorical issues, such as breast cancer. For example, New York State has initiated Breast Health Partnerships. These partnerships include "public and private business, service and social groups, nonprofit agencies and institutions, medical care providers and interested individuals."[7(p.174)] As of 1998, there were 48 Breast Health Partnerships in New York State with a total of 800 partners providing breast cancer education, outreach, screening, and support services.[7] Alternately, coalitions may form to address broader public health issues. For example, the North Carolina Community-Based Public Health Initiative was formed to: (1) improve minority health, (2) make public health education programs and services more responsive to the needs of African American communities, and (3) ensure a key role for CBO partners in shaping public health services and working with health professionals in their communities.[6] The processes of developing and building relationships among coalition partners and meeting the most urgent needs as defined by the community members were considered the primary objectives of the coalitions. Other outcomes of the coalitions included the development of a playground, a neighborhood center to offer health and economic development services, and citizen drug patrols.[6]

Community and Agency Coalition Development

In order to be responsive to the public's needs and to garner and use community expertise, it is necessary to define who is to be included from the community and bring these community members and agencies together in a coalition that creates effective programs and policies. In doing so, it is important to use already existing skills, capacities, and relationships among individuals and organizations in the community and to build new ones. Some of these tasks occur prior to the coalition development (preformation), some issues need to be considered in the initial mobilization of the coalition, and others need to be addressed in the development of coalition structures.

Preformation

Too often, public health practitioners go into community-based prevention efforts with the belief that they are going where "no man has gone before." Although everyone would like to believe that they are breaking new ground, the reality is that they are working with fields that have been planted several times, and with soil that may have either been polluted with toxins or well fertilized and ready for planting. Even with their best efforts to plant healthy plants and provide plenty of sun and water, the fruits of their labor will be affected by the conditions that existed before they began. Therefore, before even beginning to develop community coalitions, it is essential to understand the history of community relations, previous experiences with health projects, intergroup relations, and interorganizational relationships (particularly the levels of trust and respect among these individuals and groups), as well as community resources and values. These have been listed as factors that are part of what has been called community capacity or social capital.[8,9]

Those persons who are interested in learning more about the types of things to consider prior to initiating a collaborative effort should consult Goodman et al. and Kreuter et al.[8,9]

Initial Mobilization

In considering who to include in community-based public health efforts, there are several issues to consider, including breadth versus depth and agency versus community member involvement.

In terms of breadth, one type of coalition might bring together individuals who have multiple points of entry into public health. This might include individuals who work in agencies that address family violence, housing, sanitation, and access to care for the elderly, as well as health care providers. Alternately, one might be more interested in bringing together individuals concerned about youth. In that case, a coalition might include individuals from schools, religious organizations, social services agencies, smoking cessation programs, housing and family violence centers, and health care providers who work with youth. The first is more appropriate if the intent is to develop broad-based community support, determine overall community needs and assets, and plan community programs and policies based on community-defined issues and concerns. The second is more appropriate if the effort is more categorical. These are critical decisions to make at the beginning of coalition activities. If what is needed is a broad understanding of community needs, then developing a coalition with individuals who are all focused on a single issue will limit input and creativity. Alternately, if the effort is categorical and a broad-based coalition is developed, individuals will feel frustrated at being limited in the types of programs and policies that can be developed. In both cases, community support will be lessened rather than enhanced, and this will carry over to, and influence, future endeavors.

In addition to considering issues of breadth versus depth, it is important to consider the inclusion of representatives from CBOs versus community members themselves. Community members offer different perspectives than agency members. Note that it is not a single community member voice that is sought, but rather inclusion from the multiple groups and subgroups in communities. Individuals of different gender, age, abilities, class, race, ethnicity, and religion can provide different perspectives that can add to coalition activities. Inclusion of community members themselves is important, but more is needed than just an invitation. It is important to ensure that all members of the coalition have similar opportunities to influence the processes and outcomes of the coalition. In order to do this, the coalition structures must be jointly defined and established by coalition members.

Developing Coalition Structures

Once individuals have agreed to be part of a coalition, the next step is to decide how members will relate to each other. This step entails developing roles, decision-making structures, and group processes. In considering this, it is important to remember that individuals from different agencies and different community members each have different ways of engaging in these processes. Therefore, any choices regarding policies and procedures must consider the range of possibilities and include training opportunities so that all members of the coalition have the skills necessary to participate in whatever processes are decided on. These skills include cultural competence, conflict resolution, group facilitation, minute taking, agenda development, and communication structure development.

Suggestions for coalition building (including how to enhance these skills) can be found in the University of Kansas Workgroup on Health Promotion and Community Development's Community Toolbox, which can be accessed at http://ctb.lsi.ukans.edu. Johnson, Grossman, and Cassidy and Wolff and Kaye also provide helpful hints as well as worksheets to enhance community efforts at this stage.[10,11]

Deciding the Level of Integration with Other Agencies

One of the first decisions a coalition must make is to decide the level of integration it wants to have with the other agencies. This can be thought of as a continuum of integration.[6,12] On one end of the continuum is the desire of agencies and individuals to work together to identify gaps in services, avoid duplication of services, and exchange information to allow for appropriate client referral. The next level of integration involves agencies maintaining their autonomy, agendas, and resources, but beginning to use these resources to work on an issue that is identified as common to all agencies. The next level of integration involves each of the agencies lessening their level of autonomy and beginning to develop joint agendas, joint goals, and joint resources.

The level of integration that is appropriate depends on the desires of the agencies and the length of time that the coalitions have worked together. Some coalitions may decide to start at a low level of integration and move to higher levels of integration over time; others may start with attempts to engage in projects that require full integration. What is most crucial is that all agencies agree on the level of integration and jointly define their common goals as well as objectives to reach these goals.

If the decision is to move toward the more integrated involvement, the next step is to determine the appropriate issue to address and the appropriate public health actions to take. The following description of evidence-based planning is one approach to planning that incorporates community expertise with scientific expertise.

EVIDENCE-BASED PLANNING

Once individuals and agencies have agreed to work together to address a public health issue, the next step is to determine if there is sufficient evidence for public health action (in the form of a specific program or policy) and what specific action should be taken. In taking this next step, two levels of evidence should be considered. The first is to examine and collect data showing the importance of a particular health condition and its link with some preventable risk factor (Level 1 evidence). The second level of evidence focuses on the relative effectiveness of specific actions to address a particular health condition (Level 2 evidence).

Level 1 Evidence: Risk Identification

Risk identification is a process that allows community-based coalitions to review what is known about a specific issue or problem and provide information to determine if some broad action might be warranted. For example, an epidemic of lung cancer might be suspected and preventable risk factors (e.g., smoking, certain occupations) might be examined.

Issue Quantification

One of the first steps in understanding a public health problem is to examine existing data. Such descriptive data may be available from ongoing vital statistics data (birth/death records), surveillance systems, special surveys, or national studies. (See Chapter 7 for a more detailed discussion of types of public health data.) Data may be available at the national, state, or even community level, and each type of data provides different information that can increase understanding of the extent and nature of the health concern. For example, U.S. census data are one type of national data set that can be helpful because they provide information by ZIP code on a wide variety of factors that may influence health such as housing, income, employment status, and age. WONDER is another example of a national data set that may be useful to local communities. WONDER can be accessed at http://wonder.cdc.gov. This Web site contains information on the prevalence of chronic disease, cancer, and human immunodeficiency virus/acquired immune deficiency syndrome. Data on numerous other health concerns and issues including maternal and child health, sexually transmitted disease, tobacco use, occupational morbidity, injury, and tuberculosis are also available through this Web site.

In terms of statewide systems, some states have developed systems that enable community groups to assess data regarding the major health concerns in their area and determine if their area has a higher or lower rate of this health concern in comparison to the state as a whole. Similarly, some community groups have begun to either connect with state systems or develop their own systems for tracking the existence of health issues and concerns, as well as list services available to assist community members to cope with these health issues. One example can be found at the Missouri Department of Health Web site at http://health.state.mo.us.

In addition to surveillance systems, descriptive studies may be useful in quantifying the extent of a health issue. Descriptive studies can take several forms. In public health, the most common type of descriptive study involves a survey of a scientifically valid sample (a representative cross section) of the population of interest. These "cross-sectional" studies are not intended to change health status (as an intervention would), but rather they serve to quantify the prevalence of behaviors, characteristics, exposures, and diseases at some point (or period) of time in a defined population. This information can be valuable for understanding the scope of the public health problem at hand. Descriptive studies commonly provide information on patterns of occurrence according to such attributes as person (e.g., age, gender, ethnicity), place (e.g., county of residence), and time (e.g., seasonal variation in disease patterns). Additionally, under certain circumstances, cross-sectional data can provide data for use in the design of analytic studies and can be used as baseline data to compare the effectiveness of public health interventions.

Analytic studies are designed to evaluate specific scientific hypotheses, although they too may serve descriptive goals. If the objective of a given study is to quantify the degree to which a suspected risk factor contributes to the disease burden in a defined population, then case-control and cohort study designs should be considered. Results from these types of studies can be used to generate information needed to judge whether a suspected risk factor is causally related to a disease (or other outcome), thus justifying public health intervention. If such causality is established, analytic epidemiologic studies can also be used to describe quantitatively the preventive effect that could be expected if the risk factor(s) in question was reduced or eliminated in the target population (population attributable risk). On the other hand, more commonly in public health practice, the objective of the study is to change some behavior or practice that is understood to be deleterious to health. Therefore, intervention studies are designed and implemented. (See Chapter 14 for a more detailed discussion of types of public health research.) These studies may include either experimental or quasi-experimental studies, and may involve small numbers of individuals or larger population bases such as schools or entire communities.[13]

One of the challenges of quantifying a health issue or concern is to integrate the multiple sources of data available. There are several tools and processes that can assist public health practitioners in sorting through data to determine if a public health action is warranted. The next few paragraphs provide a very brief overview of five of these tools.

Public Health Surveillance. Public health surveillance involves the ongoing systematic collection, analysis, and interpretation of outcome-specific health data, closely integrated with the timely dissemination of these data to those individuals who are responsible for preventing and controlling disease or injury.[14] (See Chapter 8 for a more detailed discussion on public health surveillance systems and activities.) A viable surveillance system can provide a wealth of valuable information for decision making in public health. Public health surveillance systems should have the capacity to collect and analyze data, disseminate data to public health programs, and regularly evaluate the effectiveness of the use of the disseminated data.[15] For example, documentation concerning the prevalence of elevated levels of lead (a known toxicant) in blood in the U.S. population has been used as the justification for eliminating lead from gasoline and for documenting the effects of this intervention.[16]

Meta-Analysis. Meta-analysis is a quantitative approach that provides a systematic, organized, and structured way of integrating the findings of individual research studies.[17,18] In a meta-analysis, the study results become the unit of analysis, with the goal being to identify consistent patterns and sources of disagreement among results.[19] Meta-analysis has been used increasingly over the past two decades to synthesize the findings of multiple independent studies and has been called "possibly the most important policy-related research method that has developed in the past two decades."[20(p.229)] Detailed descriptions of how to conduct meta-analyses are described in detail elsewhere.[17,20]

Risk Assessment. Quantitative risk assessment is a widely used term for a systematic approach to characterizing the risks posed to individuals and populations by environmental pollutants and other potentially adverse exposures.[21,22] Risk assessment has been described as a "bridge" between science and policy making, and it has become an established process through which expert scientific input is provided to agencies that regulate environmental or occupational exposures.[23] In the United States, its use is either explicitly or implicitly required by a number of federal statutes, and its application worldwide is increasing. There has been considerable debate concerning U.S. risk assessment policies. The most widely recognized difficulties in risk assessment are due to extrapolation-related uncertainties, specifically, extrapolating low-dose health effects from higher exposure levels.

Economic Evaluation. Economic evaluation, commonly through cost-effectiveness studies, should be an important component of evidence-based decision making.[24] These methods provide information to help assess the relative appropriateness of expenditures on public health programs and policies. Cost-effectiveness compares the net monetary costs of an intervention with some measure of health impact or outcome, such as years of life saved.[25,26]

An example of a cost-effectiveness analysis in relation to a public health intervention was shown by Hatziandreu et al. when they assessed the benefits of regular exercise among a cohort of 1,000 35-year-old men.[27] They estimated that regular exercise would result in 78 fewer coronary heart disease deaths and 1,138 quality-adjusted life years (QALYs) gained in this cohort. The cost per QALY was favorable compared with other preventive or therapeutic interventions. In public health practice, a continuing challenge is the difficulty in measuring cost-effectiveness for community-based interventions because cost data are often not reported and indirect costs, such as lost work productivity, are difficult to measure.

Expert Panels and Consensus Conferences. Most governmental agencies, in both executive and legislative branches, as well as voluntary health organizations, use expert panels when examining scientific studies based on explicit criteria and determining their relevance to health policies and interventions.[28] Ideally, the goal of expert panels is to provide scientific peer review of the quality of the science and scientific interpretations that underlie public health recommendations, regulations, and policy decisions. When conducted well, peer review can provide an important set of checks and balances for the regulatory process. One of the successful outcomes of expert panels has been the production of guidelines for preventive medicine.[29] In related work, the Council on Linkages between Academia and Public Health Practice has concluded that "the potential benefits of public health practice guidelines are immediate and far reaching."[30,31(p.5)] These recommendations have helped to stimulate a current effort to develop a *Guide to Community Preventive Services*.[32] This guide will document the effectiveness of a variety of population-based interventions in public health through systematic review and evaluation of the scientific evidence. Information regarding the guide and its current state of development can be accessed at http://thecommunityguide.org.

A consensus conference is a related mechanism that is commonly used to review epidemiologic evidence. Expert panels can take time (sometimes years) to develop their recommendations, whereas the consensus panel must commonly make decisions within a 2½-day conference. Thus, the "consensus" of many consensus panels occurs in the middle of the night in order to meet a deadline that is imposed by the conference.[33]

Making National and State Data Sets Relevant to Local Communities

Although these surveillance systems and descriptive and analytic studies provide evidence of public health issues and concerns, it is important to note that these systems may not provide all of the information necessary to engage in community-based prevention actions. In particular, community groups may feel that these data do not accurately reflect the reality of their community because of the biases inherent in such systems. For example, some data are collected via the telephone, thus providing information only on those individuals with phones. Other information is collected via a review of hospital and health provider data, and again there are several individuals who may be ill or have health concerns who are not seen until the problem becomes acute. Hence, the data set may not reflect the importance of the issue because it is "silent" to the data collection activities.

A second concern with the validity and utility of these systems, particularly national surveillance systems, is that they focus solely on health problems, not on community assets and other aspects of the community context that may positively or negatively affect these health concerns and the ability of groups to work together to create change. The community context was discussed earlier in terms of preformation activities but is important to revisit at this stage as well. For additional information on these concepts (which have been called social capital, collective efficacy, community competence, and community capacity), see Goodman et al.; Kreuter et al.; Sampson et al.; and Eng and Parker.[8,9,34,35]

One way to address these weaknesses in existing data is through the collection of local data through quantitative and qualitative methods including questionnaires, individual or group interviews, and content analysis of local publications. These data should focus on assessing the local context, the needs of community members, and the positive social factors that enhance health and the ability of community members to work together. Coalition members can assist in ensuring that the information gathered and the methods used to gather these data are appropriate for the populations of interest.

Additional information on how to collect local data can be found in Johnson et al., Kretzmann and McKnight, and the University of Kansas Workgroup on Health Promotion and Communty Develoment's Community Toolbox, which can be accessed at http://ctb.lsi.ukans.edu.[10,36,37] Goeppinger and Baglian, Interhealth Organizations, and the National Civic League *Civic Index* may also be helpful at this stage.[38–40] State and local data (e.g., http://health.state.mo.us) may also cover some contextual data that could be useful. For example, there may be information available concerning the number of civic organizations, churches, and recreational facilities in an area.

Level 2 Evidence: Develop Program and Policy Options

Level 2 evidence provides suggestions as to what specifically should be done to address the issue of concern.

Develop an Initial, Concise, Operational Statement of the Issue

The first step in deciding the specific steps that should be taken to address an issue is to articulate the public health issue of interest clearly. The key components of an issue statement include the health condition or risk factor being considered, the population(s) affected, the size and scope of the problem, prevention opportunities, and potential stakeholders.

An example is provided for an issue that is commonly encountered in public health practice—breast cancer.

> *Background/Public Health Issue.* Based on epidemiologic data, only 45% of women aged 50 years and

older in state X are receiving mammography screening each year. Rates of screening have remained essentially constant over the past 5 years and are lowest among lower-income women.

Programmatic Issue. The state health department has been charged with developing a plan for increasing the number of women who receive mammography screening, with a special emphasis on increasing rates among low-income women.

Solutions Being Considered. Program staff, policy makers, and advisory groups have proposed numerous solutions, including: (1) increased funding for mammography services; (2) a mass media campaign to promote screening; (3) education of health care providers on how to effectively counsel for mammography screening; and (4) use of lay health advisors to work within their own communities to identify reasons for lack of compliance with screening recommendations and creation of programs and policies to address these concerns.

Determine What Is Known through the Scientific Literature

Once the issue to be considered has been clearly defined, the practitioner needs to become knowledgeable about previous or ongoing efforts to address the issue. This should include a systematic approach to identify, retrieve, and evaluate relevant reports on scientific studies, panels, and conferences related to the defined topic of interest. The most common method for initiating this investigation is a formal literature review. There are many databases available to facilitate such a review. Most common among them for epidemiology and public health purposes are MEDLARS, MEDLINE, PubMed, Current Contents, HealthSTAR, and CancerLit. These databases can be subscribed to by an organization, can selectively be found on the Internet, or sometimes can be accessed by the public through institutions (such as the National Library of Medicine [http://www.nih.nlm.gov], the Combined Health Information Database [http://chid.nih.gov)], universities, and public libraries). There are also many organizations that maintain Internet sites that can be useful for identifying relevant information, including many state health departments, the U.S. Centers for Disease Control and Prevention, and the National Institutes of Health. The methods for conducting a formal literature search can be found elsewhere.[17,41,42] In addition to these search programs and Internet sites, a *Guide to Community Preventive Services* (currently being developed), which documents the effectiveness of a variety of population-based interventions, may be useful in developing a group of potential program and policy options to consider (http://thecommunityguide.org).

Once relevant articles and reports have been identified and retrieved, an evaluation of the information should be conducted. Depending on the specific purpose of the review, this evaluation may take the form of a systematic analysis and synthesis.[17,41,42] Such a synthesis can be primarily qualitative, in which the analytic results are carefully reviewed with respect to the validity of the studies, the generalizability of the results beyond the study populations, and the applicability of the findings in the context of the specific problem definition that originated the review. As described earlier, the synthesis can also be quantitative, in the form of a meta-analysis.

In addition to reviewing existing literature and data sources, it is essential to make use of the community expertise that exists in the coalition. One step that is important to take at this point is to determine what already exists in the community to address the chosen health issue or concern. Such a review can show gaps in programs and services and illuminate policies that can assist or hinder other programmatic plans. In addition, community members and community agencies that are part of the community coalition may have many ideas about possible program and policy options. Several techniques can be used to elicit this expertise, including the nominal group process or delphi technique. Further description of how to use these processes can be found in the book, *Needs Assessment Strategies for Health Education and Health Promotion.*[43]

In considering possible program and policy options, it is also important to consider interventions at all levels of what has been described as the ecologic framework. Many community-based health promotion programs use ecologic frameworks to guide the development of their program activities. Ecologic frameworks suggest that it is important to incorporate efforts to address individual, interpersonal, community (including social and economic factors), organizational, and governmental factors because of the effect these factors have on individual behavior change, and because of their direct effect on health. Table 25–1 presents descriptions and possible interventions at each level of the ecologic framework.[4,44,45]

Programs focused on changing individual behavior may provide information and/or teach skills to enable individuals to change their behaviors. These programs may focus on changing knowledge, attitudes, beliefs, and/or behaviors. These different approaches are likely to be more or less useful depending on the individual's readiness for change.[46,47]

To address interpersonal factors, many programs include strategies to strengthen social support. As described by Israel, these programs may act to strengthen existing networks or develop new network ties, or the building of social ties may be a secondary aim of programs focusing on other types of community-based activities.[48,49] For example, a program aimed at strengthening existing networks to enhance individual behavior change might invite family members to join fitness facilities or take cooking classes together. Programs may also seek to enhance the total network through lay health advisors.[48,49] Lay health advisors are "lay people to whom others normally turn to for advice, emotional support and tangible aid."[50(p.26)] Lay health advisors may provide specific health information and information about services available to ad-

Table 25–1 Interventions at Each Level of the Ecologic Framework

Target	*Individual*	*Interpersonal*	*Community*	*Organizational*	*Governmental*
Objectives	knowledge attitudes behavior physiology abilities	practices social support social network reinforcement	programs practices policies resources facilities norms	programs practices policies resources facilities	programs practices policies legislation ordinances resource allocation regulation enforcement
Approaches	education training counseling self-regulation	develop new social ties strengthen existing ties lay health advisors peer support groups	social change media advocacy community development resource development education environmental change	organizational change consulting networking organizational development	political action lobbying policy advocacy

Source: Adapted with permission from B.G. Simons-Morton, W.H. Greene, and N.H. Gottlieb, *Introduction to Health Education and Health Promotion,* © 1995, Waveland Press.

dress different health needs, assist clients in improving their communication skills, or establish linkages with health and human service agencies for efficient and appropriate referral.[50,51]

In addition to addressing interpersonal factors, community-based health promotion programs may attempt to create changes in community factors, including social and economic factors. These efforts often focus on creating changes in community structures, processes, and policies. In terms of policy changes, these programs may, for example, focus on creating worksite smoking policies or smoke-free restaurants to support changes in individual smoking behavior and attempt to alter community norms around smoking. Alternately, efforts may be focused on creating organizational or governmental policy changes in other social, community, or economic factors such as housing, jobs, education, and the environment.[52]

Ecologic frameworks suggest that because these factors (intrapersonal, interpersonal, organizational, social, and economic) are interrelated, programs that address one level are likely to enhance outcomes at the other levels. It is important to note that ecologic frameworks are useful whether the program is categorical (e.g., focused on a particular disease process) or broadly defined (e.g., community development). For example, programs that focus on a disease category (e.g., breast cancer) and receive categorical funding to change individual behavior (e.g., mammography) will enhance their ability to influence this behavior if they consider the impact of other factors (e.g., interpersonal, economic) and intervene accordingly. This may entail providing low- or no-cost mammograms, changing the policy in the state so that more women are eligible for low- or no-cost mammograms, or developing a lay health advisor approach to enhance breast cancer screening. These different programmatic activities may occur simultaneously or sequentially.

The initial review of the scientific literature can sometimes highlight various options. More often, expert panels provide program or policy recommendations on a variety of issues. The development of these options is typically influenced by political/regulatory, economic, social, demographic, and technological considerations.[53] Of these, the assessment and monitoring of the political process is one of the most important considerations when developing policy options. "Stakeholder" input may be useful to understand fully the political ramifications of various policy options. The stakeholder for a policy might be the health policy maker; the stakeholder for a coalition-based community intervention might be a community member. In the case of health policies, supportive policy makers can frequently provide advice regarding the timing of policy initiatives, methods for framing the issue, strategies for identifying sponsors, and ways to develop support among the general public. In the case of a community intervention, additional planning data may include key informant interviews, focus groups, or coalition member surveys.[54] Several of these planning issues are also a part of the science of policy analysis.[55]

In developing options, it is useful to remember that many public health interventions are founded on the notion that action at the level of a social unit can improve health outcomes at the individual level. This notion is embodied in a *causal model*—one that leads from program inputs (programs and resources) to health outputs (changes in health behaviors or health status) if the program works as intended, and that guides program planners in designing interventions (Figure 25–1).[56] It is important for evaluation purposes that what has been termed this "small theory" of the intervention be made explicit early in the planning process.[57] The causal framework should lead toward explicit determination of mutable and immutable factors, assisting in option development.

Develop an Action Plan for the Program or Policy

This aspect of the process deals largely with strategic planning issues. Key issues are briefly covered here, with more extensive discussions by others.[58–60] Once an option has been selected, a set of goals and objectives should be developed. A *goal* is a long-term desired change in the

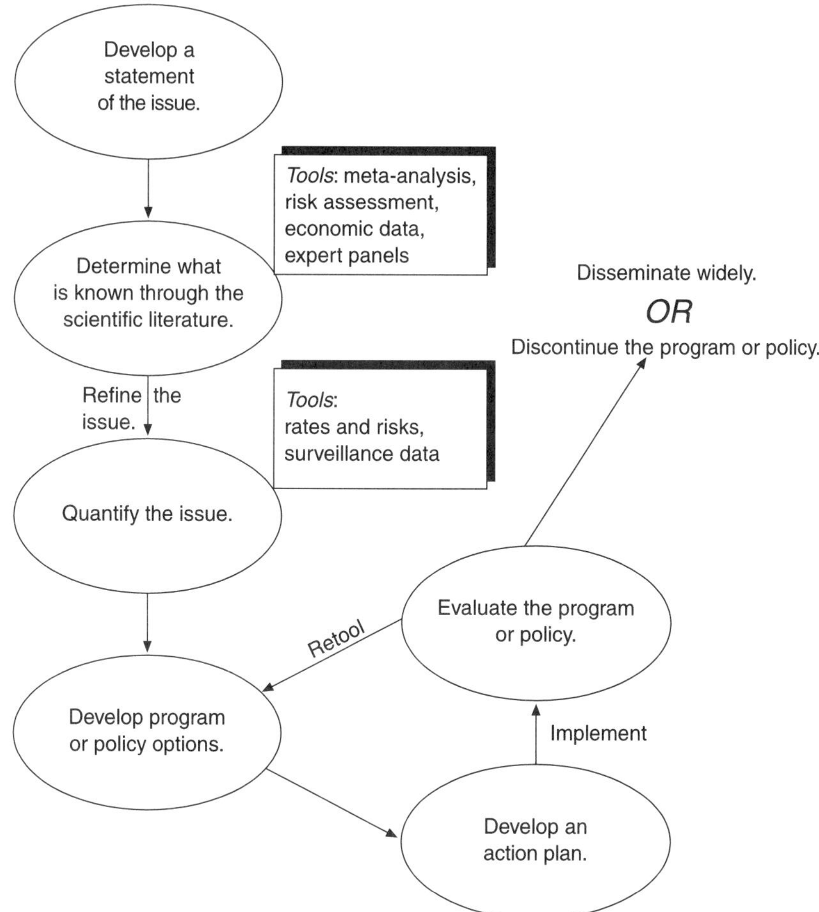

Figure 25–1 Flowchart of Community-based Prevention. *Source:* Reprinted from R.C. Brownson, J.G. Gurney, and G. Land, Evidence-Based Decision Making in Public Health, *Journal of Public Health Management and Practice,* Vol. 5, pp. 86–97, © 1999, Aspen Publishers, Inc.

status of a priority health need and an *objective* is a short-term, measurable, specific activity that leads toward achievement of a goal.[59,60] The course of action describes how the goals and objectives will be achieved, what resources are required, and how the responsibility of achieving objectives will be assigned. Excellent examples exist showing how to construct strategic goals and objectives with a "fill in the blank" format.[61] It is important that objectives are[60]

- performance, behavior, or action oriented
- precise in their language (do not use general or vague verbs)
- measurable
- results oriented, with stated outcomes
- clear in their description of content and performance
- tied to specific timetables for completion

Evaluate the Program or Policy

In simple terms, evaluation is the determination of the degree to which program goals and objectives are met. (See Chapter 13 for a more detailed discussion on different evaluation methods.) Most public health programs and policies are evaluated through "quasi-experimental" designs—that is, those lacking random assignment to intervention and comparison groups. More complete descriptions of research designs can be found elsewhere.[62,63] In general, the strongest evaluation designs acknowledge the importance of both quantitative and qualitative evaluation. Furthermore, evaluation designs need to be flexible and sensitive enough to assess intermediate changes, even those that fall short of changes in behavior. Genuine change takes place incrementally over time, in ways that often are not visible to those persons who are too close to the intervention. Several important considerations for evaluating community-based interventions are shown in Table 25–2.[56]

Measuring the impacts of a program or policy should commonly rely on three interrelated levels of evaluation: process, impact, and outcome. Potential contributions of each type of evaluation will be presented, with a more comprehensive discussion available elsewhere.[64–66] Initially, one should seek to determine which (if any) changes have occurred as the result of a particular intervention through process and impact evaluation. *Process evaluation* is the analysis of inputs and implementation experiences to track changes as a result of a program or policy.[64,66] Process evaluation occurs at the earliest stages of a public health intervention and is often helpful in determining "midcourse corrections." *Impact evaluation* can be considered a subset of outcome evaluation that assesses whether intermediate objectives have been achieved. Indicators may include changes in knowledge, attitudes, or risk factor prevalence.[64,66] The long-term measures of effects rely on *outcome evaluation* such as changes in morbidity, mortality, and quality of life. As discussed earlier, *economic evaluation* is often an important component of an overall evaluation plan. Worksheets to assist communities in developing evaluations of community-based prevention efforts can be found in Johnson et al.[10]

The usual sources of measurement error should be considered when developing and implementing an evaluation plan—that is, validity and reliability. The most useful community-based interventions show high *internal validity* (i.e., Can the observed results be attributed to the program or intervention?). Further, *external validity* relates to whether the observed results can be generalized to other settings and populations. *Reliability* (or reproducibility) refers to the extent to which the same measurement is obtained on the same occasion by the same observer, on

Table 25–2 A Summary of Evaluation Principles and Tools

Principle	*Tool*
Community programs should include an assessment of program theory.	Logic models
Instruments that are used to measure community programs must be contoured to each individual community.	Questionnaires and surveys Social indicators
Approaches should be guided by the questions asked and often require both a quantitative and qualitative orientation.	Experimental and quasi-experimental designs Qualitative designs
Evaluation should be informed by social ecology and social system concepts.	Ecology and systems designs
Community evaluation should involve local stakeholders in meaningful ways.	Participatory planning

Source: Adapted from R.M. Goldman, Principles and Tools for Evaluating Community-Based Prevention and Health Promotion Programs, *Journal of Public Health Management and Practice,* Vol. 4, pp. 37–47, © 1998, Aspen Publishers, Inc.

multiple occasions by the same observer, or by different observers on the same occasion. An additional source of error in community-based interventions may result from inadequate implementation (so-called type III error).[67]

• • •

Community-based prevention is an iterative process involving the formation and management of community coalitions that develop, implement, and evaluate programs and policies to determine if the chosen activities should be continued, modified, or discontinued in the communities served. A flowchart and program example of these activities can be found in Figure 25–1 and Exhibit 25–1, respectively. One of the factors that makes community-based prevention distinct from more traditional programs and policies is the acknowledgment that dissemination of the program or policy cannot occur with-

Exhibit 25–1 Detroit's East Side Village Health Worker Partnership

Goal of coalition: To promote and conduct collaborative, community-based prevention research that strengthens the ability of communities to address and expand the knowledge base of public health regarding the health of women and children

Steering committee members (coalition): Detroit Health Department, a managed care organization, the University of Michigan School of Public Health, community organizations (see citations for descriptions of initial mobilization and establishment of organizational structure)

Risk identification—determining what is known through the scientific literature:

- Context assessment (preformation): population descriptives including migration patterns, housing patterns, and economic base; history of union and neighborhood organizing; policy–community relationships; and past racial tensions
- Review of secondary data including crime statistics and agency referral information
- 700-household face-to-face survey developed and implemented jointly by members of the coalition and others in the community
- In-depth interviews with village health workers, health department staff, and community-based organization staff
- Analysis of newspaper clippings

Program goals:

- To design, implement, and evaluate a collaborative village health worker intervention to address the factors associated with women's and children's health in the targeted area within east side Detroit
- To identify personal, interpersonal, organizational, community, and policy factors associated with poor health outcomes for women and children on Detroit's east side
- To increase village health workers' and community members' knowledge about and participation in strategies to modify risk and protective factors to improve the health of women and children

Activities at multiple levels of ecologic framework:

- Dissemination of survey findings to community members
- Training of village health workers
- Implementation of village health worker program
- Determining policy changes that can be made at local and state level

Evaluation of activities:

- Field notes at meetings
- Pre/post testing of training of village health workers
- Focus group interviews
- Documentation records by village health workers

Note: The above outline is organized according to the constructs presented in this chapter, and not necessarily using the language used within the project materials themselves. For additional information about this project, see E. Parker et al., "Detroit's East Side Village Health Worker Partnership: Community-Based Lay Health Advisor Intervention in an Urban Area," *Health Education Quarterly 25,* no. 1 (1998): 24–45 and A.J. Schulz et al., "Conducting a Participatory Community-Based Survey," *Journal of Public Health Management and Practice 4,* no. 2 (1998): 10–24.

out regard to community context. Thus, this is a process that occurs within and across communities, and must be repeated as definitions of the community change (e.g., change in racial group, religious group, or geographic location).

Many public health practitioners are beginning to recognize the importance of developing community-based prevention programs. These programs require the development of skills to work in interdisciplinary teams and with community members who represent a variety of subgroups in the population of interest, skills in collecting and interpreting data from a variety of sources, and program and policy development skills. The types of data and information that are available to assist practitioners in these tasks are at their fingertips as never before. Practitioners should be forewarned, however. The tools and skills suggested in this chapter are necessary but not sufficient. Developing community-based prevention programs requires practitioners to not only build skills, but also to build relationships in ways that are new in the field of public health. These programs often necessitate changes in traditional public health systems such as communication systems and financial accountability systems. The blending of community and scientific expertise entails learning from each other and developing common agendas and processes to reach joint goals.

CHAPTER REVIEW

1. Community-based prevention efforts should involve both members of the community and representatives of organizations that work with, or benefit, members of the community.
2. In developing community coalitions to address public health issues, it is important to identify and use existing resources in the community, as well as to build new capacities and relationships among individuals and organizations in the community. Some of these tasks must occur prior to the coalition development (preformation), some tasks need to be considered in the initial mobilization of the coalition, and others need to be addressed during the development of coalition structures.
3. One of the first decisions a community coalition must make is to decide the level of integration it wants to have with the other organizations and individuals in the community. The level of integration that is appropriate depends on the preferences of the participants regarding autonomy and control, the extent of familiarity and trust among participants, and the degree to which participants face shared objectives, incentives, and constraints.
4. In developing community-based interventions to address health issues, two levels of evidence should be considered by decision makers within the community coalition.
   - The first level of evidence, risk identification, is based on data showing the importance of a particular health issue and its link with some preventable risk factor.
   - The second level of evidence, program and policy development, focuses on the relative effectiveness of specific interventions to address a particular health issue.
5. Key actions to be performed by the community coalition in developing programs to address health issues include the following:
   - Develop an operational statement of the health issue.
   - Identify what is known about the issue through a review of scientific literature.
   - Determine what resources and expertise already exist in the community to address the health issue.
   - Identify all possible program and policy options to address the issue.
   - Develop an action plan to address the issue, which identifies preferred options and performance objectives.
   - Develop a strategy for evaluating the program or policy.

REFERENCES

1. Institute of Medicine, *The Future of Public Health* (Washington, DC: National Academy Press, 1988).
2. J. Fielding and N. Halfon, "Where Is the Health in Health System Reform?" *Journal of the American Medical Association* 272 (1994): 1,292–1,296.
3. Committee To Review the CDC Centers for Research and Demonstration of Health Promotion and Disease Prevention, *Linking Research and Public Health Practice: A Review of CDC's Program of Centers for Research and Demonstration of Health Promotion and Disease Prevention* (Washington, DC: National Academy Press, 1997).
4. B.A. Israel et al., "Health Education and Community Empowerment: Conceptualizing and Measuring Perceptions of Individual, Organizational and Community Control," *Health Education Quarterly 21,* no. 2 (1994): 149–170.
5. J.L. McKnight, "Redefining Community," *Social Policy* Fall/Winter (1992): 56–63.
6. E.A. Parker et al., "Coalition Building for Prevention," *Journal of Public Health Management and Practice 4,* no. 2 (1998): 25–36.
7. S.J. True, "Community-Based Breast Health Partnerships," in *Community-Based Prevention: Programs That Work,* eds. R.C. Brownson et al. (Gaithersburg, MD: Aspen Publishers, Inc., 1999), 173–181.
8. R.M. Goodman et al., "Identifying and Defining the Dimensions of Community Capacity To Provide a Basis for Measurement," *Health Education and Behavior 25,* no. 3 (1998): 258–278.
9. M.W. Kreuter et al., *Social Capital: Evaluation Implications for Community Health Promotion* (Geneva, Switzerland: WHO/EURO Working Group on Evaluating Health Promotion Approaches, 1997).
10. K. Johnson et al., *Collaborating To Improve Community Health: Workbook and Guide to Best Practices in Creating Healthier Communities and Populations* (San Francisco: Jossey-Bass Publishers, 1996).
11. T. Wolff and G. Kaye, *From the Ground Up! A Workbook on Coalition Building and Community Development* (Amherst, MA: AHEC/Community Partners, 1991).
12. C. Alter and J. Hage, *Organizations Working Together: Coordination in Interorganizational Networks* (Newbury Park, CA: Sage Publications, 1992).
13. T.D. Koepsell, "Epidemiologic Issues in the Design of Community Intervention Trials," in *Applied Epidemiology: Theory to Practice*, eds. R.C. Brownson and D.B. Petitti (New York: Oxford University Press, 1998), 177–211.
14. S.B. Thacker and R.L. Berkelman, "Public Health Surveillance in the United States," *Epidemiologic Reviews* 10 (1988): 164–190.
15. S.B. Thacker and D.F. Stroup, "Public Health Surveillance," in *Applied Epidemiology: Theory to Practice*, eds. R.C. Brownson and D.B. Petitti (New York: Oxford University Press, 1998), 105–135.
16. J.L. Annest et al., "Chronological Trend in Blood Lead Levels between 1976 and 1980," *New England Journal of Medicine* 308 (1983): 1,373–1,377.
17. D.B. Petitti, *Meta-Analysis, Decision Analysis, and Cost-Effectiveness Analysis: Methods for Quantitative Synthesis in Medicine* (New York: Oxford University Press, 1994).
18. G.V. Glass, "Primary, Secondary and Meta-Analysis of Research," *Educational Research* 5 (1976): 3–8.
19. S. Greenland, "Meta-Analysis," in *Modern Epidemiology,* 2d ed., eds. K.J. Rothman and S. Greenland (Philadelphia: Lippincott-Raven Publishers, 1998), 643–673.
20. S.N. Goodman, "Meta-Analysis in Health Services Research," in *Epidemiology and Health Services*, eds. H. Armenian and S. Shapiro (New York: Oxford University Press, 1998).
21. J.M. Samet and T.A. Burke, "Epidemiology and Risk Assessment," in *Applied Epidemiology: Theory to Practice*, eds. R.C. Brownson and D.B. Petitti (New York: Oxford University Press, 1998), 137–175.
22. World Health Organization, *Assessment and Management of Environmental Health Hazards* (Geneva, Switzerland: WHO/PEP, 1989).
23. I. Hertz-Picciotto, "Epidemiology and Quantitative Risk Assessment: A Bridge from Science to Policy," *American Journal of Public Health* 85 (1995): 484–491.
24. M.R. Gold et al., *Cost-Effectiveness in Health and Medicine* (New York: Oxford University Press, 1996).
25. D.B. Petitti, "Economic Evaluation," in *Applied Epidemiology: Theory to Practice*, eds. R.C. Brownson and D.B. Petitti (New York: Oxford University Press, 1998), 277–298.
26. M.C. Weinstein and W.B. Stason, "Foundations of Cost-Effectiveness Analysis for Health and Medical Practices," *New England Journal of Medicine* 296 (1977): 716–721.
27. E.I. Hatziandreu et al., "A Cost-Effectiveness Analysis of Exercise as a Health Promotion Activity," *American Journal of Public Health* 78 (1988): 1,417–1,421.
28. R.C. Brownson, "Epidemiology and Health Policy," in *Applied Epidemiology: Theory to Practice*, eds. R.C. Brownson and D.B. Petitti (New York: Oxford University Press, 1998), 349–387.
29. U.S. Preventive Services Task Force, *Guide to Clinical Preventive Services* (Baltimore: Williams & Wilkins, 1996).
30. L.F. Novick, "Public Health Practice Guidelines: A Case Study," *Journal of Public Health Management and Practice* 3 (1997): 59–64.

31. Council on Linkages between Academia and Public Health Practice, *Practice Guidelines for Public Health: Assessment of Scientific Evidence, Feasibility and Benefits: A Report of the Guideline Development Project for Public Health Practice* (Albany, NY: University of Albany, School of Public Health, 1995).
32. M. Pappaioanou and C. Evans, "Developing a Guide to Community Preventive Services: A U.S. Public Health Service Initiative," *Journal of Public Health Management and Practice* 4 (1998): 48–54.
33. D.A. Savitz et al., "Methods in Chronic Disease Epidemiology," in *Chronic Disease Epidemiology and Control*, eds. R.C. Brownson et al. (Washington, DC: American Public Health Association, 1998), 27–54.
34. R.J. Sampson et al., "Neighborhoods and Violent Crime: A Multilevel Study of Collective Efficacy," *Science* 277 (1997): 913–924.
35. E. Eng and E. Parker, "Measuring Community Competence in the Mississippi Delta: The Interface between Program Evaluation and Empowerment," *Health Education Quarterly 21,* no. 2 (1994): 199–220.
36. J.P. Kretzmann and J.L. McKnight, *Building Communities from the Inside Out* (Chicago: ACTA Publications, 1993).
37. J.P. Kretzmann and J.L. McKnight, *A Guide to Capacity Inventories: Mobilizing the Community Skills of Local Residents* (Chicago: ACTA Publications, 1993).
38. J. Goeppinger and A.J. Baglian, "Community Competence: A Positive Approach to Needs Assessment," *American Journal of Community Psychology* 13 (1985): 507–523.
39. Interhealth Organizations, *A Guide to Community Health Needs Assessment Tools* (Atlanta, GA: 1992).
40. National Civic League, *Civic Index Workbook* (Denver, CO: National Civic League, 1987).
41. P.G. Goldschmidt, "Information Synthesis: A Practical Guide," *Health Services Research* 21 (1986): 215–237.
42. T.G. Rundall, "Conducting and Writing Research Reviews," *Medical Care Research and Review* 53 (suppl.) (1996): S132–S145.
43. G.D. Gilmore and M.D. Campbell, *Needs Assessment Strategies for Health Education and Health Promotion,* 2d ed. (Madison, WI: Brown & Benchmark Publishers, 1996).
44. K.R. McLeroy et al., "An Ecological Perspective on Health Promotion Programs," *Health Education Quarterly 15,* no. 4 (1988): 351–377.
45. M. Simons et al., *Introduction to Health Education and Health Promotion* (Prospect Heights, IL: Waveland Press, 1995).
46. J.O. Prochaska and C.C. DiClemente, "Stages and Processes of Self-Change of Smoking: Toward an Integrative Model of Change," *Journal of Consulting and Clinical Psychology 51,* no. 3 (1983): 390–395.
47. J.O. Prochaska et al., "Patterns of Change: Dynamic Typology Applied to Smoking Cessation," *Multivariate Behavioral Research* 26 (1991): 83–107.
48. B.A. Israel, "Social Networks and Health Status: Linking Theory, Research and Practice." *Patient Counseling and Health Education 4,* no. 2 (1982): 65–79.
49. B. Israel, "Social Networks and Social Support: Implications for Natural Helper and Community Level Interventions," *Health Education Quarterly 12,* no. 1 (1985): 65–80.
50. E. Eng and R. Young, "Lay Health Advisors as Community Change Agents," *Family and Community Health* 151 (1992): 24–40.
51. E. Eng and J.W. Hatch, "Networking between Agencies and Black Churches: The Lay Health Advisor Model," *Prevention in Human Services 10,* no. 1 (1991): 123–146.
52. N. Milio, "Priorities and Strategies for Promoting Community-Based Prevention Policies," in *Community-Based Prevention: Programs That Work,* eds. R.C. Brownson et al. (Gaithersburg, MD: Aspen Publishers, Inc., 1999), 20–42.
53. P.M. Ginter et al., "Keeping Strategic Thinking in Strategic Planning: Macro-Environmental Analysis in a State Health Department of Public Health," *Public Health* 106 (1992): 253–269.
54. P. Florin and J. Stevenson, "Identifying Training and Technical Assistance Needs in Community Coalitions: A Developmental Approach," *Health Education Research* 8 (1993): 417–432.
55. C. Ham and M. Hill, *The Policy Process in the Modern Capitalist State* (New York: St. Martin's Press, 1984).
56. R.M. Goodman, "Principles and Tools for Evaluating Community-Based Prevention and Health Promotion Programs," *Journal of Public Health Management and Practice* 4 (1998): 37–47.
57. M.W. Lipsey, "Theory as Method: Small Theories of Treatment," in *Research Methodology: Strengthening Causal Interpretations of Nonexperimental Data,* eds. L. Sechrest et al. (Washington, DC: U.S. Government Printing Office, 1990), 211–234.
58. J.M. Bryson, *Strategic Planning for Public and Nonprofit Organizations. A Guide to Strengthening and Sustaining Organizational Achievement* (San Francisco: Jossey-Bass Publishers, 1995).
59. B.J. Turnock, *Public Health: What It Is and How It Works* (Gaithersburg, MD: Aspen Publishers, Inc., 1997).
60. T.C. Timmreck, *Planning, Program Development, and Evaluation. A Handbook for Health Promotion, Aging and Health Services* (Boston: Jones and Bartlett Publishers, 1995).
61. American Public Health Association, *Healthy Communities 2000: Model Standards: Guidelines for Community*

Attainment of the Year 2000 Health Objectives (Washington, DC: American Public Health Association, 1991).

62. D.T. Campbell and J.C. Stanley, *Experimental and Quasi-Experimental Designs for Research* (Boston: Houghton Mifflin, 1963).
63. T.D. Cook and D.T. Campbell, *Quasi-Experimentation: Design and Analysis Issues for Field Settings* (Boston: Houghton Mifflin, 1979).
64. L.W. Green and M.W. Kreuter, *Health Promotion Planning: An Educational and Environmental Approach* (Mountain View, CA: Mayfield, 1991).
65. P.H. Rossi and H.E. Freeman, *Evaluation: A Systematic Approach* (Newbury Park, NJ: Sage Publications, 1993).
66. B.A. Israel et al., "Evaluation of Health Education Programs: Current Assessment and Future Directions," *Health Education Quarterly 22,* no. 3 (1995): 364–389.
67. R.M. Goodman and A. Wandersman, "FORECAST: A Formative Approach to Evaluating Community Coalitions and Community-Based Interventions," *Journal of Community Psychology* (CSAP special issue) (1994): 6–25.

CHAPTER 26

Environmental Health Administration

Nadia Shalauta Juzych
Thomas A. Burke

The emergence of the federal Environmental Protection Agency and many state environmental agencies during the 1970s changed the structure and function of many environmental health programs in the United States. State health agencies were no longer the sole governmental entities that addressed public health issues involving air quality, drinking water, food safety, and solid waste management. Recently, significant policy shifts are contributing to a reemergence of public health organizations as leaders on important environmental health issues. At the local level, public health organizations have multiple responsibilities related to environmental health management.

The daily headlines and nightly news reflect the ever-increasing concern about the impact of the environment on public health. From concerns about power lines to genetically modified food, mosquitoborne infections to pesticides in food, public health organizations today face unprecedented demands to evaluate and respond to environmental health risks. The management of environmental health programs presents a formidable challenge to public health administrators, who must coordinate with a multitude of regulatory and public health organizations, develop multidisciplinary expertise, communicate risks to policy makers, and garner the resources necessary to develop an effective public health response.

Recognition of the critical role of the environment in human development, health, and disease has long been fundamental to the development of prevention strategies. Figure 26–1 presents the traditional epidemiologic triad, depicting the interaction of host factors, environment, and disease agents in the causation of human disease.[1] This triad illustrates the critical importance of a healthy environment in preventing disease, and has provided a time-tested model for public health practice. The epidemiologic triad was developed during a period when infectious diseases were the primary concern in environmental health.

Although the control of infectious waterborne and foodborne outbreaks remains an essential component of environmental health, prevention efforts have shifted toward the identification and control of adverse health effects from toxic pollutants in the environment. Figure 26–2 depicts the environmental health continuum, which tracks the path of environmental hazards from their source to their impact on community health. This continuum provides a framework for hazard, exposure, and health outcome surveillance that has shaped both public health and environmental regulatory programs in environmental health.

This chapter provides an overview of the historical development of environmental health programs in the United States, with a more comprehensive review of the current approaches and structure of services designed to implement environmental health and protection programs.

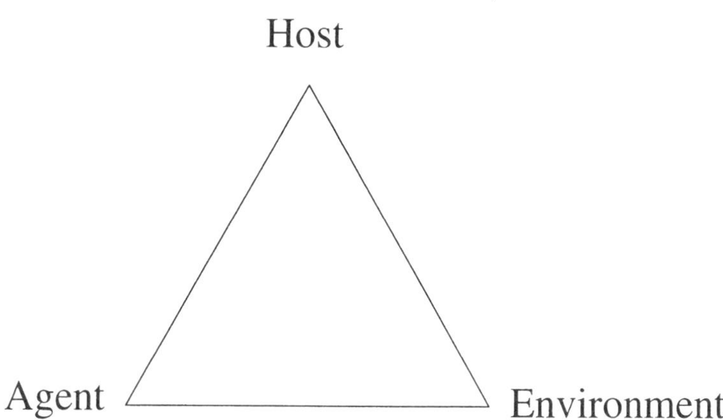

Figure 26–1 The Epidemiologic Triad. *Source:* Reprinted with permission from J. Mausner and A. Bahn, *Epidemiology: An Introductory Text,* p. 33, © 1974, W.B. Saunders Co.

The chapter also addresses the complex nature of the evolving public health work force and the challenge of training environmental health professionals. It concludes with a section on the future directions and needs for federal, state, and local public health organizations in order to achieve national environmental health goals.

THE HISTORICAL ROOTS OF ENVIRONMENTAL HEALTH

The role of environmental quality as an important determinant of public health has been recognized for many centuries. Archaeologic evidence dating as far back as 4,000 years has revealed drainage systems, bathrooms, and water delivery systems at the ancient Indian sites of Mohenjo-Daro in the Indus Valley and Harappa in the Punjab.[2] Later, Hippocrates noted the necessity of the balance between man and his environment in his book *Airs, Waters and Places*. In the book, Hippocrates first expressed the causal relationships between environmental factors and disease, and listed the factors that contribute to endemic disease in a population: climate, soil, water, mode of life, and nutrition.[2]

In the United States, early public health efforts were developed largely to address serious environmental health issues such as contaminated milk and drinking water, disease vectors, sanitation, and an unsafe food supply.[3] The 1850 *Report of the Sanitary Commission of Massachusetts* recognized the importance of environmental health and protection with the recommendation that "in laying out new towns and villages, and in extending those already laid out, ample provision be made for a supply, in purity and abundance, of light, air, and water; for drainage and sewerage, for paving, and for cleanliness."[4(p.153)]

Public health experts in Massachusetts also recommended regular surveys of health conditions and discussed the need for environmental sanitation, the regulation of food and drugs, and control of communicable disease.[5] The report thus characterized the focus of the first boards of health that were developed in major cities to concentrate on environmental sanitation.

In the 1850s in London, John Snow conducted his classic study of a cholera outbreak in which he studied the spatial pattern of disease in the population. He traced the risk to the drinking water source, and stemmed the outbreak by removing the handle of the infamous Broad Street pump.[2] This study, along with the discovery of microorganisms in the late nineteenth century, steered environmental health into microbiology and the control of infectious disease to combat epidemics of scarlet fever, diphtheria, typhoid fever, and tuberculosis.[6]

Through the early twentieth century, the sanitary movement was largely driven by the public

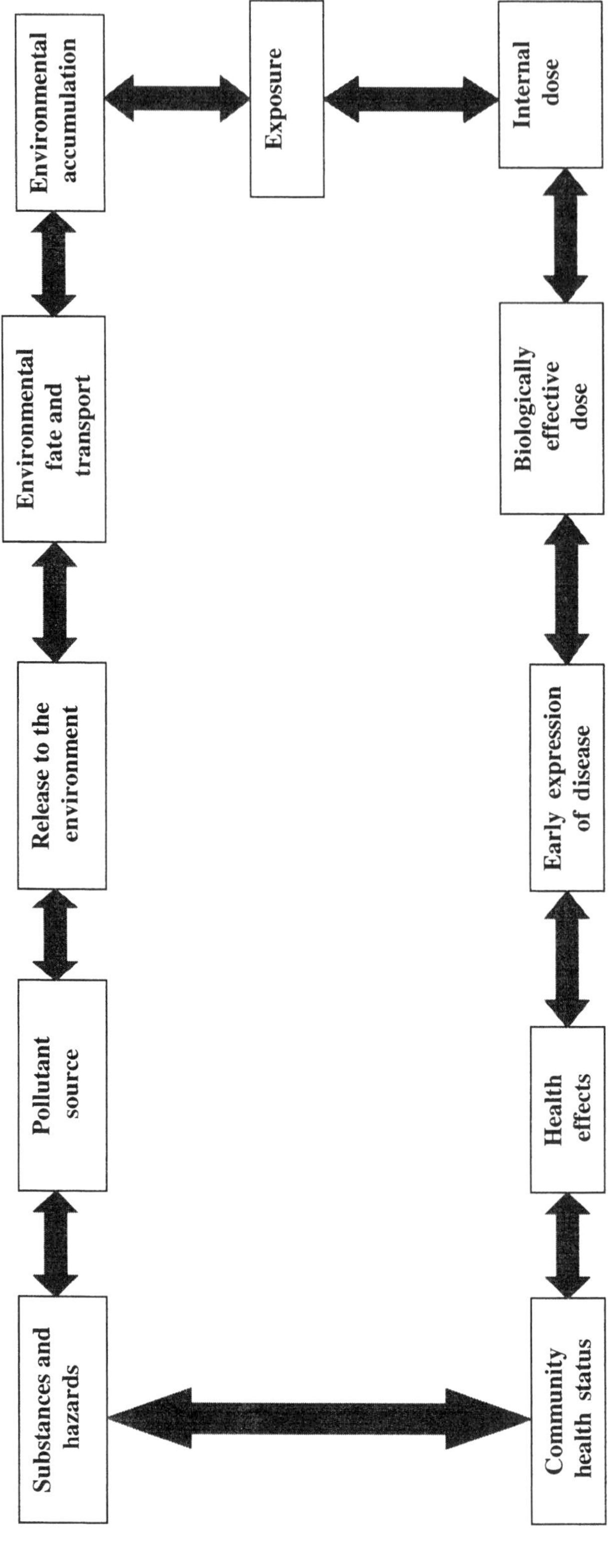

Figure 26–2 Environmental Health and Risk Management Continuum. *Source:* Adapted from K. Sexton, S.G. Selevan, D.K. Wagener, and J.A. Lybarger, Estimating Human Exposures to Environmental Pollutants: Availability and Utility of Existing Databases, *Archives of Environmental Health*, Vol. 47, No. 6, p. 339, 1992, Heldref Publications.

health community, which played a central role in the provision of sanitary water supplies, sewage disposal, and the establishment of food purity and safety programs.[7] By the 1940s and 1950s, concerns over the effects of chemicals in the food supply led to the development of standards for pesticides and pesticide residues in the Federal Food, Drug and Cosmetics Act.[8] Similarly, water pollution control efforts resulted in the passage of the Federal Water Pollution Control Act in 1948.[9] At the same time, incidents such as the emergency smog event in Donora, Pennsylvania in 1948 and the London Fog of 1952 galvanized public support for legislation addressing air quality and the control of industrial emissions, resulting in the passage of the Clean Air Act in 1955.[9]

The early 1970s in the United States brought not only the first Earth Day and the creation of the Environmental Protection Agency (EPA), but also a fundamental change in the administration and implementation of environmental health and protection services. The legislative flurry that followed the EPA's creation resulted in the formation of many state-level environmental protection agencies that took primary responsibility for environmental regulatory programs. No longer were state health departments the lead agency for the programs of clean air, drinking water, sanitation, food safety, and solid waste programs. The transition from a health-based approach for environmental health and protection programs to a regulatory approach has seen vast improvements in the quality of the environment; however, it has also contributed to the erosion of an essential public health infrastructure for environmental health. The shift of responsibilities has resulted in a detachment of public health organizations from many aspects of environmental regulation and decision making.[10]

SCOPE OF ENVIRONMENTAL HEALTH

What is meant by "environmental health?" Environmental health involves the application of multiple scientific disciplines to investigate the relationship between environmental factors and human health and prevent adverse health impacts from environmental exposures. A broad perspective that cuts across agency authorities is captured in the following description provided in *The Report on the Future of Environmental Health*.

> protection against environmental factors that may adversely impact human health or the ecological balances to long term human health and environmental quality, whether in the natural or human-made environment. These factors include, but are not limited to air, food and water contaminants; radiation, toxic chemicals, wastes, disease vectors, safety hazards, and habitat alterations.[11(p.28)]

Alternatively, the World Health Organization defined environmental health as comprising

> those aspects of human health, including quality of life, that are determined by physical, chemical, biological, social and psycho-social factors in the environment. It also refers to the theory and practice of assessing, correcting, controlling, and preventing those factors in the environment that can potentially affect adversely the health of present and future generations.[12(p.2)]

These definitions encompass both the environmental health and the regulatory aspects of the field and recognize the linkages that ultimately provide for the protection of human health. It is important to note that social and political processes are also inherent to environmental health and protection.

The Role of Public Health Organizations

The findings of a national evaluation of state environmental and public health organizations illustrate the core functions of health and environmental agencies.[10] Exhibit 26–1 presents the functions as a dichotomy divided into those functions representing primarily regulatory activities and those representing the traditional

Exhibit 26–1 The Core Functions of Environmental Health and Protection

Regulatory Functions

- Standard setting
- Permitting, registration, and licensing
- Inspection, monitoring, and enforcement
- Recordkeeping, reporting, and developing inventories
- Remediation and emergency response
- Laboratory support
- Litigation and administration

Public Health Functions

- Health surveillance and epidemiology
- Health risk assessment, toxicology, and applied research
- Communication, education, training, and consultation

Source: Adapted from T.A. Burke et al., The Environmental Web: A National Profile of the State Infrastructure for Environmental Health and Protection, *Journal of Public Health Management and Practice,* Vol. 3, No. 2, pp. 1–12, © 1997, Aspen Publishers, Inc.

public health activities.[10] The primary functions of public health organizations include health surveillance and epidemiology, applied research, communication, and training. These activities represent the traditional population-based techniques for evaluating, understanding, and responding to the control and prevention of disease and infirmity. Although public health organizations have diverse responsibilities for implementing environmental health and protection programs, it is environmental agencies that assume the lead responsibility for environmental protection in most states. At the national level, the primary functions of the EPA include activities related to permitting, licensing, enforcement, standard setting, environmental remediation, and the provision of laboratory services. These responsibilities are numerous and diverse, though they largely omit any related public health evaluations.

ORGANIZATION OF ENVIRONMENTAL HEALTH AND PROTECTION SERVICES

National Level

The decline of the role of the public health organization and the rise of the EPA as the primary regulator of the environment began with the first Earth Day in 1970. At this time, programs that had traditionally been the purview of governmental public health agencies were reorganized into environmental regulatory agencies at both state and national levels.[13] The U.S. Public Health Service, which was previously responsible for many environmental programs, witnessed a diminishing authority and a steady decline in resources for environmental health programs. The diminishing role of public health was highlighted in the 1988 Institute of Medicine (IOM) report, *The Future of Public Health*, which concluded that "the removal of environmental health authority from public health agencies has led to fragmented responsibility, lack of coordination, and inadequate attention to the health dimensions of environmental problems.[14(p.12)]

The resulting "balkanization" is evident in Figure 26–3, which presents the "environmental web" of agencies responsible for administering environmental health and protection programs.[10] The web illustrates the tremendous complexity of the national environmental health and protection infrastructure. At the same time, it demonstrates the important role of environmental health in virtually all aspects of major governmental activities. On the federal level, the legislative, judicial, and executive branches all play a major role in the shaping of policies and the implementation of environmental services. Environmental health and protection responsibilities are a part of the mission of a dozen major departments and agencies. From Defense to Housing and Urban Development, Energy to EPA, agencies with widely differing missions, separate and diverse regulatory mandates, and a plethora of organizational structures form the core of the federal efforts.

The structure and priorities of federal environmental health and protection agencies are

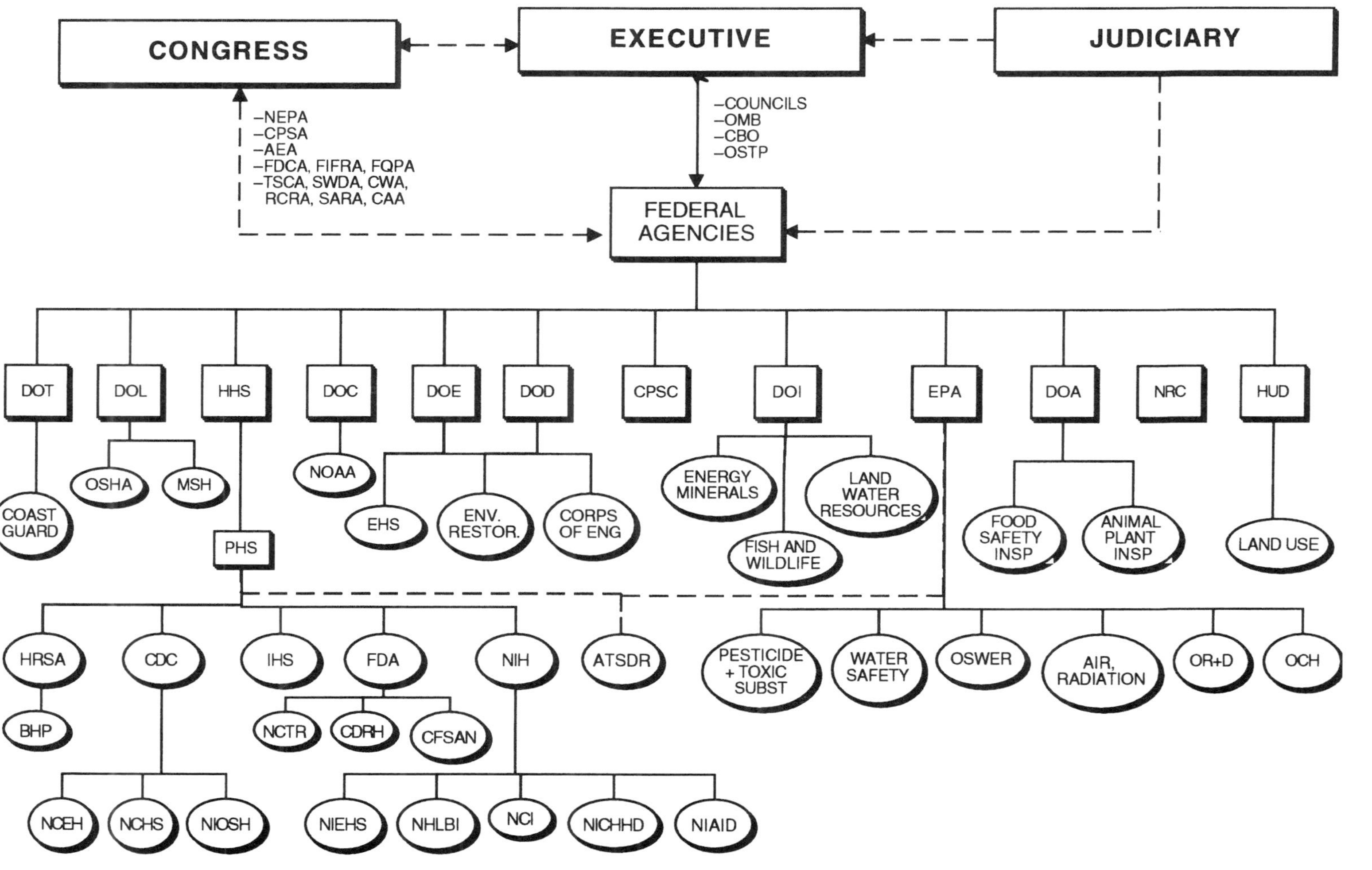

Figure 26–3 The Federal Environmental Web. *Source:* Reprinted from T.A. Burke et al., The Environmental Web: A National Profile of the State Infrastructure for Environmental Health and Protection, *Journal of Public Health Management and Practice,* Vol. 3, No. 2, p. 3, © 1997, Aspen Publishers, Inc.

Exhibit 26–2 Major Federal Environmental Statutes

- Clean Air Act
- Clean Water Act
- Food Quality Protection Act
- Federal Insecticide, Fungicide, and Rodenticide Act
- Comprehensive Environmental Response, Compensation, and Liability Act and Superfund Amendments and Reauthorization Act
- Resource Conservation and Recovery Act
- Safe Drinking Water Act
- Toxic Substances Control Act
- Occupational Safety and Health Act
- Public Health Service Act
- Federal Food, Drug, and Cosmetic Act

largely determined by the major environmental laws.[15] As listed in Exhibit 26–2, these laws have shaped the regulatory funding and authorities of the agencies. As a result, the Public Health Service continues to have important responsibilities for environmental health and protection; however, support for evaluating and addressing public health concerns is greatly lagging behind the regulatory programs. For example, support for the Agency for Toxic Substances and Disease Registry (ATSDR) public health assessment efforts under Superfund was 3.5 percent of the total monies for remediation and enforcement activities in 1998.[16]

State-Level Environmental Health and Protection Services

Because most of the actual implementation of environmental services occurs on the state level, the major federal environmental laws have provided the states with a blueprint for their organization.[15] "Mini-EPAs" have become the dominant model for state-level environmental protection agencies. The state agencies presented in Figure 26–4 do not represent any actual state organization, but rather a collective representation of the structures of state agencies involved in environmental services.[10]

In many ways, the states mirror the complexity of the federal bureaucracy but are 50 times more diverse. Although federal mandates obviously influence state organization, the state web is further complicated by the dynamic influences of state laws, policies, budget cycles, and political changes in the statehouse. In one sense, the web can be interpreted as support for the findings of the IOM report, which stated that the nation suffers from "environmental fragmentation," the result of dividing responsibility for environmental programs among hundreds of federal and state agencies.[14] However, it is perhaps more appropriate to interpret the web as an illustration of the tremendous "diversification" of environmental health and protection services that have emerged as a result of the ever-increasing recognition of the importance of the environment in virtually all aspects of government.

Although many state environmental health and protection programs stem from federal legislation, there are also many state efforts that are not derived from the statutory mandates. Such programs may be established by state law (i.e., state safe drinking water laws), be a response to nonregulatory federal guidelines (i.e., lead and radon), or represent traditional public health functions at the state level (i.e., epidemiology and sanitation). Exhibit 26–3 lists the major programs implemented by the agencies to fulfill their environmental health and protection goals.[10] The programs range from media and substance-specific programs, such as air and water pollution control and lead screening, to broad-based programs of food safety and Brownfields redevelopment.

Local Environmental Health and Protection Services

Local environmental health and protection services are administered by an even greater diversity of agencies than the federal and state programs. At the local level, governmental health departments and other agencies vary considerably and may represent a town, city, county, or district—virtually any administrative unit smaller than a state.[17] At the local level, the goals

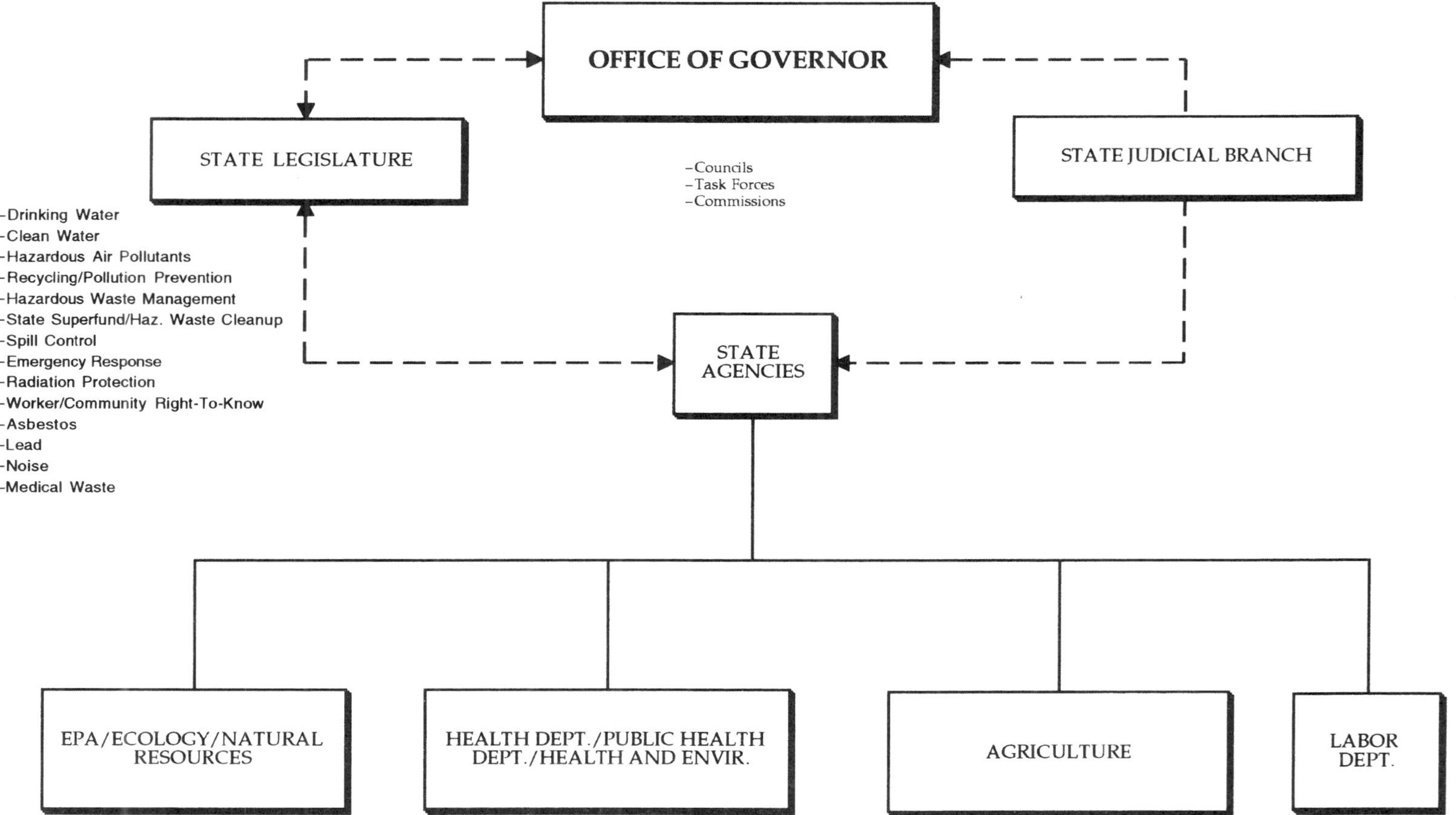

Figure 26–4 The State Environmental Web. *Source:* Reprinted from T.A. Burke et al., The Environmental Web: A National Profile of the State Infrastructure for Environmental Health and Protection, *Journal of Public Health Management and Practice,* Vol. 3, No. 2, p. 3, © 1997, Aspen Publishers, Inc.

Exhibit 26–3 Environmental Health Programs Administered by Federal, State, and Local Agencies

- Air pollution control
- Asbestos
- Asthma/allergic disease
- Brownfields
- Cancer research/registries
- Children's environmental health
- Disease prevention
- Disease surveillance
- Drinking water safety
- Education/training
- Endocrine disrupter
- Environmental epidemiology and health surveillance
- Environmentally related emergency response
- Exposure surveillance
- Farm worker protection
- Food safety
- Hazardous waste site clean-ups
- Information systems
- Indoor air quality
- Ionizing and nonionizing radiation protection control
- Lead screening and abatement
- Occupational safety and health (other than farm workers)
- Pesticides
- Pollution prevention
- Radon
- Sanitation and waste management
- Tobacco/environmental tobacco smoke
- Toxic substance-related programs/poison control
- Water pollution control

Source: Reprinted from T.A. Burke et al., The Environmental Web: A National Profile of the State Infrastructure for Environmental Health and Protection, *Journal of Public Health Management and Practice,* Vol. 3, No. 2, pp. 1–12, © 1997, Aspen Publishers, Inc.

of environmental health and protection agencies are varied and are specific to the local jurisdiction. These goals may include pollution prevention, zoning and planning, economic development, and public health. Many programs are administered with the guidance of local statutory mandates that address not only the media-specific concerns of air, water, and waste, but also noise and nuisance concerns, as well as land use and redevelopment.

Reflecting on the example of Philadelphia, there are at least six local-level agencies with responsibility for some aspect of environmental health, including the city departments of health, streets, planning, water, fire, and the mayor's office.[18] The Philadelphia Department of Health administers many environmental health and protection programs, including the Air Management Services division, which is responsible for the permitting of air pollution sources. The Streets department provides sanitation services and is responsible for cleaning up illegal dumpsites. In Philadelphia, an important environmental health role is carried out by the Department of Planning, which oversees land use activities and is involved in zoning decisions. The Department of Water ensures the quality of drinking water for the citizens of Philadelphia; the Fire Department administers the emergency response provisions of the Superfund Amendments and Reauthorization Act of 1986.[18] The mayor's office oversees the local emergency planning commission and is involved in a variety of environmental health programs in concert with the other departments. Clearly, the administration of environmental health programs requires communication, cross-agency cooperation, and an understanding of the lines of authority.

Within health departments, a broad variety of public health services are provided to ensure the health of their constituencies. According to the National Association of County and City Health Officials (NACCHO), local health agencies administer programs ranging from epidemiology and surveillance and food and milk inspection to lead abatement and screening and solid waste management.[17] In addition, they work with the state and federal agencies on cooperative agreements to implement various programs. For example, since 1994, the ATSDR has worked with communities living near hazardous waste disposal sites to develop environmental health education programs.

Local health departments (LHDs) often work with local boards of health that provide guidance and assistance to the departments. In addition, community partnerships and collaborative relationships play an increasingly large role in contemporary environmental health practice. There is increasing recognition of the importance of stakeholder interactions, which provide a means to pool resources and information. In 1997, 83 percent of LHDs reported collaboration with state health agencies, 67 percent worked with hospitals, 64 percent with nonprofit and voluntary groups, and 52 percent with universities and academic centers.[17]

The environmental health responsibilities of LHDs are very diverse. However, LHDs often lack sufficient resources to meet the many demands placed on them. Effective environmental health surveillance, which tracks potential hazards, exposures, and community health status, is key to the effective administration of environmental programs. In many cases, agencies collect extensive health data on their communities but lack sufficient resources for thorough analysis and dissemination. Thus, opportunities to use community health data to shape priorities and prevention strategies are missed.[10]

THE CONTRAST BETWEEN RISK-BASED ENVIRONMENTAL REGULATORY APPROACHES AND SURVEILLANCE-BASED PUBLIC HEALTH

The federal laws that provide EPA its mandates have resulted in tremendous improvements in the quality of air and water and have led to the restoration and preservation of many natural resources. However, the major federal environmental legislation has also compartmentalized the environment into specific media, and has led to the increased use of quantitative risk assessment as a metric for environmental decision making.[15] Although risk assessment has been used informally and intuitively for many years, the publication of the National Academy of Sciences report, *Risk Assessment in the Federal Government: Managing the Process* (commonly known as the "Red book") resulted in wide adoption of risk assessment as the basis for policy decisions.[3,19] Despite their heavy reliance on mathematical models, risk assessments have been used widely for setting standards for programs as diverse as occupational exposure and drinking water to Superfund site clean-up levels. Understanding and applying risk assessment has become an essential competency in environmental health administration.

Although both risk assessment and public health approaches share the goal of protecting public health, the increased dependence on risk assessment has resulted in a departure from human population-based studies. Quantitative risk assessment has been driven by identification of the biologic and toxicologic properties of a chemical substance, whereas the public health assessment begins with an evaluation of the human health status and subsequently attempts to elucidate causes of disease.[20] Table 26–1 presents a contrast of the regulatory risk assessment approaches and the public health approach for addressing environmental health.

The risk assessment approach is generally driven by a single hazard and is pollutant specific in its approach. In contrast, the public health approach is driven by population health impacts. As codified in 1983 in the Red book, risk assessment follows a four-step process—hazard identification, dose-response assessment, exposure assessment, and risk management.[19] This process contrasts with the core public health functions—assessment, policy development, and assurance—as defined by the IOM.[14]

The risk management step is analogous to policy development and assurance, although assurance implies a continual evaluation of interventions.[13] Risk assessment maintains heavy reliance on toxicology and mathematical modeling of exposure and of environmental fate and transport to predict risk. Cancer has been the primary health concern for many regulatory risk assessment applications, although in recent years, there is increasing concern about a broader range of health endpoints including acute respiratory, reproductive, neurological, and endocrine effects. There is also increased

Table 26–1 Comparison of the Risk Assessment and Public Health Approaches

Goal: The Protection of Public Health		
	Risk Assessment	*Public Health*
Driver	Single hazard	Population health impact
Approach	Pollutant specific	Population based
Process	Hazard identification Dose-response assessment Exposure assessment Risk characterization Risk management	Assessment Policy development Assurance
Health endpoint	Limited (cancer); changing	Diverse/multiple
Tools	Toxicology, modeling	Surveillance
Agencies	Federal/state	Local/community
Outputs	Standards, regulations	Intervention strategies
Actions	Permitting, enforcement, monitoring	Outreach, screening, treatment
Solution	High tech/pollutant specific	Low tech/broad based
Public values	No mechanism for inclusion	Essential component of intervention strategy
Decision making	Top–down	Bottom–up
Success	Regulatory compliance	Community health improvement

Source: Adapted with permission from T. Burke, N.M. Shalauta, and N.L. Tran, Strengthening the Role of Public Health in Environmental Policy, *Policy Studies Journal,* Vol. 23, No. 1, pp. 76–84, © 1995.

concern about cumulative risks from multiple exposures over a lifetime. Risk assessment is an important tool for informing regulatory and prevention strategies, but has limited application in the evaluation of actual health impacts at the community level. Despite this limitation, the capacity to conduct and apply environmental risk assessments is key to managing environmental health risks.

In contrast to the risk-based regulatory approach, the traditional public health approach largely relies on epidemiologic surveillance of population morbidity and mortality for a broad range of health outcomes. The agencies involved in the two approaches also provide a sharp contrast. Most public health programs are carried out at the local level, with strong community input and support. Risk assessment is structured by the national environmental regulations that provide for a strong federal/state partnership of regulatory agencies with limited participation of the local-level organizations. With risk assessment, the outputs are regulations and standards administered by the federal or state agency with reliance on permitting, monitoring, and enforcement, often requiring high-tech controls. Under the public health model, intervention strategies are developed with the community and the actions include outreach, screening, and treatment, which are generally low tech. Perhaps the most significant difference between the models are the measures of success. Driven by statutory mandates, environmental regulatory agencies define success in terms of regulatory compliance, whereas public health agencies measure their success in terms of improved population health status.[15]

Each of the models has its strengths and weaknesses, and ideally, the public health and risk assessment approaches draw on and complement one another. An example of success where the two approaches have been applied is illustrated by the case of lead. When the deleterious effects of lead on IQ and the development of children were identified, the EPA banned the use of lead in gasoline, established a national standard for lead in drinking water, and limited the content of lead in drinking water pipes. In coordination with these regulatory efforts, the U.S. Centers for Disease Control and Prevention (CDC) implemented a surveillance-based public health approach. The public health efforts were implemented by local health agencies and included community education on the hazards of lead and methods to control exposure, outreach efforts to educate medical care providers, identification of children at high risk for lead exposure through screening, and development of medical management approaches. These efforts have resulted in a 78 percent decrease in blood lead levels for the U.S. population.[21] Lead provides a striking example of the value of using both the regulatory risk-based approach and the public health approach in environmental health. The complementary strategy of the regulatory and public health agencies has resulted in dramatic decreases in the percentage of children who are exposed to high levels of lead in their environment, as shown by decreasing blood lead levels nationwide. The third *National Health and Nutrition Examination Survey* showed that the percentage of children with blood lead levels above 10 μg/dL fell from 88 percent in 1976–80 to 6 percent in 1988–94.[21]

The contrasting, yet complementary, roles of risk assessment and surveillance underscore the multidisciplinary nature of contemporary environmental health practice. It is essential that environmental health professionals develop an understanding of the concepts and applications of risk assessment in order to strengthen traditional approaches to managing environmental health risks, effectively meet the mandates of contemporary environmental health, and respond to ever-increasing public concerns regarding environmental risk.

CHALLENGES OF ENVIRONMENTAL HEALTH MANAGEMENT AND ADMINISTRATION

The administration of environmental health programs poses a host of managerial, political, scientific, and fiscal challenges. The following paragraphs present an overview of these challenges.

Politics

Although political pressures and considerations are a part of all aspects of public health administration, it must be recognized that the high level of public concern, increasing community development pressures, and costs of environmental regulation have combined to make environment a major political issue throughout the country. Effective administration requires recognition and response to these political pressures while maintaining a focus on the primary goal of protecting public health.

Bridging the "Cultures" of Environmental Protection and Health

Environmentalism is founded on public health principles, but includes a broader consideration of ecologic and quality-of-life considerations. Public health organizations need to recognize and endorse the values of the environmental community while acknowledging that public health practice often requires difficult trade-offs. The aerial spraying of pesticides in New York City in the fall of 1999 to control disease-carrying mosquitoes presents an example of the difficult decisions with which public health officials are faced. In September 1999, the CDC confirmed the first three cases of serious illness as a mosquitoborne viral disease, which was later identified as the West Nile virus.[22,23] The health department responded with the aerial spraying of malathion and other pyrethroid pesticides that are effective in eliminating adult mosquitoes. Malathion, however, is toxic to birds, fish, and other animals, but only slightly toxic to humans. Addressing the health risks required public health officials to consider a difficult decision that required balancing the ecologic risks posed by malathion to the human health threats posed by the West Nile virus.

Understanding the Web of Authorities and Responsibility

The complex web of agencies responsible for various aspects of environmental health and protection has been discussed. The effective administration of environmental health programs requires an understanding of these diverse roles and responsibilities, established communication protocols, and the formal development of cooperative problem-solving approaches. Agency "turf" issues are prevalent in environmental health and must be recognized and overcome.

Funding

Ensuring adequate funding for environmental health in public health organizations is a continual challenge. Little support is available for the core functions of environmental health assessment and response to public concerns. Administrators must take advantage of funding opportunities from the EPA and state environmental regulatory agencies and develop partnerships with academia and the business community. In addition, there are increasing opportunities to make the case for increased budget appropriations by capitalizing on strong public demand for preventing adverse health impacts from environmental pollution.

Setting Priorities

Clear priorities, based on sound public health principles, are essential to environmental health administration. The ideal situation is to have strong hazard, exposure, and health outcome information, supported by active stakeholder involvement to shape and support policy decisions. In reality, the current capacity to track and assess environmental and health outcome data is woefully inadequate. To avoid continually shifting "crisis of the week" priorities, it is essential to have an established priority-setting process. The community environmental health assessment process developed by NACCHO and the U.S. Department of Health and Human Services (DHHS) environmental health goals in *Healthy People 2010* can provide useful guidance.[24,25]

Measures of Success

The ability to sustain environmental health programs is ultimately dependent on the ability of administrators to demonstrate to policy makers and the public that their tax dollars have been well spent. Therefore, it is essential that environmental health programs have established performance indicators. Environmental health surveillance can provide an approach for tracking trends of environmental hazards such as air and water contamination, community exposure levels, and health outcomes such as outbreaks or trends in environmentally related diseases.

Multidisciplinary Work Force

A manager is only as good as the talent he or she is able to assemble. Environmental health requires the expertise of a multitude of disciplines including law, chemistry, toxicology, epidemiology, and environmental science. Attracting and retaining talented professionals is a continual challenge for environmental health administrators. (See Chapter 16 for a more detailed discussion of recruiting and managing human resources.) Approaches to the development of the environmental work force are presented in the following section.

Personnel and Training

What is the most appropriate educational background for a leader in environmental health or environmental protection? Physicians and public health professionals have historically provided the leadership in this field.[26] In many regards, this remains true today, particularly in the academic community. However, the change from a public health–based environmental approach to a regulatory approach for environmental programs in the 1970s had a profound influence on the environmental health and protection work force. When the programs of environment were removed from the public health agencies, the work force evolved to what is currently a work force trained in a broad range of discipline-specific specialties: from medicine to law, geology, physics, and economics. This diversification has had many positive influences on environmental progress. However, it has also resulted in a discipline whose focus has shifted away from the public health aspects of environmental health, and the proportion of professionals with formal training in public health has dramatically declined. Current strategies for addressing environmental health risks involve end-of-pipe controls that do not adequately consider possibilities for prevention.

In 1997, the Health Resources and Services Administration and the Johns Hopkins University convened the Crossroads Colloquium, a forum of leaders in environmental health and protection, to address state and federal agency work force needs.[27] The participants consisted of individuals from a variety of federal and state environmental agencies, as well as academics and private sector participants. Among the findings of the colloquium were that the current environmental health and protection work force is inadequately trained to address emerging environmental threats. Several recommendations were provided to improve the training of the work force in order to ensure that the nation will be able to fulfill its mission for the protection of populations from environmental threats in the new millennium. Among the major themes that emerged were the needs for

- providing training and education in multidisciplinary core competencies
- establishing partnerships between agencies, academia, industry, and philanthropic organizations for training students/existing work force and funding educational/training programs
- developing practical approaches that provide experiential learning for students
- redefining approaches to training that include a range of options from didactic sessions in the classroom and distance learning to hands-on experiential learning and employee mentoring

The following sections summarize the major themes of the Crossroads Colloquium.

Multidisciplinary Core Competencies. The multidisciplinary nature of the field of environmental health and protection has brought together students and practitioners with a wide variety of educational and practice backgrounds. To establish cohesive and complementary approaches for solving the nation's environmental health problems, there is a need to establish a broad-based curriculum that includes core competencies. Areas of more specialized training where students may choose an area of emphasis or expertise once core competencies have been achieved should remain a part of the curriculum. The Public Health Faculty/Agency Forum first described the need for developing a work force skilled in various disciplines and defined competencies for practitioners of environmental health and protection "to raise the level of future practice."[28] The competencies defined then have been refined and provide the fundamental skills that are desired for leaders and practitioners in environmental health and protection agencies today. Table 26–2 presents the refined list of the competencies and curricula desired for practitioners in environmental health and protection.

The four categories of competencies include technical sciences, public health sciences, political and social sciences, and risk sciences. Within each of these categories are listed more specific skills that are desirable for a practitioner of environmental health and protection. The skills and curricula listed under *technical sciences* provide a strong scientific foundation, which is necessary to understand the basis of *environmental health sciences.* The *public health sciences* provide a basis for understanding and evaluating disease in human populations. *Political sciences* provide a foundation for understanding the public policy process, which is essential to the formulation and implementation of environmental health and protection programs. Although cultural skills provide an understanding of the human context in which the policies will be implemented, *risk sciences* provide a framework for managing and organizing data and serve as an increasingly important tool in the environmental health and protection policy process.

Training in a broad core knowledge complemented by specialized advanced training is analogous to that of medical training where a core of knowledge is required for all students in medical school, after which the physicians may choose to specialize in a given field of interest. Although multidisciplinary training alone will not ensure the improved application of public health approaches in environmental protection, improving the expertise of the work force is a first step toward integrat-

Table 26–2 Core Competencies and Curricula for Environmental Health Practitioners

Core Competencies	*Core Curricula*
Technical sciences • Basic sciences • Environmental sciences • Environmental engineering/sustainable technology	• Biology, chemistry, microbiology, parasitology, physics, hydrology, toxicology • Ecology, geology, environmental fate and transport • Environmental sampling and data analysis • Environmental and occupational exposure control and prevention
Public health sciences • Epidemiology of acute and chronic diseases associated with environmental and occupational stressors • Biostatistics • Communicable disease/chronic disease	• Public health methods • Epidemiology • Biostatistics • Laboratory science
Political and social sciences • Political skills • Managerial and organizational skills • Economics/decision theory • Environment law • Ethics • Cultural issues	• Local, state, and federal agency organization and functions • Political processes and institutions • Management and organizational theory • Economics/cost–benefit evaluation • Decision theory • Environmental law • Ethics
Risk sciences • Risk assessment skills • Risk management skills • Risk and other communication skills	• Risk assessment/exposure assessment • Risk management • Risk communication and perception

Source: Adapted from N.M. Shalauta et al., *Journal of Public Health Management and Practice,* Vol. 5, No. 6, pp. 1–12, © 1999, Aspen Publishers, Inc.

ing the core functions of public health into environmental decision making.

Partnerships for Training and Funding. To address the challenge of training the environmental health and protection work force, a real need exists to develop interdisciplinary programs based on partnerships. Professionals from industry, government, and academia should be involved in teaching and advising students to increase opportunities for experiential training. Practitioners provide "real world" perspectives to learning that are invaluable to professional development. There are numerous opportunities for partnerships, including adjunct faculty appointments, internships, personnel exchanges, and on-the-job training. In addition, opportunities exist for collaboration among the agencies for providing educational and training opportunities to the work force. Various environmental agencies and industry also have needs for trained practitioners in the field of environmental health and protection. Establishing partnerships and pooling resources can provide revenue sources.

Experiential Learning. More than a decade ago, the IOM recognized that "the provision of public health services is uneven and needs strengthening across the nation, partly due to a lack of well-qualified professionals" and "some schools (of public health) have become somewhat isolated from public health practice."[14(p.15)] These findings underscore the isolation of public health education from public health practice that remains to this day. This is particularly acute in the field of environmental health and protection, where the emphasis on research in schools of public health has reduced the opportunity for students to develop practical, hands-on skills. Traditional discipline-based education does not address the realities of current environmental health practice. Cross-discipline experiential training opportunities, such as those present in programs accredited by the national Environmental Health Science and Protection Accreditation Council, must be more fully developed to prepare more personnel for the contemporary environmental health workplace. This will allow students to gain an appreciation for the interplay of science, politics, economics, law, and public values that define efforts in environmental health and protection.

Range of Training Options. Education and skill development may be achieved through various means, including formal course work for degree programs, certificate programs, on-the-job training, distance learning, and professional continuing education (Exhibit 26–4). As previously noted, most practitioners in environmental health lack formal training in public health, whereas those who have a public health background may need training in other areas, including management, economics, law, and policy. Continuing education, including distance education, can provide accessible opportunities for enhancing competencies. This range of approaches offers flexibility of content and broad options to match varying levels of available resources and time commitment.

Exhibit 26–4 Approaches for Continuing Education for Environmental Health and Protection Practitioners

- Interdisciplinary graduate programs
- Short courses
- Symposia
- Certificate series
- Distance learning
- Internships
- Interagency personnel shifts
- On-the-job mentoring
- Executive degree programs

Source: Adapted from N.M. Shalauta et al., *Journal of Public Health Management and Practice,* Vol. 5, No. 6, pp. 1–12, © 1999, Aspen Publishers, Inc.

FUTURE DIRECTIONS: THE REEMERGENCE OF PUBLIC HEALTH IN ENVIRONMENTAL PROTECTION

Thus far, this chapter has described the diminishing role of public health organizations in environmental policies over the past three decades. Recently, however, there have been a number of significant policy shifts that indicate a reemergence of public health. Exhibit 26–5 lists a number of fundamental changes in approaches to environmental policy that have occurred in the recent past. These changes have evolved gradually and have been influenced by a wide range of scientific, social, and political factors. However, one message is clear—*public health is gaining the lead as the driver of evolving environmental policies.*

Exhibit 26–5 The Reemergence of Public Health in Environmental Protection

- Interagency partnerships
- Broadening statutory mandates
- Multimedia/cross-media approaches
- Cumulative/aggregate risk guidance
- Focus on disease prevention
- Application of epidemiology and health surveillance
- Development of public health indicators
- Community-based approaches
- Increased participation of the medical community

As Exhibit 26–5 indicates, the focus of environmental policy is changing. There is a clear shift away from single-substance, single-media approaches toward a more comprehensive community health approach. Perhaps the clearest example of the change is the current Children's Environmental Health Initiative. In May 1997, the Office of Children's Health Protection was created to support the EPA's implementation of the presidential executive order and to coordinate children's health issues across the EPA. The fundamental goal of this initiative is to improve the health of children by understanding and preventing adverse effects from environmental exposures.[29] This initiative is a partnership between the EPA and the DHHS, which has combined the surveillance-based approaches of public health with the regulatory authorities of the EPA to examine the health of children and develop broader, more effective prevention strategies. This initiative has enlisted the participation of the medical and academic community by establishing academic-based centers of excellence with a strong community base.

Other examples of the shift include the current multi-agency strategies to implement the Food Quality Protection Act, the development of community-based environmental protection strategies, and the consideration of a broader range of health endpoints in regulatory decisions. The Environmental Justice Movement has refocused national attention on community health concerns, and an increasing number of studies have demonstrated the failure of media- and chemical-specific national policies to address cumulative risks on the community level. Emerging concerns regarding persistent pollutants and the human health implications of environmental endocrine-disrupting pollutants have underscored the need for improved health and exposure information. In addition, congressional efforts to bring about regulatory reform have underscored the need to provide better answers to the fundamental question: Do current environmental regulatory strategies protect public health? This question has led to increased recognition of the need for improved public health surveillance data.[30]

The application of epidemiologic methods and population health surveillance is increasing in environmental protection. Public health and exposure surveillance provided the epidemiologic basis for new Clean Air Act regulations to reduce exposure to fine particulates and ozone.[31] Concerns of the medical community regarding increasing childhood asthma were confirmed by population surveillance data, leading to a multi-agency national priority to improve childhood respiratory health. As policies shift from source regulation to preventing adverse health outcomes, integrated approaches that involve the medical and public health communities will be essential.

Exposure surveillance also represents an important interface between environmental protection and public health. As illustrated in the environmental health continuum (Figure 26–2), understanding population exposure to pollutants is essential to understanding and preventing risks to public health. Unfortunately, much of the environmental monitoring that is conducted for regulatory purposes provides little information concerning actual human exposure levels. This has hampered the epidemiologic evaluation of environmental risks, and left an essential policy question unanswered: Have our environmental laws been successful in reducing exposure to harmful pollutants? Exposure surveillance will become increasingly important as priorities shift toward cumulative risk reduction and disease prevention. The most comprehensive national evaluation of individual exposures is currently being implemented as part of the fourth *National Health and Nutrition Examination Survey (NHANES IV)*.[32] Previous *NHANES* data proved invaluable to clinicians and policy makers in reducing lead exposures and preventing lead poisoning. Expanded exposure surveillance data will provide an invaluable resource to environmental health professionals. It is an essential component of the bridge between public health and environmental protection.

Environmental health remains a vibrant and growing pillar of the nation's public health infrastructure. Although traditional public health agency roles have changed, the number and diversity of federal, state, and local agencies and their responsibilities have expanded dramatically. This has resulted in growing opportunities and challenges for environmental health professionals. Although the administration of environmental health programs presents formidable challenges, the opportunities to improve public health and preserve the quality of the environment have never been greater.

CHAPTER REVIEW

1. A dichotomy of functions exists between state environmental and public health agencies. For environmental agencies, regulatory functions predominate, including standard setting, permitting, inspection, and enforcement. For health agencies, primary functions include surveillance and epidemiology, health risk assessment, communication, and education.
2. There is a sharp contrast between the regulatory risk assessment approach of environmental agencies and the public health approach in tackling environmental problems.
   - Risk assessment is usually driven by a single hazard and relies on toxicology and mathematical modeling of exposure.
   - Public health approaches rely on epidemiologic surveillance of population health outcomes.
3. Local environmental health and protection services are administered by an even greater diversity of agencies than at the state and federal level.
4. The application of epidemiologic methods and population health surveillance is increasing in environmental protection.
5. Lead toxicity provides an example of the value of combining both the regulatory risk-based approach and the public health approach in environmental health. A dramatic decrease in the percentage of children with elevated blood lead levels has been documented.
6. The multidisciplinary nature of the field of environmental health brings together students and practitioners with diverse backgrounds. There is a need to establish broad-based training curricula to develop competencies to address the nation's environmental health problems.

REFERENCES

1. L. Gordis, *Epidemiology* (Philadelphia: W.B. Saunders Co., 1996).
2. G. Rosen, *A History of Public Health* (Baltimore: Johns Hopkins University Press, 1993).
3. L.J. Gordon, "Environmental Health and Protection," in *Principles of Public Health Practice,* eds. F.D. Scutchfield and C.W. Keck (Albany, NY: Delmar Publishers, Inc., 1997), 300–317.
4. L. Shattuck et al., *Report of the Sanitary Commission of Massachusetts* (Boston: Harvard University Press, 1850).
5. E. Fee, "History and Development of Public Health," in *Principles of Public Health Practice,* eds. F.D. Scutchfield and C.W. Keck (Albany, NY: Delmar Publishers, Inc., 1997), 10–26.
6. D.S. Blumenthal and A.J. Ruttenber, *Introduction to Environmental Health,* 2d ed. (New York: Springer Publishing Co., 1995).
7. B. Rabe, "Environmental Health Policy" in *Public Health Administration and Practice,* eds. G. Pickett and J.J. Hanlon (St. Louis, MO: Times Mirror/Mosby College Printing, 1990), 317–330.
8. Federal Food, Drug and Cosmetics Act, 21 U.S.C. 301, chapter 9, subchapter IV, section 3431. http://www4.law.cornell.edu/uscode21/ch9.html. Accessed 15 September 1999.
9. U.S. Environmental Protection Agency. "Summary of the Major Laws Implemented by the Environmental Protection Agency." http://www.epa.gov.
10. T.A. Burke et al., "The Environmental Web: A National Profile of the State Infrastructure for Environmental Health and Protection," *Journal of Public Health Management and Practice 3,* no. 2 (1997): 1–12.
11. Committee on the Future of Environmental Health, National Environmental Health Association, "The Future

of Environmental Health, Part One," *Journal of Environmental Health 55,* no. 4 (1993): 28–32.

12. U.S. Department of Health and Human Services, Environmental Health Policy Committee, Risk Communication and Education Subcommittee. "An Ensemble of Definitions of Environmental Health." http://web.health.gov/environment/DefinitionsofEnvHealth/ehdef2.htm (20 November 1998). Accessed 26 June 2000.
13. T.A. Burke, "Back to the Future: Rediscovering the Role of Public Health in Environmental Decision-Making," in *Handbook for Environmental Risk Decision-Making,* ed. C. Richard Cothern (Boca Raton, FL: CRC Press–Lewis Publishers, 1996), 93–101.
14. Institute of Medicine, *The Future of Public Health* (Washington, DC: National Academy Press, 1988).
15. T. Burke et al., "Strengthening the Role of Public Health in Environmental Policy," *Policy Studies Journal 23,* no. 1 (1995): 76–84.
16. Environmental Protection Agency, *EPA Budget 1988.* http://www.epa.gov/ocfopage/1998bib.pdf. Accessed 2 October 1999.
17. National Association of County and City Health Officials, "Preliminary Results from the 1997 Profile of U.S. Local Health Departments," *Research Brief Series* 1 (September 1988).
18. T.A. Burke and N.M. Shalauta, *Final Report for the Pilot Multi Media Environmental Health Characterization Study of South and Southwest Philadelphia.* Prepared for Region III of the Environmental Protection Agency, 1997.
19. National Research Council, *Risk Assessment in the Federal Government: Managing the Process* (Washington, DC: National Academy Press, 1983).
20. E.K. Silbergeld, "A Proposal for Overcoming Paralysis in Improving Risk Regulation," in *Regulating Risk: The Science and Politics of Risk,* eds. T.A. Burke et al. (Washington, DC: International Life Sciences Institute Press, 1993), 45–47.
21. U.S. Department of Health and Human Services, National Center for Health Statistics. *National Health and Nutrition Examination Survey II* (conducted 1976–1980) and *National Health and Nutrition Examination Survey III* (conducted 1988–1994).
22. S. Mullin and J. Gadd, *City Department Reports Three Cases of St. Louis Encephalitis (SLE) in Queens* (Press release) (New York: New York City Department of Health, Office of Public Affairs, 3 September 1999).
23. S. Mullin and J. Gadd, *Overview of the West Nile Virus Outbreak in New York City* (Press release) (New York: New York City Department of Health, Office of Public Affairs, 19 November 1999).
24. U.S. Department of Health and Human Services, *Healthy People 2010.* Conf. ed. (Washington, DC: U.S. Government Printing Office, 2000).
25. National Association of County and City Health Officials. "Protocol for Assessing Community Excellence in Environmental Health." http://www.bixler.com/naccho/GENERAL182.htm. Accessed 26 June 2000.
26. T.A. Burke, The Re-Emergence of Public Health in Environmental Protection (Paper presented at the National Leadership Forum on Environmental Education of Health Care Professionals, Washington, DC, June 11–12, 1998).
27. N.M. Shalauta et al., "An Examination of the Educational Needs for Environmental Health and Protection," *Journal of Public Health Management and Practice 5,* no. 6 (1999): 1–12.
28. A.A. Sorensen and R.G. Bialek, eds., *The Public Health Faculty/Agency Forum: Linking Graduate Education and Practice* (Washington, DC: Health Resources and Services Administration and Centers for Disease Control).
29. Environmental Protection Agency, Office of Children's Health Protection. "Our History." http://www.epa.gov/children/whowe/history.htm. Accessed 10 October 1999.
30. T.A. Burke et al., "Unanswered Questions: The Missing Link between Health and Environment." A report for the Pew Environmental Health Commission, September 20, 1999.
31. Health Effects Institute, "Particulate Air Pollution and Daily Mortality: Analyses of the Effects of Weather and Multiple Air Pollutants." The Phase IB report of the Particle Epidemiology Evaluation Project, March 1997.
32. U.S. Department of Health and Human Services, National Center for Health Statistics, *National Health and Nutrition Examination Survey IV* (in progress).

Chapter 27

Public Health Laboratory Administration

Scott J. Becker
Eric C. Blank
Robert Martin
Michael Skeels

Public health laboratories (PHLs) serve as engines of epidemiologic investigation and scientific inquiry for the public health delivery system. Imperatives for reliability, precision, timeliness, and efficiency continually challenge PHLs to improve how their work is organized and managed. As a further challenge, laboratories must interface with a broad array of health and medical care organizations in performing their core analytic activities. Public health organizations in both governmental and private settings depend on effective working relationships with the PHL system. Such relationships develop only through informed managerial decision making by laboratories and the public health organizations they serve.

The public health laboratory (PHL) has been a driving force behind the development and evolution of public health practice. The discoveries of the late nineteenth century linking microorganisms to disease, coupled with the basic epidemiologic principles developed by Snow and others, form the foundation on which public health practice is built.[1] Yet, the PHL remains an enigma to the public and even to those within public health, as well as to the larger health care community.

HISTORY OF THE PHL

PHLs are important components of the public health infrastructure in the United States, not only because all states have them, but also because they serve a crucial purpose, which is to provide scientifically valid diagnostic and analytic data for the assessment, assurance, and policy development functions of state health agencies.[2] According to Valdiserri, two key components are necessary in order for PHLs to exist: an adequate public health infrastructure *and* a strong knowledge base that supports laboratory practice as an integral part of scientific inquiry.[1] Today, these two factors are taken for granted, but they only came into being in the United States following the age of industrialization in the late 1800s. Two distinct features of that time, urbanization and population growth, created health problems that were unlike anything seen before. The health effects on society related to overcrowding, substandard housing, and the lack of proper sanitation were far greater and more pervasive than any that had previously been encountered. Cities and local governments were forced to adopt boards of health and to take direct action to address these problems. In the mid- to late 1800s, many larger cities implemented improved public health statutes and laws that provided a more "permanent administrative foundation" for public health activities by creating independent boards of health composed of physicians and sanitarians.[3]

Unlike the prompt action that was taken to create formal public health boards, the application of laboratory science to public health took much longer to develop. Scientific methods took time to root, and as new discoveries were added to the knowledge base, laboratory investigation slowly moved from the realm of the alchemist to the scientist and eventually became recognized as an essential component in scientific problem solving.[1] Late in the nineteenth century, scientists began to use laboratory-based investigations in their studies of hygiene and sanitation. In 1870, the Massachusetts State Board of Health asked a preeminent scientist, William Ripley Nichols, to "investigate the sanitary conditions of water supplies by laboratory methods."[4]

The singular scientific discovery that advanced PHLs was the germ theory of disease. Louis Pasteur's seminal work on fermentation disproved the theory of spontaneous generation and brought science to the brink of accepting the germ theory by the late 1850s.[3] Twenty years later, Robert Koch proved that the microorganism, *Bacillus anthracis*, was the cause of the disease known as anthrax.[5] Shortly thereafter, the causative agents for leprosy (1880), typhoid fever (1880), tuberculosis (TB) (1882), cholera (1883), and diphtheria (1883) were discovered.[3] In 1887, one of the first American research laboratories of bacteriology was founded at the Marine Hospital on Staten Island, New York.[6] This institution was later moved to the Washington, D.C. area, and became known as the National Institutes of Health (NIH). In 1888, Rhode Island, Kansas, and Michigan opened PHLs. By now, government had organized into public health departments and scientific knowledge had advanced to the point where the two could merge in the form of a new American institution—the PHL.

Science and Policy

PHLs grew in role and scope throughout the early 1900s, largely in response to the evolution of science, technology, and public policy. Throughout the twentieth century, advances in science and technology have provided new and improved tests for disease surveillance and diagnosis within the PHL. At the same time, public policy has changed the way that both public health and private health care are delivered. Consequently, the PHL is also evolving.

LOCAL, STATE, FEDERAL CONTINUUM

State PHLs are found now in all states and in many of the territories of the United States. Each state organizes its own "local" PHL system. In some states, this means that the state PHL operates a few branch laboratories, or, as in the case of California, state law mandates that the state provide PHL services for areas serving populations of 50,000 or more. State PHLs are an integral part of two systems: state public health systems and a "national PHL network." These systems demand uniformity of data, prompt integrated reporting, and the ability to change directions quickly with each new emerging threat to the community. State PHLs provide data to public health programs at the national, state, and local levels, and to other agencies, physicians, community health leaders, and sometimes directly to the consumer. However, PHLs do not operate as isolated institutions.

PHLs are an integral part of a public health system and must work closely with many diverse health-related programs such as TB control, lead abatement, human immunodeficiency virus (HIV)/acquired immune deficiency syndrome (AIDS), maternal and child health (MCH), and water quality monitoring, to name a few. Laboratory services for these programs must be accurate, precise, reliable, comparable, timely, cost-effective, and properly interpreted. The data derived from the laboratory analyses must be available to public health officials in a form that they can use to devise control measures to protect the public.[7] A PHL must also be involved in the initial planning and implementation of public health programs and studies to ensure that appropriate technology and quality assurance measures are used, that relevant specimens are collected, that measurements are completed in a timely manner, and that results are interpreted with suitable corrective actions.

PHLs exist at all levels of government—city, county, state, and federal. In many states today, the PHL is prescribed by state law. Even in states without statutory language concerning the PHL, policy makers have continually supported PHL services. State PHLs work most often with laboratories at the federal level, generally the U.S. Centers for Disease Control and Prevention (CDC); local laboratories work most often with the state laboratory. This local–state relationship is important so that specimens flow up to the appropriate level within the system for testing, but also so that information (and laboratory-based disease reporting) flows to all levels and back for follow-up. State PHLs serve a wider constituency than just their respective states. Each PHL is an important part of a national and global public health network that provides surveillance and data necessary for disease intervention or control. A schematic diagram of this local–state–federal continuum, also known as the national laboratory system for public health testing, can be found in Figure 27–1. Federal laboratories are operated in several federal agencies, including the Environmental Protection Agency (EPA), the Food and Drug Administration (FDA), the U.S. Department of Agriculture (USDA), NIH, and the CDC. Local and state PHLs rely on their federal counterparts for assistance during outbreaks, specialized testing, and in other situations that require expertise and capacity beyond what is available at the state level. Frequently, states also call on each other to provide surge capacity, and for testing that may not be routinely offered. In this way, each state can avoid replicating services that may be found nearby.

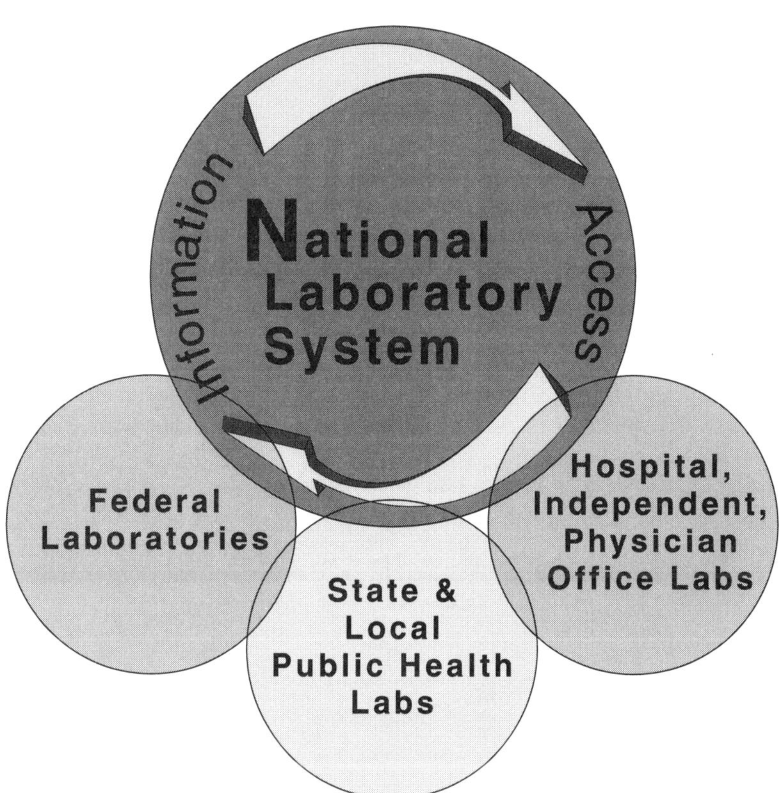

Figure 27–1 National System for Public Health Testing. *Source:* Public Health Practice Program Office, Centers for Disease Control and Prevention.

Many large cities have PHLs, which can rival state laboratories in terms of size, complexity of testing services, and in some cases, budget and/or personnel. Local PHLs are almost always organizational units within city/county health departments. Most local PHLs provide reports directly to the state laboratory or some other statistical interface within the state. One notable exception is New York City, which has a reporting function directly to the CDC for nationally notifiable diseases. There are 800–1,000 "local" PHLs in the United States.[8]

Organizational Models of State PHLs

There are three models for the organization of state PHLs in the United States today: (1) within a state health department, (2) university based or affiliated, and (3) within another state agency, known as a consolidated laboratory. The advantages and disadvantages of each model are presented in Table 27–1.

By far, the most common setting for PHLs is within a traditional health department. The Association of Public Health Laboratories (APHL) estimates that 44 state laboratories fit this general model.[8] The laboratory in this model is usually found at the same organizational level as other divisions or bureaus within the agency, such as epidemiology or MCH. It is often housed at the central health agency facility or in close proximity. This setting facilitates communication between and among laboratory scientists and program managers in the agency. In this model, the laboratory director often reports directly to the health commissioner or to a deputy

Table 27–1 Advantages and Disadvantages of Public Health Laboratory Organizational Models

Model	*Advantages*	*Disadvantages*
State health agency	– Integrated with customers because the laboratory is part of the same organization – Usually colocated or close by for ease of communication and coordination – Fully dedicated to public health	– Limited resources; competition for resources with other units in the health agency – Laboratory may be contained within another unit of the health agency, so laboratory issues, inititatives, and concerns are "buried" or not addressed – Interactions between laboratory and programs are muted by the bureaucracy
University based or affiliated	– Enriched atmosphere of science, access to libraries, and plethora of skilled employees – Isolation from political influence and vested interests of state agencies – Isolation from fiscal trimming at the state agency level – Flexibility to create separate funding streams	– Isolation from agencies' support and political processes – Agency perception that the university has excess funding; isolation from the political process and support – Location within university as an orphan with a dissimilar mission
Other state agency (e.g., consolidated laboratory for entire state)	– More diversified testing – Specialized staff – Operational efficiencies	– Laboratory support for public health is not factored into planning because the laboratory is not part of the health agency – Multiple and sometimes conflicting demands for services

commissioner. If the laboratory facility is not located jointly with the central health agency, it is often found on or near the campus of a major state university. This is not coincidental; PHLs, among many other functions, are often capable of conducting applied research. Being located or colocated with a university offers benefits to both the academician and the practitioner, and allows the PHL access to facilities the state agency may not have, such as teleconferencing, library services, and the like. This model allows for increased communication and collaboration among the "clients" of the PHL, principally the other organizational units of the health agency and local health departments (LHDs).

The second most frequent model is university based or affiliated. There are two state PHLs that have their institutional base in universities: the University Hygienic Laboratory in Iowa (University of Iowa) and the Wisconsin State Laboratory of Hygiene (University of Wisconsin-Madison). An increasing number of state PHLs are affiliated with the state university system, including Massachusetts (The University of Massachusetts-Jamaica Plain), Nevada (University of Nevada-Reno), and Nebraska, where the health agency has contracted the PHL functions to the University of Nebraska Medical Center. The academic model offers many benefits to the state laboratory. This model gives the laboratory an enriched atmosphere of science, access to libraries, and a plethora of skilled employees. Other benefits include the isolation of the lab from political influence and vested interests of state agencies and protection from fiscal trimming at state agency level. This model also allows the lab the flexibility to create separate funding streams.[9]

The third model is the consolidated laboratory, which is characterized by having its organizational home in a state governmental agency other than the health agency. The single state successfully using this model is the state of Virginia. The Virginia Division of Consolidated Laboratory Services (DCLS) is part of the Virginia Department of General Services, similar to the federal government's General Services Administration. Agencies outside of the health arena use the services of the DCLS, such as Agriculture and Consumer Services, Chesapeake Bay Assistance, Criminal Justice Services, Fire Programs, and Lottery, among others. This model affords the rapid adoption of new technology because many customers help support the infrastructure and there exists "dual use" for some equipment. A consolidated structure also requires greater attention to customer service because the laboratory may not always be "at the table" with the customer when plans are being drawn up and decisions are being made that could affect the laboratory.[10]

ROLE AND SCOPE OF PHLs

Core Functions of PHLs

PHLs provide a set of core functions that are vital to the nation's public health system, as illustrated in Exhibit 27–1. Although their specific services may vary depending on local needs and practices, PHLs share a common mission to support local, state, and federal public health programs. These programs include environmental health, disease control and prevention, MCH, epidemiology, and emergency response. Many PHLs also provide primary laboratory services for at-risk populations seen in community clinics. In addition to performing analytic testing, PHLs help ensure the quality of all medical and environmental laboratories through training, consultation, and regulatory activities. They also participate in evaluating or adapting new technologies, and in conducting epidemiologic studies and other applied research. When natural or human-caused emergencies occur, PHLs respond quickly to help identify and control public health threats.

The success of PHLs is built on a foundation of solid communications with many partners and an orientation toward delivering excellent service. One essential part of this communication is helping the PHL's constituents use laboratory services appropriately and make the most of the information generated. This can take many forms, including consultation, education, support, and outreach to the laboratory's clients. For

Exhibit 27–1 Core Functions of State Public Health Laboratories

Disease prevention, control, and surveillance

Provide accurate and timely data for the surveillance and control of infectious, genetic, and chronic diseases, and environmental exposures.

Act as the first line of defense and the center of expertise in the rapid recognition and response to communicable disease outbreaks.

Perform specialized tests for low-incidence, high-risk diseases such as tuberculosis, rabies, botulism, and plague; detect epidemiologic shifts and emerging pathogens.

Conduct population surveillance (or screening) for conditions of public health interest, such as neonatal metabolic disorders, toxic environmental exposures, antibiotic resistance, and chronic diseases.

Integrated data management

Act as the focal point for the aggregation, analysis, linkage, and dissemination of scientific information in support of public health programs.

Provide data for epidemiologists, practitioners, and other laboratories to identify health trends and sentinel events.

Reference and specialized testing

Serve as a reference microbiology laboratory for pathogens of public health importance: confirming or verifying results of other laboratories, providing oversight for quality assurance, testing epidemiologically important specimens, and fully identifying or typing disease agents referred from clinical laboratories.

Offer diagnostic testing for diseases of public health importance that are too rare or unusual for other laboratories to maintain the capacity to test.

Provide toxicology testing, including drug, alcohol, toxin, and trace metal analysis.

Environmental health and protection

Conduct scientific analyses of environmental samples (air, water, soil) to identify and monitor potential threats to human health and ensure compliance with environmental regulations.

Provide scientific data to determine the relationship between environmental hazards and human health.

Provide testing to support occupational health programs, including analyses for hazardous chemicals, microorganisms, and radioactive materials.

Food safety

Test human and food samples for pathogenic microorganisms implicated in foodborne illness outbreaks.

Analyze or monitor food samples to detect, identify, and quantify toxic chemical and radioactive contaminants.

Laboratory improvement and regulation

Promote quality assurance programs in private clinical and environmental laboratories through training, consultation, certification, and proficiency testing.

License, certify, or accredit laboratories to ensure that medical, environmental, and toxicology laboratories meet state and federal requirements.

Set a standard of analytic excellence for public and private laboratory performance and ensure the reliability of laboratory data used for communicable disease control and environmental monitoring.

Policy development

Contribute to state and federal policy development through scientific leadership and integration of laboratory science into practice.

Emergency response

Provide laboratory support as part of state and national disaster preparedness plans in response to environmental or health emergencies.

Offer rapid identification of biologic, chemical, and radiologic agents regardless of the source of exposure (accident, terrorism, or natural disaster).

Ensure the surge capacity to analyze a large volume of samples during an emergency quickly and accurately.

Public health-related research

Evaluate and implement new technologies and methods to ensure that the most accurate, cost-effective, and timely services are used to support public health and community health care.

Collaborate with academic, governmental, and private sector researchers to develop and adapt emerging technologies to public health laboratory practice.

Participate in epidemiologic and health services research to identify the distribution and determinants of disease in communities.

continues

Exhibit 27–1 continued

Training and education

Sponsor or provide training activities for working laboratorians in medical and public health laboratories in order to help maintain the highest level of scientific knowledge and technical skills.

Provide short- and long-term training opportunities to prepare scientists for careers in public health laboratory practice.

Partnerships and communication

Develop and strengthen partnerships among state, federal, and local public health agencies, business, academia, and health care organizations to promote and improve community health.

Participate in planning and policy development and communicate the role of laboratories in achieving public health goals.

Maintain ongoing communication with public health leaders, program managers, administrators, and elected officials.

Source: Adapted with permission from *Core Functions and Capabilities of State Public Health Laboratories*, © 1999, Association of Public Health Laboratories.

example, all PHLs should provide clients with a comprehensive guide to services that details the laboratory's services and how to access them, including sample collection and submission, appropriate tests to request, interpretation of results, and how to obtain additional information. This guide should be available in both hard copy and electronic formats, accessible through the PHL's Web site. In addition, the PHL should communicate proactively with its clients via the Internet, newsletters, bulletins, presentations, conferences, and personal visits, especially when there are major changes in policies or procedures. PHL staff should also be included as partners in any public health team that is planning programs and projects that have a laboratory component. PHL staff represent a valuable resource and can help identify potential problems and solutions.

PHLs can also demonstrate leadership by hosting training events and activities for laboratorians, and can use these events to provide education and outreach for the PHL's clients. PHL staff can give inservices and updates wherever key clients are gathered, such as hospital infection control meetings, public health nursing conferences, medical grand rounds, and epidemiology or environmental health staff meetings. The explosion in scientific information and technology has made it more important than ever for PHLs to take the lead in communicating with constituents.

The PHL must be perceived by its constituents as visible, approachable, and relevant. The PHL director must do everything possible to encourage active communication, responsiveness to clients, and a service orientation among all staff. For example, when new tests or methods are introduced, there must be complete communication to clients regarding their interpretation, limitations, and appropriate use. Also, PHLs must understand that their clients are often working in an urgent environment, and that test results must be communicated in "real time." PHL staff should demonstrate the same sense of immediacy when carrying out their own work and providing information. This is a challenge, because PHLs are often far removed from the point of patient care or public health intervention. However, to truly serve their constituents, PHL staff must go the extra mile to provide timely, enthusiastic support and communication.

Clinical Laboratories and PHLs

Disease surveillance and reporting are the backbone of communicable disease control, and laboratories play a central role in this system at the local, state, and federal levels.[11] Both clinical laboratories and PHLs are vitally important in reporting infectious diseases and identifying community outbreaks.

Private sector clinical laboratories contribute directly to public health efforts in at least two major ways: by diagnosing and reporting infectious diseases, and by referring microbial isolates to PHLs for confirmation and typing.[12] Clinical laboratories generate a large portion of the communicable disease reports in the United States, as well as diagnostic information for a wide array of chronic conditions of public health interest, such as toxic exposures (e.g., pesticides, lead), cancer, and cardiovascular disease. These laboratories are an integral part of community health efforts. However, the primary emphasis of clinical laboratories is diagnosing active disease for individual patient care, and cost containment pressures have made it more difficult for them to perform "extra" testing and referral for public health purposes.[12,13] This threatens their ability to work with public health departments to monitor health status and control disease outbreaks.

Contribution of PHLs

For more than a century, PHLs have been providing scientific data as a basis for public health decision making and protective actions.[14] They play a crucial role in disease surveillance by providing primary laboratory services for high-risk clients, plus specialized reference microbiology, serology, and molecular typing to identify disease clusters and sources. PHLs fill a special niche for "low-frequency, high-intensity" diseases such as rabies, plague, botulism, and anthrax. They are expected to respond to public health crises and emergencies, whether caused by floods, storms, earthquakes, or bioterrorist attacks. In addition to microbiology, PHLs provide a wide array of other analytic services, including environmental chemistry, toxicology, and neonatal metabolic screening. The nation's PHL system includes local, state, and federal laboratories working as a network to serve the entire U.S. population. The state PHLs alone test more than 20 million samples per year.

The role and scope of PHLs change constantly as new diseases emerge, technologies advance, public health priorities shift, and private sector capacity changes. Historically, PHLs have been the first to provide laboratory services to control infectious disease threats in populations, including syphilis, TB, gonorrhea, *Chlamydia*, and HIV. As diseases are brought under control, PHLs turn their attention to newly emerging threats such as *E. coli* O157:H7, hepatitis C, or antibiotic-resistant mycobacteria. They have also been the traditional providers of laboratory services for poor and uninsured clients seen in public clinics and community health centers. During the past decade, PHLs have continued these services while expanding their environmental monitoring for chemical and microbial hazards ranging broadly from volatile organic compounds to dioxins and *Cryptosporidium*.

Clinical and PHL Partnership

The public health system depends on both clinical laboratories and PHLs to protect and preserve the health of communities. Although private sector laboratories are focused mainly on the care of individual patients, they are on the front lines of detecting community illnesses, and they provide important case reports and microbial isolates for disease monitoring and surveillance. PHLs work at the population level to help identify epidemiologic trends and sentinel events, while offering specialized reference testing and primary services for vulnerable populations. It is vitally important that public and private sector laboratories work as partners to ensure high-quality scientific support for public health. See Exhibit 27–2 for a case study of PHL and clinical laboratory partnership for laboratory-based surveillance.

The PHL–clinical laboratory partnership has several dimensions and varies widely in different locales. One major component of this relationship is information exchange, both formal and informal. In their work together, PHL and clinical laboratory staff exchange day-to-day information concerning specific reference samples and significant findings. Sometimes, unique or interesting microscope slides, cultures, or digital images are shared between colleagues in PHLs and clinical laboratories. A more formal exchange of information occurs when clinical materials or cultures are referred to PHLs for epide-

Exhibit 27–2 Case Study: Laboratory-Based Disease Surveillance

Under Oregon law, certain microbial isolates in clinical laboratories must be referred to the Oregon State Public Health Laboratory (OSPHL) for typing. These include *Salmonella* and other enteric pathogens. In January 1996, an alert microbiologist at the OSPHL noticed a sudden upswing in the number of *Salmonella enterica* serotype Newport isolates being submitted, an unusual finding. He alerted epidemiologists, who soon learned that British Columbia was experiencing a similar outbreak, although no other part of the United States had reported increased Newport isolates. Foodborne illness was suspected, and the psychological profile of the vehicle suggested a widely distributed food eaten mainly by adults, perhaps preferred by women, and usually eaten away from home. The culprit turned out to be alfalfa sprouts from a 40,000 pound lot of seeds imported from the Netherlands into Kentucky, part of which was shipped to Oregon and British Columbia. To germinate, the seeds were kept warm and moist for five to seven days, creating an ideal environment for rapid bacterial growth. The mechanism of original contamination of the seeds was never determined. With the cooperation of sprout growers, distributors, and regulatory agencies, the remaining seeds and sprouted product were embargoed or recalled.

Although this outbreak resulted in at least 128 cases of salmonellosis (and perhaps hundreds more), public health agencies were able to stop the human consumption of these seeds as a result of (1) clinical laboratories isolating and referring samples to the OSPHL, (2) a well-trained and conscientious public health laboratory staff with the capacity to type and identify unusual pathogens, and (3) excellent regional, national, and international communications between laboratories, epidemiologists, the business community, and the public. This case illustrates the central role of laboratories in the early recognition, confirmation, and control of infectious disease threats to the community. Without this capacity, the outbreak might have gone on undetected to further generations of infection and other parts of the United States.

Source: Adapted with permission from Oregon Health Division, Salmonellosis Outbreak Traced to Alfalfa Sprouts—Oregon and B.C., *CD Summary,* Vol. 45, No. 4, pp. 1–2, © 1996, Center for Disease Prevention and Epidemiology, Oregon Health Division.

miologic purposes. In fact, a second major dimension of the PHL–clinical laboratory partnership is disease surveillance. Clinical laboratories are often required to refer "reportable" bacterial or viral isolates to PHLs for confirmation and typing. Also, in addition to routine disease reporting, clinical laboratories can alert PHLs and epidemiologists when they see something out of the ordinary, such as new pathogens or disease clusters. A close working relationship between the PHL and clinical laboratories makes it more likely that this will happen.

As a third aspect of this partnership, PHLs and clinical laboratories sometimes contract with each other to provide specific services. For example, PHLs may refer low-volume testing such as measles IgM serologies or biochemical confirmation of rare metabolic disorders to private reference laboratories. Similarly, clinical laboratories may contract with PHLs to provide tests that are highly specialized or unique, such as TB cultures, or tests where the high volume of public health work provides an economy of scale, such as HIV serologies. Also, PHLs can play a role in advising public health agencies that wish to contract with clinical laboratories, for example, by reviewing contracts for quality assurance requirements.

A fourth dimension of the PHL–clinical laboratory relationship is in providing technical assistance and training. PHLs vary widely in their capacity to provide training. The National Laboratory Training Network has enhanced the ability of many PHLs to host training in specific areas of laboratory practice. However, few PHLs have the ability to develop and provide training across the entire range of clinical laboratory departments. Understandably, most of the training emphasis has been in microbiology. Outside of formal workshops or bench training, PHLs are often asked to assist clinical laboratories in implementing tests or solving problems, again mainly in microbiology. This may take the form of a simple telephone call, or a visit by the clinical laboratorian to the PHL for hands-on experience. In truth, the expertise in clinical laboratories has progressed to the point that larger laboratories are no longer reliant on PHLs for technical assistance, and it is mostly smaller laboratories performing basic microbiology methods that seek this assistance.

PHL ADMINISTRATION AND QUALITY MANAGEMENT

Although the PHL is not especially different in the way it operates from other laboratories in the public or private sector, it is unique in its function and purpose. The PHL is first and foremost a laboratory, but equally as important, it is also a *public health* entity. Consequently, there is a duality of purpose and function that makes the PHL very different, if not unique, within the laboratory community. As a public health entity, the laboratory's principal reason for being is to provide scientifically valid information that can be used: (1) to assess the health status of a community, (2) to develop sound policies to protect the health of the public, and (3) to evaluate the effectiveness of those policies. As a laboratory, it derives that information from specimens and samples from individuals. Thus, as with any other laboratory, the PHL has a legal and moral obligation to the individual to provide the best testing possible in a confidential and timely manner. Unlike other laboratories, the PHL is equally obligated to provide that information to the appropriate public health unit so it can be used for assessment, assurance, or policy development. Consequently, a PHL structures its testing programs to meet the needs of the programs within the health agency. In most instances, especially at the state level, this means that PHLs perform clinical testing on specimens derived from human sources, as well as environmental testing on samples of food, water, shellfish, and dairy products, plus testing animals for rabies and other zoonotic diseases. This breadth of testing also makes the PHL unique among laboratories. Dowdle, in his article "The Future of the Public Health Laboratory," specifically defined the testing functions of a PHL not as "services," but as "essential disease assessment" that connotes far more than simply reporting test results.[15(p.658)] Boiled down to its very essence, the PHL provides information, not just test results. The laboratory director is responsible for ensuring quality, managing information to guarantee the ready availability of data, developing client relationships, defining the scope of services to be offered, and addressing funding issues.[16] Through the delegation of responsibility, the laboratory director and staff must have the requisite skills to ensure appropriate leadership and administration of the laboratory.

Management and Leadership Skills

Laboratories in general are perceived as imposing, if not intimidating or mysterious places to most people. After all, it is in laboratories where discoveries at the far reaches of human knowledge are made, where the complexities of life are unraveled, and where definitive answers regarding an individual's health status are sought. Yet few people understand how those discoveries are made, or how those answers are derived. Instead, laboratories are viewed, if acknowledged at all, as windowless edifices in which things to be analyzed go in and answers come out. In this respect, PHLs are no different from other laboratories. Also, good laboratory practice and the principles of managing a modern laboratory are no different in the public sector than in the private sector. In other words, the PHL is *operationally* no different than a private sector laboratory. However, these features make PHLs very different from most other governmental agencies, and the administration of a modern laboratory in a government milieu is a unique challenge.

In modern political terms, the PHL has no readily identifiable constituency. Its business is complicated and intimidating to most people, especially those in policy-making positions and elected officials. Its role in public health is poorly understood and neither simple nor easy to articulate. There is an expectation, held by both the public and the health agency programs, that the PHL provides the highest-quality technical services. Yet, government by its nature is deliberative, and its organizations were not established to address the needs of a scientific institution. Science and technology evolve and develop faster than public policy can be formulated. Finally, unique within government, the PHL is regulated by external agencies. PHLs must meet the requirements of the federal Clinical Laboratory Improvement Amendments of 1988 (CLIA).[17] In addition, many state and large municipal PHLs may also be regulated by the EPA under the Safe Drinking Water Act, the Clean Water Act, the Clean Air Act, or the Resource Conservation and Recovery Act.[18] If the laboratory is involved with quality assurance of the dairy industry, the FDA will regulate it. How these factors affect the management of the PHL is best shown through the following exhibits. Exhibit 27–3 deals with the seemingly simple issue of ordering a laboratory supply. Exhibit 27–4 examines the impact of CLIA on governmental civil service, or merit, systems. Exhibit 27–5 is a current example of science and technology being well ahead of the formulation of public health policy.

As can be seen from these examples, the laboratory director, and for that matter, the entire laboratory management staff, is challenged to provide the highest-quality services, but must do so within external and organizational environments that are not structured to support that activity. Consequently, there is an ever-increasing demand that the laboratory director and the laboratory management display leadership skills and practice sound management. By definition, management is getting work done through others, whereas leadership goes beyond management and requires a set of skills and abilities to influence others and take them toward a shared vision. These qualities directly affect the administration of the laboratory and are required for the successful integration of the PHL into the programmatic activities of the health agency it works for or supports, as well as into the larger health care system. This is a critical role for the PHL of the future.

Beyond leadership skills, the successful laboratory administrator must be able to promote rapid adaptability to change. Both public health and clinical laboratories have advanced significantly in recent years. The magnitude of change brought about by computer technology, rapid technology introduction, and progress in science has created a volatile environment for PHLs, with administrative challenges to match.

Laboratories were among the first to take advantage of computerization. Beyond the obvious advances related to word processing, the computerized collection and management of laboratory data presented opportunities to share information widely with a variety of groups. Not only could laboratory data be shared within state programs, but other national initiatives such as the Public Health Laboratory Information System have encouraged data sharing from around the country to detect outbreaks of disease that might

Exhibit 27–3 Newborn Screening Forms—Printing or Medical Device?

After a change in personnel in a management and budget office, a problem arose with regard to an order placed for newborn screening cards. These cards, which are used by all state newborn screening programs, contain the demographic information about the patient, child, attending physician, and hospital. In addition, a filter paper strip is attached to the end of the form. This filter paper is the blood collection device and is standardized. All newborn screening laboratories in the country use this filter paper, which has been through rigorous quality control to ensure that the volume of blood held by the filter paper does not vary from lot to lot. In this case, the budget office determined that because this was printing (e.g., the demographic information), the form must be produced by a printing business within the state. After numerous discussions and providing documentation of the fact that these cards were "medical devices" and not "forms," the appropriate contract was established. The process for reordering forms had been in place for many years, but an unpredictable change in the office of management and budget resulted in a significant expenditure of time and effort to bring the problem to resolution. The situation, even though frustrating, had to be resolved in a manner that ensured maintenance of relationships with an office on which the laboratory was dependent.

Exhibit 27–4 Public Health Laboratory Personnel and Regulations

Most public health laboratories at any level of government perform tests on specimens derived from patients and are required to be licensed under CLIA. CLIA requires all laboratories—both public and private sector—performing tests from human patients to be licensed in accordance with the variety and complexity of testing performed. In most state public health laboratories, as well as the large municipal, city, or county laboratories, there are specific personnel standards that need to be met. These standards prescribe specific education and experience for the various levels of responsibility within the laboratory. This creates several challenges for the public health laboratory.

First, the CLIA personnel standards were not completely compatible with civil service or other publicly administered personnel systems. Most such systems, to prevent potential abuses attributed to patronage or political favoritism, and to remain nondiscriminatory, begin a job series with the minimum qualifications necessary to perform a given job, then allow for advancement by experience in lieu of additional education. The CLIA requirements, especially at the higher levels of responsibility, such as laboratory director, require advanced degrees as well as specific kinds of experience. Thus, under CLIA, the faithful civil servant who has many years of experience in the laboratory, with the original bachelor's degree, or even less, could no longer be considered for these more advanced positions. This is contrary to the way many civil service systems work.

Second, public health laboratories have to compete with private sector laboratories for the same labor pool that, for some time, has been steadily shrinking. Schools of medical technology have been disappearing at a rapid rate due principally to changes in health care financing. Undergraduates seeking degrees in traditional laboratory sciences such as chemistry or microbiology tend to continue their education in graduate school and seek more lucrative positions in research. At entry levels, most governmental personnel systems are somewhat competitive with the private sector, but public sector salaries fall behind private sector salaries very quickly and most dramatically for highly skilled and experienced staff, supervisory staff, and especially, managers and directors. Thus, the public health laboratories are facing a looming shortage of experienced, skilled technical staff and, most critically, managerial staff, at the very time when science and technology are rapidly changing laboratory methods and procedures, and when all governmental functions are called on to be more efficient and accountable.

otherwise go undetected due to low frequency in any single state.

Scientific advances over the past few years abound, but probably none are as significant as the adaptation of molecular methods for both disease detection and epidemiologic purposes. One such example is the use of pulsed-field gel electrophoresis or DNA fingerprinting to determine the molecular patterns of various organisms often associated with foodborne disease, as shown in Exhibit 27–6. The CDC, state health departments, and the APHL have been collaborating to create a molecular subtyping network of PHLs called PulseNet, which is highlighted in the exhibit.[19]

Client Relationships and Partnerships

The PHL director must establish productive working relationships within his or her own organization (program staff) as well as with external clients (medical care community, local/city/state health departments, etc.). The process of developing and maintaining productive relationships is a challenge, but one that is critical to ensure an understanding of the PHL's role in public health. For example, it is important that the laboratory director work with program staff because funding is often directed to categorical programs. Grants and contracts may only refer to the assurance of the availability of certain

Exhibit 27–5 The Integration of New Technology

Like any other laboratory, the public health laboratory is at its core a scientific institution. As a governmental entity, this aspect presents complex challenges to its managers, directors, and home agency. In simplest terms, science and technology evolve and develop faster than good public policy can be formulated. The act of governing, whether at the legislative, executive, or judicial levels, is necessarily deliberative. Rapid advances in science, such as the mapping of the human genome, and emerging diseases, such as AIDS in the mid-1980s, have enormous societal and economic implications. Coupled with modern communications and a ubiquitous mass media, the time between discovery and public awareness has virtually disappeared. Consequently, even the scientists doing the research, not to mention elected officials and policy makers, have little time to contemplate the possibilities and the dangers of their discoveries. Nevertheless, the public expects, and may demand, that policies and programs be developed and administered to either take advantage of, or protect them from, these discoveries. In these cases, the public health laboratory can be caught between competing, if not conflicting interests. This is the current situation.

Beginning in the 1960s, states engaged their public health laboratories to screen newborns for inheritable errors of metabolism that, when detected within the first few weeks of life, could be effectively managed and treated. Over the years, these programs have been very successful in preventing developmental disabilities, mental retardation, and premature death in thousands of children with these diseases, in addition to saving millions of dollars in health care and special education costs. Until the mid-1990s, most states screened for at most eight of these conditions. However, new technology, using expensive, sophisticated instrumentation, has been developed and is able to screen for more than 30 conditions. This is the best available technology for many of these conditions.

The private sector can and has responded rapidly by marketing services using this technology. It can, at a moment's notice, increase the charges for this testing to capitalize the initial investment. It is potentially a very profitable enterprise because there is a very large population of newborns, the testing can be automated to reduce personnel costs, and the equipment can be depreciated over time. From the private sector perspective, this is a tremendous business opportunity.

For public health and the public health laboratory, this development is much more complicated. The screening tests performed by the public health laboratory are only one part of a state newborn screening program. The so-called "program" component of follow-up and assurance that the infants found with these conditions are being properly cared for is as critical to the overall success of these activities as is the laboratory component. However, few, if any, states have fully formulated the appropriate role of the public health agency in the area of genetics and disease prevention. Of the 30 or so conditions that can be detected by the new technology, no more than half can be treated to prevent serious consequences. Some of the remaining conditions can be managed only through intensive medical care. Several of the conditions occur so rarely in the general population that the costs of screening all newborns may exceed the benefits to the public. On the other side, the families of the afflicted children tend to be politically active and vocal. Few elected officials will oppose a program that ostensibly will improve the lives of children, but at the same time, few elected officials seek to expand public programs that will cost more money. Defining the line between what is in the domain of personal health care and what is truly a justifiable public health activity is a matter of public policy that has not yet been completely resolved in any political jurisdiction or at any level of government.

Finally, when the availability of new technology causes precipitous public policy decisions, the opportunity exists for the science, in this case, the testing technology, to outstrip the resources needed to implement public health programs that use the information from that technology. In this instance, the public health agency would have data and information, but no one available to act on it, which undermines the very reason for having a public health program in the first place.

Exhibit 27-6 Scientific Advances in Public Health Laboratory Science

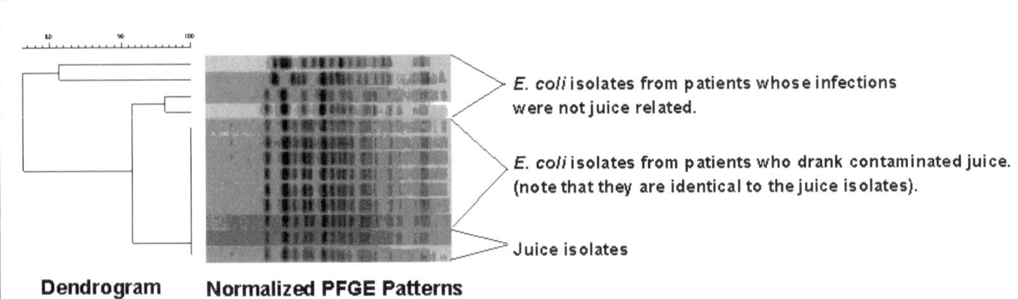

*Vertical line at 100% represents isolates that are indistinguishable from each other. Lines farther away from 100% on the dendrogram indicate isolates that have similarities to the outbreak isolates but are not a perfect match.

Pulsed-field gel electrophoresis (PFGE) is a method of molecular fingerprinting. The picture shows the relationships among PFGE patterns of *Escherichia coli* O157:H7 isolates from Washington state. The PFGE patterns of the two isolates from apple juice are identical to the patterns of isolates from patients who drank the contaminated juice, but different than those from patients whose infections were not juice related. This technology has been used to identify outbreaks of foodborne illnesses, especially those that involve clusters of cases that are too geographically or temporally scattered to come to public health attention through usual methods of surveillance.

In partnership with state health departments and the Association of Public Health Laboratories, the CDC is creating a molecular subtyping network called PulseNet, which is based on DNA fingerprinting of bacteria that cause foodborne diseases. The project is being implemented for *Escherichia coli* O157:H7 and will soon be extended to include *Salmonella enteritidis*, Typhimurium, and other foodborne pathogens. All participants will use standardized equipment and protocols, and a centralized database of DNA patterns ("DNA fingerprints") will be stored on a computer server at the CDC. Through the participation of the U.S. Department of Agriculture and the Food and Drug Administration, the database will include fingerprints of bacteria derived from contaminated foods as well as from human samples.

When outbreaks occur, participating laboratories will submit DNA fingerprints such as the ones shown in the picture for comparison with those in the database. (A fingerprint analysis can be completed at a local laboratory in 24 hours, and electronic patterns can be matched by computer within a few minutes.) If a submitted pattern matches a pattern in the database, the submitting laboratory will be able to download epidemiologic data associated with the *E. coli* strain that exhibits that pattern. If the submitted pattern is not an exact match, information on the closest matches will be provided. If the same DNA pattern is submitted by two or more participating laboratories within a short time, the CDC server will warn each participating laboratory that a multistate outbreak may be in progress.

Source: National Center for Infectious Diseases, Centers for Disease Control and Prevention.

laboratory services; therefore, it is critical that the laboratory director have early input for proposals that are submitted by program staff. Even if the laboratory services in the proposal are not to be provided by the PHL, the laboratory director can help ensure that the laboratory aspects of the proposal have been well crafted. Another critical relationship for the laboratory director is with the epidemiology program. The laboratory and epidemiology programs of state and local agencies must work closely because so much of the work of the epidemiologist is reliant on laboratory diagnosis and the quality of laboratory data.

The relationship of the state PHL to the local PHL will vary from state to state, but is, nonetheless, an important relationship to maintain. Whether or not a local governmental entity has a PHL is dependent on the resources and political nature of the LHD. For example, in some states, each county is responsible for local public health functions; in other states, counties have joined together to create health districts, thereby minimizing administrative costs. Larger counties with well-developed health departments will often have a laboratory, whereas other counties will have established relationships with other county PHLs or with the state PHL. For example, in Michigan and Tennessee, the state PHL provides certain administrative and laboratory services in a manner that ties the local and state systems together as a functional unit. Other examples undoubtedly exist, including the development of contractual relationships with independent (private) laboratories.

When decisions concerning laboratory services are made at the local level, there are a number of factors to consider. As mentioned earlier, even if a private laboratory provides certain services, it is critical to involve a PHL director in the decision-making process. Public health programs are reliant on high-quality data that can be comparable over time. When developing a contractual relationship for PHL services, one needs to be aware of the methodology being used (e.g., direct detection of an infectious agent vs. culture), hidden costs (e.g., for Lyme disease, are confirmatory Western Blots for positive EIA serology an added cost or built in to overall cost), the assurance of a requirement in the contract that if methodologies change that the client will be notified in advance, how samples will be delivered (e.g., courier, mail), what special handling factors must be considered (e.g., time delays and impact on HIV viral load), how reports will be transmitted back to the program staff (e.g., mail, fax, electronically), what confidentiality issues must be addressed, and the number of samples to be handled (e.g., in a foodborne disease outbreak when sample volume cannot be predicted, what barriers might be present that would inhibit the complete collection of information).

With the advent of several major national initiatives, including TB elimination, emerging and reemerging infectious disease, food safety initiatives, and bioterrorism, decisions concerning PHL services cannot be made without input from program staff and PHL staff. All of these initiatives are dependent on well-thought-out planning at the local level, and each has a major laboratory component.

Accordingly, relationships must also be developed and maintained with the medical community. There are many tests of public health importance that are conducted in hospital and independent laboratories. The PHL director can provide leadership by establishing relationships with the clinical laboratory community to ensure recognition of the respective roles of public health and clinical medicine. A good example can be found in the Pacific Northwest. The Washington State Clinical Laboratory Initiative (also known as the Laboratory Medicine Sentinel Monitoring Network) began in the Pacific Northwest in 1995.[20] It currently consists of 381 clinical laboratories located in Washington, Alaska, Idaho, and Oregon. The purpose of this network is to provide ongoing information, based on actual practices and experiences, related to testing quality, factors influencing the accuracy and reliability of test results, the extent and nature of laboratory-related problems and errors, access to laboratory testing services, and current trends in the practice of laboratory medicine.

Strategic Planning

As the cat in Alice in Wonderland said, "If you don't know where you are going, any road will take you there."[21(p.89)] Strategic context is crucial for all organizations, including PHLs, and the development of a strategic plan is an energizing challenge and opportunity. Strategic planning serves three purposes: first, it is a critical part of effective organizational management. Second, by having its own plan, the PHL will not have to rely on, or hope, that it will be considered within someone else's plan. Third, the planning process itself tends to encourage the inclusion of laboratory representation in other, or larger, organizational planning processes.

Public health agencies need to have reliable, service-oriented, viable PHLs. The PHL is an indispensable component of disease surveillance, outbreak investigations, and disease prevention programs. The PHL director and the senior managers cannot be viewed, nor view themselves, as simply laboratory scientists, but as public health professionals who specialize in laboratory disciplines. It is equally incumbent on the director and managers of the PHL and the administration of the public health agency to promote and take advantage of their expertise in developing and implementing public health programs.

In addition to being scientifically knowledgeable, the laboratory leadership must be skilled at modern laboratory management. The PHL must follow the same personnel rules and employment laws to which all other governmental agencies must adhere and is held to the same level of fiscal accountability as any other governmental entity. As previously noted, the PHL has to be inspected and licensed by one or more external entities, and must maintain a reputation for credibility and integrity that is beyond reproach. These attributes are common to virtually all successful laboratories in the private or public sector, but to succeed as a public health institution, the laboratory director and the senior managers must be able to articulate the role of the PHL within their jurisdiction clearly and show how their laboratory accomplishes that role. They must be able to do this as competently with the public and the elected representatives as they do within the public health agency. To improve efficiency and service, they must examine practices that work in the private sector, such as expanded use of courier systems, electronic reporting, and staggered work schedules. They must be diligent and active in engaging their colleagues within the public health agency, and those outside the public health agency, to structure and develop effective public health programs. Finally, the laboratory director and senior managers must be willing to participate in public policy discussions and debates.

These activities are essential to the survival of PHLs. Finally, the scientific and technical knowledge and expertise that reside within the PHL and its leadership are invaluable resources to the public health agency when addressing the complex policy issues that science continually presents to our society.

Laboratory Information Management

The need to share laboratory information is both a significant challenge and a tremendous opportunity. There is clearly a need for laboratory information to be transmitted as rapidly as possible to those individuals who need the data for programmatic decision making. It is not sufficient simply to develop a laboratory information system that serves the purpose of accessioning specimens and reporting results. And, because information system technology changes so rapidly, the system must be flexible enough to accommodate technological advances that enable the sharing of data. The PHL providing information for community health must also become integrated into the health care system and be seen as critical a component as the clinical laboratory that provides individual patient care.

A variety of information system options are available to PHLs. These options include the development of homegrown systems, the purchase of information systems from vendors, and sharing a system that is broadly utilized.

Regardless of the direction taken, it is critical to approach the development or improvement of information systems in much the same way one approaches strategic planning—ensure that your stakeholders are aware of your needs and that you are aware of their needs. Very often, the laboratory administrator must work cooperatively with the information services group serving a public health department or a broader community health agency. Educational efforts and a collaborative approach will be required. During the development or enhancement of a laboratory information system, the laboratory administrator must have someone on staff who can provide the appropriate expertise in both laboratory science and computer technology—and that is the order in which the expertise is most useful. That person will provide the interface with the information systems staff that is important during system development.

Personnel Administration

Work force changes are a continuing source of concern for both clinical laboratories and PHLs. As opposed to times gone by when a person might hold a single job for a lifetime, a person is now likely to have career changes. University graduates have that expectation and have interests in developing experience and expertise that will allow them to be competitive. These expectations, combined with changes brought about by economic pressures on the health care system, have resulted in job markets that vary greatly by locale. Although there are shortages of both medical technologists and cytotechnologists, there are also rapid advances in automation and technology that create an environment of uncertainty for those persons considering the field of laboratory medicine. Over the years, there have been numerous peaks and valleys related to demand and to pay scale.

Because of these unique and often conflicting factors, it is important to develop a positive working relationship with the human resources (personnel) office (see Chapter 16). Because the PHL is often a unique entity in a government's organizational structure, it is important to establish the appropriate relationships with the human resources office to ensure that there is an understanding of the nature of the work and corresponding work force needs. The PHL administrator must work closely with the human resources office to ensure that wages are competitive for the geographic area and that position descriptions for scientific positions are properly written. The staff who review position descriptions and employee applications must have interaction with laboratory staff to ensure that differences in their respective knowledge base do not hinder the hiring and retention of quality staff.

The laboratory director must also provide opportunities for internal work force development. One must provide opportunities for staff to learn through formal education and training opportunities, such as those available at scientific meetings and conferences. Although out-of-state travel is often difficult to fund, employees benefit greatly from opportunities to interact with peers from other agencies and other laboratories. Education and training are becoming increasingly available through distance learning formats, and the trend will be for those opportunities to expand due to the increasing costs of travel and the need to reduce time away from home. However, it is important to encourage participation in local and in-state professional organizations and to encourage leadership development skills.

PRODUCING RELIABLE RESULTS

A number of administrative issues critical to the operation of a PHL have been addressed in this chapter. The scientific and technical issues of administering a PHL will now be presented. It is not that quality assurance is less important than those issues presented earlier, but the issues of management and leadership skills, work force development, and laboratory information systems are important building blocks on which the laboratory technical skills are overlaid.

Quality assurance is the outcome of those activities within the laboratory that ensure that information that is generated by the laboratory is accurate. The quality assurance program must evaluate the effectiveness of the laboratory policies and procedures; identify and correct problems; ensure the accurate, reliable, and prompt reporting of test results; and ensure the adequacy and competency of the staff.[17]

CLIA

The public health and clinical laboratories are governed by a federal regulation known as CLIA, which was first implemented in 1967.[17] All laboratories performing testing on specimens of human origin (excluding forensics and drug monitoring programs) are regulated either by the federal or the state government. In 1988, the statute entitled the Clinical Laboratory Improvement Amendments (CLIA '88) was passed; it was implemented in 1992. CLIA is administered by the Health Care Financing Administration; the Division of Laboratory Systems in the Public Health Practice Program Office at the CDC is responsible for the scientific and technical input and for writing the regulations. CLIA is now considered by most people to be an important and necessary statute that governs laboratories that test human specimens. Laboratory medicine and laboratory practice are so broad and encompass so many disciplines that it has become necessary to articulate clearly the critical components and measures that must be in place to ensure that those components are addressed. Modern public health and clinical laboratories have found that it is necessary to have a quality assurance officer who reports to the laboratory director. The quality control officer monitors the various practices that have been determined critical to ensuring quality laboratory services, some of which are noted in Exhibit 27–7. These components establish a framework for the assurance of quality.

Proficiency Testing and Quality Control

Proficiency testing programs provide laboratories with an external source of testing specimens, and participating laboratories must handle these specimens in the same manner as patient samples. Laboratories must enroll in proficiency testing programs and receive challenges periodically throughout the year, each of which contains multiple test samples. They must develop corrective action plans for any proficiency test results that are incorrect. Laboratories that do not maintain appropriate performance in proficiency test programs are not allowed to continue to report patient results in that category of testing until appropriate documentation has been provided to state or federal inspectors.[17]

Exhibit 27–7 Some Components of a Laboratory Quality Assurance Program

- proficiency testing
- quality control records
- record retention
- procedure manuals
- records of establishment and verification of methods performance
- equipment maintenance
- record of corrective actions

Quality control procedures are performed on a routine basis to monitor the stability of the method or the test system. These procedures provide a basis for indirectly assessing the accuracy of patient test results. The manufacturers of test methods often provide quality control materials, but if these are not available, the laboratory must have alternative mechanisms to obtain them, or to establish alternate validation measures.

The retention of patient testing records, quality control records, corrective action records, and the like are defined within CLIA.[17] However, it is important that the quality assurance officer provide the oversight necessary to ensure adherence to the requirements. A lack of documentation and maintenance of records remains one of the often-cited deficiencies of laboratories.[17] Not only must procedure manuals be accurate reflections of step-by-step performance of the procedure, but they must also specify specimen collection and processing requirements, reporting ranges, limitations of the procedure, and protocols for reporting critical results. Any change in a procedure must be signed and dated by the laboratory director. Procedures must address preanalytic issues (clinical relevance, proper specimen collection, patient information, etc.), analytic issues (step-by-step procedure, normal values, etc.), and postanalytic issues (reporting of critical values, test interpretation, etc). Records of the establishment and verification of methods performance must be completed before reporting patient test results. Other issues to be addressed and documented include analytic sensitivity, specificity, reportable range of patient test results, reference ranges (normal values) and any other applicable performance characteristics.

Equipment maintenance records must also be maintained and made readily available for laboratory inspectors. Such records include maintenance information as defined by the manufacturer or, if using non-FDA-cleared equipment, the laboratory must establish an appropriate maintenance protocol. Records of corrective actions must be maintained. These corrective actions relate to quality control, equipment malfunction, proficiency testing, or complaint investigations. The quality assurance issues noted in Exhibit 27–7 and briefly described above are discussed in significant detail in the *Federal Register* concerning CLIA.[16]

Privatization

Beginning in the 1970s, it became common for PHLs, particularly at the state level, to charge fees for their services as a source of funding. Often, these fees took the place of state general funding or revenue. At the same time, public health agencies, also as a matter of policy, were becoming the health care provider of last resort for the indigent, uninsured, and underinsured, and they used the allowable reimbursement from the Medicaid and Medicare programs as funding sources. The PHL was often asked to provide the testing that supported the personal health care services being delivered by the public health agencies. The laboratory, in order to fulfill its main role as a public health entity, had to rely on its ability to raise revenues to support ongoing public health programs. Within government, the PHL was perceived as behaving like any private laboratory by seeking revenue through fees and reimbursement. Consequently, when the role of government became a significant political issue in the 1980s, the PHL came under very close scrutiny as a governmental function that could be conducted by the private sector.

As mentioned in previous sections, certain laboratory activities that support public health programs, especially at the local level, are often contracted out to private sector laboratories. In most instances, these laboratory activities are related to primary health care delivery through various LHD clinics (e.g., family planning or Women's, Infants', and Children's). However, the core functions of PHLs, as enumerated in Exhibit 27–1, are functions that are inherent to the protection of the public health and welfare, and in many states are implied in the enabling legislation that establishes the health department generally, or the PHL specifically. Thus, these functions cannot be delegated by contract with the private sector, or privatized, without compromising the public interest.

The most straightforward example of this would be in the area of laboratory improvement and regulation. Obviously, it would not be in the public's interest, nor would it be practical, for a private entity to oversee a regulatory program. A more complicated example would be the integrated data management function. Public health relies on data from a number of sources to assess and evaluate the health of a given community. One major source of disease surveillance information is the PHL—both in its role for reference and specialized testing, as well as its role in testing for high-risk/low-incidence diseases. Outsourcing any of those functions places that data and information outside of the control of the public health agency. It also places the essential elements of assessment, policy development, and assurance into the hands of the private provider instead of the public agency entrusted with these responsibilities.

The issue of privatization also arises as a means of reducing government spending. Here, the underlying assumption is that the private sector is more cost-efficient at delivering services, especially services that are perceived as being the same, in this case, laboratory tests. Again, referring to the core functions of PHLs in Exhibit 27–1, it can be seen that there are a number of activities of added value that are performed at PHLs, namely integrated data collection and management, statewide reference testing services, performance of high-risk/low-incidence disease testing, and population-based laboratory surveillance programs. When these activities are factored into the cost of PHL services, there is virtually no difference in private sector and public sector costs, and in fact, because of the additional data management demands, there may be increased costs in the private sector to meet those particular needs. The other potential problem with privatizing PHL services is that in the business world, especially in the laboratory sector recently, there are no guarantees that the laboratory with the contract today will be in business tomorrow, or that it will be owned by the same company next week. Under these circumstances, it is possible that what may have been a favorable contract for the state, in terms of saving money, will actually cost the state more because of the need to renegotiate and to build in the necessary contingencies should the contract laboratory fail to meet its obligations. The other important consideration in this situation is the state's inability to meet its obligations of protecting the public health while it has limited or perhaps no access to PHL services because of interruptions due to business decisions.

Although several state laboratories have had to deal with efforts to privatize all or part of their activities, for the most part, the result has been that the laboratory has remained intact as a functional unit of the state health agency. In large part, this success comes from the health agency and laboratory "making their case" regarding the critical nature of the PHL in protecting the public health and welfare. That said, it is good to be reminded that the PHL is an arm of government that is subject to overriding politics or state policy. A concerted effort in the mid-1990s to privatize the PHL in one eastern state was initiated as a result of the sitting administration's political desire to reduce the size of state government, which was a key plank in the election platform of the governor. In another state, as a matter of policy, the state PHL was required to bid for work just as any other private laboratory under that state's universal health insurance program, including the work generated through ongoing state and local public health programs. Despite these developments, both states retained their PHLs, which operate at nearly their previous levels of activities. In the first case, an intense advocacy effort involving a coalition of public health and private health care providers succeeded in establishing the PHL in statute. In the second case, the PHL adapted to the changes and continues to operate, though there remains a concern that the needs of public health are not being adequately addressed through the state-subsidized health care delivery system. Privatization will remain a significant public policy issue for PHLs in the foreseeable future, so the vital nature of the leadership and management elements discussed previously in this chapter cannot be overstated.

PHLs AND HEALTH CARE DYNAMICS

During the past decade, the U.S. health care environment has changed dramatically in ways that affect clinical laboratories, PHLs, and the programs they serve.[22] Exhibit 27–8 illustrates some of these dynamic changes. Like the rest of the public health system, PHLs must understand that they are part of a continuum of health care and population-level services. PHLs can no longer assume that being a part of government will insulate them against volatile changes in health care economics and delivery. The most profound of these changes has been the emergence of a national trend toward managed health care.

Managed care organizations and public health agencies have a common incentive to provide early preventive services that promote long-term health improvements in the populations they serve—for example, immunizations, Pap smears, sexually transmitted disease screening, and prenatal care. Much has been written about forging partnerships between managed care organizations and public health agencies.[23,24] In fact, the Managed Care Working Group of the CDC suggested in 1995 that managed care organizations could "play a powerful role in prevention" because: (1) they are rapidly becoming a major source of health care for the beneficiaries of employer-funded and publicly funded programs, (2) they historically have included prevention, and (3) they represent organized care systems that take responsibility for defined populations.[25] Thus, in a scenario where everyone is covered by health insurance (public or private) and prevention-oriented managed care is the predominant delivery model, the health of entire populations should improve over time and public health goals should be achieved. Theoretically, PHLs might see increased collaboration with private sector laboratories, with more reference test volume, better disease reporting, and formal contractual arrangements. But, in reality, are public health and managed care organizations collaborating, and are PHLs benefiting?

Exhibit 27–8 Health Care Changes Affecting Laboratories and Public Health Programs

- Consolidations, mergers, and buyouts of health care systems resulting in complex referral patterns and business relationships
- Broad move to critical path management of patients and corporate oversight of physician practices
- Inpatient care shifted increasingly to outpatient settings
- Capitated managed care emerging as the dominant form of health care delivery
- Clinical laboratories downsizing and subject to strict financial controls
- Role of clinical laboratories changing from a revenue center to a cost center
- New nonculture technologies used more widely for diagnosing infectious diseases, while fewer cultures are being typed or referred for identification beyond the needs of individual patient care
- Increased reliance on empirical antibiotic therapy

Source: Adapted with permission from M. Skeels, Public Health Labs in a Changing Health Care Landscape, *ASM News,* Vol. 65, No. 7, pp. 479–483, © 1999, American Society for Microbiology. Data from The Impact of Managed Care and Health System Change on Clinical Microbiology: A Survey Analysis, prepared by The Lewin Group for the American Society for Microbiology, June 26, 1988.

According to two separate and independent studies, the answer is "no." The inspector general of the Department of Health and Human Services (DHHS) recently found that there are very few collaborations between public health and managed care organizations, and the opportunity to build these relationships may be slipping away.[26] The DHHS report states one central conclusion: "Collaborations that address public health population-based strategies have barely begun. In fact, the current environment may mean that opportunities for realizing the potential of collaboration are fading."[26] The report goes on to say, "Very few States reported collaborations that link clinical activities of managed care organizations with population-based functions that are the responsibility of public health departments."[26] This obviously presents a challenge for PHLs, but it is also an opportunity. Of all the components of the public health system, PHLs may be among the best situated to collaborate with managed care organizations because of existing referral patterns, population screening activities, and a history of partnership with private laboratories.

However, despite this promising potential, a study by The Lewin Group showed that managed care and other health system changes are actually having *negative* effects on state PHLs and the programs they serve.[27] Selected key findings of this study included: (1) a reduction in testing volume in PHLs, (2) reduced reporting of diseases, (3) difficulty in obtaining payment for tests with associated fees, (4) few examples of contractual or collaborative agreements with managed care organizations or private laboratories, and (5) competition from large commercial laboratories for traditional public health workload. The Lewin Group found the private sector clinical laboratory market to be extremely competitive and focused on efficiency and cost reduction as a result of "overcapacity, increased outpatient testing, and intense price pressure from payers." This environment has changed the relationship between clinical laboratories, private health care systems, and PHLs, and threatens the U.S. disease surveillance system. Financial pressures have forced clinical laboratories to reduce their participation in public health activities, and lower test volumes in PHLs have made it harder for them to maintain the critical mass of staffing and other resources needed to provide population-level services that are not billable to anyone. There are also concerns that large private sector "megalabs" will fail to comply with disease reporting requirements for the many states from which they receive samples.

A NATIONAL LABORATORY SYSTEM

Clearly, the integrity of the U.S. disease control infrastructure depends on building and maintaining a cooperative network of clinical laboratories and PHLs. A recent study by the U.S. General Accounting Office (GAO) examined the nation's capacity to detect and control emerging infectious diseases.[28] Among the GAO's conclusions were: "The nation's surveillance network is considered the first line of defense in detecting and identifying emerging infectious diseases....Laboratories play an increasingly vital role in infectious disease surveillance, as advances in technology continually enhance the specificity of laboratory data and give public health officials new techniques for monitoring emerging infections."[28(p.33)] However, concluded the GAO, "Surveillance and testing for important emerging infectious diseases are not comprehensive in all states, leaving gaps in the nation's infectious diseases surveillance network."[28(p.2)]

Officials at the CDC have encouraged the development of a national laboratory system with "unique and complementary roles" for PHLs and private laboratories.[29] They warn that the nation's disease surveillance capacity is threatened by several forces: "the conflict between cost-containment efforts in administering health care and the need for essential laboratory data; a misperception that public and private sector laboratories compete and duplicate efforts; and the lack of a well-defined national laboratory system."[29(p.9)] Without such a system, the nation's public health infrastructure will remain vulnerable to shifts in health care economics and service delivery.

CHAPTER REVIEW

1. PHLs operate at local, state, and federal levels. State PHLs now operate in all states and in many of the territories of the United States. Each state organizes its own local PHL system. Federal laboratories are maintained primarily by the CDC.
2. There are three basic models for organizing state PHLs in the United States.
   - the state health department laboratory
   - the university-based or -affiliated laboratory
   - the consolidated state laboratory, which is based within a separate state agency
3. The specific services performed by PHLs vary depending on local needs and practices, but all laboratories share a common mission to support local, state, and federal public health programs. These programs include environmental health, disease control and prevention, MCH, epidemiology, and emergency response. Many PHLs also provide clinical laboratory services for at-risk populations served by community primary care clinics.
4. In addition to performing analytic testing, PHLs help ensure the quality of all medical and environmental laboratories through training, consultation, and regulatory activities. Laboratories also participate in evaluating or adapting new public health technologies, and in conducting epidemiologic studies and other applied research activities.
5. PHLs depend on strong working relationships with clinical laboratories. Although private clinical laboratories are focused mainly on the care of individual patients, they are on the front lines of detecting community illnesses, and they provide important case reports and microbial isolates for disease monitoring and surveillance. PHLs interface with clinical laboratories to help identify populationwide trends and sentinel events, and to provide specialized reference testing and clinical services for vulnerable populations.
6. Key administrative challenges for PHLs include: (1) continual evolution in computer technologies that support laboratory activities, (2) scientific advances that drive changes in laboratory technology and practice, and (3) the development and maintenance of effective relationships with a variety of clients and constituents. In addressing these challenges, laboratories must simultaneously cultivate scientific and technical expertise and an orientation toward service.
7. Successful laboratories must develop and continually improve their administrative systems for information management, personnel management, financial management, and quality management.

REFERENCES

1. R.O. Valdiserri, "Temples of the Future: An Historical Overview of the Laboratory's Role in Public Health Practice," *Annual Review of Public Health* 14 (1993): 635–648.
2. Association of Public Health Laboratories, *Core Functions and Capabilities of State Public Health Laboratories* (Washington, DC: 2000).
3. G. Rosen, "Industrialism and the Sanitary Movement," in *A History of Public Health,* ed. G. Rosen (New York: MD Publica, 1958), 192–293.
4. C.E. Winslow, "The Laboratory in the Service of the State," *American Journal of Public Health* 6 (1915): 222–233.
5. A. Sakula, "Robert Koch: Centenary of the Discovery of the Tubercle Bacillus, 1882," *Thorax* 37 (1982): 246–251.
6. National Institutes of Health, *History of NIH,* <http://www.training.nih.gov/catalog/nihhistory.html> (29 April 2000).
7. G. Anderson, *Task Force for Report on the Public Health Laboratory: A Critical National Resource* (Washington, DC: Association of State and Territorial Public Health Laboratory Directors, 1993).
8. D. Drabkowski, personal communication, December 17, 1999.
9. R. Laessig and M. Gilchrist, personal communication, December 17, 1999.
10. Commonwealth of Virginia, Virginia Department of General Services, Division of Consolidated Laboratory Services, *Making Virginia a Healthier Place To Live* [brochure] (Richmond, VA: Virginia Office of Graphic Communications, 1999).
11. M. Skeels, "Public Health Laboratories Build Healthy Communities," *Laboratory Medicine 26,* no. 9 (1995): 588–592.
12. M. Skeels, "Public Health Labs in a Changing Health Care Landscape," *ASM News 65,* no. 7 (1999): 479–483.
13. J. McDade and W. Hausler, "Modernization of Public Health Laboratories in a Privatization Atmosphere," *Journal of Clinical Microbiology* 36 (1998): 609–613.
14. K. Peddecord and R. Cada, "The Public Health Laboratory," in *Principles of Public Health Practice*, eds. F. Scutchfield and C. Keck (Albany, NY: Delmar Publishers, Inc., 1997), 350–357.
15. W. Dowdle, "The Future of the Public Health Laboratory," *Annual Review of Public Health* 14 (1993): 649–664.
16. U.S. Government Printing Office, *Clinical Laboratory Improvement Amendments of 1988,* Code of Federal Regulations, Title 42, Volume 3, Parts 430 to end, Final Rule [Revised October 1, 1998] (Washington, DC: 1998).
17. CLIA-40 CFR493.1 (Basis and Scope) and 493.3 (Applicability).
18. *Safe Drinking Water Act*, 40 CFR 141.28 and 142.10(b)(4).
19. Centers for Disease Control and Prevention, *Preventing Emerging Infectious Diseases: A Strategy for the 21st Century* (Atlanta, GA: USDHHS/CDC 1998), 23.
20. K.M. LaBeau and S.J. Steindel, *The Pacific Northwest Laboratory Medicine Sentinel Monitoring Network Final Report of Activities for Year One.* Report for Division of Laboratory Systems, Public Health Practice Program Office, Centers for Disease Control and Prevention, October 1995. http://www.phppo.cdc.gov/dls/mlp/pnlmsmn.asp.
21. L. Carroll, *Alice's Adventures in Wonderland* (New York: Avenel Books, 1865).
22. W. Check, "Managed Care Deeply Affecting Clinical Microbiology," *ASM News* 64 (1998): 495–500.
23. E. Baker et al., "Health Reform and the Health of the Public: Forging Community Partnerships," *Journal of the American Medical Association 272,* no. 16 (1994): 1,276–1,282.
24. W. Roper and G. Mays, "The Changing Managed Care-Public Health Interface," *Journal of the American Medical Association 280,* no. 20 (1998): 1,739–1,740.
25. CDC Managed Care Working Group, 1995. "Prevention and Managed Care: Opportunities for Managed Care Organizations, Purchasers of Health Care, and Public Health Agencies," *Morbidity and Mortality Weekly Report 44,* RR-14 (1995): 1–12.
26. Office of the Inspector General, U.S. Department of Health and Human Services, 1999. *Public Health and Managed Care: Opportunities for Collaboration* [DHHS OEI-01-98-00170] (Washington, DC: 1998), 1–45.
27. R. Ahn et al., *Public Health Laboratories and Health System Change* (Fairfax, VA: The Lewin Group, 1997).
28. U.S. General Accounting Office, *Emerging Infectious Diseases: Consensus on Needed Laboratory Capacity Could Strengthen Surveillance* (GAO/HEHS-99-26) (Washington, DC: 1999).
29. J. McDade and J. Hughes, "The U.S. Needs a National Laboratory System," *U.S. Medicine* 34 (1998): 9.

CHAPTER 28

Roles and Responsibilities of Public Health in Disaster Preparedness and Response

Linda Young Landesman
Josephine Malilay
Richard A. Bissell
Steven M. Becker
Les Roberts
Michael S. Ascher

Public health has broad responsibilities to prepare for and respond to disasters. Carrying out these responsibilities effectively requires a multiorganizational response. Key among these responsibilities are disaster epidemiology and assessment, which are used as managerial tools as well as instruments of scientific investigation. Public health organizations also play essential roles in managing the psychosocial effects of disasters and in managing environmental resources to ensure disaster preparedness. The emerging threat of bioterrorism creates new risks and responsibilities for public health organizations. Although the challenges of managing environmental health threats are greater in developing countries than in the United States, essential elements of public health administration—including the management of food, water, and waste—can be compromised substantially in the most devastating domestic disasters, creating imperatives for disaster preparedness.

Disasters have been defined as ecologic disruptions, or emergencies, of a severity and magnitude resulting in deaths, injuries, illness, and/or property damage that cannot be effectively managed by the application of routine procedures or resources and that result in a call for outside assistance. As the field of disaster study evolved, a common set of vocabulary emerged as well, notably distinguishing among hazards, emergencies, and disasters.[1]

- *Hazards* present the probability of the occurrence of a disaster caused by a natural phenomenon (e.g., earthquake, tropical cyclone), by failure of manmade sources of energy (e.g., nuclear reactor, industrial explosion), or by uncontrolled human activity (e.g., conflicts, overgrazing).
- *Emergencies* are typically any occurrence that requires an immediate response.[1] These events can be the result of nature (e.g., hurricanes, tornados, and earthquakes), can be caused by technological or manmade error (e.g., nuclear accidents, bombing, and bioterrorism), or can be the result of emerging diseases (e.g., West Nile virus in New York City).
- *Natural disasters* suggest rapid, acute onset phenomena (sudden-onset events) with profound effects, such as earthquakes, floods, tropical cyclones, and tornadoes. *Manmade disasters,* also called complex emergencies, suggest technological events or disasters that are not caused by natural hazards but that occur in human settlements, such as fire, chemical spills and ex-

plosions, and armed conflict. No clear demarcation exists between the two categories. For instance, fire may be the result of arson, a manmade activity, but may also occur secondarily to earthquake events, particularly in urban areas where gas mains may be damaged. With increasing technological development worldwide, a new category of disasters known as *natural–technological, or "na-tech," disasters,* has been described in the literature. Na-tech disasters refer to natural disasters that create technological emergencies, such as urban fires resulting from seismic motion or chemical spills resulting from floods.[2]

The life cycle of a disaster event is typically known as the disaster continuum, or emergency management cycle. Before (preimpact), during (impact), and after (postimpact) a disaster event, both public health and emergency management officials and the population at risk can reduce or prevent injury, illness, or death by the actions they take. The basic phases of disaster management include mitigation or prevention, warning and preparedness, response and recovery. *Mitigation* includes the measures that are taken to reduce the harmful effects of a disaster by attempting to limit impacts on human health and economic infrastructure. Although prevention may refer to preventing a disaster from occurring, such as cloud seeding to stimulate rain in fire situations, in public health terms, *prevention* refers to actions that may prevent further loss of life, disease, disability, or injury. *Warning* or forecasting refers to the monitoring of events to look for indicators that signify when and where a disaster might occur and what the magnitude might be. In *preparedness,* officials or the public itself structure a response to disasters that may occur and, in so doing, lay the framework for recovery.

In the United States, the *response* to disasters is organized through multiple jurisdictions, agencies, and authorities. The term "emergency management" is used to refer to these activities. The emergency management field organizes its activities by "sectors" such as fire, police, and emergency medical services (EMS). The response phase of a disaster encompasses relief and is followed by recovery and rehabilitation or reconstruction. *Emergency relief* focuses attention on saving lives, providing first aid, restoring emergency communications and transportation systems, and providing immediate care and basic needs to survivors, such as food and clothing or medical and emotional care. *Recovery* includes actions for returning the community to normal, such as repairing infrastructure, damaged buildings, and critical facilities. *Rehabilitation* or *reconstruction* involves activities that are taken to counter the effects of the disaster on long-term development.[3]

Domestically, there are 40–50 presidential disaster declarations per year. The Stafford Act, passed by Congress in 1988, provides for orderly assistance by the federal government to state and local governments to help them to carry out their responsibilities in managing major disasters and emergencies.[4] A disaster declaration must precede any federal aid whereby states make a request for federal assistance to activate a declaration. Most presidential declarations are made immediately following impact. However, if the consequences of a disaster are imminent and warrant limited predeployment actions to lessen or avert the threat of a catastrophe, a state's governor may submit a request even before the disaster has occurred. Although rarely used, the president may exercise his authority in certain emergencies and make a disaster declaration prior to state request in order to expedite the sending of federal resources. This presidential authority was used immediately following the 1995 bombing in Oklahoma City. Under the Stafford Act, the president may provide federal resources, medicine, food and other consumables, work and services, and financial assistance.

Disasters pose a number of unique health care problems that have little counterpart in the routine practice of emergency health care. Examples include the need for warning and evacuation of residents, widespread "urban" search and rescue, triage and distribution of casualties, having to function within a damaged or disabled health care infrastructure, and coordination among multiple jurisdictions, among levels of government, and among private sector organizations. In order to be effective managers, public health professionals must be knowledgeable about unfamiliar information such as the lexicon of emergency management and the science of engineering and must be competent in a specialized set of skills because disasters pose unique health care problems. For example, although temporary deficiencies in resources may occur at certain times in any disaster, resource problems in U.S. disasters more often relate to how assets are used or distributed rather than to deficiencies.[5] In a study of the impact of 29 major mass casualty disasters on hospitals, only six percent of the involved hospitals had supply shortages, and only two percent had personnel shortages.[6]

WHY PUBLIC HEALTH SHOULD BE CONCERNED

Public health professionals should augment their ability to respond to disasters for the following reasons:

- The occurrence of natural disasters is increasing.
- There is a ubiquitous risk across the United States.
- Disasters have negative impacts on health.
- The effects of disasters will escalate, generating an increased need for public health intervention.
- Public health has the expertise to help communities handle the most common health-related problems.

Across the globe, mankind is experiencing an increase in natural disasters, as evidenced by events in recent years.[7,8] Once a week, an average of one disaster that requires external international assistance occurs somewhere in the world. On a worldwide average, approximately 81,000 people die from natural disasters yearly. In the last two decades, as a consequence of disasters, more than 1.620 million people died, 3.5 billion lives were disrupted, and $900 billion was lost in property damage.[9]

Natural Disasters

Residents of the United States share a ubiquitous risk.[10] Across the United States, a massive number of people are at risk from three classes of natural disasters: floods, earthquakes, and hurricanes. There are more than 6,000 communities with populations of 2,500 or more persons located in flood plains that have been highly developed as living and working environments.[11] At least 70 million people face significant risk of death or injury from earthquakes because they live in the 39 states that are seismically active. In California alone, if a single major earthquake occurs, similar to nine others that occurred in the state over the past 150 years, there could be 20,000 deaths, 100,000 injuries, and economic losses totaling more than $100 billion.[12] Other parts of the country face serious risk because more than 3 million people live within a 75-mile radius of the New Madrid fault in the Midwest.[13] Even in Utah, there is a 20 percent probability that a large earthquake of a magnitude of 7.5 will occur on some segment of the Wasatch front within the next 50 years.[14]

Currently, 110 million people live in coastal areas of the United States, including the Great Lakes region. By the year 2010, the coastal population will have grown from 80 million people in 1960 to more than 127 million people—an increase of 60 percent nationwide.[15] The significance of this shift is evident when the risk posed by hurricanes alone is examined. Because of climatic changes in western Africa, hurricane activity along the Atlantic Coast and the Gulf of Mexico is expected to become as frequent as that which occurred between 1940–50.[8] During that decade, three category 4–5 hurricanes struck Miami, New Orleans, and the Gulf Coast. Since 1989, three category 4 hurricanes (Hugo, Andrew, and Opal) struck the East Coast of the United States from Florida to New England. A category 4 or greater hurricane crosses the U.S. coastline nearly once every six years.

Disasters have negative impacts on the public's health. These events result in increases in morbidity and mortality, with both physical and psychological impacts that could be reduced with adequate intervention. Following the 1993 floods in the Midwest, victims increased their use of primary health care and experienced long-term impediments to their access to health care.[16] Local health departments (LHDs) in Missouri understood the need for involvement in preparedness efforts because they experienced difficulties in collecting and using assessment information, coordination was burdensome, and there were interorganizational impediments to an effective response.[17]

Manmade Disasters

Manmade or technological disasters can also have devastating impacts on the public's health. The 1992 civil unrest in Los Angeles caused 53 deaths, more than 2,000 injuries, and destruction or closure to 15 county health centers, 45 pharmacies, and 38 medical and dental offices. There were also significant impacts to the quality of water, to hazardous materials and solid waste, and to protecting sources of food.[18] Because widespread burning, as occurred in the civil unrest, can release hazardous materials into the air, almost 3,000 sites were surveyed for release of hazardous waste.[18]

The actual and potential effects of manmade disasters will likely escalate, generating an increased need for public health intervention as the world's population grows, as population density increases, and as technology becomes more sophisticated. The need for public health information has spurred the development of readily available guidance. The National Center for Environmental Health at the U.S. Centers for Disease Control and Prevention (CDC) developed preventive guidelines, available on the CDC Web site, promoting personal health and safety for people involved in earthquakes, floods, hurricanes, and tornadoes.[19] High mortality attributed to the 1995 heat wave in Chicago demonstrated the need for standardized methodologies to make comparisons across geographic areas of the country.[20]

Public Health Personnel

Worldwide, the growing number of humanitarian emergencies has resulted in an expanding need for skilled public health professionals. The application of public health principles in a domestic response differs from public health practice in an international response, but the competencies required of the profession are the same. The tasks involved in fostering the development of community self-sufficiency are also functionally different in the United States than in international development. In developed countries, the medical response for emergency care is well organized through EMS. In developing countries, that infrastructure doesn't exist. In developing countries, public health personnel often play a key role because virtually all of the problems are related to the health of the populations. In complex humanitarian emergencies, public health personnel:

- Conduct initial assessments of health needs.
- Design and establish health activities.
- Plan for the delivery of services.
- Establish refugee camps.
- Provide and monitor food supplies.
- Supervise and monitor environmental health activities.
- Monitor the protection of human rights.

Public health can help communities handle the most common health-related problems. There are four domains where public health expertise is superior to that of other professionals involved in disaster preparedness and response. Public health officials are trained to conduct *assessments,* to survey the impacted site and determine the scope of damage and subsequent impacts on the community and the population. Using the management information systems that public health officials have developed throughout the health care industry, public health professionals are well prepared to *share information.* Some creative fine-tuning will permit public health professionals to develop procedures for capturing and sharing disaster-related information among the health community and other response organizations. Public health can build on the *triage* procedures used in emergency medicine to help other responders prioritize both medical and public health problems. Finally, public health's knowledge of *casualty distribution* will facilitate the development of procedures for disbursing casualties among available hospitals.

Disaster preparedness poses the quintessential public health dilemma—how to motivate people to prevent disaster-related health problems. It is human nature to say that "a major disaster will never happen here" and to fail to prepare. Health care organizations often don't give high priority to preparing for disastrous events, which are rare, when the general financial environment for health care is fragile. Furthermore, the benefits of preparedness often are not evident until after a disaster has occurred. In addition, economic constraints are often coupled with public apathy. Social scientists have noted that the public's perception of risk is often not correlated with actual risk, and that risks are usually downplayed. Many people continue to live in flood plains, even after repeated floods, and millions of people move to areas that are located on earthquake faults.

However, the benefits of effective prevention are demonstrated in a comparison of the morbidity and mortality statistics of Hurricane Andrew (Florida,1992) and the hurricane that struck, without warning, off the Gulf Coast of Texas in 1900. Due to successful prediction, warning, and evacuation, actual deaths following Andrew were less than two dozen. By contrast, in Texas 90 years earlier, 6,000 people were killed and 5,000 were injured.[21] Because of strong planning, the Los Angeles Department of Health provided important services following the 1994 Northridge earthquake.[22] Public health intervened when there were concerns about water and sewage, provided assessments of personal and mental health, inspected health care facilities, restored clinical operations, and educated the public about safety, health, and environmental concerns.

HISTORY OF PUBLIC HEALTH'S ROLE

Although public health is late in contributing to disaster preparedness and response, epidemiology made an early contribution to the domain of disaster research. Noji detailed the course of epidemiology's research contribution.[23] In 1957, Saylor and Gordon suggested using epidemiologic parameters to define disasters.[24] Almost a decade later, the CDC helped develop techniques for the rapid assessment of nutritional status in Nigeria. The 1970s brought the establishment of the Centre for Research on Epidemiology of Disasters in Belgium and specialized units within the World Health Organization (WHO) and the Pan American Health Organization (PAHO). The science of public health has now begun to show that variations in morbidity and mortality from one country to another are often due to differences in building standards and population density rather than the magnitude of an earthquake. This is demonstrated by a comparison of the impacts of recent hurricanes. In California, where antiseismic building and land use codes are well enforced, the Northridge earthquake of 1994 resulted in 57 deaths and almost 9,200 serious injuries.[22] In contrast, in Armenia, with poor construction and antiseismic regulations insufficient and poorly enforced, an earthquake of lesser magnitude killed 25,000 people and injured more than 100,000. The August 1999 earthquake in Turkey resulted in a variable rate of collapse of buildings that were built side by side. The standards used for construction were the determinate factor for a structure's survival.

The earliest investigations of disaster response were conducted by sociologists who studied organizational behavior under stress. Other contributions have been made by psychologists, management scientists, architects, engineers, economists, and public administrators. Since the early 1980s, there has been increased attention and interest in organizing a public health response to disasters and conducting studies within the public health discipline. The eruption of Mt. St. Helens in 1980 accelerated the involvement of the U.S. federal government in organizing a response.[25,26] The United Nations (UN) declared the 1990s as the disaster decade, International Decade for Natural Disaster Reduction, due to continued human losses across the globe.[27] The declaration for the decade spurred a broad variety of academic disciplines to develop educational and research programs in all phases of disaster management. The decade came to an end on December 31, 1999, and was succeeded by the International Strategy for Disaster Reduction as adopted by resolution 54/219 of the General Assembly of the UN.[28]

Historically, public health's response to disasters has been an ad hoc one, and on the whole, the profession has reacted slower than other disciplines in organizing professional activities. In many locales across the country, the medical/health efforts of preparedness have not been coordinated as part of the community's disaster response. Health departments were called in as an afterthought to handle problems that were part of their domain, rather than as part of the team planning the response. Other professions, such as emergency medicine, EMS, and engineering, increased training earlier in the decade to prepare their membership better for responding to disasters. The medical literature regarding disasters is full of anecdotal accounts of response.[5] However, few of these reports substantiate the *effectiveness* of the reported preparedness.

PUBLIC HEALTH'S ROLE

Public health has a natural role in disaster preparedness and response. This role is evolving as the emergency management community recognizes the skills possessed by the profession. Through increased recognition of what public health professionals can do, public health professionals are being called on more often to control injury and disease that are caused by both natural and technological hazards and to prevent infectious disease following natural disasters. State departments of health, with responsibility as a major directing unit overseeing the public's health, already work in partnership with LHDs and other appropriate federal, state, and local agencies. Disaster response is often an extension of daily tasks for public health professionals. In many states and localities, public health professionals coordinate the health response following natural and technological emergencies.[29]

Due to its impact on realms where public health is core, including health care infrastructure, Hurricane Andrew demonstrated that public health professionals must be involved in preparedness and response operations. Following Hurricane Andrew, which was categorized as "the most destructive disaster ever to affect the United States,"[30(p.243)] 175,000 Floridians were homeless and water systems were inoperable for at least a week.[21] The infrastructure of the health care system was also destroyed—59 hospitals were damaged, more than 12,000 patients needed to be examined, and pharmacies couldn't dispense medication.[31] To help in this situation, more than 850 public health nurses were deployed during the two months following the storm.[32]

With the increase in both domestic natural disasters and international complex emergencies, there is greater recognition of the need for intergovernmental experts who understand disasters. Although the calls for widespread training of the public health work force began relatively recently, there is now mainstream recognition that public health is a key player in disaster preparedness and response.[32] *Healthy People 2010* will include, as part of the core competencies, the enhancement of professional training in preparing for and responding to disasters.[33] Federal recognition of the need for public health intervention has resulted in newly directed federal funding at the end of the millennium for departments of health to improve their core abilities to respond to acts of bioterrorism, bringing public health intervention into the core of disaster preparedness and response.

WHAT IS PUBLIC HEALTH'S RESPONSIBILITY IN DISASTER RESPONSE?

The mission of public health in disaster preparedness and response includes responsibility for the following domains, referred to as "functions" within the emergency management field:

- assessment of the viability of the health care infrastructure, including the drug supply
- assessment of environmental infrastructure (food, water, sanitation, and vector control)

- assessment and provision of health care services (acute, continuity of care, primary care, and emergency care)
- preventive care
- assessment of the needs of the elderly and other special populations
- health surveillance and case identification/verification, including injury surveillance
- infectious disease control
- expert assistance in response to chemical, radiologic, or biologic hazards
- public health information
- mental health
- emergency shelter
- victim identification/body management

To fulfill these functions, public health has three major tasks.

- One task is the collection, evaluation, and dissemination of information. The other sectors that have traditionally responded to disasters are response oriented, not science oriented. Public health brings a basis for evaluating activities using a scientific method. Public health brings unique resources to the emergency management community. These include assessment and epidemiology and the capacity to analyze, make recommendations, and act on information. As an example, using Stafford Act funds, the state of Iowa established a statewide systematic electronic system for surveillance during the 1993 flood.[34]
- The second task is one of cooperation and collaboration with other disciplines. The responsibilities of public health in disaster preparedness and response are more complicated than in a typical public health response. First, the participants are from "sectors of response" (i.e., fire, EMS, emergency management) rather than from other parts of the health care delivery field. Workers have to participate as part of a multidisciplinary team that includes mostly professionals or paraprofessionals with whom they normally don't have interactions and who have little or no knowledge of public health (i.e., engineering, police, and the military/national guard). Further, the process of working together is unique. The other sectors who are involved in disaster response have a lexicon and methods that may be different than those of public health. A typical response incorporates multiple bureaucratic layers of infrastructure working together in a condensed time frame. Public health must often integrate itself into an already established response team whose members have trained together and who have clearly defined roles.
- The third task constitutes the prevention of disease and continuity of care. Public health looks at localities where a disaster has occurred, or is likely to occur, as a diseased or compromised community. No other discipline assesses how or acts to prevent disease following disaster. Public health has a major responsibility in ensuring the continuation of the delivery of all health care.

Being prepared is necessitated not only because of legal mandates, but also because of the devastating consequences if health care systems are unable to function. The Joint Commission on Accreditation of Healthcare Organizations prescribes standards and requirements that health care facilities must meet in order to remain accredited. These standards ensure that basic disaster plans are in place and that exercises of these plans are held on a regular basis.[35] The public health professional is involved in ensuring that essential health facilities are able to function after the impact of a disaster.[5,29] Essential facilities include hospitals, health departments, poison control centers, storage sites for disaster supplies, dispatch centers, paging services, and ambulance stations. The maintenance and continuation of home-based services (e.g., dialysis, intravenous antibiotics, visiting nurses services, etc.) will require creative solutions, worked out in advance. Patients in all residential care facilities (long-term care, psychiatric, rehabilitation) may need to be evacuated and placed elsewhere. Public health also initiates arrangements to ensure that routine sources of medical care will be functioning after a disaster. When physicians' offices, mental health clinics, nursing homes, pharmacies, community clinics, and urgent care centers are closed, those individuals needing routine care or medication will seek care from emergency departments based in already stressed hospitals. Following Hurricane Andrew, for example, more than 1,000 physicians' offices were destroyed or significantly damaged, greatly adding to the patient load of surviving hospitals.[32]

FUNCTIONAL MODEL OF PUBLIC HEALTH'S RESPONSE IN DISASTERS

In disaster preparedness and response, public health professionals are providers of service, scientists, and administrators. The core functions of public health have specific application to the organizational model of disaster preparedness and response, providing an opportunity for the breadth of the public health discipline to participate. In order to enter as full members of the emergency management response team, public health practitioners need to relate the framework of activities defined by the emergency management community to what public health can do. In order to provide technical assistance to communities, public health professionals must expand their lexicon to include specialized information that may not be directly related to health and seek out modalities for accessing state-of-the-art resources of other scientific fields, such as earth science, engineering, and demography. This interface between the core components of professional training and the matrix of emergency management is called the functional model of public health's response in disasters.

The functional model provides a paradigm for identifying disaster-related activities for which each core area of public health has responsibility. The functional model is composed of six phases that correspond to the type of activities involved in preparing for and responding to a disaster. The model (Table 28–1) identifies the roles and tasks for each of the core areas in each phase of a typical disaster response. This paradigm operationalizes a typical disaster response and categorizes the cycle of activities performed by the public health field. The functional model expands traditional public health partnerships with other disciplines because it requires public health professionals to collaborate with other responding sectors and to work in an integrated fashion with networks whose roles are previously well defined. The public health role for international scenarios has been independently assessed and described as if it were a conceptual fifth core area.

The components of the model follow:

- *Planning:* The goals of planning are to learn to work cooperatively with other disciplines and understand the resources, skills, and tools that public health professionals bring to the diseased community.
- *Prevention:* Prevention involves primary, secondary, and tertiary efforts and includes the activities that are commonly thought of as "mitigation" in the emergency management model.
- *Assessment:* Assessments are both short-term and long-term snapshots that help with decision making and enhance the profession's ability to monitor disaster situations. The goal of conducting assessments is to convey information quickly in order to recalibrate a system's response.
- *Response:* Response includes both the delivery of services and the management of activities.
- *Surveillance:* Surveillance includes both data collection and monitoring of disease.
- *Recovery:* Recovery has policy, political, and social implications that are both short and long term. Hurricane Floyd (1999) destroyed communities in New Jersey that had never experienced flooding. Many citizens were uninsured and received limited financial aid, making any recovery prolonged and painful.

STRUCTURE AND ORGANIZATIONAL MAKEUP OF DISASTER RESPONSE

When the health care sector responds to a disaster, it is most efficient to do so with the re-

Table 28–1 Functional Model of Public Health Responsibilities in Disaster Management

	Health Administration	*Epidemiology/ Biostatistics*	*Behavioral/ Social Sciences*	*Environment*	*International*
Planning	• Apply local public health to disaster management • Coordinate with hospital disaster plans • Help develop community disaster plan • Provide training • Determine assets	• Provide training • Analyze hazards and vulnerability • Conduct needs assessment	• Develop health promotion and disease prevention • Conduct training	• Conduct training • Analyze hazards and vulnerability	• Analyze hazards and vulnerability and develop response
Prevention Primary	• Provide immunizations • Protect and distribute food • Establish safe water and sanitation		• Educate community • Train public in first aid	• Protect and distribute food • Establish safe water and sanitation	• Provide emergency nutrition • Protect and distribute food • Establish safe water and sanitation
Prevention Secondary	• Detect and extricate victims • Provide emergency care • Manage bystander response	• Conduct care identification and surveillance • Implement infectious disease control	• Detect and extricate • Provide emergency care • Manage bystander response	• Detect and extricate • Provide emergency care • Manage bystander response	
Prevention Tertiary	• Reestablish health services • Manage emergency services • Manage injuries		• Provide long-term counseling		• Convert reponse to development

continues

Table 28–1 continued

	Health Administration	*Epidemiology/ Biostatistics*	*Behavioral/ Social Sciences*	*Environment*	*International*
Assessments	• Conduct surveillance for disease, behavioral, social, and political impacts • Assess damage to health care infrastructure • Survey assets • Conduct vulnerability analysis • Collect data for decision making	• Conduct surveillance for disease, social, behavioral, and political impacts • Assess causal factors of disease • Conduct vulnerability analysis • Conduct needs assessment • Collect data for decision making • Establish continuous monitoring	• Conduct surveillance for disease, social, behavioral, and political impacts • Collect data for decision making	• Conduct surveillance for disease, social, behavioral, and political impacts • Identify hazards and assess exposure • Conduct vulnerability analysis • Assess damage from: radiation, toxins, thermal, and water • Collect data for decision making • Do short-term cluster sampling • Establish continuous monitoring	• Conduct surveillance for disease, social, behavioral, and political impacts • Collect data for decision making • Do short-term cluster sampling
Service Response	• Administer logistics • Establish command and control, including casualty management • Identify, contain, and provide emergency treatment • Continue provision of primary care • Utilize the Federal Response Plan		• Educate to prevent illness and injury • Organize mental health services	• Identify, contain, and provide emergency equipment	• Utilize international disaster relief, United Nations agencies, International Committee of the Red Cross, and nongovernmental organizations

continues

Table 28–1 continued

	Health Administration	*Epidemiology/ Biostatistics*	*Behavioral/ Social Sciences*	*Environment*	*International*
Management Response	• Establish infection control, safe water, sanitation, and quarantine • Manage dead, biologic hazards, and waste disposal • Manage media • Utilize field skills • Establish security and protection	• Determine risk of delayed effects • Communicate risk	• Establish information systems	• Establish infection and vector control, safe water, sanitation, and quarantine • Reduce postdisaster injury (fire, nails, and electrocution) • Manage dead, biologic hazards, waste disposal • Communicate risk	• Manage dead, biologic hazards, waste disposal
Surveillance	• Establish information systems	• Utilize information systems • Look for sentinel events • Develop passive and active systems • Establish disaster informatics • Trend disease	• Establish information systems		• Monitor malnutrition
Recovery	• Use data for deployment of resources • Conduct evaluations • Plan and direct fieldwork	• Conduct evaluations • Plan and direct field studies	• Conduct evaluations • Plan and direct field studies	• Conduct evaluations • Plan and direct field studies	• Use data for deployment of resources • Conduct evaluations • Plan and direct fieldwork
Development					• Build capacity • Mobilize resources • Distribute food • Control injury and communicable disease • Provide population-based immunization • Provide primary health care, reproductive health, and transcultural care

Source: Copyright © 2000, L. Landesman.

sources already at hand. However, because disasters overwhelm the local authority's ability to respond effectively in protecting human health, local assets often need to be supplemented by resources from outside organizations. Additionally, disasters typically generate needs that are beyond the breadth of any one type of health care organization. This tension between need and availability is overcome by planning for and mounting a *multiorganizational* response, one of the key characteristics of disaster operations in the health sector. This section provides a quick overview of the organizations that are typically involved in the health sector's response to disaster, and describes how they interact with each other in disaster situations. Table 28–2 provides a listing of the most important response organizations.

Structure and Operations of the Routine EMS System

For most sudden-onset disasters, the first medical response is provided by the local or regional EMS system. The EMS system constitutes a portion of the health care delivery system that is virtually unknown to many public health professionals. Although its public health role in routine crisis management is beyond the scope of this chapter, the potential public health impact that can be contributed by EMS in times of disaster is substantial.[36] For this reason, it is important for public health emergency planners to be familiar with the organization and operations of the EMS system in both routine and disaster configurations.

In most parts of the United States, EMS is provided by semiautonomous local agencies with regional or state oversight. This service is provided under the authority of the state health department in most, but not all, states, but is not provided directly by the health department. EMS is thought to consist of

- a *public access system* by which the public notifies authorities that a medical emergency exists (In most of the United States, the 911 emergency telephone system is the backbone of this public access.)
- a *dispatch communications system* by which ambulance personnel and other emergency first responders are dispatched to respond to the person(s) in need
- *trained emergency medical responders*, commonly called emergency medical technicians (EMTs), or the higher-trained Paramedics (EMT-Ps) (EMTs and paramedics are trained to identify and field treat the most common medical emergencies and injuries, and to provide medical support to victims while they are enroute to the hospital.)
- *transportation* to definitive medical care, usually in a hospital (Ground ambulances are the vehicle of choice for most transports, but helicopters, boats, and snow cats may be used under specific circumstances. Ambulances allow for the continued medical support of patients while in transport.)
- *definitive care*, usually initiated in a hospital emergency department and followed up in a variety of health care settings (Emergency physicians and certified emergency nurses are specialists in emergency medical care in the hospital setting.)

The EMS is often discussed in terms of the prehospital system (e.g., public access, dispatch, EMTs/medics, and ambulance services) and the in-hospital system (e.g., emergency departments, inpatient care, and other definitive care facilities and personnel).

Several designs exist for the organizing authority of prehospital EMS systems: fire service, third service, private, public utility, rescue squad, and hospital based. Somewhat more than half of all EMS systems in the United States are based in local fire departments, with ambulance and fire services administered side by side.[37] In some systems, EMTs or medics are cross-trained as fire fighters with victim extrication skills, and fire fighters are cross-trained as medics. Third service systems are owned and operated by a city or county and are not run by either the fire services or the police service, therefore making them a third service. Some jurisdictions contract with private ambulance services, and some contract with a single private operator on a mo-

Table 28–2 Disaster Response Organizations

Organization	*Functions and Definitions*
Public Access System	Enables public to communicate response needs, typically through a 911 phone system.
Fire Department	Finds and extricates victims; often provides on-scene incident management.
Emergency Medical Services (EMS)	Assesses scene for medical needs, initiates triage of patients, assesses individual patients for status and treatment needs, initiates life-sustaining first aid and medical care, determines treatment destination, and transports patients to definitive care.
Incident Management System (IMS or ICS)	This is a *function*, often provided by an emergency management agency, a fire department, or multiple agencies.
Emergency Management Agency (EMA)	A state or jurisdictional agency tasked with preparedness and response for disasters and other emergencies. This is sometimes called the Office of Emergency Preparedness (OEP).
Federal Emergency Management Agency (FEMA)	The coordinating agency for all federal-level agency responses to disasters.
American Red Cross (ARC)	Private voluntary national organization tasked by government to provide mass care and shelter to disaster victims.
U.S. Public Health Services (USPHS)	The federal action agency charged with protecting the public's health.
Emergency Support Function 8 (ESF 8)	The health and medical function of the Federal Emergency Plan, which is coordinated by the USPHS Office of Emergency Preparedness.
National Disaster Medical System (NDMS)	A multi-agency response system coordinated by the USPHS-OEP with responsibility for responding to overwhelming medical needs in a disaster-struck state or territory.
Disaster Medical Assistance Team (DMAT)	A trained unit of medical response personnel available to respond with the NDMS to a disaster scene.
Private Voluntary Organization (PVO)	A broad range of functions and structures.
Substance Abuse and Mental Health Services Administration (SAMHSA)	One of the eight agencies of the USPHS; focuses on substance abuse and mental health services.
Center for Mental Health Services (CMHS)	Part of the SAMHSA; leads federal efforts to promote mental health and treat mental illness.
Emergency Services and Disaster Relief Branch (ESDRB)	Part of the CMHS; works with other agencies to provide crisis counseling and education to survivors of presidentially declared disasters.
Centers for Disease Control and Prevention (CDC)	
National Center for Environmental Health (NCEH)	Part of the CDC; assesses needs of people in disaster stricken areas and works to ensure that people receive appropriate assistance; has major responsibility for disaster epidemiology.

nopoly basis, which is called a public utility model. In some parts of eastern United States and in many rural areas, EMS is provided by volunteer independent rescue squads, or volunteer ambulance squads that are attached to a volunteer fire department. Finally, some EMS is based in local hospitals, from which they are dispatched and return. In most states, the health department has training and regulation jurisdiction over all EMS personnel regardless of their organizational affiliation. Regardless of the organizational affiliation, all EMS services work in close cooperation with fire department and specialized hazardous material teams to provide patient extrication from entrapment and dangerous situations.

The kind of medical care provided by EMS is divided into basic and advanced life support. The great majority of EMS providers are trained at the basic life support level. Basic life support prepares for the provision of fairly sophisticated noninvasive first aid and stabilization for a broad variety of emergency conditions, as well as semiautomatic defibrillation for cardiac arrest victims. Advanced life support, provided by paramedics, includes sophisticated diagnosis of patient conditions followed by initial on-site, protocol-driven medical treatment for conditions that will receive definitive treatment in hospitals. Paramedics work with a standardized pharmacopia that includes cardiac, respiratory, and blood pressure–related drugs, as well as high-potency short-acting anesthetics and analgesics. Specialized skills include endotracheal intubation, IV cannulation, surgical cricothyrotomy, intraosseous infusion, needle thoracostomy, manual defibrillation, pacing, and cardioversion.

In responding to a disaster, the function of coordinating and managing the multiple simultaneous activities, as well as managing the effective deployment of incoming resources, is of primary importance. Drabek et al. found that the coordination of multiple activities, resource inputs, and organizations was among the most difficult and crucial challenges in managing a disaster response.[38] A strong command and coordination system is imperative if emergency health services are to overcome the disruption to the normal operations of the system and to manage additional incoming resources. First published as the FIRESCOPE Program in 1982, the Incident Command System (alternatively called Incident Management System [IMS]) has become popular among fire services and EMS as a management structure that is able to maintain effective span of control, modular organization, and expandability.[39] Through a system called "sectorization," the tasks and functions of those responding, and the use of resources, are divided into manageable components. As the size or type of the operation changes, it is those sectors that allow for the IMS to be universally applied. Because of this, the IMS has become the standard operating methodology in EMS disaster response.

Organization of Public Health Emergency Response

The basis for all local public health emergency responses resides in the LHD. However, the public health sector is not nearly as uniformly organized for emergency responses as the EMS system is, with its broad variety of system designs. Although some health departments have the emergency response functions preplanned and assigned to appropriate departments, some have only designated someone to function as the emergency coordinator, and others assume that the director or his or her designee will cover any emergency contingencies. The best prepared health departments have well-designed emergency or disaster response plans, complete with a thorough risk analysis, prognostication of probable health effects, and analysis of the resources needed (and available) to provide an appropriate response. The health departments that are well prepared are likely to have coordinated their plans with other response functions in the health sector (EMS and hospitals), and with other public safety efforts, including the IMS. Regrettably, the majority of LHDs are unlikely to have comprehensive disaster response plans that are integrated with other medical response and public safety agencies.

The public health response to local-level emergencies and disasters is inevitably a multidisciplinary effort. The American Red Cross (ARC) provides emergency shelter; basic health services for those residing in shelters; food services on-site and in shelters; counseling, including mental health services or referrals; and family reunification. The public works department or a contracted commercial provider most often manages the potable water supply. Social services agencies work with the displaced, attend to psychosocial needs, and ensure that special needs populations such as the older adults, children, and individuals with disabilities receive the care required. Home nursing associations are often integrated into the emergency response plan to assist individuals with chronic diseases or special nursing needs. The health department is responsible, in most jurisdictions, for coordinating the efforts of the above-mentioned agencies on behalf of the public's health. However, the health department is only one actor in the overall emergency response, which is usually coordinated by a public safety agency such as an emergency management agency, a sheriff's office, or a fire department.

When the resources of the local jurisdiction are insufficient to meet the needs resulting from the disaster, local authorities have the option to call for additional help. The coordinating agency can seek help from surrounding jurisdictions (often referred to as mutual aid resources) or can escalate a request to the state or federal level, or both. The call for outside aid is often called "escalate upward." All states have an emergency management agency (EMA), sometimes called an office of emergency preparedness (OEP). It is the responsibility of the EMA, under the authority of the governor's office, to coordinate the efforts of all state resources used during an emergency or disaster. These resources may be expansive and include the state's health department, housing and social services agencies, and public safety agencies (i.e., state police). In disasters of this magnitude, certain federal resources are made available to the states, such as the National Guard, officers of the CDC (i.e., Epidemic Intelligence Service officers), and the U.S. Public Health Service (i.e., the Agency for Toxic Substances and Disease Registry. Local and state emergency management agencies typically convene a command center away from the disaster site whose function is to coordinate the multiorganizational response of representatives of each pertinent response agency. Health departments should plan to participate in the command center activities as a full partner.

Like a local jurisdiction, states also have the ability to escalate upward if the disaster response requires more resources than the state can quickly provide. Officials can escalate to regional mutual aid compacts or to federal resources. States in many regions of the country are forming multistate regional mutual aid compacts, such as that in the lower Mississippi River region, based on the Central United States Earthquake Consortium. These consortia can provide relatively rapid response due to geographic proximity.

Federal Response

The federal government has developed a federal response plan for the coordination of federal resources used in a disaster situation.[40] The lead agency in charge of coordinating the application of the plan is the Federal Emergency Management Agency (FEMA). The plan consists of 12 sections referred to as "Emergency Support Functions" (ESFs).

1. ESF 1: Transportation
2. ESF 2: Communication
3. ESF 3: Public Works and Engineering
4. ESF 4: Firefighting
5. ESF 5: Information and Planning
6. ESF 6: Mass Care
7. ESF 7: Resource Support
8. ESF 8: Health and Medical
9. ESF 9: Urban Search and Rescue
10. ESF 10: Hazardous Materials
11. ESF 11: Food
12. ESF 12: Energy

Although the federal response to the health needs of disaster victims is detailed in "ESF 8: Health and Medical," all other emergency support functions have both a direct and an indirect effect on the public health sector's ability to protect the health and welfare of disaster victims.

The resources covered by the federal response plan are normally accessed by a request from a state's governor or the state's EMA to FEMA, referred to earlier in this chapter as a presidential declaration. FEMA then contacts the agencies that play the lead role for each ESF. A core concept of the federal response plan is that the responding federal resources work at the behest of, and in support of, the local or state jurisdiction that is in charge of managing the disaster response.[40]

In the case of ESF 8: Health and Medical, the lead agency is the OEP. An office in the U.S. Department of Health and Human Services (DHHS), the OEP has departmental responsibility for managing and coordinating federal health, medical, and health-related social services after major emergencies and federally declared disasters. The OEP also directs and manages the interagency National Disaster Medical System (NDMS). The core of ESF 8 is the NDMS, a multi-agency program that also includes the activities of the Department of Defense, the Veterans Affairs Administration, and FEMA. The NDMS has several core functions. The first function, unrelated to domestic disasters, is to repatriate U.S. military casualties to participating U.S. hospitals where an armed conflict results in too many casualties to be adequately managed abroad. The second function, related to domestic disasters, is to provide a program whereby hospitals across the United States agree to care for civilians who have been injured in a disaster and who can't be cared for where they live. These disaster victims are transported to the participating hospitals by the NDMS. Participating hospitals are "federalized" and all charges incurred by disaster victims are paid either by insurance or by the federal government. The third and fourth functions are the result of an NDMS creation: the Disaster Medical Assistance Team (DMAT). DMATs are designed to provide on-site disaster medical assistance (third function) and to transport victims to definitive care (fourth function) while providing medical support for the transported victims. DMATs are formed locally with approximately 30 personnel, including physicians, nurses, paramedics, and logistics officers. Once trained, the team members gather enough supplies to be self-sufficient and are ready to be transported to distant disasters on short notice. These personnel are temporarily "federalized" so that they can provide services outside of their licensing jurisdiction at the level of their licensure or certification credentials without legal ramifications. There is a public health DMAT based in Rockville, Maryland.

The reach of ESF 8 is broader than just the NDMS/DMAT functions. For example, the CDC in Atlanta maintains personnel who can perform rapid needs assessments from a public health perspective. Some of these personnel are stationed at regional offices of DHHS around the country, shortening the time needed for them to respond to a disaster site.

There is also a growing network of federal, state, and local public health and security agencies working together to prepare for and coordinate the health sector response to terrorist acts using biologic, chemical, or nuclear weapons. At the time of this writing, the exact configuration of this emergency response subsystem and its relationship with existing emergency management agencies is still unclear. The OEP and the National Center for Infectious Disease at the CDC are heavily involved in coordinating the health sector participation in this effort.

Voluntary Agencies

Of considerable importance to the successful provision of good public health response to a disaster is ESF 6: Mass Care. The Federal Response Plan makes the ARC the primary agency responsible for this function, which includes sheltering, feeding, emergency first aid, family reunification, and the distribution of emergency relief supplies to disaster victims. The ARC responds first through its local chapters, then state and regional chapters, which may call on national-level ARC resources if necessary.

A vast array of other voluntary agencies participate in disaster response with functions that contribute significantly to public health outcome. Many of these are church affiliated, such as the Salvation Army, Mennonite Central Committee, and Catholic Relief Services. Some are dedicated solely to disaster-related functions, such as the International Critical Incident Stress Foundation; most have more routine public service and emergency functions that are activated according to the needs of a specific disaster.

International Agencies

A vast array of agencies stand ready to respond to requests for international assistance to protect the public's health after disasters. Multinational UN-based organizations include WHO, UNICEF, the UN High Commissioner for Refugees, and the World Food Program. The PAHO (WHO's regional affiliate for the Americas) has a highly organized Office for Emergency Preparedness and Disaster Relief Coordination, which helps coordinate international health sector response in the Americas. Many national governments have an agency that provides unilateral foreign disaster assistance, such as the U.S. State Department's Office of Foreign Disaster Assistance. Numerous voluntary agencies have gained considerable expertise in responding to postdisaster health needs across international borders. Examples include Médecins Sans Frontières, World Vision, Oxfam, and Save the Children.

A NATURAL DISASTER: A CASE STUDY

The following sections detail a realistic scenario of a major earthquake in Memphis, Tennessee. This scenario is based on research provided by FEMA, the Central U.S. Earthquake Consortium, and various Tennessee and Memphis area agencies. The scenario is as realistic as possible, given the two-dimensional format of this publication. The function of the scenario is to help illustrate how the above-described organizations would respond, to detail their responsibilities, and to provide a sense of the timeline that would evolve. Exhibit 28–1 provides a timeline for the activities that are involved.

Earthquake Hits

Suppose a 7.2 Richter scale earthquake strikes on the New Madrid fault line, with its epicenter some 75 miles north of Memphis. The earthquake hits in the early afternoon on a work day in late January, with snow on the ground and temperatures hovering a little below freezing. Much of the building stock in Memphis is constructed of unreinforced masonry, leading to massive loss of life, loss of 70 percent of hospital capacity, and a virtual total collapse of the local transport and power grids. Private housing is severely damaged, although not as completely as many of the public buildings in the downtown area.

Initial Priorities

In the first two hours after the earthquake, the local EMS and fire services agencies assess the extent of the damage and initiate the process of locating, extricating, and providing emergency medical assistance to victims. The task is overwhelming, with the sheer volume of those in need complicated by the loss of ambulances from the earthquake, the inability to traverse debris-clogged roads, and the loss of viable hospitals to take patients to. EMS immediately request mutual aid from outside agencies. Given the fact that the surrounding jurisdictions are also affected, such aid must come from much further away and be coordinated by state and federal agencies. Federal DMAT and urban search and rescue teams are requested from FEMA and dispatched within hours, but given the distances they must travel and the difficulties of logistics, such teams do not begin arriving until the following afternoon, more than 24 hours later.

Needs Assessment

During the first two-hour time period, the local and state health departments join with their respective emergency management agencies to staff the command center, an integral part of the IMS. A primary function of department personnel is to conduct an immediate needs assessment. Although the health departments dispatch some of their own personnel to the scene to report on visible signs of what the health sector needs will be, the majority of initial information comes from queries of EMS and fire department personnel, for whom initial assessments are a primary responsibility. Health department personnel contact local hospitals by radio for damage reports and information regarding the influx of victims.

Exhibit 28–1 Disaster Timeline

Disaster Event

	Pre-event Planning	Emergency Response (0–24 hrs)	Emergency Response (24–72 hrs)	Recovery (>72 hrs)
Tasks	Develop Disaster Plan interagency development hazard analysis resource analysis define concept of operations establish chain of command establish mutual aid resources integration of state and federal resources perform plan drills and exercises establish disaster training update and maintain plan establish resource/equipment caches	Activate emergency operations center Establish communications Conduct damage and needs assessment Search, rescue, and extricate Provide field triage, on-site medical care Establish casualty collection points Transport patients to definitive care Activate mass casualty hospital protocols Request mutual aid resources Mitigate occupational hazards Mitigate ongoing threats and hazards, e.g., HAZMATs, sewage	Integrate state and federal resources Continue rescue and extrication Continue health and medical care If applicable, plan and enact a medical evacuation Begin restoration of public works to essential facilities Establish shelter, potable water supplies, and the delivery of food supplies Ensure the safety of water and food Establish means of sanitation/waste disposal, minimize releases Establish disease surveillance Establish CISM services	Continue medical care Monitor public health and medical care Continue monitoring of food, water, and shelter quality and safety Monitor for disease outbreaks Establish vector control Restore public works Provide disaster grants and loans to families and businesses
Organizations	Work with • Emergency Management Agency • City/County Council • Local: Fire, EMS, Police • Social Services • Public Health • Environmental Health • Public Works • Hospitals • Nongovernmental/ Private, e.g., Red Cross, RACES	Coordinate with • Emergency Management Agency • City/County Council • Local: Fire, EMS, Police • Social Services • Public Health • Environmental Health • Public Works • Hospitals • Nongovernmental/Private, e.g., Red Cross, RACES	Seek help from • Emergency Management Agency • City/County Council • Local: Fire, EMS, Police • Social Services • Public Health • Environmental Health • Public Works • Hospitals • Nongovernmental/Private, e.g., Red Cross, RACES • State and Federal Resources: –DMATs, DMORTs –FEMA, CDC –Military	Initiate recovery activities with • Emergency Management Agency • City/County Council • Local: Fire, EMS, Police • Social Services • Public Health • Environmental Health • Public Works • Hospitals • Nongovernmental/Private, e.g., Red Cross • State and Federal Resources: DMATs, DMORTs, FEMA, CDC, Military

continues

Exhibit 28–1 continued

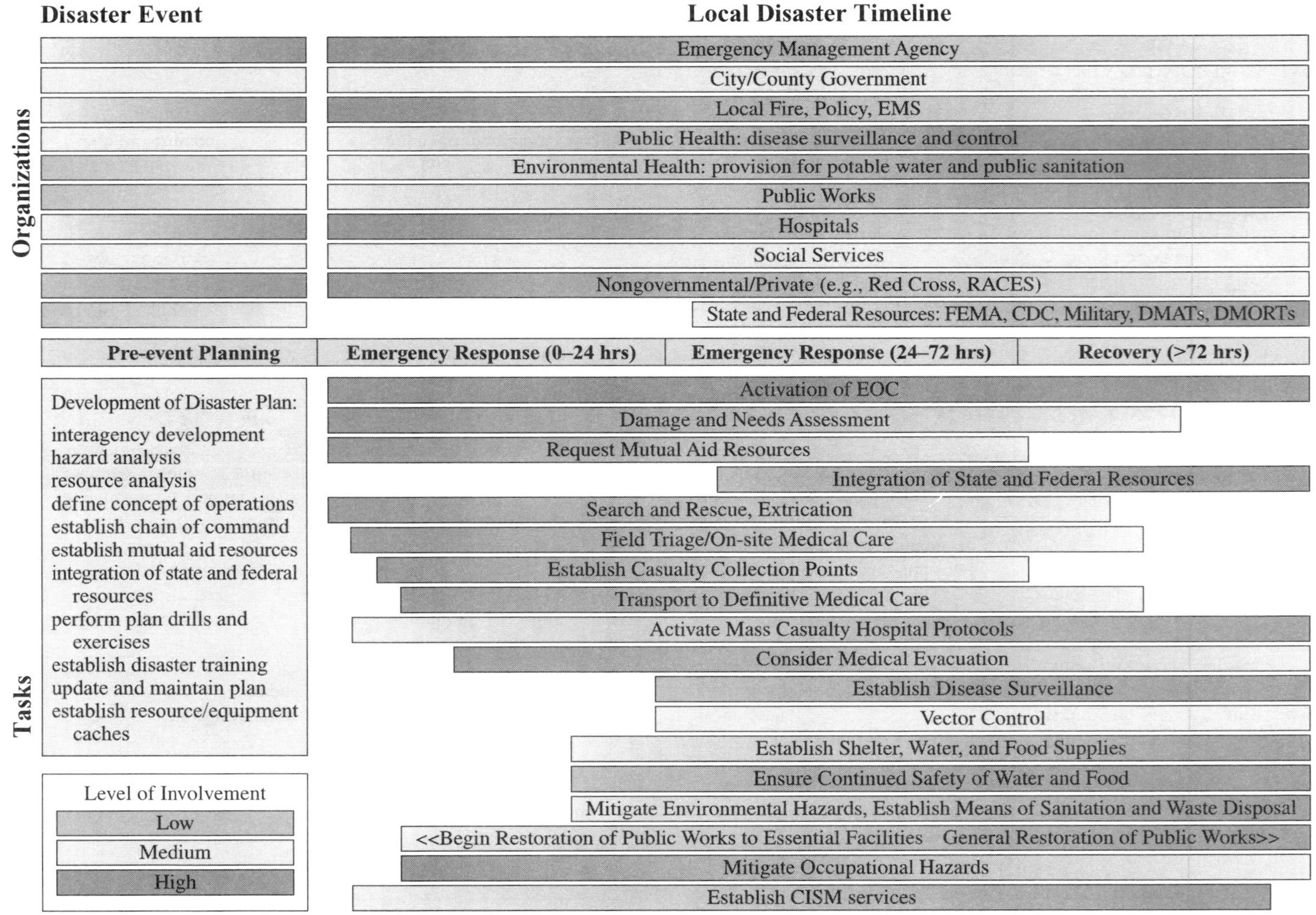

Disaster Event

Local Disaster Timeline

Organizations

Emergency Management Agency

City/County Government

Local Fire, Policy, EMS

Public Health: disease surveillance and control

Environmental Health: provision for potable water and public sanitation

Public Works

Hospitals

Social Services

Nongovernmental/Private (e.g., Red Cross, RACES)

State and Federal Resources: FEMA, CDC, Military, DMATs, DMORTs

Pre-event Planning	Emergency Response (0–24 hrs)	Emergency Response (24–72 hrs)	Recovery (>72 hrs)

Tasks

Development of Disaster Plan:
- interagency development
- hazard analysis
- resource analysis
- define concept of operations
- establish chain of command
- establish mutual aid resources
- integration of state and federal resources
- perform plan drills and exercises
- establish disaster training
- update and maintain plan
- establish resource/equipment caches

Activation of EOC

Damage and Needs Assessment

Request Mutual Aid Resources

Integration of State and Federal Resources

Search and Rescue, Extrication

Field Triage/On-site Medical Care

Establish Casualty Collection Points

Transport to Definitive Medical Care

Activate Mass Casualty Hospital Protocols

Consider Medical Evacuation

Establish Disease Surveillance

Vector Control

Establish Shelter, Water, and Food Supplies

Ensure Continued Safety of Water and Food

Mitigate Environmental Hazards, Establish Means of Sanitation and Waste Disposal

<<Begin Restoration of Public Works to Essential Facilities General Restoration of Public Works>>

Mitigate Occupational Hazards

Establish CISM services

Level of Involvement
- Low
- Medium
- High

Source: Copyright © 2000, R. Bissell.

They also seek information on the viability of the water supply system and the status of preplanned emergency shelters, usually schools. With this information, the health departments conclude that they have a truly catastrophic emergency on their hands, with the probability of many thousands of injured in need of medical care, massive loss of hospital resources, and an almost total loss of piped water. Early reports on emergency shelters reveal heavy destruction, and a cold night is rapidly approaching.

First Attempts To Meet Victims' Needs

During the next four hours (hours two to six), EMS providers find themselves out of supplies, dealing with patient needs as well as they can. Most patients cannot be transported due to road and hospital conditions, meaning that life-supporting care (including shelter and water) must be provided as well as possible at neighborhood collection points. Medics are not trained to deal with definitive care or long-term patient support needs, so improvisation is needed. Surviving private physicians' offices and facilities staffed by voluntary organization members are used. Some health department personnel scramble to consolidate hospital resources in the remaining facilities that are functional. Others work with the local emergency management agency, the ARC, and other voluntary organizations to rapidly open up and staff as many emergency shelters as possible. Other responders work with state and federal authorities to try to acquire emergency supplies of pharmaceuticals and other medical necessities. Health department epidemiologists work with fire service, EMS, and hospital personnel to try to establish a more accurate estimate of the numbers of injured, dead, and those who have other emergency medical needs (e.g., those on oxygen, dialysis, etc.).

Evolving Health Department Actions

As the first 6-hour time period evolves into the first 24, the above roles continue while others come on line. The role that health departments play in ensuring the quality of food, water, and shelter in routine times converts to one of working with multiple organizations to provide those basics, while also working to ensure quality. Emergency shelters can quickly become breeding grounds for infectious disease if proper sanitary measures are not put in place. Likewise, the safety of the emergency water supply becomes an issue of paramount importance. Health departments find themselves working with private and public utilities, housing departments, and a vast collection of private voluntary organizations in order to ensure the provision of basic necessities. Mental health and social services needs also begin to emerge at about this time, adding another layer of agency involvement and increased need for coordination.

Outside Resources Arrive

Approximately 24 hours after the first shaking was felt, many of the outside agencies begin to arrive. This includes such diverse teams as DMATs, urban search and rescue teams, assessment teams from the CDC, specialists from FEMA, emergency morgue workers, and specialists to help assess the need for hazardous materials response teams. At the same time that these broader public health functions are added to the response, the medical community is still trying to provide emergency care for the acutely injured and ill. One of the key tasks of health authorities at this point is to try to find clinicians who can replace or reinforce local clinical personnel who, by this point, are exhausted and often worried about their own families. The NDMS DMATs can help fill this role, but they are too limited in number to meet all of the needs in a catastrophic disaster.

It is the role of public health authorities to begin thinking about returning health care services to normal as soon as possible after a disaster. Although it may seem premature to start thinking about this so soon into the scenario given here, this approach is key in setting priorities during the emergency period.[41] Fire departments and EMS often deal with the complexities of managing a large emergency response by dividing the operation area up into sectors that are functional, geographic, or both. Health departments find it necessary to do the same during the early hours and days of an overwhelming disaster.

Transition from Acute Care to Primary/Preventive Care

Into days three and four, the number of new casualties found who need emergency care diminishes, but the need for acute care continues to overwhelm the restricted capacity of the health care system. Patients present with disaster-related conditions, as well as chronic illness that has become acute in a period of diminished resources. Reestablishment of primary care at this time becomes a high priority and a challenge to health authorities. This is also the period when authorities need to enforce increased vigilance for conditions that are likely to lead to outbreaks of infectious disease. Health authorities seek mutual aid from surrounding or distant jurisdictions in order to provide trained personnel to perform the core functions of case investigation, laboratory confirmation, and remedy.

The Work Continues

Despite the fact that most disasters disappear from the news headlines within a few days of their occurrence, the effects of the event take months, often years, to remedy successfully. By the end of the first week, public health authorities begin the process of planning the health sector's long-term recovery. Although many of the resources needed may not be within the control of the health department, personnel's coordination of diverse resources is crucial to successful recovery. More than ever before, the public will depend on a strong health department to coordinate effectively with the multitude of multidisciplinary agencies and voluntary organizations needed to protect the public's health while the population is struggling to pull their lives back together.

ASSESSMENT IN DISASTERS*

Public health, at the local, state, and federal levels, has a major role in assessing and monitoring the nature of disasters and their impacts on communities. These assessments are important managerial tools in preventing morbidity and mortality and in organizing a response.

Assessing the postdisaster situation requires gathering and evaluating information (critical activities in responding to a disaster), recovering from the event, and rehabilitating postdisaster conditions as they are restored to "normalcy." These processes lead to an identification of: (1) the needs of the affected community after a disaster has occurred, (2) appropriate relief goods or services for that community, (3) epidemic levels of disease or injury if indicated, and (4) resources that may be needed by health care services in the disaster zone. From objective and unbiased information produced by such an assessment, informed decisions may be made by health officials or emergency managers to direct response and recovery activities.

Measurements of Disasters

Objective measures are used to quantify environmental hazards and human impacts related to natural disasters. To indicate the severity of a disaster event, scales developed by different scientific disciplines such as seismology and meteorology to measure the disaster event are used to describe the hazard from the public health standpoint. For example, the magnitude of an earthquake is indicated by the Richter scale, which provides a measure of the total energy released from the source of the earthquake. The intensity of an earthquake is represented by the measurements on the modified Mercalli scale, which indicates a measure of the degree of damage from a particular location. Similarly, the strength of tornadoes may be measured by the Fujita scale. For hurricanes, the Saffir-Simpson scale is presently used by meteorologists, although recent storms have shown that the scale may need modification to reflect varying amounts of rain, wind, and storm surge.

Measures may also be made of the physical manifestations of a disaster event to indicate the size and severity of that event. For example, the height of a river above flood stage can signal the scope of a flood event. Levels of pollutant aerosols can represent the degree and extent of environmental exposure after uncontrolled forest fires. Levels of pesticides in drinking water or sediment after severe flooding may lead to questions about acute and chronic exposure to toxic chemicals in na-tech events.

Measures of biologic effects, that is, human health effects, indicate resulting impacts on hu-

---

**Source:* This material was published in the public domain. No copyright applies.

man health and disease. In earthquake events, age-specific injury and death rates may be calculated in cases for whom a direct health outcome is associated with the event. Among displaced persons in shelters where an infectious disease outbreak may occur, laboratory typing of organisms in biologic samples such as blood and urine may indicate exposure to a disease-causing pathogen and confirmation of disease. Similarly, biochemical testing of affected individuals exposed to toxic chemicals via oral, dermal, or inhalation routes demonstrates the presence or absence of an analyte of the chemical compound and the amount of an analyte that may be compared against a reference standard to assess exposure levels. In famine situations, anthropometric measurements, such as height to weight ratios among young children, may indicate the type and degree of malnutrition due to lack of food.

Applied Epidemiology

A systematic approach to assessing post-disaster conditions is based on the principles of epidemiology, the cornerstone of public health science. Epidemiology—derived from the Greek roots *epi* = among, *demos* = people, and *logos* = doctrine—is the study of the occurrence of diseases in human populations.[42] Epidemiology addresses disease occurrence by scientifically measuring characteristics of individuals and the relationships of people to their environments. Classically, epidemiology has been applied to infectious diseases in populations, or "epidemics," and investigators have identified microorganisms that cause diseases, determined infectiousness and immunity among humans, and recommended public health measures to thwart the spread of diseases. In recent decades, however, epidemiologic methods have been applied in many health fields, including environmental health, chronic disease, and injury control.[43]

One recent application of epidemiology is the investigation of the public health and medical consequences of natural disasters. Known as "disaster epidemiology," or "epidemiology in disaster settings," this discipline evolved as scientists realized that the effects of disasters on health were amenable to study by epidemiologic methods.[43] Some of the methods involve a comparison of people who were killed or injured with people who were not in order to learn the ways in which they differed. Epidemiologists identify risk factors with the aim of preventing the occurrence of death.

During each phase of the disaster continuum, public health assessment for a disaster event is conducted by answering the following questions:[44]

- What problems are occurring? Why are they occurring?
- Where are the problems occurring?
- Who is affected?
- What problems are causing the greatest morbidity and mortality?
- What problems are increasing or decreasing?
- What problems will subside on their own?
- What problems will increase if they are left unattended?
- What relief resources are available?
- Where are relief resources available?
- How can relief resources be used most efficiently?
- What relief activities are in progress?
- Are relief activities meeting the relief needs?
- What additional information is needed for decision making?*

Applications of epidemiology in disaster settings are conducted for many reasons. Primarily, they are used to describe the health effects of contributing factors, such as demographic characteristics and environmental parameters, and to prevent adverse health effects from occurring in a particular disaster event and in similar events in the future. After 183,000 persons died in a major tropical cyclone that struck coastal

---

**Source:* Reprinted with permission from V.W. Sidel et al., Public Health Responses to Natural and Human-made Disasters, in *Public Health and Preventive Medicine,* K.F. Maxcy, N.J. Rosenau, J.M. Last, and R.B. Wallace, eds., pp. 1173–1186, © McGraw-Hill Companies, 1992.

Bangladesh, mortality could have been further prevented by effective warnings leading to earlier response actions, access to designated cyclone shelters, and improved preparedness in high-risk communities. In particular, women and children less than 10 years of age were found to be at risk for cyclone-related deaths.[45]

Epidemiologic investigations may also provide informed advice regarding probable health effects. Following the Mt. St. Helens volcanic eruption, a comparison of people who were treated for asthma and bronchitis with healthy matched controls indicated that a history of asthma, and possibly of bronchitis, was a risk factor for contracting respiratory illness. The main exacerbating factor was the elevated level of airborne total suspended particulates, which were greater than 30,000 micrograms per cubic meter after the eruption.[46]

Epidemiologic studies may be used to identify needs in affected communities by rapid needs assessments. Using a list of needs in an affected community, public health authorities or emergency management officials can use these techniques to provide information for emergency planning, provide reliable and accurate information for relief decisions, and ultimately, match resources to needs. A needs assessment conducted two months after Hurricane Georges struck the Dominican Republic indicated the need for food, with special consideration to pregnant and lactating women and their newborns.[47] Finally, managers can employ epidemiologic applications to evaluate the effectiveness of program interventions used to provide relief.

Epidemiologic activities in the impact phase include the following techniques: (1) rapid needs assessment, (2) disease surveillance, and (3) descriptive and analytic investigations. In the immediate aftermath of a disaster, a critical concern of relief authorities is the identification of the needs of an affected community.

- Rapid *needs assessment* or rapid epidemiologic assessment, represents a collection of techniques—epidemiologic, statistical, and anthropological—designed to provide information about an affected community's needs after a disaster.[48] The objective is to obtain timely and objective information or a snapshot of a disaster-stricken community quickly so that immediate actions may be taken for relief activities.
- *Surveillance* refers to an ongoing and systematic collection, analysis, and interpretation of information linked to planning, implementation, and evaluation of public health practice, and closely integrated with the timely dissemination of these data to those who need to know.[49] Often, disease surveillance systems are implemented to signal whether outbreaks of infectious diseases are occurring in the community.
- *Descriptive and analytic investigations* may be undertaken by health authorities in situations where assessment and surveillance raise further questions and hypotheses concerning a health condition in the affected population. These investigations are designed to address questions or test hypotheses so that recommendations can be made for the prevention of any adverse health outcomes related to the disaster event.

The ultimate aim of disaster epidemiology is to determine strategies to prevent or reduce deaths, injuries, or illnesses related to the disaster. Prevention strategies are often grouped into three categories.

1. *Primary prevention*, or prevention of the occurrence of deaths, injuries, or illnesses related to the disaster event (e.g., evacuation of a community in a flood-prone area, sensitizing warning systems for tornadoes and severe storms), is an initial recommendation resulting from descriptive and analytic postdisaster investigations.
2. *Secondary prevention*, or the mitigation of health consequences of disasters (e.g., use of carbon monoxide detectors when operating gasoline-powered generators after loss of electric power after ice storms, employing appropriate occupant behavior in multistory structures during earthquakes, building a "safe room" in dwellings located in tornado-prone areas), may also be instituted when disasters are imminent.

3. *Tertiary prevention*, defined as minimizing the effects of disease and disability among the already ill, is employed in persons with preexisting health conditions and in whom the health effects from a disaster event may exacerbate those health conditions. Examples include appropriate sheltering of persons with respiratory illnesses and those prone to such conditions, particularly the elderly and young children, from haze and smoke originating from forest fires, and sheltering elderly who are prone to heat illnesses during episodes of extreme ambient temperatures.

Emergency Information Systems

Information is critical to any response effort after a disaster has occurred. The need for objective and reliable information is underscored by the nature of the postdisaster setting. First, disasters disrupt normal or existing relationships between people and their physical and social environments. Threats to health may ensue due to changes in preexisting levels of disease, ecologic changes as a result of the disaster, population displacement and movement of survivors leading to overcrowding and situations in which sanitation and hygiene are compromised, disruption of existing services such as public utilities, and disruption of normal public health programs. Moreover, the potential for communicable diseases increases for vectorborne, waterborne, and person-to-person transmission. As such, accurate and reliable information is needed in making decisions about the needs of the affected population for immediate relief efforts, short-term responses, and long-term planning for recovery and reconstruction.

There are several types of information that are collected for decision making, and each type has multiple uses. Deaths are often an initial starting point because they indicate the severity of the disaster event. Using mortality data, managers can assess the magnitude of the disaster event, evaluate the effectiveness of disaster preparedness, evaluate the adequacy of warning systems, and identify high-risk groups where more contingency planning is required. By reviewing information about casualties or the injured, emergency medical personnel and managers of critical care facilities can estimate needs for emergency care, evaluate predisaster planning and preparedness, and evaluate the adequacy of warning systems. Managers can assess information about morbidity, or disease, to estimate the types and volume of immediate medical relief needed, to identify populations at risk for disease, to evaluate the appropriateness of relief activities, and to assess needs for further planning.

In addition to information that helps public health professionals understand the health effects of disasters, information concerning public health resources, particularly from LHDs, is important for emergency information systems. Using these data, officials can estimate the types and volume of supplies, equipment, and services needed for the emergency, can assess needs for further planning, and can evaluate the appropriateness of relief interventions.

In international scenarios, managers can review information about donated goods and the overall relief effort to estimate the types and volume of supplies, equipment, and services needed over time. The goal is to match the appropriateness of the donated goods to the needs and culture of the receiving country, to evaluate the appropriateness of relief activities, and to assess needs for further planning.[50] Wool blankets are not needed in the tropics, and the donation of outdated medication presents the unwanted problem of disposal on a community that is already struggling with enough problems. One example of an information management system is SUMA (supply management program), which was developed by the PAHO and successfully applied in past disasters in Latin America. This computer-based system provides a mechanism for sorting, classifying, and preparing an inventory of relief supplies sent to a disaster-stricken country.[51]

Finally, information may be compiled for hazards, specific events related to those hazards, and health outcomes associated with those hazards. These emergency information systems monitor health events, diseases, injuries, hazards, exposures, and risk factors related to a designated event. An early warning system may forecast the occurrence of a disaster event by monitoring conditions that are likely to signal the event. An example is the Famine Early Warning System that was established by the U.S. Agency for International Development (USAID) to monitor climate and meteorology, availability of food in the market, and morbidity related to nutrition in order to predict the occurrence of famine in undeveloped countries.[52]

Surveillance

Public health surveillance is the

> ongoing and systematic collection, analysis, and interpretation of health data used for planning, implementing, and evaluating public health interventions and programs, closely integrated with the timely dissemination of these data to those who need to know. Surveillance data are used both to determine the need for public health action and to assess the effectiveness of programs. The final link of the surveillance chain is the application of these data to prevention and control. A surveillance system includes a functional capacity for data collection, analysis, and dissemination linked to public health programs.[49(p.164)]

In the postdisaster setting, surveillance provides information that can serve as the basis for action during the immediate disaster and also for planning of future activities. (See Chapter 8 for more information on surveillance activities in public health.)

Postdisaster surveillance is conducted by health authorities primarily to monitor health events. By instituting a surveillance system, one can detect sudden changes in disease occurrence, follow long-term trends of specific diseases, identify changes in agents and host factors for the diseases of interest, and detect changes in health practices for treating relevant diseases. Surveillance also provides tools for the public health practitioner in investigation and control, planning, generating hypotheses, stimulating research, testing hypotheses, and documenting disease activity.[53]

Surveillance is conducted after disasters primarily to detect any illnesses or injuries in the affected population. Information from the surveillance system is used to provide information for decision making by public health authorities. For example, measles vaccination campaigns may be launched in shelters concurrent with normal vaccination programs, with information from the surveillance indicating only sporadic cases. Surveillance is also conducted to investigate rumors, such as the occurrence of infectious disease, which commonly arise in the aftermath of a disaster event. Surveillance data can signal whether an outbreak has actually occurred. If unusual increases of disease are observed, public health workers may be deployed to investigate in order to determine the veracity of the reports and confirm diagnosis. Finally, surveillance is also conducted to monitor the effectiveness of response activities. For example, cases of acute diarrheal disease would be expected to decline with the use and implementation of water treatment interventions. A surveillance system that monitors diarrheal disease where water treatment has been implemented could indicate, as evidenced by rates of diarrheal disease, whether intervention was effective when compared to similar rates from areas without the intervention.[54]

Surveillance systems are usually one of three types: (1) hazard, (2) exposure, and (3) outcome. A *hazard* surveillance is, by definition, an assessment of the occurrence of or distribution of levels of hazards and the secular trends in levels of hazards (e.g., toxic chemical agents, physical agents, biomechanical stressors, as well as biologic agents) responsible for disease and injury. Although no strict methodology exists, a starting point for the surveillance may be to determine the parameters that affect the occurrence, quantity, and distribution of the agents and plot these through time. Alternatively, one could adapt existing information used for hazard surveillance, such as registries of use of toxic substances in compliance activities. An example of the application of postdisaster hazard surveillance is the use of a report of daily variations in respirable particulate matter (i.e., particles with a mass median aerodynamic diameter of 10 microns) after wildland fires. Thresholds can be established whereby people who are susceptible to pulmonary disease can be guided to take precautionary measures when the particles reach a certain size.

Surveillance may also be based on *exposure,* which by definition is a characteristic of interest, also known as a risk factor variable, predictor variable, independent variable, or putative causal factor. In disaster settings, exposure may be based on physical or environmental properties of the disaster event, such as "ash fall" after volcanic activity or pesticide-contaminated soil unearthed by flood water.[55] An example of postdisaster exposure surveillance is a report of daily activities, including time of exposure, of outdoor workers who are exposed to "ash fall" after a volcanic eruption.

Surveillance is more commonly based on a health *outcome,* defined as a health event of interest, usually illness, injury, or death. Outcome variables are also known as the response variable, dependent variable, or effect variable. An example of postdisaster outcome surveillance is the Health Impact Surveillance System (HISS) used by the ARC and the CDC. Using HISS, the ARC records mortality and morbidity statistics during disaster events where they are involved.[56]

Other types of surveillance systems may be based on the characteristics and objectives for establishing those particular systems. Decisions need to be made about using existing or temporary systems, hospital-based or community-based systems, and active or passive systems. When deciding to use existing systems rather than establishing temporary data collection systems, managers should consider whether existing systems, such as those for notifiable diseases, would provide adequate and timely information in the immediate aftermath of a disaster. If not, managers can set up temporary systems for the duration of the emergency period, or for the phase in which the information is desired. For hospital-based data collection versus community-based collection, one may consider whether hospital-based data would provide an accurate representation of morbidity related to the disaster. If not, data collection should be extended to include information obtained from mobile care sites or clinics. Given that resources may be finite, monitoring only at sentinel sites may be more appropriate than using a comprehensive "all-sites" approach. The critical issue is whether selected sites will provide a reasonable representation of the health outcomes being monitored. Finally, for active versus passive systems, one may decide that active solicitation of information may provide timely and appropriate information on health effects of a disaster event, in contrast to a passive surveillance system that collects data on similar health effects on a routine basis. Because of the need for information for rapid response and the myriad of health outcomes that may specifically result from a particular disaster event, active surveillance systems tend to fit more of the needs of health authorities in disaster situations.

The importance of public health surveillance may be assessed by performing the following steps:

- Determine the public health importance of monitoring selected morbidity and disaster-related mortality.
- Assess the availability of a public health response based on the data collected.
- Determine any economic impacts on the part of the institutions that will be participating in the system.
- Determine the level of public health concern for the system currently in place.

In establishing a surveillance system, the outcomes of potential importance are first determined (i.e., selected diseases, injuries, and causes of death that are important to monitor after a specific disaster event). Diseases that were endemic in the affected area prior to the disaster event should be included in the system because these would be expected to rise with increased population density, displacement, interrupted normal public health programs, and compromised sanitation and hygiene.

Case definitions for selected health outcomes should be formulated to ensure uniformity of selection in the surveillance system. A case is a unit of observation in the surveillance system with the health condition of interest. Case definitions are criteria for deciding whether a person has a particular disease or health-related condition. These definitions are standardized and are used for investigations and for comparing potential cases. The criteria are applied to individuals under investigation consistently and without bias. Three criteria are commonly used to define the cases: (1) clinical criteria, which are clinical signs and symptoms of disease; (2) laboratory criteria, which are confirmatory tests for disease; and (3) epidemiologic criteria, which place limits on person, place, and time for the development of disease. Once the criteria have been established, cases may be classified into categories: (1) confirmed, (2) probable, (3) suspect, or (4) not a case, defined as failure to fulfill criteria for confirmed, probable, possible, or suspect case. Exhibit 28–2 lists examples of a decision tree for case criteria.

Once case definitions have been established and the information for the surveillance period collected, it is important to identify data for comparison, usually from the same time period of a prior year or of the same period extending several years back, when a similar disaster event did not occur. Information from the comparison group provides a reference against which one can determine whether unusual trends or patterns are occurring in the surveillance period.

A successfully implemented surveillance system facilitates the dissemination of information. Proper dissemination would include reports in a form and with content that would alert policy and decision makers, prevention program managers, the media, and the public about information that should be linked to public health action.

Exhibit 28–2 Examples of Criteria for Case Definitions

Coccidioidomycosis after the Northridge earthquake

Confirmed case: onset of signs and symptoms consistent with acute coccidioidomycosis from January 24, 1994, until March 15, 1994, plus laboratory confirmation

Probable case: acute onset of at least four of the following features: fever, chills, cough, pleural pain, erythema nodosum, arthralgias/myalgias, same outbreak period

Possible case: acute onset of at least two of the four features, plus medical diagnosis

Suspect case: unexplained

Not a case: failure to fulfill criteria for the above

Flash flood–related deaths in Puerto Rico

Confirmed case: death that occurred as a direct result of the impact of the floods on January 5 or 6, 1992, and identified by the medical examiner's office

Probable case: death that occurred as a direct result of the impact of the floods on January 7, 1992 (e.g., cause of death would be drowning)

Possible case: death that occurred as an indirect result of the impact of the floods on January 5 or 6 (e.g., cause of death would be myocardial infarction)

Suspect case: unexplained

Not a case: failure to fulfill criteria for the above

Source: Data from (case 1) E. Schneider et al., A Coccidioidomycosis Outbreak Following the Northridge, California Earthquake, *Journal of the American Medical Association,* Vol. 277, pp. 904–908, © 1997, American Medical Association; and (case 2) C. Staes et al., Deaths Due to Flash Floods in Puerto Rico, January 1992: Implications for Prevention, *International Journal of Epidemiology,* Vol. 23, pp. 968–975, © 1994.

DATA COLLECTION

Accurate and reliable information is needed for responding to a disaster event and in planning relief and recovery activities. Such information originates from a variety of sources, including predisaster institutions and units created specifically to provide immediate response following a disaster.

Historical information of a disaster event provides a background of the hazards, risks, and vulnerabilities of a particular area. This gives the decision maker an idea about the severity of the occurrence of a disaster event. Officials may use this information for planning disaster preparedness programs, response activities, and evacuation plans. Usually, this information is available from the local civil defense office, geologic institutions, or ministries related to natural resources and the environment. Examples of background information include hazard mapping, microzonation (spatial assessment of risk), frequency and magnitude of geophysical phenomena, and vulnerability assessment. Historical information may be used by emergency managers as a reference against which to compare phenomena exhibited by the disaster event of interest.

During the relief phase, the following data provide useful information for emergency managers and public health officials to gauge appropriate relief efforts:

- demographic characteristics of the affected area and surrounding vicinities
- casualty assessment, including deaths, injuries, and selected illnesses
- assessment of the needs of the displaced population
- coordination of volunteer assistance
- management of facilities
- storage and distribution of relief materials
- communication systems
- transportation systems
- public information and rumor control
- registration inquiry services
- traffic and crowd control

Data for such information may be extracted from a variety of sources, including: (1) existing data sets (e.g., census and national health information systems); (2) hospitals and clinics (e.g., emergency department and hospital records); (3) private providers of health care (e.g., patient records); (4) temporary shelters (e.g., daily shelter census, logs at medical facility in shelter); (5) first responder logs, such as DMAT patient logs; (6) and mobile health clinics, such as those run by the military, nongovernmental organizations (NGOs), and volunteer medical groups (e.g., patient logs, records of prescription medications dispensed).

Population-based sampling techniques, when possible, should be employed if surveys are to be conducted in affected communities. The selection of an appropriate method depends on the objectives of a collection system and the existence of a sampling frame. For instance, if all of the households in an affected area are identified and mapped prior to a disaster event, a simple random sample may be appropriate for a community-based needs assessment. If a sampling frame does not already exist, then a cluster design might be more appropriate. Other designs include a systematic or stratified sampling.

Maintaining confidentiality of health records is given utmost consideration in the collection of data about an individual. If personal identifiers such as names, or identifying numbers that may link a record to a name, are recorded on a form, then the official must ensure privacy and confidentiality of the record. If data at the individual level are collected, informed consent of the patient is obtained in most cases, and information is reported in aggregate form.

Disaster Informatics

Disaster informatics is defined as the theoretical and practical aspects of processing and communicating information, based on knowledge and experience derived from processes in medicine and health care in disaster settings.[57] To date, the development of informatics in disaster settings is fragmented and specific to individual response sectors. In public health, basic computerization is gaining worldwide use, particularly in several disaster-prone developing countries. Scientific literature for public health is accessible via CD-ROMS from selected disaster centers worldwide and is also available on databases on the Internet. Surveillance activities are computer based, with EpiInfo the current software of choice for most postdisaster surveillance systems. However, networks for public accessibility have yet to be developed. Disaster informatics, like most health informatics systems, continues to adapt technology of the future, including high-capacity storage devices (CD-ROMs), networks, new user interfaces, programming tools, higher-capacity processors and increased memory, video and computer integration, voice and pen input, incorporation of a global positioning system and analytic tools for rapid analysis, and use of the Internet and Web sites for rapid access and sharing.

MENTAL HEALTH CONSIDERATIONS IN DISASTERS: PSYCHOSOCIAL IMPACTS AND PUBLIC HEALTH

When most people hear the word "disaster," they tend to picture the trail of physical destruction left in a disaster's wake. More often than not, it is images of injured people and collapsed buildings that come to mind. Yet, just as disasters can flatten trees, break bones, and tear houses apart, so too can they profoundly affect individual well-being, family relations, and the fabric of community life. Depending on the specific circumstances, the psychosocial impacts of disasters can range from mild stress reactions all the way to problems such as substance abuse, stigmatization, depression, and posttraumatic stress disorder (PTSD).

From a public health standpoint, it is important to note that the mental health sequelae of a disaster can be quite widespread. Indeed, in terms of morbidity, the social and psychological impacts of a disaster can greatly exceed the direct toll of physical injuries. Furthermore, sometimes these less-visible effects of disasters can be very long lived, affecting the functioning of individuals and communities years after a disaster strikes. Thus, any effort to help restore the health of a community that has suffered a calamity needs to incorporate mental health issues into assistance and recovery efforts. In this regard, public health professionals have a vital role to play in the prevention, assessment, and response to the mental health effects of natural and technological disasters.

Although it is not widely known, public health agencies and public health professionals are heavily involved in addressing the social and psychological impacts of disaster, and attention to these issues represents a core part of the public health profession's response to disaster.[58] In fact, at the federal level, the Public Health Service is a leader in the field of disaster mental health services. The Public Health Service's Emergency Services and Disaster Relief Branch in the Center for Mental Health Services works closely with FEMA and state and local agencies to facilitate the provision of mental health services after presidentially declared disasters. (The Emergency Services and Disaster Relief Branch and the Center for Mental Health Services are part of the Substance Abuse and Mental Health Services Administration.) Numerous other examples of public health involvement with mental health issues can be found at the federal, state, and local levels.

Mental Health Effects of Disaster

Disasters are life-changing experiences. As Myers wrote, "no one who sees a disaster is untouched by it."[59(p.1)] Similarly, Ursano et al. noted that "no one goes through profound life events unchanged."[60(p.5)] Of course, human beings and human societies are often remarkably resilient, and it is important to remember that the challenge of dealing with a disaster can produce positive responses in individuals and communities. As Tierney explained: "Research shows that, rather than being dazed and in shock, residents of disaster-stricken areas have been found to be extremely proactive and willing to help one another. Pro-social behavior, rather than anti-social behavior, is the norm. To the greatest extent possible, people respond immediately to the demands of an emergency situation, providing assistance to one another and supporting those who attempt to manage the emergency."[61]

If it is useful to note that prosocial behavior is often seen after disasters. It is also important to recognize that disasters are highly stressful, disruptive experiences for individuals, families, and entire communities. During a disaster, people may experience such stresses as loss of relatives, friends, and associates; personal injury; property loss; witnessing death or mass destruction; or having to handle bodies.[62] Loss of one's home can be an exceedingly difficult and disruptive experience. In a review of the earlier literature and a report on their own research, Gerrity and Steinglass highlighted the central importance that homes have in people's daily lives.[63] Not only do homes provide shelter, but they are also closely linked with people's sense of identity and their feelings of stability, connectedness, and safety. "Because homes have enormous psychosocial and practical importance in the lives of families, the loss of a home as a result of a catastrophic event can have a lasting impact on a family."[63(p.221)] Indeed, every aspect of a family's existence can be affected, from family roles and responsibilities to ties with the community.

More generally, survivors of a disaster may have to deal with a disturbing new sense of vulnerability. In a disaster, "the fabric of everyday existence is torn away to reveal danger and risk.... Once something of this nature has happened to a person, it is very difficult...to believe that life can ever be the same again."[64(p.1)] Severe traumas like disaster can shatter the basic assumptions people have about themselves and their world.[65]

The period after a disaster can bring additional stresses, such as grieving for lost loved ones, "adjusting to role changes such as widowhood and single-parent status, moving, cleaning and repairing property, and preparing lengthy reports associated with loss."[66(p.133–134)] Overall, experiencing a disaster "is often one of the single most traumatic events a person can endure."[58(p.101)]

People who have gone through a disaster may experience any of a range of emotional, physical, cognitive, and interpersonal effects, and the numbers of people experiencing stress reactions following a major disaster can be large. A list of common stress reactions to disaster is provided in Exhibit 28–3.

Exhibit 28–3 Common Stress Reactions to Disaster

Emotional Effects
Shock
Anger
Despair
Emotional numbing
Terror
Guilt
Grief or sadness
Irritability
Helplessness
Loss of pleasure derived from regular activities
Dissociation (e.g., perceptual experience seems "dreamlike," "tunnel vision," "spacey," or on "automatic pilot")

Cognitive Effects
Impaired concentration
Impaired decision-making ability
Memory impairment
Disbelief
Confusion
Distortion
Decreased self-esteem
Decreased self-efficacy
Self-blame
Intrusive thoughts and memories
Worry

Physical Effects
Fatigue
Insomnia
Sleep disturbance
Hyperarousal
Somatic complaints
Impaired immune response
Headaches
Gastrointestinal problems
Decreased appetite
Decreased libido
Startle response

Interpersonal Effects
Alienation
Social withdrawal
Increased conflict within relationships
Vocational impairment
School impairment

Source: Reprinted from B.H. Young et al., *Disaster Mental Health Services: A Guidebook for Clinicians and Administrators,* 1998, National Center for PTSD.

In general, the transient reactions that people experience after a disaster represent a normal response to a highly abnormal situation. As noted earlier, disasters are highly stressful, disruptive experiences. People are exposed to situations that are well outside the bounds of everyday experience, and such situations place extraordinary demands—both physical and emotional—on people. It would be remarkable, then, if individuals who experience such an extreme situation did not exhibit some physiological or emotional response.

As Myers pointed out, in general, these are "normal reactions to an extraordinary and abnormal situation, and are to be expected under the circumstances."[59(p.2)] Stated another way, "the victims of a disaster are normal persons generally capable of functioning effectively. They have been subjected to severe stress and may be showing signs of emotional strain. This transitory disturbance is to be expected and does not necessarily imply mental illness."[67(p.2)]

According to Young et al., "*mild to moderate* stress reactions in the emergency and early post-impact phases of a disaster are highly prevalent. Although stress reactions may seem 'extreme,' and cause distress, they generally do not become chronic problems."[62(p.15)] As a general rule, a majority of individuals who are exposed to a disaster do not suffer prolonged psychological illnesses.[60]

At the same time, this does not in any sense mean that common stress reactions can or should be ignored in the planning and implementation of a comprehensive public health and human service response to a disaster. On the contrary, programs and services aimed at providing "information about normal reactions, education about ways to handle them, and early attention to symptoms" represent an important opportunity for health and human services agencies to help "speed recovery and prevent long-term problems."[68(p.74)]

Although stress reactions can affect large numbers of people, most stress reactions after disaster tend to be transient. However, a portion of the population touched by a disaster may suffer more serious, persistent effects.

> Research shows that mental health problems can result from exposure to natural and technological disasters. These psychological problems include post-traumatic stress disorder (PTSD), depression, alcohol abuse, anxiety, and somatization. Other kinds of problems, including physical illness; domestic violence; and more general symptoms of distress, daily functioning, and physiological reactivity, have also been documented."[58(p.102)]

PTSD

Because PTSD has been the focus of considerable attention in recent years, it is important for public health professionals who may be involved in disaster needs assessment and response to be familiar with it. Traumatic events such as disasters are generally "dangerous, overwhelming and sudden."[69(p.41)] They "have high intensity, are unexpected, infrequent, and vary in duration from acute to chronic."[60(p.5)] In the aftermath of stressful events that are "both extreme and outside of the realm of everyday experiences," some individuals may experience a prolonged stress response known as PTSD.[70(p.29)] Unlike the transient stress reactions so often seen among disaster survivors, PTSD is associated with much greater levels of impairment and dysfunction.[62]

PTSD usually appears in the first few months after a trauma has been experienced. However, this is not always the case. Indeed, sometimes the disorder may not appear until years have passed. Likewise, PTSD's duration can vary, with symptoms diminishing and disappearing over time in some people and persisting for many years in others. It should also be noted that PTSD frequently occurs with—or leads to—other psychiatric illness, such as depression. This is known as comorbidity.[71,72]

For a diagnosis of PTSD to be made, several criteria have to be met. First, there is the nature of the traumatic event and the response it evokes: "the person experienced, witnessed, or [has] been confronted with an event or events that involved actual or threatened death or serious injury, or a threat to the physical integrity of self or others...[and] the person's response involved intense fear, helplessness or horror."[73(p.427–428)]

Second, the traumatic event is persistently *reexperienced* (e.g., recurrent distressing dreams, feeling as though the event were happening again). Third, the person persistently avoids anything that reminds him or her of the traumatic event (*avoidance*) and experiences a numbing of general responsiveness. This could involve such things as avoiding activities, places, or people that arouse recollections of the trauma, a diminished interest in activities, detachment from others, and a restricted range of affect. Fourth, the person experiences persistent symptoms of *increased arousal* after the traumatic event. Examples include sleep disturbances, irritability, difficulty concentrating, and exaggerated startle response. In addition, for a diagnosis of PTSD to be made, the duration of the disturbance must exceed one month. Finally, the disturbance must cause "clinically significant distress or impairment in social, occupational, or other important areas of functioning."[73(p.429)]

In a comprehensive review of the international literature on the epidemiology of PTSD, DeGirolamo and McFarlane reported that 16 studies assessing the prevalence of PTSD after disasters have been conducted.[74] Nine of the studies were carried out in the United States and six were carried out in other countries. In studies of natural disasters (including floods, tornadoes, earthquakes, volcanic eruptions), the PTSD prevalence rates ranged from a low of 2 percent (Mt. St. Helens) to a high of 59 percent. In studies of technological disasters, the PTSD prevalence rates ranged from a low of 5 percent to a high of 80 percent.

Although much is known about factors associated with the development of PTSD, and about factors that may reduce the likelihood of developing PTSD, the picture is far from complete. One key factor that researchers have identified is the nature of the trauma that the person experiences. "One of the best predictors of psychiatric illness after a traumatic event," wrote Ursano, Fullerton, and McCaughey, "is the severity of the trauma."[60(p.9)] The greatest risk of PTSD is in persons "exposed to life threat and perhaps, in those exposed to terror, horror, and the grotesque."[75(p.9)] According to Young et al., disaster-related variables associated with long-term adjustment problems include mass casualties, mass destruction, death of a loved one, residential relocation, and toxic contamination.[62] There is evidence that some pretrauma factors have an effect as well. Among the various pretrauma risk factors that have been identified in recent research is a history of prior exposure to trauma.

As might be expected, what happens in a disaster survivor's life after the trauma also appears to affect the risk of developing PTSD.[76] For example, it appears that in many situations, social support may play a role as a protective factor. Armed with this knowledge, and guided by an understanding of current research on PTSD, public health planners and practitioners can work to restore damaged community networks as part of a comprehensive prevention effort.

It is also important to remember that although PTSD is usually associated with primary exposure to trauma, people who have not actually experienced a disaster themselves can still develop PTSD and related symptoms. A study of the spouses/significant others (SSOs) of disaster workers after a major airline crash found that the SSOs "showed moderate levels of posttraumatic distress" even though they had not been direct victims of the crash and had not been exposed to the disaster site.[77] Among other steps, the researchers recommend involving SSOs in debriefing and education programs.[77]

In recent years, researchers have focused increasing attention on ethnocultural issues related to PTSD.[78] A number of studies of disasters in the United States have found differing rates of PTSD or other disaster-related impairment in groups of different race or ethnicity.[79] Because of these and other findings, and because "most research and clinical experience validating PTSD as a diagnostic category was carried out in Western industrialized nations," researchers now recognize "the need for culturally sensitive assessment techniques and the need to identify other posttraumatic expressions of distress...that may be particularly pertinent to non-Western individuals."[78(p.536),80(p.12),81] At the same time, the authors of a comprehensive examination of the ethnocultural aspects of PTSD recently concluded that the PTSD construct continues to have a universal dimension that makes it applicable across cultures. "There are substantive reasons to believe that the experience of trauma has similar biopsychosocial consequences in spite of the fact that different cultural traditions may define and experience reality, personhood, and trauma in different ways."[78(p.538)]

Although PTSD has been the subject of considerable research in recent years, it should be pointed out that there are also other serious problems that can develop after a disaster. Acute stress disorder (ASD) is a relatively new diagnostic category that was added to the *DSM-IV Diagnostic and Statistical Manual of Mental Health Disorders*. ASD is "characterized by posttraumatic stress symptoms lasting at least 2 days but not longer than 1 month posttrauma."[75(p.7)] In addition, "major depression, generalized anxiety disorder, and substance abuse are also well documented after exposure to traumas and disasters."[60(p.8)]

Social Impacts of Disaster

In addition to having the potential to produce PTSD, ASD, depression, and other psychological effects, it is important to bear in mind that disasters can also profoundly affect the *social* health of communities. This was dramatically illustrated in Erikson's study of the Buffalo Creek disaster.[82] The disaster occurred in West Virginia in 1972, when the collapse of a makeshift dam used by a coal mining company sent millions of gallons of waste and debris-filled flood waters roaring into a mountain hollow known as Buffalo Creek. The Appalachian mountain community was devastated: 125 people were killed, many others were injured, hundreds of homes and other buildings were wrecked, and thousands of people were displaced. Survivors, many of whom had witnessed dead and dismembered bodies, suffered a wide array of impacts including nightmares, numbing, insomnia, guilt, despair, confusion, depression, and hopelessness.

But in addition to these individual effects, the disaster, plus an ill-conceived relocation effort, effectively destroyed the fabric that held the formerly tight-knit community together. In other words, Erikson noted, the individual trauma produced by the disaster was accompanied by a collective trauma—"a blow to the basic tissues of social life that damages the bonds attaching people together and impairs the prevailing sense of communality."[82(p.154)] With the social support system that people normally depend on no longer available, recovery from individual trauma, argued Erikson, becomes difficult. Thus, postdisaster public health and human services assistance efforts need to focus not only on service delivery to affected individuals and families, but also on restoring support networks and the health of the community as a whole.

Long-Lasting Mental Health Impacts

The extent to which disasters cause serious, long-lasting mental health impacts is still a matter of some disagreement in the research community. "Studies of the victims of disasters show mixed reactions," Hartsough and Myers pointed out.[68(p.4)] "In some disasters, victims seem to fare well without long-lasting problems. In other disasters, they suffer major mental health problems both immediately and for several years after the disaster."[68(p.4)]

Erikson's sociological case study clearly falls into the "significant impacts" category, as does a long-term follow-up study of Buffalo Creek survivors that was carried out by Green and other researchers.[83,84] In that study, the researchers returned to Buffalo Creek in 1986 to conduct multifaceted diagnostic interviews with survivors. What they found was striking: even though 14 years had passed since the West Virginia disaster, the Buffalo Creek survivors still showed significantly higher rates of major depression, general anxiety, and lifetime PTSD as compared to the nonexposed group.

Studies of other disasters, though, have come to different conclusions concerning long-term mental health effects after disaster. Taylor's study of the Xenia, Ohio tornado is a case in point.[85] On April 3–4, 1974, at least 148 tornadoes hit various parts of the country in what was to be the worst outbreak of tornadoes in U.S. history. The most severely hit area was the city of Xenia, Ohio, where 33 people were killed and between 1,000–2,000 people were injured.

Employing both subjective and objective data, Taylor reported finding that although people did experience various symptoms of emotional distress, there was "an extremely low rate, if any at all, of mental illness as a consequence of the tornado."[85(p.273)] Indeed, "a large percentage of the people reported extremely positive psychological reactions to the disaster event. For example, 84 percent of the population asserted that their tornado experiences had shown them they could handle crises better than they once thought they could, and 69 percent responded that they felt they had met a great challenge and were better off for having met it."[85(p.274)]

What accounts for the dramatic difference between studies of Buffalo Creek and the Xenia study? One factor may be that whereas Buffalo Creek's tight-knit community network was for all intents and purposes obliterated by the flood, most of Xenia's extended support networks remained intact despite the damage caused by the tornado. More generally, when one considers the highly complex nature of disaster situations, the enormous variations that can exist between communities and disaster agents, the differences that exist between disciplines in terms of orientation and approach, and the fact that even the definition of the word "disaster" itself is hotly debated, perhaps it is not surprising that divergent findings have been arrived at by researchers studying different disasters.[86] Clearly, though, there is still much that is not yet fully understood concerning disaster impacts—psychosocial risk and protective factors and the effects of various actions and interventions. Rigorous public health research on these and related topics, therefore, will be critically important in the coming years.

NATURAL DISASTERS AND TECHNOLOGICAL DISASTERS

In recent years, there has been considerable discussion in the disaster research community regarding the similarities and differences between natural and manmade disasters. In practice, of course, the line between the two is not always as clear cut as one might think. If flood waters come into contact with toxic chemicals and spread them around a community, is the disaster natural or manmade? Likewise, if increases in population cause a city to expand into flood-prone areas, is the disaster that later results natural or manmade?

To the degree that natural and manmade disasters can be compared, the two, suggest Green and Solomon, "are probably more alike than different."[87(p.164)] Among the things they have in common are "the immediate threat and danger and the potential for ongoing disruption."[87(p.164)] At the same time, however, researchers have pointed to a key difference between natural and manmade disasters: the issue of control. "Manmade and natural disasters differ," wrote Ursano et al., "in the degree to which they are felt to be preventable and controllable."[88(p.xv)]

Natural disasters tend to be seen as part of the order of things, "as acts of God or caprices of nature."[89(p.142)] Such calamities are, to some extent, expected, "since we do not have, and do not expect to have, control over nature."[87(p.164)] On the other hand, manmade disasters are at least in principle preventable.[89] One expects to "be able to control technology, and thus it may be more of a blow to suffer a technological catastrophe (a loss of control), since, by definition, it could have been prevented."[87(p.164)] Thus, the issues of blame and responsibility are central in the aftermath of manmade disasters, and such disasters can produce much higher levels of anger and distrust than natural disasters.

Although many researchers accept that there may be some salient differences between natural and technological disasters, the issue of whether such differences translate into different *impacts* on people is still under discussion. Erikson maintained that the human causation associated with technological disasters brings with it additional distress.[89] People who are victimized by technological disasters, he wrote, "feel a special measure of distress when they come to think that their affliction was caused by other human beings."[89(p.129)] Weisaeth also suggested that technological disasters have a somewhat more severe psychosocial impact.[90] "Technological disasters generally cause more severe mental health problems than natural disasters when they are roughly the same magnitude."[90(p.100)] Similarly, Kliman et al. wrote that "it is harder to achieve psychological resolution and mastery of the losses incurred in human-made disaster than in natural disaster."[91(p.277)]

On the other hand, DeGirolamo and McFarlane noted that two reviews of studies on natural and technological disaster came to different conclusions about whether one type has more severe psychosocial effects than the other.[74] They suggest that the jury is still out on the issue. The "present literature review does not allow any firm conclusion on this point."[74(p.58)]

Psychosocial Impacts, Public Health, and the Challenge of Toxic Disasters

Among the most important new kinds of disaster facing public health professionals and the community as a whole are those involving hazardous materials. As the use of chemicals and radioactive materials has dramatically increased over the past 50 years, so too has the possibility of accidental release and exposure. Unfortunately, when the risks involved in the use of hazardous materials have been coupled with factors such as deficient regulation, insufficient safety and health safeguards, and inadequate emergency preparedness, the result has been serious environmental accidents.[92–94]

Chernobyl and Bhopal are probably the best known examples of these "disasters of environmental poisoning."[64] The 1986 Chernobyl nuclear accident killed 31 people, resulted in the evacuation and resettlement of several hundred thousand people, spread contaminants over a huge geographic area, and has been linked to a dramatic rise in childhood thyroid cancer.[95–97] The 1984 Bhopal chemical disaster in India killed an estimated 3,500 people and injured several hundred thousand others.[98] But in addition to Chernobyl and Bhopal, a host of less well-known chemical and radiologic accidents have taken place across the globe, ranging from relatively small releases to large-scale contamination episodes. In an increasingly complex and interconnected world, no community is immune from the threat of such accidents. Even communities that are far from industrial production or storage facilities can still be at risk from the transport of hazardous materials.

For several reasons, disasters that involve environmental poisoning present new challenges for communities, emergency planners and managers, policy makers, and public health and human service professionals.

- *community conflict:* Typically, after most disasters, people have a tendency to pull together and support one another. As Fritz explained: "The widespread sharing of danger, loss, and deprivation produces an intimate, primarily group solidarity among the survivors which overcomes social isolation, provides a channel for intimate communication and expression, and provides a major source of physical and emotional support and reassurance."[99(p.63)] But in contrast to this kind of *consensual* adaptation or "therapeutic community," toxic disasters frequently produce what Cuthbertson and Nigg called a *conflictual* adaptation.[100] Because contaminants are usually invisible, there is often great uncertainty as to who may have been exposed and who has been affected. The uneven spread of contaminants means that people who live near each other—even on the same street—can have vastly different experiences of the event. In addition, there can be enormous uncertainty as to the degree of risk involved in the present and in the longer term.[100,101] In the face of such ambiguity and uncertainty, and with high-stakes issues involved (e.g., health effects, responsibility for the accident), different understandings can lead to conflict and division. In such a "dissensus community," neighbors may be bitterly divided and vital support networks may not function.[101,102]
- *social stigma:* Although stigma may sometimes affect other types of disaster situations, the social stigma that follows environmental accidents can be remarkably powerful and pervasive. Residents of affected communi-

ties may be seen by others as "tainted" and "people to be avoided."[101,103] For example, following a radiologic accident in Goiania, Brazil, people from the city found themselves the focus of fears and discrimination. As Kasperson and Kasperson noted: "Hotels in other parts of Brazil refused to allow Goiania residents to register. Some airline pilots refused to fly airplanes that had Goiania residents aboard. Cars with Goias license plates were stoned in other parts of Brazil."[104(p.102)]

- *widespread and chronic effects:* Whereas natural disasters like a tornado generally have a low point after which things can be expected to get better, in disasters involving chemicals and radiation, there is no clear low point for those individuals who may have been affected. There is considerable uncertainty regarding the consequences of exposure, and damage (like the contaminants) may be invisible. Furthermore, long-term consequences may take many years to develop. Thus, it is not apparent whether the worst is over or is still yet to come.[105] "In a sense," Baum explained, "this pattern of influence extends the duration of victimization."[106(p.37)] Rather than an event taking place and ending, with a recovery process then commencing, the threat from toxic disasters is seen as a chronic and continuing one. People wonder whether contaminants have entered their bodies, and they worry about the health of their loved ones. Even when an accident is officially declared to be "over," it is, in an important sense, not really over for those who may have been exposed.[89] Studies show that the distress produced by toxic disasters can be quite long lived. Bromet et al. observed elevated levels of distress among mothers of young children long after the Three Mile Island nuclear accident.[107] Likewise, in studies conducted 6½ years after the Chernobyl accident, Havenaar et al. found consistently higher levels of psychological distress among people in the exposed region as compared to a control region.[108]

As Becker noted, this combination of characteristics—conflict, stigma, uncertainty, and chronic distress—can greatly complicate assistance efforts after toxic disasters.[109] At this point, many questions remain to be answered. What kinds of programs and interventions, for example, can be used most effectively to address the problem of pervasive stigma after contamination episodes? How can community fragmentation and conflict best be avoided? What interventions are appropriate for high-risk groups such as mothers with young children? Clearly, there is a pressing need for additional public health and human service research on the difficult challenges posed by toxic disasters.

Prevention As Priority

Numerous professions and disciplines (e.g., psychology, social work, psychiatry, sociology, emergency management, medicine, counseling, nursing, environmental health science, public policy, etc.) have expertise related to the social and psychosocial impacts of disaster. Working closely with those in allied fields, public health professionals have a vital role to play in developing well-integrated, comprehensive, and effective approaches for assessing and mitigating psychosocial impacts.

As in other public health domains, psychosocial assistance efforts strongly emphasize the principle of *prevention*. The primary objective is to help restore "psychological and social functioning of individuals and the community" and limit "the occurrence and severity of adverse impacts."[62(p.4)] In pursuit of this objective, public health and human service professionals generally employ a multifaceted, multilevel approach aimed at helping individuals, groups, and the community as a whole.

Psychosocial assistance services such as crisis counseling "are primarily directed toward 'normal' people responding normally to an abnormal situation, and to identifying persons who are at risk for severe psychological or social impairment due to the shock of the disaster."[62(p.4)] In this regard, outreach is vital. People generally don't see themselves as needing mental health services after a disaster. Individuals don't usually seek out such services, and they may be ambivalent or even resistant to receiving assistance.[59,62] Health and human services professionals, therefore, "must go out to community sites where survivors are involved in the activities of their daily lives."[59(p.4)] Much of the early assistance will be practical in character, ranging from providing information about how to get insurance benefits or loans to helping people with paperwork. "Some of the most important help may be in simply listening, providing a ready ear, and indicating interest or concern."[110(p.2)] Also of importance is providing people with information about what to expect in a disaster, and how to deal with it.

In thinking about public health strategies for responding to disasters, the rebuilding of support networks is absolutely critical. Figley wrote that "the family, plus the social support system in general, is the single most important resource to emotional recovery from catastrophe."[69(p.40)] Loss of homes, and evacuation and relocation, can badly disrupt social support networks just when people most need them. Therefore, it is vitally important for public health and human services workers to help bolster social support networks.[63,111]

Services Provided after a Disaster

Activities and services provided in the aftermath of disaster need to be tailored to the community being served.[59] This means involving stakeholders, community groups, and others in the development and delivery of services.[112] In addition, special services and assistance may be appropriate for vulnerable parts of the population and groups with special needs. Children, for example, require special attention and programs, as well as age-appropriate informational materials. In addition, because children spend much of their time in the classroom, mental health initiatives for children need to involve teachers and schools.[113–115] For a discussion of postdisaster public mental health interventions for children and adolescents, see Pynoos et al.[116]

Among the other groups with special needs in the aftermath of disaster are people with mental illness/psychiatric disabilities and older people.[117] Older adults may have more limited support networks, mobility impairment or limitation, or illnesses. In addition, disasters can "trigger memories of other traumas, thus adding to an increasing sense of being overwhelmed."[62(p.104)]

Also requiring special attention are disaster workers. (See the ARC series entitled "Coping with Disaster.")[118–120] According to Ursano et al., disaster workers "are often hidden victims of disasters and traumas" because "disaster and rescue workers are repeatedly exposed to mutilated bodies, mass destruction, and life threatening situations while doing physically demanding work which itself creates fatigue, sleep loss, and often risk to one's life. They also experience the stresses of their role as a help provider."[60(p.13)]

Among the prevention techniques employed in the disaster worker community are defusing and debriefing. *Defusings* are short (generally 10–30 minutes), unobtrusive, informal conversations intended to provide support, reassurance, and information.[62] *Debriefings* are a more systematic, structured attempt to help disaster workers make sense of their experiences and manage intense emotions. The Mitchell critical incident stress debriefing (CISD) model and variations of it are used in a wide range of settings.[62] Mitchell and Everly described CISD as "a group meeting or discussion about a distressing critical incident. Based upon core principles of education and crisis intervention, the CISD is intended to mitigate the impact of a critical incident and to assist the personnel in recovering as quickly as possible from the stress associated with the event."[121(p.8),122(p.118)] Despite the widespread use of CISD, and the many reports of its value, there is still no consensus in the research community as to the efficacy of CISD. Various studies to evaluate its effectiveness have come to different conclusions, with some demonstrating a positive effect, others showing no clear benefit, and a small number even suggesting a negative impact.[62] Research is continuing.

Among the numerous other activities and services that are typically provided after a disaster to deal with psychosocial concerns are telephone helplines, information and referral services, literature on the emotional effects of disaster, facilitation of self-help and support groups, crisis counseling, public education through the media, information sessions for community groups, grief support services, and advocacy services. For a more detailed discussion of social and psychological assistance efforts after disaster, see Myers, Young et al., and Raphael and Wilson.[59,62,123]

Public health professionals can also identify resources/assets (citizen groups, associations, publications, specialists at nearby universities, etc.) that exist in the community and that may not yet be linked with mental health assistance efforts.[112,124] In addition, public health professionals can work to build community capacity to address social and psychological impacts.[112,125]

Public health professionals can also work to ensure that disaster and emergency plans adequately consider the social and psychosocial dimension. The need to do so is clear. As Ursano et al. pointed out, "If disaster plans do not consider the psychological effects of trauma, the consequences can overwhelm all available services and resources, exhausting rescue workers as well as victims.... The psychological effects of a disaster, manmade or natural, can quickly overwhelm the medical and social rehabilitation resources if they are not recognized and managed."[60(p.5)] Public health professionals can work with local emergency planning committees and other relevant bodies to incorporate social/psychosocial issues appropriately in disaster plans.

Public Health Research

Finally, there is a pressing need for additional public health research on many issues related to the social and psychosocial aspects of disaster. For example, it will be important to understand the public health implications of the prolonged stress caused by chemical and radiologic contamination. (Epidemiologists and other public health researchers who carry out studies in the field should remember that people may be emotionally affected by what they see and experience, even after the disaster is "over." Just because a researcher may not be called a "disaster worker" doesn't mean that he or she is immune to the emotional effects of major disaster. Appropriate caution needs to be exercised.) In addition, because it is vitally important to understand "what works and what doesn't work," public health professionals can join with other health and human service professionals to conduct rigorous evaluation studies of mental health interventions. For a discussion of other research issues, see Gerrity and Flynn.[58]

In sum, social and psychological impacts are a significant part of the morbidity caused by disaster, making them an important public health issue. Public health professionals have much to contribute in addressing the social and psychological issues connected with disasters. Traditional public health emphases and activities, such as prevention, epidemiology, program development, and evaluation, have an important place in efforts to understand and address the mental health impacts of natural and technological disasters.

PUBLIC HEALTH ASPECTS OF ENVIRONMENTAL SERVICES DURING DISASTERS

This section addresses the environmental issues that require public health intervention during disasters. The section details methods to safeguard the population from disease related to sanitation, personal hygiene, the water supply, diarrheal disease, heating and shelter, and violence. The section concludes with guidelines for environmental surveillance.

Context

A clean environment is the foundation on which healthy populations rely. For example, most of the health benefits (lower crude mortality rate) seen in North America over the past century are due to improvements in the environment. Of the three major killers at the turn of the twentieth century in the United States—(1) influenza and pneumonia, (2) tuberculosis, and (3) gastrointestinal illness—influenza and pneumonia death rates are less than 1/10 of the 1900 rate;

the other two are less than 1/1,000th of the 1900 rates.[126] The reductions in these disease and mortality rates occurred primarily before the advent of antibiotics, and came about from improved housing, improved heating and ventilation, improved water supplies, sewage availability, improved food hygiene and refrigeration, and improved food supply (and, in the case of tuberculosis, quarantine/isolation efforts).[127] (See Chapter 1 for a more detailed history of public health.)

However, during a disaster, these "foundations of health" are often lost. The consequences of diminished environmental conditions vary widely from location to location, depending on the diseases present, the susceptibility and habits of the population, and the availability of other redundant protective measures. Diseases that are widespread and have a short transmission cycle and incubation period are the illnesses that arise most readily and rapidly. Respiratory infections and diarrhea are the primary examples. Therefore, the goal of the sanitation or environmental health specialist following a disaster is to replace or repair the existing sanitary barriers as quickly as possible.

Although the environmental actions taken in developed nations during a disaster may seem unrelated to those steps taken during crises in the world's poorest nations, the guiding sanitary principles are, for the most part, the same. In developed nations, the hazards of concern are varied and often include chemical and radioactive hazards. In undeveloped nations, the hazardous material that is usually of primary concern is human feces and the pathogens associated with it. Nonetheless, the task of the environmental health specialist is remarkably similar in these disparate settings.

General Principles

The field of environmental health is based on the concept that certain hazards move through the environment and cause harm to humans. Control measures can be focused on preventing the creation of the hazard, preventing the transport of the hazard, or preventing people from being exposed to the hazard once they encounter it. In the case of malaria control, the three areas of prevention above would correspond to preventing mosquito breeding by draining stagnant water, spraying for mosquitoes to prevent the transport of pathogens, and getting people to use impregnated bednets or insect repellent to diminish exposure opportunities. Whether the subject is diarrhea prevention or toxic waste control, these three types of preventive measures can apply.

As a general premise, no environmental measure functions perfectly 100 percent of the time. In developed countries, this is compensated for by having multiple sanitary barriers between the hazard and a population. For example, in the case of surface water supplies, source waters are protected from pollution, dramatically reducing the pathogen content of water before it reaches the treatment plant. Then, solids are settled out, removing most of the remaining pathogens. After which, water is filtered and chlorinated. If, on a given day, one of these four measures is not functioning, the others will keep the hazard to the public relatively low. Most waterborne outbreaks in developed countries occur when a series of mishaps cause several of the public health barriers to fail. The extent to which a population is free from environmental hazards depends on how aware responsible officials are of the risk and how willing they are to invest in the multiple barriers needed to keep the population's risk low.

A second sanitary principle is that distance aids safety. In general, the more dangerous a substance is and the more volume that exists, the more space that will be allotted to a site. This is because the more distance that exists between a hazard and a population, the more time will generally elapse between any inadvertent release of a hazard and the time when the population is exposed. The word release here means the intentional (e.g., a person defecating in the open) or unintentional (e.g., a break in a pipe conveying a hazardous material) deposition of a potentially hazardous material into the environment. Time allows for more opportunity for the release to be detected, and more opportunity for the population to take measures to protect themselves. Finally, most pollutants degrade or disperse over distance. Therefore, providing space for hazardous material may cut down on human exposure regardless of treatment or containment inadequacies.

Within the context of an emergency situation, where people have been displaced from their homes and may now exist in overcrowded conditions, these general premises of sanitary engineering become problematic. Resources are usually limited, and services must be established at very short notice. This makes the concept of multiple sanitary barriers seem impractical if not absurd. Moreover, displaced people are normally shunted onto the only unclaimed land available, and having "extra" space to separate people and their nearest hazard becomes an impossibility as well. Thus, the practice of environmental health becomes quite crude when applied to displaced populations and refugees. The principal hazard created within these settlements is usually feces. Because its creation is unavoidable, the task of the sanitarian is to minimize fecal transport and to minimize the population's exposure, which in the case of fecally transmitted illnesses means minimizing oral ingestion.

During natural disasters, the task of the environmental health specialist is usually either to protect or to restart the protective barriers that exist, or else to promote changes in behavior that will compensate for the disrupted sanitary barriers. Examples of such messages include orders to boil water, warnings about foods that may have spoiled during electrical outages, or announcements regarding where potable water will be provided. For displaced populations, all basic services usually need to be restarted from scratch. During natural disasters, especially in developed countries, there may be few commonalties between the same types of crises in different locations. Typically, the infrastructure to provide safe water and food is in place; it may simply be inoperative for the moment. Responding quickly and effectively is most often dependent on the local officials' organization and the prepared plans for dealing with crises.

Sanitation

Reviews of epidemiologic studies examining the causes of diarrheal illness in undeveloped countries have shown that the use of latrines or other excreta-containment facilities is more protective than any other environmental measure. Thus, during an emergency, establishing a sanitation system should be one of the first measures undertaken. The appropriate type of facility varies between settings and cultures, although several overriding concepts always apply.

- The purpose of a sanitation system is to contain human excreta at the moment of defecation so that it is not free to spread throughout the environment. Therefore, getting as many people to use the excreta-containment facilities as often as possible is an essential part of all sanitation programs. In some cultures, this may include building separate latrines for men and women or separate latrines for children. In some settings, latrines may be needed in work or gathering areas. Whatever the circumstances of a crisis, if the local workers implementing the sanitation program communicate well with the population being served and understand that their goal is for everyone to use proper facilities all of the time, an appropriate sanitation service will eventually arise.
- People's excreta poses little hazard to themselves. Some researchers have speculated that feces from one's family members is less hazardous than feces from others because families are likely to have common immunologic histories and exchange pathogens on an ongoing basis. Thus, to the extent possible, households should not share latrines or toilets with other households. Because latrine cleaning and maintenance is an unpleasant task in virtually all cultures, having one latrine per household will also increase the likelihood that the facilities will be kept clean. However, the increasing health benefit with increasing coverage needs to be balanced against the time,

effort, and expense of building excreta-containment facilities. Populations that are unstable or are expected to be moved within days, such as in complex emergencies in developing countries, are perhaps better served by a communal latrine system. Both UNHCR and UNICEF propose a minimum coverage target of 20 people per latrine, although this level of coverage is rarely achieved in transit and reception centers.

- Mortality and morbidity rates among displaced populations in the first days and weeks of a crisis are often many times higher than rates among the same population once it is stabilized. Thus, providing some sanitation facilities during the first days of a crisis is critical. This means that either latrines of some kind need to be built before the population arrives at a site (which is rare) or defecation fields need to be established. Because defecation fields need to be located away from water sources, not too far from the people who will use them, and in rainy climates downhill from living areas, reserving the proper spaces for defecation fields must be done at the outset of a crisis.
- Young children pose a particular concern for excreta-control programs. This is because children experience a disproportionate amount of diarrhea among population members, thus shedding the most hazardous feces. Also, their defecation habits are particularly difficult to control. Dealing with this problem usually involves two approaches. Educate child-care providers about proper handling of children's feces and the importance of washing their hands after cleaning the child or handling the child's feces. Second, make excreta-disposal facilities that are child-friendly available. Typically, child-friendly latrines are not dark (perhaps even have no walls) and have an opening that is smaller than in an adult latrine.
- Most latrine/toilet options perform the primary task of containing excreta whether they are above-grade barrels, pit latrines, or solar-heated composting toilets. The habits and beliefs of the served population will be the primary determinant in the effectiveness of the structures and materials provided. The process of matching the proper hardware and educational inputs to the beliefs and habits of a population is best done by that population itself. This means that having locals construct and implement sanitation facilities, especially if each household can construct latrines for themselves, is perhaps the most effective way to ensure that facilities will be used and maintained.

Sanitation Options

A brief summary of the characteristics of the most common sanitation options is presented in Table 28–3.

Personal Hygiene

No area of environmental intervention is more difficult to conduct well than personal hygiene promotion. Whether the issue is poor hand-washing practices among relief workers—which caused diarrhea during the Oklahoma City bombing—or if it is the food reheating habits of Burmese refugees, personal habits can influence a population's well-being regardless of the infrastructure and resources provided. Not only do cultural practices vary between peoples, but different languages often do not have comparable concepts for notions such as privacy or diarrhea. Therefore, as with sanitation, local professionals are best suited to develop and deliver any hygiene education program. Regardless of the setting, several basic premises are universal, specifically, soap provides protection from diarrheal illness independent of any educational program that may accompany it.[128] As people need to be able to clean themselves after defecating, materials for cleansing (paper, sticks) should be made available along with water and soap.

Hand washing, particularly after defecating and before preparing food, has been shown to be protective against fecal–oral illnesses. No studies examining the impact of personal hygiene that were included in a recent review found health benefits

Table 28–3 Sanitation Options in Disaster Response

Characteristics	*Defecation Fields*	*Latrines*	*Flush Toilets*
Physical description	An area near where people live, reserved for defecating	A pit in the ground covered with a platform; people defecate through a hole in a platform	A basin that is flushed with several liters of water to carry away the wastes through a pipe
Speed of implementation for large populations	Can be established within hours	With an organized program, a communal (shared) system can be established within days	Requires weeks or months depending on the availability of piped water and sewage treatment requirements
Typical cost	<$1 per household	$4–300 per household ($7–30 most typical)	>$50 for pour-flush >$100 for most
Most appropriate setting	Arid climates, abundant space, and a culture used to defecating with little privacy	A population accustomed to using latrines, good soils, and no high water table	Piped water available and plentiful; abundant financial resources
Main public health concerns	People will not use; people will be exposed to excreta while entering or exiting the area	Communal latrine may not be kept clean; people (especially small children) may not use	Water outages from electrical problems or water shortages; flooding can stop treatment

associated with education alone, only with documented changes in behavior.[129] Therefore, any efforts to promote hand washing should have a simple monitoring component to ensure that increased hand washing is actually occurring.

To work, educational messages should be short and focused. An educational campaign with six hygiene messages was promoted by the International Committee of the Red Cross in Tajikistan during a typhoid fever outbreak in 1997. An evaluation of the campaign found that people who received and understood the messages were as likely as those who had not to develop typhoid fever. In this case, only one of the six messages, "Boil your drinking water," had any relationship with the route by which the disease was being transmitted. All messages included in an educational campaign should promote measures known to prevent the specific health threat at hand and should focus on behaviors that are not presently practiced by a significant portion of the population.

Water Supply

Water sources fall into three general categories: rainwater, surface water, and groundwater. In general, *rainwater* collection is not reliable enough to provide water for a large population and is rarely used during complex emergencies. *Surface water* is water that is found in lakes, ponds, streams, and rivers. Surface waters have the advantages of being easy to withdraw and are of predictable reliability and volume. They have the disadvantage of generally being microbiologically unsafe, and thus require treatment. *Groundwater* sources tend to be of higher quality microbiologically, but are relatively difficult to access, and energy is needed to bring water from within the earth's crust up to the surface.

Water quality is usually evaluated based on the presence of some bacterial measure, which indicates the possible presence of feces. Because human feces typically contain tens of millions of bacteria per gram, even minute amounts of feces in water are often detectable via bacterial monitoring. Fecal coliforms are a general category of bacteria that are empirically defined to match the characteristics of bacteria found in the stool of warm-blooded mammals. Finding no fecal coliforms in untreated water is a good indication that there are no fecal–oral bacterial pathogens present, although finding fecal coliforms in water does not prove that the water is dangerous. UNHCR considers water with less than 10 fecal coliforms per 100 ml. to be reasonably safe, whereas water with more than 100 fecal coliforms is considered to be very polluted. Other indicator bacteria, such as *E. coli,* fecal streptococci, or total coliforms, operate on the same premise that absence implies water safety. Contaminated water sources should never be closed until equally convenient facilities become available.

Although water sources may be of differing water quality, in many if not most settings, the handling and storing of water by people will be the main determinant in water safety. Studies have shown that the dipping of water from household storage buckets causes considerable contamination, and that water quality deteriorates over time after the water is initially collected. The best assurance that clean water will stay clean is to add a chlorine residual to the water. This means that in unsanitary settings, or during times of outbreaks, it may be appropriate to chlorinate safe source water. Exhibit 28–4 provides additional information about surface and ground water.

Water Quantity

In developing countries, epidemiologic evidence indicates that providing people with more

Exhibit 28–4 Getting and Treating Water in a Crisis Situation

Surface Water

Bucket Collection: Where people collect water directly from water bodies in buckets, the only treatment of surface water that can easily be achieved is chlorination. Water can be chlorinated in the home or by health workers at the point of collection. Ideally, enough chlorine should be added to the bucket so that after 30 minutes, there is still at least 0.5 mg/l free chlorine in the water.

Pipe Distribution: In systems that have many broken distribution pipes or during times of disease outbreaks, attempting to have 0.5 to 1.0 mg/l free chlorine is appropriate. During crises or conflicts, pressure intermittency in pipes allows water to be drawn in through cracks, resulting in cross-contamination responsible for most major waterborne outbreaks. Monitoring of chlorine is recommended to achieve a dose allowing free chlorine throughout the system.

Groundwater

Spring: A location where groundwater flows to the earth's surface of its own accord. To protect the water from contamination, build a spring box, which is a collection basin with an outflow pipe at or below the point where the water comes to the surface.

Wells: To prevent contamination with surface water, the well usually includes a skirt around the opening of the well, or a plate sealing off the surface at the top of the well. Where there is household water contamination or high risk of a waterborne outbreak, water disinfection of wells and springs with chlorine is advisable.

Wells can be of a variety of sizes and shapes, with a variety of pumps or devices to raise the water. Although many reasons relating to siting and construction errors can cause a well to never come into service, wells that operate for a time typically fail because of lack of maintenance and repair capacity. Thus, groups planning to build wells need to budget from the outset for parts and personnel to maintain the projects until local wealth and economic activity can sustain the water system, or until the wells are abandoned.

water than they currently have is more protective against fecal–oral pathogens than is providing people with cleaner water.[129,130] UNHCR purports that people need at least 15–20 liters of water per person per day (l/p/d) to maintain human health. Although water availability is influenced markedly by the setting where one is working, more water can almost always be obtained with more resources, be they more wells, trucks, or pipes. Because the acquisition of water in arid areas is generally expensive, and the relationship between water quantity and health is somewhat stochastic, there is a tendency to not invest in enough water infrastructure because other demands seem more acute. This makes the documentation of water availability a key component of a public health program during a crisis.

Water consumption should be estimated at least weekly during a crisis. Often, the local utility or NGO providing water to a population collects these figures. Note that water consumption means what people receive, not what the water operators produce. Discrepancies frequently arise between "production" and "consumption" estimates—water can be lost or wasted during pumping and transport, and people may be prevented from getting adequate quantities because they don't have containers to hold water. Therefore, sampling that documents people's use of water (such as household interviews) or the actual collection of water at watering points is a preferable method of assessing usage than to divide the water produced at a well or a plant by the number of people served. Cholera outbreak investigations have revealed that not owning a bucket puts families at increased risk of illness or death.[131] Thus, not only should the average water consumption be 15 l/p/d or more, but there should not be anyone with very low water consumption (<5 l/p/d) in the population.

During natural disasters in areas with piped water, rapid surveys can quickly determine which areas are lacking in water service. Areas where service is expected to be cut for days or weeks are often vacated, or else water is transported to the area by vehicle. It is not common in the United States or Europe for acute water shortages to result in morbidity or mortality.

Specific Outbreak Control Strategies for Epidemic Diarrheal Diseases

For several specific fecal–oral diseases, different combinations of environmental measures have been shown to be more effective than others. This becomes important when trying to choose the one or two messages to be included in a campaign and when available staff and resources limit the environmental programs that can be undertaken. Exhibit 28–5 describes control strategies for four major diarrheal diseases.

Heating and Shelter

Although often not thought of as a health issue, heating and shelter have been essential components of disaster responses recently in Europe and the former Soviet Union. Although cold conditions are widely associated with the medical conditions of hypothermia and frostbite, symptoms of malaise and nutritional shortages probably result in more morbidity. Living in cold conditions, even with proper clothing, requires more caloric intake to maintain the same activity level. In general, approximately 1 percent more calories is needed for each degree below 20° C. Thus, someone whose house is 10° C requires 10 percent more food intake to sustain his or her activity level. Rarely does food availability or intake level increase during times of energy hardship. Thus, the metabolic response to cold is for people to slow down. Surveys in Bosnia and Armenia during the early 1990s found that many people were sleeping 18–20 hours per day.

In very cold climates, several things can be done to reduce the hardships associated with cold. High-energy foods such as oil can be made available. Plastic sheeting can be handed out to cover windows and unused doorways. Getting several people or households to share one common heated place can also be useful. In multistory buildings, the temperature in living areas can be dramatically increased by organizing structures so that each floor or apartment heats the same room, causing the heat loss from the floor below to pass into the heated room above. Blankets and sleeping bags can also help people conserve energy during hours of sleep.

Exhibit 28–5 Control Strategies for Epidemic Diarrheal Diseases

Cholera: Cholera is perhaps the most waterborne of all diarrheal diseases. Food has also been seen as the main route of transmission in many outbreaks, although foodborne outbreaks are typically less widespread and less rapidly occurring than waterborne outbreaks. Thus, the first task during a cholera outbreak is to make sure that the water people are consuming is chlorinated. In this setting, chlorinated water is considered to be water with a chlorine residual of at least 0.2 mg/l at the moment it is consumed. Where chlorination is not possible, a lemon per liter has been shown to be effective in killing the bacteria that causes cholera (*Vibrio cholerae*), as is boiling water. Because *vibrios* grow well in unrefrigerated foods, efforts to ensure that people have the fuel needed to heat their food adequately is also called for. Adding acidic sauces such as tomato sauce to foods has been shown to be protective against foodborne cholera. Educational efforts should focus on getting people to consume only chlorinated or boiled fluids and eat only hot, cooked foods or peeled fruits and vegetables. Handwashing practices among those who prepare food for others should also receive attention.

Typhoid fever: Typhoid is also a water- and foodborne disease caused by the bacteria *Salmonella typhi*. Ensuring that the water supply is chlorinated is the best assurance against a massive outbreak, as most large outbreaks are waterborne. Many smaller outbreaks are foodborne, with the hands of the food handlers being the primary hazard. Thus, food hygiene efforts should focus on hand washing among food handlers and ensuring that infected people do not prepare food for others. Although most people, once infected, stop passing the bacteria shortly after regaining their health, 10 percent of people will still be shedding three months after the onset of symptoms. Therefore, keeping food vendors with typhoid fever away from work until they are noncommunicable takes considerable effort.

Shigella: Outbreaks of *Shigella Dysentarie* Type I have become quite frequent during periods of civil unrest in recent years. Case fatality rates for this illness can exceed 10 percent. Other forms of dysentery generally follow the same transmission patterns. Because the infective dose of shigella species tends to be low, perhaps less than 100 organisms, hand-to-mouth or person-to-person transmission is more important than with many other waterborne diseases. Several epidemiologic studies have even linked shigella transmission to flies. Strategies for control need to focus on a comprehensive personal hygiene program (soap and plentiful water made available, handwashing promotion), along with water chlorination and food hygiene efforts. Secondary cases within the households of shigellosis patients are common, so outreach programs should focus education efforts on those households where cases occur.

Hepatitis E: Although hepatitis E is fairly uncommon, it disproportionately strikes refugee populations. During major outbreaks, water has been the main route of transmission, although the most common fecal–oral hepatitis, hepatitis A, is transmitted by food and other routes also. This illness is particularly lethal to pregnant women. Thus, control measures should focus on chlorinating water for the entire population and equipping and educating pregnant women about the need for personal and food hygiene.

In many areas, populations are not used to burning fuels at home as a source of heat. Moreover, during times of crisis, the quality of workmanship and materials may be less than ideal, resulting in either gas leaks or carbon monoxide buildup inside of living areas. Educational messages should warn people about the signs of carbon monoxide poisoning and how to check for gas leaks.

A second area of inexperience has to do with the actual act of burning. Many people are concerned about getting the heat from the fire into the home, and will therefore not build the fire in an insulated stove. At low temperatures (230–300° C), combustion of carbonaceous materials yields carbon monoxide, whereas at higher temperatures (400°+), combustion is generally complete and yields carbon dioxide and approximately twice as much energy. The idea that stove makers should try to keep the heat in around the combustion center is often counterintuitive and requires some education. Likewise, people without a history of burning wood rarely appreciate how important it is to let wood dry for months or years before it is burned. "Green" wood burns cooler (incompletely) because it is laden with water, energy is wasted boiling away the water in the wood, and it is more likely to lead to creosote buildup and chimney fires. Thus, it is very possible that a freshly cut piece of wood will give off less than one-third of the energy it would produce if it were burned after two years of drying.

In warmer climates, sheeting to keep people dry during rainstorms and to provide shade in the daylight can be important for improving the quality of life. Sheeting can allow for the rapid construction of shelter and is often taken by displaced populations when they return home.

Vector Control

Vector control is usually, and perhaps unfortunately, not done during crises. In the United States, mosquito spraying and mosquito monitoring can be a major component of a posthurricane public health program. In developing countries, rat control (particularly in food warehouses), mosquito spraying and eliminating breeding sites, distributing impregnated bednets, dipping cows, spraying for housefly and tsetse flies, setting fly traps, and delousing a population have all been done repeatedly among refugee settings. Usually these measures are taken because of a specific health threat. The most common measures and the most common motivations are as follows:

- Rat control is usually undertaken primarily to limit food and material losses. Rats destroy food and packaging, chew on the insulation of wires, and are generally seen as unsanitary. Thus, many if not most food warehouses will attempt to control rats with poisons, traps, cats, or some combination thereof. Rats can transmit a myriad of diseases such as plague, leptosporosis, and salmonella, although the cost-effectiveness of health improvements through rat control is largely undocumented.
- Mosquito control is often seen as an essential effort where malaria is a major cause of morbidity. Reducing breeding sites is an inexpensive and safe measure that is often undertaken either formally or informally. Efforts to distribute bednets to Burundian refugees in Tanzania were less than successful according to the International Rescue Committee; in Thailand, similar efforts were favorably evaluated. Spraying for mosquitoes has been done but is often seen as expensive or environmentally unsound.

Mosquito monitoring is widespread in the United States and can be a useful tool following storms and floods for assessing the risks of mosquitoborne illnesses. Some programs trap mosquitoes, whereas others monitor infections in sentinel animals that are placed in locations where they are readily bitten by mosquitoes.

Delousing of refugees (the killing of body lice with chemical applications) is called for when the risks of typhus are perceived to be high and where many people are infected with body lice.

Violence

Violence is becoming a more common problem during the relief phase of a crisis. Although this can be seen as a political or nonhealth issue, recent crises in Kosovo, Bosnia, and Rwanda have seen violence as the major cause of morbidity and mortality—making it THE public health issue. Thus, documenting the time, place, and extent of the violence becomes part of the responsibilities of the public health system.

For the environmental health specialist in developing countries, three facets of violence are particularly important: land mines, intentional water cuts, and protecting people as they obtain and transport water. Land mine risk happens over space. Documenting where mines have gone off and where they have been found and publicizing this information is an important task in keeping a client population safe. The intentional cutting of water supplies to a population, as occurred repeatedly in Bosnia, should be documented and reported to those UN or human rights officials who are most likely to influence the political forces causing the crisis, or to be involved in any tribunals that may occur. Finally, providing people with water in a place and fashion that minimizes their risk is becoming a greater and greater part of water provision services. This may require piping water to populations rather than having them venture into dangerous areas, or may simply mean placing taps under overhangs so that people are not exposed to snipers as they wait in the queue.

It is no longer sufficient to focus on preventing waterborne diseases when designing water supply schemes. The goal should be to prevent all water-related hazards. In Sarajevo during the 1993–94 period, the main hazard associated with the water supply was being shot by snipers while collecting water. Thus, UNICEF and the other NGOs involved in water provision appropriately began providing water to locations that snipers could not view.

Environmental Surveillance

The quantitative monitoring of services is an essential part of an effective environmental health program. The monitoring process allows for an accurate estimate of how conditions are changing over time. More importantly, having a numeric estimate of service levels or service quality often improves the service either by making the monitored workers more conscientious or by adding political impetus. Often, the process of surveying keeps workers in touch with the people being serviced and enables them to notice ancillary issues to the parameters being measured.

Monitoring information should be graphically displayed in a public location. This will increase the awareness of the efforts underway for people in other programs and the client population. Programs for which the level of indicators is favorable will help inspire other programs. Programs that are not meeting their goals may get suggestions, help, or even prodding from others, which may help the effort. Many examples have arisen where NGOs did not quantify water availability for specific populations, and the eventual measurement of insufficient quantities allowed for the acquisition of more resources to alleviate the problem. The monitoring of household levels of free chlorine by the International Federation of the Red Cross (IFRC) in Dushanbe during the latter part of 1997 through 1998 is largely responsible for the improved reliability of chlorination by the water utility and the avoidance of another widespread typhoid outbreak during 1998. When the surveillance started, less than half of the households in Dushanbe had measurable chlorine in their taps. After several months of monitoring and lively exchanges, the water utility managed to maintain a chlorine residual throughout the entire city.

Certain parameters, such as fuel and soap availability, need to be monitored only when the situation dictates. In some settings, such as when people are still in their houses and have electricity, people have all of the fuel they need and monitoring the average hours of electrical service is a more demonstrative indicator of their conditions. There are three parameters that always call for a numeric estimation.

1. *access to excreta disposal facilities:* The number of people per latrine articulates both the relative availability of latrines and the amount of sharing that is occurring.
2. *water consumption:* Estimates can be obtained by 24-hour recall interviews with a representative sample of the population or by monitoring how much water is collected at the various sources and dividing this by the number of people being served. Water consumption is always articulated as liters per person per day.
3. *percentage of people consuming safe water:* The host government or overseeing UN agency usually has a microbiologically based criteria for considering water safe. If none is available, use <10 fecal coliforms per 100 ml. water. Water with any detectable free chlorine residual should be considered safe. The fraction of

people who are getting "safe" water at the time of collection should be monitored.*

Crises tend to destroy the sanitary barriers that in times of tranquility help maintain the health of a population. In natural disasters, the general goal is to reestablish the sanitary barriers as quickly as possible. This requires planning and organization before the crisis occurs. Displaced populations always require food, water, and some type of sanitation services. Establishing these services requires a predictable set of material inputs (e.g., water, latrines, soap, food, fuel) and a set of culturally and socially appropriate messages needed to optimize the use of those materials. A primary tool for evaluating the efficacy of the services provided is environmental monitoring.

BIOTERRORISM

Bioterrorism is an emerging threat to the U.S. population. The bombings of the World Trade Center in New York City and the Murrah Federal Building in Oklahoma demonstrated to the public that terrorist activity within United States borders was a reality.[132] The likelihood of a chemical or biological warfare attack (CBW) is increasing according to a number of experts.[133] Defense Secretary William Cohen stated, "The threat is neither far fetched or far off...one that's only going to grow with time" and "The front lines are no longer overseas. It can just as well be in any American City."[133]

CBW agents can have an overwhelming impact on public health. On March 20, 1995, members of the Aum Shinriko religious cult released sarin, a nerve gas, in the Tokyo subway. Twelve people were killed, 1,000 required hospitalization, and 5,000 received medical attention.[133,134] In response to growing concerns for public safety, the Nunn-Lugar-Domenici Domestic Preparedness Program was established as part of the Defense Against Weapons of Mass Destruction Act of 1996.[135] This program was created to bolster emergency response levels at federal, state, and local levels but did not specifically address the role of public health.[132]

Although a new and demanding challenge for public health agencies, bioterrorism activity has significant historic antecedents and contemporary examples. In 1346, Tartar invaders attacked Kaffa (now Feodosia, Ukraine), a city defended by Genoese merchants. The Tartar invaders used bodies of plague victims to transmit disease by catapulting them over city walls. The plan was to spread the plague; indeed, the Genoese merchants contracted this disease, although it is unlikely the catapulting technique explained the transmission.[136,137] In 1763, Sir Jeffrey Amherst, commander of British troops in America, advocated the use of smallpox, writing: "Could it not be contrived to send the Small Pox among those Disaffected Tribes of Indians? We must on this occasion, use every Strategem in our power to reduce them."[138]

More recently, in 1984, 715 individuals became ill after two members of an Oregon sect contaminated a salad bar at a local restaurant with *Salmonella typhimurium,* ostensibly to affect the outcome of a local election.[139] A wave of anthrax scares, all hoaxes so far, is now occurring and is stressing the capacity of local public health agencies to respond appropriately. Between April 1997 and June 1999, there were approximately 200 mailed or phoned bioterrorism threats, usually claiming that the contents could transmit anthrax.[140] As a result of these incidents, local emergency responders treated more than 13,000 potential victims, sometimes requiring these individuals to strip and undergo decontamination with bleach solutions.[140]

The CDC issued a report reviewing seven bioterrorism threats that occurred in 1998.[141] Again, most of these involved claims of anthrax,

---

*Specific details on well and latrine construction can be found in other texts. *Public Health Engineering in Emergency Situation* (1994) by Medecins Sans Frontieres and *Environmental Health Engineering in the Tropics,* 2nd ed. by Cairncross S. and Feachem R. (John Wiley & Sons Ltd., 1993) are both excellent general texts for suggesting facility designs and guiding construction activities. Further information on vector control can be found in UNHCR's Vector Control in Refugee Situations PTSS/HCR, June 1996.

where laboratory tests showed no evidence of contamination by this agent.

A report by Garrett detailed one of these incidents in Wichita, Kansas. On August 18, 1998, several hundred workers were evacuated and a four-block area of downtown Wichita was cordoned off after a suspicious white powder was found in several stairwells and an elevator of an office building.[142] A threatening letter had been received in a manila envelope claiming that the substance was anthrax. Local emergency medical services and hazardous material units (HAZMAT) detained 200 potentially exposed individuals.

Testing for *B. anthracis* was performed by the U.S. Army Medical Research Institute of Infectious Diseases and a fluorescent antibody test and culture were negative. This situation reported in Wichita is far from an isolated incident, with similar scenarios in a growing number of communities.

Bioterrorism Agents

Some understanding of the specific agents that might be employed by terrorists will assist in adequate preparation for a bioterrorist incident.[136] The military weapons displayed in Table 28–4 and Exhibit 28–6 are helpful as a starting point. Of these, anthrax is most formidable in its production of mortality and is the agent of greatest concern (Table 28–5). Smallpox and pneumonic plague can also pose problems of magnitude and are contagious. Because the motives and thought processes of terrorists are difficult to understand, considering those agents that, if used, would produce the most serious consequences is advisable.[136] The CDC has developed such a list of critical agents for health preparedness (Table 28–6).[143] Category A has high impact and requires high preparedness. Category B has a lesser requirement for preparedness. Category C can be handled within current public health capacity.

Predictions of the agent used by bioterrorists are not possible, but taking the time to consider the spectrum of agents most likely to be used is helpful to public health practitioners in planning for preparedness and in developing protocols. Many of the diseases that may occur as a result of biologic terrorism are rare (inhalational anthrax, pneumonic plague) or have previously been globally eradicated (smallpox).[132] The possibly unannounced dissemination of a biologic agent may at first go unnoticed, with the exposed individuals leaving the scene and not showing signs of illness for hours, days, or weeks. This underscores the vital importance in investing in surveillance systems designed to capture local information. The first response to bioterrorism is at the local level, but subsequent public health management is coordinated at local, state, and federal levels.

The Threat List

The definition of the threat list depends heavily on who is being threatened and how the threat is perceived. The military definition focuses primarily on bacteriologic agents and toxins that have been weaponized in aerosol form by a nation to produce a large number of battlefield casualties. These are the prototypical weapons of mass destruction. The military's threat list is dynamic and depends on intelligence assessment. Thus, it is possible that an organism could be appropriate in theoretical terms as a threat but is not considered a threat because no one has developed a large-scale weapon for containment and dispersion.

The civilian threat list is much broader because the rapid onset or the effects of the diseases are not critical, and contagious diseases would also be considered effective bioterroristic agents. Many normal public health threats overlap with the agents of bioterrorism, both in the nature of the outbreaks produced, and in the nature of the response to control them. Pneumonic plague is a good example where a naturally occurring case generates a rapid and vigorous public health response to prevent further dissemination.

For purposes of this discussion, it is clear that there are relative priorities among the diseases being classified and that there are only three major categories of agents. Within these three categories, only five agents (anthrax, smallpox, plague, botulism, and tularemia) are considered

Table 28–4 Destroyed U.S. Biological Arsenal

Lethal Agents	*Incapacitating Agents*	*Anti-crop Weapons*
Bacillus anthracis	Venezuelan equine encephalitis	Wheat-stem rust
Botulinum toxin	Staphylococcal enterotoxin B	Rye-stem rust
Francisella tularensis	*Brucella suis*	Rice-blast spore
	Coxiella burnetii	

Source: Reprinted from *U.S. Army Activity in the U.S. Biological Warfare Programs,* Pub. No. B193427L, 1997, Washington, DC: U.S. Department of the Army.

serious threats. The first category of disease is that caused by an aerosolized release of bacteria. This produces respiratory or pulmonary disease. The three agents in this category are anthrax, plague, and tularemia. A second category of illness is where the dissemination is dependent on person-to-person transmission, such as smallpox. The third category of disease is that caused by contamination of food, water, or other ingested material, such as botulinum toxin.

Anthrax is considered, both in the scientific and popular literature, to be a highly efficacious biologic warfare agent for a number of reasons. First, it forms spores, which give it stability in aerosol. Second, it is relatively easy to disseminate using off-the-shelf technology. Third, if acquired by the respiratory route, the disease is frequently fatal. There are difficulties in preparing a form of the agent that is stable in aerosol, but these difficulties were apparently overcome in the course of the former Soviet Union's program, and it is possible that well-informed terrorists could replicate those procedures.

Smallpox, as mentioned previously, has the additional feature of being highly contagious in unimmunized populations, with a cycle of 10 to 14 days, an attack rate of up to 90 percent, and mortality as high as 35 percent. What makes this disease a less likely threat is that an eradication program eliminated the natural illness from the planet and only two samples of live virus remain: One is under the control of the United States at the CDC and the other is held by Russia. Some experts, therefore, consider that it would be hard for a terrorist to acquire live smallpox virus. However, it was reported in the *New York Times* (1999) that smallpox virus is held by Iraq and North Korea in addition to the two approved sites. Uncertainty underscores the potential threat and the fact that international agreements cannot be relied upon.

Plague, a respiratory-acquired illness, is also spread person-to-person. Because it occurs as an enzootic disease of rodents in the United States, it may be possible to obtain an isolate for use as a terrorist agent. Botulism is likewise an environmental organism that can be easily cultured from soil. Its toxin has the disturbing clinical feature

Exhibit 28–6 Rating System (Russian) of Bioagent Distribution According to Probability of Use as BW

- Smallpox virus
- *Yersinia pestis*
- *Bacillus anthracis*
- Botulinum toxin
- Venezuelan equine encephalitis virus
- *Francisella tularensis*
- *Coxiella burnetii*
- Marburg virus
- Influenza virus
- *Burkholderia mallei*
- *Rickettsia typhi*

Source: Reprinted from A.A. Vorobjev et al., Key Problems of Controlling Especially Dangerous Infections, in *Proceedings of an International Symposium: Severe Infectious Diseases: Epidemiology, Express-Diagnostics and Prevention,* 1997, State Scientific Institution, Volgo-Vyatsky Center of Applied Biotechnology, Kirov, Russia.

Table 28–5 Results of the Hypothetical Aerosol Dissemination of Various Infecting Agents

Agent	*Downwind Carriage*	*Deaths*	*Total Casualties*
Venezuelan Equine Encephalitis	1 km	400	35,000
Tick-Borne Encephalitis	1 km	9,500	35,000
Epidemic Typhus	5 km	19,000	85,000
Brucellosis	10 km	500	100,000
Plague	10 km	55,000	100,000
Q-Fever	>20 km	150	125,000
Tularemia	>20 km	30,000	125,000
Anthrax	>>20 km	95,000	125,000

Note: Casualty figures assume 50 kg of dried agent disseminated along a 2-km line upwind of a population center of 500,000.
Source: Data from *Health Aspects of Chemical and Biological Weapons,* © 1970, World Health Organization.

of necessitating intensive supportive care of its victims. Additionally, the treatment for it, in the form of an antitoxin, is limited in supply and availability.

Tularemia can be disseminated in water. In aerosol form it produces a severely debilitating pneumonia but without as high mortality as anthrax. Other agents are on longer threat lists. Q fever and brucella produce, in most instances, mild illnesses that would not generate large-scale stress on medical systems or produce large-scale panic. The agents in the next rank of concern are regular public health threats such as viral encephalitis, cholera, salmonella, influenza, and staphylococcal enterotoxin B.

Differences between Overt and Covert Release

It is unlikely that terrorists would use an overt release, in the form of an announced event or something that is recognized at the time, as their mode for biologic terrorism. This type of release would allow treatment before the onset of disease. There are now examples where the management of biologic threats has changed significantly. In the case of overt releases, an

Table 28–6 Critical Agents for Health Preparedness

Category A	*Category B*	*Category C*
Variola virus	*Coxiella burnetii*	All other biological agents may emerge as future threats to public health
Bacillus anthracis	*Brucellae*	
Yersinia pestis	*Burkholderia mallei*	
Botulinum toxin	*Burkholderia pseudomallei*	
Francisella tularensis	Alphaviruses	
Filoviruses and arenaviruses	*Rickettsia prowezekii*	
	Certain toxins (Ricin, SEB)	
	Chlamydia psittaci	
	Food safety threat agents (*Salmonellae, E coli* O157:H7)	
	Water safety threat agents (*Vibrio cholera,* etc)	

Source: Reprinted from *Critical Agents for Health Preparedness, Summary of Selection Process and Recommendations,* Centers for Disease Control and Prevention, National Center for Infectious Diseases, 1999.

assessment of the threat is made before the response is initiated. In many cases, announced biologic threats are considered hoaxes, and a limited and tempered response is activated. A limited response in these cases does not represent a casual response on the part of law enforcement, but rather a sophisticated analysis of the situation that allows a resolution of the incident without major difficulties.

A covert release of a biologic agent will present as illness in the community, and its detection is dependent on traditional surveillance methods. Recent federal programs have emphasized enhancing such systems and increasing the sensitivity of frontline medical practitioners to the importance of recognizing and reporting suspicious syndromes. The covert release of a contagious agent has the potential for large-scale spread before detection. A release in an airport or in a highly mobile population could disseminate a pathogen such as smallpox throughout most of the world before the epidemic would be recognized. To bring this potential epidemic under control, a major multifocal international response would need to be activated. In the case of anthrax, the treatment can be time-sensitive. If individuals are already exhibiting severe symptoms, treatment is often not effective.

Local Health Department Response

LHDs are first-line responders for incidents of bioterrorism, requiring planning for preparedness. Preparedness at the local level includes readiness assessment, expansion of surveillance and epidemiology capacity, and provisions for laboratory identification of the chemical/biologic agent.[142] Development of protocols is recommended to deal with the most likely agents to be encountered. In addition, training of personnel is needed. The foremost consideration is effective and preplanned strategies for communication with other community agencies and the public.

In planning a response strategy, LHDs should identify key responders in the community, including emergency medical services, HAZMAT, and police and fire agencies. Discussions should also take place with the directors of emergency services at local hospitals and the poison control center. In these incidents, individuals may appear at their local hospital with concerns about potential exposure. Uniform protocols between institutions, particularly with respect to prophylactic antibiotic usage, are advisable.

Linkages with a laboratory with the capability to identify agents of concern, the state public health agency, and the CDC should be accomplished in advance of any reported incident. A surveillance system to track the large numbers of potentially exposed individuals is needed and can be designed in accord with the guidance described earlier in this chapter. Methods for secure communication need to be explored. Advance discussions with the media are also advisable because extensive television, radio, and newspaper coverage of these incidents can provoke copycat episodes. In a number of recent instances, dissemination of the news has been delayed by the media in an effort to forestall repeat incidents.

The Federal Response

The Nunn-Lugar Funds provide training and equipment to 120 major cities in the United States.

Congress also provided for the establishment of Metropolitan Medical Response Systems under the public health system. These are assets that would be activated in a disaster situation involving either chemical or biologic weapons. The early federal response is deemed appropriate for a chemical event recognized by people becoming acutely ill. If terrorists wanted to have impact using biologic weapons, the last thing they would want is for the attack to be recognized and appropriate countermeasures applied, which would severely blunt the attack.

The most serious difficulty with the early federal response is that state and local public health authorities were not involved in establishment of the response systems, and the discussions were held almost exclusively in the emergency response environment. This is a problem because a biologic event would most likely present as the occurrence of a cluster of an unusual disease in the population, and the entities traditionally responsible for recognizing and responding to such an event are public health organizations. The response required for a biologic event is totally dissimilar to that required for an overt chemical event where fire, police, or HAZMAT units are the key part of the response. If a release of a contagious disease such as smallpox occurred, a number of patients would appear in emergency departments with rash illnesses that would be reported to authorities as suspect smallpox. A public health response, including quarantine and immunization, could then be activated.

National Program for the Public Health Response to Bioterrorism

Prior to fiscal year 1999/2000, no specific federal funds were set aside for a public health response to bioterrorism. In fiscal year 1999/2000, a $179 million program was established under the sponsorship of Senator Lauch Faircloth from North Carolina. The program included a significant component for central DHHS activities, and the remaining $121 million was specifically earmarked for the CDC. Approximately $51 million is allocated to a National Pharmaceutical Stockpile to detect, diagnose, and treat illnesses caused by potential bioterrorism pathogens.[132] This initiative will assist in coordinating a response and communication between local, state, and federal levels of public health and other response agencies.

A new activity was established at the CDC called the Biological Preparedness and Response Program (BPRP). During the planning, a partnership of BPRP and state and local public health programs formulated into a five-part program for the remaining $70 million. The five components of the program are planning, surveillance and epidemiologic response, a biologic laboratory network, a chemical laboratory response capability, and a health alert network. The CDC is developing public health guidelines to assist local public health agencies in developing bioterrorism preparedness plans and response protocols. These include self-assessment tools for preparedness, proficiency testing programs, attack simulation programs, and computerized resource-tracking systems. The CDC awarded $1.5 million to nine states and two cities in 1999 for preparedness and response enhancement with plans for additional funding to other jurisdictions in the following 3–5 years.[132]

The national disease surveillance systems are being upgraded to include biologic and chemical agents. In 1999, to improve state and local surveillance activities, the CDC awarded $7.8 million to 31 states and 3 large cities with further funding planned. The CDC and its public health partners are also establishing a Laboratory Response Network for Bioterrorism that will link 50 states and additional localities. The CDC has awarded a total of approximately $8.8 million in grants to 41 states and 2 large city health laboratories to improve capacity for identifying biologic agents. The CDC has also created an internal Rapid Response and Advanced Technology Laboratory to provide 24-hour availability for diagnoses of illnesses potentially secondary to agents of biologic terrorism.[132]

In developing this program, the CDC called together a group of external advisors who reviewed the biologic threat list from the public health standpoint. This advisory group reaffirmed the five highest priority agents previously mentioned and added viral hemorrhagic fevers. It also designated a second tier of organisms, for which protocols for testing are in the final stages of development.

The CDC program resulted in awards to 41 jurisdictions in the late fall of 1999. The planning component has a limited number of awards and is designed to develop templates for biologic response programs in small, medium, and large jurisdictions. The surveillance and response program, which is considered by many to be the key to the overall success of the project, includes such things as active surveillance for threat diseases, adding threat diseases to the list of reportable diseases, instituting electronic laboratory reporting, and adding staff to respond rapidly in the event of a suspected outbreak of one of these unusual diseases. The biologic laboratory network will be described in specific detail later in this chapter. The chemical laboratory network is intended to provide backup to the CDC in the event of overload. This is based on the assumption that a chemical incident would result in an expanded need for both diagnostic tests to aid in exposure assessments and medical follow-up of exposed individuals. To date, the CDC has funded four laboratories and provided mass spectrometry instruments to them.

The CDC is also building a Health Alert Network (HAN) to communicate with state and local health agencies. The HAN is the connection of all public health officers to the Internet. Under this program, a secure Web site will be established, and individuals will be trained to facilitate their effective use of this system. This national communications and distance-learning network will include high-capacity, continuous Internet connections for secure electronic communications and Web access with the ability to participate in distance learning and to receive information and guidance on bioterrorism threats. This project has the largest budget of the five program components. The CDC distributed $19 million in 1999 to state and local health departments for the development of the HAN.[132]

The Public Health Laboratory Network

The laboratory response network for bioterrorism is a CDC-sponsored program with network coordination by contract with the Association of Public Health Laboratories. All levels of laboratories are connected with built-in redundancy. The system emphasizes rapid turnaround and accuracy. The laboratories are the central points of contact for technology validation and transfer. A scientific steering group, in collaboration with the CDC, will be developing and defining priorities and protocols for new technology.

The network of public health laboratories is extensive, consisting of a program in each state and in many local jurisdictions. Using California as the example, the network concept is based on the idea of specialization rather than regionalization. There are 39 free-standing county laboratories, each with a broad range in capability and support. The local laboratories' infrastructure has undergone decay in the last few years, but they are well organized for certain things. Examples that are working in the state include the testing by one laboratory for tickborne diseases in an area of endemic occurrence, the delegation of HIV viral burden to seven major counties with the highest volume, and the establishment of computer support for rapid logistics and communication that would be an essential element of a network for response to bioterrorism as well.

The most important reason for establishing a network of public health laboratories to assist in the response to bioterrorism is that all the diseases that are threats occur naturally in the United States. For example, botulism, plague, anthrax, tularemia, and poxvirus illnesses are routinely evaluated by many public health laboratories. Not only do these diseases occur with some frequency, but the public health laboratories are in almost all cases primarily responsible for their diagnosis. While the frequency of these diseases is low, the impact is high because of the speed with which these diseases spread (i.e., pneumatic plague). The frequency of current testing is not low, and in California alone, requests for botulism testing of humans occur twice a week.

The other major premise behind establishing the network is that standard or classical microbiology technique works well for the major threat agents. The current methods of detecting bacterial agents (gram stain, culture on selective media, visual colony morphology, growth after heat shock, and confirmatory methods using phage and direct immunofluorescence) are well established for definitive recognition and diagnosis. In the case of virology, methods such as isolation in cell culture, inoculation of animals, direct fluorescence methods, and electron microscopy are well established as definitive methods.

The public health laboratory network for response to bioterrorism has four levels of performance defined as A, B, C, and D. Level A performance, in the case of bacteriology, is culture only in clinical and small public health laboratories. Level B performance is first-level confirmation using direct fluorescence or phage testing, for example. Major county and small state public health laboratories fill this role. Level C laboratories provide the second level of confirmation with more complicated methods including molecular diagnostics and are major state public health laboratories. A key task of level C laboratories in the future will be to validate new technology and pass it down to level B laboratories. Level D laboratories are federal and private partners in the Public Health Service, Department of Defense, national laboratories, and industry that can perform research on and development of new techniques for passing down to the lower levels of the network.

The laboratory network has five major tasks. The network was established to enhance the capability of level A laboratories by providing training to bench-level microbiologists in the use of algorithms so that suspect key organisms are not ignored or discarded. The network will deploy confirmatory reagents from a central stockpile to level B labs using predominantly fluorescence and phage methodology at present. Reagents will be prepared and in some cases distributed by level C laboratories, and new technology will be validated in level C laboratories, and transferred to level B laboratories after field testing. Research will be conducted in level D laboratories. Finally, a contract with the Association of Public Health Laboratories has been established to coordinate logistics and communication. This includes a secure Web site for registering laboratories, obtaining protocols, and ordering reagents. In the future, reporting of suspect threat diseases also may be done over the Internet.

This can foster the level D laboratories doing the research and development that is so important as an underpinning for this field. The laboratory network can partner with Department of Justice programs to handle environmental samples. Early in the development of this program, protocols were rapidly developed, sent around for comment, and made available on the secure Web site. The next step will be the provision of hands-on training, in some cases at the state level, and in other cases at the CDC.

If a covert event that is not recognized immediately occurs, how is the connection with the laboratory made? The occurrence of disease in the community would trigger the public health control programs to submit samples to the laboratory and report to the surveillance network. In the event of an announced threat or an overt event, the event would be reported to the Federal Bureau of Investigation (FBI), and the FBI would bring samples to the nearest appropriate laboratory resource in the network. In the case of such events, the FBI will make the determination of which laboratory will be involved.

There are four advantages for using the procedures of a public health laboratory program. First, existing tests give definitive results. Second, the procedures that are used are validated under the license of the laboratory and can be readily adapted to environmental samples such as might happen after an overt threat, or in the attribution of a source of a sample. Third, the laboratories are all certified under the Clinical Laboratory Improvement Act or CLIA, with appropriate quality assurance and quality control procedures. Finally, the personnel are highly skilled and familiar with following complex algorithms.

Using existing public health laboratories to respond to bioterrorism also has limitations. First, the final result is usually not available for a day or two, but preliminary results can be available in minutes or hours. In particular, the minimum response time for a definitive negative result with a rapidly growing organism such as anthrax may be 16 hours. More slowly growing organisms or complex procedures may take 48 hours or more. Second, these methods require a fixed laboratory facility and these techniques are not readily adaptable to a field situation.

What Is the Status of Rapid Tests?

One question that comes up frequently is what is the status of the commercial rapid hand-held assays for detection of biologic agents because the early federal response involved their purchase and dissemination. These assays are based on antibody capture technology from the 1970s and suffer from the fact that their sensitivity is not as good as culture or molecular methods by three logs or more. The specificity of these methods with stimulants has not been determined, and they can be confounded by commonly used pesticides or killed organisms. Therefore, such tests cannot be used in decision making because the sensitivity does not allow one to exclude the possibility of an event and nonspecificity does not allow one to call an event definitely. The network will evaluate and attempt to qualify these rapid test methods and for future use where appropriate.

What Countermeasures Are Available?

Preventive measures performed before the occurrence of the bioterrorist event have distinct advantages. Unfortunately, large-scale immunization of the population for smallpox has been discontinued. The response to the reintroduction of smallpox, natural or unnatural, would be a rapid large-scale immunization program to surround the outbreak. This is similar to what was done in the eradication campaign of the late 1970s. One difficulty with this strategy is that there is a limited supply of vaccine, approximately 50 million doses worldwide, and the vaccine is aging. There are plans to make a new product. This initiative has been stalled for the past few years but appears to be moving forward again. There are serious questions about how it could be licensed because there are no natural infections to prevent to conduct an efficacy trial. There are difficulties in its administration. Vaccinators require specialized training in the use of bifurcated needles. Prescreening of vaccinees for HIV may be required to prevent the occurrence of disseminated vaccinia in such immunocompromised individuals. The smallpox vaccine also has a small but significant number of complications that require the availability of an immune globulin. Vaccinia immune globulin is also in short supply and there are difficulties with plans for making more in the future.

For the major bacterial threat agents, the administration of antibiotics is the key component of the response. In the event of a release of anthrax, there are a number of possible scenarios for the large-scale administration of antibiotics. Dosing could start with the antibiotic ciprofloxacin to be replaced by penicillin once antibiotic susceptibility is determined. (The definition of the public health response to anthrax and full discussion of the use of antibiotics including use in pregnancy and pediatrics, is found in a white paper published by a working group of the Johns Hopkins Center for Civilian Biodefense in the *Journal of the American Medical Association*.) A licensed vaccine for anthrax has been administrated fairly widely to military populations. Administration of this vaccine to at-risk individuals after release of anthrax would cut down on the time of antibiotic administration required.

Antibiotics are the mainstay of the response to plague and tularemia. The description of the response to these organisms, including detail antibiotic usage, is found in the Johns Hopkins Center white papers on these particular organisms. The public health response to a botulism outbreak is a bit more complicated because the occurrence of paralysis in a number of individuals may overrun the short supply of both ventilators and intensive care beds in pulmonary units. Further, the immune globulin used in the routine treatment of both wound and foodborne botulism is in short supply, and increasing the supply would require a major effort to manufacture a large enough stockpile.

Part of the federal public health response to this problem has been the earmarking of a significant amount of money for a national stock of antibiotics and vaccine for the major bioterrorist agents of threat. The first phase of this program came online at the beginning of the year 2000. The long-term strategy for this program includes developing a "virtual supply" by contracting with manufacturers to provide large amounts of product on relatively short notice. Although this supply is called a stockpile, massive amounts of antibiotics will not actually be centrally stored.

Recent well-documented shortages of penicillin in the United States have alerted planners about the availability of antibiotics. In addition, the precursors of some antibiotics are not produced in the United States and may require the cooperation of foreign governments in the event large amounts of drugs are needed on short notice.

Appropriateness of Public Health Program for Bioterrorism Response

Cohen and colleagues[144] suggested that biologic warfare is "public health in reverse," because biologic warfare causes disease, and public health is the profession dedicated to preventing and treating disease. They suggested that the federal preparedness programs, described earlier in the chapter, are equivalent to biologic warfare itself because of the emphasis on the military response and the diversion "of resources from other, more urgently needed public health tasks." These authors claim that funding for bioterrorist initiatives has increased at the expense of existing public health budgets. However, considering the potential threat, and the fact that bioterrorism could occur anywhere, preparedness is the prudent action. Criticism of preparedness fails to acknowledge and factor in the new money that has gone to the CDC to support preparedness and response to biologic terrorism. The funds that are in this program are earmarked for dual use and will support general preparedness, response to epidemics, surveillance of syndromes, and rapid epidemiologic evaluation. In total, this program will benefit the recognition and control of many diseases of public health importance, in addition to supporting preparedness for diseases due to bioterroristic activities. It is difficult to see how this program could be anything other than a win for public health.

• • •

Public health organizations carry out a broad and complex set of responsibilities in preparing for and responding to disasters and acts of bioterrorism. Carrying out these responsibilities requires a multiorganizational effort. Disaster epidemiology and assessment are important components of the public health response, as these activities support scientific investigation as well as disaster management decision making. Public health organizations also play critical roles in preventing and controlling the psychosocial effects of disasters. The emerging threat of bioterrorism calls attention to the importance of public health organizations in disaster preparedness and response initiatives, creating new risks and responsibilities for organizations along the continuum of public health practice settings. The contemporary public health environment demands informed decision making and effective management in response to the health threats posed by manmade and natural disasters.

CHAPTER REVIEW

1. Disasters are ecologic disruptions or emergencies of magnitude resulting in deaths, injuries, and property damage exceeding the local capacity to respond and calling for external assistance.
2. The public health role in disaster is broad and includes assessment, sharing information, preparedness, triage, casualty distribution, and preventing outbreaks of infectious disease through surveillance, maintaining health care services, environmental interventions, and other measures.
3. Response to disasters are multiorganizational, with the first response at the local level.
4. Information about the acute impacts of disasters may be provided through rapid needs assessments and surveillance systems.
5. Surveillance systems are conducted after disasters to detect illnesses or injuries in the affected population and are usually one of three types.
   - hazard
   - exposure
   - outcome
6. Disasters are highly stressful, disruptive experiences for individuals, families, and entire communities. Mental health sequelae of a disaster can be widespread, exceeding the direct toll of physical injuries.
7. Most stress reactions after disaster tend to be transient. However, a portion of the population may suffer more serious, persistent effects such as PTSD.

8. Mental health measures after disaster include outreach, education, restoration of community services, crisis counseling, and rebuilding support networks.
9. Within the context of an emergency situation, where people have been displaced from their homes and are existing in overcrowded conditions, environmental factors and sanitation are key to health protection.
10. Environmental measures in a disaster situation include the provision of adequate volumes of water free from contamination, facilities to dispose of human excreta, hand washing, protection of food from spoilage, and the provision of housing and shelter.
11. Bioterrorism is an emerging threat in the United States, requiring preplanning for a coordinated first response at the local level and linkages with state and federal public health and other involved agencies.

REFERENCES

1. S.W.A. Gunn, *Multilingual Dictionary of Disaster Medicine and International Relief* (Dordrecht, The Netherlands: Kluwer Academic Publishers, 1990).
2. P. Showalter and M.F. Myers, "Natural Disasters in the United States as Release Agents of Oil, Chemicals, or Radiological Materials between 1980–1989," *Risk Analysis* 14 (1994): 169–182.
3. F. Cuny, "Introduction to Disaster Management: Lesson 2—Concepts and Terms in Disaster Management," *Prehospital Disaster Medicine* 8 (1993): 89–94.
4. *Robert T. Stafford Disaster Relief and Emergency Assistance Act,* Public Law 93–288.
5. E. Auf der Heide, *Community Medical Disaster Planning and Evaluation Guide* (Dallas, TX: American College of Emergency Physicians, 1996).
6. E.L. Quarantelli, *Delivery of Emergency Medical Care in Disasters: Assumptions and Realities* (New York: Irvington Publishers, Inc., 1983).
7. S.P. Nishenko and G.A. Bollinger, "Forecasting Damaging Earthquakes in the Central and Eastern United States," *Science* 249 (1990): 1,412–1,416.
8. W.M. Gray, "Strong Association between West African Rainfall and US Landfall of Intense Hurricanes," *Science* 249 (1990): 1,251–1,256.
9. Universite Catholique de Louvain, Brussels, Belguim, "EM-DAT: The Office of Foreign Disaster Assistance/CRED International Disaster Database." http://www.md.ucl.ac.be/cred. Accessed 20 April 2000.
10. National Research Council, *Reducing Disasters' Toll: The US Decade for Natural Disaster Reduction* (Washington, DC: National Academy Press, 1989).
11. L.R. Johnston Associates, *Floodplain Management in the United States: An Assessment Report. Volume 2 Full Report. Prepared for the Federal Interagency Floodplain Management Taskforce. FIA-18/June 1992* (Washington, DC: U.S. Federal Emergency Management Agency, Federal Interagency Floodplain Management Taskforce, 1992).
12. P.R. Berke and T. Beatley, *Planning for Earthquakes* (Baltimore: The Johns Hopkins Press, 1992).
13. J.E. Beavers, Testimony of Dr. James E. Beavers, Member, Scientific Advisory Committee of the National Center for Earthquake Engineering Research, State University of New York at Buffalo, Buffalo, NY. Testimony before the Committee on Science, Space, and Technology. U.S. House of Representatives. One Hundred First Congress First Session November 17, 1989 (No. 101). Washington, DC: U.S. Government Printing Office, 92–95.
14. Utah Earthquake Preparedness Information Center, *Earthquakes: What You Should Know When Living in Utah* (Salt Lake City, UT: Federal Emergency Management Agency).
15. T.J. Culliton et al., *50 Years of Population Change along the Nation's Coasts, 1960–2010* (Coastal Trends Series, Report 2) (Rockville, MD: National Oceanic and Atmospheric Administration, 1990).
16. C. Axelrod et al., "Primary Health Care and the Midwest Flood Disaster," *Public Health Reports 109,* no. 5 (1994): 601–605.
17. K. Gautam, "Organizational Problems Faced by the Missouri DOH in Providing Disaster Relief during the 1993 Floods," *Journal of Public Health Management and Practice 4,* no. 4 (1998): 79–86.
18. C.A. Evans, "Public Health Impact of the 1992 Los Angeles Unrest," *Public Health Reports 108,* no. 3 (1993): 265–272.
19. "Health Topics A to Z." http://www.cdc.gov/health/diseases.htm. (31 May 2000) Accessed 15 June 2000.
20. S. Whitman et al., "Mortality in Chicago Attributed to the July 1995 Heat Wave," *American Journal of Public Health 87,* no. 9 (1997): 1,515–1,518.

21. R. Lyskowski and S. Rice, *The Big One: Hurricane Andrew* (Kansas City, MO: The Miami Herald Publishing Co., 1992).
22. S.J. Carr et al., "The Public Health Response to the Los Angeles 1994 Earthquake," *American Journal of Public Health 86,* no. 4 (1996): 589–590.
23. E. Noji, ed., *The Public Health Consequences of Disaster* (New York: Oxford University Press, 1997).
24. L.F. Saylor and J.E. Gordon, "The Medical Component of Natural Disasters," *American Journal of the Medical Sciences* 234 (1957): 342–362.
25. A.S. Buist and R.S. Bernstein, eds., "Health Effects of Volcanoes: An Approach to Evaluating the Health Effects of an Environmental Hazard," *American Journal of Public Health 76,* no. 3 (suppl.) (1986): 1–90.
26. R.S. Bernstein et al., "Immediate Public Health Concerns and Actions in Volcanic Eruptions: Lessons from Mount St. Helens Eruptions, May 18–October 18, 1980," *American Journal of Public Health 76,* no. 3 (suppl.) (1986): 25–37.
27. Resolution 44/236 of the General Assembly of the United Nations, 1989.
28. Resolution 54/219 of the General Assembly of the United Nations.
29. L.Y. Landesman, ed., *Emergency Preparedness in the Healthcare Environment* (Oakbrook, IL: Joint Commission on Accreditation of Healthcare Organizations, 1997).
30. H.M. Ginzburg et al., "The Public Health Services Response to Hurricane Andrew," *Public Health Reports 108,* no. 2 (1993): 241–244.
31. P. Lewis, *Final Report: Governor's Disaster Planning and Response Review Committee* (Tallahassee, FL: Governor's Disaster Planning and Response Review Committee, 1993).
32. L.Y. Landesman, "The Availability of Disaster Preparation Courses at US Schools of Public Health," *American Journal of Public Health 83,* no. 10 (1993): 1,494–1,495.
33. Office of Disease Prevention and Health Promotion, U.S. Department of Health and Human Services, *Healthy People 2010* (Washington, DC: 1998). http://www.health.gov/healthypeople.
34. P.W. O'Carroll et al., "The Rapid Implementation of a Statewide Emergency Health Information System during the 1993 Iowa Flood," *American Journal of Public Health 85,* no. 4 (1995): 564–567.
35. Joint Commission on Accreditation of Healthcare Organizations, *Comprehensive Accreditation Manual for Hospitals: The Official Handbook* (EC 1.6, EC 2.5, EC 2.9, EC-5, EC-6, EC-12, EC-13, EC-25, EC-26, EC-49, EC-50) (Oakbrook Terrace, IL: 2000).
36. R. Bissell et al., "Health Care Personnel in Disaster Response: Reversible Roles or Territorial Imperatives?" *Emergency Medicine Clinics of North America 14,* no. 2 (1996): 267–288.
37. A. Kuehl, ed., *Prehospital Systems and Medical Oversight* (St. Louis, MO: Mosby, 1994).
38. T.E. Drabek et al., *Managing Multiorganizational Emergency Response: Emergency Research and Rescue Networks in Natural Disaster and Remote Area Setting* (Boulder, CO: Natural Hazards Information Center, University of Colorado, 1981).
39. E. Auf der Heide, *Disaster Response: Principles of Preparation and Coordination* (St. Louis, MO: C.V. Mosby, 1981).
40. "United States Government: Federal Response Plan (For Public Law 93–288, as Amended), April, 1992." [Publication no. 9230.1-PL] (Washington, DC: U.S. Government Printing Office, 1999).
41. F. Cuny, "Introduction to Disaster Management, Lesson 1: The Scope of Disaster Management," *Prehospital and Disaster Medicine 7,* no. 4 (1992): 400–409.
42. A. Ahlbom and S. Norell, *Introduction to Modern Epidemiology* (Chestnut Hill, MA: Epidemiology Resources, Inc., 1984).
43. M.F. Lechat, "The Epidemiology of Disasters," *Proceedings of the Royal Society of Medicine* 69 (1976): 421–426.
44. V.W. Sidel et al., "Public Health Responses to Natural and Human-Made Disasters," in *Public Health and Preventive Medicine,* eds. J.M. Last et al. (Stamford, CT: Appleton & Lange, 1992), 1,173–1,186.
45. C. Bern et al., "Risk Factors for Mortality in the Bangladesh Cyclone of 1991," *Bulletin of the World Health Organization* 71 (1993): 73–78.
46. P.J. Baxter et al., "Mount St. Helens Eruptions: The Acute Respiratory Effects of Volcanic Ash in a North American Community," *Archives of Environmental Health* 38 (1983): 138–143.
47. U.S. Centers for Disease Control and Prevention, "Needs Assessment Following Hurricane Georges–Dominican Republic, 1998," *Morbidity and Mortality Weekly Report* 48 (1999): 93–95.
48. M. Anker, "Epidemiological and Statistical Methods for Rapid Health Assessment: Introduction," *World Health Statistics Quarterly* 44 (1991): 94–97.
49. S.B. Thacker and R.L. Berkelman, "Public Health Surveillance in the United States," *Epidemiology Review* 10 (1988): 164–190.
50. S.F. Wetterhall and E.K. Noji, "Surveillance and Epidemiology," in *The Public Health Consequences of Disasters,* ed. E.K. Noji (New York: Oxford University Press, 1997), 37–64.
51. Pan American Health Organization, *Humanitarian Supply Management System* (Washington, DC: 1998). http://www.disaster.info.desastres.net/SUMA. Accessed 18 April 2000.

52. U.S. Agency for International Development, *Famine Early Warning* System (Washington, DC: 1985). http://www.info.usaid.gov/fews/fews.html. Accessed 18 April 2000.
53. R.I. Glass and E.K. Noji, "Epidemiologic Surveillance Following Disasters," in *Public Health Surveillance*, eds. W. Halperin and E.L. Baker (New York: Van Nostrand Reinhold, 1992), 195–205.
54. U.S. Centers for Disease Control and Prevention, Epidemiology Program Office, "Training Notes" (Atlanta, GA: 1992).
55. P.J. Baxter et al., "Mount St. Helens Eruptions, May 18 to June 12, 1980: An Overview of the Acute Health Impact," *Journal of the American Medical Association* 246 (1988): 2,585–2,589.
56. P. Duclos, *American Red Cross Disaster Database Collaborative Project: Surveillance System for Natural Disasters Using American Red Cross Records* (Atlanta, GA: U.S. Centers for Disease Control and Prevention, 1988).
57. J.H. van Bemmel and M.A. Musen, eds., *Handbook of Medical Informatics* (Houten, the Netherlands: Bohn Stafleu Van Loghum, 1997).
58. E.T. Gerrity and B.W. Flynn, "Mental Health Consequences of Disasters," in *Public Health Consequences of Disasters*, ed. E.K. Noji (New York: Oxford University Press, 1997), 101–121.
59. D. Myers, *Disaster Response and Recovery: A Handbook for Mental Health Professionals* (Rockville, MD: Center for Mental Health Services, 1994).
60. R.J. Ursano et al., "Trauma and Disaster," in *Individual and Community Responses to Trauma and Disaster: The Structure of Human Chaos*, eds. R.J. Ursano et al. (Cambridge, England: Cambridge University Press, 1994), 3–27.
61. K.J. Tierney, *Disaster Preparedness and Response: Research Findings and Guidance from the Social Science Literature* (Preliminary Paper #193) (Newark, DE: Disaster Research Center, University of Delaware, 1993).
62. B.H. Young et al., *Disaster Mental Health Services: A Guidebook for Clinicians and Administrators* (Menlo Park, CA: National Center for Post-Traumatic Stress Disorder, 1998).
63. E.T. Gerrity and P. Steinglass, "Relocation Stress Following Natural Disasters," in *Individual and Community Responses to Trauma and Disaster: The Structure of Human Chaos*, eds. R.J. Ursano et al. (Cambridge, England: Cambridge University Press, 1994), 220–247.
64. P.E. Hodgkinson and M. Stewart, *Coping with Catastrophe: A Handbook of Post-Disaster Psychosocial Aftercare*, 2d ed. (London: Routledge, 1998).
65. R. Janoff-Bulman, "The Aftermath of Victimization: Rebuilding Shattered Assumptions," in *Trauma and Its Wake: The Study and Treatment of Post-Traumatic Stress Disorder*, ed. C.R. Figley (New York: Brunner/Mazel Publishers, 1985), 15–35.
66. S.A. Murphy, "Health and Recovery Status of Victims One and Three Years Following a Natural Disaster," in *Trauma and Its Wake: Traumatic Stress Theory, Research, and Intervention*, ed. C.R. Figley (New York: Brunner/Mazel Publishers, 1986), 133–155.
67. *Training Manual for Human Service Workers in Major Disasters* (Washington, DC: Center for Mental Health Services, Substance Abuse and Mental Health Services Administration, U.S. Department of Health and Human Services, 1978, 1996).
68. D.M. Hartsough and D.G. Myers, *Disaster Work and Mental Health: Prevention and Control of Stress among Workers* (Washington, DC: Center for Mental Health Services, Substance Abuse and Mental Health Services Administration, U.S. Public Health Service, 1995).
69. C.R. Figley, "Traumatic Stress: The Role of the Family and Social Support System," in *Trauma and Its Wake: Traumatic Stress Theory, Research, and Intervention*, ed. C.R. Figley (New York: Brunner/Mazel Publishers, 1986), 39–54.
70. S.E. Hobfoll et al., "Conservation of Resources and Traumatic Stress," in *Traumatic Stress: From Theory to Practice*, eds. J.R. Freedy and S.E. Hobfoll (New York: Plenum Press, 1995), 29–47.
71. E.G. Karam, "Comorbidity of Posttraumatic Stress Disorder and Depression," in *Posttraumatic Stress Disorder: Acute and Long-Term Responses to Trauma and Disaster*, eds. C.S. Fullerton and R.J. Ursano (Washington, DC: American Psychiatric Press, 1997), 77–90.
72. K.J. Hoffman and J.E. Sasaki, "Comorbidity of Substance Abuse and PTSD," in *Posttraumatic Stress Disorder: Acute and Long-Term Responses to Trauma and Disaster*, eds. C.S. Fullerton and R.J. Ursano (Washington, DC: American Psychiatric Press, 1997), 159–174.
73. American Psychiatric Association, *Diagnostic and Statistical Manual of Mental Disorders*, 4th ed. (DSM-IV) (Washington, DC: 1994).
74. G. DeGirolamo and A.C. McFarlane, "The Epidemiology of PTSD: A Comprehensive Review of the International Literature," in *Ethnocultural Aspects of Posttraumatic Stress Disorder: Issues, Research, and Clinical Applications*, eds. A.J. Marsella et al. (Washington, DC: American Psychological Association, 1996), 33–85.
75. C.S. Fullerton and R.J. Ursano, eds., *Posttraumatic Stress Disorder: Acute and Long-Term Responses to Trauma and Disaster* (Washington, DC: American Psychiatric Press, 1997), 3–18.
76. L.S. O'Brien, *Traumatic Events and Mental Health* (Cambridge, England: Cambridge University Press, 1998).

77. C.S. Fullerton and R.J. Ursano, "Posttraumatic Responses in Spouse/Significant Others of Disaster Workers," in *Posttraumatic Stress Disorder: Acute and Long-Term Responses to Trauma and Disaster*, eds. C.S. Fullerton and R.J. Ursano (Washington, DC: American Psychiatric Press, 1997), 59–75.
78. A.J. Marsella et al., eds. *Ethnocultural Aspects of Posttraumatic Stress Disorder: Issues, Research, and Clinical Applications* (Washington, DC: American Psychological Association, 1996).
79. B.L. Green, "Cross-National and Ethnocultural Issues in Disaster Research," in *Ethnocultural Aspects of Posttraumatic Stress Disorder: Issues, Research, and Clinical Applications,* eds. A.J. Marsella et al. (Washington, DC: American Psychological Association, 1996), 341–361.
80. M.J. Friedman and A.J. Marsella, "Posttraumatic Stress Disorder: An Overview of the Concept," in *Ethnocultural Aspects of Posttraumatic Stress Disorder: Issues, Research, and Clinical Applications*, eds. A.J. Marsella et al. (Washington, DC: American Psychological Association, 1996), 11–32.
81. F.D. Gusman et al., "A Multicultural Approach and Developmental Framework for Treating Trauma," in *Ethnocultural Aspects of Posttraumatic Stress Disorder: Issues, Research, and Clinical Applications* (Washington, DC: American Psychological Association, 1996), 439–457.
82. K. Erikson, *Everything in Its Path: Destruction of Community in the Buffalo Creek Flood* (New York: Simon & Schuster, 1976).
83. B.L. Green et al., "Buffalo Creek Survivors in the Second Decade: Comparison with Unexposed and Nonlitigant Groups," *Journal of Applied Social Psychology* 20 (1990): 1,033–1,050.
84. M.C. Grace et al., "The Buffalo Creek Disaster: A 14-Year Follow-Up," in *The International Handbook of Traumatic Stress Syndromes*, eds. J.P. Wilson and B. Raphael (New York: Plenum Press, 1993), 441–449.
85. V.A. Taylor, *Delivery of Mental Health Services in Disasters: The Xenia Tornado and Some Implications* (The Disaster Research Center Book and Monograph Series #11) (Columbus, OH: Disaster Research Center, The Ohio State University, 1976).
86. E.L. Quarantelli, ed., *What Is a Disaster? Perspectives on the Question* (London: Routledge, 1998).
87. B.L. Green and S.D. Solomon, "The Mental Health Impact of Natural and Technological Disasters," in *Traumatic Stress: From Theory to Practice*, eds. J.R. Freedy and S.E. Hobfoll (New York: Plenum Press, 1995), 163–180.
88. R.J. Ursano et al., eds., *Individual and Community Responses to Trauma and Disaster: The Structure of Human Chaos* (Cambridge, England: Cambridge University Press, 1994).
89. K. Erikson, *A New Species of Trouble: The Human Experience of Modern Disasters* (New York: W.W. Norton, 1995).
90. L. Weisaeth, "Psychological and Psychiatric Aspects of Technological Disasters," in *Individual and Community Responses to Trauma and Disaster: The Structure of Human Chaos*, eds. R.J. Ursano et al. (Cambridge, England: Cambridge University Press, 1994), 72–102.
91. J. Kliman et al., "Natural and Human-Made Disasters: Some Therapeutic and Epidemiological Implications for Crisis Intervention," in *Therapeutic Intervention: Healing Strategies for Human Systems*, eds. U. Reuveni et al. (New York: Human Sciences Press, 1982), 253–280.
92. E.L. Quarantelli, "The Environmental Disasters of the Future Will Be More and Worse But the Prospect Is Not Hopeless," *Disaster Prevention and Management* 2 (1993): 11–25.
93. S.R. Lillibridge, "Industrial Disasters," in *The Public Health Consequences of Disasters*, ed. E.K. Noji (New York: Oxford University Press, 1997), 354–372.
94. International Federation of the Red Cross, "Annex III: The Role of the Red Cross and Red Crescent Societies in Response to Technological Disasters," *International Review of the Red Cross* 310 (1996): 55–130.
95. International Atomic Energy Agency/European Community/World Health Organization, *International Conference: One Decade after Chernobyl: Summing Up the Consequences of the Accident. Summary of the Conference Results, 8–12 April, 1996* (Vienna: 1996).
96. World Health Organization, *Health Consequences of the Chernobyl Accident: Results of the IPHECA Pilot Projects and Related National Programs. Summary Report* (Geneva, Switzerland: 1995).
97. Nuclear Energy Agency, *Chernobyl Ten Years On: Radiological and Health Impact: An Assessment by the NEA Committee on Radiation Protection and Public Health, November 1995* (Paris, France: Organisation for Economic Cooperation and Development Nuclear Energy Agency, 1995).
98. P. Shrivastava, "Long-Term Recovery from the Bhopal Crisis," in *The Long Road to Recovery: Community Responses to Industrial Disaster*, ed. J.K. Mitchell (Tokyo: United Nations University Press, 1996), 121–147.
99. C.E. Fritz, *Disasters and Mental Health: Therapeutic Principles Drawn from Disaster Studies* (Historical and Comparative Disaster Series #10) (Newark, DE: Disaster Research Center, University of Delaware, 1996).
100. B.H. Cuthbertson and J.M. Nigg, "Technological Disaster and the Nontherapeutic Community: A Question of True Victimization," *Environment and Behavior* 19 (1987): 462–483.

101. J.S. Kroll-Smith and S.R. Couch, "Technological Hazards: Social Responses as Traumatic Stressors," in *The International Handbook of Traumatic Stress Syndromes*, eds. J.P. Wilson and B. Raphael (New York: Plenum Press, 1993), 79–91.
102. M.R. Edelstein and A. Wandersman, "Community Dynamics in Coping with Toxic Contaminants," in *Neighborhood and Community Environments*. Vol. 9, eds. I. Altman and A. Wandersman (New York: Plenum Press, 1987), 69–112.
103. M.R. Edelstein, *Contaminated Communities: The Social and Psychosocial Impacts of Residential Toxic Exposure* (Boulder, CO: Westview, 1988).
104. R.E. Kasperson and J.X. Kasperson, "The Social Amplification and Attenuation of Risk," *The Annals of the American Academy of Political and Social Science* 545 (1996): 95–105.
105. A. Baum et al., "Natural Disaster and Technological Catastrophe," *Environment and Behavior* 15 (1983): 333–354.
106. A. Baum, "Toxins, Technology, Disasters," in *Cataclysms, Crises, and Catastrophes: Psychology in Action*, eds. G.R. VandenBos and B.K. Bryant (Washington, DC: American Psychological Association, 1987), 9–53.
107. E.J. Bromet et al., "Long-Term Mental Health Consequences of the Accident at Three Mile Island," *International Journal of Mental Health* 19 (1990): 48–60.
108. J.M. Havenaar et al., "Long-Term Mental Health Effects of the Chernobyl Disaster: An Epidemiologic Survey of Two Former Soviet Regions," *American Journal of Psychiatry* 154 (1997): 1,605–1,607.
109. S.M. Becker, "Psychosocial Assistance after Environmental Accidents: A Policy Perspective," *Environmental Health Perspectives 105,* no. S6 (1997): 1,557–1,563.
110. *Field Manual for Human Service Workers in Major Disasters* (Rockville, MD: National Institute of Mental Health, 1990).
111. S.D. Solomon, "Mobilizing Social Support Networks in Times of Disaster," in *Trauma and Its Wake: Traumatic Stress Theory, Research, and Intervention*, ed. C.R. Figley (New York: Brunner/Mazel Publishers, 1986), 232–263.
112. L.C. Leviton et al., *Confronting Public Health Risks: A Decision Maker's Guide* (Thousand Oaks, CA: Sage Publications, 1998).
113. N.L. Farberow and N.S. Gordon, *Manual for Child Health Workers in Major Disasters* (Washington, DC: Center for Mental Health Services, Substance Abuse and Mental Health Services Administration, U.S. Public Health Service, 1995).
114. L.C. Terr, "Large-Group Preventive Techniques for Use after Disaster," in *Responding to Disaster: A Guide for Mental Health Professionals*, ed. L.S. Austin (Washington, DC: American Psychiatric Press, 1992), 81–99.
115. L.T. Mega and S.L. McCammon, "Tornado in Eastern North Carolina: Outreach to School and Community," in *Responding to Disaster: A Guide for Mental Health Professionals*, ed. L.S. Austin (Washington, DC: American Psychiatric Press, 1992), 211–230.
116. R.S. Pynoos et al., "A Public Mental Health Approach to the Postdisaster Treatment of Children and Adolescents," *Child and Adolescent Psychiatric Clinics of North America* 7 (1988): 195–210.
117. *Responding to the Needs of People with Serious and Persistent Mental Illness in Times of Disaster* (Washington, DC: Emergency Services and Disaster Relief Branch, Center for Mental Health Services, Substance Abuse and Mental Health Services Administration, 1996).
118. American Red Cross Disaster Mental Health Services, *Coping with Disaster: Emotional Health Issues for Disaster Workers on Assignment* (ARC 4472) (Washington, DC: American Red Cross, 1991).
119. American Red Cross Disaster Mental Health Services, *Coping with Disaster: Emotional Health Issues for Families of Disaster Workers* (ARC 4474) (Washington, DC: American Red Cross, 1991).
120. American Red Cross Disaster Mental Health Services, *Coping with Disaster: Returning Home from a Disaster Assignment* (ARC 4473) (Washington, DC: American Red Cross, 1991).
121. J.T. Mitchell and G.S. Everly, Jr., *Critical Incident Stress Debriefing: An Operations Manual for the Prevention of Traumatic Stress among Emergency Service and Disaster Workers,* 2d ed., rev. (Ellicott City, MD: Chevron Publishing Corp., 1997).
122. G.S. Everly, Jr. and J.T. Mitchell, *Critical Incident Stress Management: A New Era and Standard of Care in Crisis Intervention* (Ellicott City, MD: Chevron Publishing Corp., 1997).
123. B. Raphael and J.P. Wilson, "Theoretical and Intervention Considerations in Working with Victims of Disaster," in *International Handbook of Traumatic Stress Syndromes*, eds. J.P. Wilson and B. Raphael (New York: Plenum Press, 1993).
124. J.L. McKnight and J.P. Kretzmann, *Mapping Community Capacity* (Evanston, IL: Center for Urban Affairs and Policy Research, Northwestern University, 1990).
125. N. Bracht, ed., *Health Promotion at the Community Level* (Newbury Park, CA: Sage Publications, 1990).
126. M.V. Melosi, *Pollution and Reform in American Cities, 1870–1930* (Austin, TX: University of Texas Press, 1980).
127. G. Rosen, *A History of Public Health* (Baltimore: Johns Hopkins University Press, 1993).
128. A.E. Peterson et al., "Soap Use Effect on Diarrhea: Nyamithuthu Refugee Camp," *International Journal of Epidemiology* 27 (1998): 520–524.

129. S. Esrey et al., "Effects of Improved Water Supply and Sanitation on Ascariasis, Diarrhoea, Dracunculiasis, Hookworm Infection, Schistosomiasis, and Trachoma," *Bulletin of the World Health Organization 69,* no. 5 (1991): 609–621.
130. "Mortality among Newly Arrived Mozambican Refugees–Zimbabwe and Malawi," *Morbidity and Mortality Weekly Report 42,* no. 24 (1992): 468–477.
131. D. Hatch et al., "Epidemic Cholera during Refugee Resettlement in Malawi," *International Journal of Epidemiology 22,* no. 6 (1994): 1,292–1,299.
132. L.D. Rotz et al., "Bioterrorism Preparedness: Planning for the Future," *Journal of Public Health Management and Practice 6,* no. 4 (2000): 45–49.
133. E. Hood, "Chemical and Biological Weapons: New Questions, New Answers," *Environmental Health Perspectives 107,* no. 12 (1999): 931–932.
134. T. Okumura et al., "The Tokyo Subway Sarin Attack: Disaster Management, Part I: Community Emergency Response," *Academy of Emergency Medicine 5,* no. 6 (1998): 613–617.
135. *The Defense against Weapons of Mass Destruction Act,* The National Defense Authorization Act for Fiscal Year 1997. Title XIV of PL (1996): 104–201.
136. T.J. Cieslak and E.M. Eitzen, "Bioterrorism: Agents of Concern," *Journal of Public Health Management and Practice 6,* no. 4 (2000): 19–29.
137. C.D. Malloy, "A History of Biological and Chemical Warfare and Terrorism," *Journal of Public Health Management and Practice 6,* no. 4 (2000): 30–37.
138. J.A. Popuard and L.A. Miller, "History of Biological Warfare: Catapults to Capsomeres," *Ann NY Acad Sci,* 666 (1992): 9–20.
139. K.B. Olson and Aum Shirikyo, "Once and Future Threat?" *Emerg Inf Dis,* 4 (1999): 513–516.
140. L.A. Cole, "Bioterrorism Threats: Learning from Inappropriate Responses," *Journal of Public Health Management and Practice 6,* no. 4 (2000): 8–18.
141. U.S. Centers for Disease Control and Prevention, "Bioterrorism Alleging Use of Anthrax and Interim Guidelines for Management," *1998 MMWR Weekly Review 48,* no. 4 (1999): 69–74.
142. L.C. Garrett et al., "Taking the Terror Out of Bioterrorism: Planning for a Bioterrorist Event from a Local Perspective," *Journal of Public Health Management and Practice 6,* no. 4 (2000): 1–7.
143. U.S. Centers for Disease Control and Prevention, National Center for Infectious Diseases, *Critical Agents of Concern, Summary of Selection Process and Recommendations* (Atlanta, GA: publisher, 1999).
144. Cohen et al. "Bioterrorism Initiatives: Public Health in Reverse?" *American Journal of Public Health 84,* no. 11 (1999): 1,629–1,631.

CHAPTER 29

Administering Effective HIV Prevention Interventions

Anton M. Somlai

Effective disease prevention and control programs are often designed to motivate behavior change at multiple levels, including those defined by the individual, family, social network, and community. The challenges that face public health organizations in designing and administering such programs are particularly acute for combating the human immunodeficiency virus (HIV)/acquired immune deficiency syndrome (AIDS) epidemic, which as yet is not amenable to vaccine. HIV prevention efforts are carried out by a constellation of loosely affiliated organizations, including AIDS service organizations (ASOs), community-based organizations (CBOs), state and local public health agencies, community health centers, academic institutions, and other health care providers. A variety of administrative strategies may be used by public health organizations in developing, coordinating, and managing these efforts to improve their effectiveness.

ADMINISTERING EFFECTIVE HIV PREVENTION INTERVENTIONS

Since the beginning of the HIV/AIDS epidemic in the early 1980s, community-based AIDS service organizations (ASOs) have been crucial providers of HIV prevention services to communities that have been affected by the disease. Initially, little was known regarding risk factors for contracting HIV infection, making education at the community level critically important. Community-based ASOs appeared shortly after AIDS was first identified as a "grassroots" response to alert and educate gay men about the emergency posed by the new disease. ASOs then expanded their programmatic efforts and activities to reach other community members with educational information concerning the spread of the HIV epidemic.

Without a vaccine, behavior change that eliminates or lessens risk constitutes the only means to prevent new HIV infections. Behavior that reduces the risk of HIV infection can occur at the individual, dyad, network, or community level. Promoting change in sexual and drug use behaviors that create risk for HIV infection is currently the most effective strategy to curtail the course of the epidemic. HIV risk reduction prevention efforts are especially critical within community populations that are most vulnerable to new infections.

Today, HIV prevention efforts are carried forth in the field by ASOs, community-based organizations (CBOs), governmental health departments, and other providers of services to at-risk individuals and populations in their communities. All of these organizations play an essential role in delivering HIV prevention programs to communities who are at risk of HIV infection. Community-

The National Institute of Mental Health Grant R01MH54935, Center Grant P30MH52776, and Wisconsin HIV Prevention Evaluation Technical Assistance and Services supported preparation of this chapter.

based nongovernmental organizations (NGOs) are distinctive in their ability to offer HIV prevention programs because most offer culturally sensitive services to traditionally underserved populations, employ staff with a direct knowledge of difficult-to-reach populations, have established trust with the communities they serve, and provide a linkage between traditional public health organizations and communities with special needs.[1] More importantly, ASOs and CBOs are able to develop HIV prevention programs that are tailored to their target populations.

Over time, the geography and topography of the HIV/AIDS epidemic has changed, resulting in the need to create innovative HIV prevention programs to reach populations at greatest risk.[2,3] Early in the epidemic, factual knowledge concerning risk for HIV infection was low among the public. ASO efforts to provide basic risk education were appropriate, essential, and in many ways, the major front-line public health initiative used in primary HIV prevention. As a result, public understanding of HIV and AIDS, practices that lead to greater HIV infection risk, and the steps needed to reduce risk, have improved. ASOs are now faced with moving beyond providing risk education programs alone, and must address the more difficult challenge of implementing programs that help at-risk persons enact and maintain behavior changes that lower their risk to HIV infection and AIDS.

The administration of these new prevention program efforts has never been more important and increasingly complex than today. An ASO/CBO administrator is not only responsible for the implementation of HIV prevention programs, but must also work with limited resources, succeed in achieving overall prevention initiatives, and counteract or remove potential barriers for program implementation. Prevention programs then become prophylactic agents aimed at impeding and preventing the spread of HIV infection through active initiatives intended to provide at-risk populations with the skills that facilitate safer levels of behavior. The effectiveness of HIV prevention program administrators is directly related to the delivery, conduct, and performance of these programs.

The purpose of this chapter is to characterize the key program elements that are important for the implementation and maintenance of initiatives to reduce HIV risk at the ASO level as well as other providers of HIV prevention services. More importantly, the goal of this chapter is to provide practical "lessons learned" from previous studies focused on bridging the gap that divides "front-line" service providers and research-based models.[4–7] Although much attention has been given science-based HIV prevention interventions, very little is known regarding ASO prevention services and access by public health service providers to those research-based HIV prevention interventions.[5]

Limited resources and the changing nature of the epidemic led to the need for strong organization and planning in the administration of HIV prevention programs and services at the local level. Community-level organizations dedicated to HIV prevention programs must understand the risk behaviors of their targeted populations and the programs that are most effective in lowering that risk. They also need to identify important organizational characteristics that facilitate the use of efficacious prevention models and strategies, especially with such hard-to-reach populations as injecting drug users (IDUs). New prevention efforts also need to deal with structural-level issues that create barriers in the provision of services to at-risk populations. And finally, HIV prevention program administrators have increasingly greater opportunities to increase the effectiveness of their organization's efforts by participating in community planning groups (CPGs) and working with state-level policy makers.

DETERMINING POPULATIONS AT NEED

Traditionally, ASOs have provided information on HIV infection and the AIDS epidemic to the general public. During the early stages of the epidemic, educational programs were necessary as the initial response to an emerging health problem filled with numerous misconceptions. As at-risk populations became more identified, specifically gay-identified men and men-who-have-sex-with-men, these educational programs needed to become more intensive, providing such skills training as condom use.

The changing nature of the HIV epidemic has resulted in the need for new and more innovative HIV prevention programs to reach persons who are presently at greatest risk.[2,3] Effective HIV prevention programs need to be based on strong theoretical risk reduction models that have been shown to be efficacious in research and effective in the field. This holds significant implications for program development, recruitment, marketing, administration, and training.

Several factors influence which at-risk populations are in need. Most importantly, the mission of the ASO should clearly identify the factors that influence the organization's provision of prevention services. This will help identify the ASO in the communities they wish to provide prevention services to as committed in helping stem the HIV/AIDS epidemic. The perceptions of prevention programs by stakeholders and users will establish a community-level awareness, identifying the ASO with public health initiatives aimed toward at-risk populations.

In determining which populations are in need of effective HIV prevention intervention programs, the ASO needs to operationalize research findings into effective "front-line" prevention efforts. To do this, the ASO needs a well-developed program implementation plan consisting of: (1) a *preoperational* phase identifying the characteristics of the at-risk population, (2) a *maintenance* phase that ensures the ongoing integrity of the program, and (3) *data collection* methods that evaluate the effectiveness of the program and provide information for future funding initiatives.

EFFICACIOUS PRIMARY AND SECONDARY HIV PREVENTION INTERVENTIONS

Although much has evolved in our knowledge about HIV infection, one fact has remained constant throughout the epidemic: behavior change constitutes the only means to prevent new infections. Therefore, behavior change interventions that are capable of effectively assisting people to reduce their risk for contracting HIV infection constitute the front line of public health efforts to prevent HIV/AIDS. A body of research in the behavioral sciences has now convincingly demonstrated the efficacy of relatively intensive, multifocused cognitive–behavioral group interventions for assisting people to change aspects of their sexual behavior that carry high risk for HIV infection.[8]

In the early 1990s, the single largest HIV prevention activity that was federally funded in the United States was counseling and antibody testing.[9] As routinely conducted, HIV counseling and testing programs are brief, providing factual information about AIDS, risk reduction recommendations, and advice to abstain from sex or to use condoms. The modal duration of counseling time offered in counseling and testing programs in the field is approximately 20 minutes.[9] A large number of studies have evaluated the behavior change effects of counseling and testing as they are routinely conducted in the field. Although some indicate modest behavior change effects,[10,11] most have found little evidence of behavior change among persons who learn that they are seronegative.[12–15] A scientific review of HIV counseling and testing programs supported by the U.S. Centers for Disease Control and Prevention (CDC) found that prevention counseling consists of a brief presentation of educational information and rarely reflects the incorporation of scientifically based behavior change principles or procedures.[9] ASOs need to adopt more substantive, behaviorally based HIV prevention programs that they can offer to their high-risk clients.

Regardless of which scientifically based intervention is chosen by an ASO, the program needs to be linked to communities and the environment(s) they live in. In front-line settings, prevention programs need to focus on either primary prevention or population strategies.

COMMUNITY PLANNING

In 1994, the CDC mandated that federally funded health departments set priorities for prevention planning efforts through the use of HIV prevention community planning.[16] Health departments are now funded in a lump sum and allocate resources as established by one or more planning groups within their jurisdiction.[17] With this change in funding, planning groups now consider the following in determining funding priorities: need, intervention effectiveness, cost-effectiveness of the intervention, scientific basis for the prevention program, community preferences, local factors, and the availability of resources.[16]

The CDC's change to a prevention community planning process has had a significant effect on the priorities of HIV prevention programs in the United States. Resources have been redistributed from counseling and testing to health education and risk reduction activities. The primary model for prevention programming has moved from counseling and testing to health education and risk reduction activities.

Community planning is now vested in a comprehensive HIV prevention model that requires a variety of interventions. Through the CDC mandate, CPGs are required to develop a comprehensive evidence-based HIV prevention plan. A number of components need to be included in this plan.

Three important factors are incorporated into CPGs' planning process: (1) sharing of expertise, (2) methodology for creating structure, and (3) a localized effort for disseminating efficacious, research-based interventions. Community-based planning increases health communications among program planners by prioritizing interventions related to sexual or drug use behavior and then building capacity resources by targeting high-risk populations that would benefit the most from this process.

ASOs benefit from this decentralized decision-making process at the local level because support is built for sound HIV prevention program planning. ASOs are then able to develop the components of a comprehensive HIV prevention program through operationalizing HIV prevention community planning and core objectives. This helps to build the essential elements of a comprehensive HIV prevention plan at the local level.

Through the CPG process, the roles and responsibilities of health departments, HIV prevention community planning groups, and local ASOs become accountable through shared responsibilities. This assists the administration of HIV prevention programs through linkages that provide information, shared resources, and capacity building in order to improve and drive better programs.

ORGANIZATIONAL MODELS FOR HIV PREVENTION

Public health agencies have traditionally provided HIV surveillance, testing, and counseling as a primary prevention strategy. However, community-based NGOs are uniquely able to contribute to HIV and sexually transmitted disease prevention efforts.[1] CBOs offer linguistically and culturally sensitive services to traditionally underserved populations. They are staffed by personnel with direct knowledge of these difficult-to-reach populations. CBOs enjoy the trust of the communities they serve. They also provide a linkage between traditional public health agencies and communities with special needs.[1]

There are two spheres of influence in the development of effective organizational structures at the local level. First, organizational construction can be developed to enhance the provision of services for people in need and/or at risk for HIV infection. Second, theoretical prevention models that drive these efforts can improve more collaborative efforts between ASOs/CBOs and researchers.

Organizational characteristics need to influence individual, network, and community barriers to efficacious prevention models and strategies. These approaches need to be flexible enough to work with such difficult populations as IDUs. An excellent model of health promotion can be found in the Ottawa Charter for Health Promotion.[18] This charter was the outcome of the first international conference on health promotion. The document identifies the basic prerequisites for health and the need to promote health through advocacy. Most importantly, the charter suggests the need for public policy to remove obstacles in creating supportive environments in nonhealth sectors. Community development and action are viewed as significant strategies in achieving better health. The responsibility for promoting health is not only the responsibility of the individual, but also of the greater social and political environmental components.

ASOs can create an ecology of health promotion by developing guiding principles that move into the arena of public health policy. Not only do they need to become active participants of their local CPGs, but they need to respond to the health gaps in society that produce rules and practices that continue to keep people at greater risk of HIV infection and AIDS. This model of HIV prevention addresses the overall quality-of-life and ecologic issues that face both people living with HIV/AIDS and those who are at risk due to a lack of compassionate public policy.

A difficult situation facing prevention programs currently in the United States is the lack of funding and support for needle exchange programs (NEPs). Policy makers at the federal level, as well as several state governments, continue to question whether NEPs reduce or maintain the spread of HIV transmission among participating IDUs. However, as early as 1994, Kaplan and Heimer found through a circulation theory of exchange that needle exchange decreased needle circulation times, leading to a reduction in the rate of new HIV infections.[19] Their analysis further suggested that HIV incidence may have reduced by more than 40 percent as a result of NEPs. Despite these findings, NEPs continue to lack support and funding from the federal government. The key then is for ASOs at the local and national level to develop prevention strategies that affect these structural barriers in promoting NEPs as a highly effective tool in the battle against the AIDS epidemic.

There are a number of environmental and contextual factors that also influence the types of models to be used by ASOs. Quality of life, living conditions, personal resources, and social pressures all impact on tailoring individual and community prevention efforts to reduce HIV risk. Nelson et al. found that a 100 percent condom campaign among young men in Thailand led to changes in sexual behavior, increased use of condoms, and lowered rates of HIV infection.[20] The program included condom distribution in commercial sex establishments, the promotion of increased condom use through the media, and an enforcement program. This environmental intervention was an effective public health strategy in a general population of young men. More importantly, the success of this structural intervention in Thailand may also demonstrate that vulnerable populations, with the proper tools and training, may be highly effective in changing sexual behavior by acting as change advocates with the general, less at-risk population.[21]

FACILITATING HIV PREVENTION MODELS: FROM RESEARCH TO SERVICE

A number of factors contribute to the gap between scientific research concerning HIV prevention interventions and prevention programs offered by applied CBOs. HIV prevention scientists ordinarily function in settings that reinforce academic productivity and scientific publication. The translation of significant HIV prevention intervention findings to service providers is not reinforced in the academic arenas of funding and promotion where most prevention scientists live.

CBOs also have barriers to new research-based HIV prevention programs, limiting efforts to improve the transfer of HIV prevention technology. CBO staff may have strong expertise in relating to community members, finding hard-to-reach at-risk populations, and culturally tailoring HIV prevention programs and yet not be familiar with the scientific principles applied to prevention. Organizations may have great investments in maintaining existing programs and be resistive to initiatives based on research findings. Scientific findings may be viewed with skepticism and thought to not directly benefit people being served by front-line service providers. Practical barriers may also exist to new prevention programs due to different organizational resources, personnel, and delivery needs.

There are a number of factors influencing the decision to use science-based HIV prevention programs at the ASO level. DiFranceisco et al. found that the adoption of small-group, risk reduction interventions based on cognitive behavioral principles was influenced by such characteristics as perceived benefits, efficacy, previous technical assistance, resource constraints, and organizational barriers.[4] Although prevention programs based on small-group, social cognitive principles can facilitate change in HIV-related sexual risk, it is likely that ASOs will need technical assistance in transferring this technology from research to the field.[4,22]

TYPES OF ASO PREVENTION ACTIVITIES AND NEW PROGRAM NEEDS

Although the CDC has used the community planning process as a tool to empower state and local organizations to implement effective HIV prevention interventions, there may be an important need to look at capacity and resources in delivering these programs. This new direction and increased support for risk reduction behavior change programs (at the individual, group, and community level) suggest that CDC-funded prevention efforts will shift more responsibility on community-based providers. In this respect, it is important to understand the types of services being provided by ASOs and the kinds of new programs that are seen as important by ASOs.

In an attempt to investigate present and future directions of HIV prevention undertaken by community-based organizations, Somlai et al. studied the types of programs being offered by ASOs to two client groups in their communities.[6] Additionally, they elicited observations from ASO prevention directors concerning the types of programs they viewed as important to meet future needs in their communities. ASOs, in this study, had modest prevention budgets, which may explain why their prevention programs focused on activities low in resource consumption, such as AIDS educational print materials and brief AIDS education sessions dedicated to providing factual information. ASO prevention directors reported wanting to move their generalist educational programs to more intensive behavior change activities with a focus on targeting specialized segments of target populations. This study also found that ASO prevention directors wanted to develop programs that addressed social, cultural, psychological, and contextual issues surrounding HIV risk behavior.[6]

ASOs reported several potential barriers to the possible implementation of new HIV prevention program efforts. ASO prevention directors had held their current positions, on average, only two years; front-line prevention staff had only one year of experience. These high levels of personnel turnover may create significant problems in prevention program continuity and limit the organization's ability to implement more complex and specialized prevention programs. The capacity of ASOs to deliver new, specialized prevention programs was severely impeded by limited budgets and inadequately trained/educated personnel and staff. This suggests that ASO prevention services will need greater technical assistance and training if they intend to broaden the nature of their HIV prevention intervention efforts.

Given the CDC's mandate that community planning groups establish HIV prevention priorities based on local needs and established on science-based evidence of program effectiveness, and the fact that ASOs are investigating new types of prevention programs, it is necessary to identify a method capable of transferring HIV prevention technology from research to service providers. Recently, Kelly et al. found that ASOs that were provided with research-based prevention intervention manuals, on-site staff training workshops, and follow-up consultation resulted in frequent program adoption.[5] The CDC has initiated the development of replicating HIV prevention interventions that were found to be effective in research trials as a first step in disseminating programs to the field.[23] The Kelly et al. study found that this approach could be made more effective with training and consultation.[5]

Historically, ASOs have operated with limited budgets and the continual danger of losing more experienced staff and management. They have also lacked the relationship with science-based investigations to receive the most effective and specialized HIV prevention programs for their greatest at-risk populations. This creates significant concerns for stemming the AIDS epidemic in the front lines of where prevention efforts are occurring. ASOs intent on delivering the most effective prevention programs will need to ensure adequate resources and funding, technical skills of manager and staff, capacity to conduct prevention programs to reach specific or hard-to-reach populations, and linkages that can build on shared resources and expertise in developing more highly effective programs. These factors are all imbedded under the umbrella of capacity, where there is a greater movement by funding sources to support programs that have proven to be effective where service providers are mandated to prove that their programs work by process- and outcome-driven evaluations.

CRITICAL ELEMENTS IN EVALUATING THE EFFECTIVENESS OF AN HIV PREVENTION PROGRAM

The primary objectives of evaluating community-based HIV prevention programs are to verify, document, and quantify the effectiveness of assisting people in changing the behavior that puts them at risk for HIV infection. The verification of a program's effectiveness is important because there are times where common sense turns out to be wrong. For example, in the early stages of the HIV/AIDS epidemic, "common sense" suggested that information regarding risk was enough to change behavior. However, it was discovered later, after efforts to verify program effectiveness, that educational-type programs focusing primarily on information were not enough to change risky behavior. Documentation of a prevention program's implementation and effectiveness provides stakeholders, funders, and communities of affected/infected people with key information regarding success and future program directions. The quantification of a program's outcomes identifies strategies that can be improved and used to determine intervention effects to advance future objectives. Because the purpose of evaluation is to benefit public health and community programs, ASOs need to ensure that prevention programs are based on foundations in such areas as behavior change theory, behavioral assessment, and quantitative methodology to determine program effects.

ASOs need to address carefully reasons that evaluation is beneficial for the implementation and maintenance of HIV prevention programs. The approaches to evaluation need to be realistic, understandable, and "doable" by agency staff. ASO staff and administration need to know the key components of effective evaluations and what the determinants of evaluation successes and challenges are. It is important to the organization to maintain a primary evaluation question for program improvement: What are we trying to learn?

Program evaluation provides ASOs with several benefits that are also incentives. The chances of reaching and serving special populations from high-risk environments are increased when programs are planned after performing a needs assessment and are monitored by progress assessments. Progress assessments will help the organization assess if the prevention program is reaching the intended at-risk population. Process evaluation provides a description of how the prevention program was implemented, and can then be used as a guide in developing or implementing similar programs. By assessing the outcome and impact of a prevention program, ASOs can find what key elements "work" with at-risk populations and suggest areas for improving the program in order to meet the desired goals. And finally, evaluation provides the opportunity to discover unanticipated benefits associated with the prevention program.

ASOs need to pay attention to special considerations that are critical in evaluating prevention programs, funding, level of intervention, and programmatic goals. CBOs compete for limited public health funding. Those organizations that provide compelling data on the "success" of their prevention programs are more likely to increase their opportunities with funders. The need to compete for funding drives the need for evaluation. Increasing public awareness of funds being spent on unevaluated programs has led policy makers to develop more stringent requirements to show the effectiveness of prevention programs. Funding, and the availability of resources, dictate whether organization prevention priorities will focus on the individual, group, and/or community level. The direction of program efforts is based on decisions that are directly related to the cost-effectiveness and utility of the level of intervention; ultimately, prevention program efforts focus on at-risk populations and have as goals the nonoccurrence, or lessening, of behaviors that place these populations at risk of HIV infection. Therefore, CBOs need to intervene at a level that can be evaluated in a manner that is consistent with the long-term goals of their prevention programs.

Although there is a strong rationale for the development of effective evaluation methodologies at the ASO level, it is quite likely that there may be significant organizational resistance to program evaluation. Staff may perceive evaluation as an unnecessary component of work and a task that impedes the process of service delivery to at-risk populations. Staff may have little "buy-in" to the evaluation process, seeing it more as an administrative function of the organization. Quite often, there is an unspoken suspicion of program evaluation coming from a concern that the collected data will be used to assess job performance, resulting in potentially negative effects such as a lack of increased salary or promotion. Organizations may also have difficulties conceptualizing prevention models and measuring behavioral change related to programmatic outcomes.

Developing an evaluation plan can enhance the framework for planning, strategic decision making, multiyear funding, resource allocation, engaging stakeholders, and increasing prevention efforts. Table 29–1 provides a model for asking questions regarding evaluation decisions and the products needed to provide the information that will help answer key questions.[24] An effective evaluation assists the organization in assessing what aspects of a prevention program are working or are in need of improvement. The organization will need to identify who the results of the evaluation are intended for and what constraints exist in completing the evaluation. This process of discovery and decision making is assisted by a clear outline of questions regarding whether the prevention program was implemented correctly, maintained appropriately, and reached the population it was meant to impact.

The collection of data and information is dependent on a retrieval plan identifying evaluation questions, instruments to be used, process, and staff that will actually conduct the evaluation. Once evaluation data have been collected, they will need to be analyzed in relationship to a norm or standard to compare against. The report plan reflects the most effective way to present

Table 29–1 Evaluation Decision Questions

Prevention Program Decisions	*Products*
1. Identify the direction of all HIV prevention programs.	Preview key evaluation issues
2. Specify programmatic questions that are important to answer.	Outline evaluation questions
3. Establish how data and information will be collected.	Data retrieval plan
4. Specify how information will be analyzed.	Analysis and report plan
5. Decide how evaluation findings will be communicated.	Dissemination plan
6. Determine who will manage and conduct the evaluation work.	Management and work plan
7. Specify how the effectiveness of the evaluation will be assessed.	Evaluation assessment plan

Source: Data from R.O. Brinkerhoff, D.M. Brethower, T. Hluchyj, and J.R. Nowakowski, *Program Evaluation: A Practitioner's Guide for Trainers and Educators,* © 1983, Kluwer-Nijhoff Publishing.

the evaluation results to stakeholders, funders, and the community receiving services from the ASO. The evaluation report will need to be disseminated in a timely manner to keep people informed regarding the effectiveness of the prevention program. A management and work plan will need to identify timelines and the amount of money, time, and staff devoted to the evaluation plan. Finally, the evaluation plan will need to be assessed regarding the standards used and the ability of the process to identify effects that either have a positive impact or provide direction for program improvement.

There are a number of issues to address in the development of an evaluation plan that will assist in making decisions about an HIV prevention program. It is important for an ASO to provide a historical perspective as to previous prevention efforts, barriers to evaluation, and potential limitations to data collection. The evaluation decision provides the story regarding how objectives for the program were chosen, the process of implementing the program, and the efforts used to maintain the program.

HIV prevention programs are inherently intended to impact a "naturally" occurring behavior that places participants at risk for HIV transmission. There is a cause and effect for at-risk behavior. Prevention programs may focus on changing the cause, lessening the effect, or both the cause and effect. Programs may also attempt to limit the enduring nature of these risk behaviors. For the most part, program participants do not know how to live without the behaviors that place them at risk for HIV infection. Evaluation assists in the examination of these relationships and the ability of the program to explain any potential "new" cause and effect behaviors that have lessened risk.

Prevention components exist in a program and are influenced by external factors such as types and experience of facilitators, targeted populations, and methods of presentation. Therefore, components break apart and decay within the context of a program over time. This necessitates the assessment of adherence to protocol, quality assurance, and fidelity issues. Evaluation looks at these components and what they are intended to do to at-risk behaviors. Program evaluation also provides a way to understand how the components will assist in reaching expected outcomes. Program evaluation provides accountability to what was promised in measurable terms. Ultimately, evaluation provides information on the quality of an ASO's HIV prevention program by identifying how the program reached the at-risk targeted population, its appropriateness for that population, and what can be said about those people who are unaffected by the program.

IDU ISSUES: ASOs MANAGING PREVENTION STRATEGIES TARGETING IDU RISK BEHAVIORS

AIDS cases and new HIV infections that are attributable to injection drug use have increased steadily and include infections contracted as a result of unsafe injection practices among IDUs, HIV transmission from infected IDUs to their sexual partners, and vertical transmission from infected women to their children. Among all AIDS cases diagnosed in the United States, 25 percent have involved injection drug use as the sole exposure route and 6 percent have been among men who report both injection drug use and male same-sex behavior as risk factors.[25] However, cumulative AIDS diagnosis data obscure more recent trends, which indicate that a majority of infections now being contracted in the United States are due to either injection drug use or sexual contact with IDUs.[26] Injection risk practices and the sexual transmission of HIV from IDUs to other individuals is driving the HIV crisis in American inner cities.

Since early in the epidemic, a variety of HIV primary prevention approaches have been undertaken to decrease injection risk practices among IDUs. Many of these approaches have yielded positive findings and have produced reductions in needle sharing and needle reuse. Among the intervention approaches studied and found to have positive effects on injection risk practices are street outreach programs in which outreach workers provide AIDS educational and harm reduction materials to IDUs in community venues as well as disseminate behavior change endorsement messages,[27–33] enhanced access to drug treatment services,[34,35] the integration of individual or small-group HIV prevention services within drug treatment programs,[36–38] and policy or structural interventions to increase the availability of clean needles and decrease the need for IDUs to reuse injection apparatus.[39–44] More recently, there has been considerable interest in social network–level interventions for HIV primary prevention among IDUs. The injection risk practices of individual IDUs are strongly influenced by normative, cultural, and behavioral factors within their social networks, as well as by characteristics of the networks themselves.[45–48] Consequently, the possibility of interventions targeted toward natural IDU social networks is now receiving considerable attention.

In contrast to evidence of change in the injection risk practices following the types of interventions just described, there is less evidence of comparable change in sexual risk behavior patterns of IDUs. Donoghoe, in a review of the literature on sexual risk behaviors of IDUs, found that changes in syringe sharing behavior are greater than those in sexual risk behavior.[49] Weissman and Brown found that only 11 percent of IDU women in the National AIDS Demonstration Research (NADR) project sample reported consistent condom use in a six-month period, 13 percent engaged in anal intercourse, and only 2 percent used condoms during this activity.[32] Stephens et al. found greater reduction in the injection risk practices of IDUs in the NADR cohort than change in condom use.[30] A survey of IDUs receiving HIV counseling and testing found that only 25 percent used condoms.[50] This is consistent with other research findings indicating that only 34 percent of IDUs used condoms at last sex,[51] that more than 60 percent of IDUs reported no condom use in the past five years,[52] and that 68 percent of IDUs did not use a condom at all in the previous month.[53] A substantial number of IDU women engage in prostitution; others use crack and cocaine, resulting in multiple encounters with risky sexual partners.[27,37]

Interventions designed to promote both injection and sexual risk behavior change among IDUs living in the community are essential for a variety of reasons. IDUs who become HIV infected and who continue to engage in unprotected sexual activities are likely to transmit infection to their sexual partners and to their newborn children through vertical transmission. IDUs who are not HIV infected often interact sexually with other drug users and are at risk for contracting HIV during these sexual episodes. As Donoghoe emphasized, new HIV infections among vulnerable inner-city populations will be reduced when more attention is directed to the sexual risk behavior practices of IDUs.[49]

Randomized trials have examined the effectiveness of individual and small-group interventions to promote sexual risk behavior change. These have employed elements including risk education; exercises to strengthen condom use attitudes, intentions, commitment, and perceived self-efficacy; behavior rehearsal exercises to teach skills such as condom use, sexual negotiation, and sexual assertiveness; goal-setting and safer sex practice assignments; and reinforcement, problem solving, and the induction of normative perceptions to support behavior change efforts. With content and procedures tailored to the risk circumstances of specific populations, intensive interventions of these kinds have produced reductions in high-risk sexual practices and increases in safer sex practices among women, gay or bisexual men, adolescents, and other populations.[54–61]

Small-group and individual risk reductions focused on injection and sexual risk behavior change have also been undertaken with IDUs, often in drug treatment settings. Colon et al. examined the impact of a single-session risk reduction skills training intervention focused on safer injection and condom use among IDUs in Puerto Rico.[62] Relative to IDUs receiving standard services, there were no significant intervention effects at seven-month follow-up in either injection risk practices or risky sex. Somewhat more promising findings were reported by Greenberg et al. in a study evaluating the impact of a group intervention for HIV positive African American IDUs.[63] In this project, IDUs participated in two-hour group sessions that addressed risk education, emotional and social coping with HIV, and strategies for enacting behavior change. Although participants who attended at least four group sessions showed some reduction in drug use and sexual behavior risk practices, one-third of the IDUs reported two or more partners in the month preceding follow-up and rates of unprotected sex with primary partners remained high. The study did not include a control group, so attribution of change to the intervention cannot be made.

Sorensen et al. undertook randomized outcome studies of a six-hour small-group HIV risk reduction intervention conducted separately with samples of methadone maintenance outpatients and heroin detoxification program clients.[64] The intervention targeted risk knowledge, attitudes, and skills related to both injection and sexual risk practices, and was evaluated relative to an AIDS education comparison group. Although participants showed change in psychosocial risk-related attitudes and behavioral skills at follow-up, there was little evidence of change at follow-up in either unprotected sex or drug use behavior.

Schilling and his colleagues also carried out a randomized outcome trial evaluating the effects of a five-session cognitive–behavioral risk reduction intervention for 91 female methadone patients.[37] The intervention, focused on sexual behavior practices, relied on skills building in areas such as condom use, sexual negotiation, and problem solving. Compared to women in a control group, intervention group women had more frequent conversations with partners concerning condom use, greater condom carrying, and greater comfort talking about sex.[37] In a long-term interview follow-up of the same participants, women who had attended the intervention reported greater use of condoms than did control group members, although a decay of effects over time was observed.[36] Although some nonrandomized trials of small-group and individual HIV prevention interventions for IDUs have found evidence of behavior change among program participants,[38,65,66] other randomized outcome trials have found little or only modest effects on behavior.[67,68]

These studies illustrate both the strengths and the limitations of small-group risk reduction interventions. On one hand, intensive face-to-face social–cognitive interventions have proven effective in promoting sexual risk behavior reduction with some populations and in some trials. On the other hand, while often producing moderate to large short-term effect sizes for sexual risk behavior change, follow-up often reveals inconsistent effects on injection risk behavior and substantial decay in effects over time of sexual behavior change.[69] This would be expected, especially when IDUs "leave" an intervention and return to a social environment that affords little natural support for maintaining sexual risk reduction behavior changes.

A large body of past ethnographic research has established that social network characteristics influence the risk behavior of IDUs. Often using participant observation in neighborhood field settings, but also open-ended interview, life history interview, injection recall interview, and direct observation of injection events, this body of ethnographic research has established a variety of ways in which IDU social network characteristics function to increase or lessen HIV risk.[70–73] For example, attendance in shooting gallery settings has frequently been shown to predict elevated HIV risk behavior.[74–76] Trotter et al. identified four types of drug-using networks based on network composition and accessibility to new members: closed, kinship, long-standing friendship, and open.[48] Closed networks were associated with the greatest, and kinship networks with the next greatest, rates of drug use risk behavior. At the same time, high levels of network turnover can also create risk. Friedman et al. found that seropositivity among IDU women was highest in social networks with high membership turnover or transience.[45] Network size is also associated with certain types of risk behavior. Rates of needle sharing are higher in large IDU social networks where more members share needles and place social pressures on other network members to share needles with them.[44]

Whether based on ethnographic field observations, the use of standardized questionnaires, or network relationship analytic approaches that permit both qualitative and quantitative data analysis, there is now considerable evidence that norms, standards, and culture within IDU social networks—as well as network type, size, density, and turnover—influence levels of HIV risk of network members.[47] This raises the possibility of intervening within networks to induce changes in network norms, including both injection practice and sexual behavior practice norms.

As early as 1989, there were reports of programs that attempted to organize IDUs living in the community into groups that would, in part, carry out peer education HIV prevention outreach efforts to other IDUs.[77] Sufian et al. and Friedman and his colleagues also described innovative efforts to promote self-organization among IDUs, including encouraging IDUs to take on roles to change IDU subcultural norms concerning the sharing and reuse of needles.[78–81]

This research also shed light on how ideas or practices are diffused through IDU social systems from person to person. Trotter et al. found that there are many more drug networks than assumed by the drug users themselves, and that these networks only minimally overlap.[48] By using an ethnographic network approach to create an outreach system for contacting high-risk individuals, prevention messages can be transmitted through key individuals to network members. One outreach program in San Francisco used this diffusion model in a word-of-mouth educational program to promote the use of bleach to clean syringes.[82] The program grew to include the distribution of bleach by outreach workers, who facilitated dissemination and acceptance of the innovation. The NADR/AIDS Targeted Outreach Model (NADR/Atom) projects used leadership models to encourage naturally occurring group leaders to model and talk about needle risk reduction with their peers. Specific efforts were made to enroll influential persons within drug-using networks into the project and have them act to influence other injection drug users to practice safer injection.[83,84] Broadhead and colleagues described a "peer driven intervention" in which IDUs are trained and provided with financial incentives for undertaking outreach HIV prevention activities to peers and engaging them to enter prevention service programs.[85] The approach was found to be as effective as traditional professional outreach methods, but considerably less costly.

Other extensions of this work have focused on the influences—and the potential basis for intervention—of IDU social networks. Because perceptions of needle-sharing social norms influence drug injection patterns among IDUs, it is likely that changes in those social and peer reference group norms can also produce changes in the risk behavior patterns of network members.[53,80,86,87] Latkin et al. reported on a randomized intervention trial that suggests that this is the case.[46] In this study, a six-session social–cognitive intervention targeting drug use risk practices was delivered—not just to individual IDUs, but also to members of that IDU's close social network. Relative to controls who received standard HIV counseling and testing, the intervention delivered to index IDUs and their social network members produced reductions in needle sharing and less frequent heroin and cocaine injection at 18-month follow-up. Sexual behavior practice outcomes were not reported in this study.

More recently, and perhaps more importantly for ASOs, community identification process methods have been applied to the challenge of understanding IDU communities. Following the methodologies outlined by others, Somlai et al. directed a set of field activities to characterize IDU communities along dimensions relevant to needle-exchange operation.[7,88,89] These field activities, conducted during a one-year period, included extensive interviews with systems representatives familiar with IDU culture (such as drug house operators, drug treatment personnel, inner-city social services agency staff, IDU outreach workers, and law enforcement personnel); interviews with key participants (IDUs purposely selected from among different injector social networks); ethnographic field observations made in venues associated with drug injection (such as drug houses, parks and street locations in targeted neighborhoods) and in other venues frequented by IDUs (bars, service agencies, shelters, and similar settings); and the development of mechanisms to gain community input and recommendations concerning harm reduction programs. In addition to supervising these field activities, the findings of this major IDU community study were integrated into a "blueprint" for how a NEP could operate most successfully. This study had several findings that are particularly relevant to CBOs attempting to develop HIV prevention programs for IDUs.

In this study, community data collection revealed three primary injection areas: the near north side (a primarily African American area), the near south side (primarily neighborhoods in transition, with a large number of new Latin American residents), and an area to the immediate west side of downtown (primarily neighborhoods with prostitution and drug trafficking). Identified venues were marked on a map that gridded the community into three geographic locations. The gridding of the data indicated 40 fixed-site drug houses on the north side, 30 drug houses on the south side, and at least 10 mobile drug purchasing sites on the west side.[7]

Gender and race/ethnicity issues related to drug use and risk were also investigated. Gender was associated with the risk behavior patterns of IDUs; women in drug houses were at particular risk because they generally traded sex for drugs or money and were viewed by men as a commodity. Male IDUs clustered into racially defined groups within the metropolitan area. African American male IDUs were primarily found on the north side of the community; Latin American male IDUs were found on the south side. African American IDUs tended to cluster in subcultures based on age and life experience. A number of older African American IDUs, usually those greater than 35 years of age, reported that they began to inject drugs while in Vietnam. These Vietnam vets had a closed IDU network that had a "club" atmosphere.[7]

There were also age-differentiated subcultures among the IDUs. For example, older IDUs generally did not want younger IDUs in their neighborhood because they perceived the younger IDUs as prone to violence and as likely to "create troubles" and bring law enforcement into the area. Older IDUs reported that discretion, and not having attention drawn to them, was extremely important. Many of the older IDUs maintained regular employment or sources of income and felt vulnerable around younger IDUs. Older IDUs also indicated that although drug quality had improved, the level of violence and crime was now a serious concern.

IDUs often shared needles and syringes because of economics. A reliable means to ensure the correct dosage of a drug was by measuring it with a syringe. By accepting a shared syringe, the IDU was given the full amount of the drug that had been purchased. Because the vast majority of IDUs were unemployed or underemployed, the cost of drugs was very important, and the most exact way of guaranteeing a full dosage was through measurement provided by the "cc" markers on the side of the syringe.

There were neighborhood differences in the types of drugs used. In the north side, predominantly African American area, IDUs were likely to inject heroin. IDUs in the south side area were more likely to inject cocaine-based combinations. The west side neighborhood was a multidrug environment where purchases were made in a more open market atmosphere. Drugs used and drug houses were associated with gang activity and control; drug houses were the distribution points for the drugs controlled by individual gangs. Specific gangs exclusively controlled drug sales in different neighborhoods of the city. Territories were tightly held by gangs, and drug supplies were closely controlled. Drug houses were generally not stable environments; many operated for only a few months before moving.[7]

Public parks and areas of prostitution were identified through ethnographic observation as sites used by IDUs. Public parks were seasonally used by IDUs given cold winters in the Midwest. Public park IDUs were older, poorer, and at significantly greater risk for arrest, personal harm, and crime than those IDUs who did not inject in parks. The public park IDUs appeared desperate, with little support or entrée to other drug environments. Some participated in homosexual acts for money or drugs. Many of these IDUs reported that they lived in shelters day to day.[7]

Using community assessment findings to inform needle exchange-operation, the Lifepoint needle exchange was implemented in early 1994.[7] Lifepoint is a mobile van-based NEP that operates in the three identified Milwaukee neighborhoods with high numbers of IDUs, drug houses, and street venues of drug use. Lifepoint exchanges needles on a one-for-one basis, provides safer sex materials and counseling, offers mobile outreach HIV counseling and testing, and refers IDUs for drug treatment and other services. In 1996, a total of 3,514 IDUs used the Lifepoint NEP.[7]

STRUCTURAL AND ENVIRONMENTAL FACTORS ASSOCIATED WITH NEP PROGRAM IMPLEMENTATION

As stated earlier in this chapter, the Ottawa Charter was an initial attempt at enabling people to increase control over and improve their health.[1] Structural and environmental interventions view health as a resource and attempt to address societal responsibility in addressing public health policy issues. If health is a resource for everyday living, it compels ASOs to create structural support for equity in the community public policy health agenda. The ASO then becomes a catalyst for community action to develop shared health promotion goals for all at-risk populations.

There are structural and environmental factors that promote the incidence of HIV. Sweat and Denison indicated that although there is greater knowledge of the relationships between structural factors and HIV/AIDS risk, there are few interventions that operate at this level.[90] Health and social problems have multiple causes, including superstructural, structural, environmental, and individual levels. Sweat and Denison identified mechanisms that need to occur at the national, international, political, community, and individual levels to address the change needed to reduce HIV incidence.[90] For an ASO attempting to implement or continue a NEP, these factors and approaches to structural change provide a template of action and point to potential methodologies and mechanisms for shaping environmental prevention efforts.

Social control and punitive mechanisms used to control the self-regulation of individuals and their networks are especially important to the public health initiatives instituted by an ASO's NEP. Fischer and Poland highlighted the governance difficulties when public health risk issues take on a moral rhetoric that excludes and stigmatizes marginalized groups.[91] The discussion of public health and punitive approaches to risk behavior is particularly appropriate for ASOs attempting to provide services for IDUs who are quite often viewed in terms of deviance and as agents contributing to societal disorder. It is the responsibility of the ASO to find a middle ground between the need for society to implement methods of self-protection and an empathetic health policy that seeks to decrease the risk of HIV infection for IDUs. Bluthenthal and his colleagues provide a compelling investigation of the relationship between law enforcement and NEPs that have a direct impact on the level of risk for HIV infection among IDUs.[92–95] ASOs that want to provide effective strategies for HIV prevention among IDUs will need to develop clear approaches based on informed policies that assess the societal benefits of denying injection equipment (thereby criminalizing injecting behaviors) and the need to provide empathetic HIV prevention programs that reduce harm and the factors associated with risk of HIV infection.

STATE AND LOCAL HEALTH DEPARTMENTS

This chapter has characterized elements important to ASOs in the implementation and maintenance of initiatives to reduce HIV risk based on research-based models. Much of the discussion centered on ASOs as the primary providers of prevention services. Although the bulk of HIV prevention work exists in the "front lines" of ASO prevention service provision, there is a web of resources and support that must work in a collaborative manner for public health initiatives to be truly effective. Public health departments at both the state and local level are invaluable in their support and involvement to the HIV community planning process. Quite often, these public agencies provide the contracted funds to ASOs and in some situations serve as sites for HIV counseling and testing, as well as education. Without the diligence, hard work, effort, and support of these public health agencies and organizations, many ASOs would be hard pressed to provide the types of services they currently have in the field. Although the focus of this chapter has not been directly on the role of governmental public health agencies, it is important to acknowledge their important and valuable contributions in support of community-level initiatives. Given the political and moral implications of this epidemic, these efforts have oftentimes been valiant and courageous.

CHAPTER REVIEW

1. The nature and progression of the HIV/AIDS epidemic changes over time, challenging public health organizations to develop innovative HIV prevention programs to reach populations at greatest risk. Today, organizations are faced with moving beyond providing risk education programs alone, and must now address the more difficult challenge of implementing programs that help at-risk persons enact and maintain behavior changes that lower their risk to HIV infection and AIDS.
2. In implementing and maintaining HIV prevention programs, public health organizations must work within tight resource constraints, balance the multiple objectives of larger prevention and health promotion initiatives, and anticipate and counteract potential barriers to program implementation.
3. HIV prevention programs require substantial and ongoing strategic planning, supported by a carefully designed organizational structure, to succeed over time. Program planning and organization are critical elements for addressing the changing nature of the epidemic and the changing constellation of organizations involved in HIV prevention and control.
4. Key steps in strategic planning for HIV prevention programs include the following:
   - Determine the populations in need.
   - Establish the overall program mission and goals.
   - Identify efficacious and cost-effective primary and secondary prevention interventions.
   - Engage relevant communities and stakeholders in program planning and priority setting.
   - Develop an effective organizational structure to support the program.
   - Design approaches for program evaluation and improvement.
5. Public health organizations must manage and coordinate multiple prevention strategies targeting the individual, family, social network, and community levels.
6. Public health organizations require strong relationships with the HIV/AIDS research community to ensure that innovations in prevention and control are rapidly developed through community-based research, and are rapidly incorporated into practice once efficacious innovations are identified.

REFERENCES

1. S.J. Klein et al., "Role of Community-Based Organizations in Control of Sexually Transmitted Diseases," *Journal of the American Medical Association* 180 (1998): 419–420.
2. R. Cain, "Community-Based AIDS Services: Formalization and Depoliticization," *International Journal of Health Services* 23 (1993): 665–684.
3. R. Cain, "Environmental Change and Organizational Evolution: Reconsidering the Niche of Community-Based AIDS Organizations," *AIDS Care* 9 (1997): 331–344.
4. W. DiFranceisco et al., "Factors Influencing Attitudes within AIDS Service Organizations toward the Use of Research-Based HIV Prevention Interventions," *AIDS Education and Prevention* 11 (1999): 72–86.
5. J.A. Kelly et al., "Bridging the Gap between the Science and the Service of HIV Prevention: Outcomes of Approaches To Transfer Effective Research-Based HIV

Prevention Interventions to Community AIDS Service Providers," *American Journal of Public Health* 90 (2000): 1082–1088.

6. A.M. Somlai et al., "Current HIV Prevention Activities for Women and Gay Men among 77 ASOs," *Journal of Public Health Management and Practice* 5 (1999): 23–33.
7. A.M. Somlai et al., "'Lifepoint': A Case Study in Using Social Science Community Identification Data To Guide the Implementation of a Needle Exchange Program," *AIDS Education and Prevention* 11 (1999): 187–202.
8. National Institutes of Health, *Interventions To Prevent HIV Risk Behavior: Consensus Development Conference Statement, February 11–13, 1997* (Bethesda, MD: NIH Office of Medical Applications of Research, 1997).
9. CDC Advisory Committee on the Prevention of HIV Infection, *External Review of CDC's HIV Prevention Strategies* (Atlanta, GA: U.S. Centers for Disease Control and Prevention, 1994).
10. T.J. Coates et al., "AIDS Antibody Testing. Will It Stop the AIDS Epidemic? Will It Help People Infected with HIV? *American Psychologist* 43 (1988): 878–885.
11. J. McCusker et al., "Effects of HIV Antibody Test Knowledge on Subsequent Sexual Behaviors in a Cohort of Homosexually Active Men," *American Journal of Public Health* 78 (1988): 462–467.
12. D.L. Higgins et al., "Evidence for the Effects of HIV Antibody Counseling and Testing on Risk Behaviors," *Journal of the American Medical Association* 266 (1991): 2,419–2,429.
13. J.R. Ickovics et al., "Limited Effects of HIV Counseling and Testing for Women: A Prospective Study of Behavioral and Psychological Consequences," *Journal of the American Medical Association* 272 (1994): 443–448.
14. M.W. Otten et al., "Changes in Sexually Transmitted Disease Rates after HIV Testing and Posttest Counseling, Miami, 1988 to 1989," *American Journal of Public Health* 83 (1993): 529–533.
15. N.S. Wenger et al., "Reduction of High-Risk Sexual Behavior among Heterosexuals Undergoing HIV Antibody Testing; A Randomized Clinical Trial," *American Journal of Public Health* 81 (1991): 1,580–1,585.
16. R.O. Valdiserri et al., "Community Planning: A National Strategy To Improve HIV Prevention Programs," *Journal of Community Health* 20 (1995): 87–100.
17. R.O. Valdiserri et al., "Determining Allocations for HIV Prevention Interventions: Assessing a Change in Federal Funding," *AIDS and Public Policy Journal* 12 (1997): 138–148.
18. International Conference on Health Promotion, *Ottawa Charter for Health Promotion* (Ottawa, Ontario, Canada: World Health Organization, Health and Welfare Canada, Canadian Public Health Association, 1986).
19. E.H. Kaplan and R. Heimer, "A Circulation Theory of Needle Exchange," *AIDS* 8 (1994): 567–574.
20. K.E. Nelson et al., "Changes in Sexual Behavior and a Decline in HIV Infection among Young Men in Thailand," *New England Journal of Medicine* 335 (1996): 297–303.
21. W. Phoolcharoen, "HIV/AIDS Prevention in Thailand: Success and Challenges," *Science* 280 (1998): 1,873–1,874.
22. National Institutes of Health, *Interventions To Prevent HIV Risk Behaviors: Consensus Development Conference Statement, February 11–13* (Bethesda, MD: National Institutes of Health Office of Medical Applications of Research, 1997).
23. E. Sogolow et al., A Public Health Approach To Move HIV Prevention Research to Practice (Paper presented to the World AIDS Conference, Geneva, Switzerland, July 1998).
24. R.O. Brinkerhoff, *Program Evaluation: A Practitioner's Guide for Trainers and Educators* (Boston: Kluwer-Nijhoff Publishing, 1983).
25. *HIV/AIDS Surveillance Report 7,* no. 1 (1995): 1–4.
26. S.D. Holmberg, "The Estimated Prevalence and Incidence of HIV in 96 Large US Metropolitan Areas," *American Journal of Public Health 86*, no. 5 (1996): 642–654.
27. R. Booth et al., "Intravenous Drug Users and AIDS: Risk Behaviors," *American Journal of Drug and Alcohol Abuse* 17 (1991): 337–353.
28. A. Neaigus et al., "Peer Culture and Risk Reduction among Street IV Drug Users," *International Conference on AIDS 6,* no. 3 (1990): 226 (abstract no. S.C. 548).
29. L. Peppas et al., "Bleachman: A Superhero Teaches AIDS Prevention," *International Conference on AIDS* 5 (1989): 1,059 (abstract no. Th.E.O.6A).
30. R.C. Stephens et al., "Comparative Effectiveness of NADR Interventions," in *Handbook on Risk of AIDS: Injection Drug Users and Sexual Partners,* eds. B. Brown and G. Beschner (Westport, CT: Greenwood Press, 1993), 519–556.
31. P.I. Thompson et al., "Promotion of HIV Prevention Outreach Activities Targeting Intravenous Drug Users in the United States," *International Conference on AIDS* 5 (1989): 849 (abstract no. T.E.P.17).
32. G. Weissman and V. Brown, "Drug-Using Women and HIV: Risk-Reduction and Prevention Issues," in *Women at Risk: Issues in the Primary Prevention of AIDS,* eds. A. O'Leary and L.S. Jemmot (New York: Plenum Press, 1995), 175–193.
33. W.W. Wiebel, "Identifying and Gaining Access to Hidden Populations," in *The Collection and Interpretation of Data from Hidden Populations,* ed. E.Y. Lambert (NIDA Research Monograph, National Institute on Drug Abuse, Rockville, MD, 1990): 4–13.

34. D. Longshore et al., "Reducing HIV Risk Behavior among Injection Drug Users: Effect of Methadone Maintenance Treatment on Number of Sex Partners," *International Journal of the Addictions* 29 (1994): 741–757.
35. K.E. Watkins et al., "High-Risk Sexual Behaviors of Intravenous Drug Users In- and Out-of-Treatment: Implications for the Spread of HIV Infection," *American Journal of Drug and Alcohol Abuse* 18 (1992): 389–398.
36. N. El-Bassel and R.F. Schilling, "15-Month Followup of Women Methadone Patients Taught Skills To Reduce Heterosexual HIV Transmission," *Public Health Reports* 107 (1992): 500–504.
37. R.F. Schilling et al., "Building Skills of Recovering Women Drug Users To Reduce Heterosexual AIDS Transmission," *Public Health Reports* 106 (1991): 297–304.
38. L. Dengelegi et al., "Drug Users' AIDS-Related Knowledge, Attitudes, and Behaviors before and after AIDS Education Sessions," *Public Health Reports* 105 (1990): 504–505.
39. D.C. Des Jarlais, *Current Findings in Syringe Exchange Research* (London: UK Department of Health, 1994).
40. D.C. Des Jarlais and S.R. Friedman, "AIDS and Legal Access to Sterile Injection Equipment," *Annals of the American Academy of Political and Social Science* 521 (1992): 42–65.
41. J. Guydish et al., "Evaluating Needle Exchange: Are There Negative Effects?" *AIDS* 7 (1993): 871–876.
42. P. Lurie et al., *The Public Health Impact of Needle Exchange Programs in the United States and Abroad* (Atlanta, GA: Centers for Disease Control and Prevention, 1993).
43. J. Normand et al., "Preventing HIV Transmission: The Role of Sterile Needles and Bleach," *Proceedings of the Commission on Behavioral and Social Sciences and Education* (Washington, DC: National Academy Press, 1995).
44. D. Paone et al., "Syringe Exchange: HIV Prevention, Key Findings, and Future Directions," *International Journal of the Addictions* 30 (1995): 1,647–1,683.
45. S.R. Friedman et al., eds., *AIDS and the Heterosexual Population* (Chur, Switzerland: Harwood Academic Publishers, 1993).
46. C.A. Latkin et al., "The Long-Term Outcome of a Personal Network-Oriented HIV Prevention Intervention for Injection Drug Users: The Safe Study," *American Journal of Community Psychology* 24 (1996): 341–346.
47. C.G. Leukefeld et al., "Community Prevention Efforts To Reduce the Spread of AIDS Associated with Intravenous Drug Abuse," *AIDS Education and Prevention* 2 (1990): 235–243.
48. R.T. Trotter et al., "Network Models for HIV Outreach and Prevention Programs for Drug Users," *NIDA Research Monograph* 151 (1995): 144–180.
49. M.C. Donoghoe, "Sex, HIV and the Injecting Drug User," *British Journal of Addiction* 87 (1992): 405–416.
50. H. Helal et al., "HIV Prevalence and Risk Behavior among Intravenous Drug Users Attending HIV Counseling and Testing Centers in Paris," *Addiction* 90 (1995): 1,627–1,663.
51. K.E. Watkins et al., "Determinants of Condom Use among Intravenous Drug Users," *AIDS* 7 (1993): 719–723.
52. A.J. Saxon et al., "Sexual Behaviors of Intravenous Drug Users in Treatment," *Journal of Acquired Immune Deficiency Syndromes* 4 (1991): 938–944.
53. S. Magura et al., "Variables Influencing Condom Use among Intravenous Drug Users," *American Journal of Public Health* 80 (1990): 82–84.
54. J.A. Kelly et al., "Behavioral Intervention To Reduce AIDS Risk Activities," *Journal of Consulting and Clinical Psychology* 57 (1989): 60–67.
55. R.O. Valdiserri et al., "AIDS Prevention in Homosexual and Bisexual Men: Results of a Randomized Trial Evaluating Two Risk Reduction Interventions," *AIDS* 3 (1989): 21–26.
56. R.J. DiClemente and G.M. Wingood, "A Randomized Controlled Trial of an HIV Sexual Risk Reduction Intervention for Young African American Women," *Journal of the American Medical Association* 274 (1995): 1,271–1,276.
57. S.E. Hobfoll et al., "Reducing Inner-City Women's AIDS Risk Activities: A Study of Single Pregnant Women," *Health Psychology* 13 (1994): 397–403.
58. J.A. Kelly et al., "The Effects of HIV/AIDS Intervention Groups for High-Risk Women in Urban Clinics," *American Journal of Public Health* 84 (1994): 1,918–1,922.
59. J.B. Jemmott et al., "Reductions in HIV Risk-Associated Sexual Behaviors among Black Male Adolescents: Effects of an AIDS Prevention Intervention," *American Journal of Public Health* 82 (1992): 372–377.
60. M.J. Rotheram-Borus et al., "Reducing HIV Sexual Risk Behaviors among Runaway Adolescents," *Journal of the American Medical Association* 266 (1991): 1,237–1,241.
61. J.S. St. Lawrence et al., "Cognitive-Behavioral Intervention To Reduce African American Adolescents' Risk for HIV Infection," *Journal of Consulting and Clinical Psychology* 63 (1995): 221–237.
62. H.M. Colon et al., "Effects of an HIV Risk Reduction Education Program among Injection Drug Users in Puerto Rico," *Puerto Rico Health Sciences Journal* 12 (1993): 27–34.
63. J.B. Greenberg et al., "A Community Support Group for HIV-Seropositive Drug Users: Is Attendance Associated with Reductions in Risk Behavior? *AIDS Care* 8 (1996): 529–540.

64. J.L. Sorensen et al., "Psychoeducational Group Approach: HIV Risk Reduction in Drug Users," *AIDS Education and Prevention* 6 (1994): 95–112.
65. S.A. Corrigan et al., "A Psychoeducational Approach To Prevent HIV Transmission among Injection Drug Users," *Psychology of Addictive Behavior* 6 (1992): 114–119.
66. S. Magura et al., "Outcomes of an AIDS Prevention Program for Methadone Patients," *International Journal of the Addictions* 26 (1991): 629–655.
67. D.A. Calsyn et al., "Ineffectiveness of AIDS Education and HIV Antibody Testing in Reducing High-Risk Behaviors among Injection Drug Users," *American Journal of Public Health* 82 (1992): 573–575.
68. J. McCusker et al., "Behavioral Outcomes of AIDS Educational Interventions for Drug Users in Treatment," *International Conference on AIDS* 7, no. 2 (1991): 70 (abstract no. TH.D. 60).
69. S.C. Kalichman et al., "Sensation Seeking as an Explanation for the Association between Substance Use and HIV-Related Risky Sexual Behavior," *Archives of Sexual Behavior* 25 (1996): 141–154.
70. P. Adler, "Ethnographic Research in Hidden Populations: Penetrating the Drug World," in *The Collection and Interpretation of Data from Hidden Populations,* ed. E.Y Lambert (Rockville, MD: NIDA Research Monograph 98, 1990), 96–112.
71. S.K. Koester, "The Context of Risk: Ethnographic Contributions to the Study of Drug Use and HIV Risk," in *The Context of HIV Risk among Drug Users and Their Sexual Partners,* eds. R.J. Batties et al. (Rockville, MD: NIDA Research Monograph 143, 1994), 202–217.
72. S.K. Koester, "Applying the Methodology of Participant Observation to the Study of Injection-Related HIV Risks," in *Qualitative Methods in Drug Abuse and HIV Research,* eds. E.Y. Lambert et al. (Rockville, MD: NIDA Research Monograph 157, 1995), 84–99.
73. W.W. Wiebel, "Identifying and Gaining Access to Hidden Populations," in *The Collection and Interpretation of Data from Hidden Populations,* ed. E.Y. Lambert (Rockville, MD: NIDA Research Monograph 98, 1990), 4–13.
74. E.E. Schoenbaum et al., "Risk Factors for Human Immunodeficiency Virus Infection in Intravenous Drug Users," *New England Journal of Medicine* 321 (1989): 874–879.
75. B.J. Page et al., "Shooting Galleries, Their Proprietors and Implications for Prevention of AIDS," *Drugs and Society* 5 (1990): 69–85.
76. D. Vlahov et al., "Association of Drug Injection Patterns with Antibody to Human Immunodeficiency Virus Type 1 among Intravenous Drug Users in Baltimore, Maryland," *American Journal of Epidemiology* 132 (1990): 847–855.
77. G. Carlson and R. Needle, *Sponsoring Addicts of Self-Organization (Addicts Against AIDS): A Case Study,* First Annual NADR National Meeting (Rockville, MD: National AIDS Demonstration Research Project, 1989).
78. M. Sufian et al., "Organizing as a New Approach to AIDS Risk Reduction for Intravenous Drug Users," *Journal of Addictive Diseases* 10 (1991): 89–98.
79. S.R. Friedman and C. Casriel, "Drug Users' Organizations and AIDS Policy," *AIDS and Public Policy* 3 (1988): 30–36.
80. S.R. Friedman et al., "AIDS and Self-Organization among Intravenous Drug Users," *International Journal of the Addictions* 23 (1987): 210–219.
81. S.R. Friedman et al., "AIDS and the Social Relations of Intravenous Drug Users," *Milbank Quarterly* 68 (1990): 85–110.
82. Institute of Medicine, National Academy of Sciences, *Assessing the Social and Behavioral Science Base for HIV/AIDS Prevention and Intervention: Workshop Summary* (Washington, DC: National Academy Press, 1995).
83. W.W. Wiebel et al., "Risk Behavior and HIV Seroincidence among Out-of-Treatment Injection Drug Users: A Four-Year Prospective Study," *Journal of Acquired Immune Deficiency Syndromes and Human Retrovirology* 12 (1996): 282–289.
84. W.W. Wiebel et al., "Prevention of New HIV Infections among Out-of-Treatment Injection Drug Users: A Four Year Prospective Study" Unpublished manuscript (1994).
85. R.S. Broadhead et al., "Drug Users vs. Outreach Workers in Combating AIDS: The Results of Peer-Driven Intervention," *International Conference on AIDS 11,* no. 2 (1996): 153.
86. D.C. Des Jarlais et al., "Risk Reductions for AIDS among Intravenous Drug Users," *Annual Review of Internal Medicine* 103 (1985): 755–759.
87. C.A. Latkin et al., "Using Social Network Analysis To Study Patterns of Drug Use among Urban Drug Users at High Risk for HIV/AIDS," *Drug and Alcohol Dependency* 38 (1995): 109.
88. D. MacKellar et al., "The Young Men's Survey: Methods for Estimating HIV Seroprevalence and Risk Factors among Young Men Who Have Sex with Men," *Public Health Reports* 111 (1996): 138–144.
89. C. Sterk and A. Long, "Formative Research as a Foundation for Intervention Development: The Community Assessment Process," unpublished manuscript (1996).
90. M.D. Sweat and J.A. Denison, "Reducing HIV Incidence in Developing Countries with Structural and Environmental Interventions," *AIDS* 9 (1995): 251–257.

91. B. Fischer and B. Poland, "Exclusion, 'Risk,' and Social Control—Reflections on Community Policing and Public Health," *Geoforum* 29 (1998): 187–197.

92. R.N. Bluthenthal et al., "Impact of Law Enforcement on Syringe Exchange Programs: A Look at Oakland and San Francisco," *Medical Anthropology* 18 (1997): 61–83.

93. R.N. Bluthenthal, "Syringe Exchange as a Social Movement: A Case Study of Harm Reduction in Oakland, California," *Substance Use and Misuse* 33 (1998): 1,147–1,171.

94. R.N. Bluthenthal et al., "Use of an Illegal Syringe Exchange and Injection-Related Risk Behaviors among Street-Recruited Injection Drug Users in Oakland, California, 1992 to 1995," *Journal of Acquired Immune Deficiency Syndromes and Human Retrovirology* 18 (1998): 505–511.

95. R.N. Bluthenthal et al., "Collateral Damage in the War on Drugs: HIV Risk Behaviors among Injection Drug Users," *International Journal of Drug Policy* 10 (1999): 25–38.

CHAPTER 30

Managed Care, Public Health, and the Uninsured

William L. Roper
Glen P. Mays

Changes in the nation's public and private health insurance systems create imperatives for public health organizations to redesign their approaches for ensuring populationwide access to health services. Managed care plans and organized health care providers have become important contributors to public health activities in many communities; nonetheless, managed care growth may complicate certain public health functions such as health care for the uninsured. Public health organizations employ a variety of strategies for working effectively with the managed care industry while also expanding access to care for vulnerable and underserved populations.

The growth of managed health care has sparked much speculation and debate about how these evolving systems of care affect the practice of public health in America. Some observers argue that the financial incentives and administrative mechanisms used by managed care plans create opportunities for integrating historically separate approaches to medical care delivery and public health practice. Managed care plans may respond to growing market imperatives for health care quality, efficiency, and consumer satisfaction by integrating traditional public health practices such as health education, clinical preventive services delivery, and epidemiologic investigation into their scope of activity. Market forces may also encourage collaboration between public health agencies and managed care plans for mutually beneficial activities such as community health status surveillance, population-based health education and training, and service delivery to vulnerable and underserved populations.[1–6] Other observers caution that managed care plans may weaken the public health infrastructure by siphoning off patients and revenues that traditionally have supported public health agencies and related safety-net providers.[7] Public health and population-based activities may fail to be incorporated in the clinical and administrative processes of managed care plans because they are not cost-effective over relatively short time horizons nor within enrollee populations that are constantly changing.[8] Similarly, some observers note that the growth of managed health care obliges public health organizations to carry out new responsibilities in monitoring the accessibility and quality of care that is provided by plans, and in ensuring consumer protection within this expanding industry.[9]

This chapter examines the evolving interface between managed health care and public health administration, with a particular focus on implications for the uninsured and other underserved populations. A key conclusion to be drawn is that interaction between public health practice and medical practice is occurring under managed care, although as yet these linkages remain relatively limited in scope and scale, and they fall far short of the integrated community health systems envisioned by some proponents.[10]

Emerging market and policy shifts pose challenges and opportunities for the practice of public health within health care environments that are increasingly shaped by managed care.[1,6] These developments suggest that population-based approaches to health improvement will continue to be adopted and used by managed care plans, but that meaningful collaboration between public health organizations and managed care plans will require new administrative strategies in the public and private sectors.

BACKGROUND

Public Health and Its Relationship to Medical Practice

The evolving relationships between managed care and public health are largely derivative of historical and contemporary trends in the practice of medicine and public health. Traditionally, these two fields of practice are distinguished by the medical care system's focus on individual patients and the public health system's emphasis on the health of populations. The New York Academy of Medicine observed in a 1997 study of medicine and public health that: "[t]he medical perspective focuses on the *individual* patient (diagnosing symptoms, treating and preventing diseases, providing comfort, relieving pain and suffering, and enhancing capacity to function)."[11] In contrast, the field of public health focuses on populations through activities such as assessing aggregate health needs and threats, developing public policies and plans to address these needs, and ensuring that populations have access to needed health services.

Public health organizations often assume primary responsibility for performing health promotion and primary prevention activities that provide protection against specific diseases (such as immunizations) and enhance overall levels of health and well-being (such as interventions involving nutrition, smoking cessation, or physical activity).[12,13] Professionals in public health and medical care typically share roles in secondary prevention activities designed to detect disease early and forestall subsequent effects on health. Common examples include cancer screening and early detection programs that are maintained both by public health agencies and by private physician practices. Tertiary prevention activities—those services aimed at limiting the effects of disease and disability, and at rehabilitation from disability—remain largely the domain of the medical profession.

The health care financing arena represents an important area of interaction between public health practice and medical practice. The most recent national estimates suggest that less than five percent of the nation's health care expenditures are devoted to population-based public health services, with the vast majority of the remaining funds devoted to medical care.[14,15] Nevertheless, some public health services are effective in reducing and preventing future medical care expenditures. For example, each dollar spent on childhood immunization services has been estimated to save more than $14 in future medical costs.[16] Other traditional public health interventions that have been found to produce a direct medical care cost offset include prenatal care services, family planning services, and sexually transmitted disease control services.[13] These examples underscore important clinical and economic relationships between public health and medical care services. Public policy decisions regarding how best to allocate scarce financial and human resources in order to improve population health clearly fall within the domain of public health.

In many cases, a public health organization's scope of practice also includes responsibilities for ensuring the availability and quality of medical care. For example, federal and state public health agencies perform inspection and licensing functions for health care facilities in order to ensure the safety and quality of care provided through institutions such as hospitals and nursing facilities. Federal and state agencies also engage in efforts to monitor the quality of health care provided to beneficiaries of governmental health insurance programs such as Medicare, Medicaid, and the State Child Health Insurance Program (S-CHIP). At the local level, some public health agencies directly provide certain medical care services to populations that cannot access these services from mainstream medical providers. In these ways, public health organizations become substantively involved in medical care issues by exercising their policy and regulatory authority and by ensuring that vulnerable populations have access to needed health services.

The numerous areas of overlap between medical practice and public health practice form the landscape in which managed care organizations and public health organizations interact. Interaction occurs in many different settings and for a variety of purposes, including

- implementing health promotion and disease prevention interventions for populations that are at risk
- delivering medical care services for vulnerable and underserved populations
- collecting and analyzing population-based health data to identify community health needs and risks and to evaluate the effectiveness of medical and public health interventions
- implementing disease surveillance and control activities to reduce the spread of disease
- ensuring the accessibility and quality of health services that are made available to populations

Both managed care plans and public health agencies exercise considerable influence over these types of activities, creating mutual dependencies between the two types of organizations. Managed care plans and public health agencies may interact explicitly or implicitly in these areas, and their exchange may be planned or ad hoc. By understanding the market and policy processes that shape this interaction, administrators in both fields of practice can better position their organizations to benefit from the exchange.

Managed Care and Public Health System Change in the United States

As a system for health care delivery and payment, managed health care has existed in the United States for nearly seven decades.[17] Throughout this period, managed care plans have operated as alternatives to the dominant approach for medical care delivery characterized by episodic, illness-driven service delivery coupled with fee-for-service payment and indemnity insurance. Since their emergence in the 1930s, the organizational forms of managed care have evolved from nonprofit, prepaid group practices to for-profit health maintenance organizations (HMOs) to an expanding array of open-ended health plans including preferred provider organizations (PPOs) and point-of-service (POS) networks. A catch-all definition for the variety of managed care plans operating today is difficult to identify, but generally these plans all function as organized systems of care that compete to assume both financial and clinical responsibility for the health of defined populations. Managed care plans use three basic types of strategies to achieve this objective (Figure 30–1).

1. *selective contracting:* Plans purposefully select the health care providers to include in their networks based on criteria such as efficiency in service delivery, service quality and patient satisfaction, service capacity, and geographic coverage (accessibility).
2. *utilization management:* Plans use both administrative and financial mechanisms to encourage efficient and effective service delivery and utilization. For example, plans often compensate health care providers using capitated payments (fixed monthly payments per member) to create financial incentives for efficient service delivery. Other common utilization management mechanisms include requirements that inpatient and specialty care be preauthorized by plan managers, and incentives for providers to follow clinical practice guidelines in delivering care (e.g., payment bonuses and withholds).
3. *competitive enrollment:* Plans compete with each other to attract purchasers and members, often on the basis of price, physician choice, covered services, and perceived quality. Plans also induce health

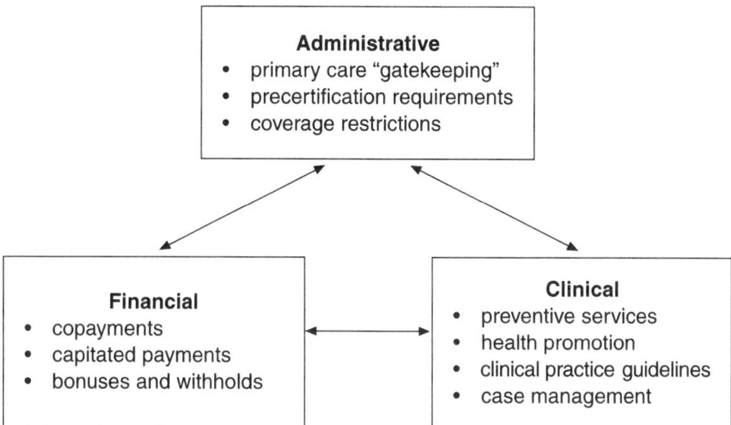

Figure 30–1 Utilization Management Strategies in Managed Care

care providers to compete with each other to obtain contracts for serving managed care members. Ideally, this competition lowers the cost of health insurance for purchasers—through the premiums that employers and governmental agencies pay to plans on behalf of their beneficiaries. At the same time, this competition potentially lowers the cost of insurance for health care consumers who must pay any premiums and copayments that are not covered by purchasers. The competition created by managed care growth may therefore increase access to health insurance coverage by making such coverage more affordable to employers, governmental insurance programs (e.g., Medicaid), and health care consumers. Managed care competition also has the potential to increase overall levels of health care quality if consumers and purchasers are able to select plans in part based on the quality of care that plans offer. In reality, many local health insurance markets are not perfectly competitive, such that consumers and purchasers have a relatively small number of plans from which to choose. Additionally, reliable information concerning health plan quality is often not readily available nor useful to health care consumers and purchasers in choosing among competing plans. Consequently, the public benefits of managed care competition may not be fully realized in practice.

Managed Care and Employer-Based Health Insurance

Managed care enrollment has grown rapidly in recent years, with more than 150 million Americans now enrolled in some form of managed care plan.[18,19] For privately insured individuals, the rapid growth in managed care enrollment dates back to the 1980s, when employers began to seek relief from rapidly escalating health care costs by purchasing employee health care coverage from these plans.[19] The rise in managed care enrollment during this period corresponded with a steady decline in the growth rate of employer health insurance costs. The double-digit annual growth rates in costs that were experienced during the 1980s were reduced to growth rates of less than three percent during the mid-1990s.[20] More recently, health insurance costs have begun to rise again as health care consumers have begun to demand health plans that can offer greater choice among providers and more immediate access to specialty services. It remains to be seen whether managed care can effectively balance consumer demands for choice and quality with purchaser demands for cost containment.

Over most of the past two decades, managed care enrollment growth has been fastest among HMOs, often regarded as the most restrictive or tightly managed form of health plan.[20] Individuals enrolled in HMOs typically do not receive any insurance coverage for services they obtain from providers outside of the HMO network. HMOs receive capitated monthly payments for each member and in return cover the full cost of all medically necessary health services needed by members. Each member of an HMO is assigned to a primary care physician or group of physicians who serve as case managers and gatekeepers for all care that the member requires. HMOs may directly employ physicians (staff model), contract on an exclusive basis with multispecialty physician groups (group model), or contract on a nonexclusive basis with a number of groups and independent physician practices (network and independent practice association [IPA] models).

A less-restrictive alternative to the HMO, the PPO, consists of a network of health care providers who agree to serve health plan members on a discounted fee-for-service basis. PPO members incur lower deductibles and copayments when they obtain care from providers in the network, but they can also access providers outside the network by paying higher fees. Both HMOs and PPOs use utilization management mechanisms such as preauthorization requirements and primary care gatekeeper models to encourage efficiency in health care delivery.

A third type of managed care plan, the POS plan, is a hybrid of the HMO and PPO models. POS members can access services from within their HMO network without incurring substantial out-of-pocket expenses, but they can also seek care from out-of-network providers by paying established deductible and copayment fees. Enrollment in all three forms of managed care continues to grow substantially, but the most rapid rates of growth since the mid-1990s have occurred among PPO and POS plans.[18–20]

The various organizational models of managed care can be distinguished by the extent to which health plans' health care providers are integrated within a common institutional and financial structure, and by the degree to which plans can influence clinical practice (Figure 30–2). The staff model HMO, in which providers are employees of the plan, creates a relatively high degree of integration and influence. By comparison, under the PPO model providers op-

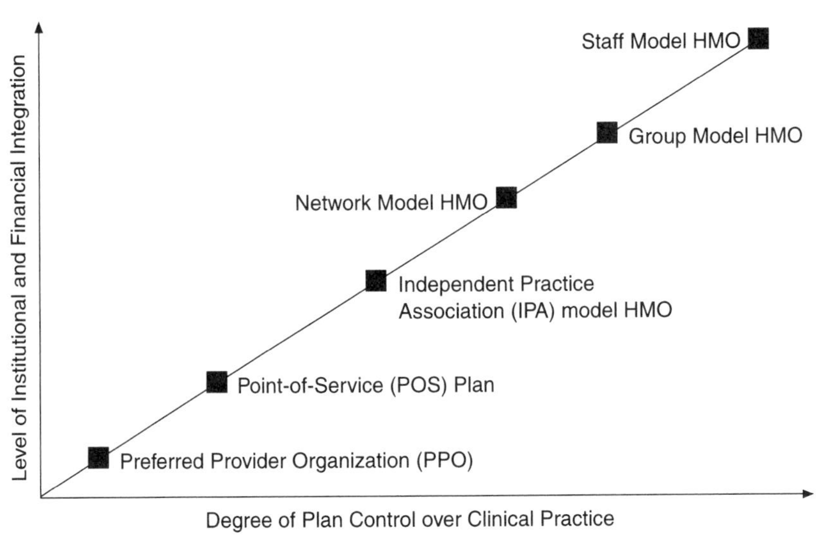

Figure 30–2 Types of Managed Care Plans

erate relatively independently of the health plans with which they contract.

Enrollment in managed care plans grew rapidly during the 1990s (Figure 30–3), and this growth has introduced new competitive dynamics to the nation's health care industry. Competitive managed care markets create pressures for health plans to develop and adopt innovations in health care processes and technology that will allow them to demonstrate enhanced efficiency and effectiveness to their consumers and purchasers. The current heterogeneity within the nation's managed care industry reflects this trend—health plans are adopting a wide range of clinical and managerial innovations in their efforts to earn market share by offering value to purchasers and consumers.[21,22] The recent public and media backlash against the managed care industry that erupted in 1997 and 1998 has created additional pressures for health plans to respond to consumer and purchaser demands for greater choice and greater value in managed care plans.[23] Examples include

- the growing number of health plans offering POS options, which expand consumer choice by allowing enrollees to seek care from providers who are outside of the plan's network.[18]
- the growing number of plans offering direct access to specialists, in response to consumer demand.[18]
- the growing involvement of health plans in medical outcomes research, using targeted studies of health care processes to develop evidence-based guidelines that ensure quality of care. (Increasingly, these efforts are being conducted through partnerships among health plans, and between plans and leading scientists at major universities and federal agencies such as the U.S. Centers for Disease Control and Prevention [CDC].)[6]
- the increased use of clinical practice guidelines and other mechanisms for educating health care providers about proven strategies for enhancing quality of care, and for informing them of innovations in technology and practice.[18]
- the increased use of financial incentives to encourage efficient and effective clinical practices among providers. (These incentives include capitated payments to provid-

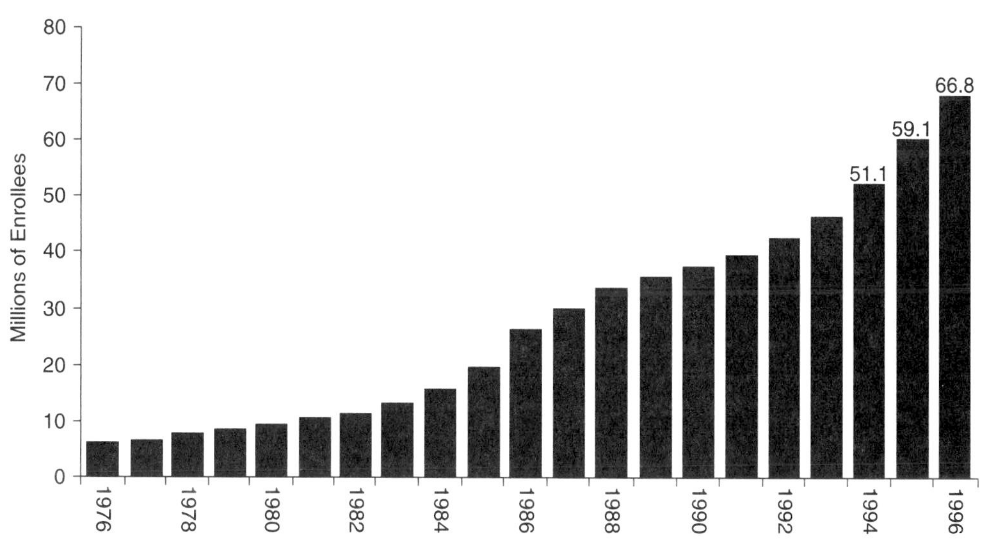

Figure 30–3 Growth in HMO Enrollment. *Source:* Data from 1997, American Association of Health Plans; and 1997, Interstudy.

ers and payment incentives that are linked to elements of clinical performance such as rates of hospitalization, childhood immunization, or patient satisfaction.) For example, a 1994 study conducted for the Physician Payment Review Commission found that 55 percent of network- and IPA-model HMOs adjust their physician payments based on the results of patient satisfaction surveys.[24]

- continued improvements in the clinical information systems used by health plans to provide feedback to providers regarding the quality and efficiency of their health care delivery practices. These systems create powerful mechanisms through which clinicians can continually improve on their methods of practice.

Medicare Managed Care

Following the experience of employers, many government-operated health insurance programs now rely heavily on managed care plans for serving their beneficiaries efficiently with limited public funds. Managed care enrollment among Medicaid recipients and Medicare beneficiaries dates back to the mid-1980s in some areas, but enrollment since 1990 accounts for most of the managed care growth within these government programs (Figure 30–4).[18] The federal Medicare program allows beneficiaries to opt out of the traditional fee-for-service program and voluntarily enroll in a Medicare-approved HMO, provided that the beneficiary resides in an area that is served by one or more Medicare-approved HMOs. In comparison to the fee-for-service program, Medicare HMOs typically offer a broader range of benefits (such as coverage for prescription drugs and some preventive services) and lower beneficiary cost-sharing provisions. Approximately 18 percent of the nation's 38 million Medicare beneficiaries are now enrolled in managed care plans.[25] Provisions passed as part of the federal Balanced Budget Act of 1997 are intended to expand Medicare managed care enrollment further by allowing other forms of managed care plans to participate in Medicare, including PPOs and plans sponsored by Medicare providers such as hospitals and medical groups.[26] However, efforts to expand enrollment may be complicated by the recent decisions by some HMOs to discontinue their participation in Medicare or to reduce their service areas in response to recent Medicare payment changes.

Medicaid Managed Care

Regulations established in the original federal Medicaid legislation have long enabled Medicaid beneficiaries to enroll voluntarily in managed care plans.[27] Problems with an early voluntary enrollment program in California during the early 1970s motivated several additional federal and state regulations regarding voluntary Medicaid managed care programs. These regulations restricted voluntary enrollment primarily to federally qualified HMOs that meet stringent requirements for submitting financial audits and reports, maintaining specified levels of financial reserves, and serving sufficient numbers of privately insured enrollees.[28] During the 1980s, a few states created incentives for Medicaid beneficiaries to enroll voluntarily in these plans, or for plans to aggressively seek Medicaid enrollment. Studies of voluntary enrollment programs operating during the 1980s largely indicated that these programs failed to produce significant cost savings, often because individuals with the highest levels of service utilization chose not to enroll in managed care plans.[29–31] As a result, many states have moved to secure the legal authority necessary to mandate managed care enrollment—at least for some groups of Medicaid beneficiaries. Many states have continued to operate voluntary enrollment programs for certain groups of Medicaid beneficiaries, such as the disabled and elderly populations that traditionally have not been served through managed care plans.

To implement mandatory managed care programs, state governments historically have had to obtain one of two types of waivers from federal Medicaid regulations.[27] One type of waiver, authorized by Section 1915(b) of the Social Security Act as amended in 1981, allows the federal government to suspend the freedom-of-choice provisions of the Medicaid program in

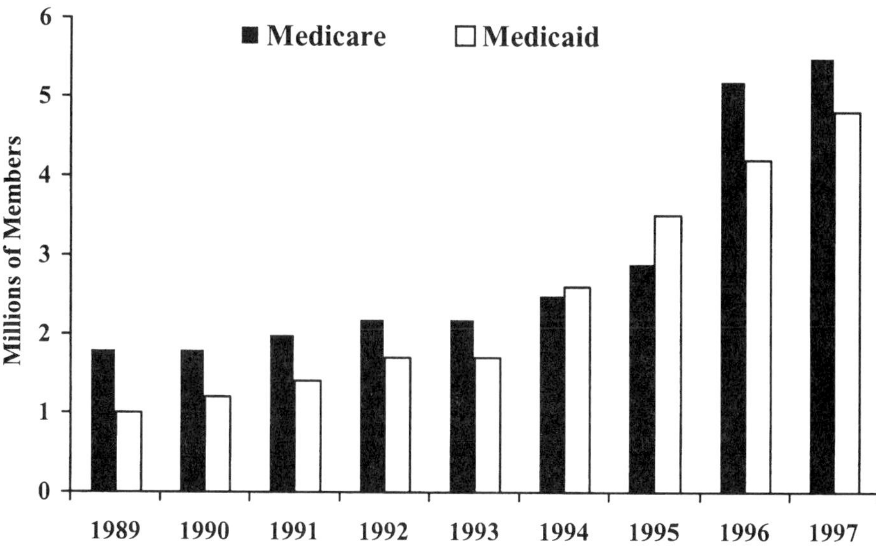

Figure 30–4 HMO Enrollment among Medicare Beneficiaries and Medicaid Recipients. *Source:* Data from 1996–1997, Interstudy Competitive Edge.

order to enable states to mandate enrollment in managed care plans for certain groups of Medicaid beneficiaries. States that secure a §1915(b) waiver for their Medicaid managed care programs must abide by all other federal Medicaid regulations, such as eligibility requirements, mandated benefits, and provider qualification standards.[32]

The second type of Medicaid waiver, authorized by Section 1115 of the Social Security Act, allows the federal government to suspend numerous provisions of federal Medicaid law, including eligibility standards, benefit levels, provider qualification standards, and administrative requirements.[27] States that have secured §1115 waivers use this authority for purposes such as expanding Medicaid eligibility to uninsured populations, limiting Medicaid coverage for certain medical services, and enabling organizations that are not licensed health insurance corporations, such as provider-sponsored organizations, to operate as full-risk or partial-risk health plans under capitated payment systems.[32,33]

As of mid-1998, 17 states operated Medicaid managed care programs under §1115 waivers granted by the U.S. Department of Health and Human Services.[34] Eight of these states implemented their mandatory-enrollment managed care programs on a statewide basis, with the remaining states requiring managed care enrollment only in certain geographic regions within the state.[32] Another 32 states launched programs through §1915(b) waivers. Most of these states established mandatory enrollment policies only for specified geographic regions within their states. These regions were often defined to include only urbanized areas that have existing managed care plans operating within them. Only the state of Alaska has yet to experiment with Medicaid managed care through one of the federal waiver programs.

The Balanced Budget Act of 1997, which took effect in October of 1997, now allows states to implement certain types of Medicaid managed care programs without obtaining federal waivers.[35] These types of programs include mandatory-enrollment case management programs and mandatory-enrollment capitated programs that offer a choice among at least two competing managed care plans. Provisions of this act also give states more flexibility in the types of managed care plans with which they may contract without a federal waiver. Managed care plans participating in Medicaid programs are no longer required to maintain at least 25 percent of their membership from privately insured enrollees. Similarly, provider-sponsored organizations and county-owned health-insuring organizations that are not licensed as HMOs can participate in state Medicaid managed care programs without a federal waiver. Finally, provisions in the Balanced Budget Act of 1997 allow states to implement certain Medicaid managed care benefit features without a federal waiver.[35] For example, states may provide up to six months of guaranteed Medicaid eligibility for Medicaid recipients who enroll in managed care plans—a benefit that historically could be provided only through a federal waiver.

Beneficiary Groups. Most state Medicaid managed care programs originally required managed care enrollment only for specified subgroups of Medicaid beneficiaries.[27,31] Most commonly, these groups included low-income pregnant women and families who participated in the federal Aid to Families with Dependent Children (AFDC) Program (now the Temporary Assistance for Needy Families [TANF] Program). States used these beneficiaries for testing their mandatory managed care programs because they typically have fewer complex medical and social needs than other beneficiaries and they appear most similar to the privately insured individuals who most managed care plans have experience serving. Medicaid eligibility expansions that occurred during 1990–92 created other eligibility categories that are often included in mandatory managed care programs. These categorically eligible recipients include uninsured children and pregnant women who do not meet the income-based eligibility requirements for participation in the AFDC Program.

More recently, many states have begun to encourage the enrollment of other types of Medicaid beneficiaries in managed care plans. As of year-end 1996, 21 states and the District of Columbia operated either mandatory or voluntary enrollment programs for disabled individuals who are eligible for Medicaid through the Supplemental Security Income Program or similar state programs.[32] Several other states have begun to encourage managed care enrollment among elderly beneficiaries of the Supplemental Security Income Program. Most of these states expanded the types of Medicaid beneficiaries to be enrolled in managed care plans only after several years of successful program operation among low-income families, pregnant women, and children. A few states, however, immediately initiated mandatory managed care enrollment for all of their Medicaid beneficiaries—including Arizona in 1982 and Tennessee in 1994. Nationwide, 54 percent of all Medicaid recipients are now enrolled in some type of managed care program.[36]

Delivery and Financing Mechanisms. State Medicaid managed care programs use several different approaches to deliver and pay for health services through managed care plans. Two of these approaches rely on managed care plans to use utilization management practices to improve efficiency and quality. Under one approach, private physicians and other primary care providers contract with the state Medicaid office to serve as primary care case managers.[27,31] As part of their Medicaid contract, these providers agree to provide case management and utilization review services for the Medicaid beneficiaries who choose to enroll with them. Recipients are required to receive all or most primary care services from their chosen provider, and to receive prior authorization from their provider for all hospital and specialty services. Providers participating in these programs continue to receive fee-for-service payment for services rendered to Medicaid beneficiaries. In addition, providers receive a small, monthly per-enrollee fee for serving as the designated case manager.

A second model used by some states allows primary care providers to provide primary care and case management services to enrolled beneficiaries in exchange for a capitated, per-member per-month payment from the state Medicaid office.[27,31] This partial-risk model operates much like the primary care case management model, except that the capitated payment system allows providers to assume the risk of financial loss associated with the demand for primary care services.

Both the case management model and the partial-risk model depend primarily on the utilization management practices of primary care physicians to secure cost savings for state Medicaid programs. Unlike the case management model, the partial-risk model uses capitated payment schedules to create financial incentives for physicians to employ effective utilization management strategies for primary care services. Neither model includes strong incentives for utilization management of hospital and specialty services.[31] Furthermore, neither model relies on the ability of managed care plans to secure price discounts through selective contracting.

A third and increasingly prevalent Medicaid managed care model allows managed care plans to contract with the state Medicaid office on a capitated payment basis to provide the full range of covered health services to enrolled beneficiaries.[27,31] Under this full-risk model, managed care plans are able to employ selective contracting strategies in negotiating price discounts from the providers and facilities that contract with plans to serve their enrollees. Additionally, managed care plans in this model are financially responsible for the cost of all covered health services that are used by their enrollees, including hospital services and other specialized medical services. Consequently, these plans face strong financial incentives for engaging in effective utilization management practices.

Many states initially used case management and partial-risk models in designing their Medicaid managed care programs because these models represented the smallest departure from the Medicaid fee-for-service systems.[27] More recently, most states have begun to implement full-risk models for at least some portion of their Medicaid population because these types of programs have been shown to offer greater potential for cost savings.[31]

Children's Health Insurance Programs

A relatively new avenue of governmental involvement in managed care exists in the S-CHIP that was enacted in 1997 as part of the Balanced Budget Act of 1997.[35] Through the S-CHIP, states receive federal funding to provide health insurance coverage for the nation's 11 million low-income uninsured children. Annual funding allotments to each state are based on the number of low-income children (below 150 percent of the federal poverty level) and the number of uninsured low-income children in the state. A majority of states have designed their S-CHIPs to function as part of their Medicaid programs, with the primary difference being a higher income eligibility ceiling.[37] More than half (26) of the states have established eligibility ceilings at 200 percent of the federal poverty level or higher. Fifteen states have constructed separate S-CHIPs to cover uninsured children. Even among states with separate S-CHIPs, most state health agencies have chosen to use one or more of the common Medicaid managed care delivery models in providing health insurance coverage to low-income children—primary care case management, partial-risk capitation, and full-risk capitation. An estimated 2.7 million children have been enrolled in the S-CHIP as of September 1999.[37]

THE INTERFACE OF MANAGED CARE AND PUBLIC HEALTH ADMINISTRATION

The nation's public health system is highly sensitive to the policy and marketplace trends that occur within the field of managed health care. The interface between the public health system and the managed care industry can be distilled into three interrelated domains.

1. Public health organizations and managed care plans face an array of shared interests and common resource needs that can be addressed through collaboration. These shared interests include those related to health promotion and disease prevention approaches, population health data needs, and systems of care for vulnerable populations.
2. Public health organizations at all levels of government face an array of policy development and regulatory issues that are inextricably linked to the evolving managed care industry in the public and private sectors. These include issues of consumer protection, quality assurance, and health

care accessibility and affordability under managed care—all of which fall within the purview of the public health system to some extent.

3. Managed care plans give rise to a series of indirect effects on the public health system that need to be recognized in formulating public health policy and implementing public health programs. These indirect effects create both opportunities and challenges for the public health system, and include changes in medical practice, safety-net providers, teaching and research institutions, and aggregate health insurance coverage.

Important implications for policy and managerial decision making arise in each of these domains of interaction.

Interaction for Shared Interests and Resource Needs

A number of recent studies have documented a growing involvement of managed care plans in traditional public health activities. A 1996 study of collaborative activities maintained between medical care and public health organizations—part of the Medicine–Public Health Initiative supported by the American Medical Association and the American Public Health Association—revealed more than 400 such efforts across the United States, many of which involved participation by managed care plans.[11] Other recent studies have examined in detail the content of these relationships.[5,9,10,38] Together, these studies suggest that key skills and resources can be shared through partnerships between managed care plans and public health agencies, including

- *technical and scientific expertise:* Public health agencies maintain expertise in areas such as disease surveillance; population-based strategies for health education, health promotion, and disease prevention; and outreach to vulnerable and underserved population groups. These skills may be valuable to health plans seeking to improve the delivery and management of care for their enrolled populations. At the same time, health plans maintain expertise that may be useful to public health agencies as they respond to health system changes, including utilization management strategies, quality measurement and improvement processes, health marketing, and contract development.
- *individual-level and population-based interventions:* Health plans may contract with public health agencies for specific types of services such as family planning, communicable disease diagnosis and treatment, immunization delivery, and health education and counseling services. Public health agencies may seek the assistance of health plans in launching population-based interventions using the defined networks of enrollees and providers maintained by these plans.
- *administration and management skills:* Health plans and public health agencies may share expertise in managing complex interorganizational initiatives such as health education programs and community health assessment projects.
- *legal and regulatory authority:* Local and state health agencies have statutorily defined powers that can be used in developing local policies and regulations concerning health issues of interest to health plans and other providers, such as tobacco control and environmental health risks.
- *convening power:* Public health agencies can often be helpful in securing the participation of public officials and community representatives in community health efforts. Health plans often have the power and stature to serve as effective conveners of local health professionals and organizations involved in health care delivery, financing, and purchasing.
- *influence with policy makers, professionals, and the public:* Both public health agencies and health plans have strengths in these areas. Governmental public health agencies may offer strong ties with policy makers and community representatives; health plans often maintain strong connections with local medical professionals.

- *data and information systems:* Public health agencies traditionally have led the way in the collection of birth, death, and disease surveillance statistics. More recently, health plans have taken the lead in developing population-based clinical data systems that capture service quality, consumer satisfaction, health outcomes, and costs. Promising opportunities exist for sharing data and developing collaborative approaches for expanding the availability of community health information.
- *human and capital resources:* Arrangements for shared staff, equipment, and facilities may enable public health agencies and managed care plans to address critical resource shortages and to realize gains in efficiency for tasks such as community health assessment, disease surveillance, health education and counseling, and community outreach.

Types of Interaction

Linkages between managed care plans and public health agencies can occur for a variety of purposes, but much of the interaction that currently exists can be distilled into one of three basic activities.

1. the delivery of personal health services
2. the exchange of health data and information
3. the development and implementation of community interventions and policies

For activities involving *personal health services delivery*, Medicaid beneficiaries and other vulnerable and underserved populations are typically the focus of these collaborative efforts.[5,9,10] Activities may coordinate the delivery of personal health services offered by managed care plans and public health agencies, or they may involve the development of formal referral networks and service contracts between the two types of organizations. Most often, health plans contract with public health agencies to provide a set of specialized public health services such as family planning and communicable disease services; however, some agencies are able to provide a comprehensive range of primary care and case management services to managed care enrollees. In some communities, health plans hire public health agencies to provide health assessment and wellness services to a broad range of managed care members who are not limited to Medicaid beneficiaries.

For activities involving *health data and information*, collaborative efforts may range from the simple exchange of existing data to the joint collection and management of data through new surveillance strategies and information systems.[5,9,38] Some plans and agencies establish data-sharing agreements that ensure that clinical information is reported back to the health plan whenever enrollees access services from public health agencies. These mechanisms allow health plans to track accurately the utilization of preventive health services like immunizations or mammograms, and to learn quickly about any new health conditions that are detected by public health clinics. In other communities, health plans and public health agencies jointly sponsor population-based surveys of behavioral risk factors and access to care in order to obtain a better picture of health status and health risks within their service areas. In still other areas, plans and agencies collaborate in the development and management of childhood immunization registries that potentially allow the organizations to identify and target underimmunized children in health plans and the community at large.[5]

For activities involving *community interventions and policies*, collaborative efforts may involve a broad array of jointly sponsored initiatives such as mass media campaigns, health fairs, community health clinics, and community planning projects.[5,9,38] In some cases, health plans may engage in these efforts primarily for the purposes of marketing and community relations. Nevertheless, these activities often have the potential to achieve larger public health goals by raising awareness about health issues, risks, and community health resources. Collaborative interventions may target health care consumers in an effort to raise awareness about health issues or influence health-related decision making and behavior in areas such as nutrition, physical activity, safety, or preventive services utilization. Additionally, collaborative interventions may target health care professionals in an effort to influence clinical practice. For example, health plans and public health agencies may jointly sponsor educational interventions that address topics such as appropriate immunization delivery and storage procedures and communicable disease diagnosis and treatment practices.

Mechanisms of Interaction

Public health organizations and managed care plans may interact through a variety of structural mechanisms. These mechanisms reflect the diversity of organizational roles, financing structures, and managerial approaches that can be maintained jointly by managed care plans and public health organizations. Two basic structural approaches to interaction are apparent in most communities: a *service-shedding* approach in which activities in a given functional area are terminated by the public health organization and transferred completely to managed care plans, and an *alliance-building* approach in which public health agencies develop collaborative structures with plans for the joint performance of selected activities.[39] Within each of these alternative approaches, several different structural models exist (Figure 30–5). Each model

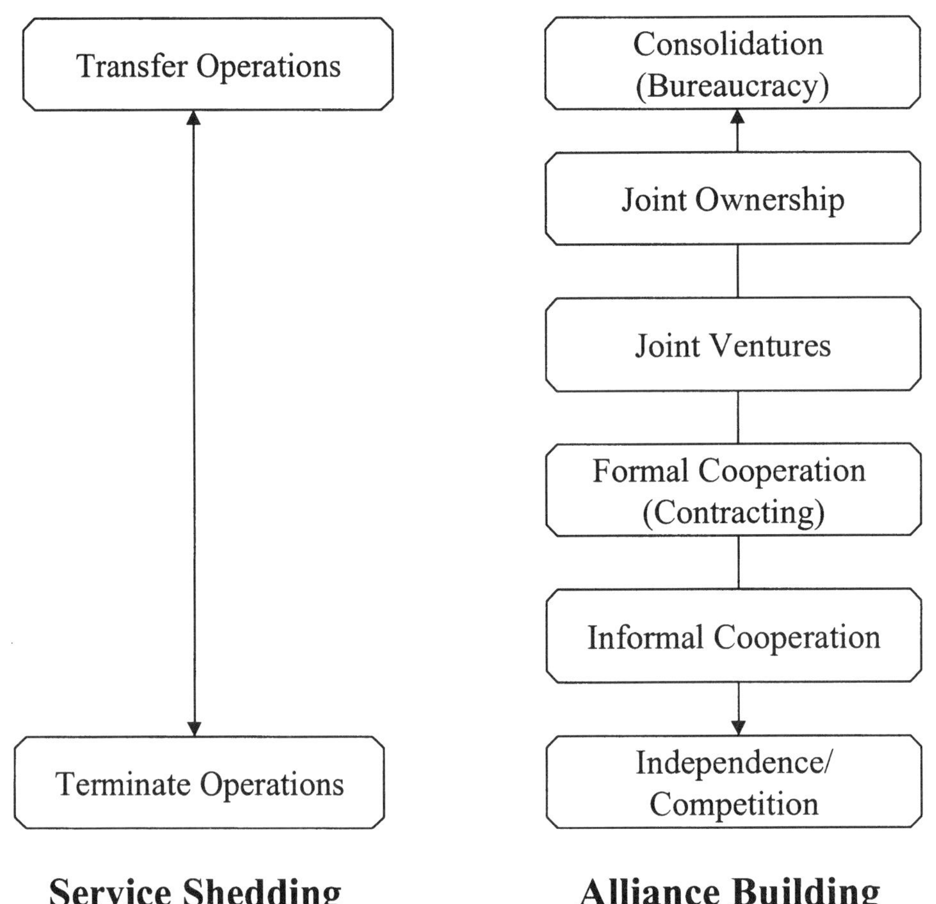

Figure 30–5 Structural Models of Interaction between Public Health Organizations and Managed Care Plans. *Source:* Reprinted from P.K. Halverson, A.D. Kaluzny, G.P. Mays, and T.B. Richards, Privatizing Health Services: Alternative Models and Emerging Issues for Public Health and Quality Management, *Quality Management in Health Care,* Vol. 5, No. 2, p. 6, © 1997, Aspen Publishers, Inc.

entails a unique set of costs and benefits from both organizational and societal perspectives.

Service-Shedding Models. Interaction between managed care plans and public health organizations may be achieved by completely devolving the responsibilities of providing selected public health services to private managed care plans.[39] Under this approach, responsibilities for the organization, operation, and management of selected public health services are assumed by one or more managed care plans, while public health involvement in these activities terminates. Public health organizations may initiate this activity simply by *ceasing operations* in a given service area, or by *transferring operations* to plans through formal agreements. Ideally, the first model of ceasing operations is employed only when sufficient capacity and expertise exists among existing managed care plans for adequately delivering services that were previously provided in the public sector. In implementing this model, public health providers must ensure that this capacity and expertise is present among the local network of managed care plans, and that the full spectrum of community members understands the intricacies of accessing services from these plans. Consequently, a large public health effort in community assessment, education, and outreach may be required before this model can be implemented successfully.

Under the cessation model, managed care plans may experience substantial changes in the sociodemographic characteristics, service delivery needs, and utilization patterns of the populations they serve. Plan responses to these changes may be diverse and volatile without a communitywide action plan in place to guide and coordinate the actions of managed care plans in assuming responsibility for public health services that were formerly performed in public settings. The public sector's role in facilitating the development of such a plan prior to implementation of the model is critical in ensuring an adequate transition from public to private service delivery.

A second model of service shedding involves the transfer of operations from public to private ownership. Typically, these exchanges include the purchase or lease of public health facilities and equipment, as in the private acquisition of a public health clinic. This model may afford a less disruptive transition process compared with the cessation model because services often continue to be provided in the same locations and facilities as they were prior to the exchange. Greater levels of planning and coordination often occur under this model as well because the transfer of service responsibility occurs explicitly between two organizations.

Conflicts in organizational mission and culture may emerge under the service-shedding model. The organizations that assume responsibility for public health services may hold organizational priorities and strategies that differ from those of the internal and external stakeholders of the public health organizations that formerly provided these services. Employees, patients, community members, and other public and private health care providers may hold expectations about the public health service that run counter to those of the new leadership. As a result, newly privatized public health services may give rise to operational problems in areas such as internal productivity and efficiency, community outreach and marketing, recruitment and retention of clinical and administrative staff, and interorganizational cooperation. As in any institutional merger, conflicting organizational cultures may create challenges for the effective management of public health services that are transferred to private managed care plans.

At face value, the service-shedding approach to interacting with managed care plans offers an element of managerial simplicity. Whether implemented by ceasing operations or transferring operations, these models potentially allow public health organizations to reduce their responsibilities in direct service provision. These approaches do not, however, allow organizations to reduce their responsibilities in carrying out core public health functions. Public health organizations using service-shedding approaches must find indirect ways of ensuring that necessary population-based health services and interventions are available, accessible, and effective for the populations they serve. Consequently, service-shedding models entail significant risks and costs from a public health perspective. The devolution of direct responsibility in a service area severely limits opportunities for ongoing public involvement in ensuring adequate financial and organizational access to services, and in monitoring and evaluating quality. For these reasons, alliance-building approaches may offer distinct advantages for public health organizations seeking to establish effective relationships with managed care plans.

Alliance-Building Models. Alliance-building models allow public health organizations and managed care plans to share responsibilities in the performance of public health activities within the community. At a minimum, these models preserve a role for the public sector in the management and oversight of service delivery responsibilities that may be transferred to private plans. Many alliance models allow public and private organizations to share responsibilities both in direct service provision and in evaluation and management activities. Strategic alliances are proving effective in accomplishing many of the objectives that are central to collaborative public health initiatives, such as sharing the costs associated with service delivery, improving efficiency, reducing duplication, sharing responsibilities and risks in service delivery, and improving the quality of public health services and their delivery mechanisms.

Strategic alliances encompass a range of structural models that specify the relationships among participating organizations. These models can be compared with regard to the level of integration achieved among organizations, which may vary between the extremes of complete independence (the free market) and complete consolidation (the bureaucracy).[40] Recent evidence suggests that alliances achieving higher levels of organizational integration may realize greater levels of clinical and financial performance.[41,42] At the same time, more integrated alliance structures may entail greater sacrifices of organizational control and autonomy.[43] A clear trade-off exists for public health agencies considering strategic alliances with managed care plans. Fortunately, a range of interorganizational alliance models lies along the continuum between free-market exchange and single-firm consolidation, offering a number of options for achieving public health objectives (Figure 30–5).

In the absence of cooperation, public health organizations and managed care plans carry out their efforts in health promotion and disease prevention independently. In some environments, plans and public health agencies may even become competitors for serving defined populations. Competition between the two types of organizations most commonly arises under Medicaid managed care programs. In some cases, public health organizations that provide clinical services may directly compete with managed care plans to enroll and serve Medicaid recipients. Such competition may be beneficial if it motivates both the plans and the public health organizations to improve the quality and efficiency of their services. However, such competition may be harmful if unnecessary duplication of services results, or if animosity and mistrust develop among the competing organizations so as to preclude cooperation for other purposes. In other cases, Medicaid recipients that have enrolled in managed care plans may continue to seek clinical services from public health organizations not affiliated with these plans. If plans do not reimburse public health organizations for their expenses in these cases, then plans realize lower medical costs from such behavior while public health organizations incur higher costs for uncompensated care. Without a cooperative solution to this type of problem, public health organizations may experience limitations in their ability to serve uninsured populations and to maintain other activities that do not generate revenue. These types of difficulties create strong incentives for public health organizations to seek cooperative relationships with managed care plans.

Informal cooperation typically occurs among organizations that maintain relatively high levels of mutual understanding and trust. Under these arrangements, organizations engage in collaborative efforts such as sharing supplies, equipment, and staff on an as-needed basis and with little monitoring or oversight. These efforts are structured and governed mainly by interorganizational trust and interpersonal relationships, rather than through formal mechanisms such as contracts or agreements. For example, a county health department and a large HMO in the state of Washington share medical supplies on an as-needed basis to avoid the need for large supply inventories and reduce the risk of supply shortages.[5] The success of this informal model hinges on the existence of close working relationships between the organizations involved. In the absence of such strong relationships, more formalized alliance structures may be required to initiate and sustain cooperative action.

Alliances based on formal cooperation are less reliant on personal relationships and tacit understanding in undertaking collective action. These relationships are typically based on contractual agreements between organizations for providing services, purchasing supplies, or sharing resources. Performance expectations, evaluation criteria, and management responsibilities may be explicitly identified through the contracts. In executing public health initiatives through these structures, public health organizations may assume ongoing roles in monitoring and evaluating the performance of managed care plans that contract to deliver health services.

Contracts between health departments and managed care plans are becoming increasingly prevalent under the Medicaid managed care programs now operating in 49 states. These contracts typically occur at two levels: (1) a contract between health plans and the state Medicaid agency, which specifies health plan responsibilities in enrolling and serving Medicaid beneficiaries and (2) contracts between health plans and local public health organizations, which typically specify provisions for delivering public health services to Medicaid recipients that are enrolled in the health plans. In most states, the state Medicaid contract exists as the key vehicle for building quality assurance and performance measurement criteria into Medicaid managed care programs. As the primary guarantor of access to public health services at the community level, public health organizations have a clear interest in helping to shape the Medicaid managed care contracts negotiated at the state level. Public health organizations potentially can play important roles in ensuring that these contracts contain adequate provisions for monitoring the accessibility and quality of care delivered by plans, and for providing coverage for health promotion and disease prevention services. Unfortunately, in many states, local public health organizations are not formally included in the state Medicaid contract design and negotiations processes.[5] These same concerns are present when public health organizations are involved in negotiating local service delivery contracts with managed care plans. In developing and executing these local contracts, public health organizations face the added concerns of ensuring that they are able to code and bill for public health services that are often not specified in managed care contracts with medical care providers, such as health education and counseling services. Most often, managed care plans negotiate contracts with local public health organizations for the delivery of specific clinical services such as childhood immunizations, sexually transmitted disease treatment, family planning services, and prenatal care services.

In some cases, public health organizations and managed care plans use *joint ventures* to produce programs and services collectively.[38] Whereas simple contractual relationships allow managed care plans to purchase selected services from local public health organizations, joint ventures allow plans and public health organizations to produce and manage services jointly. Typically, the organizations participating in joint ventures share in contributing the staff, resources, and funding necessary to sustain the program or service line. This arrangement allows both public health organizations and managed care plans to engage in the production and the oversight of the service. As a consequence, this arrangement requires participating organizations to tolerate a greater level of shared authority and control than is required under simple contractual relationships. Examples of programs and services produced through joint ventures between managed care plans and public health organizations include childhood immunization registries, telephone health information lines, and community health assessment and planning initiatives.[38]

Several other structural models of alliance-building are possible,[44] but to date these models have not been used frequently by public health organizations in forming relationships with managed care plans. Under the *shared ownership* model, collaborating organizations create a new corporate entity to assume responsibility for providing a range of programs and services. Rather than supporting a single product or service, the participating organizations share ownership of a new organization that performs an array of activities of mutual interest. The shared ownership model has been used by several public health organizations in developing managed care plans for serving Medicaid beneficiaries. For example, the local public health agency serving Multnomah County, Oregon developed such a managed care plan in collaboration with a local hospital and several community health centers.[38] The *consolidation* model takes the strategy of integration a step further, such that collaborating organizations fully merge their operations within a single organizational structure. This model has been used by public health organizations to formalize their relationships with organizations such as hospitals, community health centers, and neighboring public health organizations. To date, however, this model has not been employed to merge the operations of managed care plans and public health organizations.

Of all of the structural models considered here, the shared ownership and consolidation models entail the highest levels of shared control and shared financial risk among participating organizations. As a result, these models may offer the greatest potential for realizing gains in efficiency by creating a single organization through which a range of programs and services are produced. The consolidated organizational structures created under these models may offer organizations increased leverage in contracting and purchasing activities, as well as economies of scale and scope in the use of human and capital resources. Less integrated structures for interorganizational cooperation may fail to realize these types of efficiencies and synergies. However, both the joint ownership model and the consolidation model require the public health organization to cede substantial organizational autonomy and control to its partners, and to place itself at risk for the liabilities and limitations of these partners. For these reasons, these models of alliance-building are likely to succeed only among organizations that are highly compatible in their mission, organizational culture, operations, and populations served.[44,45] Without such similarities, the costs of integration and consolidation may far outweigh the benefits.

Interaction for Public Health Policy and Regulatory Issues

As fields of practice, public health and managed care intersect for another set of activities that involve the development and implementation of public policies designed to protect and improve health at the population level. Public health agencies at state and federal levels carry out broad policy implementation responsibilities that include ensuring the accessibility and quality of health services needed by the populations residing in their jurisdictions. These responsibilities are distributed among an array of governmental agencies, including those responsible for public health, Medicaid, insurance, and labor and employment activities. (See Chapter 3 for a discussion of these types of agencies and their public health contributions.) In addressing issues of health care accessibility and quality, these governmental agencies must respond simultaneously to the often competing objectives of: (1) expanding health insurance coverage through policy and market mechanisms that enhance the affordability of public and private insurance coverage, and (2) ensuring the safety and quality of health care that is delivered to populations with public and private health insurance coverage. To pursue these objectives through policy development and implementation, public health organizations must become involved either directly or indirectly in the managed care marketplace and in the economic and political processes that influence health insurance coverage.

A primary driver of managed care growth during the 1990s has been the potential for cost containment and efficiency gains within the nation's health care industry. Governmental health insurance programs such as Medicaid, Medicare, and S-CHIP have readily adopted managed care models as strategies for containing costs and thereby expanding these public programs to cover larger numbers of the uninsured than could be covered under traditional fee-for-service systems. From the perspective of quality improvement and consumer protection, however, managed care models offer another compelling advantage over traditional fee-for-service systems—accountability. Under the fee-for-service arrangements for financing medical care services that dominated before the rise of managed care, no single individual or organization is accountable for the clinical and financial outcomes experienced by health care consumers as a result of receiving, or not receiving, needed services. Under these arrangements, clinical accountability is diffused across the multiple health care providers that may render services to individual patients—including physicians, hospitals, and subacute care facilities—with few if any provisions for ensuring coordination and comprehensiveness across these settings.

Under managed care, a single organization assumes responsibility for managing the delivery of a comprehensive range of health services that may be needed by its enrollees, and this organization can be held accountable for the clinical and financial outcomes that result. In health care markets characterized by competing health plans and adequate information concerning the comparative performance of these plans, health care purchasers, consumers, and even public health regulators can hold plans accountable for their performance by basing their enrollment and purchasing decisions on this information.[46] Such informed decision making was not possible in the traditional fee-for-service setting. It must be noted, however, that managed care plans assume explicit clinical and financial accountability only for their enrolled members, and not for individuals that fall outside their membership. From a public health perspective, therefore, managed care plans assume only partial accountability for the health of communities and broadly defined population groups—an accountability that is limited by health insurance coverage and health plan market share.

Policy Options for Purchasing and Regulating Health Care Delivery

In carrying out their responsibilities to promote and protect health care quality, governmental public health agencies face the challenge of capitalizing on the opportunities for accountability that are created by managed care systems while guarding against their potential limitations. As purchasers of health care services for millions of Americans under such programs as Medicare, Medicaid, and S-CHIP, state and federal health agencies have direct and straightforward responsibilities to carry out in ensuring the quality and accessibility of care delivered to public program beneficiaries under managed care systems. Like employers and other purchasers in the health care industry, these governmental agencies hold the primary authority and responsibility to establish performance objectives, reporting requirements, incentives and penalties, and other contract provisions with the health plans they select to serve program beneficiaries. For these programs, the government's challenge is to identify the most effective ways of ensuring accountability and encouraging quality among the health plans with which it contracts.

At the federal level, the U.S. Health Care Financing Administration (HCFA) has continued to make progress in this task throughout its three decades of involvement in the managed care arena. Recent actions include requiring Medicare HMOs to report measures from the National Committee for Quality Assurance's (NCQA's) performance measurement system, the *Health Plan Employer Data and Information Set (HEDIS);* requiring Medicare and Medicaid HMOs to conduct consumer satisfaction surveys, to report physician risk-sharing arrangements, and to carry stop-loss insurance for physicians in risk-sharing arrangements; and regulating the marketing practices of Medicare and Medicaid HMOs. Similarly, state health agencies have developed an array of effective performance measurement systems for monitoring access and quality among the managed care plans that participate in Medicaid and S-CHIP programs—many of them based on the *HEDIS* system and on HCFA's Quality Improvement System for Managed Care Programs.[47]

The appropriate governmental strategies for encouraging quality and accessibility within the private health care marketplace are less clear. Traditionally, individual states have maintained responsibility for regulating the practices of private health insurance organizations through state insurance agencies. State and local public health agencies may or may not have a voice in the regulatory actions of state insurance agencies, depending on the formal and informal mechanisms of intergovernmental communication and coordination that exist within individual states. Additionally, private organizations have taken the lead responsibility for reviewing the organizational practices and capacities of health plans as part of accreditation and certification programs. The most prominent accreditation programs for health plans include those maintained by the NCQA and the Joint Commission on Accreditation of Healthcare Organizations. The leading industry trade group for health plans, the American Association of Health Plans, has also made substantial contributions to these private sector accountability efforts by developing industrywide policies for its 1,000 member organizations on topics including consumer information disclosure, physician–patient communication, emergency care utilization, and mastectomy care. Increasingly, state agencies rely on the performance measures and accreditation standards developed by these private organizations in assessing the quality and accessibility of health services delivered through managed care plans.[48]

Recent legislative activity has given the federal government new and unprecedented responsibilities in regulating private markets for managed care and health insurance.[49] These new responsibilities include requiring plans to offer enrollees a minimum of 48 hours of hospital stay for childbirth; limiting health plan exclusions for preexisting conditions; guaranteeing renewable health insurance policies for employers, regardless of their size; and requiring large employers to adopt mental health insurance coverage limits that are equal to the limits that are imposed for medical care insurance.[50] Some policy analysts argue that, despite worthy intentions, these new federal roles inevitably fall short of their intended purpose of ensuring quality within the evolving health insurance industry. It is a near impossible task to forge a comprehensive framework for quality improvement from piecemeal regulations regarding the processes of care. The complexities of medical decision making, in combination with the rapid pace of innovation in health care processes and technologies, overwhelm even the most informed and efficient policy-making bodies. For this reason, some observers argue that attempts to legislate the processes of health care delivery under managed care will be at best ineffective, and at worst disruptive to the quality improvement efforts these policies seek to support.[49] Moreover, direct federal interventions in health care delivery may attenuate or even distort the potentially powerful incentives for innovation and efficiency that are created by the competitive managed care marketplace.

Market-Based Options for Ensuring Accessibility and Quality in Managed Care

Policy theorists and health care analysts have long recognized the potential value of the health care marketplace in motivating continuous improvements in the quality and efficiency of health care delivery. Some theorists suggest that if health care consumers and providers are able to interact in competitive and equitable health care markets, natural incentives for cost containment and quality improvement will shape the delivery of health care.[46] The existence and influence of such market-based incentives depend on several critical characteristics of the health care market: (1) the ability of purchasers and consumers to hold a single entity—the health plan—accountable for the clinical and financial outcomes of its members, (2) the existence of competitive markets in which multiple plans vie to assume responsibility for the health care needs of defined populations, and (3) the availability of comparative information on health plan performance that can be used by consumers and purchasers in making their health care decisions.

A market-based approach to ensuring quality in health care, therefore, needs to ensure the existence of these three conditions within local health care markets. Rather than devising a regulatory scheme to reach every doctor and hospital, a market-based approach establishes an incentive system to correct for imperfections in the health care marketplace, and then allows competition to generate improvements in health care quality, efficiency, and accessibility. This approach eliminates the need for government to become involved in monitoring and regulating specific elements of health care quality and accessibility. Instead, these elements are continually developed and revealed through the process of market competition.

Market-based approaches to health care quality are not without limitations, however. First and foremost, the processes of ensuring sufficient market competition and adequate flows of information on quality are far from perfect. Governmental agencies must rely on inexact sciences—imperfect methods of evaluating and supporting competition in local health care markets—and primitive but improving measures of quality that can be used to characterize health plan performance. However, when compared with the alternative and much more daunting task of regulating the specifics of health care quality, the responsibilities of ensuring competition and information flows often appear more feasible.

In determining the appropriate roles for public health policy and regulation within an increasingly market-based health care industry, the strengths and weaknesses of governmental health agencies must be recognized. One of the government's greatest strengths in the health care market is its ability to act as a convening and mobilizing force for major stakeholders within the industry. The visibility, stature, and power of federal and state health agencies confer on them the unique ability to bring together diverse public and private sector actors and facilitate the levels of collaboration, consensus building, and decision making that ultimately result in improved health care practice and policy.

The governmental roles of convening and facilitating become critically important in the context of market-based approaches to quality improvement. In the absence of direct regulatory intervention, these roles are vital in establishing systems to encourage competition in local markets and to collect and disseminate relevant information on health care quality. In carrying out these roles, no other entities within the health care industry are comparable to federal agencies such as HCFA, the CDC, the National Institutes of Health (NIH), and the Agency for Healthcare Research and Quality. These agencies are indeed uniquely qualified for convening diverse and powerful health care stakeholders at the national level, including health professions associations, insurers, employers, consumer groups, organized labor, and state and local governments.

Governmental health agencies also have inherent weaknesses that limit their effective involvement in quality improvement efforts within the health care industry. First and foremost, these agencies often lack the organizational agility necessary to keep up with the pace of innovation that is now occurring within the health care industry. The bureaucratic structure necessary for careful policy development and equitable regulatory enforcement is simply incompatible with a dynamic organizational structure that supports rapid decision making and immediate responsiveness to industry shifts. It is the absence of such dynamic structures within governmental bureaucracy that necessarily limits the effectiveness of direct governmental intervention in health care quality improvement. Recognizing this inherent weakness of the governmental health agencies, policy makers may need to incorporate market-based approaches for ensuring quality improvement in health care.

Balancing Market and Governmental Approaches for Ensuring Access and Quality in Managed Care

Perhaps the most promising strategy for ensuring quality and accessibility in health care uses the capacities of the evolving health care market as well as the tested strengths of governmental health agencies. Governmental and market-based approaches are not mutually exclusive, bur rather complementary strategies for creating effective public health policies to address issues of access and quality in the managed care marketplace. Three approaches for developing and implementing these complementary strategies appear promising.

First, federal and state health agencies can assume lead roles in protecting and encouraging the natural market processes supporting innovation development and diffusion for quality improvement.[49] These roles involve working across multiple state and federal governmental agencies to encourage health care policy making at all levels of government that helps rather than hinders the market-driven incentives for innovation and quality improvement. Additionally, health agencies should consider appropriate policies and incentives to encourage greater levels of competition within markets that traditionally have experienced difficulty in supporting multiple, competing health care providers.

Second, federal and state health agencies need to assume leading roles in expanding the availability of standardized, comparative information on health plan performance to health care consumers. Such information should allow consumers to make valid comparisons across health plans in areas such as health outcomes; performance of preventive health services; policies for provider choice, access to specialists, and cost sharing; and information regarding member satisfaction and rates of disenrollment. The federal government's role should also include efforts to identify new methods of measuring quality and new approaches to widespread information dissemination. However, in order to ensure sufficient expertise and organizational agility to respond to rapid innovations in health care quality, the entity responsible for managing the process of quality measurement and dissemination should come from within the health care industry and outside the governmental sphere. This private sector approach to the measurement of quality is often compared to the highly successful approach that is used within the accounting profession, wherein a privately funded body known as the Federal Accounting Standards Board establishes the performance standards that are implemented industrywide.[51]

Third, a successful market-based approach to quality improvement will require widespread acceptance of the quality measurement standards and protocols that are established by a recognized body within the health care industry. Another key role of governmental health agencies, therefore, lies in using their leverage as health insurance purchasers and public health leaders to encourage industrywide acceptance of and compliance with these standards as they are developed.[49] Such industrywide compliance will not only expand the availability of health plan information, but will also ensure a level playing field for the diversity of competing plans within the industry. In developing a market-based approach to quality improvement, the health care industry should take advantage of the substantial developmental work on quality measurement that is already underway through projects such as the NCQA's *HEDIS* system for performance measurement. Already, this work has entailed industrywide collaboration by federal and state health agencies as well as private and public sector health care providers, purchasers, and insurers. More than 330 health plans across the country have used this system, and a recent survey of 400 U.S. employers suggests that more than half of large employers take into account *HEDIS* performance measures when making health care purchasing decisions.[52]

Although existing public and private sector capacities for quality improvement are encouraging, substantial challenges remain to be faced in adopting public health policies that incorporate effective market-based approaches for ensuring quality and accessibility in health care. Such approaches run counter to the traditional bureaucratic culture of control and regulation within most governmental health agencies. These approaches may also conflict with political processes that favor incremental policy development at federal, state, and local levels. Nonetheless, the progress already underway within the health care system is substantial, suggesting that sustained approaches for ensuring health care accessibility and quality are achievable through the synergies of market dynamics and responsible leadership in public health policy development.

Indirect Interaction between Managed Care and the Public Health System

The interface between public health practice and managed health care delivery is not always direct and intentional, as it is in the realm of governmental regulation. These two fields of practice come into contact explicitly when public health agencies collaborate with health plans to pursue shared interests, and when these agencies participate in policy development and regulatory enforcement activities that target the managed care industry. The evolving managed care industry also influences public health practice indirectly through several mechanisms of effect. Some of these indirect effects offer opportunities for strengthening the public health system, as when managed care programs induce greater numbers of private health care providers to serve public program recipients, or to adopt more prevention practices and higher standards of clinical quality. Other indirect effects of managed care growth pose challenges for public health organizations, as when managed care programs redirect important revenue sources that support safety-net providers, health professions training programs, and clinical research activities. Even public health organizations that do not engage explicitly in interaction with managed care plans will eventually face opportunities and challenges that are precipitated indirectly by trends in the managed care marketplace. By recognizing and anticipating these indirect effects, public health organizations can respond effectively to changes in the health care marketplace.

Effects on Medical Practice

Medical practice is changing rapidly in response to managed care growth, and these changes appear to have substantial implications for public health organizations. For example, Medicaid and S-CHIP managed care programs in several states appear effective in encouraging larger numbers of private medical providers to serve recipients of these public programs.[53] In many cases, these managed care programs allow private physicians and hospitals to receive higher payment levels than were available under the traditional fee-for-service Medicaid programs, which historically paid fees that were often less than 50 percent of the usual and customary rates charged by private providers. By delivering medical care services more efficiently through managed care arrangements, many governmental health insurance programs are now able to offer providers more competitive payment levels. The higher payment levels offered through managed care programs may take the form of additional case management fees offered to primary care physicians or capitated payments and bonuses that reward efficient health care delivery.

The growing participation of private providers in public health insurance programs may have the positive effect of reducing the administrative and financial burdens that many public health organizations face in providing personal health services to underserved populations—thereby freeing resources that can be applied to population-based public health activities. Unfortunately, in some cases, this expanded private participation may also have the adverse effect of reducing an important revenue stream for public health organizations, forcing these organizations to pursue other avenues for funding public health activities and infrastructure.[54] Consequently, managed care programs may create some short-term financial instability for public health organizations that depend heavily on patient care revenue from sources such as Medicaid and S-CHIP. Nevertheless, the long-term effects of such changes are likely to be beneficial for the public health system if these changes ultimately allow public health organizations to enhance their focus on population-based health interventions.

Additionally, the growing presence of managed care plans potentially creates incentives for medical care providers to become more active in offering health promotion and disease prevention services to their patients, and in improving the clinical quality of care that they provide.[55] The capitated payment systems used by many managed care plans create financial incentives for providers to deliver services that forestall the need for future costly medical care—including many preventive services such as immunizations, prenatal care, and disease screening and early detection services. Moreover, a growing number of managed care plans use administrative and financial mechanisms to encourage providers to follow clinical practice guidelines that detail standards of quality for common medical conditions.[20] These mechanisms include provider reminders and prompts, provider report cards and performance profiles, and provider payments and bonuses based on performance. Efforts to monitor and compare quality of care across competing managed care plans—such as *HEDIS*—create additional incentives for plans to improve the quality of care delivered by their medical providers. If these types of activities persist among managed care plans, they promise to expand the availability and accessibility of preventive health services while reducing medical errors and other gaps in medical care quality. Despite these optimistic signals, however, it largely remains to be seen whether the incentives created by the managed care industry are sufficiently strong and widespread to change medical practice and thereby enhance public health. In practice, the incentives for prevention and quality may be dominated by the short-run financial imperatives that health plans must meet to remain solvent, or they may be diminished by high turnover in the enrolled populations that many health plans serve.[8]

Effects on Safety-Net Providers

Managed care growth within the public and private health insurance markets is likely to affect the ability of health care providers to serve vulnerable and underserved populations. Historically, health care providers have used the revenues they generate from serving insured patients to cross-subsidize care for the uninsured and other underserved populations.[56,57] By encouraging competition among health care providers and efficiency in medical care delivery, managed care plans potentially reduce the financial margins earned by health care providers in serving privately insured patients. Several recent studies of hospitals and private physician practices suggest that these providers may reduce their involvement in providing care to the uninsured as their involvement in managed care contracting and competitive health care delivery increases.[56–61] Although far from conclusive, these studies suggest that managed care growth may place added burdens on safety-net providers such as community health centers and public health clinics that provide access to care regardless of insurance status and ability to pay.

Many safety-net providers are now participating in managed care programs for Medicaid and S-CHIP recipients, creating concerns about their continued ability to provide care for the uninsured. The selective contracting practices used by managed care plans may exclude some safety-net providers from the provider networks of these plans. These practices potentially reduce the revenue that safety-net providers obtain from serving publicly and privately insured patients—thereby reducing their ability to cross-subsidize free and reduced-fee care for the uninsured. Even if not excluded from managed care networks, safety-net providers that successfully negotiate contracts with managed care plans may experience reductions in the payments they receive for serving Medicaid recipients. The utilization review practices used by some managed care plans may also adversely affect safety-net providers if these practices motivate managed care enrollees to seek free and reduced-fee care from safety-net providers when these enrollees encounter administrative or financial barriers to care within their plans. In this way, increased demand for free and reduced-fee care from managed care enrollees could further reduce the ability of safety-net providers to finance care for the uninsured.

The evidence to date suggests that at least some types of providers are able to balance their safety-net roles with the marketplace imperatives of managed care. A recent longitudinal analysis of the nation's federally funded community health centers indicates that centers participating in capitated managed care contracts are able to maintain and expand their delivery of care to the uninsured—a finding that stands in contrast to recent studies of private physicians.[61] One reason for the successful performance of health centers under capitated contracting appears to be their extensive use of nonphysician clinical labor to improve production efficiency—a strategy that may not be easily followed by private physicians serving large numbers of privately insured patients.

Safety-net providers that fail to secure managed care contracts appear to face the greatest difficulties in fulfilling their mission of providing care to the uninsured. Efforts to ensure the viability of safety-net providers under managed care should therefore focus on the providers least likely to be selected into these contracts, and on the tractable organizational and policy characteristics that may influence this selection. For example, recent evidence suggests that safety-net providers offering nonmedical services in addition to primary care services are significantly less likely to obtain managed care contracts, whereas providers offering inpatient physician services are more likely to obtain these contracts.[61] Managed care plans may be reluctant to contract with providers that offer nonmedical services because these services may attract patients with greater health service needs to their membership, a phenomenon known as adverse patient selection.

One important consequence of these findings is that access to nonmedical services may decrease over time in medically underserved communities as safety-net providers reduce their scope of services in order to secure contracts with managed care plans. To preserve health center involvement in nonmedical service provision, new policies may be required to induce managed care plans to contract with providers offering a broad scope of services. For example, state Medicaid managed care contracts may be designed to include dental and mental health care coverage under a single capitated contract, rather than "carving out" these services through separate service contracts. Such inclusive contracts may increase demand among managed care plans for providers that offer both medical and nonmedical services. Some states are already using or considering strategies for integrated coverage of medical and mental health services in light of evidence that integrated mental health care may produce offsets in medical care costs.[62]

Safety-net providers with limited clinical capacity also appear less likely to secure managed care contracts. This finding is consistent with the view that managed care plans seek economies of scale and lower transaction costs by contracting with providers having the capacity to serve large numbers of plan members.[63–64] Several policy and managerial strategies may assist safety-net providers in securing managed care contracts. First, policies to increase the number of physicians practicing in safety-net institutions—such as expansions of the National Health Service Corps educational loan repayment program and the J-1 visa program for noncitizen physicians—could be effective in helping these institutions obtain managed care contracts. Such policy expansions may be particularly effective if they target safety-net providers with limited physician capacity, such as providers with less than three full-time equivalent physicians on staff. Additionally, small providers may increase their participation in managed care contracts by developing multi-institutional provider contracting organizations with other safety-net providers and private physician practices.[65] These organizations allow providers to pool their clinical capacity and offer managed care plans access to a large number of providers with broad geographic coverage through a single contracting instrument. Small safety-net providers in some states have joined together on a regional or statewide basis to develop their own managed care plans, which in turn contract with each participating health center.[66] These plans are likely to entail larger resource commitments and greater regulatory oversight than provider contracting organizations, but they potentially offer health centers greater control and predictability in securing managed care contracts. The Balanced Budget Act of 1997 recently relaxed federal restrictions on provider-sponsored organizations' participation in state Medicaid programs, thereby reducing regulatory barriers to developing these types of organizations.

Several Medicaid policy options may also increase the selection of safety-net providers into managed care contracts and thereby increase provider survival and uncompensated care delivery. Recent evidence suggests that safety-net participation in managed care contracting is higher in states that enroll a broad range of their Medicaid caseload in managed care plans—such as categorically eligible Medicaid recipients and individuals who are eligible for Medicaid through expansion-waiver programs—compared with states that limit managed care enrollment to recipients who are eligible for Medicaid through AFDC (now TANF).[61] In these states, managed care plans are more likely to serve recipients with chronic diseases, disabilities, and complex social services needs.[67] Managed care plans operating in expanded-enrollment states may therefore face greater incentives for contracting with public health clinics and other safety-net providers because of these providers' expertise in serving high-risk populations. At the same time, safety-net providers operating in expanded-enrollment states face fewer opportunities for serving Medicaid recipients on a fee-for-service basis, thereby creating greater incentives for providers to pursue managed care contracts. In these ways, policies that expand the types of Medicaid recipients enrolled in managed care plans may help to achieve compatibility between the contracting incentives faced by managed care plans and those faced by safety-net providers. It should be recognized, however, that expanded-enrollment policies may also affect quality of care and health outcomes for high-risk populations. Several states have chosen not to implement expanded-enrollment policies because of concerns that disabled, aged, and chronically ill populations may experience poorer health outcomes in managed care arrangements as compared with fee-for-service settings.[68–71]

Medicaid HMO payment policies offer additional strategies for increasing safety-net participation in managed care contracts. Some evidence suggests that safety-net providers are more likely to participate in managed care contracts in states that offer higher capitated Medicaid payments to HMOs.[61] Higher capitated payments may reduce the incentives that managed care plans face to contain costs through selective contracting, thereby reducing the risk of contract exclusion for safety-net providers. Higher Medicaid payments may also allow managed care plans to offer higher payments to safety-net providers, thereby increasing the likelihood that providers will accept contract offers from plans. One policy option used in several states involves offering higher Medicaid payment rates only to managed care plans that contract with community health centers and other safety-net providers.[72] Conditional payment policies may therefore offer promising strategies for reducing safety-net contract exclusions and improving the performance of safety-net providers.

Effects on Teaching and Research Institutions

The growth of managed health care also influences the public health system through its effects on academic health institutions, which provide vital educational and training opportunities for the nation's health work force while supporting most of the nation's clinical and health services research activities. Traditionally, these institutions charge higher prices for the patient care services they provide in order to subsidize the costs of health professions education, training, and research.[73] With the rise of managed care, many academic health centers are actively seeking strategies to improve operating efficiency in order to compete more effectively for managed care contracts and thereby avoid large losses of patients and revenues. In some cases, these strategies may require institutions to scale back their training and research activities in order to offer competitive prices for patient care services. Recent studies confirm that medical schools located in advanced managed care markets secure fewer research awards from NIH, and their faculty members publish fewer research articles than those from schools in less-developed markets.[73,74] Faculty and staff in these advanced markets appear to have more patient care responsibilities and fewer protected hours for research.[75] Moreover, medical students and residents within these markets appear to face fewer opportunities for training in health services research, resulting in a declining number of new clinical researchers entering the field.[76] These findings suggest that the growing managed care industry may create unintended, adverse effects on the production of the future health professions work force and the discovery of new biomedical knowledge and applications.

The challenges faced by academic health centers under managed care are substantial, and likely defy any potential solution that falls short of a comprehensive reform of the financing mechanisms for clinical and health services research. Market-based approaches to health care delivery that are designed to promote quality and efficiency through competition cannot be relied on to produce adequate levels of public goods such as research and training without explicit payment systems to support these activities. Using patient revenues to cross-subsidize clinical research activities no longer appears to be a viable strategy for health care institutions in a competitive health care environment. To protect the vital public health roles these organizations play in research and training, academic health centers need to be funded fully and explicitly for their efforts in these areas.

As public goods, research and work force training should be financed through a system that allows the beneficiaries of the research and the work force to share equally in its cost. One simple approach would involve a small surcharge or tax on patient care revenues, which could then be directed to researchers and training programs, including academic health centers, for research purposes on a competitive basis. This approach could ensure that academic centers are not disproportionately saddled with the burden of supporting research and training activities through patient revenues. Rather, all providers, payers, purchasers, and consumers would share in the costs as well as the benefits of these activities. This explicit, rational approach to financing clinical research activities has broad appeal within the health care industry, and has received endorsements from organizations such as the Association for Health Services Research and the American Association of Health Plans.[77]

Effects on Health Insurance Coverage

The managed care industry also influences the public health system through its effect on aggregate health insurance coverage and affordability. During the 1990s, the United States experienced an unprecedented reduction in the growth rate of health insurance costs, and much of this reduction was attributable to the growth in managed care enrollment. By keeping health insurance coverage affordable, the managed care industry played an important indirect role in helping Americans maintain their insurance coverage and in reducing the indigent care burdens shouldered by public health agencies. A 1997 study by The Lewin Group estimated that managed care growth saved purchasers of private insurance between $23.8 billion and $37.4 billion in 1996, representing an average savings of between $304 and $406 per family for families headed by a person under age 65.[78] The Lewin Group further estimated that without the managed care growth that was experienced between 1992–96, there would have been between 3.1 and 5.0 million more persons without insurance than there actually were in 1997. These findings offer evidence that managed care has indirectly benefited the public health system and its systems of care for the uninsured. It remains an open question as to whether these benefits outweigh the potential public health challenges precipitated by managed care growth.

NEW DEVELOPMENTS SHAPING THE PUBLIC HEALTH–MANAGED CARE INTERFACE

Recent marketplace and policy trends within the health care field have important implications for the interface between public health and managed care. The practice of managed care and public health has changed markedly over the past few years, calling into question some of the assumptions that have been made about how these fields may interact. It is important that public health decision makers examine these trends and anticipate how they may affect the current and future relationships between managed care and public health.

The Evolving Nature of Managed Care

One critically important trend is the evolving nature of managed health care. Health plans must be highly responsive to consumer and purchaser preferences as well as to the regulatory environments in which they operate. Changes in market demand and in regulatory requirements cause health plans to adjust their organizational structures and operational strategies to address these imperatives. Recently, dramatic growth in open-ended managed care products has occurred in response to consumer demands for greater choice among providers. These demands have also encouraged the growth of plans that allow direct access to specialists. Current and proposed health plan regulations at state and federal levels promise to create additional shifts in plan organization and operation.[21,79] As the dynamics among health plans and their members and providers change, so too will the roles that these plans can play in public health initiatives.

Continued Transformations in Public Health Organizations

Public health organizations are also undergoing dramatic changes in their mission, organization, and operation as they seek to improve population health within their jurisdictions and remain responsive to changes within the larger health systems in which they operate. Many public health agencies have begun to diminish their involvement in personal health care delivery as this capacity develops among other community providers.[54] These agencies are placing more emphasis on population-based activities such as assessing community health needs and risks, developing policies and plans to promote and protect health, and ensuring the availability and quality of health services that are provided in the community. As they undertake these changes, many public health organizations are developing capacities in areas such as outcomes measurement, continuous quality improvement, performance-based contracting, and decision analysis.[80] These changes will undoubtedly affect the ways in which public health agencies interact with managed care plans. Agencies may reduce their involvement as service providers within managed care plans, but they may need to increase involvement with these plans for assessment and policy development activities.

Changes in Access to and Use of Health Information

Trends regarding the availability and use of health information are also likely to shape relationships between public health agencies and managed care plans. Both health plans and public health agencies face growing pressures to demonstrate their performance in addressing population health needs and their accountability for public and private investments in health.[5,9,10] These developments create incentives for collaboration in developing population-based health information systems that can be used to monitor performance and demonstrate accountability. Moreover, as growing numbers of health care consumers and purchasers receive access to this information, health plans and public health agencies face urgent needs to ensure that the public can make appropriate use of this information in their health-related decision making. Therefore, another key area of collaboration may involve joint efforts to disseminate community health information and to assist consumers and purchasers in making effective use of this information.

An important component of these efforts involves addressing the difficult problem of health literacy in communities. Along with the flood of health information, consumers are being asked to assume more responsibility in decision making about health and health care. However, educational, language, and cognitive barriers prevent many individuals from effectively using health information for activities such as choosing among providers and health plans or following treatment protocols and self-care strategies.[81] Health plans and public health agencies share a compelling interest in addressing these health literacy issues and supporting optimal personal decision making in health care.

Additionally, health plans and public health agencies both face the need to address privacy and confidentiality concerns regarding health data and information. Both types of organizations depend on a free flow of information to support population-based health assessment and health management activities. Joint efforts to address these issues through smart information technology and smart information policy will become increasingly urgent.

Changes in Systems of Care for Vulnerable and Underserved Populations

Finally, the systems for ensuring access to health care for vulnerable and underserved population groups continues to evolve, and these shifts have important implications for the interface of managed care and public health. Recent evidence suggests that nationally, growing numbers of commercial managed care plans are reducing or discontinuing their participation in Medicaid programs as they face the difficult realities of serving these often hard-to-reach populations with very low Medicaid payment rates.[82] Those plans that continue to serve these populations often appear very different in structure and function from the traditional commercial managed care plans. Many are provider-sponsored organizations that specialize in serving Medicaid beneficiaries—and many do not meet the regulatory requirements and accreditation standards that cover HMOs and other types of health plans. The types of relationships that are needed and that are possible with these types of plans are likely to be substantially different from public health relationships with commercial health plans.

As managed care systems continue to develop for Medicaid beneficiaries and other traditionally underserved population groups, public health agencies and other safety-net providers are reevaluating their roles in serving these groups. Most of these agencies are following one of three general strategies.[10]

1. Discontinue the delivery of personal health services as health plans assume this responsibility.
2. Reorganize to become managed care providers.
3. Organize with other providers to form their own managed care plans.

This last strategy may give rise to competitive pressures between public health agencies and health plans, whereas the first strategy may allow population health issues and strategies to assume priority in relationships between health plans and public health agencies.

STRATEGIES FOR MANAGING THE INTERFACE OF PUBLIC HEALTH AND MANAGED CARE

Marketplace and policy shifts create both challenges and opportunities for establishing viable and effective relationships between managed care plans and public health organizations. Recent experiences and observations suggest that two basic managerial approaches are possible in this context.[1,5,10]

Passive Management

The first approach is classified as passive management because the relationships require minimal attention and maintenance, even in the face of substantial marketplace and policy changes. These relationships involve organizations that

- Collaborate with similar organizations having shared missions and common incentives.
- Engage in collaborative initiatives that do not require changes in usual clinical or administrative practices.

- Invest slack resources that are not needed for other purposes in collaboration.
- Limit the collaboration to planning and assessment activities that are easily reversed, terminated, or ignored.

These types of relationships are perhaps the most common form of interaction among managed care plans and public health agencies today. Although easy to develop, these efforts are unlikely to produce meaningful and sustained improvements in population health. Moreover, these types of relationships are perhaps the most vulnerable to the types of marketplace and policy shifts that are currently occurring in the health care environment. If organizations do not make substantial investments in collaborative efforts for public health, then they have little incentive to continue to monitor and nurture these efforts in the face of larger health system changes. In this case, incurring substantial sunk costs in collaborative efforts may actually be beneficial if they provide motivation and rationale for sustained community health engagement.

Active Management

A second approach, involving active management of the public health–managed care interface, requires substantially greater investments of time, resources, and expertise in developing and maintaining relationships between public health organizations and managed care plans. These relationships require the participating organizations to

- Manage the competing missions and incentives of dissimilar organizations.
- Redesign and reprioritize clinical and administrative processes in relation to those of its partners.
- Invest core organizational resources in collaboration, and accept the risks and opportunity.
- Move beyond planning and assessment activities by implementing promising health improvement strategies.

Without achieving these types of commitments, the interface between public health and managed care will remain largely an unfulfilled promise about collaboration for population health. Meaningful improvements in health cannot be achieved through collaborative efforts without engaging at these much more difficult levels. Addressing society's most persistent health issues will require more institutional commitment, resource investment, and evidence-based coordination and management in the fields of public health practice and managed health care. Effective health improvement strategies must go beyond biomedical causes and interventions in approaching population health issues. Underlying social, cultural, and economic processes must be addressed at the population level through interdisciplinary approaches. Medicine and public health are natural allies for these types of interventions, and managed care provides a vehicle for this interaction.

Strategies for Health Plans

Public health organizations will not always serve as the initiating and sustaining forces for population-based, interorganizational efforts in health. Health plans must also be willing to assume leadership positions in these efforts and to create the conditions in which they can develop. For managers of health plans, several preliminary actions are necessary for engaging effectively in public health initiatives.

- Health plans must know the public health resources, skills, and leadership that are available within their service areas. Without this knowledge, plans can hardly anticipate what types of collaborative activity may be possible and desirable.
- Health plans must work to educate the public health community about their plan's objectives, skills, and methods for health improvement. These activities will help to overcome the inevitable negative images that some individuals in public health maintain about managed care, and allow public health agencies to realize shared interests with health plans.
- Health plans must identify specific areas of operation that can benefit from public

health knowledge and expertise. These may include activities involving clinical prevention, health education, lifestyle/behavior change, disease management, and surveillance and data systems. Health plans that do not already recognize the value of these types of activities in managing the health of populations will likely have difficulty in identifying meaningful areas of interaction with public health.

- Health plans must invest in relationship building around the identified areas that require public health knowledge and expertise. Effective relationships do not always emerge naturally and voluntarily from given circumstances. Organizations and their leaders must invest time, effort, and resources in building meaningful relationships that span the boundaries between managed care and public health.

• • •

Managed care is now the dominant form of health care delivery in the private and public sectors. As such, it shapes the nature and structure of relationships between medical practice and public health practice. The growing involvement of managed care plans in rural areas suggests that few public health organizations will be left unaffected by the evolving managed care industry. Managed care creates both opportunities and challenges for public health organizations. Effective managerial decision making in public health organizations is critical to protect essential public health functions and to forge new initiatives in public health improvement within the evolving health system. A variety of organizational structures and strategies can be used by public health organizations to manage their relationships with managed care plans effectively. The optimal mix of these arrangements is context specific and depends heavily on the objectives and incentives of the public health organizations and managed care plans involved.

The interaction between public health organizations and managed care plans entails both direct and indirect effects that must be considered carefully when developing and managing interorganizational relationships. Access to health care for the growing numbers of uninsured individuals is key among these indirect effects. The evolving health care marketplace and health policy environment create complex incentives for both managed care plans and public health organizations. Consequently, public health administrators must continually reexamine their relationships with plans and other stakeholders within the health care system. Among the institutions that comprise this system, public health organizations are uniquely situated to mobilize population-based improvements in managed care and in systems of care for the uninsured.

CHAPTER REVIEW

1. Managed care plans are organized health care systems that compete to assume clinical and financial responsibility for the health care needs of defined populations. Defining characteristics of managed care plans include
   - *selective contracting:* Plans select health care providers to include in their networks based on criteria such as efficiency in service delivery, service quality and patient satisfaction, service capacity, and geographic coverage (accessibility).
   - *utilization management:* Plans use both administrative and financial mechanisms to encourage efficient and effective service delivery and utilization patterns.
   - *competitive enrollment:* Plans compete with each other to attract purchasers and members, often on the basis of factors such as price (premiums and copayments), physician choice, covered services, and perceived quality. Plans also induce health care providers to compete for health plan contracts on the basis of efficiency and quality.

2. Public sector health insurance programs increasingly rely on managed care plans to control program costs and expand insurance coverage. Several states have expanded Medicaid coverage and benefit levels through managed care programs. More recently, the federal S-CHIP has allowed states to extend insurance coverage for previously uninsured children through managed care programs.
3. Most types of interaction between public health organizations and managed care plans can be distilled into three basic functional areas.
   - delivery of personal health services
   - exchange of health data and information
   - development and implementation of population-based interventions, policies, and regulations
4. A growing number of public health organizations interact with the managed care industry by carrying out policy implementation responsibilities designed to ensure the accessibility and quality of health services. Some governmental organizations carry out these responsibilities as purchasers of health services for public health insurance programs such as Medicaid and S-CHIP. Additionally, public health organizations interact with the managed care industry through the exercise of regulatory and licensing authority. Public health organizations participate in quality assurance and consumer protection initiatives carried out at federal and state governmental levels, as well as those carried out through industry-based efforts.
5. Managed care plans may affect public health organizations indirectly through their ability to influence the behavior of health care providers, consumers, and purchasers. Important indirect effects include
   - changes in medical practice precipitated by managed care plans, which may encourage improvements in clinical preventive services delivery and disease management
   - changes in the financial performance of health care providers, which may compromise their ability to provide care to the uninsured and other underserved populations
   - changes in the financial performance of academic health centers, which potentially constrain their ability to conduct clinical research and provide training to health professionals
   - changes in the availability and affordability of private health insurance coverage due to managed care growth, which may help to reduce the uninsured and underinsured populations

REFERENCES

1. W.L. Roper et al., "Public Health in the New American Health System," *Frontiers of Health Services Management 10,* no. 4 (1994): 32–36.
2. E.L. Baker et al., "Health Reform and the Health of the Public," *Journal of the American Medical Association 272* (1994): 1,276–1,282.
3. H.H. Schauffler and F.D. Scutchfield, "Managed Care and Public Health," *American Journal of Preventive Medicine 14,* no. 3 (1998): 240–241.
4. J. Showstack et al., "Health of the Public: The Private-Sector Challenge," *Journal of the American Medical Association 276,* no. 13 (1996): 1,071–1,074.
5. P.K. Halverson et al., *Managed Care and Public Health* (Gaithersburg, MD: Aspen Publishers, Inc., 1998).
6. U.S. Centers for Disease Control and Prevention, "Prevention and Managed Care: Opportunities for Managed Care Organizations, Purchasers of Health Care, and Public Health Agencies," *Morbidity and Mortality Weekly Review* RR-14 (1995): 1–13.
7. T. Citrin, "Topics for Our Times: Public Health—Community or Commodity? Reflections on Healthy Communities," *American Journal of Public Health 88,* no. 3 (1998): 351–352.
8. B.E. Dowd, "Financing Preventive Care in HMOs: A Theoretical Analysis," *Inquiry* 19 (1982): 68–78.
9. F.D. Scutchfield et al., "Managed Care and Public Health," *Journal of Public Health Management and Practice 4,* no. 1 (1998): 1–11.

10. W.L. Roper and G.P. Mays, "The Changing Managed Care–Public Health Interface," *Journal of the American Medical Association 280,* no. 20 (1998): 1,739–1,740.
11. R.D. Lasker, *Medicine and Public Health: The Power of Collaboration* (New York: New York Academy of Medicine, 1997), 2.
12. B.J. Turnock, *Public Health: What It Is and How It Works* (Gaithersburg, MD: Aspen Publishers, Inc., 1996).
13. U.S. Public Health Service, *For a Healthy Nation: Return on Investments in Public Health* (Washington, DC: U.S. Government Printing Office, 1994).
14. R.E. Brown et al., *National Expenditures for Health Promotion and Disease Prevention Activities in the United States* (Washington, DC: Medical Technology Assessment and Policy Research Center, 1991).
15. U.S. Department of Health and Human Services, Office of Disease Prevention and Health Promotion, *Health Care Reform and Public Health: A Paper Based on Population-Based Core Functions* (Washington, DC: U.S. Government Printing Office, 1993).
16. C.C. White et al., "Benefits, Risks and Costs of Immunization for Measles, Mumps and Rubella," *American Journal of Public Health 75,* no. 7 (1995): 739–744.
17. H. Luft, *Health Maintenance Organizations: Dimensions of Performance* (New York: John Wiley & Sons, 1981).
18. Interstudy, *The Competitive Edge 9.1: HMO Industry Report* (St. Paul, MN: 1999).
19. Hoechst Marion Roussel, *HMO-PPO Digest* (New York: 1998).
20. American Association of Health Plans, *HMO-PPO Trends Report* (Washington, DC: 1996).
21. D.W. Moran, "Federal Regulation of Managed Care: An Impulse in Search of a Theory?" *Health Affairs 16,* no. 6 (1997): 7–21.
22. J.C. Robinson, The Future of Managed Care Organizations," *Health Affairs 18,* no. 2 (1999): 7–24.
23. R.J. Blendon et al., "Understanding the Managed Care Backlash," *Health Affairs 17,* no. 4 (1998): 80–94.
24. M. Gold et al., *Arrangements between Managed Care Plans and Physicians: Results from a 1994 Survey of Managed Care Plans* (Washington, DC: Physician Payment Review Commission, 1995).
25. U.S. Health Care Financing Administration, *Medicare Managed Care Enrollment Report* (Washington, DC: 1999).
26. P. Neuman and K.M. Langwell, "Medicare's Choice Explosion? Implications for Beneficiaries," *Health Affairs 18,* no. 1 (1999): 150–160.
27. D.A. Freund and R.E. Hurley, "Medicaid Managed Care: Contribution to Issues of Health Reform," *Annual Review of Public Health* 16 (1995): 473–495.
28. A. Schneider and J. Stern, "Health Maintenance Organizations and the Poor: Problems and Prospects," *Northwestern University Law Review 70,* no. 1 (1975): 90–138.
29. A. Leibowitz et al., "A Randomized Trial To Evaluate the Effectiveness of a Medicaid HMO," *Journal of Health Economics 11,* no. 3 (1992): 235–257.
30. S. DesHarnis, "Enrollment in and Disenrollment from Health Maintenance Organizations by Medicaid Recipients," *Health Care Financing Review 6,* no. 3 (1985): 39–50.
31. R.E. Hurley et al., *Managed Care in Medicaid: Lessons for Policy and Program Design* (Ann Arbor, MI: Health Administration Press, 1993).
32. S. Rosenbaum et al., *Negotiating the New Health System: A Nationwide Study of Medicaid Managed Care Contracts* (Washington, DC: George Washington University Medical Center, 1997).
33. J. Holohan et al., "Insuring the Poor through Section 1115 Medicaid Waivers," *Health Affairs 14,* no. 1 (1995): 199–217.
34. U.S. Health Care Financing Administration, *1998 National Summary of State Medicaid Managed Care Programs* (Washington, DC: 1999).
35. U.S. Health Care Financing Administration, *Medicare and Medicaid Provisions of P.L.105–33: Balanced Budget Act of 1997* (Washington, DC: 1998).
36. U.S. Health Care Financing Administration, *1998 Medicaid Managed Care Enrollment Report* (Washington, DC: 1998).
37. National Governor's Association, *1999 State Children's Health Insurance Program Annual Report* (Washington, DC: 1999).
38. G.P. Mays et al., "Collaboration To Improve Community Health: Trends and Alternative Models," *Joint Commission Journal on Quality Improvement in Health Care 24,* no. 10 (1998): 518–540.
39. P.K. Halverson et al., "Privatizing Health Services: Alternative Models and Emerging Issues for Public Health and Quality Management," *Quality Management in Health Care 5,* no. 2 (1997): 1–18.
40. P. Lorange and J. Roos, *Strategic Alliances: Formation, Implementation, and Evolution* (Cambridge, MA: Blackwell, 1993).
41. S.M. Shortell et al., "The New World of Managed Care: Creating Organized Delivery Systems," *Health Affairs* 13 (1994): 46–64.
42. J.B. Goes and C.L. Zhan, "The Effects of Hospital-Physician Integration Strategies on Hospital Financial Performance," *Health Services Research* 30 (1995): 507–530.
43. C. Alter and J. Hage, *Organizations Working Together* (Newbury Park, CA: Sage Publications, 1993).
44. A.D. Kaluzny et al., *Partners for the Dance: Forming Strategic Alliances in Health Care* (Ann Arbor, MI: Health Administration Press, 1995).

45. J.B. Christianson et al., "The Structure of Strategic Alliances: Evidence from Rural Hospital Networks," in *Partners for the Dance: Strategic Alliances in Health Care*, eds. A.D. Kaluzny et al. (Ann Arbor, MI: Health Administration Press, 1995), 99–117.
46. A.C. Enthoven and C.B. Vorhaus, "A Vision of Quality in Health Care Delivery," *Health Affairs 16,* no. 3 (1997): 44–57.
47. S. Felt-Lisk and R. St. Peter, "Quality Assurance for Medicaid Managed Care," *Health Affairs 16,* no. 3 (1997): 248–252.
48. P.J. Silberman, "Ensuring Quality and Access under Managed Care," in *Managed Care and Public Health,* eds. P.K. Halverson et al. (Gaithersburg, MD: Aspen Publishers, Inc., 1998), 321–332.
49. W.L. Roper, "Regulating Quality and Clinical Practice," in *Regulating Managed Care: Theory, Practice, and Future Options,* eds. S.H. Altman et al. (San Francisco: Jossey-Bass, 1999), 145–159.
50. "Interim Rules for Health Insurance Portability for Group Health," *Federal Register 62,* no. 67 (1997).
51. L. Etheredge, "Promarket Regulation: An SEC-FASB Model," *Health Affairs 16,* no. 6 (1997): 22–25.
52. Watson Wyatt Worldwide and the Washington Business Group on Health, *Getting What You Pay For: Purchasing Value in Health Care* (Washington, DC: Watson Wyatt Worldwide, 1996).
53. S. Felt-Lisk et al., *Medicaid Managed Care: Does It Increase Primary Care Services in Underserved Areas?* (Washington, DC: Mathematica Policy Research, 1997).
54. S. Wall, "Transformations in Public Health Systems," *Health Affairs 17,* no. 3 (1998): 64–80.
55. G.P. Mays et al., "Health Promotion and Disease Prevention in Managed Care: Examining Strategies for Coverage, Delivery, and Use," *Compensation and Benefits Management 15,* no 4 (1999): 37–46.
56. P.J. Cunningham et al., "Managed Care and Physician's Provision of Charity Care," *Journal of the American Medical Association 281*, no. 12 (1999): 1,087–1,092.
57. J.M. Mann et al., "A Profile of Uncompensated Hospital Care, 1983–1995," *Health Affairs 16,* no. 4 (1997): 223–232.
58. M.A. Morrisey, "Movies and Myths: Hospital Cost Shifting," *Business Economics 30,* no. 2 (1995): 22–25.
59. D.A. Banks et al., "Uncompensated Hospital Care: Charitable Mission or Profitable Business Decision?" *Health Economics 6,* no. 2 (1997): 133–143.
60. J. Gruber, "The Effect of Competitive Pressure on Charity: Hospital Responses to Price Shopping in California," *Journal of Health Economics* 13 (1994): 183–212.
61. G.P. Mays, "Managed Care Contracting and Community Health Center Performance" (PhD dissertation, The University of North Carolina at Chapel Hill, Chapel Hill, NC, 1999).
62. M. Olfson et al., "Mental Health/Medical Care Cost Offsets: Opportunities for Managed Care," *Health Affairs 18*, no. 2 (1999): 79–90.
63. A.E. Roussel et al., "Primary Care Physicians' Participation in Managed Care Networks," *Journal of Ambulatory Care Management 22*, no. 2 (1999): 27–40.
64. M.R. Gold et al., "A National Survey of the Arrangements Managed-Care Plans Make with Physicians," *New England Journal of Medicine 333*, no. 25 (1995): 1678–1683.
65. G.P. Mays, "Case Study: Reconfiguring Memphis' Public Health System for Managed Care," in *Managed Care and Public Health,* eds. P.K. Halverson et al. (Gaithersburg, MD: Aspen Publishers, Inc., 1998), 243–251.
66. G.P. Mays, "Case Study: Integrated Public and Private Health Care Systems in Denver, Colorado," in *Managed Care and Public Health,* eds. P.K. Halverson et al. (Gaithersburg, MD: Aspen Publishers, Inc., 1998), 201–221.
67. D. Rowland et al., *Medicaid Managed Care: Lessons from the Literature* (Washington, DC: Kaiser Commission on the Future of Medicaid, 1995).
68. D.G. Safran et al., "Primary Care Performance in Fee-for-Service and Prepaid Health Care Systems: Results from the Medical Outcomes Study," *Journal of the American Medical Association 271*, no. 20 (1994): 1,579–1,586.
69. J.E. Ware, Jr. et al., "Differences in 4-Year Health Outcomes for Elderly and Poor, Chronically Ill Patients Treated in HMO and Fee-for-Service Systems," *Journal of the American Medical Association 276,* no. 13 (1996): 1,039–1,047.
70. R.H. Miller, "Does Managed Care Lead to Better or Worse Quality of Care?" *Health Affairs 16,* no. 5 (1997): 7–25.
71. R.A. Dudley et al., "The Impact of Financial Incentives on Quality of Health Care," *Milbank Quarterly 76*, no. 4 (1998): 511, 649–686.
72. T.A. Coughlin et al., "A Conflict of Strategies: Medicaid Managed Care and Medicaid Maximization," *Health Services Research 34*, no. 1, Part II (1999): 281–294.
73. L.I. Iezzoni, "Major Teaching Hospitals Defying Darwin," *Journal of the American Medical Association 278,* no. 6 (1997): 520.
74. E. Moy et al., "Relationship between National Institutes of Health Research Awards to US Medical Schools and Managed Care Market Penetration," *Journal of the American Medical Association 278,* no. 3 (1997): 217–221.
75. E.G. Campbell et al., "Relationship between Market Competition and the Activities and Attitudes of Medical School Faculty," *Journal of the American Medical Association 278,* no. 3 (1997): 222–226.

76. J.N. Thompson and J. Moskowitz, "Preventing the Extinction of the Clinical Research Ecosystem," *Journal of the American Medical Association 278,* no. 3 (1997): 241–244.

77. M. Meyer et al., "Clinical Research: Assessing the Future in a Changing Environment: Summary Report of Conference Sponsored by the American Medical Association Council on Scientific Affairs, Washington, DC, March 1996," *American Journal of Medicine 104*, no. 3 (1998): 264–271.

78. J.F. Sheils and R.A. Haught, *Managed Care Savings for Employers and Households: Impact on the Number of Uninsured* (Washington, DC: The Lewin Group, 1997).

79. S.H. Altman et al., *Regulating Managed Care: Theory, Practice, and Future Options* (San Francisco: Jossey-Bass, 1999).

80. G.P. Mays et al., *Local Public Health Practice: Trends and Models* (Washington, DC: American Public Health Association, 2000).

81. "Health Literacy: Report of the Council on Scientific Affairs," *Journal of the American Medical Association 281,* no. 6 (1999): 552–557.

82. R.E. Hurley and M.A. McCue, *Medicaid and Commercial HMOs: An At-Risk Relationship* (Princeton, NJ: Center for Health Care Strategies, 1998).

EPILOGUE

Population-Based Management and the Emerging Public Health System

Modern public health organizations manage change continuously. Very few elements of the contemporary public health environment remain static for any length of time. The health status of communities and population groups evolves in response to emerging disease risks, evolving patterns in human behavior, demographic shifts, and environmental and climactic turbulence. Chronic diseases are now our nation's leading causes of death, but new outbreaks such as the recent West Nile virus demonstrate the continued threats posed by emerging infectious diseases. Meanwhile, the professional knowledge and technology available to prevent and control disease continues to expand as the biomedical and behavioral sciences advance. For example, the public health profession now stands on the brink of a vast new knowledge base for disease prevention and control that has been made available by the sequencing of the human genome. Public health organizations also navigate a political and economic landscape that shifts rapidly and often unpredictably as public health issues compete with a variety of other interests for resources and public attention. All of these forces interact to create a volatile environment for carrying out public health activities within communities.

Public health organizations are uniquely skilled in using population-based approaches to manage change within the health environment. Although originally developed to control infectious disease epidemics, the basic principles of population-based management are being used on a much larger scale today, and by a much broader range of organizations and professions. These principles are now proving useful for purposes as varied as preventing and managing chronic diseases, reducing the incidence and effects of violence and unintentional injury, preparing for and responding to disasters, encouraging the delivery of clinical preventive services among medical care providers, and addressing the health care needs of the uninsured.

Perhaps even more importantly, the principles of population-based management are beginning to be applied across individual programs, organizations, interventions, and risk groups in order to create coordinated public health delivery systems. Increasingly, successful public health organizations use these principles to manage an intricate web of relationships with other institutions that influence community health—including medical care providers, health plans, employers and other health care purchasers, community-based organizations, consumer groups, and policy makers. The skills and strategies needed to manage these types of alliances are often far different from the management approaches that work in traditional bureaucratic settings. Organizations must make decisions and acquire the resources necessary for action without the clear lines of authority and control that exist within public and private bureaucracies. Managing peers rather than subordinates requires a new set of skills, especially in areas such as communications, constituency building, marketing, performance measurement, and leadership. To support new multi-institutional efforts, public health organizations must also transform their internal management approaches, including their strategies for financial management, human resources management, work force development, strategic planning and assessment, and organizational design and evaluation. Increasingly, these tasks must be oriented toward systemwide goals and objectives rather than the performance of individual programs and interventions.

The chapters in this text describe in detail the concepts and strategies of population-based management that empower public health organizations to improve community health. In applying these concepts to specific organizational and community settings, several recommendations may warrant special attention by public health decision makers.

- Carefully identify stakeholders and the entities to which the public health system is accountable. The public health system is ultimately accountable to the population it serves. To ensure that the system meets the needs and expectations of this population, public health organizations must maintain an open dialogue with the individuals and institutions that represent society's interest in health, including community-based organizations, elected political representatives, public and private purchasers of public health services, and consumer groups. Public health structures and activities should be designed to be optimally responsive to these important stakeholders.
- Seek out peers and potential partners using broad and inclusive criteria. Successful public health organizations may often find it necessary to "manage" partners that maintain considerably more resources and influence than they do, and that pursue vastly different institutional objectives. Public health administrators should not allow such differences to dissuade them from interorganizational cooperation and management. For-profit health care providers and multinational corporations, for example, should not be ruled out as potential public health partners. Rather, public health organizations should identify shared interests and then leverage their unique skills and resources to achieve these interests through the broadest possible forms of collaboration.
- Clearly define the values, goals, objectives, and activities (products) of the public health system. Public health organizations require a clear understanding of the objectives pursued by the public health system, and the services and activities performed by the system. This clear understanding and delineation is critical to the effective management of public health systems, particularly as these systems take on a complex array of multi-institutional partnerships and alliances. It is the public health organization's responsibility to ensure that all participants in the public health system share in this understanding of system objectives and activities.
- Use a broad set of administrative tools to manage partnerships and alliances. Traditionally, public health organizations have relied heavily on purchasing and regulatory authority to manage their relationships with external organizations. In the emerging public health system, organizations will need to manage a growing number of partnerships that extend beyond the simple purchase of goods and services and beyond the regulatory authority of governmental public health agencies. Public health organizations must rely on a broader set of strategies for interacting with partners and influencing their behavior and performance. Increasingly, public health organizations will need to use entrepreneurial strategies in marketing, communications, constituency development, resource development, and performance monitoring to establish effective partnerships for community health improvement.
- Monitor the output and outcomes of the public health system to support continual improvement. Like other organizations in the health system, public health organizations must have a clear understanding of

what the public health system is producing and how these products are affecting community heath status. Monitoring public health output and outcomes becomes an increasingly challenging yet increasingly important task as delivery systems become more complex through interorganizational partnerships. Consequently, partnerships should be designed with a monitoring and evaluation function in mind.

- Seek out innovations in public health management and practice through research, evaluation, and prototypes. Finally, public health organizations face an imperative to identify new and better ways of improving health continually at the population level. Without such innovations, public health organizations can have no hope of keeping pace with the rapid changes in population health needs and health system structures. Practice-based research and evaluation allow organizations to continually improve public health institutions and interventions using empirical measures of performance. In translating scientific findings into practice innovations, organizations can use small-scale prototypes and demonstrations to test innovations within real-world settings. Successful innovations can be expanded while failures can be discontinued with little risk and expense.

The fundamental question facing the public health system of the future is the capacity of the population-based approach to achieve further gains in community health outcomes. Can the earlier public health successes in sanitation and immunization be replicated in reducing the risk behaviors responsible for the bulk of otherwise preventable mortality? Are complex psychosocial problems such as violence, unintended pregnancies, racial and ethnic disparities in health, and mental illness amenable to population-based strategies? The emerging public health system appears increasingly well positioned for populationwide approaches to these health issues. Increasingly, we have the information, expertise, and organizational capacity necessary to develop and sustain such approaches. The remaining challenge lies in the ability of public health decision makers to manage these collective health resources and skills appropriately at the population level so as to achieve gains in community health. Population-based management offers the perspective and the process to make these gains possible.

Glossary

Account: a federal program under consideration by the congressional appropriations process.

Accreditation: the periodic issuance of credentials and endorsements to organizations that meet a specified set of performance standards. Several states have developed accreditation processes for local public health agencies.

Adjusted rates: numerical measures of disease risk or health outcomes that are statistically transformed to adjust for the effects of a characteristic that may influence risk. The most common adjustment is for age.

Administrative procedure acts: policies established by both state and federal legislatures that govern the deliberative processes that public agencies must undertake in issuing rules.

Agent: a causal factor associated with disease. The agent can be infectious, toxic, or environmental.

AIDS service organizations (ASOs): community-based organizations that provide educational information concerning the spread of the HIV epidemic, as well as support for persons with AIDS and HIV.

Alliance: a cooperative relationship formed between two or more organizations to accomplish a shared objective or pursue a common interest. Alliances may or may not be formalized through contractual agreements (see also *partnership*).

Annual appropriations: provide new budget authority for the particular fiscal year for which they were enacted.

APHA: American Public Health Association, a national membership organization of public health professionals, researchers, educators, and advocates.

Appropriations bills: legislative proposals that determine spending levels for programs and that are specifically prohibited from creating programmatic changes.

Assessment: the process of regularly and systematically collecting, assembling, analyzing, and making available information on the health needs of the community, including statistics on health status, community health needs, and epidemiologic and other studies of health problems. Assessment is one of the three core functions of public health agencies as identified by the Institute of Medicine.

Assessment Protocol for Excellence in Public Health (APEXPH): an assessment and planning tool designed to help public health organizations identify operational strengths and weaknesses within their institutions and to identify and prioritize health risks and health resources within the communities they serve. The tool assists organizations in developing action plans to address internal weaknesses and to respond to opportunities and threats in the community. The tool was developed by the National Association for County and City Health Officials in cooperation with CDC.

Assurance: process of assuring that a population has access to the health services that are necessary to achieve agreed-upon health status goals. Public health organizations may carry out this process by encouraging the efforts of other service providers (private or public sector), by requiring such actions through regulation, or by providing services directly.

ASTHO: Association of State and Territorial Health Officials, a membership organization composed of the senior administrators of state and territorial public health agencies.

ASTLHLO: Association of State and Territorial Local Health Liaison Officials, a membership organization composed of state officials that provide information, assistance, and advocacy for local public health agencies within their state.

Attribute data: health, social, and environmental information that can be linked with other types of data using geographical location information.

Autonomy: the right of individuals to behave according to their own reason.

Bias: a systematic error in measuring the effect of an intervention or the statistical associations among variables of interest. The three most common sources of bias in public health research involve the selection of observations (e.g., cases and controls), the classification of observations, and the treatment of confounding variables.

Biostatistics: the application of statistical theories and methods to the study of biomedical and health processes at the individual and population levels.

Bioterrorism: the malicious release of biological agents into the environment to affect human health adversely.

Bivariate analysis: statistical methods for examining statistical associations between two variables of interest.

Block grant: a mechanism for allocating governmental funds to support programs operated at lower governmental levels, such that considerable discretion in use of funds is given to grantees within broadly defined program areas.

Board of health: a body of individuals appointed to advise or provide oversight to the governmental public health agency. Boards may be appointed by local elected officials to serve local agencies and by state officials to serve state agencies. Appointees often include health professionals, community representatives, and elected officials.

BRFSS: the behavioral risk factor surveillance system, maintained by the Centers for Disease Control and Prevention to collect information from U.S. adult residents about health-related behavior, health status, and health care access.

Budget authority: federal rules established by congressional law that govern the extent to which federal agencies can incur financial obligations.

Budget conferencing: meetings held between elected officials in the U.S. Senate and U.S. House of Representatives to resolve differences in the budget resolutions passed by each legislative body.

Budget reconciliation: process of legislative negotiation and decision making whereby elected officials balance the financial needs of authorized governmental programs with the realities of governmental budget levels.

Budget resolution: blueprint to establishing budget priorities and define parameters for all subsequent budgetary actions for that year.

Buffering: feature of GIS analysis where polygons are created based on the distance from a target object. This can be used to identify risk of exposure to environmental hazards.

Capitation: a compensation method commonly used by managed care plans for paying health care providers, in which a flat monthly fee is paid to the provider for each plan member that enrolls with the provider, regardless of the amount of health care resources used by the member.

Categorical grant funding: governmental grant-in-aid programs that specify detailed requirements regarding how funds are to be used by the grant recipient, including specifications for the types of services to be produced and the types of population groups to be served.

Census Bureau: federal agency charged with designing and implementing surveillance systems to collect demographic, economic, and social statistics on the U.S. population.

Centers for Disease Control and Prevention (CDC): the federal government's leading public health agency, charged with conducting research on the detection, prevention, and control of diseases and causes of injury; maintaining surveillance systems to track diseases, health risks, and health care trends in the U.S. population; and maintaining programs, resources, and interventions that protect the public's health. The CDC consists of 11 centers, institutes, and offices.

Centralized-authority public health system: a means of allocating governmental public health authority and control at the state level such that local public health agencies operate under the direct authority of the state government and therefore function as administrative units of the state health agency.

Chairman's mark: a legislative budget proposal created by each federal budget committee chair.

Channels of communication: methods by which organizations or individuals exchange information.

Chloropleth map: a map displaying geographic variation in a characteristic of interest using shading or colors.

Coalition: a group of individuals and/or organizations that join together for a common purpose.

Combination funding: the use of more than one method to allocate financial resources to public health agencies. Usually this involves per capita funding for basic public health services in combination with specific grants for discrete local activities or local staff.

Community engagement: strategies for attracting the interest of community members in public health issues and motivating these members to participate in the design, implementation, and evaluation of public health interventions.

Community health centers: not-for-profit ambulatory care centers that provide an array of primary care and preventive health services to communities and population groups that are underserved by mainstream medical providers. Most centers provide care without regard to the client's ability to pay for services. Many centers receive financial support from federal grant programs administered by the U.S. Health Resources and Services Administration.

Community Health Improvement Process (CHIP): a model developed by the Institute of Medicine for identifying community health needs and developing interventions to address these needs. The CHIP model uses a broad definition of health and proceeds with a community effort to maintain and improve health with progress measured by performance indicators.

Community-based organizations: organizations formed and directed by members of a community to address needs and issues within the community.

Community-based programs: public health interventions that are designed, implemented, and evaluated with the participation of community representatives and with the guidance of professional expertise.

Competitive enrollment: the process by which managed care plans compete with each other to attract purchasers and enrolled members, often on the basis of price, physician choice, covered services, and perceived quality.

Comprehensive health planning (CHP): formalized processes for identifying community health resource needs, priorities, and allocation strategies, initially carried out by local and state planning agencies under the Comprehensive Planning Act of 1966 and the National Health Planning and Resource Development Act of 1974.

Conference report: a final report of legislative appropriations actions proposed for a federal program by leaders in the U.S. House of Representatives and U.S. Senate. This report is sent back to each legislative body for final passage.

Constituencies (for public health organizations): organizations and individuals that have an interest in the activities performed by the public health organization. Constituencies are often defined to include clients of public health programs, staff, community residents, policymakers, governing board members, health-related organizations and professionals in the community, and area businesses and employers.

Continuing resolution: permits Congress to continue funding for a federal program at current levels through a specified time period.

Contract funding: the use of a negotiated contract to fund the public health services provided at the local level. Usually local health departments annually submit a funding application to the state health agency to receive funds available through funds allocated for local public health services.

Core public health functions: activities regarded as essential elements of public health practice at local, state, and national levels. The Institute of Medicine identified three core functions in its 1988 review of the U.S. public health system: (1) assessment, (2) policy, and (3) assurance.

Cost-benefit analysis: an economic analysis in which the total costs and total benefits of an intervention are measured and valued in monetary terms and then compared.

Cost-effectiveness analysis: an economic analysis in which the total costs of an intervention are measured in monetary terms and then compared with the outcomes achieved by the intervention (such as lives saved or quality-adjusted life-years produced). The cost-to-outcome ratio indicates the total cost of achieving a particular outcome of interest using the intervention under study. This ratio can be used to compare the cost-effectiveness of the intervention with that of other interventions that produce the same outcome.

Crude data/statistics/rates: data (or statistics or rates) that are based on simple counts of events and that are not adjusted for confounding variables.

Cultural competency: the ability to communicate acceptance, understanding, and responsiveness to the needs and concerns of members of diverse cultural populations. A thorough knowledge of the values, traditions, and customs of diverse cultures is often required to communicate effectively with members of these cultures.

Decentralized-authority public health system: a means of allocating governmental public health authority and control at the state level such that local public health agencies operate under the direct administrative authority of local governments rather than state governments.

Declaration of Helsinki: published by the World Medical Association in 1964, this initiative developed principles to guide research involving human subjects, including principles for obtaining the informed consent of research participants.

Determinants: broad causal factors involved in influencing health and illness, including social, economic, genetic, perinatal, nutritional, behavioral, and environmental characteristics.

Disasters: ecological disruptions, or emergencies, of a severity and magnitude that result in significant death, injury, illness, or property damage that cannot be effectively managed by the application of routine public safety procedures and resources and that result in a call for outside assistance.

Discretionary programs: federal programs for which funding levels are determined annually through the congressional appropriations process. Funding levels are determined through 13 general appropriations bills and several other special purpose appropriations bills, including those for emergency appropriations.

Earmarking: legislative processes for ensuring that appropriated funds are spent for a specific project or in a specific location.

Ecologic fallacy: making false assumptions about the nature of association between an exposure and an outcome by attempting to make individual-level inferences from group-level data (e.g., populations residing in a geographic area). The fallacy occurs by assuming that results based on group data can be applied to individuals who comprise the group.

Effectiveness: the extent to which a program or other intervention produces intended outcomes in actual practice settings rather than under optimal conditions.

Efficacy: the extent to which a program or other intervention produces intended outcomes under the controlled conditions of an experiment or controlled trial.

Emergencies: any health threat that requires an immediate response. These events can be the result of nature (e.g., hurricanes, tornadoes, and earthquakes), caused by technological or manmade error (e.g., nuclear accidents, bombing, and bioterrorism), or the result of emerging diseases (e.g., West Nile virus in New York City).

Empowerment evaluation: a process for both assessing and improving the performance of a program or intervention. Steps include examining the program's operational strengths and weaknesses, identifying its primary goals and achievements, developing self-initiated strategies to achieve goal fulfillment, and determining the type of evidence that will document credible progress.

Enforcement: the process of ensuring that governmental laws and regulations are followed by the individuals and institutions who are covered by them. Most governmental public health agencies are given the enforcement authority to inspect premises and businesses, investigate health-related complaints, and monitor the activities of organizations and individuals who fall under the health and safety statutes and administrative rules of the governmental jurisdiction.

Entitlement programs: programs that require funding levels to be set such that specified benefits can be paid to the persons, states, governments, or other entities eligible for such benefits under the authorizing law.

Environmental health: the application of multiple scientific disciplines to investigate the relationship between environmental factors and human health, and to prevent adverse health events that result from environmental exposures.

Environmental health continuum: the path that environmental hazards follow from their sources to their effects on community health.

Epidemic: the occurrence of a disease or other health event in a population at levels that exceed normal occurrence.

Epidemiologic triad: the interaction of host factors, environment, and disease agents in the causation of human disease.

Epidemiology: the study of disease mechanisms and health processes in populations, including disease etiology, disease transmission, disease prevention, and disease control. The discipline of epidemiology focuses on the interaction of host factors, disease agents, and environmental conditions in determining disease transmission and progression.

Epidemiology Program Office (CDC): supports the development and use of epidemiologic surveillance systems, analytic methods, and tools throughout the CDC and the public health organizations with which it interacts. Among other activities, this office maintains the National Notifiable Diseases Surveillance System, which tracks the incidence of 52 high-priority infectious diseases among U.S. residents.

Essential Public Health Services: a descriptive categorization of core activities used by public health organizations and professionals in carrying out population-based health promotion and disease prevention efforts. The categorization, identified by a work group convened by the U.S. Department of Health and Human Services, includes 10 essential services.

Evaluation: the process of critically examining the inputs, processes, outputs, and outcomes of a program or other intervention—usually in relation to established goals, objectives, and standards—to determine its operational strengths and weaknesses. Evaluations produce information about which programs work and also which program components work most effectively. Information obtained from evaluations is most often used for program appraisal, management, and improvement.

Evidence-based planning: a process for planning and designing public health interventions in which two levels of scientific evidence are considered: (1) evidence about the importance of a particular health condition and its link with some preventable risk factor in the population of interest; and (2) evidence about the relative effectiveness of specific actions to address the health condition of interest.

Experimental designs: studies that measure the effect of an intervention by comparing the outcomes observed among a group of subjects treated with the intervention (the treatment group) with outcomes observed among an equivalent group of subjects not treated with the intervention (the control group). Equivalent treatment and control groups are typically constructed by randomly assigning study participants to each group.

Externality: harmful or beneficial side effects created by the production or consumption of a commodity and borne by those who are not directly involved in the production or consumption of the commodity.

Federal budget: a comprehensive accounting of the federal government's spending revenues and borrowing. The budget reflects the nation's priorities for spending on public programs.

Federal Register: a daily report of all public documents issued by the President and federal agencies that describes actions taken and actions proposed by the executive branch of government.

Federalism: the separation of governmental power and authority into federal and state jurisdictions. New federalism refers to the recent trend of delegating authority to states that formerly resided in the federal government, through the actions of executive, legislative, and judicial bodies at the federal level.

Filibuster: a series of legislative procedures undertaken to slow the pace of legislative activity.

Formative evaluation: the earliest stage of process evaluation consists of preliminary assessments before a traditional program evaluation. Qualitative methods are often used such as focus groups and structured interviews to understand a process or system.

Formula funding: the distribution of funds to local health units based on a formula that incorporates variables indicating demographic, economic, social, and health characteristics within the population. The formulas include variables such as population size, per capita income, assessed land value, health insurance coverage, and disease rates.

Free-standing agency: one of two basic organizational structures for state public health agencies in which public health activities are organized within an agency that is administratively separate from governmental agencies responsible for other health and social services programs, that is headed by an administrator who reports directly to the state's governor.

Geocoding: the process of assigning geographic location information to attribute data that are to be used for analytic purposes.

GIS: geographic information systems that are computer-based processes for capturing, linking, summarizing, and analyzing data containing geographical location information. These systems are particularly useful in supporting visual analysis and communication of data using maps that display the geographic distribution of data.

Hazard: the probability of an occurrence of a disaster caused by a natural phenomenon (e.g., earthquake, tropical cyclone), by failure of manmade technology (e.g., nuclear reactor meltdown, industrial explosion), or by uncontrolled human activity (e.g., warfare, overgrazing).

Health information system (HIS): a collection of computer-based processes for collecting, storing, searching, retrieving, analyzing, reporting, and communicating health-related information both within and between organizations. The system includes processes for linking multiple data sources.

Health Maintenance Organization (HMO): often regarded as the most restrictive form of managed care plan, HMOs provide health insurance coverage only for health services that members of the plan obtain from providers that are affiliated with the plan. HMOs receive capitated monthly payments for each plan member and in return cover the full cost of all medically necessary health services provided to members by network providers. HMO members typically pay small copayments for each visit to a health care provider. Each member of an HMO is assigned to a primary care physician or group of physicians who serve as case managers and gatekeepers for all care that the member requires. HMOs may directly employ physicians (staff model), contract on an exclusive basis with multispecialty physician groups (group model), or contract on a nonexclusive basis with a number of physician groups and independent physician practices (network and independent practice association [IPA] models).

Health promotion: any combination of educational, organizational, environmental, and economic interventions designed to encourage behavior and conditions of living that are conducive to health.

Health status objectives: established goals and specific targets for health improvement at the population level. Usually objectives are linked to specific health status measures that are used to track progress toward the goal.

Healthy Communities projects: broad-based initiatives to improve health status within defined communities. Many of these initiatives can be traced to the 1986 meeting of the World Health Organization (WHO), where the development of the WHO Europe Healthy Cities Project launched a series of efforts to improve the quality of life in European cities. The role of local government in establishing the conditions of a healthy city coupled with a contemporary notion of health promotion has resulted in the implementation of a variety of health improvement initiatives in European cities. In the United States, projects have received support from state governments and from a partnership between the U.S. Office of Health Promotion and Disease Prevention and the National Civic League. As of mid-1995, more than 200 self-proclaimed Healthy Cities and Healthy Communities initiatives have been launched in the United States.

Healthy People 2000: a publication of the U.S. Department of Health and Human Services establishing national health promotion and disease prevention goals and objectives to be accomplished by the year 2000.

Healthy People 2010: an update of the Healthy People 2000 document, establishing national health promotion and disease prevention goals and objectives to be accomplished by the year 2010.

HEDIS: Health Plan Employer Data and Information Set, the most widely used set of performance measures for managed care plans.

Hold (legislative): a legislative mechanism used by individual members of the U.S. Senate to block a bill or nomination from consideration by the full Senate.

Home rule authority: governmental powers delegated to local governments that allow them to adopt their own constitutions and exercise a broad range of powers that are otherwise reserved for state governments, such as levying and collecting taxes to support local programs and services.

Host: an individual who is potentially susceptible to a disease.

Incidence: the number of new cases of disease occurring in a defined population during a specified time period.

Indicator: an element used to measure health status, risk, or outcome.

Infant mortality rate: the annual number of live-born infants who die during their first year of life, expressed per 1,000 live births.

Information Network for Public Health Officials (INPHO): a national program supporting electronic communication and exchange of health-related information among state and local public health officials, sponsored by the CDC.

Infrastructure: basic support for the delivery of public health activities such as work force, information systems, physical plant and equipment, and organizational structures.

Institutional Review Boards (IRBs): committees established at research institutions and health services organizations to review research proposals to ensure the safety of the research proposed and to ensure the adequacy of the process by which researchers propose to obtain informed consent from research participants.

Labor-H Bill: the bill that funds most health programs included in the federal budget, except for entitlement programs.

Leadership: behavior that goes beyond required performance expectations within an organization or community to provide direction and motivation for the behavior of others.

Local funding: reliance on locally collected funds and grants to support public health services.

Logic model: a description of the logical sequence of events that connect an intervention to the desired effect. This is useful in evaluating complex interventions or simple interventions in complex causal chains.

Low birth weight (LBW): weight at birth of less than 2,500 grams; very low birth weight is defined as weight at birth of less than 1,500 grams.

Managed care: a system of health care delivery and financing in which organized health care plans compete to assume both clinical and financial responsibility for the health care needs of defined populations. Plans within this system play active roles in (a) selecting the providers that deliver services to plan member, (b) negotiating the prices paid to health care providers, (c) establishing the conditions under which specific types of health services are covered by the plan, and (d) monitoring the delivery practices of providers and the utilization patterns of patients to encourage efficient and appropriate service delivery.

Mandatory spending: expenditures that the federal government is obliged by law to incur, including interest on debt and funding for entitlement programs such as Medicare and Social Security.

Manmade disasters: occurrences that involve technological events or disasters that are not caused by natural hazards but that occur in human settlements, such as fire, chemical spills and explosions, and armed conflict. Also called complex emergencies.

Marketing (in public health): processes for shaping awareness of and attitudes about specific public health issues and interventions to influence individual health behavior and to mobilize public support for core public health policies and institutions.

Mark-up: legislative committee amendments to a committee chairperson's federal budget proposal.

Medicaid: the largest joint federal/state entitlement program. Provides payment for health care services for certain groups of low-income individuals. Encompasses three distinct funding areas: (1) long-term care for chronically ill, disabled, and aged persons; (2) comprehensive medical care for low-income children and families; and (3) payments to assist hospitals that serve disproportionate shares of uninsured and publicly insured patient populations.

Medicare: a federal health insurance program covering individuals who are 65 years or older, who are permanently disabled, or who have end-stage renal disease.

Merit or Civil Service System: a body of protocols commonly used by governmental agencies in recruiting, hiring, and advancing employees. Protocols are designed to help minimize patronage that can exist in political organizations. Provisions include competitive examinations, probationary periods, and protection from political pressures.

Meta-analysis: a method for integrating and summarizing findings from multiple individual research studies to draw conclusions about the body of evidence as a whole. Individual study results are used as the unit of analysis to identify areas of consensus and divergence among the results.

Misclassification bias: measurement error that occurs when data elements are incorrectly grouped (or classified) during the data collection phase.

Mixed-authority public health system: a means of allocating governmental public health authority and control at the state level such that some local public health agencies within the state function as administrative units of the state health agency whereas other local agencies function under the authority of local governments.

Mobilization: stimulating and organizing people and resources for active involvement in a public health activity.

Modeling: a spatial analysis process that can identify risk factors for disease.

Morbidity: characteristics of disease severity, progression, and burden, including the disease's biomedical, functional, and psychological effects on health status.

Mortality rate: a measure of the number of people dying with a disease in a population over a specified period of time.

Multidisciplinary core competencies: the collection of knowledge and skills needed for effective public health practice, including concepts from the natural sciences, social sciences, and public health sciences.

Multivariate analysis: statistical methods that allow the researcher to control for the effects of multiple variables in predicting an outcome or describing an association.

NACCHO: National Association of County and City Health Officials, a membership organization composed of the administrators of local public health agencies throughout the nation.

NALBOH: National Association of Local Boards of Health, a membership organization representing individuals appointed to serve on governing and advisory boards for local public health agencies.

National Center for Chronic Disease Prevention and Health Promotion (CDC): fields research and development activities involving chronic disease prevention and early intervention for health issues such as cancer, cardiovascular disease, diabetes, arthritis, and the special health concerns of maternal, infant, and adolescent populations. Among other activities, this center fields the Behavioral Risk Factor Surveillance System, which collects periodic national and state-level data on adult health risk factors.

National Center for Environmental Health (CDC): fields research and intervention efforts designed to forestall illness, disability, and death due to human interaction with harmful environmental substances such as indoor and outdoor air pollutants, hazardous wastes, waterborne pathogens and pollutants, foodborne pathogens, and lead exposure.

National Center for Health Statistics (CDC): functions as the nation's public health data repository by fielding national surveys of health status, health behavior, and health care practices and by maintaining vital and health statistics databases. Among the periodic national surveys and surveillance systems fielded by the center are the National Health Care Survey, the National Immunization Survey, the National Health Interview Survey, and the National Health and Nutrition Examination Survey. The center also maintains efforts for tracking national statistics on prenatal care, births, and deaths through the National Vital Statistics System.

National Center for HIV, STD, and TB Prevention (CDC): administers surveillance and disease prevention and control programs that target the transmission of the serious and often interrelated communicable diseases of human immunodeficiency virus (HIV), other sexually transmitted diseases (STDs), and tuberculosis (TB).

National Center for Infectious Diseases (CDC): sponsors research and program development activities designed to prevent and control a wide array of existing, emerging, and resurgent infectious diseases, including those that pose unique health threats due to drug resistance or intentional transmission through bioterrorist acts.

National Center for Injury Prevention and Control (CDC): designs and fields research and intervention programs that focus on the prevention of both unintentional and intentional injuries occurring outside the workplace.

National Commission for the Protection of Human Subjects of Biomedical and Behavioral Research: established by the National Research Act of 1974, this body of experts issued the report "Ethical Principles and Guidelines for the Protection of Human Subjects of Research," which is also known as the Belmont Report.

National Immunization Program (CDC): oversees national and state-based efforts to expand age-appropriate vaccination coverage rates for children, adolescents, and adults. This agency has been heavily involved in the development of immunization registries and tracking systems at the provider level, the community level, and the state level.

National Institute for Occupational Safety and Health (CDC): supports scientific investigations of workplace health threats and designs prevention and control programs to improve safety and wellness and reduce health risks within occupational settings.

Natural disasters: rapid, acute onset events having widespread effects, such as earthquakes, floods, tropical cyclones, and tornadoes.

Natural–technological disasters: natural events that create technological emergencies, such as urban fires resulting from seismic motion or chemical spills resulting from floods.

Notifiable Disease Reporting: federal and state surveillance processes that require health professionals and laboratories to report information on confirmed cases of diseases to designated public health agencies. The CDC defines notifiable diseases as those for which regular, frequent, and timely information regarding individual cases is considered necessary for the prevention and control of disease. Currently, approximately 50 notifiable diseases are defined by CDC; other diseases are defined by individual state health agencies.

Obligations: requirements that governmental agencies must meet as a condition of entering into contracts, employing personnel, and purchasing goods and services.

Observation bias: measurement error that occurs when either the research subjects or the research investigators are not blinded to the exposure status of the subjects.

Omnibus appropriations: a consolidated federal bill that includes spending provisions for multiple federal programs if Congress runs out of time to consider each of the 13 appropriations bills separately.

Outlays: the actual payment for obligations incurred by governmental agencies, usually in the form of electronic transfers or checks from the Treasury Department.

Partnership: a cooperative relationship formed between two or more organizations to achieve a shared goal or pursue a common interest.

Passback: notification of pending federal budget decisions.

Paternalism: governmental activities that purport to advance the welfare and health of a defined population by imposing restrictions on the rights and freedoms of individuals within the population.

PAYGO rules: federal legislative rules that apply to new bills involving direct spending and revenue collection activities, such that Congress and the President are held accountable for any increase in the federal spending deficit as a result of legislative action.

Per capita funding: the distribution of state funding to local health units based solely on the population base served by the local health units.

Performance measurement: an analytic approach used to track the work produced and results achieved by public health organizations, often in relation to established goals and standards. Performance measures can be specified to monitor and compare the inputs, processes, outputs, and outcomes of public health organizations. Organizations use the results of performance measurement activities to improve the effectiveness and efficiency of their operations and to demonstrate accountability for public funds.

Performance standard (in public health): an expectation of the work to be produced or the outcomes to be achieved by public health organizations. Expectations may be based on expert opinion or scientific evidence concerning best practices in public health. Standards are used to evaluate measures of public health performance and to identify performance gaps in need of improvement.

Point of order: a legislative rule prohibiting the U.S. Senate from considering any direct spending or revenue legislation that would violate the PAYGO requirements by increasing the deficit.

Point of service plan (POS): a hybrid of the HMO and PPO managed care plans. POS members can access services from providers within their HMO network without incurring substantial out-of-pocket expenses, but they can also obtain care from out-of-network providers by paying established deductible and coinsurance fees.

Police power: the inherent authority of the state (and, through delegation, local government) to enact laws and promulgate regulations to protect, preserve, and promote the health, safety, and general welfare of the people.

Policy development: processes by which public health organizations formulate policies and plans to address priority health issues for the populations they serve, and advocate for the adoption and implementation of these policies by legislative and regulatory bodies and by private sector institutions. Policy development processes typically involve planning and priority-setting efforts that include broad participation by community members as well as health-related professionals and institutions.

Population-based intervention: a strategy for preventing and controlling disease by targeting groups rather than individuals, and thereby addressing the population-level processes that influence disease. Target groups are defined by behaviors, environmental exposure, geographic location, or other risk factors.

Population-based management: an administrative strategy that seeks to maximize expected health and well-being across an entire community or population, rather than maximizing outputs and outcomes within specific programs and organizations. Population-based management requires public health professionals to make optimal decisions across multiple interventions, institutions, and risk groups—rather than within them.

Practice guideline: a standardized set of information describing best practices for addressing health problems commonly encountered in public health practice. Information is based on scientific evidence of the effectiveness and efficiency of the practices described. Where such evidence is lacking, guidelines are often based on the consensus opinions of public health experts.

PRECEDE: a model of health education to influence voluntary health behaviors with specific planning phases.

Preferred provider organization (PPO): a managed care plan consisting of a network of health care providers who agree to serve health plan members on a discounted fee-for-service basis. PPO members incur lower deductibles and coinsurance when they obtain care from providers included on this network, but they also receive insurance coverage for services obtained from non-network providers, in exchange for higher coinsurance fees.

Prevalence: the number of cases of disease present in a community at a particular time or in a specified time period. This number is related both to the incidence and the duration of the disease.

Prevention Research Centers: federally funded research centers operated by academic health institutions to conduct scientific investigations about preventive health interventions. The development of the Prevention Research Centers (PRCs) marks a significant federal effort to unite the academic missions with public health and community interests. In 1984 Congress enacted Public Law 98–551, legislation that authorized the creation of the Health Promotion and Disease Prevention Center Program designed to establish a national network of academic centers for prevention research. These centers, 23 at the present and implemented through the CDC, include multidisciplinary faculty emphasizing community-based training in health promotion. The multidisciplinary public health expertise and the community involvement are distinguishing.

Primary prevention: the prevention of a disease by mechanisms that prevent its initiation including by modifying the environment (assurance of water quality) or reducing the susceptibility of the individual (immunization).

Privatization: the process of transferring part or all responsibility for performing selected governmental activities to private sector organizations. Most often this transfer occurs through a contract negotiated between the governmental agency and the private sector vendor(s). Some local health departments have contracted out entire personal health programs to private providers, while maintaining a monitoring oversight role.

PROCEED: a model of health promotion that includes health education at its core along with other types of organizational and regulatory interventions.

Process evaluations: methods for assessing the operation and output of a program, where a relationship is assumed between program outputs and outcomes, possibly based on previous research.

Public good: a commodity for which consumption by one individual does not reduce its availability to other individuals, such that the benefits of the commodity can accrue to a broad cross section of the population that has access to it.

Public health approach: health interventions and activities that are designed to achieve population-level improvements in health rather than individual health improvement. These activities typically involve one or more of the core public health functions of assessment, policy development, and assurance.

Public health authority: an independent governmental unit authorized by state charter to deliver specified public health services through contracts and agreements with local governments. Authorities operate relatively independently of state and local elected officials, although they rely on both state and local revenue sources. Authorities typically operate under more flexible purchasing and personnel rules than those that cover county and state governmental units.

Public health education: uses a combination of methods and learning opportunities designed to facilitate voluntary adaptations of behavior conducive to health.

Public health laboratories (PHLs): conduct biological, chemical, and environmental analyses to support epidemiologic investigation and scientific inquiry by public health organizations. Laboratories are operated at federal, state, and local levels.

Public health law: study of the legal powers and duties of the state to ensure the conditions for people to be healthy and the limitations on the power of the state to constrain the interests of individuals including autonomy and privacy.

Public Health Practice Program Office (CDC): performs research, technical assistance, program development, and evaluative activities designed to strengthen the nation's public health infrastructure and improve the organization and operation of state and local public health systems. This office sponsors initiatives that target the development of state and local public health agencies and administrators, public health laboratories, public health information systems, and global public health work force and infrastructure capacities.

Public health system: the network of organizations and professionals that participate in producing public health serves for a defined population or community. This network includes governmental public health agencies as well as relevant health care and social service providers, community-based organizations, and private institutions with an interest in population health.

QARR: specific quality assurance reporting requirements designed to examine managed care performance.

Quasi-experimental designs: research studies that rely on comparisons between treatment and control groups that may not be equivalent because they were not prospectively and randomly selected. Statistical methods such as multivariate analysis are used to control for baseline differences between control and treatment groups. The evidence produced by these studies is not as definitive as that yielded in experimental designs.

Regional Medical Planning (RMP): a federally sponsored planning program legislated in 1965 with the goal of coordinating federally funded programs. This program was directed at the not-for-profit sector. Planning consisted of cooperative teaching and research activities centered in the medical schools and their hospitals.

Registries: listings maintained and updated of individuals with specific diseases or health problems. Passive registries accept reports but do not update or confirm information. Active registries seek data and use follow-up to obtain more reliable and complete information.

Reimbursement funding: a mechanism used to allocate financial resources to public health organizations such that the organizations are reimbursed for the estimated cost of providing a specific set of services.

Relative risk: a measure of disease incidence among individuals who were exposed to the characteristic of interest, relative to the incidence among unexposed individuals. The relative risk provides an indication of the strength of an association between the characteristic and the exposure.

Reliability: the degree to which an indicator consistently measures the concept of interest.

Report language: an explanation of the intent of a specific legislative provision. This language does not have the force of law, but is useful in establishing a legislative history.

Reportable Diseases: collection of data at national, state, and local levels on selected diseases.

Research synthesis: the process of summarizing and integrating research findings identified from a comprehensive literature review so that they can be translated into practice and policy. Meta-analysis is a specific type of research synthesis that quantifies the degree of consensus existing among research findings.

Revenue measures: taxation programs used by governments to collect financial resources.

Rider: a legislative provision attached to appropriations bills that does not affect spending levels but rather changes policy.

Risk assessment: a systematic approach to quantifying the risks posed to individuals and populations by environmental pollutants and other potentially harmful exposures.

Risk factor: a factor associated with the occurrence of disease. This is an association and not necessarily causal.

Risk reduction objectives: goals and targets for reducing behaviors that lead to increased risk for health problems.

Risk-Based Regulatory Approach: the development and enforcement of regulatory provisions that target a specific type of hazard or pollutant and that follow a four-step process: (1) hazard identification, does-(2) response assessment, (3) exposure assessment, and (4) risk management.

Safety-net providers: health professionals and institutions that specialize in providing routine medical care services to populations who lack access to mainstream medical providers due to their insurance status, income, language and cultural characteristics, or geographic location.

Sample: a collection of observations drawn from a larger population of observations so as to be representative of the larger population.

Sanitary reform: prevention of infectious disease by providing quality drinking water, effective sewage and solid waste disposal, and other sanitation measures.

Secondary prevention: the prevention of disease by detecting and intervening in early or preliminary stages of disease progression such as by screening programs (e.g., mammography to prevent breast cancer mortality).

Segmentation: dividing a larger population group into smaller, more homogenous groups so that communications and marketing messages can be more effectively targeted to these groups.

Selection bias (or sampling bias): measurement error that occurs when the control group used in research is not representative of the population of interest. For example, selection bias occurs when low-income or under-served population groups are less likely to participate in the intervention under study. The resulting difference may not reflect the intervention but the greater social advantage in the intervention group.

Selective contracting: methods by which managed care plans purposefully select the health service providers to include in their networks based on criteria such as efficiency in service delivery, service quality and patient satisfaction, service capacity, and geographic coverage (accessibility).

Sensitivity to change: assesses an indicator's ability to measure change that might be attributed to the intervention being evaluated.

Sentinel surveillance: collection of a targeted set of health-related information—usually disease-specific information—from a purposefully selected sample of health care providers. Information is typically designed not to produce population estimates of disease burden but rather to track disease transmission patterns and monitor disease severity.

Service and Protective objectives: goals and targets for implementing beneficial health services and prevention activities within a population of interest.

Shared-authority public health system: a means of allocating governmental public health authority and control at the state level such that some activities carried out by local public health agencies are subject to the administrative authority of the state health agency, whereas other activities are subject to the authority of the local government.

Social marketing: the development and implementation of information dissemination activities designed to influence changes in individual health behavior.

Socioeconomic gradient: the concept that health problems are generally more prevalent among individuals with lower socioeconomic status.

Spendout rate: the rate at which legislative budget authority becomes outlays in a fiscal year. This varies across an agency's financial accounts depending on the timing of the programs supported by each account.

Stakeholders: organizations and individuals that are involved in a specific activity because they participate in producing, consuming, managing, regulating, or evaluating the activity.

Standardization of data: methods used to prepare data derived from multiple sources so that they may be compared. Steps include developing comparable variable definitions, identifying comparable time periods, and examining quality assurance procedures used in data collection activities.

Standardized mortality (morbidity) ratio: a ratio of the observed outcome measure to the expected outcome measure in a given population, where the expected outcome measure is typically predicted from a multivariate analysis of outcomes observed in multiple populations. An SMR of greater than 1 indicates that the outcome measure (e.g., disease incidence) was higher than expected in the population of interest.

State funding: mechanisms through which state health agencies provide financial resources for public health services delivered at the local level.

Statistical power: the likelihood that an evaluation will be able to detect the effect of the intervention. Statistical power is driven by two factors: (1) sample size and (2) effect size, a quantitative measure of program's impact, such as a 10 percent improvement in immunization rates.

Statistical significance: the likelihood that observed differences between treatment and control groups in a study are not due chance.

Super-agency: one of two basic organizational structures for state public health agencies, in which public health activities are organized within an administrative unit that is part of a larger department housing units for other health and social services programs. Under this structure, the public health agency director typically reports to the department secretary rather than reporting directly to the governor.

Surveillance: the process of collecting health-related data that are representative of a population of interest, for use in assessing trends in disease and other health conditions, measuring the prevalence of health risk factors and health behaviors, and monitoring the use of health services.

Target populations: the identification of people at risk or most affected by a health problem. Identification can be by community, age, occupation, or other characteristic.

Tertiary prevention: prevention of further disability and limitation from disease already developed such as rehabilitation and exercise programs for individuals receiving treatment for ischemic heart disease.

TIGER: the topographically integrated encoding and referencing system, a set of computer-based methods for linking geographic location information with population attribute data using U.S. Census Bureau data.

Total Quality Management (TQM): an administrative process to stimulate continuous improvements in work systems based on the active participation of the involved workers in monitoring performance, identifying problems, designing and implementing innovations, and evaluating innovations.

Univariate analysis: statistical methods for examining the distributional properties of measures.

Universal health care coverage: a condition in which all members of a defined population have a specified level of health insurance coverage for an identified set of health care services.

Utilization management: administrative and financial mechanisms used by managed care plans to encourage efficient and effective service delivery and utilization. For example, capitated physician payments may be used to create financial incentives for efficient service delivery. Other common utilization management mechanisms include preauthorization requirements for inpatient and specialty care, and inducements for providers to follow clinical practice guidelines in delivering care (e.g., payment bonuses and withholds).

Validity: an indicator's capacity to measure the intended concept.

Views and Estimates: comments filed by members of the U.S. Congress about federal budget proposals, which are then used to draft and report budget resolutions to the appropriate body of Congress.

Vital statistics: information compiled by state health agencies concerning births, deaths, marriages, divorces, fetal deaths, and abortions.

WONDER: a computer-based, Internet-accessible information system for generating county-level and state-level demographic and health statistics from multiple national sources. Maintained by the CDC.

Workforce diversity: the degree to which workplaces reflect variation in population characteristics such as ethnicity, culture, gender, religious background, age, and disability status.

Years of Potential Life Lost (YPLL): a measure of the years of life lost from premature death before a specific age (usually 75), which provides a measure of the impact of specific diseases and injuries on the population of interest.

Index

A

D

E

G

H

I

N

O

P

Q

R

W

Y